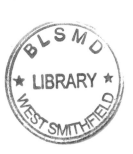

Principles and Practice of Clinical Virology

FIFTH EDITION

Principles and Practice of Clinical Virology
FIFTH EDITION

Edited by

Arie J. Zuckerman

Royal Free and University College Medical School, London, UK

Jangu E. Banatvala

Guy's, King's and St Thomas' School of Medicine, London, UK

John R. Pattison

Department of Health, London, UK

Paul D. Griffiths

Royal Free and University College Medical School, London, UK

Barry D. Schoub

National Institute for Communicable Diseases, Sandringham, South Africa

John Wiley & Sons, Ltd

First published 1987; Second Edition published 1990; Third Edition published 1994; Fourth Edition published 2000

Copyright © 1987, 1990, 1994, 2000, 2004   John Wiley & Sons Ltd,
The Atrium, Southern Gate, Chichester,
West Sussex PO19 8SQ, England

Telephone (+44) 1243 779777

Email (for orders and customer service enquiries): cs-books@wiley.co.uk
Visit our Home Page on www.wileyeurope.com or www.wiley.com

Reprinted October 2004

This publication is designed to provide accurate and authoritative information in regard to the subject matter covered. It is sold on the understanding that the Publisher is not engaged in rendering professional services. If professional advice or other expert assistance is required, the services of a competent professional should be sought.

Other Wiley Editorial Offices

John Wiley & Sons Inc., 111 River Street, Hoboken, NJ 07030, USA

Jossey-Bass, 989 Market Street, San Francisco, CA 94103-1741, USA

Wiley-VCH Verlag GmbH, Boschstr. 12, D-69469 Weinheim, Germany

John Wiley & Sons Australia Ltd, 33 Park Road, Milton, Queensland 4064, Australia

John Wiley & Sons (Asia) Pte Ltd, 2 Clementi Loop #02-01, Jin Xing Distripark, Singapore 129809

John Wiley & Sons Canada Ltd, 22 Worcester Road, Etobicoke, Ontario, Canada M9W 1L1

Wiley also publishes its books in a variety of electronic formats. Some content that appears in print may not be available in electronic books.

British Library Cataloguing in Publication Data

A catalogue record for this book is available from the British Library

ISBN 0-470-84338-1

Typeset in 9/11pt Times by Dobbie Typesetting Ltd, Tavistock, Devon.
Printed and bound in Great Britain by Antony Rowe Ltd, Chippenham, Wilts.
This book is printed on acid-free paper responsibly manufactured from sustainable forestry in which at least two trees are planted for each one used for paper production.

Contents

Contributors

Jangu E. Banatvala *Emeritus Professor of Clinical Virology, Guy's, King's and St Thomas' School of Medicine, Lambeth Palace Road, London SE1 7EH, UK*

Jennifer M. Best *Reader in Virology, Guy's, King's and St Thomas' School of Medicine, Lambeth Palace Road, London SE1 7EH, UK*

Nigel K. Blackburn *Senior Consultant Virologist, National Institute for Communicable Diseases, Sandringham, South Africa*

Judith Breuer *Reader and Consultant in Virology, Skin Virus Laboratory, St Bartholomew's and the Royal London School of Medicine and Dentistry, 25–29 Ashfield Street, London E1 1BB, UK*

Kevin E. Brown *Senior Investigator, Virus Discovery Group, Hematology Branch, National Heart, Lung and Blood Institute, Bethesda, MD, USA*

David Cavanagh *Principal Scientist, Institute for Animal Health, Compton Laboratory, Compton, Newbury, Berks RG20 7NN, UK*

Graham M. Cleator *Reader in Medical Virology, Laboratory Medicine Academic Group, Department of Virology, 3rd floor, Clinical Sciences Building, Manchester Royal Infirmary, Oxford Road, Manchester M13 9WL, UK*

John Collinge *Head, Department of Neurodenegerative Disease and Director, MRC Prion Unit, Institute of Neurology, University College London, London, UK*

Dorothy H. Crawford *Professor of Medical Microbiology and Head of the School of Biomedical and Clinical Laboratory Sciences, The University of Edinburgh, Hugh Robson Building, George Square, Edinburgh EH8 9XD, UK*

Angus G. Dalgleish *Professor of Oncology, St George's Hospital Medical School, Cranmer Terrace, London SW17 0RE, UK*

Inger Damon *Chief, Poxvirus Section, Division of Viral and Rickettsial Diseases, National Center for Infectious Diseases, Centers for Disease Control and Prevention, 1600 Clifton Rd NE, Mailstop G-18, Atlanta, GA 30333, USA*

Ulrich Desselberger *Consultant Virologist and Director, Clinical Microbiology and Public Health Laboratory, Addenbrooke's Hospital, Hills Road, Cambridge CB2 2QW, UK*

Kristina Dörries *Senior Scientist and Group Leader, Institute for Virology and Immunobiology, Julius-Maximilians-University Würzburg, Versbacher Strasse 7, D-97078 Würzburg, Germany*

Geoffrey M. Dusheiko *Professor of Medicine, Department of Medicine, Royal Free and University College Medical School, Rowland Hill Street, London NW3 2PF, UK*

Marcela Echavarria *Assistant Professor of Microbiology, Centro de Educación Médica e Investigaciones Clínicas, CEMIC University Hospital, Galvan 4102, (C1431FWO), Buenos Aires, Argentina*

Susan P. Fisher-Hoch *Professor of Biological Sciences, University of Texas, Houston School of Public Health at Brownsville, 80 Fort Brown, Brownsville, TX 78520, USA*

Ursula A. Gompels *Senior Lecturer in Molecular Virology, Pathogen Molecular Biology Unit, Department of Infectious and Tropical Diseases, London School of Hygiene and Tropical Medicine, University of London, Keppel Street, London WC1E 7HT, UK*

Jim Gray *Head, Enteric Virus Unit, Enteric, Respiratory and Neurological Virus Laboratory, Specialist and Reference Microbiology Division, Health Protection Agency, 61 Colindale Avenue, London NW9 5DF, UK*

Paul D. Griffiths *Professor of Virology, Royal Free and University College Medical School, Rowland Hill Street, London NW3 2PF, UK*

Caroline Breese Hall *Professor of Pediatrics and Medicine in Infectious Diseases, University of Rochester School of Medicine, 601 Elmwood Avenue, Box 689, Rochester, NY 14642, USA*

Tim J. Harrison *Reader in Molecular Virology, Royal Free and University College Medical School, Royal Free Campus, Rowland Hill Street, London NW3 2PF, UK*

Cornelia Henke-Gendo *Clinical Virologist, Department of Virology, Hannover Medical School, Carl-Neuberg Strasse 1, 30625 Hannover, Germany*

Shigeo Hino *Department of Virology, Faculty of Medicine, Tottori University, 86 Nishi, Yonago 683-8503, Japan*

Colin R. Howard *Vice-Principal for Strategic Development and Professor of Microbiology, Royal Veterinary College, University of London, Royal College Street, London NW1 0TU, UK*

Peter Jahrling *USAMRIID, Fort Detrick, Frederick, MD 21702-5001, USA*

Katie Jeffery *Consultant Virologist, Department of Microbiology, John Radcliffe Hospital, Headington, Oxford OX3 9DU, UK*

Sebastian Johnston *Professor, Department of Respiratory Medicine, National Heart and Lung Institute, Imperial College, London, UK*

Paul E. Klapper *Consultant Clinical Scientist and Honorary Senior Lecturer, Health Protection Agency, Leeds Laboratory, Bridle Path, York Road, Leeds LS15 7TR, UK*

James LeDuc *Director, Division of Viral and Rickettsial Diseases, National Center for Infectious Diseases, Centers for Disease Control and Prevention, 1600 Clifton Road, Mail-stop A-30, Atlanta, GA 30333, USA*

Pauli Leinikki *Professor, Department of Infectious Diseases Epidemiology, National Public Health Institute (KTL), Mannerheimintie 166, FIN-00300 Helsinki, Finland*

Graham Lloyd *Head, Special Pathogens, Centre for Applied Microbiology and Research, Porton Down, Salisbury, Wiltshire SP4 0JG, UK*

Clive Loveday *Clinical Director, International Clinical Virology Centre, Great Missenden, UK*

Brian W. J. Mahy *Senior Scientific Research Advisor, National Center for Infectious Diseases, CDC, 1600 Clifton Road, Mailstop C12, Atlanta, GA 30333, USA*

Dennis McCance *Department of Microbiology and Immunology, Head, Virology Unit, University of Rochester, Box 672, 601 Elmwood Avenue, Rochester, NY 14642, USA*

Philip D. Minor *Head, Division of Virology, National Institute for Biological Standards and Control, Potters Bar, Hertfordshire, UK*

Peter Muir *Health Protection Agency South West, Myrtle Road, Bristol BS2 8EL, UK*

Nikolaos G. Papadopoulos *Lecturer, Allergy Unit, 2nd Department of Pediatrics, University of Athens, Greece*

Deenan Pillay *Reader in Virology, Royal Free and University College Medical School, Windeyer Building, 46c Cleveland Street, London W1P 6DB, UK*

Chris W. Potter *Emeritus Professor, University of Sheffield, Division of Genomic Medicine, School of Medicine and Biomedical Sciences, F Floor, Beech Hill Road, Sheffield S10 2RX, UK*

Stelios Psarras *Research Associate, Allergy Unit, 2nd Pediatric Clinic, University of Athens, Greece*

Philip Rice *Consultant Virologist, St George's Hospital Medical School, Cranmer Terrace, London SW17 0RE, UK*

Sibylle Schneider-Shaulies *Institute for Virology and Immunobiology, University of Würzburg, Versbacher Strasse 7, D-97078, Würzburg, Germany*

Barry D. Schoub *Executive Director, National Institute for Communicable Diseases, Sandringham, South Africa*

Thomas F. Schulz *Head of the Department of Virology, Hannover Medical School, Carl-Neuberg Strasse 1, 30625 Hannover, Germany*

Robert Swanepoel *National Institute for Communicable Diseases, Sandringham, South Africa*

Graham P. Taylor *Senior Lecturer/Honorary Consultant, Department of Genito-urinary Medicine and Communicable Diseases, Faculty of Medicine, Imperial College, London, UK*

Volker ter Meulen *Institute for Virology and Immunology, University of Würzburg, Versbacher Strasse 7, D97078 Würzburg, Germany*

Anthea Tilzey *Clinical Senior Lecturer, Virology Section, Department of Infectious Diseases, Guy's, King's and St Thomas' School of Medicine, St Thomas' Campus, UK*

Abel Viejo-Borbolla *Postdoctoral Fellow, Department of Virology, Hannover Medical School, Carl-Neuberg Strasse 1, 30625 Hannover, Germany*

Mary J. Warrell *Research Associate, Centre for Tropical Medicine, John Radcliffe Hospital, Oxford OX3 9DU, UK*

Robin A. Weiss *Professor of Viral Oncology, University College, London, UK*

Arie J. Zuckerman *Professor of Medical Microbiology, Royal Free and University College Medical School, Rowland Hill Street, London NW3 2PF, UK*

Preface

The knowledge and practice of clinical virology continues to expand. The first edition of *Principles and Practice of Clinical Virology*, published in 1987, contained 16 chapters and 590 pages. Each of the subsequent editions became progressively larger. This edition has 902 pages and 38 chapters, including seven within the section on the *Herpesviridae*, each of which is comprehensive.

Rapid progress in the field has occurred between the fourth and fifth editions. There are now two new editors and a number of new authors, which will increase international representation. In addition, each of the remaining chapters has been extensively revised or rewritten, taking into account knowledge accumulated in molecular biology with its applications for laboratory diagnosis, immunisation and antiviral chemotherapy. Each chapter also highlights the clinical features and epidemiological patterns of infection. Between this new edition and the last, much concern has been focused on the global threat posed by new viruses. Consequently, a new chapter on 'Emerging Infections' is included.

There is also a new chapter on 'Hospital-acquired Infections', which will be of benefit to those who have to deal with the day-to-day management of patients in hospital. This chapter also includes some advice relating to SARS. However, fresh knowledge about SARS continued to accumulate as the fifth edition was in preparation, and further information is included, not only in the chapter on 'Emerging Infections' but also in the one on 'Coronaviruses'.

In comparison with the fourth edition, additional colour plates have been included, and, as in previous editions, an attempt has been made to limit references to key publications.

A. J. Zuckerman
J. E. Banatvala
J. R. Pattison
P. D. Griffiths
B. D. Schoub

Preface to the Fourth Edition

It is now 13 years since the first edition of *Principles and Practice of Clinical Virology* was published. A comparison of the first and fourth editions testifies to the rapid expansion in virology during the intervening years, including major developments in technology, the application of these to clinical practice and advances in the treatment of viral infections with an increasing number of antiviral drugs. Indeed, such has been the progress in the field of clinical virology even within the period between the third and fourth editions that we have asked a number of new authors to contribute chapters. These include the chapters on rhinoviruses, viruses associated with acute diarrhoeal disease, and human polyomaviruses. Of the remaining chapters, virtually all have been revised substantially. The chapter on the *Herpesviridae* has been expanded considerably, particularly in relation to *Human herpesviruses 6, 7* and *8*; new authors have contributed to these sections. The chapter on hepatitis viruses reflects the considerable expansion of information relating to hepatitis E and C as well as the role of such newly recognised agents as GB and the new human virus, TTV.

Advances in diagnostic methods, particularly molecular biological techniques and their application to clinical problems, are reflected in a new chapter on 'Diagnostic Approaches', which presents an overview of the value and limitations of established and more recently developed techniques. Advances in serological techniques as well as in virus identification are emphasised. This chapter also includes an important section on assays for determining antiviral drug resistance.

Most of the chapters reflect advances in patient management, including—where appropriate—antiviral chemotherapy. As expected, the chapters on hepatitis viruses and human retroviruses have been expanded considerably in the light of continuing and rapid advances in these fields. Both chapters now include a component by authors with everyday practical experience in the management and treatment of patients with these infections.

In comparison with the third edition, more coloured plates have been included, which we hope our readers will appreciate. As in previous editions, we have attempted to limit the reference lists to key publications.

A. J. Zuckerman
J. E. Banatvala
J. R. Pattison

Preface to the Third Edition

Principles and Practice of Clinical Virology was first published in 1987; a third edition within 7 years of the first attests to the continuing and rapid progress in the field of clinical virology.

All the chapters have been revised and some completely rewritten, reflecting the increasing knowledge of viruses or groups of viruses included in the various chapters. Thus, the chapter on hepatitis viruses now contains sections on hepatitis A and E viruses as well as individual contributions on hepatitis B, D and C. The previous edition contained two chapters on viral haemorrhagic fevers but this section now includes separate chapters for the flaviviruses, alphaviruses, *Bunyaviridae*, arenaviruses and filoviruses. The chapters on arenaviruses and filoviruses have been contributed by new authors.

New authors have also contributed the chapter on herpes simplex virus infections and the chapter on the more newly-recognised herpesviruses now includes a section on *Human herpes virus 7*.

As expected, rapid developments continue to occur in the field of human retroviruses, particularly the human immunodeficiency viruses, and this chapter reflects the accumulation of new and important data in this area. The chapter on human prion disease has been almost entirely rewritten to reflect many of the substantial advances in prion research.

Most of the authors stress the developments and application of molecular biological techniques which are leading not only to improved methods of diagnosis but also to an increased understanding of viral pathogenesis.

Rather than burden readers with a large number of references, we have aimed to include most of the key ones.

Finally, we are grateful for the helpful comments which we received from many of our readers; some of their suggestions have been incorporated into the third edition.

A. J. Zuckerman
J. E. Banatvala
J. R. Pattison

Preface to the Second Edition

In the preface to the first edition of *Principles and Practice of Clinical Virology* we stated that it was our intention, with new editions, to remain up-to-date as the subject advanced. Such is the pace of development in clinical virology that plans were laid for a new edition within a few months of the first being published, and this second edition is appearing only two and a half years after the first. Each chapter has been revised, many extensively, to take account of progress in the understanding of the epidemiology, pathogenesis, diagnosis, management and prevention of virus infections. Perhaps the greatest single recent contribution to the subject has been made by the application of molecular biological techniques, and each of our authors has highlighted the contribution of this rapidly developing discipline to clinical virology.

Human herpesvirus 6 is now the subject of a new chapter, and we have also added a new chapter on haemorrhagic fevers to include much new information on their pathogenesis. As expected, the extensive accumulation of new information relating to infection by human retroviruses has resulted in extensive updating of this chapter, not only to include much more information on human immunodeficiency viruses but also on HTLV-1 and -2. The chapter on hepatitis has been separated into two sections: the first on hepatitis A and the viruses causing non-A, non-B hepatitis, two of which have been identified as hepatitis C and E, and the second on hepatitis B and D (delta agent).

As before, we were aware when organising the book that no single arrangement is entirely satisfactory. We have chosen to arrange the chapters on the basis of individual viruses or groups of viruses. General chapters on virus structure, taxonomy and pathogenesis are not included, but the information on these aspects necessary for an understanding of the practice of clinical virology is included in the individual chapters.

Such factors as the likely discovery of yet new viruses, improvements in the rapidity and sensitivity of diagnostic techniques, and the development of new vaccines, which are likely to involve recombinant techniques and progress in antiviral therapy, will ensure that thought will be given to revision and preparation of another edition.

A. J. Zuckerman
J. E. Banatvala
J. R. Pattison

Preface to the First Edition

There has been a spectacular increase during the last 30 years in our knowledge of virology. This has taken place to such an extent that virology can now be regarded as an umbrella term encompassing a variety of distinct but related disciplines. There are fundamental connections with biochemistry, genetics and molecular biology, and each of these aspects would be worth a treatise in itself. Clinical virology is that aspect which is concerned with the cause, diagnosis, treatment and prevention of virus infections of man. It too has acquired a substantial body of knowledge and accumulated experience over the past 30 years and this book is intended to be an authoritative account of the present situation. Formerly virological diagnosis was time consuming, retrospective and rarely influenced the management of the patient. During the past 10–15 years the picture has changed dramatically. Newly recognised diseases such as AIDS and some haemorrhagic fevers, which have very serious consequences for individuals and populations, have been shown to be due to viruses. In the clinical virology laboratory there has been a change in emphasis towards rapid diagnostic techniques. Finally, effective antiviral chemotherapy is a reality at least for some virus infections and there has been an expansion in the use of immunoprophylaxis. Thus the current principles and practice of clinical virology are concerned with rapid laboratory diagnosis leading to appropriate patient management which might involve specific therapy and/or infection control measures at a hospital, a national and occasionally at an international level.

In organising the book we were aware that there is no single arrangement that is entirely satisfactory. We have chosen to arrange the chapters on the basis of individual viruses or groups of viruses. General chapters on virus structure, taxonomy and pathogenesis are not included but the information on these aspects necessary for an understanding of the practice of clinical virology is included in the individual chapters.

Clinical virology is a subject which continues to evolve. This is usually for one of two reasons, either the need to apply new technology or the need to study new diseases or epidemiological situations. We have therefore invited authors who are specialist investigators into each of the viruses to contribute up-to-date, stimulating accounts of the practice of clinical virology and provide a framework for the assimilation of imminent advances. One chapter has already had to be significantly updated during the time of preparation of the book and it is our intention, with new editions, to remain up-to-date as the subject advances.

A. J. Zuckerman
J. E. Banatvala
J. R. Pattison

PLATE I   xvii

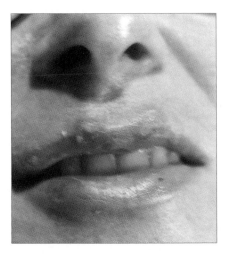

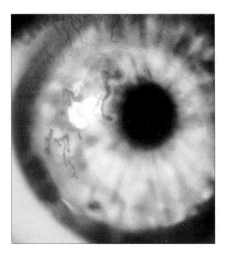

Figure 2A.2 'Cold sores' at the pustular and crusting stages

Figure 2A.3 Rose Bengal staining of herpes simplex virus dendritic ulceration in a grafted cornea. (Kindly provided by R. E. Bonshek and A. B. Tullo)

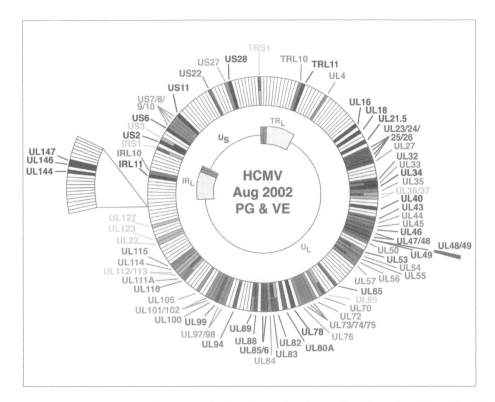

Figure 2C.4 Proteins of CMV which have been mapped to date. UL = unique long region; US = unique short region; TR = terminal repeat; IR = inverted repeat. The genome is linear within the virus but has been circularized for convenience. Open reading frames of known function are coloured according to the following code: orange = transactivators; pink = DNA replication; green = capsid and/or assembly; red = tegument; pale blue = envelope; dark green = immune evasion; dark blue = miscellaneous

PLATE II   xviii

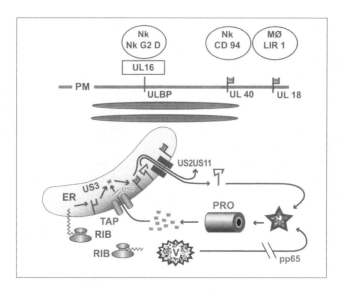

Figure 2C.8   Schematic representation of the ways viruses can interfere with presentation of HLA-peptide complexes at the plasma membrane. Rib, ribosome; ER, endoplasmic reticulum; V, virus-encoded protein; PRO, proteosome; PM, plasma membrane; TAP, transporter associated with antigen presentation. Peptides derived from virus-infected cells are generated in the proteosome and actively transported by TAP into the lumen of the ER. A ribosome is shown producing a protein with a signal peptide, which folds in the ER to produce the HLA Class I chain. This should normally associate with peptide and be transported to the plasma membrane. Misfolded HLA molecules can be re-exported from the lumen of the ER back into the cytosol where they are degraded by the proteosome. Virus-encoded genes interfere with this process as follows: the proteins may be inherently insusceptible to proteosome digestion (EBNA of EBV) or may be modified to reduce their digestion (pp65 acts on MIE protein of HCMV). Proteins may block the function of TAP (ICP47 of HSV; US6 of HCMV). Proteins may bind mature class I molecules within the ER and so sequester them (E3-19K protein of adenoviruses; US3 protein of HCMV; m152 protein of MCMV). Two proteins of HCMV (US2 and US11) facilitate the re-export from the ER to the cytosol of mature HLA class I molecules. If all of these mechanisms are completely successful, the level of HLA display at the PM will be insufficient to prevent NK cells or macrophages recognising the cell as being abnormal and so destroying it. Proteins/peptides encoded within HCMV (UL18) or MCMV (m144) are presented at the plasma membrane to act as a decoy for NK cells by providing a negative signal. In addition, HCMV UL16 blocks transmission of a positive signal to another group of NK cells

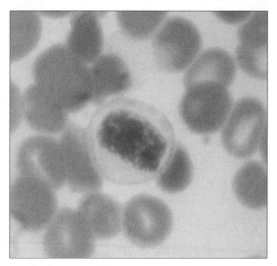

Figure 2D.7   Photomicrograph of a May–Grunwald–Giemsa-stained peripheral blood film from acute infectious mononucleosis. An atypical mononuclear cell is illustrated (**x** 1000)

PLATE III   xix

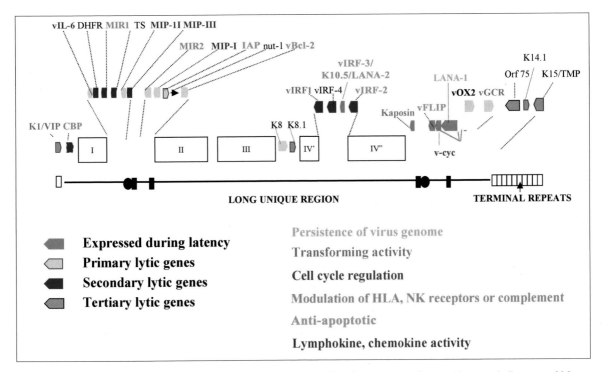

Figure 2F.5   Genome diagram of KSHV. Open boxes with Roman numbers denote groups of structural or metabolic genes which are conserved among γherpesviruses and also many other herpesviruses. The solid line represents the long unique (coding) region, open and filled rectangles internal or terminal repeat regions. Solid circles represent originas of lytic relication [ori-(L), ori-(R)]. The position and transcriptional orientation of viral genes discussed in the text is indicated by pointed boxes. A red shading indicates genes known to be expressed in latently infected spindle cells and PEL cells (see text), light blue, dark blue and green shading refers to genes expressed in the different stages of the lytic cycle (see text). Colour coding of the names of individual viral genes refers to their presumed function, as indicated (see also text)

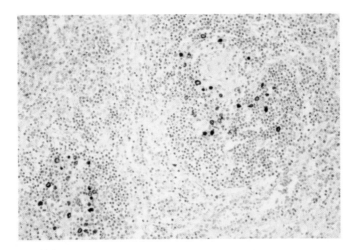

Figure 2F.6   Expression of vIL-6 in B cells of Multicentric Castleman's Disease. vIL-6 is expressed in a small number of KSHV-infected B cells, but may affect others through paracrine action (see text). Photograph kindly provided by Drs Y. Chang and P. Moore

PLATE IV   XX

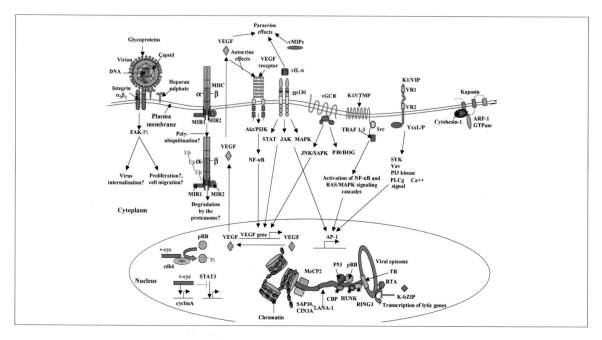

Figure 2F.7   Overview of some KSHV–encoded proteins that may contribute pathogenesis. Vital proteins are coloured in red, interacting cellular proteins in grey. See text for a detailed explanation of the pathways and receptors engaged by KSHV proteins

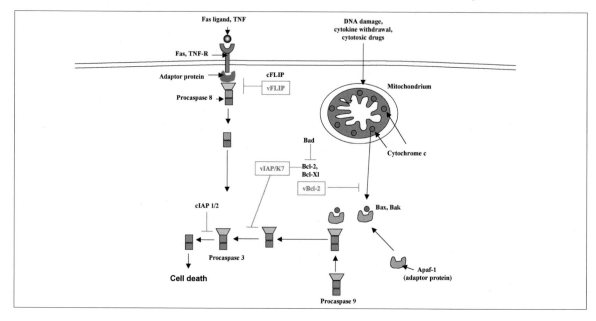

Figure 2F.8   KSHV–encoded proteins involved in the control of apoptosis. Two apoptosis pathways exist in human cells and are regulated by a number of cellular and viral components. The extrinsic pathway is initiated by Fas-L or tumour necrosis factor (TNF) and assembly of the procaspase 8 complex is inhibited by FLIP (FLICE–inhibitory protein; see text). A KSHV–enclosed FLIP homologue, vFLIP, acts in a similar manner. The intrinsic pathway is triggered by DNA damage, cytokine withdrawal, cytotoxic drugs and regulated by the Bcl/Bad/Bax group of proteins. A viral bcl-2 homologue, vbcl-2, acts at this stage. Finally, vIAP acts in the intrinsic pathway and on procaspase 3, as discussed in the text

PLATE V

xxi

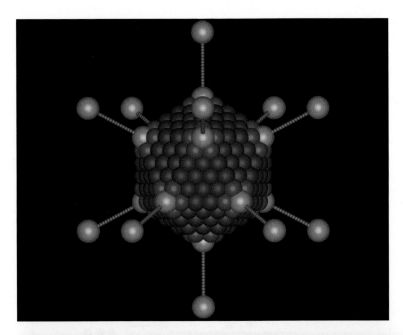

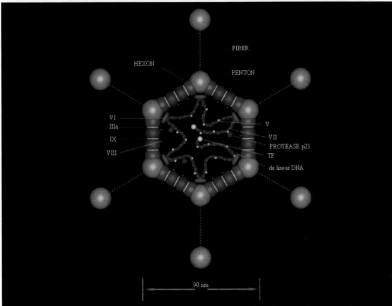

Figure 8.1 Schematic graphic of adenovirus particle

PLATE VI   xxii

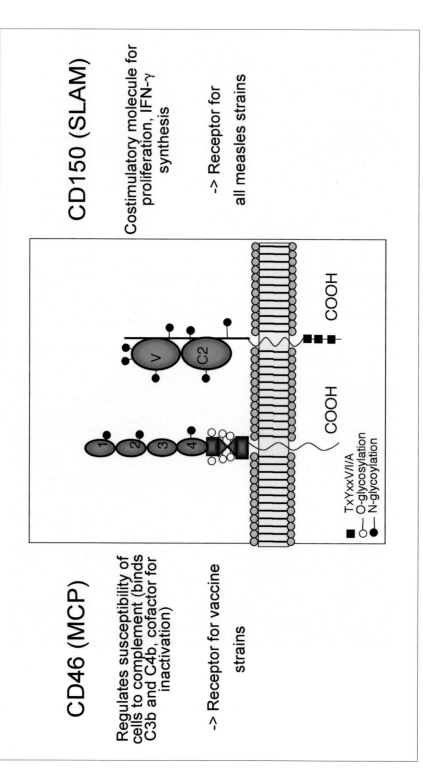

Figure 11.3 A schematic representation of CD46 (MCP, membrane cofactor protein) (left), the major protein receptor for attenuated MV strains. MV binding sites are located within the short consensus repeat (SCR) domains 1 and 2, whereas complement components C3b/C4b bind to SCR 3 and 4, respectively. Proximal to the transmembrane domain, oligo-saccharide-rich serin/threonine/proline (STP) domains are located. CD150, a member of the Ig superfamily, (right) is the receptor of all MV strains tested as yet. MV binding occurs at the membrane distal domain (the V domain). Glycosylation sites in the extracellular domains are indicated as are residues in the cytoplasmic domain identified as important for signaling

PLATE VII   xxiii

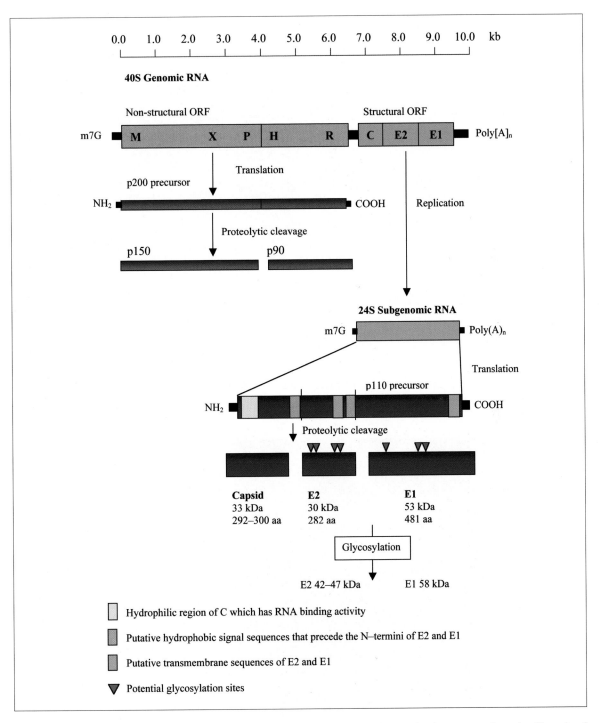

Figure 12.2 Schematic representation of the replication and translation of rubella virus structural and non-structural proteins. (Reproduced from Best, Cooray & Banatvala, Topley and Wilson, 10th edition)

PLATE VIII   xxiv

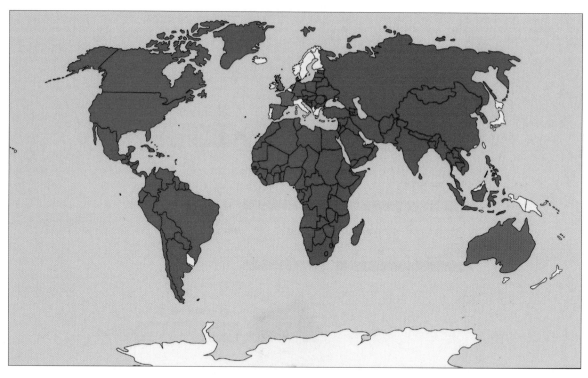

Figure 21.3   World distribution of rabies. Rabies free areas are white; red indicates terrestrial rabies with or without bat rabies, and countries with only bat lyssaviruses are green

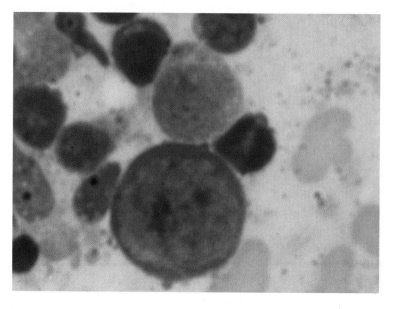

Figure 24.4   Giant pronormoblast

PLATE IX xxv

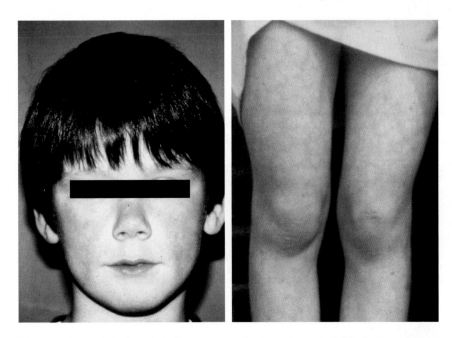

Figure 24.5   Children with characteristic slapped cheek appearance and reticular lacy rash of fifth disease

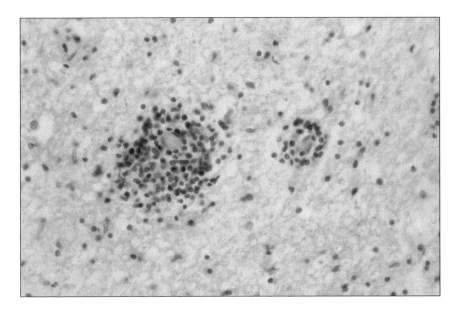

Figure 25A.8   Perivascular lymphocytic infiltration in the central nervous system. (Courtesy of Dr Margaret Esiri)

PLATE X   xxvi

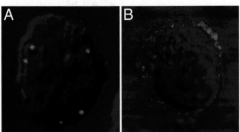

In an isolated HTLV-I infected CD4 lymphocyte HTLV-I gag p15 (red) is unpolarized (A) whilst HTLV-I env gp46 (red) accumulates at the cell surface (B)

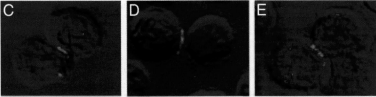

40 minutes after contact with an uninfected CD4 lymphocyte HTLV-I p15 (C), p19 (D) and gp46 (E) polarize at the cell-cell junction

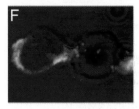

HTLV-I gag p19 (red) from the infected (CSFE stained- green) CD4 lymphocyte is transferred to the uninfected CD4 lymphocyte

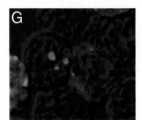

The transfer of HTLV-I genome (red) from the CFSE stained infected CD4 lymphocyte to the uninfected control CD4 cell can be demonstrated by PNA-FISH after 120 minutes.

(PNA-FISH – peptide nucleic acid – fluorescence in-situ hybridization)

Figure 25A.9   Using unstimulated, uncultured peripheral blood lymphocytes from a patient with HTLV-I associated myelopathy the accumulation of viral proteins at the cell-cell junction and subsequent transfer of gag proteins and HTLV-I nucleic acids to a CD4 lymphocyte from an uninfected donor is demonstrated (courtesy of Professor Charles Bangham)

PLATE XI   xxvii

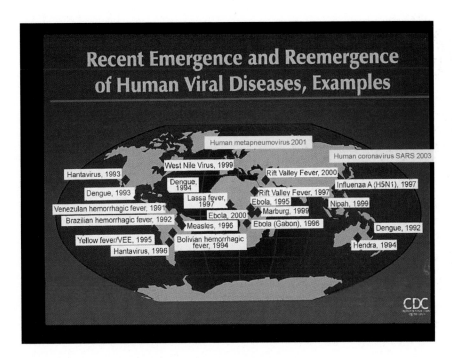

Figure 28.3   Recent Emergence and Reemergence of Human Viral Diseases, Examples

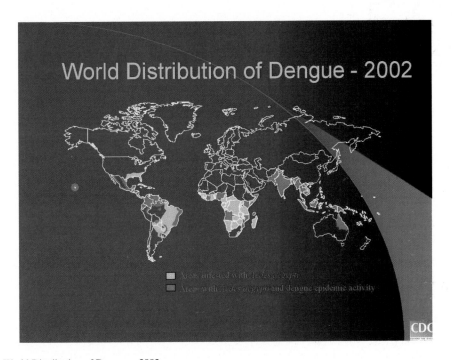

Figure 28.4   World Distribution of Dengue – 2002

PLATE XII   xxviii

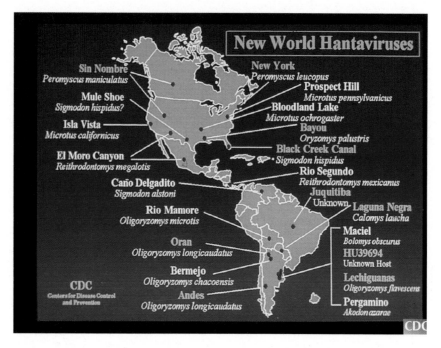

Figure 28.5   New World Hantaviruses

1

Diagnostic Approaches

Katie Jeffery[1] and Deenan Pillay[2]

[1]*John Radcliffe Hospital, Oxford, and*
[2]*Royal Free and University College Medical School, London, UK*

INTRODUCTION

If clinical virology in the 1980s was characterised by the widespread use of enzyme-linked immunosorbent assay (ELISA) technology, then there is no doubt that the 1990s will be seen as the time when molecular methods of virus detection entered routine diagnostic use. Following on from this development, the first few years of the twenty-first century will be seen as the period when real-time PCR and virus quantitation came of age, along with increasing automation of molecular diagnostics. Concurrently, the emphasis and priorities of diagnostic virology laboratories have shifted in response to: the availability of rapid diagnostic methods; the identification of new viruses, many of which are non- or poorly cultivatable; the increasing availability of effective antiviral agents; the emergence of antiviral resistance; the increasing number of immunocompromised patients, in whom opportunistic viral infections are life-threatening; and new cost pressures on pathology services.

This chapter provides an overview of diagnostic techniques against this background, and highlights those clinical scenarios of particular importance to virologists in a diagnostic setting.

TECHNIQUES—AN OVERVIEW

Virus Isolation

Many of the advances in clinical virology have come about because of the ability to propagate viruses in the laboratory. Historically, viruses were propagated in laboratory animals and embryonated eggs, although most virus isolation techniques now rely on cultured cells. With appropriate specimens and optimal cell lines, this technique can be highly sensitive and specific, and a presumptive diagnosis made on the basis of a characteristic cytopathic effect (CPE), confirmed by immunostaining. The judicious use of two or three cell lines, such as a monkey kidney line, a human continuous cell line and a human fibroblast line, will allow the detection of the majority of cultivatable viruses of clinical importance, such as herpes simplex virus (HSV), varicella zoster virus (VZV), cytomegalovirus (CMV), enteroviruses, respiratory syncytial virus (RSV), adenovirus, parainfluenza viruses, influenza viruses and rhinoviruses. In addition, the ability to grow virus from a clinical specimen demonstrates the presence of viable virus (albeit viable within the chosen cell line)—this is not necessarily the case with detection of viral antigen or genome. For example, following initiation of antiviral therapy for genital herpes, HSV antigen can be detected from serial genital swabs for longer than by virus propagation in cell culture. This infers that antigen persists in the absence of viral replication and underlines the importance of correct interpretation of laboratory results. Nevertheless, virus isolation has now been shown to be less sensitive than molecular amplification methods for this and other viruses (see later).

The advantages of virus isolation include: the ability to undertake further examination of the isolate, such as drug susceptibility assays (see later) or typing (Table 1.1); the provision of epidemiological information on

Principles and Practice of Clinical Virology, Fifth Edition. Edited by A. J. Zuckerman, J. E. Banatvala, J. R. Pattison, P. D. Griffiths and B. D. Schoub
© 2004 John Wiley & Sons Ltd   ISBN 0 470 84338 1

Table 1.1 Virus isolation

Advantages	Disadvantages
Sensitive	Slow (conventional cell culture)
'Catch-all'	Labour-intensive
Generates isolate for further study	Multiple cell lines required
Detects 'viable' virus	
Adaptation for rapid result	

viruses of public health importance; and the culture and identification of previously unrecognised viruses, e.g. human metapneumovirus (van den Hoogen *et al.*, 2001) and SARS-associated coronaviruses (Drosten *et al.*, 2003). However, routine cell culture techniques available in most laboratories will not detect a number of clinically important viruses such as gastroenteritis viruses, hepatitis viruses, Epstein–Barr virus (EBV), *Human herpesvirus 6, 7* and *8* (HHV-6, -7, -8), and/or human immunodeficiency virus (HIV). Other than HSV, for which most isolates will grow in human fibroblast cells within 3 days, the time for CPE (or, for example, haemadsorption) to develop for most clinical viral isolates is between 7 and 21 days. For this reason, a number of modifications to conventional cell culture have been reported, to provide more rapid results. These include centrifugation of specimens on to cell monolayers, often on cover slips, and immunostaining with viral protein-specific antibodies at 48–72 h following inoculation (Shell Vial Assay) (e.g. Stirk and Griffiths, 1988). Such techniques can also be undertaken in microtitre plates (O'Neill *et al.*, 1996).

The role of conventional cell culture for routine diagnosis of viral infections is diminishing and is a subject of active debate within the virology community (Carman, 2001; Ogilvie, 2001). Many laboratories are discontinuing or downgrading virus isolation methods in favour of antigen or genome detection for the rapid diagnosis of key viral infections (usually those that are treatable, such as CMV and VZV). Nevertheless, it is important for large laboratories to maintain the ability to employ this methodology for the reasons given above. Where primary diagnosis is undertaken by cell culture, there will be increasing pressure to generate quicker results by use of the many rapid techniques that have been reported.

Antigen Detection

Immunofluorescence

One of the most effective rapid diagnostic tests is indirect or direct immunofluorescence (IF). Initially undertaken with polyclonal antisera, and then subsequently with pools of monoclonal antibodies, this method uses either indicator-labelled antibody or a labelled antispecies antibody (indirect) to directly visualise viral antigens in clinical specimens. Usually, the label used is fluorescein. The indirect method is more sensitive, since more label can be bound to an infected cell. Results can be available with 1–2 h of specimen receipt. The most common use of this technique is for the diagnosis of respiratory viral infections whereby a panel of reagents are utilised to detect RSV, parainfluenza viruses, influenza A and B and adenovirus in multiple wells of a microscope slide. This technique is sensitive compared to cell culture, especially for the detection of RSV. The ideal specimen for such testing is a nasopharyngeal aspirate, most usually obtained from infants with suspected bronchiolitis, for whom a rapid result is essential for correct clinical management and implementation of infection control measures. However, detection can also be made from a well-taken throat/nasal swab. There is increasing evidence that community or nosocomial acquired respiratory viruses lead to severe disease in immunocompromised patients (for review, see Ison and Hayden, 2002), and it is important that bronchoalveolar lavage specimens from such patients with respiratory disease are also tested for these viruses in addition to the more common pathogens, such as CMV. Respiratory virus antigens are expressed within the epithelial cells, and the success of the technique depends on an adequate collection of cells. A particular advantage of IF, compared to the commercial rapid antigen tests available for RSV and influenza, is that microscopic examination of the fixed cells can determine the presence of adequate cell numbers for analysis (Table 1.2). IF has been used widely for the direct detection of HSV and VZV in vesicle fluid, and has advantages over electron microscopy in both sensitivity and specificity. IF methods have also been used to detect more unusual viruses, such as Lassa fever (Wulff and Lange, 1975). An important limitation of IF is that well-trained microscopists are required for interpretation, which remains subjective.

Table 1.2 Antigen detection by immunofluorescence

Advantages	Disadvantages
Rapid	Requires skilled staff
Sensitive for some viruses (e.g. RSV)	Variable sensitivity
	Dependent on high-quality specimen

Detection and semi-quantitation of CMV antigen-containing cells in blood can also be undertaken by direct IF (CMV/pp65 antigenaemia assay). This technique involves separation of peripheral blood mononuclear cells (PBMCs) and fixing on a slide, followed by staining with a monoclonal antibody directed against the matrix protein pp65. The frequency of positive cells can predict CMV disease in the immunocompromised patient (van der Bij *et al.*, 1989), and is used in a number of laboratories. However, it is labour-intensive, needs large numbers of PBMCs (making it unsuitable for all patient populations) and requires a rapid processing of blood specimens if a reduction in sensitivity of detection is to be avoided (Boeckh *et al.*, 1994). Therefore, PCR is rapidly replacing antigenaemia as the method of choice for qualitative and quantitative detection of CMV.

ELISA/Latex Agglutination for Antigen Detection

Solid phase systems for antigen detection are now used widely. ELISAs are based on the capture of antigen in a clinical specimen to a solid phase via a capture antibody, and subsequent detection using an enzyme-linked specific antibody. Variation in capture and detector antibody species has increased the sensitivity of these assays, which are widely used for hepatitis B virus (HBV) surface antigen detection (HBsAg) and, more recently, for hepatitis C core antigen in donor blood-testing laboratories (Peterson *et al.*, 2000). ELISA-based systems for the diagnosis of, for example, RSV, influenza and HSV may be appropriate in some contexts for point-of-care testing, although often at the expense of sensitivity when compared to IF and/or virus culture.

Small latex particles coated with specific antibody can be agglutinated in the presence of antigen, which can then be observed with the naked eye. This rapid assay is used for rotavirus diagnosis, with an equivalent sensitivity to electron microscopy. Capture of antibody, rather than antigen, can also be undertaken, although latex assays for CMV and VZV antibodies may lack sensitivity and specificity compared to ELISA systems (see below).

Electron Microscopy

Electron microscopy (EM) is the only technique available for directly visualising viruses, and therefore has many applications beyond purely diagnostic purposes. The major role of EM in a clinical setting is in the diagnosis of viral gastroenteritis, for which many of the aetiological agents are non-cultivatable, and analysis of skin lesions for herpes, pox and papillomaviruses.

Preparation of specimens and the technique of negative staining are straightforward and quick, and the method is a 'catch-all' approach to detecting viruses. Nevertheless, it has a limit of sensitivity of approximately 10^6 viral particles per millilitre of fluid. Vast numbers of virions are present during acute skin and gastrointestinal disease, and a diagnosis is easily made. This becomes more difficult later in the course of infection, when viral shedding is reduced below the level of detection. Sensitivity can be enhanced by antibody-induced clumping of virus (immune EM) or ultracentrifugation; however, it is unrealistic to undertake these methods routinely. The advantages and disadvantages of electron microscopy are summarised in Table 1.3.

The survival of EM within the routine clinical virology laboratory hinges on the availability of alternative, more sensitive methods of diagnosis. Many centres already use latex agglutination for rotavirus diagnosis, and polymerase chain reaction (PCR) is more sensitive for the detection of herpesviruses in vesicular fluid (Beards *et al.*, 1998). Currently, EM in diagnostic virology laboratories is used primarily for outbreak investigation. Now that PCR-based methods of Norovirus detection are established (Green *et al.*, 1995), show increased sensitivity with respect to EM (O'Neill *et al.*, 2001) and can be adapted for real-time PCR detection (Miller *et al.*, 2002), the future of EM in clinical virology is in doubt. One of the first indications for electron microscopy was for the rapid diagnosis of smallpox; in the era of bioterrorism, EM will continue to play a role in specialist centres in the event of a bioterrorist attack, such as confirming VZV infection in cases of vesicular rash.

Table 1.3 Electron microscopy

Advantages	Disadvantages
'Catch-all'	Requires skilled staff
Economical running costs	Poor sensitivity
Detects unculturable viruses	Large capital outlay
Adaptable, e.g. immunoelectron microscopy confirms cytopathic effect	

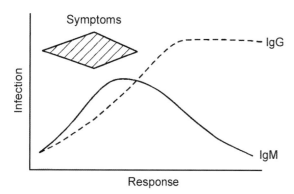

Figure 1.1 Typical evolution of antibody responses following an acute viral infection

Histology/Cytology

Direct microscopic examination of stained histology or cytology specimens can on occasion provide the first indication that a virus may be responsible for a pathological process; e.g. the intranuclear (early) or basophilic (late) inclusions seen in interstitial nephritis in renal transplant biopsies due to BK polyoma virus; changes in cervical cytology seen in association with human papillomavirus (HPV); and the nuclear inclusions seen in erythroid precursor cells in parvovirus B19 infection.

Serology

All viral infections generate a humoral response, and this can be used for diagnostic purposes. The classical pattern of response following an acute infection is illustrated in Figure 1.1. The functional nature of this response is extremely variable. In some instances, these antibodies are neutralising and can be assessed for this activity (e.g. polioviruses). However, many infections are controlled more effectively by T cell responses, and antibody detection is used as a surrogate of infection. Traditionally, methods of antibody detection did not distinguish between IgG and IgM responses, and diagnosis was based on seroconversion or a significant rise in antibody titre between acute and convalescent samples (10–14 days apart). The complement fixation test was used widely in this respect; however, assay insensitivity and the cross-reactivity of many antigens used within the assay limited its clinical usefulness. Most importantly, a diagnosis could only be made after the time of acute illness. Currently, the major use of this assay is for the diagnosis of 'atypical' pneumonia (*Chlamydia psittaci/pneumoniae*, *Coxiella*

or *Mycoplasma*), since there are few alternative serological methods. Other serological techniques include haemagglutination inhibition, latex agglutination and immunofluorescence (used most widely for EBV diagnosis). Serum is the specimen of choice for most serological assays, but oral fluid can be used as a non-invasive alternative for the detection of a number of different antibodies, which may be useful for surveillance studies or in children (Perry *et al.*, 1993; Parry *et al.*, 1989). In patients with viral central nervous system infections, the cerebrospinal fluid (CSF) may be tested for virus antibodies, and the antibody ratio compared with serum to confirm intrathecal antibody synthesis.

Increasingly, solid-phase ELISAs are used in diagnostic laboratories. Recent technological advances, e.g. using synthetic peptides or recombinant antigens instead of whole viral lysates, and improvements in signal detection have led to more sensitive, specific and rapid methods for measuring virus specific antibody levels. The ELISA format is extremely versatile, and new assays can be designed quickly to cope with clinical demands, e.g. the investigation of new viruses, such as severe acute respiratory syndrome (SARS)-associated coronaviruses. Many of these assays are available commercially, and can be automated. They are essentially of three types (Figure 1.2):

- *Indirect assays.* Viral antigen is immobilised onto a solid phase, specific antibody in the patient serum sample binds to this antigen and, after a washing step, this antibody is detected by an enzyme-labelled antihuman immunoglobulin. In this way, either specific IgG or IgM can be detected, depending on the indicator immunoglobulin (Figure 1.2a,b). Clearly, detection of IgM species is dependent on the prevailing level of IgG, such that a high level of specific IgG reduces the sensitivity of an IgM assay for the same virus. If rheumatoid factor is present in the clinical sample, it may lead to false-positive IgM results (Figure 1.2c).
- *Capture assays.* IgG or IgM species are captured onto the solid phase by antihuman immunoglobulin, followed by addition of antigen and then labelled antibody. With regard to IgM assays, this method reduces the potential interference of rheumatoid factor, and is used increasingly for a number of IgM species (Figure 1.2d).
- *Competitive assays.* In this case, a labelled antibody in the ELISA system competes for binding to immobilised antigen with antibody in the clinical sample. This assay improves both the specificity and sensitivity of the assay (Figure 1.2e).

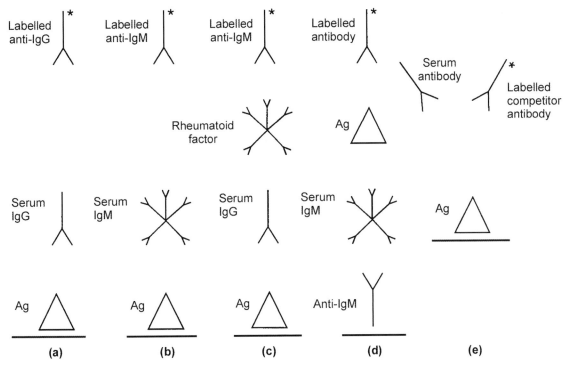

Figure 1.2 ELISA formats: (a) indirect IgG assay; (b) indirect IgM assay; (c) rheumatoid factor interference in IgM assay (indirect); (d) IgM capture assay; (e) competitive assay. Note that the solid horizontal line represents the solid phase

Serological diagnosis of acute infection is best suited to situations in which detection of the virus itself is difficult, time-consuming or where virus excretion is likely to have ceased by the time of investigation, such as hepatitis A, rubella or parvovirus B19. There are situations, however, where IgM is produced over a prolonged period, or in response to reinfection, as is the case for rubella. In these cases, past infection can be distinguished from recent infection by antibody avidity tests. These are based on the principle that antibody responses mature over time, such that high-avidity antibodies predominate at a later stage. By using a chaotropic agent (e.g. urea) during the ELISA washing stage, low-affinity antibodies (representing recent infection) will be preferentially dissociated from antigen, compared to higher-affinity antibodies (Thomas and Morgan-Capner, 1991).

Immunoblot methods can be used for confirmation of HIV (Western blot) and hepatitis C virus (HCV) infection. These methods are based on the detection by antibodies within a serum sample of multiple epitopes blotted on to a membrane. Non-specific reactions within ELISAs are often clarified in these systems, since possible cross-reacting antibodies can be identified by non-viral antigenic epitopes. Immunoblot assays are expensive and technically demanding.

Serology is also essential for the diagnosis and screening of persistent infections where antibodies are detectable in the presence of virus replication, such as HIV and HCV. The availability of sensitive assays allows widespread screening for immunity against, for example, HBV, rubella, VZV and hepatitis A.

Finally, for HIV infection, combined p24/antibody assays have been developed, for which a signal indicates the presence of either/both components. This is of advantage for a first-line screening assay, since p24 antigen is detectable prior to antibodies following primary infection, and thus leads to a shorter window period (Hashida *et al.*, 1996).

Despite these more recent advances in serological techniques, there remain some inherent limitations with this form of virological diagnosis (Table 1.4). It is highly dependent on the ability of the individual to mount appropriate immune responses to infection. Thus, serological methods have a limited role for diagnosing viral infections in the immunocompromised patient (Paya *et al.*, 1989) and every effort must be made to detect the virus itself. Transfusion or

Table 1.4 Serology

Advantages	Disadvantages
Specific IgG assays good indicator of prior infection	Retrospective (e.g. rising CFT titres) CFTs insensitive, especially to assess previous infection
Capture IgM assays good indicator of recent infection	
Allows retrospective diagnosis if no acute clinical specimen obtained	Cross-reactivity and interference
	Insensitive for diagnosing some congenital infections (e.g. CMV)
Rapid	Not appropriate for immunocompromised
Automated	Spurious results possible following receipt of blood products
Diagnosis of unculturable or poorly culturable viruses	
Can utilise non-invasive clinical samples, e.g. saliva, urine	

CFT = complement fixation test.

receipt of blood products may also lead to spurious serological results, e.g. leading to a false interpretation that seroconversion indicates acute infection. The major role of serology in transplant patients is in identifying immune status at baseline in order to ascribe a risk to primary infection, reinfection or reactivation during subsequent immunosuppression (see Table 1.10).

Interpretation of Serological Assays

Viral serology results should be interpreted carefully, taking into account the patient's history and symptoms. The diagnosis of a primary virus infection can be made by demonstrating seroconversion from a negative to a positive specific IgG antibody response, or by detecting virus-specific IgM. A four-fold rise in IgG antibody titre between acute and convalescent samples can also be indicative of a primary infection (e.g. by complement fixation test). Detection of virus-specific IgG in a single sample, or no change in virus antibody titre between acute and convalescent phase sera, indicate exposure to the virus at some time in the past. Results of serological assays can be complicated by a number of factors; the age of the patient (the production of serum IgG or IgM antibodies can be absent or impaired in the immunocompromised, neonates and the elderly); receipt of blood products with passive antibody transfer; maternal transfer of IgG antibodies; and non-specific elevation of certain virus antibodies due to recent infection with other viruses. This last point is particularly common with herpesvirus infections, which have group-specific cross-reacting epitopes. IgM antibodies may persist for extended periods of time following primary infection, and may also be produced as a result of reactivation of latent infection, although not reliably so (e.g. CMV, EBV). The production of virus-specific

intrathecal antibody (requires demonstration of an intact blood–brain barrier) can confirm the diagnosis of viral CNS infection, e.g. subacute sclerosing panencephalitis. Serological assays may be complemented and confirmed by molecular assays, e.g. PCR for HCV RNA in the presence of hepatitis C antibody, and PCR for HIV, used in the diagnostic setting for the investigation of infants of HIV-seropositive mothers.

NUCLEIC ACID DETECTION

The area of most rapid development in diagnostic virology relates to molecular amplification assays to provide qualitative and quantitative results. PCR and other similar molecular assays have been applied to the diagnosis of virtually all human viruses. In general, the sensitivity of these assays far exceeds that of other virus detection systems, and subsequent interpretation of results in a clinical setting may be very difficult. A number of commercial kits and automated systems are now available, with the advantage of standardisation improving quality control and inter-laboratory variability. These issues will be discussed following a brief review of the techniques available.

Polymerase Chain Reaction

This technique uses a thermostable DNA polymerase to extend oligonucleotide primers complementary to the viral DNA genome target (Saiki *et al.*, 1988). Consecutive cycles of denaturation, annealing and extension result in an exponential accumulation of target DNA. This is limited only by substrate (nucleotide) availability and possible competition between target genome and non-target amplicons for reaction components (Figure 1.3). RNA genomes require transcription to complementary DNA (reverse

Step

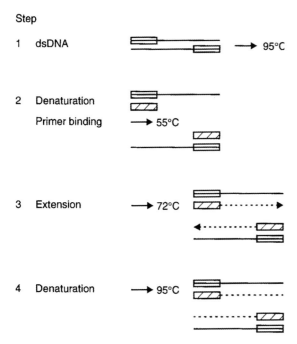

1 dsDNA → 95°C

2 Denaturation

Primer binding → 55°C

3 Extension → 72°C

4 Denaturation → 95°C

Figure 1.3 Polymerase chain reaction

transcription) prior to the PCR reaction. Undertaking a second PCR round on the first round amplicon can increase the overall sensitivity of detection (nested PCR). This uses a different set of PCR primers internal to the first set, and therefore can act as a confirmation of the correct amplicon produced by the first round reaction.

Primers

The correct choice of primers is an important determinant of the success of any PCR. Clearly, the nucleic acid sequence of at least a part of the viral genome needs to be known, and primers must target a well-conserved region. This can be done using multiple alignment programmes; however, the final success of the PCR depends on the availability of sequence data from a range of different viral isolates. Since unusual viral variants may not be detected by an established PCR technique, it is important for the clinical virologist to have knowledge of the primer targets in order to interpret results correctly. This issue is equally as important for commercial assays as it is for 'in-house' assays, as has been demonstrated regarding suboptimal HIV subtype detection by a commercial quantitative PCR assay (Arnold *et al.*, 1995). The appropriateness of primers also requires continual re-evaluation in the light of new selective pressures on

viral evolution, such as antiviral drug resistance. Other important aspects of primer design include the avoidance of secondary structure, or complementarity between primers (leading to so-called primer–dimer amplification artefacts). Computer programs used to design primer sequences address these aspects.

Preparation of Clinical Specimen

Viral gene detection methods do not require the maintenance of viral infectivity within the clinical specimen. Thus, specimens can be transported and stored in the refrigerator or freezer prior to analysis, with more flexibility than that required for virus isolation. This is a major advantage over traditional methods of virus detection. However, of particular concern is the susceptibility of RNA to nucleases, which are present in all biological material. In addition, certain specimen types, e.g. intraocular fluids (Wiedbrauk *et al.*, 1995) and urine (Chernesky *et al.*, 1997), are intrinsically more susceptible to false negative results. Thus, specimens for qualitative and, especially, quantitative PCR require careful preparation and assays need to be evaluated for individual specimen types and patient groups. The anticoagulant heparin is contraindicated for blood samples because it inhibits the PCR reaction. Currently, it is recommended that ethylenediaminetetraacetic acid (EDTA) blood for HIV RNA quantitation is separated as soon as possible, after which the plasma can be stored frozen until analysis. If multiple tests are to be undertaken on one sample, it should be aliquoted on receipt to avoid multiple freeze–thawing. A number of different nucleic acid extraction methods are available, and their use depends on the nature of the clinical specimen and whether the target is RNA or DNA.

Detection of Product

The PCR product of any specific reaction has a known size, and can therefore be detected on an agarose gel in comparison to a molecular weight ladder. However, more than one band may be seen, or the band may not be in precisely the correct position. For this reason, specific detection of the product by hybridisation with a nucleic acid probe is to be encouraged. This can be undertaken within a microtitre plate format, with a colorimetric end-point, and read in a standard spectrophotometer, e.g. Gor *et al.* (1996). Many commercial PCR assays employ this system. The addition of such a

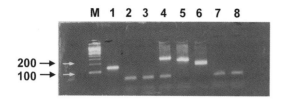

Figure 1.4 A 2% agarose gel of ethidium bromide-stained products from a multiplex PCR for HSV, VZV and CMV. Lanes: M, size markers (the 100 and 200 bp markers are indicated on the left); 1, isolate of HSV; 2, 3, 7 and 8 are negative specimens; 4, CMV control; 5, VZV control; 6, HSV control

step enhances further the specificity of the assay, and may also improve sensitivity.

Multiplex PCR

Since more than one viral target is often sought in one specimen, efforts have been made to combine multiple sets of primers, against different targets, within one PCR reaction (Jeffery *et al.*, 1997). Each set of primers requires specific conditions for optimal amplification of the relevant target, and the development of a multiplex system requires a detailed evaluation of these conditions to ensure that the efficiency of amplification for any one target is not compromised. Identification of the specific product in this system may be based on different sized amplicons, or use of different probes. Figure 1.4 illustrates a multiplex PCR for HSV, VZV and CMV with agarose gel-based detection.

Quantitation

Conventional PCR is inherently a qualitative assay. Initial attempts to produce quantitative information involved the simultaneous analysis of samples with known target genome copy number, and comparing the intensity of bands on an agarose gel with that of the test specimen. However, the efficiency of amplification within any one PCR reaction is exquisitely sensitive to changes in condition, or indeed inhibitory factors within the clinical specimen, as above. It is therefore important that internal standards (within the same PCR reaction) are used for quantitative competitive (qcPCR) assays. These control sequences should mimic the target genome as closely as possible, yet be detectable as a distinct entity on final analysis. This can

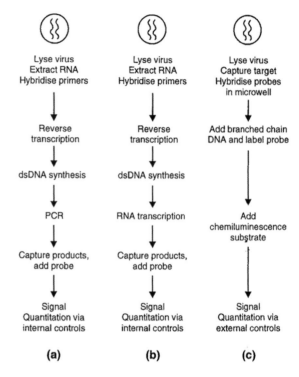

Figure 1.5 Quantitative molecular methods for HIV plasma RNA. (a) PCR; (b) NASBA; (c) bDNA

involve the incorporation of restriction enzyme sites, whereby the control amplicon, but not target sequence, can be cleaved subsequently (Fox *et al.*, 1992), or merely a control sequence of different size (Piatak *et al.*, 1993). Commercial assays often use a jumbled sequence as a control, with subsequent use of probes against both control and target sequences. In all cases, since the number of input control genomes is known, simple proportions can be applied to the signals to generate a quantitative value for the clinical specimen (Figure 1.5a).

These assays are inherently variable, due to both laboratory and biological variation. Many commercial qcPCR assays are associated with a variation of $0.5 \log_{10}$, and this must be considered in the clinical interpretation of results (Saag *et al.*, 1996). The dynamic range of these assays is determined by the linearity of the reaction. Variability is more likely at the extremes of this range, and this variability determines the lowest value (lower limit) at which the user can be confident that the value given approximates to the truth. The lower limit of sensitivity for quantitative HIV PCR can be increased by initial ultracentrifugation of plasma to concentrate virus.

Real-time PCR

The type of PCR reaction discussed above depends on end-point detection of product, with the aim of maximising the amplification reaction. More sensitive detection methods allow the kinetics of the amplification to be measured, and require fewer cycles of amplification for product to be detected.

Real-time PCR systems allow the reactions to be undertaken within a closed system, and fluorescence generated by the assay is measured without further manipulation. These systems produce very rapid temperature cycling times and, together with removal of post-PCR detection procedures, PCR reactions can be completed within minutes. Many of the signalling technologies rely on energy transfer between a fluorophore and a proximal quencher molecule (fluorescence resonance energy transfer). In the 'TaqMan' system, a specific probe binds to the relevant amplicon, and subsequent hydrolysis of this probe produces an increase in fluorescence (Morris *et al.*, 1996). The 'LightCycler' system allows product detection by the incorporation of an intercalating dye into double-stranded DNA, with an increase in fluorescence as product accumulates (Wittwer *et al.*, 1997). Specificity of this reaction for the correct product (rather than artefacts) is provided by analysing a decrease in fluorescence at the melting temperature specific for that product. These commercial systems are under constant review, with new systems and applications for

the diagnostic laboratory coming on-line (e.g. the 'iCycler iQ real-time PCR detection system'). A number of probe systems are also available to generate sequence-specific fluorescence signals (reviewed in Mackay *et al.*, 2002).

The major advantage of real-time PCR is that it is inherently suitable for quantitative PCR, based on the number of temperature cycles required for a threshold fluorescence signal to be reached, usually in comparison with an external standard curve. An example of real-time detection of a calibration series for the detection of hepatitis C is shown in Figure 1.6. The dynamic range of real-time PCR of at least 8 $\log_{10}$ copies of template surmounts the problems encountered by many qcPCR reactions, of an inability to quantitate high virus loads while maintaining sensitivity at the lower end of the assay. In addition, intra- and inter-assay variability is reduced in comparison with qcPCR (Locatelli *et al.*, 2000; Abe *et al.*, 1999).

The disadvantages of real-time PCR in comparison with conventional PCR include an inability to monitor the size of the amplicon or to perform a nested PCR reaction without opening the system, incompatibility of some systems with some fluorescent chemistries, and currently limited capability with multiplexed reactions because of the limited number of fluorophores available. Recent advances in the design of hairpin primers, hairpin and nuclease oligoprobes and novel combinations of fluorophores will allow discrimination of an increasing number of targets in single rapid reactions

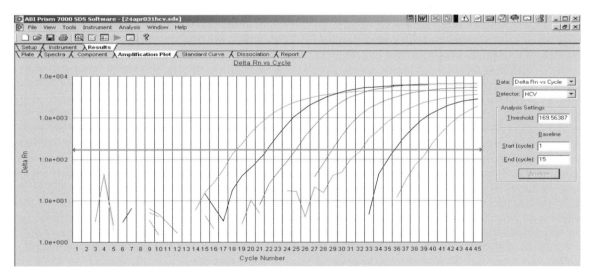

Figure 1.6 Real-time PCR detection of a hepatitis C calibration series from 10 million IU/ml down to 10 IU/ml in 1 log steps. *x* axis = cycle number; *y* axis = log fluorescence. The sample with the highest virus load (10^7 IU/ml) crosses the baseline at cycle 18, whereas that with the lowest virus load (10 IU/ml) requires 39 cycles of PCR before reaching a detectable level. Results obtained by Dr Jeremy Garson

Table 1.5 PCR—recommended controls

Negative controls
- Extraction control —to control for contamination during extraction
  —mimic clinical sample
- Reagent control —to control for contamination of reagents
  —use solvent in which extracted nucleic acid is suspended

Positive controls
- Extraction control —use positive clinical specimen
- Control genome —to control for PCR efficiency, specifically to assess sensitivity
- Alternate target —to control for inhibition of reaction

in future (Mackay *et al.*, 2002; Vet *et al.*, 1999). In addition, the start-up costs of real-time PCR may be prohibitive. Despite these difficulties, real-time PCR is now used routinely in many diagnostic virology laboratories, for both qualitative and quantitative applications. As with conventional PCR, real-time PCR has proved to be cost-effective in high-throughput laboratories in comparison with traditional culture-based methods of viral diagnosis.

PCR Contamination and Control Reactions

PCR is highly susceptible to contamination from amplified products generated in a previous reaction, from target sequences cloned in plasmid vectors and from other positive clinical specimens. By contrast, a false negative result can arise from inadequate nucleic acid extraction from a sample and inhibitory factors in the PCR reaction. Similarly, the sensitivity of the assay may be reduced but not completely inhibited. Relevant controls within each PCR run are essential for a correct interpretation of a positive or negative result, and these are highlighted in Table 1.5. The limit of sensitivity for any one assay must be assessed. This can be undertaken by serial dilutions of a tissue culture fluid of known median tissue culture infective dose (TCID$_{50}$), purified viral genome, tissue culture fluid with known virion concentration (by EM) or plasmid containing the target genome. Many laboratories are reluctant to introduce plasmids into the molecular biology area because of the risk of widespread contamination.

There are two specific procedures designed to reduce PCR contamination. First, extraneous DNA within PCR reagents can be inactivated by subjecting 'clean' PCR reagents to ultraviolet irradiation. This introduces thymidine dimers into the DNA chain, rendering it unamplifiable. More effective is the substitution of dUTP for dTTP in the PCR reaction (Longo *et al.*, 1990); this does not affect specific product detection. In subsequent PCR reactions, the addition of uracil DNA glycosylase prevents DNA polymerisation of any uracil-containing DNA, but has no effect on thymidine-containing DNA template. Thus, any contaminating DNA from a previous reaction is not amplified.

Physical Organisation of the Laboratory

The physical requirements for undertaking 'in-house' PCR reactions are demanding (Victor *et al.*, 1993). A 'clean room' is required, in which preparation and aliquoting of reagents occurs. This must be isolated from any possible contamination with viral nucleic acid. A separate area is also required for nucleic acid extraction, although this can be undertaken in a diagnostic area. A dedicated PCR room is required for setting up reactions and siting of thermal cyclers. Finally, another room is required for post-PCR analysis, such as gel running and genome detection. Dedicated laboratory coats and equipment are required for each of these areas, and strict adherence to protocol by all staff is essential (Table 1.6).

Clearly, the provision of such a dedicated set of rooms for molecular biology is a challenge for busy diagnostic virology laboratories. Nevertheless, it is of paramount importance that diagnostic PCR reactions are undertaken with minimal risk of contamination, and every effort must be made to provide the relevant space if such assays are to enter the routine diagnostic armamentarium. Some of the newer automated commercial assays incorporate some of the above steps within a self-contained machine. However, it is unwise to use such assays outside of a molecular biology environment in which staff are well trained in this type of work.

Table 1.6 PCR—physical separation

1. Preparation of reagents
   —'clean' room (no nucleic acid)
   —separate room
2. Nucleic acid extraction
3. Amplification reactions (in cases of nested reactions, second round PCR should be further separated
4. PCR product analysis

Quality Control

Molecular biology is expensive compared to more traditional virological methods, making it difficult for each laboratory to undertake comprehensive evaluations of each PCR assay. For this reason, there is an urgent requirement for standardised methodologies and, at least in this respect, the availability of commercial assays is welcome. There is also a need for external quality control (QC) schemes, since major clinical and therapeutic decisions are made on the basis of molecular assay results, many of which have been developed 'in house' (Valentine-Thon, 2002). QC programmes such as Quality Control for Molecular Diagnostics (www.qcmd.com) provide QC schemes for blood-borne viruses and other pathogens, such as CMV and enterovirus; however, such programmes are still under development in terms of repertoire, and participation can represent a significant expense for diagnostic laboratories.

Other Amplification Systems

Other amplification systems include the ligase chain reaction (LCR) which, as with PCR, requires a thermal cycler. Technical innovations in molecular amplification allow techniques such as nucleic acid sequence-based amplification (NASBA), transcription mediated amplification (TMA), strand displacement amplification (SDA) and branched chain DNA (bDNA) to detect minute quantities of nucleic acid without the use of a specialised thermal cycler.

Ligase Chain Reaction

LCR involves hybridisation of two oligonucleotide probes at adjacent positions on a strand of target DNA which are joined subsequently by a thermostable ligase. The reaction also takes place on the complementary strand, so multiple rounds of denaturation, annealing and ligation lead to an exponential amplification of the viral DNA target (Hsuih et al., 1996). RNA targets require prior reverse transcription.

Nucleic Acid Sequence-based Amplification

This technique uses RNA as a target, utilising three enzyme activities simultaneously: reverse transcriptase (RT), RNase H, and a DNA-dependent RNA polymerase (Guatelli et al., 1990). A DNA primer incorporating the T7 promoter hybridises to the target RNA and is extended by RT. RNase degrades the RNA strand, and the RT utilising a second primer produces double-stranded DNA. T7 polymerase then forms multiple copies of RNA from this DNA template. This method is suited to the detection of RNA viruses, or mRNA transcripts of DNA viruses. In addition, it can be modified to a quantitative assay using internal controls (Figure 1.5b). Different detection formats for the amplified RNA product have been developed, including electrochemiluminescence and molecular beacon detection technologies, and adapted for rapid detection of many viruses, e.g. West Nile and St Louis encephalitis (Lanciotti and Kerst, 2001). Transcription-mediated amplification (TMA) techniques are very similar. Detection of the amplicon is commonly performed with detection systems such as the Hybridization Protection detection system, which uses a chemiluminescent signal, as in Gen-Probe© systems. TMA is widely used to detect HIV and HCV nucleic acid sequences.

Strand Displacement Amplification

Strand displacement amplification technology has been established in a fully automated system known as BDProbeTec©. In SDA technology, an oligonucleotide primer containing a restriction enzyme site binds to its complementary (target) nucleic acid. An exonuclease-deficient DNA polymerase (exo-) is used in the presence of dGTP, dATP, dUTP and a dCTP containing an α-thiol group (dCTP αS) to produce double-stranded DNA containing a restriction enzyme site. Upon binding, the restriction enzyme nicks the strand without cutting the complementary thiolated strand. The exo-DNA polymerase recognises the nick and extends the strand from the site, displacing the previously created strand. The recognition site is repeatedly nicked and restored by the restriction enzyme and exo-DNA polymerase with continuous displacement of DNA strands containing the target segment. The process becomes exponential with the addition of an antisense primer containing the appropriate recognition site.

Branched Chain DNA

A number of hybridisation methods for detecting viral genome have been developed and used extensively since the 1980s. These are based on the hybridisation of a labelled oligonucleotide probe to a unique complementary piece of viral genome, and can be undertaken either on a solid phase or *in situ*. These short probes are 20–30 bases in length and can be RNA (riboprobe) or DNA. Many solid-phase assays are of the dot–blot or slot–blot type, and have been widely used for HPV diagnosis and typing. The bDNA assay is a modification of probe assays. This method uses a signal amplification system rather than amplifying target genome. Single-stranded genome (RNA or DNA) is hybridised to an assortment of hybrid probes, which are captured in turn onto a solid phase by further complementary sequences. Branched DNA amplifier molecules then mediate signal amplification via enzyme-labelled probes with a chemiluminescent output. This method can also provide quantitative results (Dewar *et al.*, 1994; van Gemen *et al.*, 1993) (Figure 1.5c).

Table 1.7 Clinical use of molecular amplification techniques

- Diagnosis of infection
- Diagnosis of disease
- Virus genotyping
- Prediction of disease/staging of infection
- Monitoring antiviral therapy
- Prediction of transmission
- Confirming transmission events
- Epidemiology of infection

Clinical Use of Molecular Techniques

The application of qualitative and quantitative molecular analysis to human viral infections has provided new insights into the natural history of human viral infections, such as HIV, HBV, HCV and the herpesviruses. This includes the nature of viral persistence and latency, viral replication and turnover rate, and an understanding of the response to antiviral therapies. It follows that molecular diagnostic assays do not merely offer an increase in sensitivity over alternative methods; rather, their correct interpretation demands an understanding of our transformed knowledge. These issues are discussed further below (Table 1.7).

Diagnosis of Infection

Infection is defined by the presence of virus in a clinical specimen. The infection may be asymptomatic or symptomatic (disease). However the key determinant for correct diagnosis is the sensitivity of the assay, with a goal of detecting viral genome if it is present at any level. A sensitive qualitative assay is relevant, for instance, in the diagnosis of HIV in infants (proviral DNA in PBMCs) (Lyall *et al.*, 2001) or HCV (serum RNA) infection (Zeuzem *et al.*, 1994). Before introducing such an assay into routine use, the sensitivity and specificity of the new test must be established, according to the formulae in Table 1.8. Note that, in

Table 1.8 Evaluation of a new diagnostic assay

Parameter	Description	Formula
Sensitivity	Proportion of true positives correctly identified by test	$\dfrac{\text{positive results}}{\text{true positives}}$
Specificity	Proportion of true negatives correctly identified by test	$\dfrac{\text{negative results}}{\text{true negatives}}$
Positive predictive value	Proportion of patients with positive test results who are correctly diagnosed	$\dfrac{\text{sensitivity} \times \text{prevalence}}{\text{sensitivity} \times \text{prevalence} + (1 - \text{specificity}) \times (1 - \text{prevalence})}$
Negative predictive value	Proportion of patients with negative test results who are correctly diagnosed	$\dfrac{\text{sensitivity} \times (1 - \text{prevalence})}{(1 - \text{sensitivity}) \times \text{prevalence} + \text{specificity} \times (1 - \text{prevalence})}$
Likelihood ratio	Indicates how much a given diagnostic test result will raise or lower the pretest probability of the target disorder	$\dfrac{\text{sensitivity}}{(1 - \text{specificity})}$

this instance, these parameters are compared to an existing gold standard assay (true positives or negatives) and therefore relate purely to a comparison between assays. Since molecular assays are usually more sensitive than existing assays, it is often necessary to confirm that those samples positive solely by the molecular assay are indeed true positives. This can be done by confirming the identity of the PCR product, correlation with another marker of infection (e.g. seropositivity, where appropriate) or the clinical background. Thus, an expanded gold standard, including positives by both existing and new assay, is used for sensitivity and specificity calculations. A useful concept in evaluating a diagnostic test is the likelihood ratio (Table 1.8), which indicates how much a given diagnostic test result will raise or lower the pretest probability of the target disorder (Altman and Bland, 1994).

Diagnosis of Disease

As discussed above, the nature of viral disease has had to be redefined in the light of qualitative and quantitative molecular data. Increasingly, it is possible to detect the presence of infectious agents at low copy number in the absence of symptoms. This makes the interpretation of positive results problematic and requires close clinical–virological liaison. Three approaches are possible:

1. Qualitative detection of viral genome at a site which is normally virus-free. A good example is the diagnosis of viral encephalitis, in which detection of HSV, CMV, VZV or enterovirus genome is diagnostic (Jeffery et al., 1997). Indeed, it has been very difficult traditionally to propagate herpesviruses in cell culture from CSF samples. It is unclear whether this is a reflection of a low level of virus, or whether there is a preponderance of disrupted, non-infectious virus produced from brain tissue into the CSF. Qualitative PCR offers significant advantages in terms of speed over traditional methods of viral diagnosis. Early diagnosis and treatment of central nervous system infection can improve prognosis in herpes simplex encephalitis (Raschilas et al., 2002), or can reduce unnecessary treatment and hospitalisation, as in the case of enteroviral meningitis (Nigrovic and Chiang, 2000).

2. Qualitative detection of virus without an exquisite level of sensitivity. This is important for instances in which low-level viraemia may occur in the absence of disease, and which does not predict disease. An example is CMV infection following transplantation. The sensitivity of a diagnostic qualitative PCR must be chosen with care in order that the results are predictive of disease (Figure 1.7).

3. Quantitative detection of virus at a level associated with disease. For many persistent virus infections with transient or continual low-level viraemia, the onset of disease is related to a higher viral replication rate. This provides the rationale for identifying levels of viraemia that are predictive of disease. HHV-6 and HHV-7 infections can be used as examples. These herpesviruses are acquired commonly in early childhood, and primary infections are associated with erythema infectiosum and febrile seizures in a small proportion of infants, with the majority of infections remaining asymptomatic (Hall et al., 1994). These persistent infections can be detected by PCR in the saliva and blood of many seropositive individuals, so that a qualitative PCR is not helpful in diagnosis of symptoms specifically associated with these infections. By contrast, application of a quantitative PCR to such clinical specimens demonstrates that febrile seizures are specifically associated with higher systemic viral loads (Clark et al., 1997). Quantitative molecular data on CMV disease in transplant patients (Boeckh et al., 1996), those with the acquired immune deficiency syndrome (AIDS) (Spector et al., 1998) and BK polyomavirus-associated nephropathy in renal transplant recipients (Limaye et al., 2001) also demonstrates the usefulness of this approach. Clear diagnostic definitions of diseases will depend on the assay

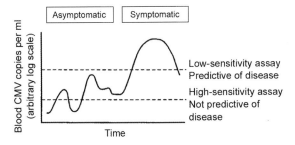

Figure 1.7 The relevance of PCR sensitivity for CMV diagnosis following transplantation. A very sensitive assay for detection of persistent/latent viruses, such as CMV, may not provide clinically useful information. This is because low levels of viraemia may occur without causing disease. With regard to CMV, the threshold for detection of virus in whole blood should have a higher level

itself and the patient group concerned. Large prospective studies are therefore required in each case. Standardisation within commercial assay systems will help in this respect.

Genotyping

HCV is a genetically heterogeneous virus with six major genotypes (Simmonds *et al.*, 1993). Interestingly, some genotypes (viz. types 2 and 3), have a more favourable response to interferon-based treatment (Chemello *et al.*, 1994), and therefore genotyping has become central in the management of HCV infection. Sequencing is the reference method of HCV genotyping, and is becoming increasingly automated (e.g. Trugene™ HCV 5′NC genotyping test). Another widely used genotyping technique is based on a genotype-specific probe with reverse hybridisation (INNO-LIPA HCV II™).

Hepatitis B is a similarly heterogeneous virus. Several studies have recently shown that genotype B (prevalent in the Far East) is associated with both a better overall prognosis (Sakugawa *et al.*, 2002; Kao *et al.*, 2002) and a higher rate of IFN-induced HBeAg clearance, compared with hepatitis B genotype C (Wai *et al.*, 2002). Stratification for HBV genotypes is likely to be used clinically in future.

Sequence-based genotyping assays are in clinical use for the typing of HIV and HPV. Over 70 genotypes of HPV are recognised, but only a few of these types have the potential to cause lesions that may progress to malignancy.

Prediction of Disease/Staging of Infection

Preemptive therapy entails the initiation of therapy in those at highest risk of disease, and is an approach that is used commonly for CMV infection in bone marrow and solid organ recipients. The capacity of a positive laboratory test to predict disease must be established by detailed prospective surveillance protocols, in order to generate positive and negative predictive values (Table 1.8). Since the natural history of viral infections (relationship between replication and disease) may be influenced by factors such as the length and nature of immunosuppression, these parameters should be determined separately for different patient groups, such as bone marrow recipients, solid organ recipients and patients with AIDS.

A similar approach has now been established for HIV infection. The large Multicentre AIDS Cohort Study (MACS) clearly demonstrated a relationship between plasma HIV RNA load and risk of disease progression. In this analysis, CD4 cell count was also an independent predictor, and both measurements together provided the best prognostic indicator (Mellors *et al.*, 1997). Data from the MACS study have shown that a high virus load predicts a faster rate of decline of $CD4^+$ cells (Mellors *et al.*, 1996). Subsequently, this prognostic capability has been transformed into guidelines for initiating antiviral therapy. The decision on when to initiate therapy for HIV disease is complex. Recent guidelines (BHIVA, 2001; Dybul *et al.*, 2002) have moved away from recommending initiation of therapy based on plasma HIV RNA load alone and suggest that therapy should be deferred until the CD4 cell count is 200–350 cells/μl. Recent studies in the era of highly active antiretroviral therapy (HAART) showed that HIV plasma RNA levels prior to starting therapy were not predictive of response to HAART independently of the CD4 count (Sterling *et al.*, 2001).

A similar analysis of HCV viral load has been undertaken which suggested that high viral load could be used to predict disease stage (Gretch *et al.*, 1994). However, a large natural history study found three independent risk factors that predicted the rate of progression of hepatic fibrosis; age at infection older than 40 years, daily alcohol consumption of 50 g or more and male sex. Virological factors (HCV genotype and viral load) were not independently associated with fibrosis progression (Poynard *et al.*, 1997).

A detailed understanding of the virological natural history of HBV using sensitive quantitative molecular assays is required before prognostic criteria can be applied to this infection. As discussed above, there is increasing evidence that HBV genotype influences both prognosis and response to treatment. A recent multivariate analysis in patients with hepatocellular carcinoma in the context of hepatitis B infection identified the level of serum HBV-DNA and tumour size at diagnosis as independent and significant prognostic factors (Ohkubo *et al.*, 2002).

Use of Molecular Assays to Monitor Antiviral Therapy

The relationship of HIV RNA quantitation to prognosis supports the thesis that the 'disease activity' is reflected in overall viral replication rate. It follows that antiviral-induced reduction in plasma RNA is likely to

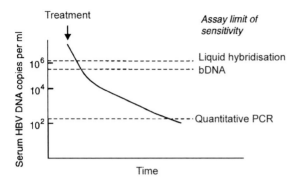

Figure 1.8 Quantitative assays for HBV: their relevance in assessing response to antiviral drugs. A relatively modest reduction in HBV viral load in response to therapy is required in order for HBV DNA levels to become undetectable by an insensitive assay. Important information on the rate and extent of viral suppression is missed by the liquid hybridisation assay

translate into clinical benefit. This has now been confirmed in a number of clinical trials. For example, a virological analysis of the AIDS Clinical Trial Group 241 trial (zidovudine, lamivudine with/without nevirapine) showed that for each 1 $\log_{10}$ reduction of HIV RNA between baseline and week 8, there was an incremental reduction in clinical progression of death at week 48 (Hughes *et al.*, 1997). The virological goal of HIV therapy is to reduce HIV RNA to undetectable levels (<50 RNA copies/ml of plasma), and optimal therapy should achieve this by 16–24 weeks following initiation of therapy (Dybul *et al.*, 2002). Commercially available assays have a limit of sensitivity of around 50 copies/ml. Clinical trial data suggest that reduction of viral load to below this level predicts the durability of the antiviral response (Montaner *et al.*, 1998; Powderly *et al.*, 1999). The main use of regular monitoring of plasma HIV RNA levels is, therefore, to monitor the success of therapy, and current protocols recommend subsequent tests at 3–4 month intervals (Dybul *et al.*, 2002).

Quantitation of serum HBV DNA has been an important tool in assessing response to treatment. HBV DNA quantitation has traditionally been undertaken by a relatively insensitive liquid hybridisation assay (limit of sensitivity approximately 10^6 copies/ml), with results expressed as pg/ml. More recently, nucleoside analogues (lamivudine, famciclovir) and nucleotide analogues (adefovir) have demonstrated potent anti-HBV activity, e.g. Lai *et al.* (1998). Using more sensitive quantitative assays, such as bDNA or PCR, four log reductions in HBV viral load have been

observed (defined as copies/ml or genome equivalents/ml). These new assays can provide important information on the potency of drugs, the development of drug resistance and the dynamics of response (Figure 1.8).

The HCV genotype and the widespread availability of qualitative HCV RNA PCR are now central to the planning and monitoring of antiviral therapy, but the role of quantitative PCR for monitoring therapy requires further clarification. Recent data suggest that with combination treatment (pegylated interferon and ribavirin) in genotype 1 disease, if at 12 weeks the HCV RNA load has not fallen by >2 $\log_{10}$ units, the likelihood of a sustained viral response is very low and treatment could be discontinued, with the benefits of cost savings and a reduction in the inconvenience and side-effects of treatment (Davis, 2002).

Virological monitoring of patients receiving anti-CMV therapy is important. Not only does a high viral load predict CMV disease in a number of risk groups, such as solid organ transplant recipients (Fox *et al.*, 1995), HIV-infected patients (Spector *et al.*, 1998) and congenitally infected newborn infants (Revello *et al.*, 1999), but persistent viraemia following the onset of therapy, or virological relapse on therapy, is associated with continuing disease. Conversely, in bone marrow transplant recipients treated with ganciclovir preemptively, clearance of viraemia can be used as a guide to stop therapy (Einsele *et al.*, 1995). Controversy exists over optimum methods for monitoring for CMV disease (qualitative vs. quantitative), ideal specimens (plasma or whole blood/leukocyte fraction), and defining threshold values that correlate with active disease rather than latent infection. These issues need to be taken into account for each risk group in choosing an appropriate method of monitoring.

In all cases of antiviral drug monitoring using qualitative or quantitative molecular assays, a rebound in viral load or failure to suppress viral replication may reflect reduced drug susceptibility. In these cases, it may be appropriate to undertake drug susceptibility assays, and these are described later.

Prediction of Transmission

It is reasonable to assume that a high viral load within an individual will predict transmission to another. Studies on vertical HIV transmission suggest that the mother's viral load is a better indicator of vertical transmission than CD4 cell count (O'Shea *et al.*, 1998). The HIV viral load has been shown to be the main predictor of heterosexual transmission in a study of

HIV-discordant couples in Uganda (Quinn *et al.*, 2000). A high HIV load in genital secretions is also associated with efficient heterosexual HIV transmission (Chakraborty *et al.*, 2001). Mother-to-infant hepatitis C transmission is independently associated with a high hepatitis C virus load (Dal Molin *et al.*, 2002), and similarly, in a study of 155 HIV and HCV co-infected women, the maternal plasma HCV RNA was significantly higher in those who transmitted HCV to their offspring compared to those who did not (Thomas *et al.*, 1998). Hepatitis B e antigen (HBeAg) has long been used as a surrogate marker of a high HBV virus load, and therefore high risk of mother-to-infant transmission, in pregnant women. Increasingly studies are detecting significant levels of HBV DNA in HBeAg-negative individuals (Berger and Preiser, 2002). Following a number of incidents of transmission of hepatitis B from HBeAg-negative health care workers (HCWs), recent guidance (HSC 2000/020) has extended the role of HBV DNA monitoring in the UK, as HCWs with a DNA load of $> 10^3$ genome equivalents/ml are now excluded from practising exposure-prone procedures.

Use of Viral Genetic Analysis for Transmission Events and Epidemiology

Viral genome sequencing is now a standard method for establishing transmission events. This uses the nature of viral quasispecies, in that genetic relatedness between viruses is sought against a background of variation. In such investigations, the choice of gene targets to amplify and sequence is important, and results must be subject to the correct statistical and phylogenetic analysis if strong evidence for a transmission event is to be demonstrated. This approach is particularly important in the investigation of HCWs infected with blood-borne viruses, such as HBV (Ngui and Teo, 1997; Zuckerman *et al.*, 1995) and HIV (Blanchard *et al.*, 1998).

Sequence relatedness between different virus isolates is also essential for virus classification. The data used to generate phylogenetic trees are usually derived from conserved genes, such as those coding for viral enzymes or structural proteins. This type of analysis has been used recently to develop a new classification of the *Retroviridae* (http://www.ncbi.nlm.nih.gov/ICTVdb/Ictv/fs_retro.htm).

Antiviral Drug Resistance

Resistance has been documented to virtually all compounds with antiviral activity, and the emergence of antiviral resistance in clinical practice should come as no surprise. Drug susceptibility is a biological concept, and defined by the concentration of drug required to inhibit viral replication. Thus, drug resistance is not 'all-or-none' but rather a quantitative measure. The genetic basis of this resistance is becoming well understood, and thus specific viral genetic mutations are associated with resistance.

As the use of these drugs increases, there will be increasing pressure on diagnostic laboratories to provide assays to determine the cause of drug failure, of which drug resistance is one. Laboratory assays for drug resistance fall into two major categories:

Table 1.9 Advantages and disadvantages of phenotypic and genotypic antiviral drug resistance assays

	Advantages	Disadvantages
Phenotype	Represents sum of all mutations Quantitative assessment of resistance (IC_{50}, IC_{95}) Can assess cross-resistance	Expensive Labour-intensive Slow Selection of culture-adapted strains (not with recombinant virus assay)
Genotype (a) Selective (e.g. point mutation assay, line probe)	Quick Relatively inexpensive (PMA) Semiquantitation (PMA)	Difficult to interpret single mutation in absence of other information
(b) Sequencing	Rapid Comprehensive information Background polymorphisms detected	Expensive Labour-intensive Expertise in genomic analysis required Simultaneous mutations not necessarily on same genome

phenotypic and genotypic assays. Their relative advantages and disadvantages are summarised in Table 1.9.

Phenotypic Assays

The plaque reduction assay is used widely for herpesviruses and remains the gold standard for detecting HSV, CMV and VZV drug resistance. In essence, a specific titre (plaque-forming units) of virus is inoculated onto a permissive cell monolayer, usually within a multiwell plate. These monolayers are overlaid with increasing concentrations of drug in a semisolid medium, thus preventing extracellular virus spread. The plaque reduction associated with drug inhibition can then be calculated, with results expressed as IC_{50} or IC_{90} (concentrations of drug required to inhibit virus production by 50% and 90%, respectively). Alternative methods for HSV include the dye uptake method which quantitates viable cells within a viral infected monolayer. The time-consuming nature of VZV and CMV culture techniques has led to the development of rapid culture methods, using viral antigen detection or genome detection to assess drug efficacy (Pepin et al., 1992). All these assays produce different IC_{50} values on the same isolates, and standardisation is therefore required.

Plaque assays have also been developed for HIV, making use of a CD4-expressing HeLa cell line (Chesebro and Wehrly, 1988). This assay is easy to use but is limited to syncytium-inducing isolates and cannot be used to assess protease inhibitor activity. The most standardised of HIV susceptibility assays uses PBMCs in which to grow the isolate in question, in the presence of drug. The end-point in this primary cell assay is p24 production (Hollinger et al., 1992). However, this is a very labour-intensive assay, which is impractical for routine clinical use. A more interesting development in the area of HIV susceptibility assays is the recombinant virus assay, whereby PCR product amplified directly from plasma virus is recombined with an HIV clone lacking the relevant gene (Hertogs et al., 1998). These fragments can include the RT gene protease gene and gag cleavage sites, and the resulting recombinant can then be screened for susceptibility to a range of drugs. Since the background clone of virus used grows rapidly in culture, this method is more rapid than conventional phenotypic assays, and holds much promise for the future. Appropriate phenotypic assays will require development as new classes of antiretroviral drugs become available, targeting such stages as viral fusion with the host cell.

Phenotypic assays are clearly important, since they reflect global determinants of drug resistance. A criticism is that they require propagation of a virus stock before the assay is undertaken. This process is selective itself, and may lead to the final susceptibility assay being carried out on an unrepresentative species. On the other hand, PCR-based phenotypic assays suffer from the same genetic selection limitations as genotypic methods.

Genotypic Assays

An understanding of the genetic basis of drug resistance and the availability of automated and non-radioactive methods of nucleic acid sequencing have enabled widespread assessment of clinical isolates with reduced viral susceptibility. These methods are used most commonly for HIV drug resistance, and will become important for poorly cultivatable viruses, such as HBV and HCV. Genotypic assays for drug resistance in CMV have also been developed (Bowen et al., 1997).

Detection of individual mutations. A number of groups have described selective PCR or point mutation assays (PMAs) for HIV, HBV and CMV resistance-associated mutations. In the selective PCR assays, PCR primers are synthesised that selectively hybridise to a wild-type or mutant target (Kozal et al., 1993). The PMA is based on the specific detection (by radioactivity or colorimetry) of one of four bases extending the 3′ end of a primer, complementary to the wild-type or mutant sequence (Kaye et al., 1992). One particular advantage of the PMA is the ability to detect mixtures of genotypes within a viral population with a sensitivity of less than 10%. These assays are most appropriate when the mutation in question is clearly associated with resistance, such as the detection of lamivudine-resistance mutations in HBV by a real-time PCR method (Cane et al., 1999). Since multiple mutations may be associated with resistance, especially in the context of combination therapy for HIV, the implications of a single mutation may change, making interpretation of a PMA difficult. To some extent this can be overcome by the application of a range of PMAs to one PCR product. Further, the ability to detect small proportions of a particular mutation within a viral quasispecies is a further advantage of these assays.

Table 1.10 A typical protocol for virological monitoring of transplant recipients

Pretransplant	Donor serology:	HIVAb, HCVAb, HBsAg, HBcoreAb, CMVAb, EBVAb	
	Recipient serology:	HIVAb, HCVAb, HBsAg, HBcoreAb, CMVAb, EBVAb, HSVAb, VZVAb	
Posttransplant	Weekly surveillance (3 months):	CMV viraemia (PCR, antigenaemia)	
Symptoms	*Specimens*	*Possible causes*	*Techniques*
Respiratory	Throat swab	CMV, HSV, influenza	Virus isolation/PCR
	BAL	RSV, parainfluenza	Immunofluorescence/virus isolation
	Blood	Adenovirus, CMV	PCR
Gastrointestinal	Biopsy, stool, blood	CMV, HSV	Virus isolation/PCR
		Adenovirus	PCR and EM
		Rotavirus (rare)	
CNS	CSF	CMV, JC (rare)	PCR
	Blood	CMV	PCR
Urinary tract (haemorrhagic cystitis)	Urine	Adenovirus, BK	PCR, EM

BAL, bronchoalveolar lavage.
Risk factors for specific viruses differ between transplant groups.
Significance of CMV viraemia during routine surveillance depends on nature of prophylaxis given.

Line probe assays. These assays are available commercially for HIV mutations. An RT-PCR product is hybridised to multiple probes attached along a solid-phase strip. The visual signal generated by such hybridisation allows a range of possible mutations to be detected and compared with a standard (Stuyver *et al.*, 1997). Problems with this assay include a lack of signal due to viral genome polymorphism in the hybridisation region. In addition, strips need almost constant updating in order to detect mutations conferring resistance to new drug combinations.

Restriction fragment length polymorphism assays. Based on the common ganciclovir resistance mutations within the UL97 (kinase) gene of CMV, a system has been devised involving two PCR reactions and restriction digests of the products to detect one or more of these mutations from clinical isolates. This system detects some 70% of currently recognised UL97 mutations, and can function as a useful screening assay (Chou *et al.*, 1995).

Nucleic acid sequencing. Recent advances in automated sequencing, such as the use of capilliary sequencers, allows for high throughput within a clinical laboratory setting. This has been most widely utilised for HIV drug resistance assays, but is appropriate for all functions such as the study of nosocomial transmission events. The biggest challenge that this technique provides is the manipulation and analysis of the data provided. Sequence editing is required, and subsequent sequence interpretation. With regard to HIV drug resistance, the identification

of key resistance mutations and interpretation of drug susceptibility pattern is variable, depending on the software systems utilised. When based on PCR-amplified product from the plasma, as they usually are, these techniques provide information only on the majority population within the quasispecies and cannot identify specific linkages between two or more mutations, i.e. they cannot exclude different mutations existing on separate genomes.

RECOMMENDED INVESTIGATIONS

Making an accurate virological diagnosis is critically dependent on receiving adequate and appropriate specimens relative to the onset of symptoms and the clinical presentation. All swabs and tissue samples should be placed into virus transport media, and if sample transport is delayed, samples should be stored at 4°C or on wet ice (for a maximum of 24 h). It is the role of the clinical virologist to decide on the most appropriate investigations for any given clinical scenario. Laboratory request forms are important in this respect, and should encourage documentation of full clinical details. The practice of sending a serum sample to the virology laboratory accompanying a request for a 'screen' should be strongly discouraged. In the light of assay developments and identification of new viruses, clinical protocols require constant updating. There is an increasing emphasis on direct and rapid detection of viral causes of disease, in contrast to retrospective serological diagnosis, and this is to be encouraged. Not only is this important for clinical management, but it also leads to a higher rate of positive identifications.

A special emphasis on the immunocompromised patient population is required, since they may experience life-threatening viral infections, which may present atypically. Ongoing antiviral prophylactic therapy may also distort the nature and timing of presentation. Table 1.10 highlights a typical set of protocols for the monitoring of transplant recipients. Precise protocols will depend on the patient group concerned, availability of laboratory facilities and, of course, budgetary constraints. Nevertheless, in the context of high-risk patients, such as those receiving long-term chemotherapy or transplants, the overall cost of virological investigations will be relatively small.

The time of retrospective viral diagnosis has gone, to be replaced by rapid techniques which impact directly on patient management. More competition for health care resources means that new techniques are introduced at the expense of more traditional methods with limited clinical use. Clinical virologists are having to work more closely with their clinical colleagues to establish new diagnostic criteria, develop protocols for use of antiviral drugs, and for monitoring of those patients with persistent infections. The diversity of diagnostic methods now available makes communication between physicians and clinical virologists more important than ever before.

REFERENCES

Abe A, Inoue K, Tanaka T *et al.* (1999) Quantitation of hepatitis B virus genomic DNA by real-time detection PCR. *J Clin Microbiol*, **37**, 2899–2903.

Altman DG and Bland JM (1994) Diagnostic tests 2: Predictive values. *Br Med J*, **309**, 102.

Arnold C, Barlow KL, Kaye S *et al.* (1995) HIV type 1 sequence subtype G transmission from mother to infant: failure of variant sequence species to amplify in the Roche Amplicor Test. *AIDS Res Hum Retroviruses*, **11**, 999–1001.

Beards G, Graham C and Pillay D (1998) Investigation of vesicular rashes for HSV and VZV by PCR. *J Med Virol*, **54**, 155–157.

Berger A and Preiser W (2002) Viral genome quantification as a tool for improving patient management: the example of HIV, HBV, HCV and CMV. *J Antimicrob Chemother*, **49**, 713–721.

BHIVA (2001) British HIV Association guidelines for the treatment of HIV-infected adults with antiretroviral therapy. *HIV Med*, **2**, 276–313.

Blanchard A, Ferris S, Chamaret S *et al.* (1998) Molecular evidence for nosocomial transmission of human immunodeficiency virus from a surgeon to one of his patients. *J Virol*, **72**, 4537–4540.

Boeckh M, Gooley TA, Myerson D *et al.* (1996) Cytomegalovirus pp65 antigenemia-guided early treatment with ganciclovir versus ganciclovir at engraftment after allogeneic marrow transplantation: a randomized double-blind study. *Blood*, **88**, 4063–4071.

Boeckh M, Woogerd PM, Stevens-Ayers T *et al.* (1994) Factors influencing detection of quantitative cytomegalovirus antigenemia. *J Clin Microbiol*, **32**, 832–834.

Bowen EF, Johnson MA, Griffiths PD and Emery VC (1997) Development of a point mutation assay for the detection of human cytomegalovirus UL97 mutations associated with ganciclovir resistance. *J Virol Methods*, **68**, 225–234.

Cane PA, Cook P, Ratcliffe D *et al.* (1999) Use of real-time PCR and fluorimetry to detect lamivudine resistance-associated mutations in hepatitis B virus. *Antimicrob Agents Chemother*, **43**, 1600–1608.

Carman B (2001) Molecular techniques should now replace cell culture in diagnostic virology laboratories. *Rev Med Virol*, **11**, 347–349.

Chakraborty H, Sen PK, Helms RW *et al.* (2001) Viral burden in genital secretions determines male-to-female sexual transmission of HIV-1: a probabilistic empiric model. *AIDS*, **15**, 621–627.

Chemello L, Alberti A, Rose K and Simmonds P (1994) Hepatitis C serotype and response to interferon therapy. *N Engl J Med*, **330**, 143.

Chernesky MA, Jang D, Sellors J *et al.* (1997) Urinary inhibitors of polymerase chain reaction and ligase chain reaction and testing of multiple specimens may contribute to lower assay sensitivities for diagnosing *Chlamydia trachomatis* infected women. *Mol Cell Probes*, **11**, 243–249.

Chesebro B and Wehrly K (1988) Development of a sensitive quantitative focal assay for human immunodeficiency virus infectivity. *J Virol*, **62**, 3779–3788.

Chou S, Guentzel S, Michels KR *et al.* (1995) Frequency of UL97 phosphotransferase mutations related to ganciclovir resistance in clinical cytomegalovirus isolates. *J Infect Dis*, **172**, 239–242.

Clark DA, Kidd IM, Collingham KE *et al.* (1997) Diagnosis of primary human herpesvirus 6 and 7 infections in febrile infants by polymerase chain reaction. *Arch Dis Child*, **77**, 42–45.

Dal Molin G, D'Agaro P, Ansaldi F *et al.* (2002) Mother-to-infant transmission of hepatitis C virus: rate of infection and assessment of viral load and IgM anti-HCV as risk factors. *J Med Virol*, **67**, 137–142.

Davis GL (2002) Monitoring of viral levels during therapy of hepatitis C. *Hepatology*, **36**, S145–S151.

Dewar RL, Highbarger HC, Sarmiento MD *et al.* (1994) Application of branched DNA signal amplification to monitor human immunodeficiency virus type 1 burden in human plasma. *J Infect Dis*, **170**, 1172–1179.

Drosten C, Gunther S, Preiser W *et al.* (2003) Identification of a novel coronavirus in patients with severe acute respiratory syndrome. *N Engl J Med*, **348**(20), 1967–1976. E-pub, 10 Apr 2003.

Dybul M, Fauci AS, Bartlett JG *et al.* (2002) Guidelines for using antiretroviral agents among HIV-infected adults and adolescents. Recommendations of the Panel on Clinical Practices for Treatment of HIV. *Morbid Mortal Wkly Rep Recomm Rep*, **51**, 1–55.

Einsele H, Ehninger G, Hebart H *et al.* (1995) Polymerase chain reaction monitoring reduces the incidence of cytomegalovirus disease and the duration and side effects of antiviral therapy after bone marrow transplantation. *Blood*, **86**, 2815–2820.

Fox JC, Griffiths PD and Emery VC (1992) Quantification of human cytomegalovirus DNA using the polymerase chain reaction. *J Gen Virol*, **73**(9), 2405–2408.

Fox JC, Kidd IM, Griffiths PD et al. (1995) Longitudinal analysis of cytomegalovirus load in renal transplant recipients using a quantitative polymerase chain reaction: correlation with disease. *J Gen Virol*, **76**(2), 309–319.

Gor D, Lee D and Emery VC (1996) Detection of human cytomegalovirus polymerase chain reaction products using oligonucleotide probes directly conjugated to alkaline phosphatase. *J Virol Methods*, **61**, 145–150.

Green J, Gallimore CI, Norcott JP et al. (1995) Broadly reactive reverse transcriptase polymerase chain reaction for the diagnosis of SRSV-associated gastroenteritis. *J Med Virol*, **47**, 392–398.

Gretch D, Corey L, Wilson J et al. (1994) Assessment of hepatitis C virus RNA levels by quantitative competitive RNA polymerase chain reaction: high-titer viremia correlates with advanced stage of disease. *J Infect Dis*, **169**, 1219–1225.

Guatelli JC, Whitfield KM, Kwoh DY et al. (1990) Isothermal, *in vitro* amplification of nucleic acids by a multienzyme reaction modeled after retroviral replication. *Proc Natl Acad Sci USA*, **87**, 7797.

Hall CB, Long CE, Schnabel KC et al. (1994) Human herpesvirus-6 infection in children. A prospective study of complications and reactivation. *N Engl J Med*, **331**, 432–438.

Hashida S, Hashinaka K, Nishikata I et al. (1996) Earlier diagnosis of HIV-1 infection by simultaneous detection of p24 antigen and antibody IgGs to p17 and reverse transcriptase in serum with enzyme immunoassay. *J Clin Lab Anal*, **10**, 213–219.

Hertogs K, de Bethune MP, Miller V et al. (1998) A rapid method for simultaneous detection of phenotypic resistance to inhibitors of protease and reverse transcriptase in recombinant human immunodeficiency virus type 1 isolates from patients treated with antiretroviral drugs. *Antimicrob Agents Chemother*, **42**, 269–276.

Hollinger FB, Bremer JW, Myers LE et al. (1992) Standardization of sensitive human immunodeficiency virus coculture procedures and establishment of a multicenter quality assurance program for the AIDS Clinical Trials Group. The NIH/NIAID/DAIDS/ACTG Virology Laboratories. *J Clin Microbiol*, **30**, 1787–1794.

Hsuih TC, Park YN, Zaretsky C et al. (1996) Novel, ligation-dependent PCR assay for detection of hepatitis C in serum. *J Clin Microbiol*, **34**, 501–507.

Hughes MD, Johnson VA, Hirsch MS et al. (1997) Monitoring plasma HIV-1 RNA levels in addition to CD4$^+$ lymphocyte count improves assessment of antiretroviral therapeutic response. ACTG 241 Protocol Virology Substudy Team. *Ann Intern Med*, **126**, 929–938.

Ison MG and Hayden FG (2002) Viral infections in immunocompromised patients: what's new with respiratory viruses? *Curr Opin Infect Dis*, **15**, 355–367.

Jeffery KJ, Read SJ, Peto TE et al. (1997) Diagnosis of viral infections of the central nervous system: clinical interpretation of PCR results. *Lancet*, **349**, 313–317.

Kao JH, Chen PJ, Lai MY and Chen DS (2002) Genotypes and clinical phenotypes of hepatitis B virus in patients with chronic hepatitis B virus infection. *J Clin Microbiol*, **40**, 1207–1209.

Kaye S, Loveday C and Tedder RS (1992) A microtitre format point mutation assay: application to the detection of drug resistance in human immunodeficiency virus type-1 infected patients treated with zidovudine. *J Med Virol*, **37**, 241–246.

Kozal MJ, Shafer RW, Winters MA et al. (1993) A mutation in human immunodeficiency virus reverse transcriptase and decline in CD4 lymphocyte numbers in long-term zidovudine recipients. *J Infect Dis*, **167**, 526–532.

Lai CL, Chien RN, Leung NW et al. (1998) A one-year trial of lamivudine for chronic hepatitis B. Asia Hepatitis Lamivudine Study Group. *N Engl J Med*, **339**, 61–68.

Lanciotti RS and Kerst AJ (2001) Nucleic acid sequence-based amplification assays for rapid detection of West Nile and St. Louis encephalitis viruses. *J Clin Microbiol*, **39**, 4506–4513.

Limaye AP, Jerome KR, Kuhr CS et al. (2001) Quantitation of BK virus load in serum for the diagnosis of BK virus-associated nephropathy in renal transplant recipients. *J Infect Dis*, **183**, 1669–1672.

Locatelli G, Santoro F, Veglia F et al. (2000) Real-time quantitative PCR for human herpesvirus 6 DNA. *J Clin Microbiol*, **38**, 4042–4048.

Longo MC, Berninger MS and Hartley JL (1990) Use of uracil DNA glycosylase to control carry-over contamination in polymerase chain reactions. *Gene*, **93**, 125–128.

Lyall EG, Blott M, de Ruiter A et al. (2001) Guidelines for the management of HIV infection in pregnant women and the prevention of mother-to-child transmission. *HIV Med*, **2**, 314–334.

Mackay IM, Arden KE and Nitsche A (2002) Real-time PCR in virology. *Nucleic Acids Res*, **30**, 1292–1305.

Mellors JW, Munoz A, Giorgi JV et al. (1997) Plasma viral load and CD4+ lymphocytes as prognostic markers of HIV-1 infection. *Ann Intern Med*, **126**, 946–954.

Mellors JW, Rinaldo CR Jr, Gupta P et al. (1996) Prognosis in HIV-1 infection predicted by the quantity of virus in plasma. *Science*, **272**, 1167–1170.

Miller I, Gunson R and Carman WF (2002) Norwalk-like virus by light cycler PCR. *J Clin Virol*, **25**, 231–232.

Montaner JS, Reiss P, Cooper D et al. (1998) A randomized, double-blind trial comparing combinations of nevirapine, didanosine, and zidovudine for HIV-infected patients: the INCAS Trial. Italy, The Netherlands, Canada and Australia Study. *J Am Med Assoc*, **279**, 930–937.

Morris T, Robertson B and Gallagher M (1996) Rapid reverse transcription-PCR detection of hepatitis C virus RNA in serum by using the TaqMan fluorogenic detection system. *J Clin Microbiol*, **34**, 2933–2936.

Ngui SL and Teo CG (1997) Hepatitis B virus genomic heterogeneity: variation between quasispecies may confound molecular epidemiological analyses of transmission incidents. *J Viral Hepatol*, **4**, 309–315.

Nigrovic LE and Chiang VW (2000) Cost analysis of enteroviral polymerase chain reaction in infants with fever and cerebrospinal fluid pleocytosis. *Arch Pediatr Adolesc Med*, **154**, 817–821.

Ogilvie M (2001) Molecular techniques should not now replace cell culture in diagnostic virology laboratories. *Rev Med Virol*, **11**, 351–354.

Ohkubo K, Kato Y, Ichikawa T et al. (2002) Viral load is a significant prognostic factor for hepatitis B virus-associated hepatocellular carcinoma. *Cancer*, **94**, 2663–2668.

O'Neill HJ, McCaughey C, Wyatt DE *et al.* (2001) Gastroenteritis outbreaks associated with Norwalk-like viruses and their investigation by nested RT-PCR. *BMC Microbiol*, **1**, 14.

O'Neill HJ, Russell JD, Wyatt DE *et al.* (1996) Isolation of viruses from clinical specimens in microtitre plates with cells inoculated in suspension. *J Virol Methods*, **62**, 169–178.

O'Shea S, Newell ML, Dunn DT *et al.* (1998) Maternal viral load, CD4 cell count and vertical transmission of HIV-1. *J Med Virol*, **54**, 113–117.

Parry JV, Perry KR, Panday S and Mortimer PP (1989) Diagnosis of hepatitis A and B by testing saliva. *J Med Virol*, **28**, 255–260.

Paya CV, Smith TF, Ludwig J and Hermans PE (1989) Rapid shell vial culture and tissue histology compared with serology for the rapid diagnosis of cytomegalovirus infection in liver transplantation. *Mayo Clin Proc*, **64**, 670–675.

Pepin JM, Simon F, Dussault A *et al.* (1992) Rapid determination of human cytomegalovirus susceptibility to ganciclovir directly from clinical specimen primocultures. *J Clin Microbiol*, **30**, 2917–2920.

Perry KR, Brown DW, Parry JV *et al.* (1993) Detection of measles, mumps, and rubella antibodies in saliva using antibody capture radioimmunoassay. *J Med Virol*, **40**, 235–240.

Peterson J, Green G, Iida K *et al.* (2000) Detection of hepatitis C core antigen in the antibody negative 'window' phase of hepatitis C infection. *Vox Sang*, **78**, 80–85.

Piatak M Jr, Luk KC, Williams B and Lifson JD (1993) Quantitative competitive polymerase chain reaction for accurate quantitation of HIV DNA and RNA species. *Biotechniques*, **14**, 70–81.

Powderly WG, Saag MS, Chapman S *et al.* (1999) Predictors of optimal virological response to potent antiretroviral therapy, *AIDS*, **13**, 1873–1880.

Poynard T, Bedossa P and Opolon P (1997) Natural history of liver fibrosis progression in patients with chronic hepatitis C. The OBSVIRC, METAVIR, CLINIVIR, and DOSVIRC groups. *Lancet*, **349**, 825–832.

Quinn TC, Wawer MJ, Sewankambo N *et al.* (2000) Viral load and heterosexual transmission of human immunodeficiency virus type 1. Rakai Project Study Group. *N Engl J Med*, **342**, 921–929.

Raschilas F, Wolff M, Delatour F *et al.* (2002) Outcome of and prognostic factors for herpes simplex encephalitis in adult patients: results of a multicenter study. *Clin Infect Dis*, **35**, 254–260.

Revello MG, Zavattoni M, Baldanti F *et al.* (1999) Diagnostic and prognostic value of human cytomegalovirus load and IgM antibody in blood of congenitally infected newborns. *J Clin Virol*, **14**, 57–66.

Saag MS, Holodniy M, Kuritzkes DR *et al.* (1996) HIV viral load markers in clinical practice. *Nature Med*, **2**, 625–629.

Saiki RK, Gelfand DH, Stoffel S *et al.* (1988) Primer-directed enzymatic amplification of DNA with a thermostable DNA polymerase. *Science*, **239**, 487–491.

Sakugawa H, Nakasone H, Nakayoshi T *et al.* (2002) Preponderance of hepatitis B virus genotype B contributes to a better prognosis of chronic HBV infection in Okinawa, Japan. *J Med Virol*, **67**, 484–489.

Simmonds P, Holmes EC, Cha TA *et al.* (1993) Classification of hepatitis C virus into six major genotypes and a series of subtypes by phylogenetic analysis of the NS-5 region. *J Gen Virol*, **74**(11), 2391–2399.

Spector SA, Wong R, Hsia K *et al.* (1998) Plasma cytomegalovirus (CMV) DNA load predicts CMV disease and survival in AIDS patients. *J Clin Invest*, **101**, 497–502.

Sterling TR, Chaisson RE and Moore RD (2001) HIV-1 RNA, CD4 T-lymphocytes, and clinical response to highly active antiretroviral therapy. *AIDS*, **15**, 2251–2257.

Stirk PR and Griffiths PD (1988) Comparative sensitivity of three methods for the diagnosis of cytomegalovirus lung infection. *J Virol Methods*, **20**, 133–141.

Stuyver L, Wyseur A, Rombout A *et al.* (1997) Line probe assay for rapid detection of drug-selected mutations in the human immunodeficiency virus type 1 reverse transcriptase gene. *Antimicrob Agents Chemother*, **41**, 284–291.

Thomas DL, Villano SA, Riester KA *et al.* (1998) Perinatal transmission of hepatitis C virus from human immunodeficiency virus type 1-infected mothers. Women and Infants Transmission Study. *J Infect Dis*, **177**, 1480–1488.

Thomas HI and Morgan-Capner P (1991) Rubella-specific IgG1 avidity: a comparison of methods. *J Virol Methods*, **31**, 219–228.

Valentine-Thon E (2002) Quality control in nucleic acid testing—where do we stand? *J Clin Virol*, **25**(suppl 3), 13–21.

van den Hoogen BG, de Jong JC, Groen J *et al.* (2001) A newly discovered human pneumovirus isolated from young children with respiratory tract disease. *Nature Med*, **7**, 719–724.

van der Bij W, van Son WJ, van der Berg AP *et al.* (1989) Cytomegalovirus (CMV) antigenemia: rapid diagnosis and relationship with CMV-associated clinical syndromes in renal allograft recipients. *Transplant Proc*, **21**, 2061–2064.

van Gemen B, Kievits T, Nara P *et al.* (1993) Qualitative and quantitative detection of HIV-1 RNA by nucleic acid sequence-based amplification. *AIDS*, **7**(suppl 2), S107–110.

Vet JA, Majithia AR, Marras SA *et al.* (1999) Multiplex detection of four pathogenic retroviruses using molecular beacons. *Proc Natl Acad Sci USA*, **96**, 6394–6399.

Victor T, Jordaan A, du Toit R and Van Helden PD (1993) Laboratory experience and guidelines for avoiding false positive polymerase chain reaction results. *Eur J Clin Chem Clin Biochem*, **31**, 531–535.

Wai CT, Chu CJ, Hussain M and Lok AS (2002) HBV genotype B is associated with better response to interferon therapy in HBeAg(+) chronic hepatitis than genotype C. *Hepatology*, **36**, 1425–1430.

Wiedbrauk DL, Werner JC and Drevon AM (1995) Inhibition of PCR by aqueous and vitreous fluids. *J Clin Microbiol*, **33**, 2643–2646.

Wittwer CT, Herrmann MG, Moss AA and Rasmussen RP (1997) Continuous fluorescence monitoring of rapid cycle DNA amplification. *Biotechniques*, **22**, 130–131, 134–138.

Wulff H and Lange JV (1975) Indirect immunofluorescence for the diagnosis of Lassa fever infection. *Bull WHO*, **52**, 429–436.

Zeuzem S, Ruster B and Roth WK (1994) Clinical evaluation of a new polymerase chain reaction assay (Amplicor HCV) for detection of hepatitis C virus. *Z Gastroenterol*, **32**, 342–347.

Zuckerman MA, Hawkins AE, Briggs M *et al.* (1995) Investigation of hepatitis B virus transmission in a health care setting: application of direct sequence analysis. *J Infect Dis*, **172**, 1080–1083.

2

The Herpesviridae

Graham M. Cleator[1] and Paul E. Klapper[2]

[1]*Manchester Royal Infirmary and* [2]*Health Protection Agency, Leeds, UK*

The *Herpesviridae* are a large family of enveloped double-stranded DNA viruses. To date, more than 130 members of the family have been identified. These viruses have been found in almost every species in which they have been actively sought, including both warm- and cold-blooded species, vertebrate and invertebrate. Some species appear to be the host of only one member of the *Herpesviridae*, whilst others harbour multiple viruses (e.g. 16 herpesviruses have been found in cercopithecine spp., and nine equid herpesviruses are known). The viruses are clearly ancient pathogens which have co-evolved with man and other species over more than 200 million years (McGeogh and Davidson, 1999).

Viruses included in the family *Herpesviridae* have a double-stranded DNA genome of 80–150 million Da molecular weight. The DNA has up to 200 potential open reading frames, and functional characterisation of these viral genes by the generation of virus mutants and observation of the resultant change in phenotype has been extensively explored in order to further understanding of herpesvirus replication and pathogenesis (Wagner *et al.*, 2002). The genome, tightly wound in the form of a torus, is enclosed within an icosadeltahedral capsid (triangulation number, $T = 16$), 100–110 nm in diameter. The capsid is composed of 12 pentavalent capsomers and 150 hexavalent capsomers. The hexagonal capsomeres (7.5 × 12.5 nm in size) have a central channel 4 nm in diameter running from the surface to the inside of the nucleocapsid. An envelope surrounds the nucleocapsid. This has a typical trilaminar appearance in thin section electron microscopy. Numerous glycoprotein spikes project from the envelope, these being more numerous and shorter than are found on the surface of other enveloped viruses. The glycoprotein spikes provide important antigenic determinants that distinguish individual members of the group. Between the nucleocapsid and the envelope is an amorphous electron dense area, the tegument. This is believed to have an ordered structure and contain proteins that are important to the virus in controlling host cellular functions immediately following virus penetration of the host cell. The overall diameter of the enveloped particle is 120–300 nm, depending upon the particular virus and the preparation method utilised for examination in the electron microscope.

Following infection of their natural host, the viruses establish a latent infection that persists for the life of the host. In the latent state only a small subset of the viral genes are expressed. Reactivation, with expression of viral proteins and production of progeny virus, may occur at intervals to produce recurrent infection. This allows virus transmission to new, susceptible hosts. Individual members are well adapted to their natural host and exhibit little or no ability to cause cross-species infection. The viruses encode an array of enzymes involved in nucleic acid metabolism (e.g. thymidine kinase, DNA polymerase, ribonucleotide kinase) and in processing of proteins (e.g. protein kinases). The replication and assembly of progeny virus occurs in the host cell nucleus and capsids are enveloped as they transit through the nuclear membrane. The host cell is ultimately lysed as a result of virus infection.

Several members of the *Herpesviridae* have strong oncogenic associations, the most notable among the human herpesviruses being the associations of *Human*

Principles and Practice of Clinical Virology, Fifth Edition. Edited by A. J. Zuckerman, J. E. Banatvala, J. R. Pattison, P. D. Griffiths and B. D. Schoub
© 2004 John Wiley & Sons Ltd   ISBN 0 470 84338 1

Table 2.1   Properties of the human herpesviruses

Virus	Site of latency	G+C (moles %)	Genome (kb pairs)	Sequence*
Human herpesvirus 1	Sensory nerve ganglia	68	152	X14112
Human herpesvirus 2	Sensory nerve ganglia	69	154	Z86099
Human herpesvirus 3	Sensory nerve ganglia	46	125	X04370
Human herpesvirus 4	Leukocytes, epithelial cells	60	172	V01555
Human herpesvirus 5	B lymphocytes	57	229	X17403
Human herpesvirus 6A	T lymphocytes (CD4$^+$), epithelial cells	43	159	X83413
Human herpesvirus 6B	T lymphocytes (CD4$^+$), epithelial cells	43	162	AF157706
Human herpesvirus 7	T lymphocytes (CD4$^+$)	36	153	AF037218
Human herpesvirus 8	B lymphocytes, epithelial cells	59	170	U75698**

*European Molecular Biology Laboratory Accession Numbers (http://www.embl-heidelberg.de).
**Sequence lacks a 3 kb region at the right end of the genome that was refractory to cloning.

herpesvirus 4 (Epstein–Barr virus) with nasopharyngeal carcinoma and Burkitt's lymphoma, and *Human herpesvirus 8* with Kaposi's sarcoma and abdominal cavity B cell lymphomas in AIDS patients.

The Herpesvirus Study Group of the International Committee on the Taxonomy of Viruses divided the *Herpesviridae* family into three subfamilies, the *Alpha-*, *Beta-* and *Gammaherpesvirinae* (Roizman *et al.*, 1995), broadly on the basis of differences in the biological properties of the various viruses (Tables 2.1 and 2.2). This classification was made before the DNA sequence of individual members of the *Herpesviridae* was known. The Study Group subsequently classified a small number of herpesviruses into genera based on more objective parameters, such as: the conservation of genes and gene clusters and their relative position in the genome; the presence and distribution of nucleotides that are subject to methylation; and genome sequence arrangements (Figure 2.1). The latter difference is particularly distinctive: six different structural forms of virion DNA have been identified among members of the *Herpesviridae* (reviewed by Roizman and Pellet, 2001), differing in the presence and location of reiterations of terminal sequences of greater than 100 base pairs.

A formal binomial nomenclature is not currently applied in classification of the *Herpesviridae*. The International Committee on the Taxonomy of Viruses (van Regenmortel *et al.*, 2000; ICTVdB, 2002) agreed that herpesviruses will be described by serial number and the family or subfamily in which the natural host of the virus is classified (e.g. *Bovine herpesvirus 1*, *Cercopithecine herpesvirus 1*). Each subfamily is divided into a series of subgenera. The subfamily *Alphaherpesvirinae* contains two genera—*Simplexvirus*, exemplified by *Human herpesvirus 1*; and *Varicello-virus*, exemplified by *Human herpesvirus 3*. The subfamily *Betaherpesvirinae* contains three genera—

Table 2.2   Biological properties of *Herpesviridae*

Common properties

- Large, linear, double-stranded DNA genome
- Synthesis of DNA and assembly of capsid within the nucleus, acquire envelope by budding through nuclear membrane
- Specify a large array of enzymes involved in nucleic acid metabolism and synthesis
- Production of progeny virus results in destruction of the host cell
- Establish latency in their natural host

Alphaherpesvirinae

- Variable host range
- Short reproductive cycle
- Rapid spread in cell culture
- Efficient destruction of infected cells
- Establish latency primarily but not exclusively in sensory ganglia

Betaherpesvirinae

- Restricted host range (a non-exclusive property of this subfamily)
- Long reproductive cycle
- Infection progresses slowly in culture, frequently forming enlarged (cytomegalia) cells
- Latency in secretory glands, lymphoreticular cells, kidneys, and other tissues

Gammaherpesvirinae

- Experimental host range limited to family or order of natural host
- *In vitro* replication in lymphoblastoid cells
- *In vivo* replication and latency in either T or B lymphocytes

Cytomegalovirus, exemplified by *Human herpesvirus 5* (human cytomegalovirus); *Muromegalovirus*, exemplified by *Murid herpesvirus 1*; and *Roseolovirus*, exemplified by *Human herpesvirus 6*. The subfamily *Gammaherpesvirinae* contains two genera—*Lympho-cryptovirus*, exemplified by *Human herpesvirus 4*

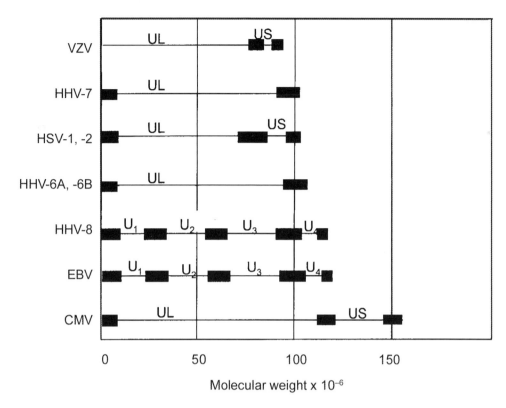

Figure 2.1 Diagram to illustrate the arrangement of sequences found in human herpesviruses. The blocks indicate reiterated sequences, the single lines are unique sequences designated as UL for unique long sequence, and US for unique short sequence or U1–4 illustrate the four unique regions found in HHV-8 and EBV genomes

Table 2.3 Classification of the Human herpesviruses

Official name	Subfamily	Genus	Trivial name and abbreviation
Human herpesvirus 1	*Alphaherpesvirinae*	*Simplexvirus*	Herpes simplex virus type 1 (HSV-1)
Human herpesvirus 2	*Alphaherpesvirinae*	*Simplexvirus*	Herpes simplex virus type 2 (HSV-2)
Human herpesvirus 3	*Alphaherpesvirinae*	*Varicellovirus*	Herpes varicella zoster virus (VZV)
Human herpesvirus 4	*Gammaherpesvirinae*	*Lymphocryptovirus*	Epstein–Barr virus (EBV)
Human herpesvirus 5	*Betaherpesvirinae*	*Cytomegalovirus*	Human cytomegalovirus (CMV)
Human herpesvirus 6A	*Betaherpesvirinae*	*Roseolovirus*	HHV-6A
Human herpesvirus 6B	*Betaherpesvirinae*	*Roseolovirus*	HHV-6B
Human herpesvirus 7	*Betaherpesvirinae*	–	HHV-7
Human herpesvirus 8	*Gammaherpesvirinae*	*Rhadinovirus*	Kaposi's sarcoma-associated herpesvirus (KSHV)

(Epstein–Barr virus); and *Rhadinovirus*, exemplified by *Samiirine herpesvirus 2*.

There are presently nine members of the *Herpesviridae* known to infect man (Table 2.3). These viruses are distributed worldwide and no animal reservoirs of infection have been identified for any of these viruses. The official names, *Human herpesviruses 1–8*, are seldom utilised, with the exception of *Human herpesviruses 6A, 6B, 7* and possibly *8*, and the viruses are more usually known by their vernacular (common) names (i.e. HHV-1 and 2, herpes simplex virus types I and 2; HHV-3, herpes varicella zoster virus; HHV-5, human cytomegalovirus; HHV-4, Epstein–Barr virus). One further member of the

Herpesviridae, Cercopithecine herpesvirus 1 (common name 'B' virus), is known to occasionally infect man (Huff and Barry, 2003). Transmitted by the bite of an infected monkey, the virus may cause an ascending myelitis that can progress to a fulminant demyelinating encephalopathy.

The reclassification of *Human herpesvirus* 6 as two distinct species was based upon the finding that all HHV-6 strains analysed could be segregated into one of two subtypes. Type B is the major aetiologic agent of exanthem subitum while type A has no clear association with human disease. The subtypes differ in *in vitro* cell tropism, reactivity with monoclonal antibodies and T cell clones, and in nucleotide sequence. Subtypes of other herpesviruses have been described, e.g. Epstein–Barr virus (HHV-4; EBV). The two EBV variants, EBV-1 and EBV-2, differ only in a small number of genes and the variants do not occupy discrete ecologic niches. By contrast, HHV-6A and HHV-6B show differences across their entire genomes; they differ in their epidemiology and association with disease, and recombination between viruses has not been described in nature.

REFERENCES

Huff JL and Barry PA (2003) B-virus (*Cepcopithecine herpesvirus 1*) infection in humans and macaques: potential for zoonotic disease. *Emerg Infect Dis*, **9**, 246–250.

ICTVdB (The Universal Virus Database of the International Committee on Taxonomy of Viruses) (2002) *http://www.ncbi.nlm.nih.gov/ICTVdb/index.htm.*

McGeogh DJ and Davison AJ (1999) The molecular evolutionary history of the herpesviruses. In *Origins and Evolution of Viruses* (eds Domingo E, Webster R and Holland J), pp. 441–465. Academic Press, New York.

Roizman B and Pellett PE (2001) The family *Herpesviridae*: a brief introduction. In *Field's Virology* (eds Fields BN, Knipe DM and Howley PM), pp. 2381–2397. Lippincott-Williams and Wilkins, Philadelphia.

Roizman B, Deroisiers RC, Fleckenstein B *et al.* (1995) Herpesviridae. In *Sixth Report of the International Committee on Taxonomy of Viruses* (eds Murphy FA, Fauquet CM, Bishop DHL *et al.*), pp. 1–586. *Arch Virol* (suppl 10). Springer Verlag, New York.

van Regenmortel MH, Fauquet CM, Bishop DHL *et al.* (2000) *Virus Taxonomy: The Classification and Nomenclature of Viruses. The Seventh Report of the International Committee on Taxonomy of Viruses*, pp. 1–1167. Academic Press, San Diego.

Wagner M, Ruzsics Z and Koskinowski UH (2002) Herpesvirus genetics has come of age. *Trends Microbiol*, **10**, 318–324.

2A

Herpes Simplex

Graham M. Cleator[1] and Paul E. Klapper[2]

[1]*Manchester Royal Infirmary and* [2]*Health Protection Agency, Leeds, UK*

THE VIRUSES

Human herpesvirus 1 (herpes simplex virus type 1; HSV-1) and *Human herpesvirus 2* (herpes simplex virus type 2; HSV-2) are members of the family *Herpesviridae*, subfamily *Alphaherpesvirinae*, genus *Simplexvirus*. Man is the only natural host, although a wide range of primates and non-primates can be infected under artificial (laboratory) conditions. Infection with either virus may be clinically inapparent or may produce symptoms which range from the mild and trivial to those of severe disease. During this infection, the virus establishes latency in the nuclei of nerve cells in the local dorsal root ganglion. At intervals throughout the life of the host the virus may reactivate (i.e. produce recurrent infection) and is either shed silently or produces overt symptoms. In immunocompromised individuals both primary infection and recurrent infection may be severe and life-threatening.

Morphology

The morphology of the viruses as seen by electron microscopy (EM) is similar for all members of the *Herpesviridae* (Figure 2A.1). By negative staining, transmission electron microscopy (EM) the virus particle often appears to be pleomorphic. However, the pseudo-replica EM technique reveals a spherical virus particle 150–200 nm in diameter with four structural elements:

- An electron-opaque core.

- A protein capsid, surrounding the virus core, comprised of 162 capsomeres.
- An amorphous tegument surrounding the capsid.
- An outer envelope with spikes on its surface.

The core is composed of linear double-stranded DNA packaged in the form of a torus. Data derived from electron micrographs suggests that the DNA is physically stabilised within the capsid by a series of protein fibrils embedded on the inner surface of the capsid and passing through the central hole of the torus. The ends of the genome are probably held in close proximity within the capsid, since the DNA rapidly circularises soon after it enters the host cell nucleus.

The viral capsid (100–110 nm in diameter) is a closed shell in the form of an icosadeltahedron ($T = 16$) with 162 capsomers arranged as 12 pentamers (vertices) and 150 hexamers (face and edges). Using high-resolution cryo-EM and computer image reconstruction techniques, the three-dimensional structure of empty capsids of HSV-1 has been determined to a resolution of approximately 8.5 Å (Zhou *et al.*, 2000). There appear to be four viral proteins (VPs 5, 19c, 23 and 26) aggregated as pentons and hexons that are associated with polypeptide triplexes to form the nucleocapsid. The interior of the capsid is accessible via trans-capsomeric channels (tubes) formed by the polypeptide arrangement of the pentons, hexons and holes at the base of each triplex. These openings are postulated to play a role in the transport of genomic DNA and scaffolding proteins during capsid morphogenesis.

Between the capsid and envelope is the tegument, an amorphous structure as visualised in thin section EM,

Principles and Practice of Clinical Virology, Fifth Edition. Edited by A. J. Zuckerman, J. E. Banatvala, J. R. Pattison, P. D. Griffiths and B. D. Schoub
© 2004 John Wiley & Sons Ltd   ISBN 0 470 84338 1

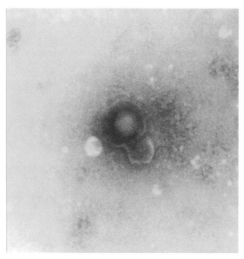

Figure 2A.1   Enveloped virus particle, HSV-1

but with a fibrous appearance on negative staining. The tegument contains at least 12 proteins that are believed to have important functions in the early stages of virus replication following penetration of the host cell by the virion.

The virus envelope has a typical trilaminar appearance and is thought to be derived from patches of host cell nuclear membrane modified by the insertion of virus glycoprotein spikes. Numerous such spikes may be observed on the surface of the envelope, with lengths ranging from 8 to 24 nm (Stannard *et al.*, 1987).

REPLICATION

The viruses are characterised by a short (18–24 h) replicative cycle that is cytolytic. Initial attachment and penetration of the host cell is mediated via the glycoprotein spikes of the virus envelope. These spikes have been extensively investigated (Table 2A.1) and the major antigenic differences between HSV-1 and HSV-2 relate to the type-specific epitopes found on certain of these glycoproteins (Bergstom and Trybala, 1996).

Studies with deletion mutants, purified glycoproteins, peptides and monoclonal antibodies show that *in vitro*, at least four of the 11 virion glycoproteins are essential for virus entry to a host cell and for egress from the infected cell. Initial attachment of HSV-1 appears to be mediated via glycoprotein C (and to a lesser extent by glycoprotein B) and initial attachment of HSV-2 by glycoprotein B (Chesenko and Herold, 2002). These glycoproteins bind to glycosaminoglycan moieties of cell surface heparan sulphate or, on cells

Table 2A.1   HSV glycoproteins

Glycoprotein nomenclature[1]	Gene[2]	Essential for virus infectivity[3]	Function
gB	$U_L 27$	Yes	gB is essential for viral entry. It forms a dimer and induces neuralising antibody
gC	$U_L 44$	No	Involved in cell attachment and may have a role in blocking the host response to infection
gD	$U_S 6$	Yes	Required after attachment of virus to cell, to allow virus entry into the cell
gE	$U_S 8$	No	Complexes with gI. Binds Fc portion of antibodies
gG	$U_S 4$	No	Involved in entry, egress and spread from cell to cell
gH	$U_L 22$	Yes	Forms complex with gL. Role in entry, egress and cell–cell spread
gI	$U_S 7$	No	gI and gE form a complex for transport to plasma membrane where the Fc receptor is expressed
gJ	$U_S 5$	No	Minor glycoprotein reported role in blocking apoptosis
gK	$U_L 53$	No	Required for efficient egress (viral exocytosis)
gL	$U_L 1$	Yes	Forms complex with gH, which is required for transport of gH and gL to plasma membrane and for viral entry mediated by gH
gM	$U_L 11$	No	Necessary for efficient encapsidation and exocytosis

[1]Viral glycoproteins are named sequentially by letter as glycoprotein A, glycoprotein B, etc. The missing sequence letters (e.g. gA, gF) reflect earlier misidentification of precursors of glycoprotein species as the actual virion glycoprotein. There are a further two (the products of genes $U_L 20$ and $U_L 34$), and possibly more, non-glycosylated viral proteins inserted in the membrane.
[2]Gene or transcriptional unit: U_S = unique short sequence of the genome; U_L = unique long sequence.
[3]Information from *in vitro* experimentation with HSV-1. All glycoproteins are essential in wild-type virus. In cell culture only some functionality can be dispensed with. Requirement of glycoprotein, non-essential in routine cell culture, can be demonstrated under specialised conditions, e.g. gC is essential for attachment to the apical surface of polarised MDCK cells; gI is essential for basolateral spread of virus in polarised cells.

devoid of heparan sulphate, equivalent glycosamino-glycan moieties of other cell surface proteoglycans, such as chondroitin sulphate. Initial attachment is followed by the binding of glycoprotein D to a co-receptor belonging to one of several cell surface molecules (including a member of the tumour necrosis factor family, members of the immunoglobulin super-family or an *O*-sulphated form of heparan sulphate).

Attachment to the host cell activates a process mediated by the virion surface glycoproteins that induces a pH-independent fusion of the virion envel-ope and cell plasma membrane. This process probably involves several, if not all, of the virion surface glycoproteins. Fusion results in the introduction of tegument proteins and viral nucleocapsid into the cell cytoplasm. Subsequently host macromolecular meta-bolism is rapidly and efficiently shut down. Host DNA synthesis ceases, protein synthesis declines rapidly, ribosomal RNA synthesis is reduced and host protein glycosylation ceases. There are at least 12 tegument proteins, and whilst the function of a number of these is not understood, they are all believed to act directly or indirectly to produce early shut-off of host macromolecular synthesis and to contribute to the early events of replication. The virion-associated host shut-off protein (vhs) appears to remain in the cytoplasm, where it causes the disaggregation of polyribosomes and degradation of cellular and viral RNA. Conversely, some tegument proteins are believed to facilitate attachment of the nucleocapsid to nuclear pores and facilitate release of viral DNA.

The nucleocapsid is transported through the cyto-plasm to a nuclear pore via microtubules of the cell cytoskeleton. On arrival at a nuclear pore, virus DNA is released from the capsid into the nucleus of the cell, where it immediately circularises. To initiate transcrip-tion, the circularised DNA binds a host cell protein (OCT-1), the tegument protein α-trans inducing factor (α-TIF), an additional host cell factor designated C1, and other transcriptional factors to promote the expression of α (or 'immediate early') genes—the first set of viral genes to be transcribed (Roizman and Knipe, 2001). Viral gene expression is regulated and sequentially ordered as a cascade (α→β→γ). The five α gene products are regulatory proteins, their expression is required for the production of all subsequent polypeptide groups. The proteins serve to *trans*-activate β and γ gene expression and to turn off both α and early γ gene expression (other domains of the viral genome are transcribed under 'α' conditions including the 'latency-associated transcript' LAT-1; see below). Viral DNA is transcribed throughout the replicative cycle by host RNA polymerase II.

The expression of the β genes results in the production of enzymes involved in nucleic acid metabolism (ribonucleotide reductase, thymidine kinase, thymidilate synthetase, alkaline DNase, dUT-Pase, etc.) and in DNA synthesis (DNA polymerase, helicase, primase, etc.). Peak rates of synthesis of β gene products are observed 5–7 h post-infection, and when sufficient levels of these proteins have accumu-lated within the infected cell, viral DNA replication commences. Early (α) gene expression is significantly reduced following the start of DNA replication, while late genes begin to be expressed at high levels. HSV DNA is believed to replicate by a rolling circle mechanism, yielding a concatomer that must be subsequently cleaved to package genome lengths of DNA within the nucleocapsid.

The synthesis of nucleocapsid and all other struc-tural proteins occurs when γ gene expression is induced by β gene products. HSV capsids are assembled around viral scaffolding proteins in the nucleus, and other viral proteins then interact with replicated viral DNA to allow DNA encapsidation. The tegument proteins also migrate to the cell nucleus and form patches underneath the modified nuclear membrane. The DNA-filled capsids proceed to associate with tegument (matrix) proteins near the nuclear mem-brane. Virus glycoproteins undergo extensive post-translational modification during transit through the Golgi apparatus; they then become inserted in the nuclear and other cellular membranes. Mature nucleo-capsids bud through the nuclear membrane at these points and acquire their envelope and tegument. The virion is released from the infected cell by transit through the cisternae of the rough endoplasmic reticulum of the Golgi apparatus and cytoplasmic transport vesicles. Productive infection of a cell results in the destruction of the host cell, through the major structural and biochemical changes induced by the replication of the virus.

PATHOGENESIS

Terminology

A *primary infection* refers to the first experience of HSV-1 or HSV-2 infection by a susceptible individual. If a person already infected with one type of virus (e.g. HSV-1) becomes infected with the other virus type (e.g. HSV-2), then the infection is described as an *initial infection*. During primary infection and during initial infection the virus establishes a *latent infection* of sensory nerves at the local dorsal root ganglion.

Subsequent reactivation of latent virus results in *recurrent infection*. If someone already infected with HSV becomes infected with the same strain of virus but at a different site to the usual site of recurrent infection (e.g. transfer of HSV-1 from a cold sore to the eye), then the infection at the new site is described as an *endogenous reinfection*. Finally, it is possible that a person already infected with HSV may be reinfected with the same type of virus. Infection in this case is described as *exogeneous reinfection*.

Overview

Man is the only natural host of HSV. While animal studies have provided, and continue to provide, significant insights into the pathogenetic mechanisms of HSV infection of humans, it is important to appreciate that no animal model can exactly mimic human HSV disease.

The transmission of HSV requires direct contact between a susceptible individual (usually antibody-negative) and a person actively shedding the virus. Transfer of virus is achieved by infection of mucosal surfaces or by entry through abrasions or cuts in the skin. Virus replication occurs at the site of infection and produces a short-lived viraemia. This primary infection is usually inapparent, but in a minority of cases may lead to localised and even systemic symptoms. The site of infection is mainly determined by the route of transmission of the virus from the infected to the susceptible host. For HSV-1 it is the buccal cavity and oropharynx, and for HSV-2 the genital mucosa. However, HSV-1 and HSV-2 may infect at either of these sites.

Latency is central to the success of HSV as a human pathogen; it permits persistence of the virus in the presence of a fully developed immune response and life-long infection of the host. As a result of periodic reactivation of latent virus and the production of recurrent infection, virus shedding and transmission of infection to susceptible individuals occurs at intervals throughout life, allowing the virus to persist in populations with high levels of herd immunity.

During the primary or initial infection, the virus comes into contact with the cutaneous receptors of local sensory nerves. It attaches to and penetrates the nerve cell via these receptors. Once internalised, the nucleocapsid moves to the perikaryon, utilising the normal cellular retrograde axoplasmic flow. Viral DNA is released, enters the nucleus and immediately circularises. Viral gene expression is then tightly restricted, so that the usual cascade of gene expression and the cytopathic results of productive infection do not occur. A latent infection of the nerve cell is established. In the latent state the virus is believed to exist as extrachromosomal circularised DNA (analogous to plasmids). No virions can be detected and no viral antigens appear to be expressed on or within the latently infected cell. The host immune response to infection rapidly eliminates virus and virus-infected cells from peripheral sites but does not recognise latently infected nervous tissue as harbouring virus, since no viral antigens are expressed.

The site of virus latency is related to the site of primary infection; for HSV-1 the trigeminal ganglia, and for HSV-2 the sacral ganglia, are the most common sites. Other dorsal root ganglia, including the superior cervical, vagal and geniculate ganglia, may also harbour virus. Although primary HSV-1 infection of the genitalia and primary HSV-2 infection of the oropharynx are often reported, recurrent infection of the genitalia by HSV-1 and recurrent orofacial infection by HSV-2 are uncommon. Infrequent reactivation is not thought to be due to a failure by HSV-1 to establish latent infection in cells of the sacral ganglia, or of HSV-2 to fail to establish latent infection in cells of the trigeminal ganglion, since the respective genomes of the viruses have been detected at these sites. The inhibition seems to be at the level of effective viral gene expression in relation to the particular environment of these sites. Sensory nerve ganglia may not be the only sites of latency of HSV. Using molecular techniques for the detection of viral nucleic acid, evidence for latency within the cornea, brain and other (non-neuronal) sites is accumulating.

Latently infected neurones apparently contain no viral protein but do contain numerous virus-specified RNA transcripts—the so-called latency-associated transcripts (LATs). Mutant viruses that do not produce LATs (i.e. LAT⁻) are also capable of establishing latency. Thus, the production of LAT transcripts alone is insufficient to explain the establishment of latency. The maintenance of the HSV genome in latently infected neurones appears to be passive, in that it does not require any other viral gene expression or gene product. In latently infected individuals, 0.2–4.3% of neurones in the human trigeminal ganglia have been found to harbour viral DNA (Cohrs and Gilden, 2001) and latently infected neurones seem to harbour more than one viral genome per cell. It is possible that low levels of replication of the viral genome occur, since in animal experiments the numbers of copies per cell appears to increase with time. Such low-level replication may be important for the maintenance of latency and to allow reactivation. A host-dependent origin of DNA replication has been identified within the viral genome (Sears and Roizman, 1990) and thus host cell enzymes could effect viral protein expression-independent replication of the viral DNA in latently infected neurones.

The LAT intron is stable within the latently infected cell nucleus and, whilst LAT-negative viruses are capable of establishing latency, these viruses, which can lack LAT, a LAT promoter, or a 348 bp sequence in the 5' end of LAT, exhibit reduced efficiency of reactivation. However, a full understanding of the role of LATs and of other molecular events involved in latency remains elusive. Among the many functions ascribed to the LAT introns are: downregulation of genes that are lytic; blocking the transcription of the gene encoding ICP0 (a potent gene transactivator); enabling reactivation from the latent state; maintenance of virus in the latent state; and protection of neurones from apoptosis.

Reactivation of latent virus produces recurrent infection. A variety of non-specific 'triggers' for this process have been described, e.g. injury to tissue innervated by the latently infected neurones, emotional or physical stress, menstruation, ultraviolet light, hormone imbalance. However, the molecular basis of such 'triggering' is not understood. A conceptual difficulty is that productive herpes simplex infection is cytolytic. If the usual process of virus replication were followed in nervous tissue, then an individual experiencing frequent reactivation over a period of years might be expected to experience local loss of sensation through the progressive depletion of sensory nerves. The damage might also be compounded through the action of the immune system, because in a productive infection virus antigens are expressed on the infected cell surface, rendering the infected cell 'visible' to the immune system. Various models have been proposed to explain this process, although none is entirely satisfactory. It seems likely that, upon reactivation, virus replication is so thoroughly controlled that only a few virions are produced, with no expression of virion glycoproteins on the cell surface (thereby permitting the cell to escape immune-mediated cytolysis). Viral genes interfere with apoptosis to prevent cell death and the cytopathology associated with normal productive infection is thereby prevented. In this way the neurone may be able to survive repeated episodes of reactivation.

Studies of HSV-1 infection of cultured human embryonic dorsal root ganglion cells (Lycke et al., 1988) suggest that egress of virus from sensory nerves is accomplished via anterograde axoplasmic flow in transport vesicles. The released virus infects adjacent skin cells, replicates, and infects further cells by cell-to-cell passage, leading to the distinctive lesions of recurrent HSV infection.

The Immune Response to Infection

Data derived from animal experimentation suggests that the host genetic make-up has an important role in determining immune responsiveness and disease pathogenesis. In man, despite numerous reports that have alternately suggested or refuted human leukocyte antigen (HLA) associations with HSV infection, there is no firm evidence to either confirm or deny HLA involvement in disease pathogenesis. Recovery from HSV infection and the control of reactivated virus infection involves all components of the immune system, acting in concert as an immune 'network' (Jerne, 1976). Macrophages, specific T cell populations, complement, specific antibodies and lymphokine and cytokine responses all have an important role in the immune response to HSV infection.

Humoral Immunity

Western blot and radio-immune precipitation experiments show that serum from patients recovering from severe HSV infection may contain antibody to all the structural (virion) proteins of HSV. The actual number and quantity of antibodies detected correlate with the severity of infection and in mild infection only a restricted number of antibodies may be detectable.

The immune response is principally directed to the glycoprotein spikes (Table 2A.1) found on the virion envelope and on the surface of virus-infected cells. Neutralising and cytolytic antibodies may be detected, glycoprotein D being the most potent inducer of neutralising antibody. In a primary infection, an IgM subclass response is detected just before, or at the same time as, an IgG and IgA immune response. The response is relatively short-lived but IgM antibody may also be detected during recurrence, rendering serological differentiation of primary from recurrent infection difficult. Both IgG and IgA antibody persist, although the IgG antibody response is of greater magnitude. Repeated HSV recurrences lead to a gradual boosting of antibody levels but individual reactivation events or even reinfection may not result in a significant increase in circulating antibody. The presence of serum antibody may not protect from reinfection, and neither the quantity nor the range of reactivity (i.e. the lack of antibody to a particular virus protein) appears directly to influence either the frequency or severity of reactivation events.

The early immune response to HSV is relatively type-specific but 'later' antibody is more broadly cross-reacting. Monoclonal antibody studies show that both type-common and type-specific epitopes may be found on virion glycoproteins. As a major part of the humoral immune response is directed to virion glycoproteins, the change from type specificity with time presumably reflects temporal changes in the relative preponderance of antibodies to type-specific and subsequently type-common epitopes on the virion glycoproteins.

Cell-mediated Immunity

The cellular immune response to infection involves a complex interaction of natural killer cells, macrophages, T lymphocytes and associated cytokines. During initial or primary infection, the appearance of non-specific inflammatory changes coincide with the peak of viral replication. Delayed type hypersensitivity reactions may be detected that are followed by a cytotoxic T lymphocyte (CTL) response and the appearance of IgM and IgG specific antibodies. When virus reactivates from latency and produces lesions, there is a swift infiltration of natural killer cells and CD4 T cells, followed by CD8 T cells. High levels of β-chemokines and T cell cytokines are also found. CTL activity peaks with CD4 activity and correlates with viral clearance (Koelle and Corey, 2003).

The majority of adults can be shown to be HSV-seropositive and are therefore presumed to harbour latent virus. About 45% of this population give a history of herpes labialis. Some may recall only one recurrence, whilst others report frequent episodes. If seropositive persons with no history of herpes labialis are monitored, silent virus shedding may be shown to occur at intervals. Differences in humoral immune status fail to explain these observations. In a comparison of persons with infrequent recrudescence of orofacial herpes and those with frequent recurrence (10 or more episodes per year), only differences in HSV-specific T cell proliferation, interferon-γ production and levels of HSV-specific IgE could be demonstrated between the two groups (McKenna *et al.*, 2001). In those suffering frequent recurrence, the immune response is apparently both delayed and less effective than those with infrequent recurrences and is manifest as less effective control of HSV in the periphery following reactivation from latency. The reasons for the appearance or non-appearance of clinical symptoms

and the severity of these symptoms are therefore probably explained in terms of an early and effective local cellular immune response. Support for this hypothesis is found in patients with known cellular immune deficiencies, where herpes labialis occurs frequently and is a very much more severe and prolonged disease.

Virus-induced Modulation of the Immune Response

In cell culture experiments *in vitro* and in animal experiments, HSV-1 has been shown to be capable of preventing apoptosis in differentiated cells. Premature death of a virus-infected cell presents one of a range of possible host responses to prevent the spread of virus to other, as-yet uninfected, cells. The products of genes that map to the long unique component of the viral genome, particularly the γ34.5 gene (Chou and Roizman, 1994), appear to be involved in this process. The viral glycoproteins expressed on the surface of the infected cell provide further modulators of the immune defence. The complex of glycoproteins E and I (Table 2A.1) produces an Fc receptor which binds monomeric IgG molecules. Glycoprotein E, by itself, provides a further type of Fc receptor binding polymeric IgG molecules. Glycoprotein C has been shown to bind the C3b component of complement, possibly through mimicry of the C3b receptor CR1. The effect of these molecules is presumably to interfere in antibody interaction with infected cells and virions and complement-mediated and antibody-dependent cytotoxic T cell destruction of virus-infected cells. A further effect of HSV is to prevent the induction of CD8$^+$ T lymphocytes. It is known that HSV-induced epithelial lesions contain a disproportionately high number of CD4$^+$ cells and relatively few CD8$^+$ cells. It appears that the product of the α47 gene of HSV renders cells resistant to the activity of CD8$^+$ lymphocytes by retaining MHC class 1 molecules in the cytoplasm, resulting in a lack of peptide presentation on the cell surface (York *et al.*, 1994). In addition, a wide variety of HSV-induced mechanisms operate to interfere in antigen presentation and processing, in modulating interferon production and in interfering with its action and that of other chemokines and cytokines (reviewed by Koelle and Corey, 2003).

Pathogenesis in Immunocompromised Patients

Congenital deficiencies in humoral immunity (hypo-gammaglobulinaemia, or even agammaglobulinaemia) do not appear to be significant risk factors for serious primary or recurrent HSV disease. Congenital deficiencies in CMI may, however, be associated with severe HSV disease. The risk of serious disease varies with the particular immune deficit, e.g. patients with congenital athymic aplasia (Di George syndrome) do not appear to be at particular risk, whilst those with severe combined immune deficiency, such as the Wiskott–Aldrich syndrome, are. These differences emphasise the complex interplay of the immune network in controlling HSV infection. Severe HSV disease is also observed in infants, children and adults with deficiencies in CMI induced by 'therapy'. These include recipients of cytoxic chemotherapy (e.g. for cancer) and recipients of major organ grafts. The severity of HSV disease in these patients is related to the type and degree of immunosuppression. Severe primary and recurrent HSV infections also occur in patients with AIDS.

EPIDEMIOLOGY

HSV has a worldwide distribution and is endemic in all human population groups examined. There do not appear to be any animal reservoirs for the infection. The rate of infection and the timing of primary infection differs for HSV-1 and HSV-2, reflecting the differences in the major modes of transmission of the two viruses.

Primary HSV-1 Infection

Primary HSV-1 infection usually occurs when a susceptible individual comes into close, intimate contact with an individual who is actively shedding the virus. Thus, infants become infected when their parents or relatives kiss them; adolescents who escape infection in infancy are usually infected later by kissing. Infection in an infant is likely to be missed or dismissed as 'teething'. In adolescents, infection is more commonly symptomatic but rarely severe. Because the majority of primary infections are asymptomatic, epidemiological data collected by observation of clinically apparent disease provide only a partial measure of its true incidence. For accurate data collection, serological studies must be employed.

The broad principles of the sero-epidemiology of primary HSV-1 infection were established in the classic study of Burnet and Williams (1939) and have since been confirmed in numerous studies. Burnet and Williams showed that in the first 6–9 months of life, infants escape infection by virtue of passively transferred maternal immunity. Later, infants become infected and develop HSV IgG antibody. The majority of these seroconversions occur during the first 5 years of life and those who escape infection in infancy undergo seroconversion during adolescence or early adulthood. A relationship between the age of acquisition of the virus and socioeconomic status was also found. Populations associated with a low socioeconomic environment collectively exhibited earlier acquisition of HSV infection than more affluent populations, although in both groups 90–95% infection rates were observed by early adulthood and primary HSV-1 infection was a rare event in those of > 30 years of age.

In recent years sero-epidemiological studies have shown that in developed countries there has been a lowering in the overall prevalence of HSV-1 antibody (rates of 70% or lower are often reported among 30–40 year-old adults). However, even within individual countries, there are wide variations of seroprevalence, e.g. inner city residents generally exhibit higher seroprevalence rates than those from rural areas. The major mediator of seroprevalence is the frequency of direct person-to-person contact. In crowded areas (e.g. disadvantaged inner city areas) seroprevalence is highest; in affluent, rural areas, seroprevalence is lowest. On a worldwide basis, however, overall rates of 90–95% seroprevalence are still commonplace in adult populations.

Primary HSV-2 Infection

HSV-2 transmission is apparently less efficient than that observed for HSV-1. The principal route of transmission is sexual activity. Although some infants acquire HSV-2 infection, in most cases primary infection is delayed until the onset of sexual activity in adolescence and early adulthood. At this time the majority will have already experienced primary infection with HSV-1 (i.e. infection with HSV-2 often causes an *initial* rather than a *primary* infection). Because of the shared antigenicity of HSV-1 and HSV-2, HSV-1 immunity may be partially protective and not all those exposed to HSV-2 will necessarily become infected. Also, since transmission usually involves sexual contact, the number of exposures to the virus will inevitably be lower than the number of exposures to HSV-1 infection.

A major problem in determining the sero-epidemiology of HSV-2 infections has been the lack of well-characterised methods to differentiate HSV-1 and HSV-2 antibody. Only very recently have relevant assays become available on a commercial basis (see section on Diagnosis, below). The data collected to date suggest that the major influence on acquisition of HSV-2 infections is, as might be expected for a sexually transmitted virus, the number of sexual partners. Rates of up to 95% seroprevalence have been reported in some female commercial sex workers. In the general population there are wide differences in seroprevalence between different patient groups and even between apparently similar social groups in different cities. Women are generally infected at an earlier age than men, and rates of infection in women are higher for all age groups up to and including those of 45 or more years of age. Studies among genitourinary medicine clinic attendees suggest that only in homosexual men do the rates of infection with HSV-2 match those found in women. Although even in this context, it is not until age 40–45 that equivalent rates are observed. The majority (80% or more) of those found to be HSV-2 antibody-positive cannot recall primary infection with the virus and either do not recall, or are unaware of, recurrent genital herpes, emphasising that, as with primary HSV-1 infection, the majority of primary infections are mild and clinically 'silent' (Van de Laar *et al.*, 1998).

The Changing Sero-epidemiology of HSV Infections

The changing sero-epidemiology of HSV-1 infections in developed countries has meant that primary eye infections with HSV are now infrequent in children but much more frequent in young adults. Young adults entering the world of work are also more frequently susceptible to primary herpes. In addition, HSV-1 is now much more commonly seen in association with genital herpes. In some UK studies 40–60% of isolates of HSV from first-episode genital herpes have been found to be due to HSV-1.

Recurrent HSV-1 and HSV-2 Infections

Both silent and overt (i.e. symptomatic) recurrences of HSV-1 and HSV-2 infection occur. Thus, without continuous monitoring of a cohort (by virus isolation studies), accurate data on rates of recurrence cannot be obtained. Only 38–45% of an adult population (in whom seroprevalence rates of 90–95% are reported) will give a history of recurrent herpes labialis.

The frequency of recurrence of genital HSV-2 infection (up to 60%) is higher than that observed in HSV-1 herpes labialis, although the number of lesions produced per episode and their duration are generally shorter. The rate of recurrence is believed to be slightly higher in men than in women, with rates of up to 2.7 and 1.9 episodes per 100 patient-days, respectively.

Endogenous and Exogenous Reinfections

Reinfection, recognised by the appearance of lesions at another body site, e.g. infection of the finger (herpetic whitlow), can occur at any age. Differentiation of endogenous and exogenous reinfection can only be accomplished by examination of viruses obtained from distinct sites and demonstration of genetic polymorphism by restriction enzyme analysis or sequencing of a region of their respective DNAs.

CLINICAL FEATURES

Oropharyngeal and Orofacial Infection

In a symptomatic, primary, HSV infection of the oropharynx, gingivostomatitis is the most common symptom. The incubation period ranges from 2 to 12 days, with a median of 4 days, and the duration of clinical illness is 2–3 weeks. The spectrum of severity ranges from the trivial, involving the buccal and gingival mucosa, to severe, painful, ulceration of the mouth, tongue, gingivae and fauces. In severe disease, shallow ulcers on an erythematous base evolve from vesicles and often coalesce, particularly on the mucosa of the cheeks and under the tongue. The ulcers are observed on the hard rather than the soft palate—a feature that may help differentiate herpetic ulcerations from those caused by the coxsackieviruses ('herpangina'). In young children the skin around the mouth is frequently involved. Submandibular lymphadenopathy and fever (39–40°C) are common and may produce febrile convulsions in children. A moderate lymphocytosis (up to 7000/mm^3) and mild neutropenia are frequently observed. Elevated liver enzymes are noted in occasional cases. Acute gingivostomatitis is a self-limiting disease and resolution begins abruptly. The lesions become painless and inflammation subsides. Intraoral ulceration progresses to healing, although crusting of lesions, as seen in resolving cutaneous HSV infection, is not usually observed. The patient becomes afebrile and symptoms regress rapidly, although lymphadenopathy may persist for several weeks.

Other symptoms that may be associated with primary infection include sore throat, mild conjunctivitis, nausea and vomiting, myalgia and abdominal discomfort. Dehydration and anorexia may result through the pain and oedema of the mucosal membrane infection, with its associated mouth discomfort and difficulty in swallowing. Older patients may experience a pharyngitis associated with a mononucleosis syndrome (up to 20% atypical lymphocytes) and submandibular lymphadenopathy. The tonsils are also frequently found to be ulcerated during this pharyngitis.

The oral disease can be associated with lesions elsewhere. Herpetic dermatitis, nasal herpes, ocular herpes, herpetic whitlows and even genital herpes are not infrequent complications of primary HSV infection of the mouth. These probably represent endogenous reinfections caused by auto-inoculation from the site of primary infection.

Recurrent infection, triggered by a variety of apparently non-specific stimuli (such as fever, stress, cold, menstruation and ultraviolet radiation) appears as a fresh vesicular eruption termed 'herpes labialis', 'herpes febrilis', 'fever blisters' or 'cold sores'. The most frequent site is at the border of the lips but lesions may appear elsewhere, e.g. on the chin, cheek and on or inside the nose. Their appearance is usually preceded by a prodrome of tingling or itching at the site where recurrence will occur. In the immunocompetent, the area of involvement is usually small and vesicles progress to the pustular and crusting stage within 3–4 days (Figure 2A.2). The time for complete healing is variable (5–12 days, mean 7.5 days).

Asymptomatic oral shedding of HSV can occur and is occasionally preceded by a prodrome similar to that associated with overt herpes labialis. Recurrent intraoral ulcers are only rarely caused by HSV. In the few instances where reactivation of HSV is responsible, lesions are limited to the gingivae and the hard palate. Severe cellular immune deficiency can, however, lead to extensive ulceration of the mouth and involve the pharynx and oesophagus.

Genital Infection

In comparison to primary infection of the oropharynx, primary genital infection is often a more severe clinical disease that may last for up to 3 weeks. Fever, dysuria associated with urethritis and cystitis (with urinary retention in a proportion), localised inguinal adenopathy and malaise are common. A prominent feature of primary genital herpes is pain, which, especially in women, may be severe. In women the lesions are located principally on the vulva but the vagina and cervix are almost always involved. The lesions may extend to the perineum, upper thigh and buttocks. In men, vesicular lesions with an erythematous base are observed on the glans of the penis or on the penile shank. Perianal and anal infections, producing proctitis, are common in homosexual men. Secondary microbial infections often follow primary genital HSV infection and their occurrence necessitates appropriate antimicrobial therapy.

Rarer complications of genital HSV infection include aseptic meningitis and sacral radiculomyelitis with urinary retention and attendent neuralgia. Primary (maternal) genital herpes occurring at or around the time of birth may produce severe neonatal infection (see below).

In recurrent genital herpes a limited number of vesicles are produced and their appearance is usually associated with a localised irritation, rather than with significant pain. In comparison to herpes labialis, recurrent lesions in the perineal area tend to be more numerous and can persist longer than their oral counterparts. New vesicles often appear during the course of a recurrence, and delay healing. The mean healing time in recurrent genital herpes may be up to 15 days, compared to an average of 7.5 days in recurrent oral disease. Complications (neurological or systemic) associated with recurrent infections are rare. Although HSV-1 is increasingly found as a cause of genital infection, recurrence of genital HSV-1 is infrequent, averaging about one episode per year in the first year and reducing thereafter. This contrasts with calculated rates of recurrence of HSV-2 genital herpes of 3–9 episodes per year. Overall, about 60% of patients known to have had primary infection will report recurrence, although, as serological surveys of HSV-2 seroprevalence indicate, this is probably an overestimate, since many of those shown to be HSV-2-seropositive are not aware of their infection.

Ocular Infection

The early symptoms of herpes keratitis are of a unilateral or bilateral conjunctivitis, with pre-auricular lymphadenopathy. The most common first presentation is, however, of a unilateral, characteristic, dendritic (branching) ulcer (Figure 2A.3). The normal course of the disease is 3 weeks but if ulcers are large, healing can be slow. Mild systemic disturbances, blepharitis and circumocular herpetic dermatitis are commonly present during the primary infection. Infection may occur as a part of a primary infection but most cases are thought to represent an endogenous reinfection caused by auto-inoculation from the site of a recurrent infection. Almost all cases are due to HSV-1. In the UK new HSV infections of the eye are estimated to occur at a rate of 8.4/100 000 person-years, the overall incidence of new and recurrent ocular HSV is 20.7/100 000 person-years and the prevalence of ocular HSV is 1.5 cases/1000 population.

A single recurrence of ophthalmic infection is observed in 20–30% of patients within 2 years of the first infection. Subsequent recurrences are less common but if a second recurrence does occur, then further recurrences will be observed in 40–45% of these cases. There are several forms of recurrent ophthalmic infection that may occur in combination. Dendritic or larger 'geographic' ulcers are usually the first manifestation of recurrence, with the patient complaining of ocular irritation, lacrimation, photophobia and sometimes blurring of vision. Infection is usually confined to the superficial layers of the cornea and stromal involvement is absent or only relatively mild. Days or weeks after the recurrent infection, the corneal epithelium may ulcerate to form a nondescript ovoid ulcer, known as post-infectious or metaherpetic keratitis. Virus replication does not appear to be directly responsible for the production of this ulcer. If the ulceration is prolonged (weeks and months) collagenolytic activity may appear, leading to stromal melting and perforation.

Repeated and severe epithelial disease recurrence or chronic epithelial keratitis leads to involvement of the deeper layers of the cornea, producing interstitial or disciform keratitis. Neo-vascularisation and scarring may ultimately lead to loss of vision. In developed countries, ocular HSV disease is the most common cause of corneal blindness (Liesegang, 1989).

The observation of recurrent infection of the cornea raises questions as to extraneuronal sites of latency of HSV. Restriction endonuclease analysis of viral DNA isolated from successive ocular recurrences suggests that the same strain of virus is involved in each recurrence. Repeated auto-inoculation of the virus from a cold sore seems unlikely and virus latency in the ophthalmic division of the trigeminal ganglion, and spread to the cornea in the tear film might not explain the recurrence of virus infection in the same region of the cornea in each episode. Thus, extraneuronal virus latency within the cornea has been suggested. Using the polymerase chain reaction (PCR) it has proved possible to demonstrate HSV DNA within corneal cells of both normal and diseased corneal tissues obtained at keratoplasty. Moreover, infectious virus has been isolated using co-cultivation techniques from corneas obtained from patients with stromal herpes keratitis. These observations do not in themselves prove that corneal latency of HSV occurs (they might reflect low-grade virus persistence, rather than latency) and further work will be required to allow firm conclusions to be drawn.

The influence of the immune response in control of ocular infection is an additional area of interest in the pathogenesis of ocular HSV infection. Because of the unique anatomy and physiology of the eye, the local immune response to infection may differ from that occurring at, for example, cutaneous sites. The lack of, and/or relative overproduction of, individual components of the immune response undoubtedly influences disease pathogenesis at this site.

Recurrent iridocyclitis and occasionally panuveitis may be caused by HSV. Iridocyclitis, produced by intraocular inflammation, is often observed in association with active herpes keratitis. It may be due to direct involvement of the virus or may be secondary to the irritative effects of keratitis. Acute retinal necrosis caused by HSV-1, or less commonly by HSV-2, is a severe ocular inflammatory syndrome associated with a poor (visual) prognosis. The presentation is usually unilateral but will progress to involve the fellow eye, even after extended periods of time. Suppressive antiviral therapy is therefore warranted for all patients suffering this complication of HSV infection of the eye.

Ophthalmic disease associated with intrauterine and neonatal infection with HSV can present as keratoconjunctivitis or later as chorioretinitis. However, cataract, corneal ulceration, anterior uveitis, vitritis, optic atrophy, nystagmus, strabismus, microphthalmia and retinal dysplasia have all been reported in association with such infection. Ocular manifestations are more common in those infected *in utero* than in those infected intra- or post-partum.

Neonatal Herpes

The reported incidence of neonatal herpes varies from extremes of 1 case in 2500 live births (Alabama, USA; Whitley, 1993) to 1.65 per 100 000 live births reported in a UK survey (Tookey and Peckham, 1996). In many parts of the world neonatal herpes is, or has been, predominantly caused by HSV-2. In a recent European review, however, 73% of cases were found to be due to HSV-1 (Gaytant et al., 2002). The difference between the incidence of neonatal herpes and the type of virus causing neonatal herpes observed in Europe was not explained in terms of the seroprevalence of HSV-1 and HSV-2 antibodies among pregnant women. The frequency of neonatal herpes did not increase over an observation period of 17 years when rates of genital herpes simplex infection were increasing. Furthermore, under-reporting of cases of neonatal herpes was thought unlikely, as the number of clinical virology laboratories serving the population increased more than two-fold during the period. Factors other than genital herpes must presumably be involved. The difference in rates of HSV-1-caused and HSV-2-caused neonatal herpes perhaps reflects the changing sero-epidemiology of HSV infections (see above), with increasing numbers of primary HSV-1 infections occurring at term and increases in post-natal acquisition of virus. In the largest US systematic study of neonatal herpes, involving the monitoring of more than 58 000 live births over a 17 year period to 1999 (Brown et al., 2003), 18 cases were identified, eight due to HSV-1 and 10 due to HSV-2.

Primary or initial maternal infection during the first or second trimester of pregnancy is not associated with significant risk to the developing foetus. However, congenital infection has been documented, the risk increasing when infection occurs during the third trimester. This intrauterine infection can lead to foetal loss or an infant born with overt disease. Premature rupture of the membranes can lead to ascending infection from an infected birth canal, and again an infant can be born with overt disease. Most commonly, infection is acquired during passage through an infected birth canal and disease is evident 3–21 days (mean 12 days) post-delivery. Infection can also occur as a result of transmission of oral herpes from the mother, her relatives or hospital staff in the immediate post-delivery period. In this situation disease may appear up to 28 days post-partum.

Symptoms at presentation can range from the very severe, associated with high mortality, to the relatively mild, which nonetheless can be a cause of significant residual morbidity. Most mothers bearing children who develop neonatal herpes *do not* have genital lesions at delivery and in up to 50% of cases the neonate may have no obvious skin lesions. American studies (Whitley, 1990) suggest that there are three types of disease presentation: those presenting with lesions of the skin, eye and mouth (evident 4–5 days

post-partum); those with neurological symptoms (appearing by day 17–18); and those with disseminated disease (apparent 11–12 days post-partum). The latter form of the disease carries the highest mortality, sometimes presenting as a picture of fulminant liver failure or as multi-organ failure, including CNS, lung, liver, adrenals, eyes and skin. Skin, eye and mouth disease may progress to involve the CNS or become disseminated. In the absence of specific antiviral therapy, mortality exceeds 80% in disseminated disease and exceeds 50% in those with CNS symptoms only. Both forms of disease are associated with severe morbidity. Babies exhibiting only skin, eye and mouth infection may suffer permanent ocular damage and most will, if followed for a sufficient period of time, eventually show some sign(s) of neurological impairment. All HSV infections identified in the neonatal period therefore warrant antiviral therapy.

The diagnosis of neonatal herpes must not rely solely upon examination of CSF. Investigation of CSF for HSV DNA in the skin, eye and mouth form of the disease is positive in only 24% of cases. This rises to 76% in neonatal herpes presenting as CNS symptoms and 93% in those with disseminated disease. Appropriate investigation of a potential case of neonatal herpes entails examination of blood, urine and skin or vesicle swabs, as well as CSF.

Primary maternal genital herpes poses the greatest threat to the neonate, although recurrent genital herpes is also a risk. In the study of Brown et al. (2003) four of the eight neonates with HSV-1-caused neonatal herpes were due to primary maternal HSV-1 infection and four were due to recurrent HSV-1. Of the 10 with HSV-2-caused disease, seven were due to primary or initial HSV-2 infection and three to recurrent maternal HSV-2 infection.

Herpes Simplex Encephalitis

The most common presentation of herpes simplex encephalitis (HSE) is of a focal encephalopathic process with signs and symptoms that localise to the frontotemporal and parietal areas of the brain. As the disease progresses, symptoms increase in severity and there is progressive decrease in consciousness, leading, in severe cases, to coma and death. In the majority of patients there is a history of a 'flu-like' illness occurring at some time in the 2 weeks preceding the appearance of neurological symptoms. Herpes encephalitis occurs in all age groups and with the same frequency in both men and women. There is no seasonal variation in incidence and cases occur sporadically. Because of under-reporting, precise estimates of the incidence of HSE are not possible, but estimates range from about 1 case per million population per year to 1 case per 200 000. Most cases are caused by HSV-1, with HSV-2 causing 2–6.5% of cases. In the immunocompromised, 'classical' herpes encephalitis appears to occur at the same rate as in the immunocompetent, although in AIDS patients an atypical, subacute encephalitis associated with either HSV-1 or -2 has been identified in 2% of cases studied at autopsy, usually in association with a concurrent CMV infection of the CNS (Cinque *et al.*, 1998).

The onset of disease may be either abrupt or insidious. In the early stages, signs and symptoms of the infection may not be distinctive. Electroencephalographic examination (EEG) will usually reveal non-specific slow-wave activity during the first 5–7 days of illness. Later, more characteristic paroxysmal sharp waves or triphasic complexes with a temporal predominance can be found. Low-density lesions are demonstrable by X-ray computed axial tomography (CAT) in about 70% of cases, within 5 days of the onset of neurological illness. Proton magnetic resonance imaging (MRI) has the potential to detect abnormalities that may not be revealed by routine CAT. MRI may show fronto-basal and temporal lesions, as hypointense lesions on T1-weighted images and hyperintense lesions on proton density and T2-weighted images at an earlier stage than changes can be detected by CAT.

The histopathological changes associated with severe HSE consist of acute inflammation that evolves to produce haemorrhagic and necrotising lesions. The lesions are characteristically located in the temporal lobes and orbital surface of the frontal lobes, but adjacent frontal, parietal and occipital lobes and the cingulate gyri may also be involved. Clinically, herpes encephalitis ranges in severity from a mild encephalitis of low mortality and morbidity to severe necrotising encephalitis associated with both high mortality (70–90% in the absence of specific antiviral chemotherapy and expert neurological care) and high morbidity (with only 10% of survivors returning to normal neurological function in the absence of antiviral chemotherapy). Herpes encephalitis is, however, a treatable disease and prompt initiation of chemotherapy, using the antiviral drug aciclovir combined with intensive neurological nursing care, results in a reduction of mortality to less than 20% with up to 40% of survivors returning to apparently normal neurological function. In some patients there may be residual neurological deficit; this may be severe, with impairment or complete loss of short-term memory being the most commonly observed sequelae.

In contrast to several other enveloped viruses, including herpes varicella zoster, Epstein–Barr virus and human cytomegalovirus (CMV), HSV does not seem to be a significant cause of perivascular leukoencephalopathy ('post-infectious encephalitis'). However, this disease has been reported to occur in a minority of patients recovering from acute herpes encephalitis. Five days to 3 weeks after apparent recovery from acute encephalitis, the patient suddenly develops a 'relapse' and a further bout of encephalitic illness. In the small number of cases examined by brain biopsy, no virus antigen has been detected and histopathologically lesions are similar to those seen in post-infectious encephalitis triggered by other virus infections (i.e. significant demyelination and immune cellular infiltration). Viral DNA is usually not detected in the CSF and most patients survive and recover to at least their level of disability following acute herpes encephalitis.

The pathogenesis of herpes encephalitis remains enigmatic. The structure of the vasculature within the brain, together with the meninges surrounding the brain, represent, in the physiologically normal host, a significant barrier to virus entry to brain parenchyma. Haematogenous spread of virus to the brain is usually prevented by these blood–brain and blood–CSF barriers. To gain access to the brain, the virus must circumvent the physiological/anatomical barriers. The virus may achieve this by transit from the periphery within nerve cells. Various pathways have been proposed, although in all probability no one route explains all cases of herpes encephalitis.

During the early stages infection is principally of neurones, with only occasional involvement of astrocyte and glial cells. The frontal and temporal lobes, together with the associated limbic structures of the brain, appear to be the primary targets of the infectious process (Esiri, 1982) and has led to the suggestion that this localisation reflects the particular neurochemical and perhaps local neuroimmunological environment of the limbic region (Damasio and Van Hoesen, 1985). However, such localisation is not observed in all cases and virus may spread to involve other regions of the brain. The amount of HSV DNA found in CSF appears to be correlated with prognosis, in that the higher the viral load detected during the acute stages of infection, the poorer the outcome.

Disease in the Immunocompromised

Patients who are immunocompromised through deficits in CMI are at risk of severe HSV infection, with the possibility of life-threatening, disseminated infection. Oral HSV infection can progress to extensive necrotic mouth ulceration, with bacterial super-infection or haemorrhage in those with thrombocytopenia. Equally severe, progressive genital HSV infections may occur. Auto-inoculation may result in initial infection at sites distant from the original focus. Cutaneous dissemination can take place and may be clinically indistinguishable from varicella. Visceral dissemination is also possible, with hepatitis, pneumonia and encephalitis. Primary, recurrent and exogenous reinfections all pose a significant threat to such patients. In organ transplant recipients, progressive disease may involve the oesophagus, respiratory tract and even the gastrointestinal tract, the severity of disease observed in such patients being linked with the degree of immunosuppression. In patients with HIV infection, recurrent HSV infection may occur, with high frequency at multiple sites, widespread cutaneous distribution may occur and markedly prolonged times to healing of lesions are observed. Prolonged viraemia in such patients leads to multi-organ distribution, including dissemination to the CNS.

Prophylactic antiviral chemotherapy is now routinely given to those receiving organ graft transplants and HSV has effectively ceased to be a major problem in this group of patients, although antiviral drug resistance has emerged as a significant difficulty. In patients with HIV, combination anti-HIV therapy has significantly reduced the prevalence of active herpes. For those patients with HIV suffering frequent recurrence of infection, suppressive antiviral therapy is used selectively (see section on Treatment, below) as there is some evidence that active HSV infection, in common with other herpesviruses, can act as a co-factor in AIDS, activating HIV and making it easier for HIV to infect certain cells.

Herpes Simplex Meningitis

Herpes meningitis occurs in 4–8% of cases of primary genital herpes. Women appear to be more frequently affected than men. Symptoms include headache, fever, stiff neck, vomiting and photophobia. The meningitis usually resolves without complications within 2–7 days. HSV-2 is the most common cause, although occasional cases of HSV-1 are reported in association with primary genital HSV-1 infection. The use of PCR for examination of CSF in diagnosis of cases of suspected HSV meningitis has radically improved the efficiency of diagnosis. PCR has also provided evidence that most cases of Mollaret's meningitis—a benign recurrent aseptic meningitis characterised by three to 10 episodes of fever and meningeal irritation occurring over a period of years—are due to HSV-2 recurrent infection. For the management of such cases, which are rare, patient-initiated specific antiviral therapy or suppressive antiviral therapy may be appropriate.

Herpes Simplex Dermatitis; Herpetic Whitlows; Traumatic Herpes; Herpes Gladiatorum

Herpetic dermatitis is a complication of primary infection. Perioral or periorbital herpes simplex regularly accompanies more severe primary gingivostomatitis or primary/initial herpes keratitis. In babies, seeding of the virus can involve large areas of the face and, when transferred to the anogenital area by scratching, may involve the whole napkin area. In primary HSV vulvovaginitis, vesicles readily appear on the perineum and thigh.

In patients with atopic eczema or with Darier's disease, the normal resistance of the skin to HSV infection is reduced and primary, recurrent and possibly both endogenous and exogenous reinfection may produce eczema herpeticum. Eczema herpeticum as a primary infection carries a small but significant mortality through progression to severe generalised disease.

Under normal circumstances HSV does not readily penetrate healthy skin, but when the dermis is breached a portal of entry is created. Health care personnel are at particular risk of perforation injuries. Direct inoculation of virus into the fingers of those who constantly manipulate in the oral cavity (dentists, dental nurses, intensive care doctors, nurses and anaesthetists) lead to herpetic whitlows, inflammation of the nail folds. A similar condition is seen in children and adolescents who transfer their own oral virus through nail biting. In other situations, workers such as hairdressers, dressmakers and laboratory personnel can be infected by accidental stab injuries with contaminated needles or broken glassware (traumatic herpes).

Herpes gladiatorum and 'scrum pox' are conditions spread among wrestlers through bites or 'mat burns', and among rugby players through bites and facial scraping. The appearance of herpetic vesicles at 'unusual' sites can sometimes be explained by an inquiry into the individual's athletic pursuits!

A distinct form of cutaneous infection, 'zosteriform herpes simplex', is an infrequent presentation of herpes simplex but is recognised when the distribution of HSV lesions accords with a dermatome and otherwise resembles zoster. Unlike zoster, nerve root pain is not a feature.

Erythema Multiforme

Erythema multiforme is regarded as a hypersensitivity phenomenon precipitated by a variety of infectious agents, immunisations and drugs. The clinical lesions are characteristic; acrally distributed erythematous papules which evolve into concentric 'target' lesions; annular plaques and bullae may also be produced. Although usually mild and self-limiting, the disease can be recurrent, progress to toxic epidermal necrolysis, or to severe mucous membrane involvement (Stevens–Johnson syndrome). *Mycoplasma pneumoniae* and HSV are the infectious agents most commonly associated as precipitants. Up to 65% of patients with recurrent erythema multiforme give a preceding history of herpes labialis, on average 11 days before the lesions of the disease appear. Infectious virus cannot be cultured from the lesions but immunofluorescence studies have shown HSV glycoprotein B located around keratinocytes in the viable epidermis, PCR studies have detected HSV DNA in cutaneous lesions, and *in situ* hybridisation has been used to demonstrate HSV nucleic acids within the epidermis.

Erythema multiforme does not respond directly to antiviral chemotherapy (HSV replication is apparently a precipitant of the disease but not a direct cause of the pathology) but cases of recurrent HSV-associated erythema multiforme can be prevented by prophylactic use of aciclovir. Some cases of idiopathic recurrent erythema multiforme (i.e. where antecedent herpes labialis is not suspected) also respond to prophylactic use of aciclovir. This is perhaps consistent with a preceding 'silent' recurrence of HSV.

DIAGNOSIS

The ability of HSV to establish latent infection inevitably complicates diagnosis. A clinical role for the virus in causation of disease is not established simply because it is recovered from a patient. To achieve *meaningful* diagnosis, a close collaboration between clinic and laboratory is always necessary.

Light and UV Microscopy

In diagnostic virology, direct light microscopic examination of clinical material is now seldom used to provide a diagnosis of HSV infection, although histopathological examination remains an important technique in the differential diagnosis of infection. Staining of relevant tissue sections with specific antibodies tagged with enzymes provides rapid and specific localisation of virus. Rapid detection of HSV in clinical material may be achieved by direct or indirect immunofluorescence (IF) microscopy. Scrapings from vesicles, impression smears or cryostat sections of tissue biopsies all provide suitable specimens.

Electron Microscopy

Transmission electron microscopic examination of negatively stained vesicle fluid presents one of the most rapid methods for the detection of HSV. Although not available in all diagnostic laboratories, this procedure can be very helpful in establishing a rapid, early diagnosis, particularly for immunocompromised patients or their contacts. The morphology of HSV is characteristic, although HSV-1, HSV-2 and herpes varicella zoster virus cannot be differentiated by such direct examination. As the clinical management of cutaneous lesions is similar, this is an academic rather than a practical problem (exact typing can be achieved by complementary techniques, such as immunofluorescence or PCR). The technique is relatively insensitive and a specimen must contain at least 10^6 or more particles per millilitre to allow detection of virus. In practice, vesicle fluid from primary infections will usually yield sufficient virus. Thin section electron microscopy, sometimes combined with immunological staining using gold-labelled specific monoclonal antibody, has a role in the examination of histological material.

Virus Culture

HSV-1 and HSV-2 are among the easiest of viruses to cultivate and propagate in the laboratory. A wide range of both primary and continuous monolayer cell cultures can be infected with HSV. Cytopathic effect (CPE) develops within 1–7 days of inoculation. Both ballooning degenerating cells and polykarocytes may be observed. The CPE of HSV-1 and HSV-2 may be rapidly differentiated by immunofluorescence staining of infected cells with type-specific monoclonal antibodies.

Virus isolation in cell culture provides a highly sensitive method for the detection of HSV but its efficiency depends on the method of specimen collection and the preservation of virus infectivity between the patient and the laboratory. Vesicle fluid is usually rich in virus, provided that the fluid is collected from a 'fresh' vesicle. Virus is rarely isolated from crusted vesicles. A cotton wool bud is used to swab ulcers or mucous membranes in order to detach virus-containing cells. To reduce loss of infectious virus between the patient and laboratory, the swab is then placed in a suitable transport medium. If there is delay in transportation, the material should be maintained at $+4°C$ or immersed in liquid nitrogen. Cerebrospinal fluid (CSF), biopsy or necropsy specimens are collected into dry sterile containers and require no special transport media. Such specimens should be transported and maintained at $+4°C$; they should not be frozen. On arrival in the laboratory, they are inoculated onto at least two different cell types. Biopsy or necroscopy specimens are homogenised in a small amount of transport medium prior to their inoculation onto cell cultures. As for human cytomegalovirus (DEAFF test), detection of virus growth in tissue culture can be accelerated if the specimens are centrifuged onto cells cultivated on small cover slips and the cells are stained after 24 h with a monoclonal antibody directed to HSV early antigen. Isolates of virus may be readily typed as HSV-1 or HSV-2 by the use of specific monoclonal antibodies tagged with fluorescein.

Immunoassay

A number of ELISA procedures are available for the rapid detection of HSV. Whilst the specificity of these procedures is high (ca. 98%) their sensitivity for the detection of virus in acute vesicular lesions is only about 80% and with material from crusting lesions may reduce to less than 60%. In comparison to culture, immunoassays offer an advantage where suboptimal transportation of specimens to the laboratory has resulted in loss of virus infectivity. This is because they are not reliant upon the detection of infectious virus.

Nucleic Acid Detection

Direct hybridisation of clinical samples with radio- or enzyme-labelled oligonucleotides has been used for the direct detection of HSV but these techniques are now seldom utilised, apart from in the examination of histopathological materials (see section on *In Situ* Hybridisation, below). A number of alternative nucleic acid amplification or signal amplification techniques have been applied to the diagnosis of HSV infection but it is nucleic acid amplification, particularly the polymerase chain reaction (PCR), that is most widely applied. A wide variety of PCR techniques have been used, including single, semi-nested and nested PCR techniques with product detection via gel electrophoresis, Southern blotting or ELISA-like hybridisation. More recently, 'real-time' PCR procedures have been utilised. These allow direct detection of the products of amplification 'in real time', are quantitative and usually allow typing of HSV-1 and HSV-2 within the same test.

Rigorous quality control and attention to detail are essential for routine application of these techniques. Many types of clinical samples contain substances that prove inhibitory to the PCR reaction which, if not efficiently removed, will result in the production of false negative test results. The use of internal control molecules within PCR tests is used to monitor for test failure through test sample inhibition. Where internal molecules are not available, the same check may be performed by 'spiking' a sample with a known amount of HSV or by checking for an alternative human gene always expected to be present within a clinical sample.

The intra- and extra-laboratory contamination of samples with virus or amplicons may give rise to false positive PCR results. This represents a significant practical problem and requires careful consideration in the design of PCR protocols. A particular consideration in herpesvirus PCR is the possible detection of DNA from (asymptomatic) recurrent herpesvirus infections. This may create difficulties in defining the clinical significance of a test result.

Sequencing of the products of PCR is a useful method for the comparison of strains of virus detected, e.g. from different bodily sites or from different persons, and provides a more rapid method for epidemiological investigation than the technically demanding restriction-fragment polymorphic analyses previously applied in such studies.

PCR has been most widely applied in the diagnosis of herpes encephalitis and herpes meningitis. In retrospective studies conducted using stored samples of CSF from proven cases of herpes encephalitis with CSF taken during the acute stages of illness (<10 days after onset of neurological illness), PCR was found to have a sensitivity of 95–100% and a similarly high specificity of 98–100%. In extended prospective studies it is recognised that the PCR is not infallible and negative results may be obtained with samples taken early in the disease course (days 1–3 after onset of neurological illness) or where aciclovir therapy has been instituted prior to lumbar puncture. Caution is therefore warranted in the interpretation of results and an algorithm (Cinque *et al.*, 1996; reproduced as Figure 2A.4) emphasised the necessity of repeating the lumbar puncture wherever negative test results were obtained and the diagnosis was still in doubt. The

algorithm further mentioned the necessity of repeating the lumbar puncture at the end of therapy to ensure full clearance of viral nucleic acid from the CSF. It is important to emphasise that antiviral chemotherapy and/or an intrathecal immune response may clear viral DNA from the CSF, and the reliability of PCR in diagnosis of herpes encephalitis declines rapidly in the second week of diagnosis. PCR is thus a valuable method during the acute stages of illness, but its usefulness reduces 10–12 days after onset, when measurement of specific intrathecal antibody

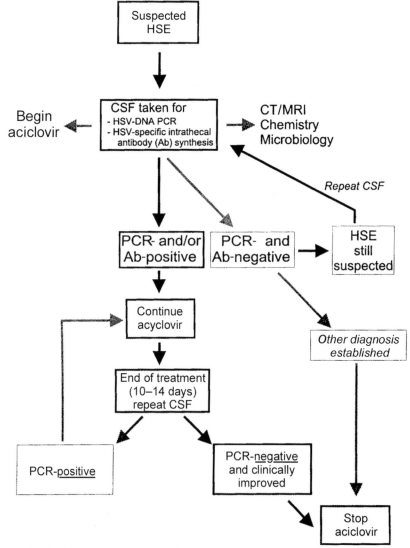

Figure 2A.4 Diagnostic algorithm for management of patients with suspected HSE. As patients may present with raised intracranial pressure, immediate lumbar puncture may not be possible. In these circumstances commencement of aciclovir therapy prior to lumbar puncture is warranted. Reproduced from Cinque *et al.* (1996), with permission from the BMJ publishing group

responsiveness (see below) may be a more appropriate diagnostic procedure.

The application of real-time PCR for the diagnosis of herpes infection of the CNS has shown that a sensitivity of 10–25 genome equivalents (copies)/ml CSF is necessary to detect all cases of HSV infection of the CSF. Initial CSF viral load varied between 2×10^2 and 2×10^7 for HSV-1 and 9×10^3 and 6×10^5 for HSV-2 in one study (Linde *et al.*, personal communication). The amount of HSV DNA detected in the initial CSF has been shown to correlate with disease severity. None of nine patients with an initial viral load of $> 10^5$ genome equivalents/ml returned to normal neurological function, compared to five out of six whose initial viral load was $< 10^5$ genome equivalents/ml (Domingues *et al.*, 1998), providing further emphasis of the role of PCR in the diagnosis and management of HSV infection of the CNS.

The availability of simplified and automated methods for sample extraction and assay set-up, coupled with improved assays employing internal control molecules to monitor possible sample-induced inhibition of PCR, has led to the more widespread uptake of PCR in diagnosis of other HSV infections. This use of automation coupled with real-time PCR procedures has allowed PCR to become price-competitive with virus culture. One of the major uses of viral isolation in cell culture has been for confirmation of a diagnosis of genital HSV infection. Increasingly PCR is being utilised to supplant culture, providing more rapid and sensitive detection and typing of virus than can be achieved by cell culture.

In Situ *Hybridisation and* In Situ *PCR*

HSV nucleic acids may be detected in biopsy or necroscopy material by *in situ* hybridisation. Paraffin-embedded tissue sections are dewaxed, rehydrated and digested with proteinase K. After a denaturing step, a labelled DNA fragment or 'probe' (an oligonucleotide produced synthetically or a cloned, plasmid-amplified, fragment of HSV DNA) is incubated with the tissue section. The section is then washed to remove unhybridised probe DNA. The probe may be detected by radiological, enzymatic or chemiluminescent methods appropriate to the label utilised. Where particularly small amounts of viral DNA are present in a clinical sample, *in situ* PCR methods are available to allow detection. The technical complexities of this procedure currently preclude its application, except in research settings.

Serology

Peripheral Blood

A large number of techniques are available to detect and quantitate the humoral immune response to HSV infection including complement fixation tests (CFTs), immunofluorescence tests and tests for neutralising antibody. Differences in both specificity and sensitivity are observed between the different techniques and different assays. These tests have now been largely replaced by commercially available ELISA tests. In most clinical situations assay of HSV-specific IgG antibody is sufficient. In primary infection seroconversion is readily detected in adequately spaced samples (14 or more days). In a primary infection IgG production can be detected at around the same time as an IgM response. Differentiation of primary and reactivated infection may be possible by measurement of HSV-specific IgG avidity. In recent infection IgG avidity will be low, while in reactivated infection IgG avidity will usually be high.

IgM antibody to HSV can be detected using a suitable enzyme-labelled antiglobulin in the standard indirect ELISA technique or, with superior specificity, by IgM 'capture' immunoassay. The detection of IgM antibody does not always allow differentiation of a primary infection and a reactivation event. During reactivation an IgM response can often be detected. The magnitude of the response can vary from individual to individual, thus the results of IgM immunoassays must be interpreted with caution.

The type common epitopes of HSV-1 and HSV-2 ensure that most conventional ELISA techniques are adequate for the detection of seroconversion to either virus. Co-terminal seroconversions to herpes varicella zoster virus are occasionally observed and may be due to an anamnestic immune response, or possibly because of synchronous reactivation ('dual reactivation') or synchronous infection ('dual infection').

ELISA procedures utilising 'whole virus' preparations representative of the complete antigenic spectrum of HSV provide the most sensitive assays for HSV antibody. However, to differentiate HSV-1 and HSV-2 serological responses, ELISA procedures that utilise type-specific purified virion glycoproteins, peptides and/or recombinant antigens to distinguish HSV-1-specific and HSV-2-specific antibodies are necessary. Such assays are commercially available and are useful in epidemiological studies and in specialised situations, such as determination of the serostatus of the partner of a newly diagnosed case of genital herpes.

Cerebrospinal Fluid

Demonstration of a peripheral blood HSV antibody response is not in itself diagnostic of CNS infection. Such a response may merely reflect reactivation of latent HSV secondary to neurological disease of unrelated aetiology. Detection of HSV IgM in HSV IgG-negative patients or in patients with very low levels of specific HSV IgG is suggestive of a primary infection, although false positive IgM reactions are known to occur, making follow-up serology necessary.

Serological diagnosis of CNS infection requires proof of intrathecal synthesis of specific antibody. To determine whether specific antibodies are produced intrathecally and not passively transferred from serum, the integrity of the blood–CSF barrier (BCB) must be assessed. A variety of methods are available (Linde *et al.*, 1997). The most accurate are believed to be those in which the ratio of antibody quantitated in both serum and CSF are compared to the distribution of a reference protein such as albumin or, where antigen-mediated capillary blotting is performed, after isoelectric focusing of serum and unconcentrated CSF (Monteyne *et al.*, 1997).

In the former technique, the most reliable of several formulae applied to determine intrathecal synthesis was determined to be that of Reiber (1994). Here, locally produced IgG is differentiated from polyclonal IgG derived from peripheral blood circulation by dividing the unit ratio by 'Q$_{Lim}$' ('Q$_{Lim}$' representing the fraction of antibody in CSF originating from serum, i.e. Q$_{Lim}$ = 0.93[(QAlb + 6 × 10^6) − 1.7 × 10^3]. Q$_{Lim}$ can be estimated for IgG, IgM and IgA using Reiber's (1994) diagrams.

The antigen-mediated capillary blot technique, performed after isoelectric focusing of serum and unconcentrated CSF, provides an alternative and sensitive method for the detection of specific intrathecal synthesis of antibody. The presence of two or more anti-HSV oligoclonal IgG bands present only in CSF is considered to provide a definite diagnosis.

MANAGEMENT

Outside the natural host, HSV has only a short half-life and is readily inactivated by a variety of physical and chemical agents, including detergents, common disinfectants (phenolics, formaldehyde, glutaraldehyde, hypochlorite, quaternary ammonium compounds) and solvents (e.g. 70% alcohol). Standard methods of sterilisation, including autoclaving, dry heat, UV- or

γ-irradiation and ethylene oxide sterilisation, are all equally effective for the decontamination of medical equipment. In the controlled environment of a hospital, prevention of host-to-host transmission is achieved by simple hygiene. In the home, or other social contexts, prevention of transmission by avoidance of contact with a person with evidence of recurrent infection (cold sores or genital herpes) is only partially effective. This is because infectious virus is often excreted before the appearance of overt symptoms of recurrent infection and 'silent' recurrent infections also occur.

Antiviral Chemotherapy

A large number of compounds with anti-HSV activity have been described in *in vitro* experiments. Few have progressed to clinical trial and fewer still have gained a place in clinical practice. The major 'antiherpetic' in current use is aciclovir, although newer antivirals, such as penciclovir or the pro-drugs of aciclovir and penciclovir, valaciclovir and famciclovir, offering better systemic bio-availability following oral administration, are now in use (Waugh *et al.*, 2002).

Aciclovir (Zovirax™)

The structure of aciclovir is shown in Figure 2A.5. The compound is an acyclic nucleoside analogue. The mode of action of aciclovir is illustrated in Figure 2A.6. Virus-infected cells appear to be slightly more permeable to aciclovir than non-infected cells but the compound is only entrapped and selectively concentrated within virus-infected cells. Within the infected cell, a virus-specified enzyme, thymidine kinase, effects the monophosphorylation of aciclovir. The resulting aciclovir monophosphate cannot traverse the cellular membranes and is consequently localised within the virus-infected cell. Host cell kinases (including host cell-derived thymidine kinase) do not appear capable of catalysing this reaction to any significant degree.

The active antiviral drug is aciclovir triphosphate and conversion of aciclovir monophosphate to the active triphosphate form is accomplished by host cell kinases. The triphosphate form of aciclovir has much greater affinity for virus-specified, as opposed to host cell-derived, DNA polymerase. Aciclovir triphosphate binds to host-derived DNA polymerase, leading to the inactivation of this enzyme's activity. Thus, viral DNA replication is inhibited, whilst normal host cell DNA metabolism remains virtually unaffected. An additional

Aciclovir

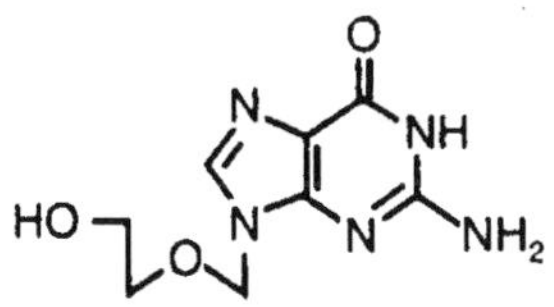

2-Amino-1,9-dihydro-9-[(2-hydroxyethoxy)methyl]-6*H*-purin-6-one (MW 225.21)

Valaciclovir

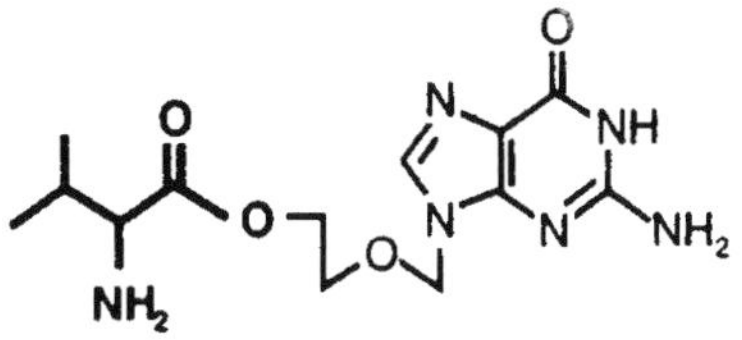

L-Valine, 2-[(2-amino-1,6-dihydro-6-oxo-9*H*-purin-9-yl)*m*-ethyoxy]-ethyl ester, monohydrochloride (MW 360.80)

Penciclovir

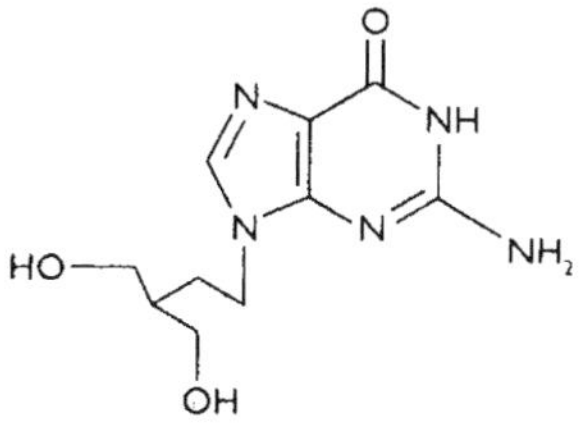

9-[4-hydroxy-3-(hydroxymethyl) butyl] guanine (MW 253.26)

Famciclovir

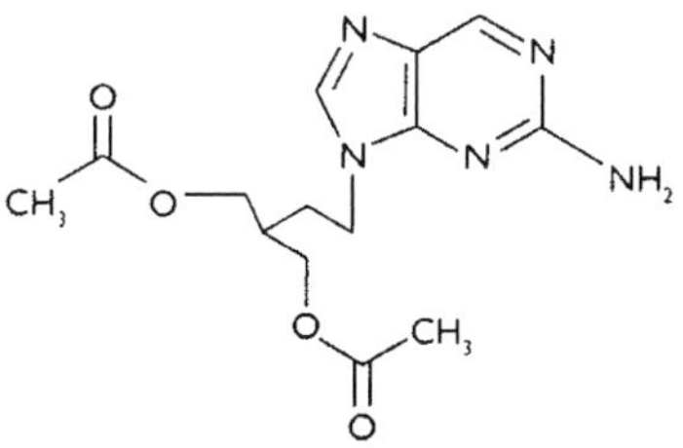

2-[2-(2-amino-9*H*-purin-9-yl) ethyl]-1,3-propanediol-acetate (MW 321.3)

Figure 2A.5 Antiviral drugs

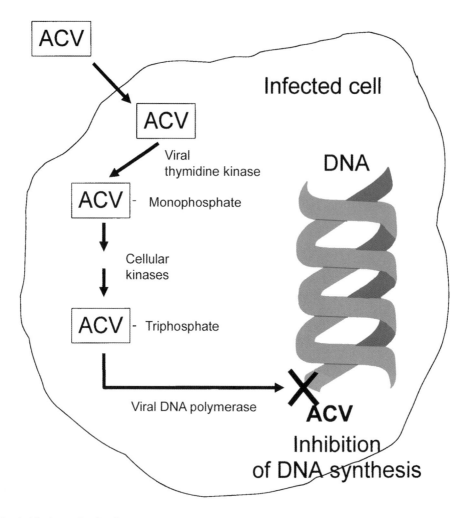

Figure 2A.6   Aciclovir: mode of action

but less significant antiviral action is via chain termination through incorporation into the growing viral DNA chain (absence of 2′ and 3′ carbons of guanosine).

Valaciclovir (Valtrex™)

The oral bio-availabilty of aciclovir is relatively low and for this reason a prodrug, the L-valyl ester of aciclovir, called valaciclovir, was developed (Figure 2A.5). Valaciclovir hydrochloride is rapidly adsorbed from the gastrointestinal tract and rapidly and almost completely converted to aciclovir and L-valine by first-pass intestinal and/or hepatic metabolism. The mode of action, safety profile and clinical spectrum of

activity of valaciclovir are believed to be identical to those of aciclovir. The plasma concentrations of aciclovir achieved after oral administration of valaciclovir are believed to be equivalent to those achieved by intravenous administration of aciclovir and are three- to five-fold greater than are achieved with oral administration of aciclovir. Valaciclovir can therefore provide a much more convenient dosing regimen of once, twice, or three times daily, in comparison to the five times daily for aciclovir.

Penciclovir (Denavir™)

Penciclovir is an acyclic nucleoside analogue (Figure 2A.5) whose mode of action and safety profile are essentially identical to those of aciclovir. However, the drugs differ in their rate of cellular uptake, phosphorylation rate, stability of the intracellular triphosphate and inhibitory concentration for HSV DNA polymerase (100-fold higher for penciclovir triphosphate than for aciclovir triphosphate). The intracellular half-life of the active antiviral (penciclovir triphosphate) is substantially longer (7–20 h) than that of aciclovir triphosphate (0.7–1 h), which compensates for the slightly lower activity of the drug.

Famciclovir (Famvir™)

Famciclovir (Figure 2A.5) is the diacetyl 6-deoxy prodrug of penciclovir. Famciclovir achieves high levels of systemic bio-availability following oral administration. Following administration, the drug is deacetylated and oxidised to form penciclovir. The mode of action and clinical spectrum of activity are thus identical to those of penciclovir.

Other Antivirals

Ganciclovir {[9-(1,3-dihydroxy-2-propoxy)methyl] guanine} has good activity against HSV-1 and HSV-2. It has higher toxicity than the aforementioned drugs, its main side-effect being myelosuppression. The L-valyl ester valganciclovir allows oral administration of the drug.

The pyrophosphate analogue foscarnet (trisodium phosphonoformate), an inhibitor of DNA polymerase, is utilised in severe HSV infections refractory to aciclovir therapy. Slow intravenous infusion of the drug is necessary because of its poor oral bioavailability and potential for nephrotoxicity. An alternative is the nucleotide analogue cidofovir. This compound, like foscarnet, has dose-dependent nephrotoxicity and must be given with oral probenecid to reduce cidofovir accumulation in the renal tubules. The drug's extraordinary intracellular half-life means that only one intravenous infusion every 1–2 weeks is required.

Drug Resistance

Prolonged use of aciclovir can result in the development of drug-resistant strains of HSV. Thymidine kinase mutants have been reported with either altered substrate specificity (i.e. aciclovir is no longer recog-

nised as a substrate for virus-specified enzyme) or with loss of thymidine kinase (TK) activity. These mutants arise through nonsense, frame-shift or missense mutations in the TK gene and are thus readily generated both in vivo and in vitro. A third type of mutant has altered DNA polymerase, such that aciclovir triphosphate no longer binds with high affinity to the virus-encoded enzyme (altered substrate specificity). The consequence of alteration in TK is a failure of the virus-infected cell to phosphorylate and thereby selectively concentrate aciclovir. Alteration in DNA polymerase results in a much reduced antiviral activity, since the only antiviral action of the drug resides in the ability of aciclovir triphosphate to induce chain termination.

The emergence of drug resistance gives rise to concern but is currently limited to patients who are immunocompromised; about 4% of HSV isolates from patients with AIDS and up to 18% of isolates from recipients of bone marrow transplants are resistant to aciclovir. Among immunocompetent individuals, a very low rate (< 0.5%) of resistance to aciclovir is observed. Most aciclovir-resistant strains of virus are also likely to be found to be resistant to penciclovir, valaciclovir and famciclovir. Most drug-resistant isolates have an altered or deleted thymidine kinase, and thus drugs which act directly upon the viral DNA polymerase, such as foscarnet or cidofovir, are effective as second-line treatments. Multiple drug resistance has, however, been documented. Drug susceptibility assays should be performed in immunocompromised patients with unresponsive herpes simplex infection in order to distinguish drug resistance from problems such as poor compliance or maladsorption of drug.

Transmission of drug-resistant HSV is extremely rare. This may be related to a requirement of thymidine kinase for replication of virus within nervous tissue. Resistant virus shed in cold sores will revert back to wild-type in subsequent reactivations.

Immunisation

Active Immunisation

The short time interval between loss of passively acquired maternal immunity and acquisition of primary infection, together with the high level of HSV infection in the general population, means that effective prevention of HSV-1 infection by vaccination is problematic. However, the changing sero-epidemiology of HSV-1 infections suggests that, at least in developed countries, application of a vaccine against HSV-1 becomes a feasible possibility. Due to the psychosocial problems associated with HSV-2 infection, immunisation against this virus has been much more actively sought. At the present time, two strategies are being investigated: classical immunisation, which aims to produce so-called 'sterilising immunity' (i.e. a broad and durable immune response which will be effective in preventing HSV entry via genital mucosa, facial mucosa or the eye) prior to virus exposure; and immunotherapy; modification of the immune response by vaccine administration designed to potentiate immunity and improve control of, or prevent, recurrent infection.

The production of effective vaccines against HSV have been actively pursued since the 1920s. A very wide range of vaccines have been explored as both 'sterilising' and immunotherapeutic vaccines (Table 2A.2). As yet no vaccine has progressed beyond Phase II/III clinical evaluation. The evidence from the many studies performed suggests that cellular rather than humoral immune responses are important in protecting against both infection and recurrence. Many of the vaccines produced thus far have been able to stimulate humoral immunity, but the antibodies developed have not been accompanied by an effective co-stimulus of cell-mediated immunity and have not proved to be protective. Improved knowledge of the viral determinants necessary to stimulate protective cellular immunity appear to be key to the future development of immunisation against HSV.

Table 2A.2 Active immunisation against HSV

Auto-inoculation of live virus	Inoculation of an individual's own vesicle fluid in an attempt to treat recurrence
Attenuated live virus	e.g. R7020 and HSV-1 strain with thymidine kinase deletion plus insertion of glycoproteins of HSV-2; disabled infectious single cycle virus; genetically attenuated (e.g. Medimmune, AURx)
Inactivated virus	Formalin, phenol or UV-inactivated
Non-specific DNA vaccines	Vaccinia, BCG
Subunit vaccines	e.g. HSV-2 glycoprotein B + D + adjuvant; gD2 + alum; Skinner vaccine—mixed glycoproteins of HSV-1
Immunostimulatory complexes	
Peptide vaccines	

Passive Immunisation

Passive immunisation using hyperimmune HSV-specific immunoglobulin has not been widely utilised and normal immune globulin is ineffective. In neonatal disease, and possibly in immunocompromised patients, trials of therapy using human recombinant monoclonal antibodies are planned, since such therapy might have a role in helping to prevent virus dissemination by viraemia.

SPECIFIC MANAGEMENT

Primary or Initial Infection

Primary or initial infection with HSV is, in the majority of cases, inapparent or only associated with mild symptoms and, as the aetiological diagnosis may not be clear, antiviral therapy is not given. If the diagnosis is apparent, as in severe cases, then oral antiviral therapy can be given and there is some evidence of marginal shortening of duration of pain and time to healing in children with gingivostomatitis and in patients with primary or initial genital herpes. Bicarbonate- or chlorhexidine-containing mouthwashes combined with simple analgesia may be helpful in gingivostomatitis. Saline bathes, and in severe cases topical anaesthetic agents, may provide relief in primary/initial genital herpes. Aciclovir and penciclovir creams are available for direct application to skin lesions; however, a more effective treatment is oral administration of aciclovir (given in 200 mg doses five times daily), valaciclovir (500 mg twice daily), or famciclovir (250 mg, three times daily) for 5 days unless new lesions appear, when continued therapy should be contemplated. Intravenous therapy is indicated if the patient cannot swallow or tolerate oral administration because of vomiting.

In theory, antiviral treatment of primary or initial infections may impact upon the subsequent frequency of reactivation. By reducing viral load during the acute infection, the efficiency of colonisation of sensory nerves may be decreased, which in turn lowers the frequency of reactivation from these sites. In support of this hypothesis is the finding that severe primary or initial infections are associated with a higher frequency of (symptomatic) reactivation. In practice, the large majority of primary/initial infections are undiagnosed and in those that, are the peak of viral replication may already have passed before antiviral therapy can be commenced. Secondary bacterial and fungal infection is common in severe symptomatic primary and initial HSV infection and requires appropriate antimicrobial therapy.

Steroid treatment in general increases the severity of disease, and where patients are receiving high doses of steroids (e.g. in the treatment of eczema) the appearance of HSV infection is an indication for temporary cessation or reduction of steroid dosage. In other cases of iatrogenic immunosuppresion (e.g. for organ transplantation), HSV infection is an indicator for temporary reassessment of the dosage of the immunosuppressive therapy. Primary HSV infection in the immunocompromised host always gives cause for concern because of the possibility of the development of generalised multi-organ infection. Serious HSV infections require not only the prompt initiation of specific antiviral chemotherapy but also full medical and nursing intervention. Generalised infection in the immunocompromised produces osmotic imbalances, endocrine dysfunction, circulatory and respiratory failure which necessitate an aggressive approach to intensive care.

Recurrent Infection

Recurrent HSV infections inconvenience the host but are rarely serious in the immunocompetent individual. Patients with only occasional recurrences often develop their own preferred self-treatment, the dabbing of perfume or alcohol on cold sores or the use of aciclovir cream. Frequent or severe recurrences may require oral or systemic antiviral chemotherapy. The most effective episodic treatment requires a 5 day course of oral antiviral therapy initiated as soon as prodromal symptoms are observed. In a recurrent episode, the earlier the treatment is started, the more effective it proves in reducing the severity and duration of the recurrent episode.

Since the maintenance of latent virus infection appears to be independent of virus replication, antiviral chemotherapy cannot 'cure' recurrent virus infection. Patients with frequent recurrences (defined as more than six episodes per year) should be considered for continuous suppressive therapy. Aciclovir (200 mg four times daily or 400 mg twice daily), valaciclovir (500 mg daily or 250 mg twice daily), or famciclovir (250 mg twice daily) are believed to be effective. Usually a 6–12 month period is chosen for continuous therapy and the necessity for therapy is then reassessed.

Ocular Infection

The majority of cases of ocular HSV infection are thought to result from an endogenous reinfection (i.e. transfer of virus from the site of a recurrent infection to the eye). Misdiagnosis of the condition has frequently led to the administration of corticosteroids to the eye. Unfortunately, such treatment may exacerbate and prolong the infection. Endogenous reinfections or primary infections of the eye should not be treated with steroids. Conservative treatment is warranted, with application of specific antiviral chemotherapy (aciclovir ophthalmic ointment) and possibly debridement of the cornea. Oral or systemic antiviral therapy (see above) should be given in severe disease. Secondary bacterial infection may occur, necessitating appropriate antimicrobial therapy. Recurrent ocular HSV infections are managed in a similar fashion except that the indication for antiviral chemotherapy is more pronounced.

Long-term suppressive oral aciclovir therapy (400 mg twice daily) has been shown to be of benefit in patients with prior HSV stromal keratitis (Herpetic Eye Study Group, 2000) but of lower benefit in preventing recurrence of epithelial keratitis. Steroid therapy is almost certainly indicated in stromal herpes keratitis and possibly also in iridocyclitis, since most damage is believed to result from an inflammatory reaction rather than the direct action of virus replication in corneal tissues. Severe stromal scarring necessitates corneal transplantation. One small study has shown that postoperative oral aciclovir reduces the rate of recurrence of dendritic keratitis and improves graft survival (Tambasco et al., 1999).

CNS Infection

Treatment of herpes encephalitis requires the early administration of antiviral chemotherapy (Cinque et al., 1996). Antiviral chemotherapy should also be given in herpes meningitis, since the sequelae of this infection are not defined but do include the possible development of recurrent meningitis. The currently accepted antiviral treatment for herpes encephalitis is a 10 day intravenous course of aciclovir at 10 mg/kg given every 8 h. Aciclovir therapy should be approached with caution in patients with impaired renal function, since build-up of excessive serum concentrations of aciclovir has been associated with (reversible) neurotoxicity.

Specific antiviral chemotherapy is not the only important factor in the treatment of CNS infection.

Brain oedema is believed to represent the major cause of mortality in herpes encephalitis, hence reduction in intracranial pressure is an important consideration in the overall treatment regime and necessitates careful management in close collaboration with the clinical virology laboratory (Cinque *et al.*, 1996).

Neonatal Infection

HSV-1 and HSV-2 can both cause neonatal infections. The difficulty in early recognition of infection and consequent delay in the institution of antiviral therapy for HSV have been identified as major factors in the outcome of infection. Studies have nevertheless demonstrated the benefit of high-dose aciclovir therapy (60 mg/kg/day administered intravenously in three divided doses) for a period of 21 days (Kimberlin *et al.*, 2001). Despite aciclovir therapy, progressive disease can occur, with recurrence of herpetic lesions or relapse of neurological or retinal disease. A Phase III placebo-controlled trial to examine the benefits of prolonged (6 months) oral aciclovir therapy in infants with treated neonatal herpes is currently under way to determine whether suppressive therapy is of benefit in prevention of these late sequelae.

Primary maternal genital infection appears to pose the greatest threat to the neonate, although recurrent maternal infection is also a risk. Current UK guidelines (MSSVD, 1999) suggest that genital herpes acquired in the first or second trimester of pregnancy should be treated with oral or intravenous aciclovir as appropriate to the clinical condition. Continuous aciclovir during the last 4 weeks of pregnancy should then be considered, as this has been shown to reduce the risk of recurrence at term. Where a genuine primary or initial genital infection is identified in the third trimester, caesarean section should be considered, particularly in those developing infection after 34 weeks of gestation. If vaginal delivery cannot be avoided, aciclovir treatment of both mother and baby may be indicated. In mothers suffering recurrent disease, suppressive aciclovir therapy during the last 4 weeks of pregnancy may reduce the risk of recurrence at term. If recurrent lesions are evident at the time of delivery, it is current UK practice to perform caesarean section. The latter advice is somewhat controversial, since no randomised controlled trial has been performed, caesarean section is not absolutely protective from risk of neonatal herpes and there is risk to the mother in caesarean section procedure.

In the US study of Brown *et al.* (2003), cultures for HSV were attempted at term for 40 000 women; subclinical (i.e. no overt maternal lesions) virus shedding was detected in 128 women, 10 of whom transmitted the infection to their babies. However, viral culture at term was not an absolute predictor of risk of neonatal herpes, in that negative viral cultures were reported in six women whose babies developed neonatal herpes.

It has been suggested that the new type-specific serological assays for HSV-1 and HSV-2 could be used to identify mothers who are seronegative for HSV-1 or HSV-2 or both and their discordant partners. Appropriate counselling could then be given to avoid risk during the third trimester. Such a strategy may, however, be difficult to implement and would not prevent all cases of neonatal herpes. Improved sexual health counselling with respect to the risk of acquiring genital herpes infection during pregnancy, coupled with heightening of clinical awareness, remain the current mainstays for prevention of this infection.

REFERENCES

Bergstrom T and Trybala E (1996) Antigenic differences between HSV-1 and HSV-2 glycoproteins and their importance for type-specific serology. *Intervirology*, **39**, 176–184.

Brown ZA, Wald A, Morrow RA *et al.* (2003) Effect of serologic status and cesarean delivery on transmission rates of herpes simplex virus from mother to infant. *J Am Med Assoc*, **289**, 203–209.

Burnet FM and Williams SW (1939) Herpes simplex: a new point of view. *Med J Aust*, **1**, 637–641.

Chesenko N and Herold BC (2002) Glycoprotein B plays a predominant role in mediating herpes simplex virus type 2 attachment and is required for entry and cell to cell spread. *J Gen Virol*, **83**, 2247–2255.

Chou J and Roizman B (1994) Herpes simplex virus 1 γ34.5 gene function which blocks the host response to infection maps in the homologous domain of the genes expressed during growth arrest and DNA damage. *Proc Natl Acad Sci USA*, **91**, 5247–5251.

Cinque P, Cleator GM, Weber T *et al.* (1996) The role of laboratory investigation in the diagnosis and management of patients with suspected herpes encephalitis: a consensus report. *J Neurol Neurosurg Psychiat*, **61**, 339–345.

Cinque P, Vago L, Marenzi R *et al.* (1998) Herpes simplex virus infections of the central nervous system in human immunodeficiency virus-infected patients: clinical management by polymerase chain reaction assay of cerebrospinal fluid. *Clin Infect Dis*, **27**, 303–309.

Cohrs RJ and Gilden DH (2001) Human herpesvirus latency. *Brain Pathol*, **11**, 465–474.

Damasio AR and Van Hoesen GW (1985) The limbic system and the localisation of herpes simplex encephalitis. *J Neurol Neurosurg Psychiat*, **48**, 297–301.

Domingues RB, Lakeman FD, Mayo MS and Whitley RJ (1998) Application of competitive PCR to cerebrospinal fluid samples from patients with herpes simplex encephalitis. *J Clin Microbiol*, **36**, 2229–2234.

Esiri MM (1982) Herpes simplex encephalitis: an immuno-histological study of the distribution of viral antigen within the brain. *J Neurol Sci*, **54**, 209–226.

Gaytant MA, Steegers EA, van Laere M *et al.* (2002) Seroprevalences of herpes simplex virus type 1 and type 2 among pregnant women in The Netherlands. *Sex Transm Dis*, **29**, 710–714.

Herpetic Eye Study Group (2000) Oral acyclovir for herpes simplex virus eye disease: effect on prevention of epithelial keratitis and stromal keratitis. *Arch Ophthalmol*, **118**, 1030–1036.

Jerne NK (1976) The immune system: a web of v-domains. *Harvey Lectures*, **70**, 93–110.

Kimberlin DW, Lin CY, Jacobs RF *et al.* and the National Institute of Allergy and Infectious Diseases Collaborative Antiviral Study Group (2001) Safety and efficacy of high-dose intravenous acyclovir in the management of neonatal herpes simplex virus infections. *Pediatrics*, **108**, 230–238.

Koelle DM and Corey L (2003) Recent progress in herpes simplex immunobiology and vaccine research. *Clin Microbiol Rev*, **16**, 96–113.

Liesegang TJ (1989) Epidemiology of ocular herpes simplex. Natural history in Rochester, MN, 1950 through 1982. *Arch Ophthalmol*, **107**, 1160–1165.

Linde A, Klapper PE, Monteyne P *et al.* and the European Union Concerted Action on Virus Meningitis and Encephalitis (1997) Specific diagnostic methods for herpesvirus infections of the central nervous system: a consensus review by the European Union Concerted Action on Virus Meningitis and Encephalitis. *Clin Diagn Virol*, **8**, 83–104.

Lycke E, Hamark B, Johansson M *et al.* (1988) Herpes simplex infection of the human sensory neuron. An electron microscope study. *Arch Virol*, **101**, 87–104.

McKenna DB, Neill WA and Norval M (2001) Herpes simplex virus-specific immune responses in subjects with frequent and infrequent orofacial recrudescences. *Br J Dermatol*, **144**, 459–464.

Monteyne P, Albert F, Weissbrich B *et al.* and the EU Concerted Action on Virus Meningitis and Encephalitis (1997) The detection of intrathecal synthesis of anti-Herpes simplex IgG antibodies: comparison between an antigen-mediated immunoblotting technique and antibody index calculations. *J Med Virol*, **53**, 324–331.

MSSVD (1999) National guidelines for the management of genital herpes. Clinical Effectiveness Group (Association of Genitourinary Medicine and the Medical Society for the Study of Venereal Diseases). *Sex Transm Infect*, **75**(suppl 1), S24–S28.

Reiber H (1994) Flow rate of cerebrospinal fluid (CSF)—a concept common to normal blood–CSF barrier function and to dysfunction in neurological diseases. *J Neurol Sci*, **122**, 189–203.

Roizman B and Knipe DM (2001) Herpes simplex viruses and their replication. In *Field's Virology* (eds Fields BN, Knipe DM and Howley PM), pp. 2231–2295. Lippincott-Williams and Wilkins, Philadelphia.

Sears AE and Roizman B (1990) Amplification by host factors of a sequence contained within the herpes simplex virus 1 genome. *Proc Natl Acad Sci USA*, **87**, 9441–9445.

Stannard LM, Fuller AO and Spear PG (1987) Herpes simplex virus glycoproteins associated with different morphological entities projecting from the virion envelope. *J Gen Virol*, **68**, 715–725.

Tambasco FP, Cohen EJ, Nguyen LH *et al.* (1999) Oral acyclovir after penetrating keratoplasty for herpes simplex keratitis. *Arch Ophthalmol*, **117**, 445–449.

Tookey P and Peckham CS (1996) Neonatal herpes simplex virus infection in the British Isles. *Paediatr Perinat Epidemiol*, **10**, 432–442.

Van de Laar MJW, Termorschulzen F, Slomka MJ *et al.* (1998) Prevalence and correlates of herpes simplex virus type 2 infection: evaluation of behavioural risk factors. *Int J Epidemiol*, **27**, 127–134.

Waugh SML, Pillay D, Carrington D and Carman WF (2002) Antiviral prophylaxis and treatment (excluding HIV therapy). *J Clin Virol*, **25**, 241–266.

Whitley RJ (1990) Herpes simplex viruses. In *Field's Virology* (eds Fields BN and Knipe DM), pp. 1843–1888. Raven Press, New York.

Whitley RJ (1993) Neonatal herpes simplex virus infections. *J Med Virol*, (suppl 1), 13–21.

York IA, Roop C, Andrews DW *et al.* (1994) A cytosolic herpes simplex virus protein inhibits antigen presentation to CD8[+] T lymphocytes. *Cell*, **77**, 525–535.

Zhou ZH, Dougherty M, Jakana J *et al.* (2000) Seeing the herpesvirus capsid at 8.5 Å. *Science*, **288**, 877–880.

Varicella Zoster

Judith Breuer

St Bartholomew's and the Royal London School of Medicine and Dentistry, London, UK

INTRODUCTION

Two common diseases are caused by *Human herpesvirus 3*, commonly called varicella zoster virus (VZV): chickenpox (varicella) and shingles (herpes zoster). Nobody appears to know for sure what the word 'chicken' has to do with chickenpox but one possible derivation of the term 'chicken'-pox is from the Old English 'gican' (itch), designating it the 'itchy' pox to differentiate it from diseases such as smallpox. The words 'zoster' and 'shingles' are derived from Greek and Latin words, respectively, meaning a belt or girdle, and are obviously descriptive of the characteristic distribution of the rash.

Chickenpox is the manifestation of primary infection with VZV and is one of the commonest communicable diseases worldwide. Its characteristic presentation in the majority of cases is as familiar to laymen as it is to doctors and is usually of little concern to either. However, it has also been long recognised that chickenpox can have serious consequences in adults and in immunosuppressed individuals. Shingles is the manifestation of VZV reactivation and although rarely a life-threatening disease, it is perhaps of more concern community-wide because of the pain, not only of the acute lesion but also of the frequent post-herpetic neuralgia, which can be very debilitating and is notoriously difficult to treat.

The common aetiology of varicella and herpes zoster was first recognised at the beginning of the century by clinicians who noticed that a case of zoster in a household was often followed by an outbreak of varicella in the younger members of the family and their friends. Furthermore, it was shown that vesicle fluid taken from cases of herpes zoster could induce chickenpox when inoculated into young volunteers. Virus particles were first observed in vesicle fluids by electron microscopy in 1943 and definitive evidence that the two diseases are due to the same virus came with the isolation of the virus in cell culture by Weller in 1953 (Weller *et al.*, 1958). It has now been confirmed by analysis of viral DNA in sequential isolates from the same individual that the same virus causes varicella, upon primary infection, and later causes zoster as a manifestation of reactivation.

There is currently considerable interest in VZV infections, which partly stems from the increasing problems encountered with these infections and partly from the recent advances in prevention and treatment. It is likely that the medical significance of VZV infections will continue to increase in industrialised countries as a direct result of demographic changes in the population. The size of the aged population is increasing, which will result in increasing incidence of herpes zoster. The success of treatment regimens that are immunosuppressive in the fields of oncology and transplantation surgery, as well as the increasing numbers of individuals who are infected with HIV, are creating an ever-increasing number of patients who are at risk of contracting the severe forms of varicella and herpes zoster. At the same time, VZ vaccines have been licensed for mass infant

Principles and Practice of Clinical Virology, Fifth Edition. Edited by A. J. Zuckerman, J. E. Banatvala, J. R. Pattison, P. D. Griffiths and B. D. Schoub

Capsid (Three forms exist: A (empty), B (intermediate) and C (mature). Assembly proteins present in the B form are lost during DNA insertion to produce the C form

Tegument A complex mass of proteins surrounding the capsid. Contains enzymes controlling virus replication and regulating cell function

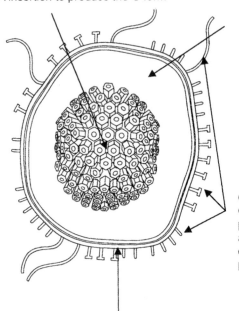

Glycoprotein 'spikes'
Glycoproteins gE, gB, gH, gI, gC and gL project through the lipid envelope, allowing the virus to interact with its environment. gE/gI and gH/gL are present as complexes

Envelope A complex membranous structure derived from cellular membranes of the trans-Golgi network

Figure 2B.1 Structure of the VZV particle (virion). When intact, the particle is spherical and approximately 200 nm in diameter. Amorphous forms may be seen using traditional electron microscopy. From *The Sourcebook of Medical Illustration*. Parthenon Press

immunisation in some countries (e.g. the USA) and targeted immunisation in others, including the UK.

THE VIRUS

Structure

Varicella zoster virus has the characteristic morphological appearance of a herpesvirus (Figure 2B.1), which has been described in detail in Chapter 1. However, because VZV is quite difficult to grow and particularly difficult to purify, less is known about its proteins and genome organisation than is known about those of herpes simplex virus (HSV). In fact much of the knowledge about VZV has been obtained by parallels with HSV. The complete DNA sequence of VZV was published in 1986 by Davison and Scott. A

general review of the molecular biology of VZV is given by Davison (1991). The genome is a linear double-stranded DNA molecule with a molecular weight of 80×10^6 (approximately 125 kilobase pairs, bp) and is thus among the smallest of all herpesviruses studied. Buoyant density estimations, as well as the sequence data, show a $(G+C)$ content of 46%, which is much lower than most herpesviruses, e.g. 67% in herpes simplex 1 (HSV) and 58% in cytomegalovirus (CMV) DNA. Within the genome there are, however, $(G+C)$-rich regions, notably the repeat regions. The organisation of the VZV genome (summarised in Figure 2B.2) shows distinct similarities with HSV DNA and the two viruses have sufficient sequence homology to permit hybridisation under non-stringent conditions. However, there is substantial local variation in the extent of this homology, most notably in the almost complete loss of the repeats around the long unique sequence in VZV, which accounts for much of

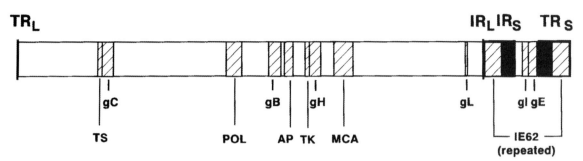

Figure 2B.2 Gene map showing the organisation of the VZV genome and the location of genes (hatched) encoding the viral glycoproteins, the major capsid antigen (MCA), the DNA polymerase (POL), the thymidine kinase (TK), the thymidylate synthetase (TS) and the assembly proteinase/protein (AP). The unique long (U_L) and unique short (U_S) regions are identified, as are the terminal repeat (TR_L and TR_S) and inverted repeat regions (IR_L and IR_S). TR_L and IR_L are 88 bp long, while TR_S and IR_S (black boxes) are 7300 bp long

the size difference between the genomes of these two viruses. The similarities between the HSV and VZV genomes would be compatible with a common ancestry, and a model for this has been proposed (Davison and McGeoch, 1986). The VZV genome is divided into two main coding regions: a unique long region (ca. 105 000 bp) which is flanked by inverted repeat elements (at 88 bp, far shorter than those of HSV), and a unique short region (ca. 5200 bp), also flanked by inverted repeat sequences (7300 bp). The short region can be found in either of two orientations relative to the long region, producing two isomeric forms of the genome which occur in equal proportion. Inversion of the long region is rare. By contrast, in HSV and CMV both regions invert at equal frequency, resulting in four isomeric forms. An inherent size variation of the genome of approximately 2% (2500 bp) has been demonstrated in clinical isolates, concentrated in five variable regions. Restriction endonuclease cleavage patterns show some DNA polymorphism between clinical isolates, and strain differences in circulating viruses are now becoming apparent which may make such analyses a useful tool in epidemiological studies (see below).

Seventy unique open reading frames (ORFs) have been identified on the VZV genome, of which three are repeated, two are spliced and two are located entirely within other genes. Over 70 RNA transcripts have been demonstrated in VZV-infected cells but the majority of these appear to contain more than one ORF. The genes that have been identified to date account for virtually the whole genome, although the presence of overlapping genes does allow for further

ORFs to be identified. The list of genes that have been identified, mostly by analogy with HSV, is shown in Table 2B.1. Five of the VZV genes, including a gene for a thymidylate synthetase, are not found in HSV, while three HSV genes have no VZV equivalent. In common with other herpesviruses, the synthesis of VZV proteins broadly involves three phases, designated immediate-early (α), early (β) and late (γ). More than 30 virus-coded polypeptides can normally be detected in VZV-infected cells, ranging in molecular weight from 7 kDa to over 200 kDa. Among these, at least six groups of glycoproteins can be identified with molecular weights ranging from 38 kDa to 118 kDa, which correspond to the gene products of VZV glycoproteins E, B, H, I, C and L (Table 2B.2). VZV gE is the major glycoprotein expressed on VZV infected cells and mediates IgG Fc-binding in a complex with VZV gI. Two signal sequences within the gE cytoplasmic domain interact with cellular proteins to transport gE complexed with gI to the trans-Golgi network, where post-translational processing occurs before expression on the cell surface. The other glycoproteins, including gB, which is present in virions as a disulphide-linked complex of 140 kDa molecular weight, and gH, which is chaperoned by gL are also directed to the trans-Golgi network of membranes (TGN) to be processed before expression at the cell surface. Glycoproteins C and I have been shown in the SCID hu mouse animal model (see below) to be important for infection of skin cells (Moffat *et al.*, 2002). In addition to the glycoproteins, a range of non-glycosylated proteins have been identified. These include the main protein

Table 2B.1 VZV genes for which functional products have been identified

Gene	HSV homologue	Protein identity (%)	Translation product (kDa)	Function
1	No homologue		12.1	Membrane protein
4	U_L54	29	51.5	Transcriptional activator (IE protein)
5	U_L53 (gK)	28	40	gK, E^b
6	U_L52	37	122.5	DNA helicase/primase component
8	U_L50	25	44.8	Deoxyuridine triphosphatase
9A	$U_L49.5$	Low	9.8	Stearoylated membrane protein
10	U_L48 (VP16)	60	50	Transactivator, tegument protein, NE
13	No homologue		34.5	Thymidylate synthetase
14	U_L44	23	61.4	Membrane glycoprotein gC (gp V)
16	U_L42	21	46.1	Associated with DNA polymerase
17	U_L41	32	51.4	Host shut-off
18	U_L40	54	35.4	Ribonucleotide reductase small subunit
19	U_L39	30	86.8	Ribonucleotide reductase large subunit
28	U_L30	52	134.0	DNA polymerase
29	U_L29	50	132.1	Binds single-stranded DNA
31	U_L27	45	98.1	Membrane glycoprotein gB (gpII)
33	U_L26	34	66.0	Assembly protease
33.5	$U_L26.5$	24	32.8	Assembly protein
36	U_L23	28	37.8	Pyrimidine deoxyribonucleotide kinase
37	U_L22	25	93.6	Membrane glycoprotein gH (gpIII)
40	U_L19	52	155.0	Major capsid antigen
47	U_L13	33	54.3	Protein kinase
48	U_L12	29	61.3	Deoxyribonuclease
49	U_L11	26	8.9	Myristoylated protein
51	U_L9	44	94.4	ori_s binding protein
52	U_L8	28	86.3	DNA helicase/primase component
55	U_L5	56	98.8	DNA helicase/primase component
59	U_L2	39	34.4	Uracil-DNA glycosylase
60	U_L1	19	17.6	Membrane glycoprotein gL (gpVI)
61	IE110	Local only	50.9	Transcriptional repressor (IE protein)
62/71	IE175	Complex	140.0	Transcriptional activator (IE protein)
63/70	U_s1	Local only	30.5	Transcriptional activator (IE protein)
66	U_s	33	43.7	Protein kinase
67	U_s7	23	39.4	Membrane glycoprotein gI (gpIV)
68	U_s8	22	70.0	Membrane glycoprotein gE (gpI)

Table 2B.2 VZV

VZV gene	HSV homologue (% protein identity)	Primary transcript (kDa)	Glycosylation pathway (where known)	Mature form (kDa)
gE (gpI)	gE (22)	73	—— 81 —— 90 —— N-linked O-linked sialylation	98
gB (gpII)	gB (45)	100	—— 126 —— 130 —— 140 —— N-linked O-linked Sialylation Proteolysis Sulphation	66, 68
gH (gpIII)	gH (25)	79	—— 98 —— N-linked O-linked	118
gI (gpIV)	gI (23)	35	———————	60
gC (gpV)	gC (23)	58	———————	100
gL (gpVI)	gL (18)	18	———————	20

component of the nucleocapsid (major capsid antigen or MCA, 155 kDa), an assemblin proteinase/assembly protein complex produced from gene 33, and the IE62 protein (175 kDa), an immediate-early translational activator analogous to the HSV ICP4 protein, which is present in the virions. Many of the other proteins of VZV are involved in virus replication. These include the thymidine kinase and thymidylate synthetase enzymes, several virus-specified protein kinases, a range of DNA-binding proteins, including the viral DNA polymerase, and five transcriptional regulators produced from ORFs 4, 10 and 61–63 (see Table 2B.1).

Replication

VZV attaches to the outer membrane of the cell, and this is followed by membrane fusion and entry of the viral core into the cell. This process is mediated primarily by the glycoproteins, projecting from the virus particles although some tegument proteins may also play a role in viral penetration. Attachment is thought to involve binding, predominantly of gB to heparan sulphate proteoglycan on the cell surface. This binding is followed by attachment of mannose-6-phosphate (M-6-P) oligosaccharides, present on the surface of VZV particles, to M-6-P-specific receptors on the host cell (Zhu et al., 1995).

The tegument proteins prepare the cell to produce virus and separate from the nucleocapsid during transportation of virus particles to the nucleus. Once within the nucleus, the linear DNA genome circularises.

In common with other herpesviruses, the replication cycle is coordinately regulated. There are three basic stages of gene expression and protein synthesis: immediate-early (IE), early (E) and late (L). The first viral proteins (IE) can be detected 4–6 h post-infection. Structural proteins (L) such as the major capsid protein and viral glycoproteins are not detected until 18 h post-infection. Viral protein synthesis appears to reach maximum levels at 46–48 h post-infection in some cell culture systems.

IE transcripts are translated in the cytoplasm and the IE (regulatory) proteins are then transported back into the nucleus, where they induce the early gene expression and downregulate further IE gene transcription. The early (E) proteins include those that are required for VZV DNA replication, such as viral DNA polymerase, viral thymidine kinase and protein kinases. As with the IE proteins, the early proteins are not generally present in the virus particles and only detected in virus-infected cells.

The late proteins can be subdivided into two categories: the early-late proteins, which do not require the synthesis of viral DNA, and the late-late proteins, which are dependent on new viral DNA synthesis. DNA synthesis occurs by the movement of the DNA polymerase around the circularised genomic DNA, producing head-to-tail polymers of the viral genome (concatamers). This is referred to as a 'rolling circle' mechanism. After translation of late mRNA, the structural proteins that will form the viral capsid are transported back to the nucleus and are assembled around a core of the viral assembly protein. The newly transcribed DNA genome is inserted into the assembled capsid, concurrent with the loss of at least some of the assembly proteins (Harper et al., 1995). Capsids acquire a 'temporary envelope' from the inner nuclear membrane and move to the TGN, where the final stages of assembly take place. The nucleocapsid acquires an envelope containing the viral glycoproteins, to which the tegument proteins are bound. In the normal course of events it appears that a second membrane derived from TGN forms a transport vesicle around the mature virions, which then leave the infected cell by a process of exocytosis. In some cells, however, the virions appear to be aberrantly processed and are transported to digestive lysosomes, which possibly accounts for the very low level of cell-free infectious virus found in VZV-infected cell cultures (see below).

Growth in Cell Culture

Varicella zoster virus replicates with varying degrees of success, in cultures of most cells of human and several of simian origin. Cells from non-primates are generally resistant to infection but the virus has been adapted to embryonic guinea-pig cells and passage in these cells was an early stage of the attenuation of the virus used in the current live vaccine. The behaviour of VZV in cell culture can be regarded as being intermediate between that of herpes simplex virus (HSV), which will grow in nearly all cell cultures, and cytomegalovirus (CMV) which will grow only in few cell types of human origin. In other respects, VZV behaves more like CMV, e.g. it grows slowly even in the most sensitive cell systems, with the cytopathic effect (Figure 2B.3) taking from 3 days to over 2 weeks to appear. This process may be mediated by apoptosis rather than direct cell killing. VZV remains even more strongly

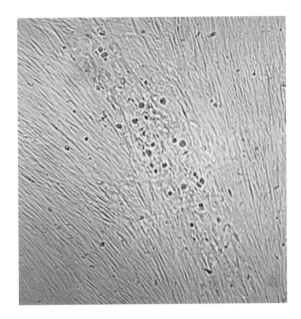

Figure 2B.3 The typical early ovoid cytopathic effect of VZV seen in unstained human embryo lung cells

cell-associated than CMV, and with most systems passage can be achieved only by transfer of infected cells. Cell-free virus can be obtained by a number of procedures, which typically include sonication of the infected cells. Additionally, protective storage media may be used to increase the yield of infectious virus. Higher yields of infectious cell-free virus can be obtained from the media of infected cultures of human thyroid or malignant melanoma cells, which may reflect the release of a high proportion of defective virus particles in other cell culture systems as noted above.

The cytopathic effect in most cell systems is so characteristic that no further means of identification may be required. Because of the strong cell association of the virus, the lesion it produces is typically focal and slowly extends into the surrounding cell sheet, due to the spread of virus between contiguous cells. Viral antigen can be detected much more rapidly than cytopathic effect. Typically, antigens can be detected in the cytoplasm and nuclei of infected cells within 2–4 h after infection and in neighbouring cells after 8–18 h, depending on cell type and the type of antigen targeted. The shape of the lesion is dependent on the architecture of the cell sheet. The typical elongated ovoid shape of the lesion in human embryo lung fibroblasts is shown in Figure 2B.3. Enlarged cells can frequently be seen in the lesion and staining reveals

that these are multinucleated, resulting from virus-induced cell fusion. Staining of the affected cell sheet reveals another feature of VZV cytopathology, namely that many of both the mononuclear and the multi-nucleated cells have irregularly shaped intranuclear inclusions (Figure 2B.4). With time, the infection ultimately spreads to involve the whole cell sheet.

Strain Variation and Antigenic Properties

The nucleotide diversity of the VZV genome as a whole has been estimated at 0.063%, which is comparable to that of human DNA but may be less than that of HSV (0.2–0.5%). As with all herpesviruses, the VZV genome contains blocks of repeated nucleotide sequences, in this case five (R1–5). R1, R2 and R3 are gC-rich and are located in the coding sequences of genes 11, 44 and 22, respectively. R4 (which is present in both of the inverted repeat regions (TR_L and IR_L) flanking the unique long region) and R5 are non-coding. Variation in the number of repeat elements within these regions has been used to distinguish one strain of virus from another, either by means of restriction endonuclease sites generated or lost or by variations in the length of the cleaved fragments (Hawrami *et al.*, 1996). Other restriction sites and single nucleotide polymorphisms (SNPs) throughout the genome have also proved useful for typing of clinical isolates and this has led recently to the identification of at least four main genotypes, currently designated A, B, C and J. Genotypes are geographically segregated, with type A predominating in Africa, Asia and the Far East, type J in Japan and types B and C in Europe and the USA. Mixing of genotypes and intertypic recombination has been observed where migration has occurred, e.g. in London and Rio de Janeiro. Single nuclotide polymorphisms (SNPs) generating restriction sites have been used to distinguish the Oka vaccine virus from wild-type strains. A *Pst*1 restriction site in gene 38 and a *Bgl*1 restriction site in gene 54 have been used to distinguish most UK and US wild-type viruses from the Oka vaccine strain, but in 30% of cases, were unable to discriminate between wild-type Japanese strain and Oka. More recently, a *Sma* restriction site in ORF62, which is present in all wild-type viruses but absent in Oka, has been identified. These SNPs are used to determine whether cases of chickenpox and zoster following vaccination are due to Oka vaccine virus or wild-type virus.

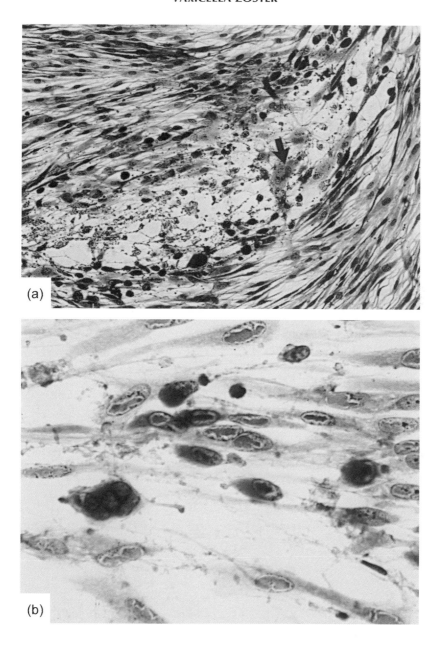

Figure 2B.4 (a) Stained VZV-infected human embryo lung fibroblasts. Note the rounded and multinucleated cells (arrow) (H & E stain). (b) High-power view with many affected cells showing typical intranuclear inclusions

Worldwide, experience suggests that antibody produced against any strain of VZV is protective against clinical disease and this is the basis for immunisation with the live attenuated Oka vaccine. However, well-documented clinical reinfection has been described in up to 13% of children (Hall *et al.*, 2002) and pregnant women with low antibodies (Martin *et al.*, 1994). Protein differences have also been observed in the amino-terminal region of ORF10 (a tegument protein), which may be useful for identifying strains of Japanese origin, including the Oka vaccine strain. Most recently a wild-type strain of VZV called MSP, in which a single glutamate to aspartame mutation in IgE abrogates binding of the 3B3 monoclonal antibody that is commonly used used for diagnostic immunofluorescence, has been isolated. MSP-VZV appears to replicate and spread more aggressively in tissue culture and animal models, such as the SCID hu epithelial mouse.

Some serological cross-reaction with HSV does occur, indicating that these two viruses share common antigens. It has not been shown conclusively on which of the viral proteins the responsible epitope (or epitopes) is situated. The gB glycoproteins of VZV and HSV have cross-reacting epitopes but it has been difficult to demonstrate any significant cross-reactivity with other proteins, in spite of the sequence homologies between the two viruses. More likely is that infection with one virus boosts the levels of antibody to any different but antigenically related virus strains previously encountered, so-called 'original antigenic sin'. This theory cannot entirely explain the heterologous reactions between VZV and HSV, since it is known that a small number of children, with no previous exposure to VZV but who are experiencing primary HSV infection, go on to develop low levels of antibody transiently which react with VZV. The converse has also occasionally been observed with patients experiencing primary VZV infection. It is not known whether this cross-reactivity extends to cellular immune responses or whether it confers any cross-protection between the two viruses.

It is also known that there is appreciable cross-reaction between VZV and simian viruses which cause varicella-like illnesses (see below). The level of cross-reactivity between these viruses is such that administration of live human varicella virus will prevent the development of clinical illness in animals subsequently infected with the simian virus.

Host Response to Infection

Following infection with VZV, antibodies are produced to the various structural and non-structural proteins of VZV. Up to 30 protein bands can be detected with convalescent sera by radioimmunoprecipitation or immunoblotting. The predominant immunogenic components of the virus appear to be the glycoproteins, the major capsid protein and the assembly protein complex (Harper et al., 1988). Both IgG and IgM antibodies react with these proteins (Figure 2B.5). Typically, sera from cases of zoster react more strongly and reveal a wider range of proteins

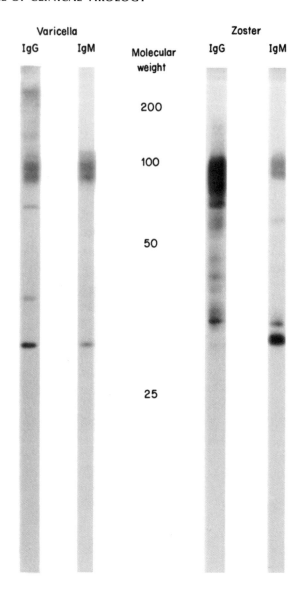

Figure 2B.5 Typical immunoblot patterns for IgG and IgM antibodies obtained with early convalescent sera from varicella and zoster cases. The viral proteins were separated on a 9% polyacrylamide gel, electroblotted onto nitrocellulose and reacted with the sera. IgG and IgM antibodies were detected with ^{125}I-labelled sheep antihuman IgG or IgM. The bands revealed by zoster sera are more numerous and more intense

compared to varicella. gE, gH and the tegument protein IE62 are the major targets for the cell-mediated immune response against VZV, although T lymphocyte responses are also measured against epitopes in gI, gB and gC, as well as the transcriptional regulator IE63, and the products of ORF4, ORF10 and ORF29 genes (Arvin *et al.*, 1991). Although specific antibody against VZV may protect against or attenuate infection, control of primary infection and clearance of virus appears to depend on cellular immunity. The incidence of complications and death from primary infection are higher if there is underlying impairment of cell-mediated immunity.

Pathogenicity for Animals

Animals other than man are reputed not to be susceptible to VZV but there are reports of successful infection of primates such as gorillas and chimpanzees as well as marmosets. It has also been shown that guinea-pigs can be infected with virus which has been passaged in embryonic tissue obtained from these animals, leading to virus replication in the nasopharynx, viraemia and an immune response, but without a rash. Hairless guinea-pigs have been reported to develop a papular rash frequently after inoculation but this model remains challenging to use. Some progress has recently been made on studies of VZV latency (see below) using VZV-infected rats in which latent virus appears to behave in a fashion similar to that seen in human ganglia. However, no *in vivo* reactivation is observed in this model. Recently the use of SCID hu mice with thymus/liver or epithelial implants have greatly facilitated studies of virus tropism for and replication in T cells and skin, respectively. Outbreaks of varicella-like illness have been reported in several specimens of monkeys from primate centres throughout the world and viruses which are similar to VZV have been isolated from these monkeys. These viruses, which are immunologically indistinguishable from one another, are partially related to VZV, showing 70–75% DNA homology across the genome, and are currently being evaluated in an attempt to establish a useful model of VZV infection in man. Studies of simian varicella virus continue to identify similarities to human VZV (Pumphrey and Gray, 1995) but the applicability of data obtained from such a model directly to man is limited.

Pathogenesis

Knowledge about the pathogenesis of VZV-induced diseases, particularly the primary infection, is still limited due to the difficulty in growing the virus and the paucity of suitable animal models.

Surprisingly little is known about the source and route of transmission of the virus. The skin lesions are certainly teeming with infectious virus, even at the maculopapular stage. Airborne transmission from skin lesions is therefore highly likely, especially since VZV DNA is readily detected by polymerase chain reaction (PCR) in the air surrounding patients with VZV infection. It is virtually impossible to isolate infectious virus at any stage from the upper respiratory tract of cases of varicella, although viral DNA may be detectable by PCR. Nevertheless, it is widely believed that transmission occurs from this site, probably from asymptomatic oral lesions which are present before the skin eruption appears. Whatever the case, VZV undoubtedly is transmissible via an airborne route and does not require close personal contact. The clinical attack rate of varicella in outbreaks is typically in the range 70–90% of susceptible individuals, which is slightly less than other viruses transmitted via the respiratory route, e.g. 90% for measles.

The proposed model for the pathogenesis of varicella is shown in Figure 2B.6. It is presumed, as with the vast majority of human virus infections, that the respiratory tract is the portal of entry. Again it is presumed that after an initial phase of replication at the site of entry, the virus spreads to a distant site, the lymphoid system, where a second phase of replication takes place. What is certain is that after a period of about 14 days the virus arrives at its main target organ, the skin, and the final phase of replication occurs there. It is likely that the virus spreads to and replicates in many other organs of the body, particularly the lung. In most cases, the infection at these sites does not manifest clinically, presumably because little or no damage results from it. However, in those cases when extensive infection involves organs such as the lung or brain, serious disease can result.

There is considerable clinical evidence in support of this proposed model for the pathogenesis of varicella and leukoviraemia has been demonstrated during the incubation period in healthy as well as immunocompromised patients. For a full discussion of this subject, see Grose (1987).

Histological examination of the skin lesions of both varicella and zoster shows focal degenerative changes in the epidermis. The affected cells are swollen and many of these contain well-defined eosinophilic intranuclear inclusions. Multinucleated cells, also with intranuclear inclusions, are characteristically seen at the base of the lesion (Figure 2B.7). The histology of the skin lesions is thus essentially similar to the cytopathology seen in cell culture. The lesion extends and its centre fills at first with clear fluid, which then

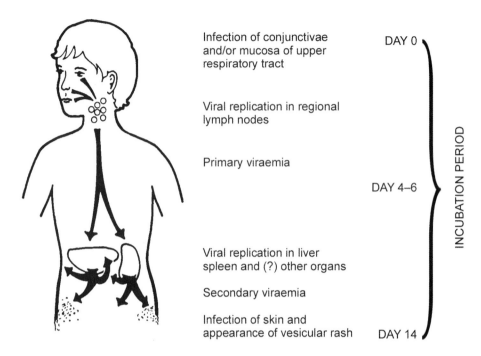

Figure 2B.6 Proposed model for the pathogenesis of varicella. Reprinted from Grose (1981), © 1981, American Academy of Pediatrics

becomes cloudy due to the influx of inflammatory cells.

Termination of the infection at this site is indicated by the drying up of the pustules, which is followed by separation of the scabs and regeneration of the epithelium. Termination must be brought about by both the humoral and the cellular immune responses and it appears likely that the latter is the more important. The presence of large amounts of free and cell-associated virus in the lesion, as well as degenerating cells showing all the characteristic features of VZV infection, strongly suggests that the damage results from a lytic effect of the virus. The lesions in the immunocompromised are not modified in any way other than being more extensive and this makes it unlikely that immunopathology is playing an important part in their genesis.

Recovery from the primary infection results, in most people, in life-long immunity to exogenous infection, although clinical reinfection has been described in up to 13% of children and in some pregnant women with low antibody titres (Martin *et al.*, 1994; Hall *et al.*, 2002). Subclinical reinfection may be even more common, since it has been demonstrated that seropositive individuals who are in contact with varicella can occasionally show significant rises in the level of specific antibodies and boosting of cell-mediated responses (Gershon *et al.*, 1996). Furthermore, viral DNA can be detected by PCR in nasopharyngeal secretions of immune individuals who are in close contact with chickenpox, suggesting that localised reinfections may occur (Connelly *et al.*, 1993). Asymptomatic systemic spread of virus is also suggested by reactivation of UK viral strains in patients whose primary infections occurred in Africa (Quinlivan, 2002). It is probable that such re-exposures to VZV throughout life help to maintain effective immunity to varicella. Recent epidemiological data also confirm the hypothesis that exposure to varicella protects against subsequent zoster (Brisson, 2002).

Latency

Following the primary infection, the virus remains latent in one or more posterior root ganglia. The trigeminal and thoracic ganglia are most frequently involved but ganglia at multiple sites may contain VZV DNA, including ganglia not directly connected with the skin (Furuta *et al.*, 1997). VZV can also infect T lymphocytes and this is likely to be the

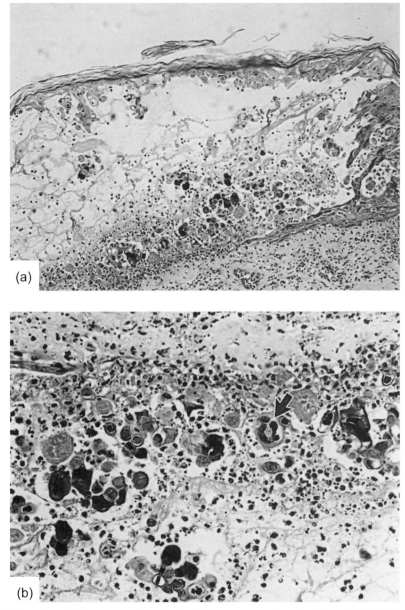

Figure 2B.7 VZV skin lesions. (a) Low-power view showing inflammatory exudate into the vesicle. (b) High-power view showing multinucleated cells (arrow). Many of the affected cells have typical intranuclear inclusions

route of infection of at least some ganglia. In up to 20% of individuals a single recurrent infection occurs, usually several decades after the primary infection. The virus reactivates in the ganglion and then progresses peripherally down the sensory nerve to produce the typical skin lesions of herpes zoster, which are restricted to the dermatome supplied by the nerve.

Less is known about VZV latency and reactivation than is known about the corresponding processes with HSV. During latency the viral DNA appears to exist in episomal form, with fused genome termini. Latent virus is located predominantly in the neurons within the ganglia (2–5%), with a much smaller proportion (less than 0.1%) of non-neuronal satellite cells being infected. Unlike HSV, there is no evidence that VZV

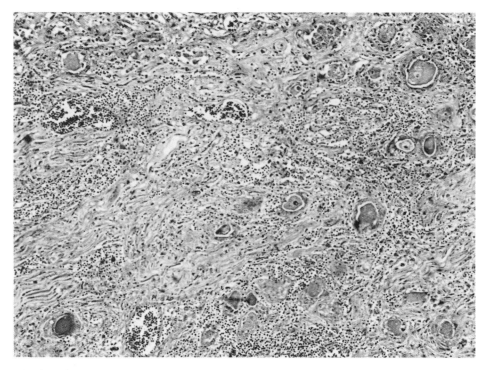

Figure 2B.8 Section of a posterior root ganglion obtained from a patient with herpes zoster. Note the intense inflammatory exudate and degenerate neurons (H & E stain)

encodes latency-associated transcripts. Instead, *in vitro* studies have shown that the majority of the VZV genome is inactive during latency, and only transcripts from ORFs 63 (which is most abundant), 21, 29, 62 and, to a lesser extent, 4 and 18 are detectable. ORF63 is the most abundant transcript and there is evidence that, unlike the situation with HSV, protein products of ORFs 4, 21, 29, 62 and 63 are produced during latency (Mahalingam *et al.*, 1996) and are present in the cytoplasm as well as the nucleus, as expected, of both neuronal and non-neuronal cells.

Reactivation of virus is associated with intense destructive inflammatory changes in the involved ganglion (Figure 2B.8) and this may be reflected in the severe pain which is frequently experienced in association with zoster. The failure of the host defence mechanisms to contain the virus in the ganglia after such prolonged periods of time is not understood. In immunocompetent individuals it is probably due to the decline of the effectiveness of previously acquired *cell-mediated* immunity to VZV. In particular, T cell responses to IE 63 have been proposed to protect against reactivation. Inadequacy of cell-mediated immunity is likely to be of critical importance, since not only the elderly but patients with Hodgkin's

lymphoma, HIV and similar diseases are also more likely to experience zoster. These patients are also more likely to experience more than one attack of the disease or they may develop the *disseminated* form of the disease. The term 'disseminated' implies that the virus spreads through viraemia from the affected dermatome to infect the skin or other organ at some distal site, producing lesions that are similar to those of varicella in their appearance and distribution. In recent years it has also been shown that the appearance of zoster correlates with increasing immunodeficiency in patients infected with human immunodeficiency virus (HIV), which primarily affects cellular immunity.

Most cases of zoster occur spontaneously but trauma and stress have also been proposed as triggers of reactivation. Anecdotal case reports suggesting that re-exposure to varicella or vaccination with Oka may trigger zoster have yet to be confirmed.

EPIDEMIOLOGY

Cases of varicella are seen throughout the year but they occur more frequently in the winter and early

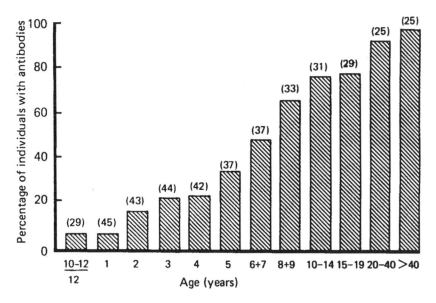

Figure 2B.9 Age prevalence of antibodies to VZV. The antibodies were detected by both RIA and indirect immunofluorescence procedures. The numbers of each age group tested are given at the end of the columns. These results were obtained in a collaborative study with Dr J Cradock-Watson, Withington Hospital, Manchester

spring months. The seasonal incidence of the disease is therefore roughly similar to that of other systemic diseases such as measles and rubella and the respiratory viral infections, but quite unlike that of the enteroviruses. Because of the comparatively small variation in the seasonal incidence of varicella, it is preferable to regard it as a disease which shows variation in seasonal endemicity, rather than as an epidemic disease. Annual variation in incidence also occurs with higher than average incidence in 3–4 year cycles. Herpes zoster, in contrast, occurs sporadically and evenly throughout the year.

Varicella is one of the most common communicable diseases worldwide and is predominantly a disease of childhood. However, different parts of the world can show significant variations in the age distribution of infection. In *temperate areas* it is one of the classic diseases of childhood. In the past the highest incidence of varicella occurred in the age group 4–10 years (Figure 2B.9). Recent serological surveys and data from surveillance general practices (Royal College of General Practitioners) have shown that the peak age of primary infection in Western countries occurs in children aged under 5 years, which is presumably related to an increased use of day-care and playgroup facilities, leading to greater exposure at a younger age. In general, varicella is highly communicable in temperate countries, with a reported attack rate of

up to 96% in close contacts (i.e. household or play-friend), and therefore most people become infected before adulthood. Seroprevalence studies generally show that less than 10% of young adults are still susceptible to varicella (Figure 2B.9) and, despite a temporary increase in the incidence and overall proportion of cases in adults (aged over 15 years) (Fairley and Miller, 1996), this remains the case today.

It is not known what role different environmental and social factors or different virus strains (see below) may play in determining the epidemiology of varicella, but the patterns of infection and disease can be very different in *tropical regions* compared to those of temperate regions. In many tropical countries, varicella is predominantly a disease of adults, with a mean age of 20–25 years, or even as high as 38 years reported from St Lucia. Studies from the Indian subcontinent, south-east Asia and the Caribbean have shown that 25–60% of adults aged over 15 years are susceptible to varicella. It appears that less transmission occurs amongst the young children in these areas and this may reflect patterns of social mixing between infected cases and susceptible contacts. The effects of temperature and humidity at these latitudes on a naturally labile virus has also been proposed to explain lower rates of infection, but is partially discounted by evidence of a childhood pattern of infection in countries with similar climatic conditions, such as

Hong Kong and Northern Australia. The effect of low population density in a rural setting leading to lower rates of transmission is supported by the lower rates of VZV seropositivity for subjects living in rural Bengal and rural Brazil, as compared with their age-matched urban counterparts. Other theories include competition with other viruses infecting the respiratory tract. Asymptomatic infection occurring in infants protected by maternally transferred antibodies is also possible, with the virus failing to establish latency and some individuals thus remaining susceptible later in life.

It is important in hospital practice in temperate climates to be aware of the fact that staff who were born in tropical countries are more likely to be susceptible to varicella.

Molecular Epidemiology

Using restriction fragment length polymorphisms (RFLPs) and PCR, strains of VZV in the USA have been shown to be related and distinct from strains circulating in Japan (Takada *et al.*, 1995). Restriction analysis has also been used to prove that the virus causing chickenpox in an individual was the same as that reactivating as zoster some years later and that Oka vaccine strain can be distinguished from wild-type viruses in the USA (Adams *et al.*, 1989). Most RFLPs are generated by variations in the numbers and sequence of repeats in the five (gC)-rich repeat regions, R1–R5, in the genome. RFLP differences between the Oka vaccine strain and wild-type American strains have been described (Adams *et al.*, 1989), while PCR across a *Bgl*1 restriction site in gene 54 and a *Pst*1 site in gene 38 has simplified the identification of Oka which, unlike VZV in USA, is $Pst1^- Bgl1^+$. The Oka strain also differs from all UK strains tested but is genetically indistinguishable from about 3% of wild-type Japanese strains. It is probable that, as with herpes simplex, geographical variations reflect selection by host factors. However, there is also evidence for transcontinental spread and recombination of strains. (Barrett-Muir *et al.*, 2002).

CLINICAL FEATURES

Varicella—the Primary Infection

The incubation period of varicella is approximately 2 weeks but a range of 7–23 days has been quoted. A shortened incubation period can be encountered,

particularly in immunocompromised patients. A potential source of error in these estimates will be the infections that are acquired from asymptomatic cases.

The illness usually commences with the appearance of the rash but occasionally there are prodromal symptoms that resemble an influenza-like illness. These symptoms appear a few days before the rash and are seen more frequently in adults than in children.

The rash is characteristically centripetal in distribution and is seen mainly in areas that are not exposed to pressure, such as the flanks, between the shoulder blades and in the axillae. It is generally sparse in the antecubital and popliteal fossae and is rarely seen on the palms or the soles. This distribution is markedly different from the more centrifugal distribution of the smallpox rash, a distinction which used to be of considerable diagnostic importance. Other differentiating features are that the lesions of smallpox are rounder and deeper than the more superficial and irregular shaped lesions of varicella.

The skin lesions progress fairly rapidly through the stages of macules and papules to vesicles, which rapidly break down with crust formation. The vesicle with its surrounding area of erythema is the most characteristic feature of the rash. The lesions appear in a series of crops, so that all stages in their genesis can be seen at any one time. This is very different from smallpox, where the lesions are always at the same stage. Patients with varicella are generally considered to be infectious from a couple of days before the rash until new vesicle formation has ceased and existing vesicles have crusted. This usually occurs 5–7 days after onset but may be longer in the immunocompromised. The crusts separate usually within 10 days, revealing healthy skin, but a minor degree of scarring is common. The general constitutional symptoms of the illness are typically mild, particularly in children.

Complications of Varicella

Sepsis

Secondary bacterial infection is by far the most common complication of varicella, especially in children, and causes increased scarring of the skin. Streptococci group A and staphylococci are most frequently involved and may be life-threatening in the immunocompromised. Of those children requiring hospitalisation for pneumonia associated with VZV, over 30% may have bacterial pathogens.

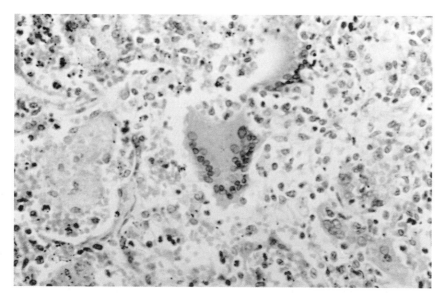

Figure 2B.10 Varicella pneumonia. Area of consolidated lung with typical multinucleated cells. (H & E stain)

Viral Pneumonia

Symptomatic varicella pneumonia occurs in 1 in 200 000 cases of varicella in children, rising to 1 in 200 in immunocompetent adults, although radiological changes may be found in 10 times this number. In pregnant women the incidence of pneumonitis is increased to 9% whilst 10% of smokers develop this complication. Those most at risk are the immunocompromised, including children with leukaemia, in whom up to 32% develop pneumonitis with a mortality of up to 25% (Feldman and Lott, 1987). Adults with malignant disease of the lymphoreticular system who have received organ transplants and patients taking systemic steroids are also at increased risk.

Pneumonia complicating varicella begins 1–3 (range 1–6) days after the onset of rash and the clincial features include dry cough, dyspnoea and tachypnoea with chest pain, haemoptysis and cyanosis occurring less frequently. Over 90% of patients with chest symptoms will develop pneumonitis and all such patients should be admitted to hospital for antiviral therapy. Histological examination of an area of lung affected by VZV shows alveoli filled with oedema fluid, a few foamy macrophages and other round cells. The absence of an extensive outpouring of polymorphonuclear leukocytes is a feature that distinguishes this disease from bacterial pneumonia. The presence of multinucleated giant cells with intranuclear inclusions

(Figure 2B.10) is pathognomonic, although somewhat similar cells are seen in measles pneumonia. It is important to realise that these multinucleated cells are not always seen but large swollen mononuclear cells, similar to cytomegalic cells but without the dominant intranuclear inclusion, are always present. Clinical diagnosis is confirmed by chest X-ray changes and direct immunofluorescence of vesicle fluid and nasopharyngeal secretions, using a fluorescein-conjugated monoclonal antibody. PCR of vesicle fluid and respiratory secretions and specific IgM antibodies in the serum are also be useful.

The illness runs a fulminating course if not treated early with high-dose intravenous aciclovir and is the single most common cause of varicella-associated death in the immunocompromised. Surviving patients may recover completely but others develop fibrosis of the lungs, with permanent respiratory impairment.

Haemorrhagic Chickenpox

Haemorrhagic symptoms sometimes occur during the course of varicella and usually make their appearance on the second or third day of the rash. Haemorrhage typically occurs into the skin but epistaxis, malaena or haematuria may be additional presenting features. The haemorrhage may be so severe as to be life-threatening. This complication is more commonly seen

in immunocompromised patients such as renal transplant recipients, in whom a thrombocytopenia and/or
consumptive coagulopathy may also develop. Other
clinical features in these cases often include hepatitis
and gastrointestinal bleeding or distention. Treatment
is with high-dose intravenous antivirals (aciclovir) and
intensive care. Intravenous immunoglobulin, although
it has not formally been evaluated, is also commonly
used. The addition of steroids is more controversial.

Encephalitis

Varicella meningoencephalitis necessitating admission
to hospital occurs in 3–4 cases per 100 000 children and
more commonly in adults. Cerebral symptoms are
more common in adults, whilst cerebellar ataxia occurs
in children. In the majority of cases symptoms begin
4–8 days after onset of rash. CSF examination may be
normal or reveal a lymphocytosis, with a high cell
count and protein level being more likely in encephalitis than in cerebellar disease. Typical cases of
encephalitis presenting with headache and vomiting
and proceeding to coma are rarely seen but carry a
high mortality. By contrast, most patients with
cerebellar disease recover fully, although it may take
some months. Other neurological disorders, including
meningitis, transverse myelitis and Guillain–Barré
syndrome, have also been associated with the disease.

As with varicella pneumonia, CNS involvement
occurs much more frequently in immunocompromised
patients and is another important factor contributing
to the increased mortality of the disease in these
patients.

Other Unusual Manifestations and Complications of Varicella

As mentioned in the section on Pathogenesis, above,
VZV infection may involve virtually any organ of the
body but, apart from in the skin and occasionally the
lung and brain, it is unusual for infection at other sites
to manifest clinically. Nevertheless, myocarditis,
arthritis, hepatitis and both renal and ureteric damage
associated with varicella have been reported.

Reye's syndrome is a serious and frequently fatal
form of encephalopathy which is secondary to liver
damage occurring in children with varicella or
influenza and is associated with ingestion of aspirin.
The incidence of this has fallen with strictures on the
use of salicylates in children.

Varicella in Pregnancy

From Figure 2B.9 it can be seen that approximately
10% of women of childbearing age are still susceptible
to varicella, but this figure may be as high as 20% in
communities with a high proportion of immigrants
from India and Africa. The incidence of varicella in
adults aged 15–44 years has been estimated at 3 cases
per 1000, which would result in about 2000 cases/year
in pregnant women in England and Wales. In areas
with immigrant populations from India and Africa, the
incidence may be over twice as high. Varicella in
pregnancy can present two quite distinct problems,
depending on whether the infection is contracted in the
early or in the very late stages of the pregnancy. For a
review of varicella in pregnancy, see Hanshaw et al.,
(1985).

Varicella in the Early Stages of Pregnancy

Congenital varicella syndrome occurs in fewer than
1% of foetuses where maternal infection occurs before
13 weeks of gestation, but this rises to 2% if maternal
infection occurs between weeks 13 and 20 (Pastusak
et al., 1994; Enders et al., 1994). The main features of
this syndrome are shown in Table 2B.3. Certain
defects, such as those involving the brain and eye,
are similar to those seen in congenital infections caused
by rubella virus and cytomegalovirus but other
features are quite different. Scarring of the skin,
which can be extensive, is a unique feature of the
varicella syndrome and indicates that VZV is derma-
totrophic even in utero. Other unique features are
hypoplasia of the limbs and rudimentary or even
missing digits, indicating that VZV intrauterine infection has a marked propensity for the musculoskeletal
system. Gastrointestinal abnormalities are also
described. The pathogenesis of the unique lesions of
the congenital varicella syndrome is not fully understood but it is probable that they result from foetal
zoster following the initial VZV infection. The very
short latency period is explained by poorly developed
cell-mediated immunity in the foetus.

Table 2B.3 Clinical features of the congenital varicella
syndrome

Scarring of the skin
Hypoplasia of the limbs, muscular atrophy, rudimentary digits
Cortical atrophy, psychomotor retardation
Choreoretinitis, cataracts

All of the reported cases in the literature were seriously affected and less than half of them survived beyond 20 months. In addition, a few cases have been reported in the literature of babies born with severe disseminated varicella acquired as late as the 25th week of gestation.

Varicella in the Late Stages of Pregnancy

In common with other viruses (e.g. poliovirus), varicella is known to cross the placenta in the late stages of pregnancy, causing congenital infection of the foetus, and infection acquired in this way can result in the child developing varicella. Varicella occurring within 10 days of delivery is evidence of intrauterine infection. The risk of a child acquiring varicella in this way is dependent on the rapidity with which the mother develops and transfers humoral immunity across the placenta and also the time interval between the date of onset of the rash in the mother and the date of delivery. This period is important because it affects the management of these cases. From numerous clinical observations it has now become consistently apparent that if the onset of the rash in the mother occurs 7 days or more before delivery, sufficient immunity will have been transferred so that, even if infection has occurred *in utero*, it will subsequently be mild or even inapparent. In contrast, if the onset of the mother's rash is 6 days or less before delivery, the child will be exposed to infection without the protection of maternally transferred antibody. Young children infected in this way may experience severe fatal disseminated forms of the disease. Case-fatality rates of approximately 30% have been reported for untreated neonatal varicella. Also at risk of severe infection are babies born to seronegative mothers who contract varicella in the neonatal period, as no passive immunity will have been transferred from the mother. The administration of VZIG to attenuate infection (see below) is therefore recommended for all children in contact with varicella within the first 28 days of birth where the mother is seronegative. Infected children born to seropositive mothers are usually protected, although it is worth noting that this protection is not complete, since cases of mild varicella have been reported in babies born to seropositive mothers. The protective efficacy of the maternal antibodies is maximal during the first 2 months of life. Children born before 32 weeks gestation may not have acquired maternal immunity, even if the mother has antibodies to VZV. In such cases, and indeed in all cases where a prematurely born infant is exposed to varicella whilst in hospital, it is advisable to test the infant for varicella antibody and administer prophylactic VZIG if it is absent.

As stated above, the pathogenesis of varicella is not fully understood. The behaviour of VZV in pregnancy does, however, shed some light on this. First, the fact that intrauterine infection occurs at all provides further evidence that primary infection must have a viraemic phase. Of greater significance is the observation that serious congenital varicella will occur only if the onset of the maternal rash is within 7 days of delivery. This clearly indicates that humoral immunity can affect the course of infection.

Herpes Zoster—the Recurrent Infection

This is the recurrent form of VZV, which typically affects a single dermatome of the skin. The average annual incidence is 0.2% and it can occur at any age. Over 50% of cases occur in individuals aged over 50 years but the incidence rises sharply from far fewer than 1/1000 in the under-50s to 3–4/1000 in those aged over 50 and 8–10/1000 in those aged 65 years and above. Zoster is rare in children, although maternal varicella and varicella acquired during infancy have been identified as predisposing factors.

The disease is a result of the virus reactivating in a single sensory ganglion and then proceeding peripherally down the associated sensory nerve to infect the skin supplied by that nerve. The location of the skin lesions are therefore dependent on the ganglion involved. The ophthalmic branch of the trigeminal nerve, as well as the lower cervical (in children especially), thoracic and lumbar (T5–L2) posterior root ganglia are those that are most frequently involved. The eruption is usually preceded by abnormal sensations and, perhaps, by burning or shooting pains in the involved segment, and the skin may be exquisitely tender to the touch (hyperaesthesia). This is followed by the familiar unilateral 'strap' of vesicles on the trunk. This can be accompanied by muscle weakness in the affected or adjoining limb. The density of the vesicles is very variable, being often sparse in children but densely packed in adults. Definitive involvement of the eye in ophthalmic shingles is signalled by vesicles appearing at the tip of the nose, which is supplied by the nasopharyngeal branch of the nerve (Hutchinsons's sign). Where the sacral ganglia may be involved, the skin lesions may be associated with retention of urine or symptoms suggestive of urinary tract infection, and sometimes there is frank haemorrhagic cystitis. Facial palsy associated with vesicles in the external auditory meatus is known as the Ramsay–Hunt syndrome and is thought to be a form of zoster involving the geniculate ganglion of the seventh nerve. It is often accompanied by hearing loss and vertigo. However, the pathology of this form of zoster is disputed and it is preferable to refer to this disease as 'aural zoster' rather than by its eponymous title or even 'geniculate herpes'. VZV reactivation has also been implicated as a cause of facial Bell's-type palsy without vesicles or other symptoms but this association is difficult to prove. A form fruste of herpes zoster (zoster sine herpete), in which dermatomal pain is present without lesions, has been shown to be associated with high IgG antibody titres to VZV, and VZV DNA is detectable by PCR in circulating lymphocytes (Gilden et al., 1994) and in the naso-pharyhngeal secretions (Furuta et al., 2001).

As with primary VZV infection, herpes zoster is a far greater problem in immunocompromised patients. In these individuals it frequently occurs earlier in life and second attacks, which are virtually unknown in the immunocompetent, are sometimes seen. Moreover, the disease process is frequently prolonged in immuno-compromised patients and they are most likely to experience the *disseminated* form of zoster. If any patient with zoster is examined carefully it is not uncommon to find isolated vesicles in areas of the skin far away from the main lesion. This means that a minor degree of dissemination must occur quite frequently. In one study, asymptomatic VZV viraemia was detected in 19% of bone marrow transplant recipients, using PCR (Wilson et al., 1992). In the immunocompromised patient, however, extensive dis-semination of the virus can occur so that the appearance is identical to varicella but with the addition of the zoster lesion. Such patients are frequently extremely ill, often with visceral involvement, but with antiviral therapy there is rarely a fatal outcome.

Herpes zoster, unlike varicella, does not usually present a problem during pregnancy. The disease is typically mild in pregnant women and transmission to the foetus is not described. Herpes zoster near term is not associated with serious neonatal infection, pre-sumably because of the protection afforded by maternal antibodies.

Complications of Herpes Zoster

Infection

As with varicella, secondary bacterial infection of the skin can occur and occasionally can lead to impetigo

or cellulitis, but with appropriate antibiotic therapy this is rarely a serious problem.

Neuralgia

Pain lasting more than 4 weeks after the onset of the rash has been termed post-herpetic neuralgia. Since the pain is usually a continuum of the pain occurring during the acute phase, a more modern terminology is zoster-associated pain (ZAP). Prolonged ZAP is the most common complication of zoster, occurring in 15% of cases overall and up to 40% of those aged 60 years and over. Nearly all patients experience severe acute pain at the site of the lesion, although the severity and duration increase with age. The pain may be present before the onset of the rash but in just over 85% of cases it remits within 2–3 weeks. It may consist of a constant pain, an intermittent stabbing pain or paraesthesia. Worsening of the pain on touch, allodynia, is also characteristic. In some patients severe disabling chronic pain occurs. The cause of the pain is not clear but is associated with ganglionic destruction and scarring with perturbation of type C nociceptor function (Rowbotham and Fields, 1996). Symptoms may be precipitated by temperature change and are often worse at night. Age and, when that is controlled for, severity of pain at the onset of zoster are the factors which most strongly predict severe ZAP. Female gender and ophthalmic location of the rash are also associated with more severe and prolonged pain. Treatment with antiviral drugs will reduce the incidence, duration and severity of ZAP if started within 72 h of the onset of rash, especially in those aged over 50 years. The level of active drug, both peak values and total dose (area under the curve), have also been shown to be inversely correlated with severity and duration of ZAP (Beutner et al., 1995) and more recently the presence of virus in the blood at presentation was found to correlate with prolonged ZAP (Scott et al., in press). Post-herpetic neuralgia is rarely seen in children.

Meningitis Encephalitis and Myelitis

Neurological complications due to VZV may be more common than hitherto thought. PCR of CSF has determined that VZV is amongst the most frequently detected viruses in patients with aseptic meningitis. VZV may also cause encephalitis, usually in the presence of lesions but sometimes, in immunosuppressed patients, in the absence of visible rash. Typically the rash, if present, involves the cranial or upper cervical nerves. It is fortunately very rare and little is known about its pathogenesis.

A number of clinical observations have strongly suggested that motor as well as sensory neurons may be involved in cases of herpes zoster. Ptosis associated with ophthalmic zoster and paralysis of the intrinsic muscles of the hand associated with skin lesions of the deltoid region are examples of this. The phenomenon is thought to be due to centripetal spread of the virus from a ganglion into the central nervous system and thence into a motor neuron. It is possible that facial palsy with aural herpes, referred to above, may be mediated in this way rather than through involvement of the geniculate ganglion. Most of the motor neuropathies are fortunately transient and serious sequelae are rarely seen. Guillain–Barré syndrome and transverse myelitis with ascending paralysis have been reported in small numbers of cases and appear to be more common in HIV-positive patients. A rare but serious complication, particularly associated with ophthalmic zoster, is contralateral hemiparesis. This is caused by a granulomatous inflammatory process in the brain with infarction of the cerebral arteries.

Ocular

The presentation of ophthalmic zoster is complex because of the many structures of the eye and its surrounds which can be involved, such as the eyelid, conjunctiva, sclera, cornea and iris. Consequently the risk of complications is high, even in immunocompetent individuals. The risk of complications is particularly high if the nasociliary branch of the fifth cranial nerve is involved. Iritis and keratitis are the most common complications. Blindness following ophthalmic zoster is, however, rare.

Varicella Retinitis

Acute retinal necrosis due to reactivation of VZV has been described, and is characterised by focal, well-demarcated necrotising retinitis occurring predominantly unilaterally. Treatment with intravenous aciclovir produces improvement within 48–72 h and prevents the development of ragged retinal holes and retinal detachment. A similar picture can be produced by herpes simplex virus, usually in association with encephalitis. The clinical complexities of ophthalmic

zoster have been reviewed by Marsh (1976) and Culbertson (1986).

In patients with the acquired immunodeficiency syndrome (AIDS), rapidly progressive herpetic retinal necrosis due to VZV infection has been recognised. First described as progressive outer retinal necrosis (PORN), the condition is characterised by outer retinal opacification and absence of inflammatory changes in the eye bilaterality and multifocality. The signs are rapidly progressive and are distinct from the retinal infiltration and haemorrhages seen in CMV retinitis. Untreated, PORN quickly progresses to bilateral total blindness. VZV is the most common cause of this condition and is diagnosed by PCR of fluid from the anterior chamber. Treatment with intravenous aciclovir or ganciclovir may halt the progression of the lesions but will not usually affect the loss of visual acuity. Foscarnet has also been used, both alone and in combination with a nucleoside analogue, either aciclovir or ganciclovir. Foscarnet and ganciclovir have been given as intravitreal injections.

Zoster and HIV

Zoster occurs in up to 30% of patients with HIV infection and in parts of Africa 85% of patients with zoster aged less than 45 years are HIV-1-positive. Most episodes of zoster occur early in the HIV disease process, before the CD4 cell count has fallen, and tend to be uni-dermatomal. Zoster occurring after the onset of AIDS is associated with disseminated and multi-dermatomal zoster. Recurrent zoster is common as the CD4 cell count falls, occurring in up to 30% of patients. Up to 10% of patients will also experience an episode of zoster following the start of antiretroviral therapy. This reactivation can be triggered by immune reconstitution. Some HIV positive patients may develop a chronic form of zoster with atypical verrucous-like skin lesions, which have been associated with decreased expression of VZV gE and gB (Nikkels et al., 1997).

DIAGNOSIS OF VZV INFECTION

The clinical presentations of both varicella and herpes zoster are usually so typical that laboratory confirmation is rarely required. Notwithstanding, in one series of shingles diagnosed clinically in the community, 15% turned out to be due to HSV infection or non-herpetic (Breuer et al., 2001). Where the distinction between

HSV infection and herpes zoster is difficult, such as in a generalised vesicular rash occurring in an immuno-compromised patient or where atypical lesions occur, laboratory confirmation should be sought. Similarly, laboratory diagnosis may also be useful for some of the less common CNS and ocular complications affecting immunocompromised patients. The VZV antibody status of an individual is also commonly required, now that treatment and prophylactic measures are readily available and also because of the increasing problem of nosocomial varicella outbreaks which require prompt intervention.

Direct Demonstration Techniques

The main advantage of these techniques is that they are rapid, usually giving results on the same day that the specimen is received.

Electron Microscopy (EM)

Typical herpesvirus particles can be seen in profusion in fluid taken from early vesicles of either varicella or zoster. The particles can also be seen in emulsions of material scraped from the base of lesions. The particles are more difficult to see when the specimens are taken late in the disease. EM unfortunately will not distinguish between VZV and HSV infection unless combined with immunological techniques.

Cytology

Smears of scrapings of the base of the lesions, stained by Papanicolaou's method or, for quickness, methy-lene blue, will reveal characteristic multinucleated giant cells (Figure 2B.11), also known as Tzanck cells. Although not a routine procedure, microscopic examination of biopsies of the lesion will also reveal these giant cells as well as the other characteristics of the histology which have been described above. Again, neither cytology or histology will distinguish between HSV- and VZV-induced lesions.

Immunofluorescence Cytology

A more specific diagnosis can be made if immuno-fluorescence or immunoperoxidase examination of the

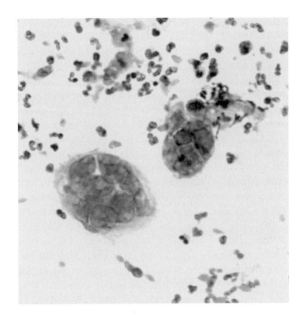

Figure 2B.11 Scraping of the base of a lesion of herpes zoster. Note the typical multinucleated cells (Papanicolaou stain)

smears is carried out. Even cells from crusted lesions contain viral antigen in abundance, allowing easy detection. This method is therefore particularly useful at a time when EM or virus isolation (see below) may not be reliable. Direct detection of VZV in cells scraped from the base of a vesicle is now easily achieved using the FITC-conjugated monoclonal 3B3 antibody, which is directed against an epitope in gE. This simple method has replaced indirect immuno-fluorescence.

Detection of Viral DNA

The polymerase chain reaction (PCR) is more sensitive than immunofluorescence, EM and culture for the detection of VZV in vesicle fluid. For this reason it is the method of choice where the vesicular viral load is low and a diagnosis is required, e.g. where the rash is old, following antiviral treatment and where recurrent varicella infection is suspected. PCR of vesicle fluid is also used to confirm verruciform zoster occurring in HIV-positive patients, and has been shown to detect VZV in up to 10% of simplex-like rashes. PCR is most extensively used for the diagnosis of VZV CNS and ocular disease. Using PCR, VZV was the commonest virus (29%) detected in 3231 Finnish patients with suspected meningoencephalitis. This result is borne out by other studies, confirming that VZV is a significant cause of viral meningitis and encephalitis in both immunocompetent and immunocompromised patients. VZV viral load in the blood may be useful for the detection of visceral zoster infection, which may present in immunocompromised patients as abdominal pain in the absence of rash. PCR of vitreous fluid is also used to confirm the diagnosis of ARN and PORN.

More recently PCR has been used to demonstrate the presence of viral DNA in throat swabs from patients with zoster and zoster *sine herpete*. PCR of vesicle fluid is also the method of choice for differentiating the Oka vaccine virus from wild-type strains in rashes occurring in subjects who have been immunised.

Virus Isolation

This remains the gold standard for diagnosing VZV infections; however, isolation of virus is difficult and recovery rates in most laboratories are generally less than 50%. Human fibroblast cultures are used in most laboratories as they can be maintained for the 21 days required for some isolations.

Vesicle fluid or material swabbed from the base of fresh lesions are the specimens most suitable for isolation attempts. Supernatants from emulsion of affected organs, such as the lung, obtained at post-mortem or by biopsy, can also be used. Virus can rarely, if ever, be recovered from crusted lesions, the upper respiratory tract or blood.

With virus-containing specimens, the characteristic cytopathic effect of VZV will ultimately be produced (see Figure 2B.3). Occasionally, clinical isolates only show a restricted CPE on primary isolation and require 'blind passage' onto fresh fibroblast cultures before the classical CPE develops.

It is possible to increase the speed of isolation by centrifugation-enhanced infection ('shell-vial' culture). In addition, immunological staining techniques utilising monoclonal antibodies can be used to detect viral antigens in cell cultures within 24–48 h after inoculation, before a cytopathic effect becomes apparent (Figure 2B.12).

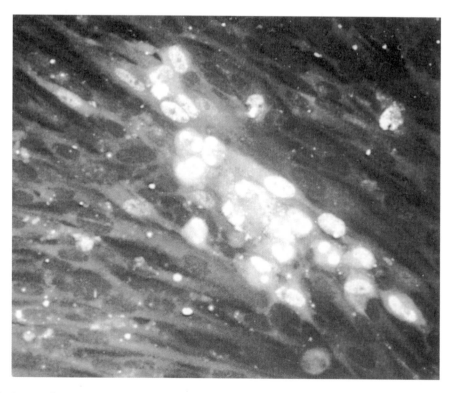

Figure 2B.12 Immunofluorescence staining of a cell sheet of human embryo lung fibroblast cells infected with VZV. An indirect method with monoclonal antibody was used

Identification of Isolates

Many laboratories do not undertake further identification of isolates because the cytopathic effect of VZV is so characteristic. This is not unreasonable provided that there is awareness that the early changes in the culture may not be too dissimilar from the early cytopathic effect of both HSV and CMV.

The definitive identification of an isolate has traditionally involved tedious methods in which a crude antigen preparation is prepared from the affected cell sheet and reacted with a standard VZV antiserum in serological tests such as the complement fixation test. However, staining with VZV monoclonal antibodies (Figure 2B.12) or detection of viral DNA, e.g. by PCR, now provide simple and rapid means of identification.

Serological Diagnosis

A number of different methods are currently available for the serological diagnosis of VZV infection, but perhaps the most important use of this technology is the determination of the immune status of patients prior to the administration of prophylaxis.

The serological diagnosis of varicella using acute and convalescent sera is easily accomplished but is less reliable for herpes zoster. Sera obtained in the early stages of varicella are either devoid of or contain only low levels of specific antibody, whereas these antibodies are present in high titre in sera taken in the convalescent period. Whilst significant rises in antibody titre in paired sera can be demonstrated in cases of zoster, this is generally only possible if the first serum is taken soon after the onset of the rash, for the reason that pre-eruption sera will always contain some specific antibodies and the titres rise very rapidly after onset. In cases of zoster it is not uncommon to see a drop in the pre-eruption antibody level around the time of onset, so that the antibodies may barely be detectable in sera taken within the first 2 days after appearance of the rash. Testing for avidity of IgG antibodies provides a means of distinguishing between primary and anamnestic antibody responses.

The sharing of antigens between VZV and HSV (discussed above) sometimes makes the interpretation of serological results difficult. It is quite frequently found that levels of antibodies to both VZV and HSV will have shown significant rises in association with a particular illness; however, without additional information, such as virus isolation data, it may be impossible to determine which of these viruses was responsible for the infection.

Complement Fixation (CF)

This test is now all but obsolete for the diagnosis of VZV as it is too slow, not sensitive enough for the determination of immune status and more susceptible to cross-reaction between VZV and HSV than other tests.

Immunofluorescence (IF)

This method provides a sensitive determination of serological status to VZV but has now been superseded by enzyme immunoassays in most diagnostic laboratories. In IF tests, serial dilutions of sera are reacted with VZV-infected culture cells, and any specific antibodies attaching to these cells are detected with a fluorescein-conjugated anti-human IgG serum. There are two variants of this basic test. One is the standard IF procedure, in which sera react with acetone-treated culture cells, and is therefore capable, at least theoretically, of detecting antibodies to all virus-induced proteins. This method is no more sensitive than most commercially produced EIAs. The fluorescent antibody to membrane antigen (FAMA) technique uses unfixed or glutaraldehyde-fixed cells and is designed to detect only antibodies to viral antigens that appear on the surface of infected cells. Consequently, FAMA should in theory specifically detect those antibodies that are concerned with protection. FAMA together with the GP ELISA (see below) are the most sensitive assays available for the detection of VZV antibody.

Enzyme Immunoassays (EIA)

In general, the commercially available assays for varicella zoster antibodies are less sensitive than FAMA. Currently commercial tests may fail to detect protective vaccine induced in up to 30% of immunised individuals. The gpELISA that has been developed by Merck and which uses VZV glycoproteins as antigen is as sensitive as FAMA. A level of 5 units or above in the gpELISA has been shown to correlate with protection against breakthrough infection following vaccination. The gpELISA is only available at one or two reference centres. Latex agglutination is more sensitive than most commercially available EIAs but can be difficult to interpret. Although assays of the indirect solid phase kind are used most frequently a competitive type assay has also been described, which should not, theoretically, be affected by cross-reacting antibodies to HSV.

Neutralisation

Theoretically, this should be the method of choice for determining VZV immune status, since it measures antibodies concerned with protection. However, current procedures are technically very difficult to carry out, due mainly to the difficulty of obtaining a consistent supply of challenge virus, since virus infectivity is so highly cell-associated. It is also an insensitive test. For these reasons, it has no role in routine diagnosis. Antibody detected by FAMA and gpELISA correlates well with neutralising antibody.

Detection of VZV-specific IgM Class Antibodies

This class of antibody can be detected using the indirect IF or immunoassay procedures, in which the labelled antibody used in the system is directed against human IgM class antibodies. Procedures in which the IgM antibodies are captured onto the solid phase (MACRIA or MACEIA) can also be used. VZV IgM may not initially be detectable in sera from patients with varicella but is present in 100% of convalescent sera, and it can be detected for about 3 months from the onset of the illness. Tests for specific VZV IgM are therefore useful for diagnosing recent infection when the only sera available are those taken late or after the termination of the illness.

Unfortunately it is not possible to use these tests to distinguish reliably between primary and recurrent VZV infection, since specific IgM antibodies are also induced in most cases of herpes zoster. In these patients, however, the amount of IgM antibody is generally lower than that found in varicella cases and is also of shorter duration (Figure 2B.13).

VZV IgM can also be detected in some congenital varicella infections.

MANAGEMENT

Varicella

Varicella in healthy individuals is generally mild and complications are rare. Where treatment is indicated, the drug of choice is aciclovir, a nucleoside analogue that blocks viral replication. VZV is less susceptible to aciclovir than is HSV and requires approximately a 10-fold higher concentration of the drug for effective inhibition. The inhibitory concentration (ID_{50}) of aciclovir for VZV in cell culture is usually in the range 2–$20\,\mu M$, depending on the cell type and virus strain used. It is possible to obtain adequate inhibitory concentrations in the blood if a dose of $10\,mg/kg$ (or $500\,mg/m^2$ for children aged <12 years) is given intravenously over a 1 h period every 8 h. This dosage maintains plasma levels in the range 10–$90\,\mu M$. Duration of treatment is normally 5–10 days, depending on the severity and progression of the disease, but a minimum of 7 days is recommended for immunocompromised patients and adults with visceral complications. Oral aciclovir is poorly absorbed and the recommended dose of $800\,mg$, 5 times a day, will give blood levels of 4–$8\,\mu M$, which are only just at the ID_{50} concentration for VZV. Studies in children (Dunkle et al., 1991) and adults (Wallace et al., 1992) have shown that antiviral treatment must be started within 24 h of the onset of rash to be effective. In immunocompetent patients, the duration of rash and fever are reduced by treatment with aciclovir but none of the studies have had the power to show whether treatment reduces the risk of complications.

The nucleoside analogues famciclovir (Famvir™) and valaciclovir (Valtrex™), are both better absorbed orally (50–70%) than aciclovir (20%) and metabolised to produce blood levels of active drug equivalent to intravenous aciclovir. However, these have not yet been licensed for the treatment of varicella.

A detailed review and recommendations for the management of varicella in different patient groups have recently been prepared by the UK Advisory Group on Chickenpox for the British Society for the Study of Infection (Carrington and McKendrick, 1998).

Varicella in Children

For the typical childhood case, no treatment is required apart, perhaps, from soothing lotions for itching and antibiotics if there is any question of secondary infection. There is some evidence that

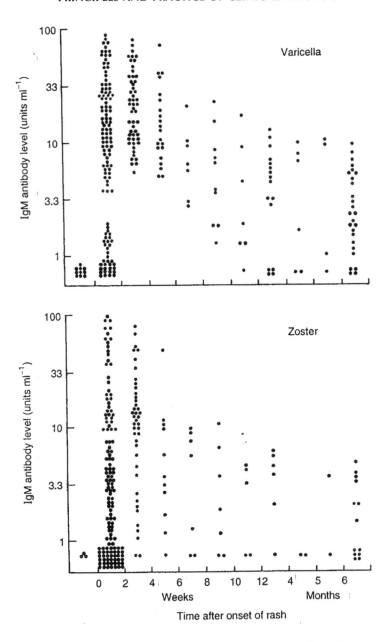

Figure 2B.13   Detection and duration of the specific IgM response in patients with varicella and herpes zoster. MACRIA was used for the antibody determinations

secondary cases of varicella acquired within a family are more severe and treatment of such cases, particularly adolescents, is advocated by some, although the current UK consensus is not to use oral aciclovir routinely in healthy children. Children on inhaled or intranasal steroids are not considered to be at special risk but such cases should be considered individually. No great pressure is usually exerted on parents even to quarantine affected children and, indeed, there are some who advocate that it is preferable for children to contract the disease to ensure that immunity is acquired at an early age.

Varicella in Adults

One in 200 adults will develop clinical pneumonitis and approximately 1 in 2000 will require intensive care. Those most at risk include smokers, patients with severe chronic lung conditions and those with more dense rashes. Aciclovir commenced within 24 h of the onset of symptoms does reduce viral shedding and new lesion formation by 0.5 days, and accelerates rash healing by 1–2 days (Wallace *et al.*, 1992). Pregnant women are also at increased risk of pneumonitis but aciclovir is currently not licensed for use in pregnancy. However, it has been used successfully in numerous pregnant women to treat serious VZV disease without ill-effect and there is no evidence to date that it is teratogenic, although it is known to cross the placenta and can be detected in the urine from infants of mothers who have been treated. It is not known at present whether treatment with aciclovir has any beneficial effect on foetal varicella syndrome. Current UK recommendations are therefore to treat varicella presenting within 24 h in otherwise healthy adult smokers, patients with chronic lung conditions (including adults on inhaled steroids) and pregnant women in the second half of pregnancy (Carrington and McKendrick, 1998). Adults presenting more than 24 h after the onset of the rash should have their clinical progress assessed. Those who appear to be deteriorating, e.g. with recurrent fever or progressive rash or who develop chest symptoms or signs, should be admitted for chest X-ray, gases and assessment as to whether they need intravenous aciclovir and antibiotics. For detailed algorithms for the management of varicella in adults, see Wilkins *et al.* (1998).

Varicella in the Immunocompromised Patient

Varicella in the immunocompromised can be a serious, even fatal, illness and consequently its management in these patients is different from that in a previously healthy individual. Immunocompromised patients, including those on systemic steroids (including for up to 3 months previously), should be aware of their immune status and, where possible, i.e in all except those with lymphoreticular malignancies, immunised with live attenuated Oka vaccine. Where this is not possible, patients should be counselled against contact with patients with varicella or zoster as well as being advised to seek medical help immediately if contact occurs. Where the patient has no immunity and significant exposure has occurred, measures should be taken to prevent or attenuate the infection (see below). Significant exposure has been defined arbitrarily by the American Academy of Paediatrics and by the UK Joint Committee on Vaccination and Immunisation. Broadly, there is consensus that 'significant contact' constitutes living in the same house as a case of zoster or chickenpox, indoor contact with a case of zoster or chickenpox for a period of time (15 min or more in the UK) and face-to-face contact with a case of chickenpox.

Aciclovir has been shown to be effective in preventing varicella in the immunocompetent if given between 7 and 9 days post-exposure. Post-exposure aciclovir prophylaxis is not effective if given earlier than 7 days, presumably because it interferes with the primary viraemic phase, which primes the specific T cell responses.

Herpes Zoster

The main aims of therapy in acute herpes zoster occurring in a previously healthy individual are to heal the rash rapidly, alleviate acute pain, prevent postherpetic neuralgia and reduce the risks of ophthalmic and neurological complications.

Antiviral Drugs

Several drugs are currently licensed for use in the UK for treatment of acute shingles, including topical idoxuridine, aciclovir, famciclovir and valaciclovir. Idoxuridine was the first antiviral drug to be used for this purpose. It is too toxic to be used systemically but can be administered topically as a 40% suspension in dimethyl sulphoxide. This form of treatment is cumbersome and has now been replaced by systemic or oral treatment with the newer antiviral compounds.

Patients given high-dose aciclovir (800 mg orally, five times/day) for acute shingles have been shown, in placebo-controlled studies, to have faster resolution of the rash (by up to 2 days), have less acute pain, reduced viral shedding (by 1–3 days) and fewer ophthalmic complications. Several studies have also shown a reduction in the incidence, severity and duration of persistent ZAP in those most at risk, i.e. over the age of 50 years, when aciclovir is given within 72 h of the onset of rash. Valaciclovir (a pro-drug of aciclovir) and famciclovir (a pro-drug of penciclovir) give higher blood levels of the active drug, and thus allow easier treatment regimens on account of their improved oral bioavailability. In addition, penciclovir and its derivative, famciclovir, have a significantly longer intracellular half-life compared to aciclovir. A dosing schedule of famciclovir of 250 mg three times/day or valaciclovir 1000 mg t.d.s. are as effective as high-dose aciclovir for treatment of zoster. The newer pro-drugs also have the potential to prove more effective than aciclovir in reducing the severity and duration of ZAP (Beutner et al., 1995; Cirelli et al., 1996). Valaciclovir has also been shown to have an effect if given later than 72 h after the onset of rash.

Other new drugs that have been developed for the treatment of zoster include Sorivudine (BVaraU) and Brivudin (BVDU). Both these agents are particularly active against VZV when taken orally, and result in accelerated rash healing. Brivudin has been licensed in Germany. Furthermore, when administered in combination with 5-fluorouracil, Sorivudine has caused the deaths of a number of patients. Brivudin is also contraindicated in this situation.

Adjunctive Treatment

Oral prednisolone in addition to aciclovir slightly reduces acute symptoms but does not protect against prolonged ZAP more than aciclovir alone. Oral steroids are generally not used, as the risks are felt to outweigh the benefits. A retrospective case control study showed that amitriptyline given acutely reduced the severity and duration of pain. Other treatments, such as sympathetic nerve blocks, have been reported anecdotally to reduce pain and require proper trials to assess adequately.

Treatment of Established ZAP

During the acute attack of zoster, paracetamol, with or without mild opiate analgesics, is recommended. Non-steroidal analgesics are less effective. Low-dose tricyclic antidepressants such as amitriptyline, the dose of which is titrated against side-effects and pain relief, can also be given for 4–8 weeks, particularly if sleep loss is a problem. The anticonvulsant gabapentin has also been shown to be effective in patients with pain of 3 months duration or more. Other recommendations for pain relief include ice packs, topical local anaesthetic (e.g. Lidocaine patches), capsaicin and, if necessary, stronger opiates. Patients with intractable pain should be referred for specialist pain management advice.

Ophthalmic Zoster

Management of patients with ophthalmic zoster should include topical aciclovir applied to the eye and oral aciclovir (800 mg five times/day), whatever the patient's age. Treatment should, however, be started as soon as possible to be effective and preferably within 72 h of onset. It is currently not known how effective aciclovir or the newer antivirals are in treating chronic complications such as anterior uveitis and stromal keratitis. Early referral of patients with ophthalmic zoster to an ophthalmologist is desirable and topical steroids should in no case be administered without specialist consultation.

Herpes Zoster in Immunocompromised Patients

The more severe, and particularly the disseminated, forms of herpes zoster are seen in those who are immunocompromised and may be life- or sight-threatening. Patients at high risk should be educated to recognise shingles and to seek medical advice early. Highly immunocompromised patients should initially receive intravenous aciclovir followed by oral aciclovir if necessary. Treatment should be continued until the lesions crust, approximately 5–7 days later. Less severely immunocompromised patients with localised shingles can be given oral aciclovir or one of the newer pro-drugs.

Antiviral Drug Resistance

VZV resistance to aciclovir has been described in immunocompromised patients, particularly those infected with HIV. There is currently no evidence that such resistant virus strains are transmissible but they can present a considerable challenge to treatment and are therefore of much concern. Almost all the resistant strains that have been characterised to date have had reduced TK function as a result of mutations in the thymidine kinase gene (Talarico et al., 1993), although some DNA polymerase mutants have also been found (Kamiyama et al., 2001). Mutations in the TK gene have been identified as either (a) deletions or point mutations leading to a truncated protein, or (b) single point mutations leading to amino acid substitutions. Mutations involved in resistance to aciclovir have been demonstrated in different positions in the gene and are not only restricted to the ATP or nucleotide binding sites on the protein. Some aciclovir-resistant strains have also been shown to be cross-resistant to other TK-dependent drugs, including penciclovir and Sorivudine. However, such resistant strains are generally found to be sensitive to foscarnet, a broad-spectrum antiviral drug which directly inhibits viral DNA polymerase and thus provides an alternative treatment. AIDS patients with aciclovir-resistant VZV infections have been successfully treated with foscarnet (40 mg/kg every 8 h in a 1 h infusion over 10 days) in an open study (Safrin *et al.*, 1991) but the optimal dose and duration of treatment are not yet defined.

PREVENTION

Prevention of VZV disease is important in those who are at risk of contracting the severe forms of the disease. An increase in adult susceptibility to varicella (see section on Epidemiology, above) also has serious implications for hospital infection control, since medical staff without immunity may become infected following contact with zoster patients and can, sometimes with disastrous consequences, transmit the infection to patients who are immunocompromised.

Many immunocompromised patients will cope normally with varicella, but the possibility of administering varicella zoster immune globulin (VZIG) and/or antiviral drugs prophylactically to these patients should always be considered if they come in contact with VZV. At the moment there is, unfortunately, no means of preventing herpes zoster.

Antiviral Drugs

Acyclovir is now routinely used for prophylaxis against HSV infections in immuncompromised patients and may also provide some benefit against VZV. However, studies have not yet been performed to demonstrate the efficacy of such a strategy. Oral aciclovir has been shown to prevent or modify varicella in young immunocompetent household contacts given a 7 day course (40 mg/kg in divided doses), beginning 7–9 days after the contact with the index case, i.e. during the presumed phase of secondary viraemia. Administration within 7 days following contact, i.e. during primary viraemia, was not as effective, possibly because early priming of T cells is reduced.

Passive Immunisation

Human immunoglobulin preparations with high titres of antibody to VZV are an established means of attempting to prevent varicella. Such preparations were originally prepared by cold ethanol precipitation from the blood of patients recovering from shingles and were consequently designated 'zoster immuno-globulin' (ZIG). Current preparations are obtained by processing preselected sera from blood donors with high titres of antibody to VZV. These preparations are referred to as 'varicella zoster immune globulin' (VZIG) or 'human anti-varicella zoster immuno-globulin'. VZIG preparations are frequently in short supply but antibody concentrations in the blood as high as those with VZIG have been obtained with intravenous normal human immunoglobulin (iv-NHIG) preparations and these may be used empirically as an alternative when VZIG is not available. NHIG given intramuscularly has been shown not to be effective and plays no role in the prevention of varicella.

VZIG is recommended for any susceptible 'at-risk' individual (Table 2B.4) who has *significant* exposure to varicella or herpes zoster. It should be administered as soon as possible after contact, preferably within 96 h, although some studies have shown VZIG to have a beneficial effect when given up to 10 days after contact. The immune status of the patient should be assessed by testing for specific antibodies in the serum before administration of VZIG whenever possible. Since tests with the appropriate sensitivity (see section on Diagnosis, above) are generally only available in specialist laboratories, the administration of VZIG

Table 2B.4 Underlying or associated conditions which place patients at risk of contracting the severe forms of varicella

Leukaemias, Hodgkin's disease and other neoplasms of the lymphoreticular system, whether or not treatment is being given

Other cancers that are being treated with cytotoxic drugs or other regimes that are immunosuppressive

Primary immunodeficiency syndromes

Bone marrow transplant recipients, irrespective of their own or the donors' VZV status

Diseases requiring systemic steroids at a dosage equivalent to at least 2 mg prednisone/kg/day

Susceptible pregnant women in close contact with VZV

Newborn infants of women who contracted varicella ≤ 7 days before or after delivery

Premature infants whose mothers have no history of varicella or any infant whose birth weight was < 1000 g

should not be delayed past 7 days after the initial contact while waiting for the test result. A convincing history of varicella or zoster is a reasonably reliable indicator of immunity and usually obviates the need to administer prophylactic agents. Nevertheless, it is recommended that an antibody test is performed to confirm the immune status in immunocompromised patients, even if a past history of VZV infection is given. The true efficacy of VZIG has not been established in well-controlled trials and differences in the results of different studies may reflect different potencies of the preparations used. It is known that VZIG gives incomplete protection against infection. In a study carried out in the UK it was shown that of 27 seronegative children who were in contact at home, 18 (67%) became infected—14 (52%) with symptoms—in spite of receiving VZIG. Therefore, the rationale for administering VZIG to those at risk is not so much to prevent infection but to prevent the serious forms of the disease with visceral involvement. There are numerous studies, based on case series, showing the beneficial effects of VZIG in reducing morbidity and mortality compared to historic controls or untreated patients. Unfortunately, there are also reports of correctly administered VZIG failing to prevent fatal varicella in immunocompromised patients. Feldman and Lott (1987) reviewed the impact of varicella in 280 children with cancer and the effectiveness of various forms of management. In their study group, passive immunization significantly reduced both the incidence and mortality of pneumonitis compared to untreated children. Even so, pneumonitis developed in 11% of children who received VZIG, requiring intensive additional antiviral chemotherapy.

It is important, particularly in a hospital environment, to be aware of the shortcomings of VZIG and to be alert to the possibility that an inoculated patient might develop varicella and become a source of infection for others.

It is also recommended that VZIG be given to susceptible pregnant women in close contact with VZV infection at any stage of the pregnancy, in the hope that it will reduce the risk of transmission of infection to the foetus and also to ameliorate any potentially serious VZV disease which can occur in pregnant women. Maternal varicella can still occur despite VZIG prophylaxis but a large prospective study has shown that even in such cases, the risk of foetal infection during the first 20 weeks of pregnancy, and subsequent foetal damage, may be reduced (Enders et al., 1994). Should a woman contract varicella perinatally, it is important to administer VZIG to the newborn baby (Table 2B.4).

The recommended dosages for VZIG preparations available in the UK are as follows: 0–5 years, 250 mg; 6–10 years, 500 mg; 11–14 years, 750 mg; and 15 years or more, 1000 mg. A second dose can be given after 3 weeks if necessary.

Active Immunisation

Although individual cases of varicella may be prevented or modified by VZIG or with antiviral drugs, control of varicella in the community can only be achieved by widespread vaccination. Active immunisation also has the advantage in individual 'at-risk' patients by offering long-term protection. Varicella vaccines based on the attenuated Oka strain of VZV have been available since 1974, when it was first developed in Japan (Takahashi et al., 1974). The original vaccine was derived from VZV isolated from vesicles of a 3 year-old child with typical varicella and was attenuated by serial passage in guinea-pig cells and human embryo lung cells. Biologically, vOka grows less well than wild-type virus at 37°C and better at 33°C. Replication in the SCID hu mouse epithelial cells is also reduced. Comparison of the sequence of the vaccine Oka strain and wild-type strains, including parental Oka, has identified approximately 30 amino acid changes unique to vOka. Eight of these are located in the IE 62 protein and reduce its ability to transactivate the expression of early VZV proteins (Gomi et al., 2002).

The vaccine is clinically attenuated, as evidenced by the less severe rash, the rarity of secondary transmission (three cases in 15 million doses given) and the lower rates of reactivation (2% vs. 15% following wild-type infection in leukaemic children) (reviewed in Breuer 2002a). Clinical studies in Japan, the USA and Europe have shown the vaccine to be effective; 95% of healthy children seroconvert after one dose of the vaccine, while leukaemic children immunised during maintenance therapy, and healthy adults, require two doses to achieve 90% seroconversion. Clinical protection against subsequent (breakthrough) varicella appears to be good, although estimates of protection within the first 10 years vary between 65% and 97%, depending on the potency of the vaccine preparation used. In a study of 4042 healthy children and adolescents, protection appeared to correlate with the titre of VZV-specific antibody at 6 weeks post-vaccination. However, breakthrough infections are higher in adults and immunosuppressed patients. Antibody levels decline with time but long-term follow-up studies spanning 20 years in Japan and 10 years in the USA have shown that over 90% of vaccinated children retain protective immunity. Fewer than 5% of recipients develop a mild varicella-like rash after vaccination and fever is rare. Genotyping of virus shows that vaccine-related rashes occurring within the first 2 weeks of immunisation are wild-type in origin, while those occurring after 2 weeks are vaccine-related. No data are available for the GSK vaccine. In vaccinated leukaemic children, the incidence of adverse events in the first 6 weeks after immunisation is higher than in healthy children, and this, coupled with a reluctance to interrupt chemotherapy for immunisation, has led to other approaches to preventing serious varicella in immunosuppressed children. To this end, the vaccine has been licensed for the immunisation of seronegative household contacts of children suffering with leukaemia and cancer.

Since 1995 the Oka vaccine has been given to all children in the USA at age 12–15 months. This has resulted in a fall in circulating varicella and a reduction in associated hospitalisations (Seward et al., 2002). Other countries have licensed the vaccine for use in adults and in children undergoing treatment for leukaemia. In the UK, considerable doubts about the economic benefits of preventing varicella in healthy children remain, especially if the costs of time lost from work by parents caring for sick children are not considered in the analysis (reviewed in Breuer, 2002b). Moreover, modelling of the consequences of vaccination against VZV have shown that eradication of circulating wild-type chickenpox would be likely to lead to an upsurge in the incidence of zoster. These data were based on hypothesis, but more recently concrete evidence for the affect of contact with circulating varicella in boosting immunity to the VZV virus and indirectly preventing its reactivation to cause zoster has emerged. Two studies have independently shown that contact with children, a surrogate for contact with varicella, is inversely related to the incidence of zoster (Brisson et al., 2002; Thomas et al., 2002). Such data, when included in economic models, severely prejudice the likelihood of mass vaccination against varicella alone being medically or economically beneficial. Notwithstanding the vaccine has recently been licensed in the UK for use by seronegative health care workers and seronegative household contacts of immunosuppressed children.

The vaccine is potentially useful for post-exposure prophylaxis and is licensed for this in the USA. Antibody responses usually do not appear until 3–5 weeks after vaccination, but cell-mediated immune responses develop within 4 days after vaccination in approximately 50% of recipients and have been shown in controlled trials to confer protection after contact.

There is also considerable interest in the possibility of vaccinating seropositive adults with the aim of preventing zoster. This arises from the observation that the vaccine can effectively boost both antibody levels and cell-mediated immunity in elderly patients (Sperber et al., 1992). A double-blind prospective case control study of vaccine in subjects aged over 60 years is under way in the USA and the results will be available in the next couple of years.

REFERENCES

Adams SG, Dohner DE and Gelb LD (1989) Restriction fragment differences between the genomes of the Oka varicella vaccine virus and American wild-type varicella-zoster virus. J Med Virol, 29(1), 38–45.

Arvin AM, Sharp M, Smith S et al. (1991) Equivalent recognition of a varicella-zoster virus immediate early protein (IE62) and glycoprotein 1 by cytotoxic T lymphocytes of either CD4 or CD8 phenotype. J Immunol, 146(1), 257–264.

Barrett-Muir W, Nichols RA and Breuer J (2002) Phylogenetic analysis of varicella zoster virus; evidence of intercontinental spread of genotypes and recombination. J Virol, 76(4), 1971–1979.

Beutner KR, Friedman DJ, Forszpaniak C et al. (1995) Valaciclovir compared with acyclovir for improved therapy for herpes zoster in immunocompetent adults. Antimicrob Agents Chemother, 39(7), 1546–1553.

Breuer J, Leedham-Green M and Scott FT (2001) Pathogenesis of postherpetic neuralgia should be determined. Br Med J, 322(7290), 860.

Breuer J (2002a) Live attenuated vaccine for the prevention of varicella-zoster virus infection: does it work, is it safe and does really need it in the UK? Rev Med Microbiol, (in press).

Breuer J (2002b) Monitoring the virus after varicella zoster infection: is there a need and what might be the affect of vaccination. Commun Dis Rep, (in press).

Brisson M, Gay NJ, Edmunds WJ and Andrews NJ (2002) Exposure to varicella boosts immunity to herpes zoster; implications for mass vaccination against chickenpox. Vaccine, 20(19–20), 2500–2507.

Carrington D and McKendrick MW (1998) Varicella Supplement 1998 and consensus guidelines for management. J Infect, 36(suppl 1), 1–83.

CDC (1996) Prevention of varicella: recommendation of the Advisory Committee on Immunization Practices (ACIP). MMWR (p 1–6).

Choo PW, Donahue JG, Manson JE and Platt R (1995) The epidemiology of varicella and its complications. J Infect Dis, 172(3), 706–712.

Cirelli R, Herne K, McCrary M et al. (1996) Famciclovir: review of clinical efficacy and safety. Antiviral Res, 29(2–3), 141–151.

Connelly B, Stanberry LR and Bernstein DI (1993) Detection of varicella zoster DNA in nasopharyngeal secretions of immune household contacts. *J Infect Dis*, **168**(5), 1253–1255.

Culbertson WW, Blumenkranz MS, Pepose JS *et al.* (1986) Varicella-zoster virus is a cause of the acute retinal necrosis syndrome. *Ophthalmology*, **93**(5), 559–569.

Davison AJ (1991) Varicella-zoster virus. The Fourteenth Fleming Lecture. *J Gen Virol*, **72**(3), 475–486.

Davison AJ and McGeoch DJ (1986) Evolutionary comparisons of the S segments in the genomes of herpes simplex virus type 1 and varicella-zoster virus. *J Gen Virol*, **67**(4), 597–611.

Dunkle LM, Arvin AM, Whitley RJ *et al.* (1991) A controlled trial of acyclovir for chickenpox in normal children. *N Engl J Med*, **325**(22), 1539–1544.

Enders G, Miller E, Cradock-Watson JE *et al.* (1994) Consequences of chickenpox and herpes zoster in pregnancy; a prospective study of 1739 cases. *Lancet*, **343**(8912), 1548–1551.

Fairley CK and Miller E (1996) Varicella-zoster virus epidemiology—a changing scene? *J Infect Dis*, **174**(suppl 3), S314–S319.

Feldmann S and Lott L (1987) Varicella in children with cancer: impact of antiviral therapy and prophylaxis. *Pediatrics*, **80**, 465–472.

Furuta Y, Ohtani F, Sawa H *et al.* (2001) Quantitation of varicella-zoster virus DNA in patients with Ramsay–Hunt syndrome and zoster sine herpete. *J Clin Microbiol*, **39**(8), 2856–2859.

Furuta Y, Takasu T, Suzuki S *et al.* (1997) Detection of latent varicella-zoster virus infection in human vestibular and spiral ganglia. *J Med Virol*, **51**(3), 214–216.

Gershon AA, La Russa P, Steinberg S *et al.* (1996) The protective effect of immunologic boosting against zoster; an analysis of leukaemic children who were vaccinated against chickenpox. *J Infect Dis*, **173**(2), 450–453.

Gilden DH, Wright R, Schneck SA *et al.* (1994) Zoster sine herpete, a clinical variant. *Ann Neurol*, **35**(5), 530–533.

Gnann JW Jr, Crumpacker CS, Lalezari JP *et al.* (1998) Sorivudine versus acyclovir for treatment of dermatomal herpes zoster in human immunodeficiency virus-infected patients: results from a randomized, controlled clinical trial. Collaborative Antiviral Study Group/AIDS Clinical Trials Group, Herpes Zoster Study Group. *Antimicrob Agents Chemother*, **42**(5), 1139–1145.

Gomi Y, Sunamachi H, Mori Y *et al.* (2002) Comparison of the complete DNA sequences of the Oka varicella vaccine and its parental virus. *J Virol*, **76**(22), 11447–11459.

Grose C (1981) Variation on a theme by Fenner: the pathogenesis of chicken pox. *Pediatrics*, **68**(5), 735–737.

Grose C (1987) Varicella-zoster virus: pathogenesis of the human disease, the virus and viral replication, and the major viral glycoproteins and proteins. In *Natural History of Varicella-Zoster Virus* (ed. RW Hyman), Chapter 1. CRC Press, Boca Raton, FL.

Hall S *et al.* (2002) Second varicella infections: are they more common than previously thought? *Pediatrics*, **109**(6), 1068–1073.

Hanshaw JB, Dudgeon JA and Marshall WC (1985) Varicella-zoster infections. In *Viral Diseases of the Fetus and Newborn* (p 161). W.B. Saunders, Philadelphia.

Harper DR *et al.* (1988) Serological responses in varicella and zoster assayed by immunoblotting. *J Med Virol* **25**(4): 387–98.

Harper DR, Sanders EA and Ashcroft MA (1995) Varicella-zoster virus assembly protein p32/p36 is present in DNA-containing as well as immature capsids. *J Med Virol*, **46**(2), 144–147.

Hawrami K, Harper D and Breuer J (1996) Typing of varicella zoster virus by amplification of DNA polymorphisms. *J Virol Methods*, **57**(2), 169–174.

Izurieta HS, Strebel PM and Blake PA (1997) Postlicensure effectiveness of varicella vaccine during an outbreak in a child care center. *J Am Med Assoc*, **278**(18), 1495–1499.

Kamiyama T, Kurokawa M and Shiraki K (2001) Characterization of the DNA polymerase gene of varicella-zoster viruses resistant to acyclovir. *J Gen Virol*, **82**(11), 2761–2765.

Kennedy PG, Grinfeld E and Gow JW (1998) Latent varicella-zoster virus is located predominantly in neurones in human trigeminal ganglia. *Proc Natl Acad Sci USA*, **95**(8), 4658–4662.

Mahalingam R, Wellish M, Cohrs R *et al.* (1996) Expression of protein encoded by varicella-zoster virus open reading frame 63 in latently infected human ganglionic neurones. *Proc Natl Acad Sci USA*, **93**(5), 2122–2124.

Marsh RJ (1976) Ophthalmic herpes zoster. *Br J Hosp Med*, **15**, 609–618.

Martin KA, Junker AK, Thomas EE *et al.* (1994) Occurrence of chickenpox during pregnancy in women seropositive for varicella-zoster virus. *J Infec Dis*, **170**(4), 991–995.

Moffat J, Ito H, Sommer M *et al.* (2002) Glycoprotein I of varicella-zoster virus is required for viral replication in skin and T cells. *J Virol*, **76**(16), 8468–8471.

Nikkels AF, Rentier B and Pierard GE (1997) Chronic varicella-zoster virus skin lesions in patients with human immunodeficiency virus are related to decreased expression of gE and gB. *J Infect Dis*, **176**(1), 261–264.

Ooi PL, Goh KT, Doraisingham S and Ling AE (1992) Prevalence of varicella-zoster virus infection in Singapore. *SE Asian J Trop Med Publ Health*, **23**(1), 22–25.

Pastusak AL, Levy M, Schick B *et al.* (1994) Outcome after maternal varicella infection in the first 20 weeks of pregnancy. *N Engl J Med*, **330**(13), 901–905.

Pumphrey CY and Gray WL (1995) DNA sequence of the simian varicella virus (SVV) gH gene and analysis of the SVV and varicella-zoster gH transcripts. *Virus Res*, **38**(1), 55–70.

Quinlivan M, Hawrami K, Barrett-Muir W *et al.* (2002) The molecular epidemiology of varicella zoster virus: evidence for geographical segregation. *J Infect Dis*, **186**(7), 888–894.

Rentier B, Piette J, Baudoux L *et al.* (1996) Lessons to be learnt from varicella-zoster virus. *Vet Microbiol*, **53**(1–2), 55–66.

Rowbotham MC and Fields HL (1996) The relationship of pain, allodynia and thermal sensation in post-herpetic neuralgia. *Brain*, **119**(2), 347–354.

Safrin S, Berger TG, Gilson I *et al.* (1991) Foscarnet therapy in five patients with AIDS and aciclovir-resistant varicella-zoster virus infection. *Ann Intern Med*, **115**(1), 19–21.

Scott FT, Leedham-Green ME, Barrett-Muir W *et al.* (2002) Study of shingles and the development of postherpetic neuralgia in East London. *J Med Virol* (in press).

Seward JF *et al.* (2002) Varicella disease after introduction of varicella vaccine in the United States, 1995–2000. *JAMA*, **287**(5), 606–611.

Sperber SJ, Smith BV and Hayden FG (1992) Serologic response and reactogenicity to booster immunization of healthy seropositive adults with live or inactivated varicella vaccine. *Antiviral Res*, **17**(3), 213–222.

Takada M, Suzutani T, Yoshida I *et al.* (1995) Identification of varicella-zoster virus strains by PCR analysis of three repeat elements and a *Pst*I-site-less region. *J Clin Microb*, **33**(3), 658–660.

Takahashi M, Otsuka T, Okumo Y *et al.* (1974) Live vaccine used to prevent the spread of varicella in children in hospital. *Lancet*, **2**(7892), 1288–1290.

Talarico CL, Phelps WC and Biron KK (1993) Analysis of the thymidine kinase genes from acyclovir-resistant mutants of varicella-zoster virus isolated from patients with AIDS. *J Virol*, **67**(2), 1024–1033.

Thomas SL, Wheeler JG and Hall AJ (2002) Contacts with varicella or with children and protection against herpes zoster in adults: a case-control study. *Lancet*, **31**(360; 9334), 678–682.

Wallace MR, Bowler WA, Murray NB *et al.* (1992) Treatment of adult varicella with oral acyclovir. A randomized, placebo-controlled trial. *Ann Intern Med*, **117**(5), 358–363.

Weller TH, Witton HM and Bell EJ (1958) The etiological agents of varicella and herpes zoster. Isolation, propagation and cultural characteristics *in vitro*. *J Exp Med*, **108**, 843–863.

Wilkins EG, Leen CL, McKendrick MW and Carrington D (1998) Management of chickenpox in the adult. A review prepared for the UK Advisory Group on Chickenpox on behalf of the British Society for the Study of Infection. *J Infect*, **36**(suppl 1), 49–58.

Wilson A, Sharp M, Koropchak CM *et al.* (1992) Subclinical varicella-zoster virus viremia, herpes zoster, and T lymphocyte immunity to varicella-zoster viral antigens after bone marrow transplantation. *J Infec Dis*, **165**(1), 119–126.

Zhu Z, Gershon MD, Ambron R *et al.* (1995) Infection of cells by varicella-zoster virus: inhibition of viral entry by mannose-6-phosphate and heparin. *Proc Natl Acad USA*, **92**(8), 3546–3550.

Cytomegalovirus

Paul D. Griffiths

Royal Free and University College Medical School, London, UK

INTRODUCTION

Cytomegalovirus (CMV) infections were first described in the early years of the twentieth century when the typical 'owl's eye' intranuclear inclusions were found by histopathologists in tissues from foetuses stillborn following cytomegalic inclusion disease. These strange inclusions were thought to result from a protozoan infection and, in 1910, one group of workers even proposed the name *Entamoeba mortinatalium* for the supposed agent. In the 1920s, the similarity of the inclusions to those produced by varicella were noted and the guinea-pig form of CMV was transmitted by salivary gland extracts passed through a Berkefeld N filter. Despite these two pieces of evidence suggesting a viral aetiology, reports were still occurring in the late 1940s attributing the disease to a strange protozoan infection. In 1956, three laboratories simultaneously isolated CMV, having successfully developed cell culture technology, so that the true nature of the infectious agent was apparent. One of these three investigators, Weller, gave the virus its name from the effects produced in cell culture, so CMV is named after its cytopathic effect.

THE VIRUS

Morphology

Electron micrographs of cytomegalovirus reveal a typical herpesvirus appearance (Figure 2C.1). The central DNA-containing core is surrounded by a capsid composed of 162 capsomeres, each of which is a hollow hexagon in cross-section. The capsid is in turn surrounded by a poorly demarcated area, the tegument, which is itself surrounded by a loosely applied envelope.

When CMV is propagated in cell cultures, two additional morphological forms are produced from the virus-specific proteins and envelope. The first is termed a 'dense body' and appears as a large amorphous structure without nucleocapsid or DNA. The second has been termed a 'non-infectious enveloped particle' and consists of an empty capsid surrounded by a lipid envelope.

Nucleic Acid

CMV strain AD 169 contains 235 kb double-stranded DNA. The structure of the DNA is similar to that of herpes simplex virus (HSV) in that long and short unique sequences are bounded by terminally repetitive segments. Each long and short sequence can be orientated in one of two directions so that four DNA isomers are produced by cells in culture. The whole genome of strain AD169 has been sequenced (Chee *et al.*, 1990). The genes are numbered according to their relative positions on one of these four isomers, termed the prototype configuration. By international agreement, the proteins they encode are designated by *p* (for protein); *gp* (glycoprotein); or *pp* (phosphoprotein), followed by the gene number. This formal terminology may then be followed by a trivial name, e.g. *gpUL75* (*gH*) is glycoprotein H, the product of gene number 75 in the unique long region.

Principles and Practice of Clinical Virology, Fifth Edition. Edited by A. J. Zuckerman, J. E. Banatvala, J. R. Pattison, P. D. Griffiths and B. D. Schoub
© 2004 John Wiley & Sons Ltd ISBN 0 470 84338 1

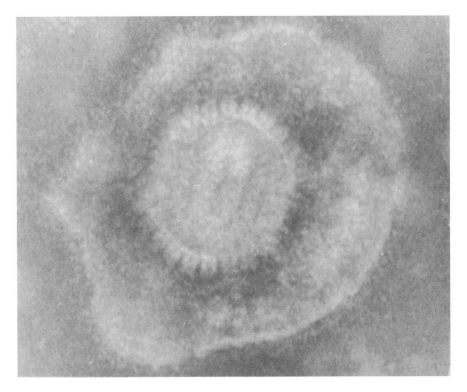

Figure 2C.1   The typical electron microscope appearance of cytomegalovirus. Photograph kindly prepared by Mr J. A. Bishop

Productively infected cells produce linear genomes from concatameric precursors. Cleavage is accomplished by an endonuclease (terminase) coincident with packaging. *pUL89* is part of this complex, and there are thus similarities between the cleavage/packaging of herpesvirus DNA and that of bacteriophage T4, supported by sequence conservation of the terminase genes. The physical state of the CMV genome during latency in myeloid precursors is episomal.

Some areas of the genome are homologous with regions of human chromosomal DNA, which has practical importance for the selection of CMV DNA probes. Distinct transforming regions of DNA have been identified. One maps to a previously unrecognised open reading frame, UL111A, which is expressed in transformed cells (reviewed in Doniger *et al.*, 1999). The UL111A protein binds *p53* and is spliced to two other exons within UL111A to form another protein, which binds to the cellular IL-10 receptor. It is not known whether the transformation is linked to the expression of the IL-10 homologue (Kotenko *et al.*, 2000). In addition, CMV induces specific breaks in chromosome 1 when infection occurs during the S phase of the cell cycle (reviewed by Fortunato and Spector, 2002). While such experiments are interesting, it must be emphasised that, at present, there is no evidence that CMV is naturally oncogenic.

The DNA can be digested with restriction endonucleases so that, following gel electrophoresis, oligonucleotide patterns characteristic of distinct CMV strains are produced. This technique cannot prove that two strains are identical but if strains fail to show different patterns after digestion with at least two restriction endonucleases then it is very likely that they are identical (Huang *et al.*, 1980). Use of restriction enzyme analysis can provide useful epidemiological information, but there is no consistent evidence to suggest that any one strain is associated with any particular type of clinical presentation.

Genetic changes also occur in the genome without acquisition of new cleavage sites for commonly used restriction enzymes. The polymerase chain reaction (PCR) followed by sequencing can be used to explore genetic variation at the fine molecular level for particular regions of interest, e.g. where viral variants acquire resistance to antiviral drugs.

Control of Genome Expression

Expression of the CMV genome is controlled by a cascade synthesis of proteins. The first proteins to be synthesised (α or immediate-early) are required for the transcription of the messenger RNA (mRNA) for the second group of proteins (β or early). The early proteins allow DNA replication to proceed and this is followed by the appearance of the last proteins (γ or late). This cascade sequence is depicted in Figure 2C.2, which also shows the stages at which metabolic inhibitors can be employed to manipulate the cascade. If cell cultures are prepared and infected with CMV in the presence of an inhibitor of protein synthesis, then relatively large concentrations of α-mRNA build up behind the metabolic block. When this block is released by refeeding the cultures, synthesis of α-proteins will occur within minutes. To prevent α-proteins inducing β-mRNA and then β-proteins, inhibitors of transcription should be incorporated into the refeeding medium. To allow β-protein expression without inducing γ-proteins, the cultures can be refed with an inhibitor of DNA synthesis. Finally, fresh medium without added inhibitors can be used to induce the cells to produce γ-proteins. It should be emphasised that this cascade synthesis dictates that at each time after infection the appropriate proteins, together with their preceding proteins, are present in the infected cells. It is therefore not possible to produce cells containing only β-proteins or only γ-proteins by

means of infection; to achieve this, individual genes must be cloned and expressed separately.

Note that some γ-genes are transcribed at early times but are only translated after DNA replication has occurred. These are sometimes termed 'leaky-late' genes to differentiate them from true late genes, which are only transcribed after DNA replication. Some latency-associated transcripts which map in both sense and antisense orientation to the major immediate-early region of CMV have been described (Kondo *et al.*, 1996). Some of these have unique expression at immediate-early and late times and so have been classified as λ-genes. The term 'virion RNAs' refers to transcripts packaged within the virus which are delivered to an uninfected cell (Bresnahan and Shenk, 2000). It remains to be proven that such RNAs are specifically packaged and play the postulated role of producing viral proteins before the onset of genomic transcription.

The mechanism(s) which control genome expression are not fully understood. Certainly, there is no evidence for a canonical sequence upstream of β-genes which could be activated directly by α-proteins. This suggests that α-proteins mediate their effects through activation of endogenous transcription factors. Cellular transcription factors such as SP1 and NF-κB have been implicated so far.

Some control of expression is also exerted at the translational level. The DNA polymerase (*pUL54*) has an untranslated leader region which suppresses trans-

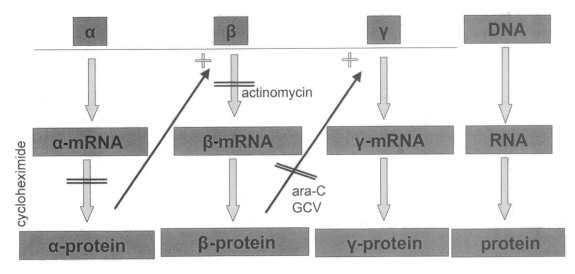

Figure 2C.2 Cascade genome expression of herpesviruses. Genes labelled α (immediate-early), β (early) or γ (late) are transcribed into messenger RNA and then translated into proteins. Inhibitors of protein synthesis (cycloheximide), transcription (actinomycin-D) or DNA replication [cytosine arabinoside (ara-C) or ganciclovir (GCV)] can be used to interrupt genome expression, as discussed in the text

lation. Furthermore, the presence of upstream AUG codons, which, according to the ribosome scanning hypothesis, allow production of short peptides in preference to the authentic proteins, appears to restrict early expression of some transcribed leaky-late mRNA.

Proteins

The CMV genome is sufficiently large to encode over 200 proteins of average size, and sequencing of one strain has identified 204 predicted open reading frames (Chee *et al.*, 1990). Of these, approximately 189 may be unique proteins, since others are found in duplicate in the repeat regions of the genome.

One expression unit has been studied in great detail: that encoding the major immediate-early (MIE) proteins of CMV. As shown in Figure 2C.3, this genetic unit is expressed via differential splicing to produce four α-proteins of distinct M_r. The protein of M_r 86 000 (*IE86*) interacts with the basal transcriptional machinery, especially the TATA binding protein, to enhance formation of pre-initiation complexes. It also cooperates with the M_r 72 000 protein to synergistically increase expression of its own, and heterologous, promoters, probably through activation of endogenous transcription factors and/or by bridging between their binding sites and the TATA binding protein. The M_r 55 000 protein has minor stimulatory effects, either alone or in combination with either of the other two larger proteins. The smallest protein

(M_r 18 000) is expressed during replication in differentiated monocytes.

The largest of these proteins downregulates its own synthesis and so is autoregulated (Stenberg and Stinski, 1985). This downregulation is mediated by a distinct region in the carboxy-terminus, which is shown stippled in Figure 2C.3. This region is also present in a late protein of M_r 40 000 embedded within this region, and it is likely that activation of its promoter at late times leads to downregulation of the major immediate-early region. *IE86* also binds cellular *p53* which may decrease *p53*-induced apoptosis. *IE86* also interacts with the protein product of *UL84*, which is a transdominant inhibitor of *IE86*. Some of the latency-associated transcripts found in the bone marrow of normal donors code for proteins which are recognised by infected humans (Kondo *et al.*, 1996). Their function is obscure but, by analogy with HSV, they may play important roles in the establishment or regulation of the latent state. Expression of the MIE region was found in multiple tissues of transgenic mice containing a *lacZ* gene which correlated well with the cell types in which CMV replication is found *in vivo* (Baskar *et al.*, 1996). Thus, in summary, expression and regulation of the MIE region are remarkably complex, with the potential for exquisite control of virus replication.

Other immediate-early genes are of interest. Genes *UL36–37* encode transactivators which are essential for DNA replication and which represent a molecular target for antiviral chemotherapy. Likewise, TRS1 is required for DNA replication. *pUL69* is present in the tegument of the virion, as is *ppUL83*. Although the

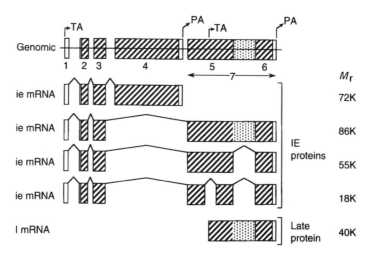

Figure 2C.3 Proteins encoded within the major immediate-early region of CMV. Exons are numbered 1–7. TA, transcriptional activation; PA, polyadenylation; ie, immediate-early; l, late

latter is a late protein, in combination, these two proteins appear to play a similar role to the α-transinducing factor of herpes simplex virus, which is released into the cell during the process of uncoating and is then able to interact with a cellular transcription factor to upregulate the major immediate-early promoter.

Early proteins mainly provide essential enzymic functions within the cell, e.g. *pUL54*, DNA polymerase, and *pUL97*, a protein kinase which phosphorylates antiviral nucleosides such as ganciclovir (GCV) or aciclovir (ACV), so starting their anabolism to the functional nucleoside triphosphate inhibitors of *pUL54*.

Late proteins generally play a structural role in virion formation, e.g. surface glycoproteins are potentially important because of their interaction with the immune system. Neutralising epitopes have been described on *gB* and *gH*. *gH* requires *gpUL115* (glycoprotein L) to facilitate surface expression. Much of the neutralising activity of serum samples can be absorbed by recombinant gB, suggesting that this protein contains dominant neutralising sites (Britt *et al.*, 1990). *gB* forms the active component of some vaccine preparations which have reached the stage of Phase I clinical testing.

Note that an alternative nomenclature system terms gB 'glycoprotein complex I' (*gCI*) and gH 'glycoprotein complex III' (*gCIII*) (Gretch *et al.*, 1988). The protein products of individual genes which combine to form these complex glycoproteins are summarised in Table 2C.1.

A variety of other proteins have been identified and mapped to the genome (see Figure 2C.4), important examples of which will be mentioned briefly. A total of 11 proteins are required in *trans* to effect replication (see Table 2C.2). Many of these perform similar functions to HSV proteins except that CMV does not have an identified origin binding protein and requires transactivators. *pUL80A* and *pUL80.5* encode the protease and assembly protein, respectively. Protease,

Table 2C.1 HCMV envelope glycoproteins

Complex in envelope	Constituent proteins	Mapped ORFs
gCI	gB homodimer	gpUL55
gCII	gM (IMP)	gpUL100
	gN	gpUL73
gCIII	gH	gpUL75
	gL	gpUL115
	gO	gpUL74

ORF, open reading frame; IMP, integral membrane protein.

Table 2C.2 Eleven loci required for HCMV replication

DNA-*pol*	*UL54*
pol-Associated protein	*UL44*
ssDNA BP	*UL57*
Helicase-primase	*UL70*
	UL105
	UL101–102
Transactivators	*UL36–37*
	IRS1 (or *TRS1*)
	IE1/2
	UL112–113
Binds IE86 protein	*UL84*

Data from Pari *et al.* (1993).

which is not packaged into the virion, is responsible for cleaving the original polyprotein at four distinct sites. The assembly protein facilitates formation of B-capsids and entry of DNA, being lost from the capsid in the process. Four genes (US27, US28, UL33, UL78) are homologous to G-protein-coupled receptors and so may be involved in signal transduction. The US28 gene facilitates entry of HIV into CD4$^+$ cells, which are otherwise not susceptible to HIV infection (Pleskoff *et al.*, 1997), and also confers chemotactic mobility on arterial smooth muscle cells, which may be relevant to the pathogenesis of atherosclerosis (Streblow *et al.*, 1999).

In addition, open reading frames with predicted similarities to known proteins have been identified from the sequenced genome of AD169. It will be important to determine rigorously that these proteins are actually expressed and that they have the predicted function.

Note also the 22 extra genes depicted outside the main circle of Figure 2C.4. These are not present in AD169 but are found in other strains of CMV with a lower passage history (Cha *et al.*, 1996). Presumably, they have been lost during the process of adapting CMV to grow in fibroblast cell lines which led to the strain termed AD169. This strain is popular with researchers because it grows rapidly to relatively high titre and releases many extracellular virions. Wild strains of CMV lack these properties and so are difficult to work with in the laboratory. As a result, one has to question whether AD169 is fully representative of CMV strains *in vivo* and the presumed loss of these 22 genes illustrates this issue. None of the 22 genes has homology with known herpesvirus proteins. Many appear to encode glycoproteins and vaccine candidates containing these genes are being studied. One gene (UL146) encodes an α-chemokine.

Growth *In Vitro*

The only cells which replicate CMV to high titre *in vitro* are human fibroblasts, although wild strains can also be propagated in endothelial cells, macrophages and smooth muscle cells. This finding is in complete contrast to that *in vivo* where, at post mortem, cells infected with CMV are found in organs of epithelial origin (kidney, liver, bile ducts, salivary gland, gut epithelium, lung parenchyma, pancreas) as well as in endothelial cells. This observation again suggests that the virus propagated in the laboratory should not be assumed to be an authentic model of the wild-type virus. The genetic changes which confer tropism for endothelial cells and for polymorphonuclear leukocytes have not yet been defined (Gerna *et al.*, 2002). The cell surface proteins which act as receptors for CMV have not been identified although several candidates have been proposed.

In fibroblast cell cultures, encapsidation occurs in the nucleus. The products of genes UL50 and UL53 combine to digest the structural lamins which form the inner nuclear membrane (Muranyi *et al.*, 2002) and the virus envelope is then acquired by budding through this membrane. Enveloped virions are found within vesicles in the cytoplasm and these appear to fuse with cellular membranes to allow egress of the mature virus particles. Dense bodies also mature and are released from the infected cell in the same way as virions, so that they contain virus-specific glycoproteins.

At late times after infection, CMV induces the appearance in infected fibroblasts of an Fc receptor which has high affinity for human IgG, but not other human immunoglobulin isotypes, and has low affinity for rabbit IgG or mouse IgG (Keller *et al.*, 1976). Recent results show that one Fc receptor is encoded by gene TRL11 and its duplicate ILR11, while a second is formed by a UL119–UL118 fusion protein. The Fc receptor is found in the Golgi apparatus which enlarges to form a perinuclear inclusion body in the concavity of the reniform nucleus. It has been suggested that HSV produces an Fc receptor so that antibody attached by its Fab portion to a virus protein can be bound by its Fc portion back onto the virion. This would have the effect of preventing immune effector mechanisms, which require an intact Fc portion after opsonisation. Whether such a mechanism is operative for CMV remains to be defined. However, the production by CMV of Fc receptors *in vivo* might allow opsonised bacteria or fungi to gain access to cells which they cannot normally infect; this might explain why CMV infection is often associated with secondary bacterial and fungal infections. A similar process might operate for HIV coated in non-neutralising antibody.

Unlike HSV, CMV does not switch off host macromolecular synthesis but actually stimulates cellular DNA, RNA and protein synthesis. The overall effect is to push the cell towards the S phase of the cell cycle without allowing cell division to occur. One cellular function which is stimulated as a result is thymidine kinase activity. It is tempting to suggest that CMV has learned to increase cellular uptake of thymidine by switching on the host enzyme responsible, whilst HSV has used a different tactic, the production of a novel thymidine kinase to achieve the same objective. Likewise, CMV induces cellular topoisomerase II and may package this enzyme into extracellular virions. Recent results have also shown that human complement is bound to the virion but not activated. Host cell complement regulatory proteins were detected in virions and might explain this phenomenon (Spiller *et al.*, 1997). Thus, like HIV (reviewed in Ott, 2002), the mature virion may contain host proteins of potential importance for understanding pathogenesis.

EPIDEMIOLOGY

Cytomegalovirus must be acknowledged as one of the most successful human parasites. It has learned to survive in its human host by infecting both vertically and horizontally; the virus can be transmitted by either route during primary infection, reinfection or reactivation; at all times the virus causes minimal disability, allowing infected individuals to remain active and so maintain the maximum opportunity of encountering susceptible contacts; the virus is excreted from multiple sites, so contact of varying degrees of intimacy can lead to transmission.

Infection may be acquired during delivery following ingestion of infected maternal genital secretions or soon afterwards by ingestion of breast milk containing CMV (Stagno *et al.*, 1980). These two means of perinatal transmission combine to infect 2–10% of infants by the age of 6 months in all parts of the world.

Throughout the rest of childhood, close contact is known to be required for transmission, although the precise route of infection is not known. As a result, CMV may transmit readily within family groups. The possibilities for infection must be increased where individuals are crowded together in unhygienic circumstances, and this probably explains why CMV infection is most common in societies which are socially disadvantaged. Infection is transmitted less well in the general community, apart from child-to-child transmission, which has been documented in play groups (Pass *et al.*, 1986). Once infected, such children can transmit CMV to their parents (Pass *et al.*, 1986) and so represent a potential threat to a future sibling should the mother be pregnant.

In populations of poor socioeconomic background, the vast majority of children have experienced primary CMV infection by the onset of puberty. In countries with good social circumstances, roughly 40% of adolescents have been infected and, as shown in Figure 2C.5, seroprevalence increases by approximately 1%/year thereafter (Griffiths and Baboonian, 1984). Such primary infection can lead to vertical transmission if the individual is pregnant when she becomes infected.

The prevalence of CMV IgG antibodies in organ transplant recipients reflects their socioeconomic grouping. The same applies to individuals who acquired HIV infection via blood (or blood products), heterosexually or through contaminated needles used for intravenous drug use. In contrast, HIV-positive male homosexuals have a very high prevalence of CMV IgG antibodies (typically 95%).

At whatever age primary infection occurs, the virus is not eradicated from the host but persists for the rest of the life of the individual. Occasionally, however,

CMV reactivates from its latent state and infectious virions appear in the saliva and/or urine. These reactivations of CMV are entirely asymptomatic but form an important means by which CMV can spread horizontally. Reactivations can also lead to vertical transmission of CMV. This finding came as something of a surprise, since it was assumed that a woman who possessed antibody against CMV before becoming pregnant would be immune to intrauterine transmission. However, not only can reactivation of latent maternal infection lead to congenital infection but more foetuses are infected worldwide by this route than are infected as a result of primary maternal infection. Congenital CMV infection thus has its highest incidence in the poorest communities of the world, since most women in poor societies are infected before reaching child-bearing age. Note, however, that primary CMV infection in the mother represents a greater risk to the foetus than recurrent maternal infection (Fowler *et al.*, 1992), so the burden of congenital disease is greatest in developed countries.

Finally, 'immune' hosts can also be reinfected with another or, possibly, the same strain of CMV. Epidemiologically, it is important to distinguish between reinfection and reactivation of latent infection but, in clinical practice, the term 'recurrent infection' is often used to cover both possibilities.

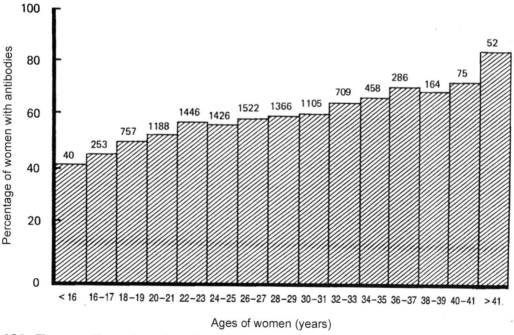

Figure 2C.5 The age-specific prevalence of complement-fixing serum antibodies against cytomegalovirus. The number of women in each group is shown above each column of the histogram. Reprinted from Griffiths and Baboonian. A prospective study of primary cytomegalovirus infection during pregnancy: final report, 307–315 (1984) with permission from Elsevier

ROUTES OF INFECTION

Intrauterine Infection

As is the case with rubella, intrauterine infection is assumed to follow maternal viraemia and subsequent placental infection, although this has not been proved formally. Due to the lack of maternal illness it has not been possible to identify a series of pregnant women with primary CMV infection and show that viraemia is a risk factor for congenital infection. If viraemia is responsible for transmission, then it must be determined whether cell-free virus or leukocyte-associated virus is required for placental infection. Intrauterine transmission of CMV occurs in only one-third of pregnant women with primary infection but we remain ignorant of how the majority prevent the virus from infecting the foetus. It may be that the placenta acts as a form of barrier, but representation of this organ as a sieve which may or may not trap CMV must surely be simplistic. Ultrastructural studies of the placenta emphasise the importance of macrophage-mediated defence against potential virus infections.

Perinatal Infection

Perinatal infection is acquired predominantly from one of two sites: infected maternal genital secretions or breast milk. During delivery, the foetus is surrounded by copious quantities of genital secretions, which may contain high titres of CMV as a result of recurrent maternal infection. Under these conditions, infection has been described as occurring 'during passage through the Sea of Cytomegalovirus'.

Breast milk, especially colostrum, has also been shown to be a good source of CMV. Although virus titres are relatively low, large quantities of milk are imbibed, so a heavy viral inoculum can be ingested. Clinical studies have demonstrated that it is not just the presence of CMV in breast milk which is required but that this milk must also be fed. Women whose only site of CMV excretion was from the breast were studied. Perinatal infection occurred only when breast-feeding took place, not when such women gave formula feeds (Stagno et al., 1980). Having ingested CMV, infection might be established in the neonate by infection of buccal, pharyngeal, respiratory, salivary gland or oesophageal mucosa.

Postnatal Infection

The absence of symptoms associated with postnatal CMV infection makes it impossible to implicate with certainty the routes of transmission, although evidence exists to support salivary transmission.

Saliva containing CMV has been recovered from toys at day-care centres and this would seem to be an ideal means by which the virus could be transmitted among young children unable to conform to basic standards of hygiene (Pass et al., 1986). Likewise, occasional cases of CMV mononucleosis are seen in young adults and, by analogy with EBV, the infection has been dubbed a 'kissing disease' (see Chapter 2D).

The prevalence of CMV IgG antibodies in developed countries increases at 1%/year from puberty to middle age (see Figure 2C.5). It is often stated that these infections result from sexual exposure but this remains unproven. Certainly they result from contact with an infected individual, but whether this contact takes place at the level of oral or genital mucosa is a matter of speculation. Evidence can be found to support the concept of venereal transmission, since CMV is found in semen and on the cervix. However, this is only circumstantial evidence; we do not talk of brain-to-brain transmission of poliomyelitis or urinary transmission of mumps just because these viruses may be found at particular sites. Sexual contact is almost invariably preceded by oral–oral contact. Thus, even if CMV is shown to be transmitted by intimate contact, it may have resulted from salivary rather than from venereal exposure. This issue is important because we may need in the future to target CMV vaccines to particular mucosal sites in order to prevent infection, and parents may be less reluctant to vaccinate their adolescent children against a 'kissing disease' than against a perceived 'sexually transmitted' infection.

One setting in which sexual transmission of CMV does occur, however, is between male homosexuals, who have a high prevalence of CMV infection, and those who are initially seronegative run a high risk of primary infection during follow-up. At least one study has implicated rectal intercourse as an independent risk factor for CMV seroconversion, implying that the rectal mucosa provides less of a barrier to the high titres of virus found in semen than is provided by the stratified squamous epithelium of the vagina.

Blood Transfusion

In the early 1960s, when extracorporeal blood perfusion was introduced to facilitate open heart surgery, a syndrome of leukopenia, pyrexia and atypical leukocytosis was recognised which was termed the post-perfusion syndrome. In the mid-1960s, Finnish workers showed that the syndrome was attributable to primary CMV infection acquired by blood transfusion.

Transmission of CMV by blood transfusion was first recognised in these patients for three reasons. First, they received large quantities (typically 10 units) of blood both during priming of the pump and after the operation. Second, the blood was transfused to replenish heat-labile clotting factors and so was used as soon as possible after donation, a procedure which would increase the likelihood of transferring viable virus. Third, the patients were being carefully followed up, so that the appearance of the new syndrome in convalescence was likely to be recognised by the attendant physicians.

Although it has been established that CMV can be transmitted by blood transfusion, it is clear that this is an uncommon event, since only 1–5% of blood units taken from seropositive donors leads to infection of seronegative recipients. To date, it has not been possible to determine which donors have a high risk of transmitting the virus. It is presumed that the virus exists in the blood of healthy donors in a latent state within monocytes (Soderberg-Naucler et al., 1997) and that CMV is reactivated following transfusion when these cells encounter an allogeneic stimulus (reviewed in Roback, 2002). In contrast, CMV can be grown from the peripheral blood of immunocompromised patients and *pp65* antigen is found in polymorphonuclear leukocytes and macrophages. However, this is clearly a different pathogenetic situation from that found in healthy blood donors and could be the result of the phagocytic scavenging activity of these cells.

Organ Transplantation

Several studies have shown that seronegative patients undergoing renal transplantation can be divided into two risk groups according to the serological status of the donor. Those receiving a kidney from a seronegative donor have a virtually zero risk of acquiring primary infection, whereas a seropositive kidney may transmit the virus in 60–80% of cases. Molecular typing of CMV strains excreted by multiple recipients of organs from a single donor proved that the donor organ was the source of CMV (Wertheim et al., 1983). Since both organs from a single donor are usually concordant for transmission, the infectivity must be bilateral; either parenchymal cells or infiltrating leukocytes are prime suspects. Interestingly, the same techniques showed that donor virus could also infect seropositive individuals and cause CMV disease (Grundy et al., 1988). Thus, recipient natural immunity acquired prior to immunosuppression cannot prevent but may alleviate CMV infection, a finding which has implications for the development and evaluation of CMV vaccines. Several studies have shown the same results following all types of solid organ transplants, so all organs from seropositive donors should be regarded as potentially infectious.

In contrast, typing of virus strains showed that the virus causing disease after bone marrow transplant is derived from the recipient and not from the donor (Winston et al., 1985). Seropositive donors have been reported to adoptively transfer immunity to recipients (Grob et al., 1987). This has only been reported in recipients of T cell-depleted marrow, so it is tempting to speculate that this process removes the cells containing CMV while leaving intact immunocommitted non-T cells which can function in the recipient.

PATHOGENESIS

Risk Factors for CMV Disease

Comparison of the results from pregnancy, from recipients of solid organ transplants, from bone marrow transplants and from patients with HIV infection reveal some interesting parallels, despite the different organs involved in CMV disease (Table 2C.3). Thus, primary infection is a major risk factor during pregnancy and for recipients of solid organ transplants but not for bone marrow transplant or AIDS patients. Viraemia has been repeatedly shown to be a risk factor following solid organ or bone marrow transplantation (Meyers et al., 1990) and the same is true for AIDS patients (Bowen et al., 1997). A high CMV virus load was initially shown to be important in neonates with congenital infection (Stagno et al., 1975b) and more recently in renal transplant (Cope et al., 1997b), liver

Table 2C.3 Risk factors for CMV disease

Factor	Pregnancy	Solid transplant	Bone marrow transplant	AIDS
Primary infection	+	+	−	−
Viraemia	No data	+	+	+
Increased load	+	+	+	+

+, Factor that has been shown to correlate with risk of CMV disease.

Table 2C.4 Univariate and multivariate assessment of prognostic variables for CMV disease after renal transplant

Parameter	Univariate			Multivariate		
	OR	95% CI	*p*	OR	95% CI	*p*
Viral load (per 0.25 log)	2.79	(1.22–6.39)	0.02	2.77	(1.07–7.18)	0.04
Viraemia	23.75	(3.69–153)	0.0009	34.54	(0.75–1599)	0.07
Recipient seropositive	0.22	(0.05–0.95)	0.05	0.92	(0.002–446)	0.98

OR, odds ratio; CI, confidence interval. Reproduced by permission from Cope *et al.* (1997b).

transplant (Cope *et al.*, 1997a), bone marrow transplant (Gor *et al.*, 1998) and AIDS patients (Bowen *et al.*, 1996). Furthermore, multivariate statistical analyses show that, for renal transplant patients, once virus load in urine has been controlled for as a marker of poor prognosis, the other recognised risk factors of viraemia and donor/recipient serostatus are no longer statistically associated with CMV disease (Table 2C.4). This demonstrates that high CMV load is the determinant of CMV disease and that viraemia and donor/recipient serostatus are markers of CMV disease, simply because of their statistical association with a high virus load. Similar multivariate studies in liver transplant and bone marrow patients confirm that high CMV load in blood explains the association with donor/recipient serostatus (Cope *et al.*, 1997a; Gor *et al.*, 1998). Furthermore, in all groups of transplant patients, a threshold association with CMV disease is apparent (see Figure 2C.6) showing that low viral loads are tolerated by the host.

All of these results provide insight into the pathogenic stages leading to CMV disease. Figure 2C.7 illustrates the concepts, using the flow of water from a tap into a bath with an open drain. This is analogous to virus-infected cells at a peripheral organ (such as kidney or salivary gland) producing CMV virions. Their number may be controlled by local immune responses (drain) but, if these are inadequate, the number of virions will increase. If they overwhelm the local immune responses, virions will overflow into the systemic circulation, causing viraemia. The same process is then repeated in the target organ (e.g. liver, retina), whose local immune responses may be able to prevent virus load reaching the critical levels required to cause disease. This explains why viraemia is a strong predictor of CMV disease, but does not guarantee that it will occur. Finally, the model suggests that different cellular mechanisms of pathogenesis may be activated at different virus loads. Thus, immunopathology may be triggered by low virus loads, while high virus loads may be required to damage sufficient cells by lysis to cause clinically recognised disease.

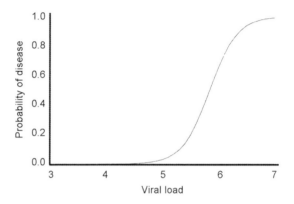

Figure 2C.6 The threshold concept: non-linear relationship between increasing viral load and the risk of CMV disease. Reproduced from Cope *et al.* (1997b)

Speculatively, some disease may be produced when cells are bombarded with very high virus loads without requiring replication, e.g. binding of gB and gH can activate release of transcription factors (Yurochko *et al.*, 1997).

Based on the model in Figure 2C.7, it has been possible to conduct clinicopathological studies to define the dynamics of CMV replication (Emery *et al.*, 1999). Remarkably, serial measures of viral load in blood show that CMV replicates with rapid dynamics, giving a doubling time (viral load on the increase) or half-life (viral load on the decrease) of approximately 1 day. This information has been used to predict the emergence of resistant strains of CMV during prolonged ganciclovir treatment and explain why conventional cell culture assays frequently fail to detect this (Emery and Griffiths, 2000). The perspective of CMV replication and pathogenesis given by this application of modern molecular biology highlights the misleading impressions given about CMV when studied by fibroblast cell cultures (see Table 2C.5).

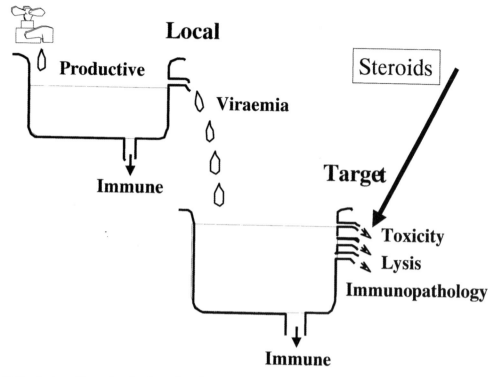

Figure 2C.7 Cartoon illustrating the dynamics of CMV production leading to disease in a target organ. The tap represents production of virions by virus-infected cells. The drain represents the ability of local immune responses to control CMV accumulation

Table 2C.5 Misleading impressions about CMV

Impression	Fact
• *In vitro* strains represent those found *in vivo*	• AD169 strain has 22 missing ORFs; Towne strain has 19
• Live attenuated vaccine can be prepared in fibroblasts	• No protection against CMV infection from Towne, ↓ severity of disease
• *In vitro* assays correctly identify susceptibility of CMV to antivirals	• Failed to detect clinically important susceptibility to ACV
• CMV is a slowly replicating virus	• CMV replicates rapidly
• GCV-resistant strains occur infrequently in immunocompromised patients	• Resistance is more common. Cell cultures select against detection of resistant strains

Incubation Periods

Examination of three settings in which the date of infection and date of onset of virus excretion can be reliably predicted gives an estimate of 4–8 weeks for the 'incubation period' of primary infection. The three informative clinical settings are where infection is acquired perinatally or is transmitted by organ allograft or blood transfusion.

In contrast, it is not clear whether congenital infection involves a foetal incubation period as well as a maternal one. Maternal seroconversion at different stages of pregnancy has been documented in several studies, with gestational stage recorded as the duration of pregnancy at which maternal seroconversion occurred. However, even if it is assumed that the placenta is infected following maternal viraemia at the time of seroconversion, it is not known whether the foetus can be infected immediately or whether replication in the placenta provides an intrauterine incubation period before viral dissemination to the foetus can occur. This point is important, as the damage to the foetus should be described according to its developmental maturity when infected rather than to the length of the mother's amenorrhoea; this has implications for the timing of diagnostic amniocentesis (see later).

Allograft recipients typically have recurrent CMV infections in the second or third month following transplantation. Studies of pregnant and non-pregnant women as well as male homosexuals have shown that up to 10% of seropositive individuals may be excreting CMV from saliva or urine, or from the cervix in females. Excretion rates are, however, very low after the age of 30 years, suggesting that a host response required for suppression may 'mature' at about this age.

Earlier reports showed that virus excretion from the cervix increased as pregnancy progressed and this was interpreted as being a response to some 'immunosuppressive' effect of pregnancy. A later study, however, showed that CMV excretion was actually suppressed during early pregnancy, so the increase seen in virus isolation towards the end of pregnancy only brought the rate up to the level seen in non-pregnant women (Stagno et al., 1975a). All studies to date have been cross-sectional rather than longitudinal, so person-to-person differences in CMV excretion could account for these results.

Host Defences

The defences mounted by the host against different types of CMV infection will be outlined. In combination, these responses in people with normal immunity keep CMV suppressed into a latent state in most individuals for most of the time. Abrogation of these responses permits CMV replication, with full expression of its potential pathogenicity in some cases. Since severe CMV disease is restricted to individuals with impaired cell-mediated immunity, it can be concluded that this arm of the immune response provides most protection against disease. Nevertheless, several lines of evidence suggest that humoral immunity may contribute towards control of CMV: (a) a randomised trial of prophylactic CMV immunoglobulin reports that CMV disease was reduced compared to patients receiving placebo; (b) neonates who acquire CMV from blood products have reduced disease if they are born to seropositive women, showing that transplacental antibody from their mothers protects against disease (but not infection); (c) recent results with rituximab, a humanised mouse monoclonal reactive

against CD22, report severe CMV disease secondary to profound B cell immunodeficiency.

Humoral Immunity

Antibodies of IgG class are produced promptly at the time of primary infection and persist for life. IgM class antibodies are produced on primary but not recurrent infection of immunocompetent individuals and persist for 3–4 months. Immunocompromised patients may fail to produce IgM antibodies with primary infection and one-third of them have IgM detectable with recurrent infections. With intrauterine infection, IgM antibodies are produced by the foetus, together with an IgG class response which only becomes detectable as passively acquired maternal IgG antibody is catabolised.

Intrauterine CMV infection represents less of a risk to a foetus if it has been transmitted by means of recurrent maternal rather than primary maternal infection (Fowler et al., 1992). Women with primary CMV infection who transmit the virus in utero have higher levels of total IgG but lower levels of neutralising antibodies and lower avidity than women who do not transmit (Boppana and Britt, 1995). While all of this information is compatible with the concept that immune responsiveness can be protective, it does not prove that antibody is the beneficial component. For example, cytotoxic T cells may be protective and the ability to mount this response promptly may correlate with the ability to mount a humoral immune response. Likewise, the postulated humoral defect in women experiencing primary infection during pregnancy may be a relative failure of T helper responses rather than of B cells.

There is evidence to show that enhanced humoral immune responsiveness in the foetus correlates with poor prognosis. Cord blood levels of specific IgM, total IgM and rheumatoid factor are positively correlated with symptomatic rather than asymptomatic congenital infection. This effect has been shown to be independent of virus titre at birth and so is not simply secondary to a high virus load in symptomatic infants. Although this suggests that foetal antibody is responsible for immunopathology, it could equally well be that there is another response of the foetus which is damaging and which indirectly correlates with the humoral immune response.

The beneficial or adverse effects of humoral immunity could be discerned better if reactivity against a particular virus-coded protein could be shown to correlate with prognosis. Many CMV proteins are recognised by the humoral immune system and work to date has not been able to identify such a pattern in congenitally and perinatally infected infants. The ability of serial sera to immunoprecipitate radio-labelled virus-coded proteins has simply shown that symptomatic infants are more likely to have reacted to multiple virus proteins and that their sera will precipitate more of any given virus protein than will asymptomatic infants. These results are therefore compatible with heightened immune responsiveness leading to disease production.

Cell-mediated Immunity

For studies of cell-mediated immunity (CMI), the lymphocyte blastogenic response to CMV antigen has mainly been used supplemented recently with tetramer assays. Most seropositive adults have a positive test result, with a surprisingly high proportion of total CD8 cells (e.g. 1%) recognising tetramers containing epitopes from the ppUL83 (pp65) protein. This proportion is suppressed for at least 6 months in transplant recipients, in direct correlation with the dose of immunosuppressive drugs received (Hassan-Walker et al., 2001).

The lymphocyte blastogenic response is suppressed in congenitally or perinatally infected infants. This failure recovers with time and there is a direct correlation between cessation of viruria and acquisition of immune responsiveness at 3–5 years of age (Pass et al., 1983). The defect is known not to be one of generalised T cell immunosuppression, for three reasons. First, CMV-infected infants who also acquire HSV infections generally mount good responses against HSV but not against CMV. Second, these infants respond normally to both killed and live vaccines. Third, the suppressor (CD4) and helper (CD8) T cell lymphocyte subsets remain entirely normal.

Recent work, summarised in Figure 2C.8, has identified complex but plausible mechanisms which, in combination, allow the CMV-infected cell to evade lysis by T cytotoxic, macrophage and natural killer (NK) cells. Immediately after uncoating, the tegument protein ppUL83 (pp65) is available in the cell to phosphorylate the IE72 isoform of the major immediate-early protein and so prevent its presentation as a target epitope. At immediate-early times, pUS3 retains Class I HLA molecules within the endoplasmic

reticulum (ER). Once the virus-infected cell has moved into the early phase of CMV gene expression, pUS2 and pUS11 act to re-export Class I HLA molecules back from the lumen of the ER into the cytoplasm, where they are degraded in the proteasome. At both early and late times, pUS6 blocks the activity of the transporter associated with antigen presentation so that epitopes derived from CMV proteins cannot be presented as targets. All of these functions might, in combination, decrease surface HLA display to such an extent that the cell becomes a target for NK cells or macrophages which recognise the absence of these normally ubiquitous molecules. To prevent this, CMV has evolved a series of distinct strategies. HLA-E normally presents leader peptides from Class I molecules at the plasma membrane to indicate cellular health. Gene UL40 contains the same peptide which upregulates HLA-E and is displayed to provide a negative signal to NK cells via their CD94 molecule. CMV also encodes another protein, pUL18, which is structurally strongly homologous to Class I HLA molecules and acts as a decoy to prevent macrophages attacking the CMV-infected cells. The pUL18 ligand on macrophages is leukocyte immunoglobulin-like receptor 1. Another protein, pUL16, is not membrane-bound but interferes with the ability of cellular proteins (termed UL16-binding proteins) to activate NK cells via their NKG2D receptors.

From the description above, it will be apparent that CMV has evolved a series of genes (coloured dark green in Figure 2C.4) which act in a coordinated way to abrogate cell-mediated immune responses specific for the virus. There is much to be learned about the mechanistic aspects of how this objective is achieved. For example, the expression of UL18 is not blocked by the action of the set of US genes which normally reduce Class I expression and, remarkably, US2 is able to block Class II expression as well as Class I. Thus, many responses may be initiated but are unable to detect their cellular targets during the initial round of replication. However, when the virus leaves the first cell to initiate infection in a second cell, it is vulnerable to display of epitopes before downregulation of HLA can be effected in that cell. Accordingly, the dominant effector cell-mediated immunity is directed against ppUL83 (pp65), revealed when the input virion is uncoated, thus explaining why CMI is focused on this late protein rather than those formed earlier in the viral cascade. However, it is possible that epitopes from other proteins may make contributions as well, with the major immediate-early proteins being prime contenders.

Possible Interactions with HIV

The multiple mechanisms by which HIV may interact with herpesviruses are reviewed elsewhere (Griffiths, 1998). Many studies have shown *in vitro* that CMV infection (or transfection of particular genes) can transactivate HIV (reviewed in Ghazel and Nelson, 1993). Under some circumstances, CMV can also downregulate HIV replication, but CMV is more likely to stimulate HIV when the latter has an integrated provirus and when CMV is not actively replicating (Moreno *et al.*, 1997).

All of the postulated mechanisms of interaction would require close contact between HIV and CMV, either in the same cell or in neighbouring cells. Studies of human autopsies have shown that CMV and HIV frequently co-infect the same organs and that individual cells can be found infected with both viruses.

Epidemiological studies report that the presence of active CMV infection or high quantities of CMV are associated with more rapid progression of HIV infection to AIDS or AIDS to death. It is therefore possible that CMV (and other herpesviruses) may act as co-factors to accelerate HIV disease but this hypothesis remains unfashionable and the reader is referred elsewhere for more details (Griffiths, 1998).

CLINICAL FEATURES

Congenital Infection

7% of congenitally infected babies are born with symptoms. They are said to have 'cytomegalic inclusion disease' and their prognosis is poor. The remaining 93% appear to be normal at birth but about 15% develop sequelae on follow-up (Stagno, 1990).

Those Symptomatic at Birth

The classic presentation is one of intrauterine growth retardation, jaundice, hepatosplenomegaly, chorioretinitis, thrombocytopenia and encephalitis, with or without microcephaly. It is often difficult, even for experienced paediatricians, to differentiate solely on clinical grounds between the several agents causing chronic intrauterine infection; laboratory tests for CMV, rubella, syphilis and toxoplasmosis are therefore invaluable. Most of the pathology outside the central nervous system (CNS) is self-limiting, although severe thrombocytopenic purpura, hepatitis, pneumo-

nitis and myocarditis are occasionally protracted and life-threatening. The CNS involvement may present as microcephaly, hearing loss, encephalitis, seizures, apnoea or focal neurological signs. As regards congenital malformations, inguinal hernia in males, first branchial arch abnormalities, anophthalmia, diaphragmatic eventration or cerebellar hypoplasia have all been reported. However, these occur sporadically and so may be merely coincidental. There is therefore no evidence that CMV acts as a teratogen to impair normal organogenesis. Most of the clinically apparent sequelae can be attributed to destruction of target organ cells once they have been formed.

In 20% of these cases (1% of all those congenitally infected) the damage caused by the virus is so severe that they die during infancy. If a neonate survives, it is almost certain to have serious abnormalities for life, especially if there is microcephaly or if abnormalities are seen by computerised axial tomography (Noyola *et al.*, 2001). On follow-up, clinically apparent extraneural damage is rare but brain damage may manifest as microcephaly, mental retardation, spastic diplegia or seizures, and perceptual organ damage such as optic atrophy, blindness or deafness. Any of these abnormalities may occur alone or in combination. These defects may appear in children who do not have signs of CNS involvement at birth (including CSF examination). Milder forms of CNS damage, such as defects in perceptual skills, learning disability, minor motor incoordination or emotional lability, may be noticed as the child becomes older.

Those Asymptomatic at Birth

Long-term follow-up of such children has revealed that approximately 15% are likely to have hearing defects or impaired intellectual performances when compared to control children. The mean intelligence quotient of infected children has been reported to be significantly lower than controls. Other investigators have not noted these defects but their studies have often, although not always, failed to follow the children for a sufficient length of time, or have failed to use matched controls. There has been scepticism about the reliability of hearing tests in young children but there is now sufficient evidence to prove that the hearing loss can occur in a child born with normal hearing. In addition, a plausible pathogenesis for progressive hearing loss is apparent. Figure 2C.9 shows a histological preparation of inner ear structures from a fatal case of congenital CMV infection,

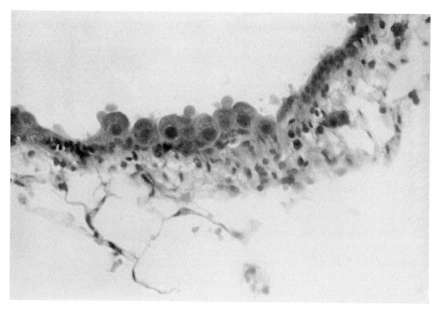

Figure 2C.9 Histological preparation of an inner ear structure from a fatal case of congenital CMV infection showing cell–cell extension of CMV accompanied by an inflammatory response. Courtesy of Dr S. Stagno, Alabama

demonstrating virus spread by the cell-to-cell route to produce a focus of infection surrounded by inflammation. It is tempting to suggest that this represents the infectious process in the inner ear causing progressive damage to the organ of Corti and decreased ability to perceive sound.

Perinatal Infection

Despite the continued excretion of virus for many months, the vast majority of perinatally infected infants appear not to develop acute symptoms. The initial titres of CMV in the urine are significantly lower than those found in neonates with congenital CMV infection or disease (Stagno *et al.*, 1975b), which is compatible with the virus load hypothesis of CMV disease induction. Occasional cases of infantile pneumonitis have been attributed to perinatal CMV infection. This would appear to be an uncommon event, although CMV is a frequent pathogen in those few infants who do develop pneumonitis in the first 3 months of life. Disease may occur in preterm neonates (<1500 g birth weight). One study reported transmission of CMV in 17% of cases (Yeager *et al.*, 1983), while a more recent publication reported transmission in 37% (Hamprecht *et al.*, 2001). In both papers, individual cases of neutropenia were temporally

associated with CMV acquisition, sometimes accompanied by a clinical picture of sepsis with negative bacterial cultures.

Postnatal Infection

The commonest clinical outcome of primary or recurrent postnatal infection is a mild course without the production of symptoms. Most individuals identified by prospective serological studies as having seroconversions express surprise when told that they have experienced a virus infection.

Occasionally, however, primary infections are accompanied by the syndrome of infectious mononucleosis. This is similar to the syndrome produced by EBV except that lymphadenopathy is uncommon and that the Paul–Bunnell test is invariably negative. Sometimes, the hepatic component of CMV mononucleosis is prominent, so a diagnosis of viral hepatitis is considered initially. Within a few days, however, the full clinical picture becomes clear, with persisting pyrexia and atypical lymphocytosis. The post-perfusion syndrome, described earlier, is essentially CMV mononucleosis acquired by blood transfusion.

CMV is such a common virus infection that primary infection tends to occur by co-incidence with a variety of medical conditions. In addition, since CMV is an opportunist, it will tend to reactivate when a patient becomes debilitated as a result of some underlying condition. If the underlying disease is esoteric and has an unknown aetiology, a case report tends to appear describing the association. By scanning through PubMed, internet surfers will be able to find literally dozens of such spurious associations, but they should be reassured; CMV is not the cause of all known diseases.

Immunocompromised Patients

Immunocompromised patients may respond to primary or recurrent CMV infections by remaining entirely asymptomatic. More frequently, they will develop a spiking pyrexia which resolves after a few days. Some may develop viraemia with fever and leukopenia, which is sometimes termed 'CMV syndrome'. This may progress to pneumonitis or this complication may supervene directly. In either case, once pneumonitis has become established, the prognosis is poor (mortality 80–90%). Some patients present with virus dissemination to the retina without other signs. Any part of the gut may be the site of CMV replication, which may be asymptomatic or may be associated with ulceration which can, in extreme circumstances, cause erosion of neighbouring blood vessels, with catastrophic haemorrhage. Patients with AIDS may develop an encephalopathy of either a subacute progressive dementia or an acute presentation with cranial nerve palsies caused by necrotising ventriculitis. Alternatively, AIDS patients may present with a syndrome of weakness of the lower limbs, bladder paralysis and a polymorphonuclear CSF response which is termed polyradiculopathy. At post mortem examination, AIDS patients often have CMV adrenalitis. Finally, CMV may induce an immunosuppressive syndrome in which the patient becomes unable to deal with superinfecting bacteria or fungi. In this instance, and in some of the other clinical presentations (pneumonia, hepatitis, gut ulceration, septicaemia), the underlying nature of the CMV infection is often not recognised by the clinical staff, who are understandably distracted by the more easily recognised superinfecting organisms.

The major clinical diseases associated with CMV are summarised in Table 2C.6, according to the type of immunocompromised patient. Some complications, such as gastrointestinal involvement, are found in all patient groups. Some are found in all but predominate in one group; for example, 85% of CMV disease

Table 2C.6 CMV diseases in the immunocompromised

Symptoms	Solid transplant	Bone marrow transplant	AIDS
Fever/hepatitis	+ +	+	+
Gastrointestinal	+	+	+
Retinitis	+	+	+ +
Pneumonitis	+	+ +	
Immunosuppression	+		
Myelosuppression		+ +	
Encephalopathy			+
Polyradiculopathy			+
Addisonian			+
Immunosuppression	+	?	?
Rejection/GvHD	+	?	
Atherosclerosis	+		
Death		+	+

presents as retinitis in AIDS patients compared to less than 5% in transplanted patients. While this observation remains unexplained, it is hypothesised that CMV pneumonitis in allograft patients is an immunopathological condition caused by an aggressive cell-mediated response against a lung target antigen coded by, or revealed by, CMV infection. Accordingly, AIDS patients may be relatively spared pneumonitis because, by the time they are sufficiently immunocompromised to permit CMV dissemination to the lung, they have insufficient T cell responsiveness to mount the postulated immunopathological response. Likewise, the myelosuppressive CMV disease results when CMV replicates in stromal supporting cells releasing cytokines and producing a milieu unfavourable for haematopoiesis.

These observations concerning the different CMV diseases found in distinct patient groups, combined with the increasing knowledge about the importance of CMV viraemia and viral load, lead to a potential explanation for the diversity of CMV diseases. CMV viraemia may be a prerequisite for CMV disease at any target site. Increasing viral load may increase the chance that CMV may penetrate tissues to cause disease. Other organ-specific changes, distinct for each patient group, may then dictate in which organ CMV localises, e.g. the marrow suppression is presumably found only after bone marrow transplant because these new cells are receptive to CMV replication.

Indirect Effects

Several studies consistently associate CMV with allograft rejection, secondary fungal or bacterial infections and accelerated atherosclerosis after heart transplant. The results (discussed later) from double-blind placebo-controlled trials of antiviral agents demonstrate that each of these is significantly reduced by preventing CMV disease, so supporting the hypothesis that CMV causes these conditions in some patients. There are no clinical features to distinguish CMV-associated graft rejection/secondary infection/atherosclerosis from the cases that are not prevented by anti-CMV drugs.

DIAGNOSIS

As with all viruses, there are two potential strategies for providing a diagnosis: the detection of virus or the demonstration of a specific immune response.

Detection of Virus

Collection of Specimens

Urine must be fresh and can be obtained by mid-stream collection, by urine bags in neonates or by urinary catheter. Samples can be collected at any time of day and should be sent to the laboratory without additives, since CMV is stable in urine.

Saliva should be allowed to soak onto a plain cotton-tipped swab, which is then shaken in virus transport medium and broken off.

Heparinised blood samples should be collected with care, since heparin inhibits CMV replication and the phenolic preservatives found in proprietary pathology bottles may be toxic to cell cultures. Some 10 ml of peripheral blood should be mixed gently with 500 units of preservative-free heparin. For PCR, acid citrate–dextrose or EDTA is preferred to heparin.

Tissue biopsies should be placed into plain sterile containers with no additives. Fluid and cells obtained by bronchoalveolar lavage should similarly be placed in a plain sterile container.

Amniotic fluid should be collected into a plain sterile container without any additives.

All specimens should be sent to the laboratory without delay. If delay of more than a few hours is anticipated, then all samples should be sent refrigerated, or on wet ice, but under no circumstances should any specimen be frozen at any temperature.

Selection of Sites for Examination

To diagnose congenital or perinatal infection, urine or saliva samples are usually collected. More invasive procedures, such as lumbar puncture or liver biopsy, are sometimes performed but identification of CMV at these sites has not been shown to have any prognostic value.

If adults with mononucleosis or hepatitis are being investigated, then urine and blood are the best samples. It should be possible to detect CMV from all urine samples collected within a few weeks of onset, whilst viraemia is often detected in the first few days of illness. The identification of urinary CMV excretion in a patient with such symptoms might be coincidental but the detection of viraemia strongly supports the diagnosis of CMV mononucleosis or hepatitis.

If pregnant women have symptoms, they should be investigated for viraemia. Amniotic fluid can be tested by PCR and culture but amniocentesis should not be performed before 21 weeks because foetal renal function must be established to allow CMV to appear in foetal urine and then amniotic fluid. In addition, amniocentesis performed within 6 weeks of primary infection may give false negative results for CMV because of the postulated placental incubation period, which delays the transfer of CMV from the maternal to the foetal compartment. However, there is no advantage in actively screening asymptomatic women. Investigations involving the culture of urine, genital secretions, saliva and breast milk have been carried out but the results are not predictive of which women will have babies with congenital or perinatal infection. Since the 'patient' in these examples is the neonate, not the woman herself, samples should not routinely be collected from any maternal site.

Immunocompromised patients should be investigated by means of surveillance samples, taken at least weekly, of blood and possibly also urine or saliva. This must be done as routine on all patients, rather than waiting for symptoms to develop. CMV excretion from urine and saliva is very common in allograft recipients so the relative risk for future disease is typically 3. In contrast, PCR viraemia is detected less frequently in allograft patients but, when it does occur, is indicative of a relatively poor prognosis, with a relative risk of about 10. However, even the detection of viraemia does not guarantee that CMV is the cause of, say, the patient's hepatitis or pneumonitis. Ideally, samples should be collected from these target organs whenever possible.

An alternative way of detecting viraemia is through detection of antigenaemia in preparations of peripheral blood mononuclear cells as targets (van den Berg et al., 1991). These are reacted with monoclonal antibodies against ppUL83 (pp65) followed by immunoperoxidase staining (see Figure 2C.10). Note that the monoclonal

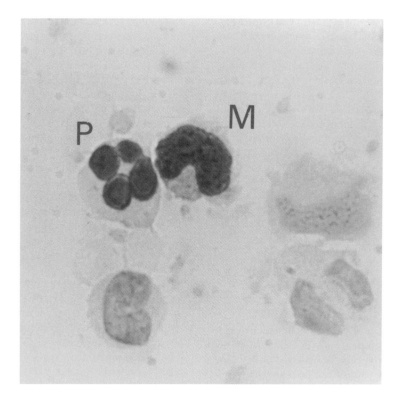

Figure 2C.10   Direct detection of cytomegalovirus in peripheral blood leukocytes. M, monocyte; P, polymorphonuclear leukocyte. Kindly provided by Professor H. Thé

antibody required for this assay does not recognise the immediate-early proteins as originally described. Presumably, the phagocytic activity of the leukocytes shown in Figure 2C.10 has led them to ingest virus-infected material, among which *ppUL83* is prominent. It is tempting to speculate that this may derive from dense bodies, since *ppUL83* is a major component of these aberrant forms. In practice, antigenaemia is useful where samples can be processed by the laboratory within a few hours and where the leukocyte count is relatively normal, e.g. in recipients of solid organs.

Histopathology

Cytomegalovirus can be recognised in histological preparations by its characteristic 'owl's eye' inclusions. These Cowdry type A intranuclear inclusions have a surrounding halo and marginated chromatin. They can be found in kidney tubules, bile ducts, lung and liver parenchyma, gut, inner ear and salivary gland but are less prominent in brain tissue (see Figures 2C.9 and 2C.13 for examples).

Although histopathology provides a specific diagnosis, it is known to be insensitive. One study showed that CMV can be cultured from tissue six times more frequently than typical inclusions can be seen, while a later study showed that organs with inclusions have a median viral load 2 logs higher than those in which inclusions could not be seen (Mattes *et al.*, 2000).

Tissue Immunofluorescence

Some biopsy samples (e.g. liver, lung) may contain cells infected with CMV which can be visualised by staining frozen sections with antisera to CMV. Alternatively, the tissue can be disrupted and the cells fixed to glass slides before staining. Broncho-alveolar lavage fluid contains a suspension of cells exfoliated from the respiratory tract, which can be centrifuged, washed to remove adherent mucus and then air-dried and fixed to microscope slides before staining.

Cell Cultures

For conventional cell cultures, human fibroblasts are used routinely. Foreskins or embryo lungs may be employed as a source of fibroblasts and must be used only at low passage (<25).

To detect wild strains of CMV reliably, the cultures must be cared for obsessionally. The medium must be drained, 0.2 ml of each clinical specimen inoculated and incubated at 37°C for 1 h to permit virus adsorption. The cultures should then be refed with maintenance medium to reduce the toxic effects of the inoculum. This is especially important in the case of particulate samples, such as blood and tissue homogenates. For the detection of viraemia, buffy coat or unseparated heparinised blood can be inoculated into cell cultures. If toxicity is observed, denuded areas of the monolayer can be repaired by the addition of fresh fibroblasts.

All cultures should be observed at least twice weekly for the typical focal cytopathic effect (CPE) of CMV (Figure 2C.11). Occasionally, urine samples from cases of congenital infection produce widespread CPE within 24–28 h which resembles that of HSV. Usually, however, the CPE evolves only slowly, so the cultures must be maintained for a minimum of 21 days before being reported as negative. This delay in obtaining an answer has stimulated research into more rapid ways of detecting CMV, which are discussed below.

Electron Microscopy

Samples of urine from infants infected congenitally or perinatally contain high titres (10^3–10^6 $TCID_{50}$/ml) of CMV. Using the pseudoreplica electron microscopy technique, it has been possible to demonstrate this viruria. Several authors have reported that approximately 80% of infected infants can be detected, with the false negative results being clearly attributable to low-titre urine samples ($<10^3$ $TCID_{50}$/ml). The viral specificity of the technique has been reported at 100%, simply because it would be most unusual for any other herpesvirus to be found at such high titre in urine from infants.

Electron microscopy cannot be used in immunocompromised patients for several reasons. First, the titre of CMV found in clinical samples from adults is generally lower than that found in infants. Second, all

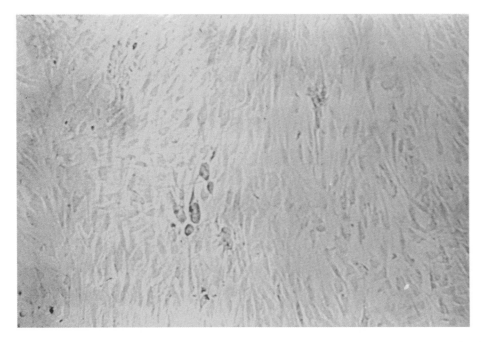

Figure 2C.11 The local cytopathic effect typical of cytomegalovirus seen in monolayer cultures of human embryo lung fibroblasts. Photograph kindly prepared by Ms A. Grzywacz

human herpesviruses frequently infect immunocompromised patients and cannot be distinguished from each other by electron microscopy. Since different antiviral therapy may be required for each herpesvirus, the results of electron microscopy would not be specific enough to influence patient management.

Detection of Early Antigen Fluorescent Foci (DEAFF)

The technique of DEAFF was developed as a means of retaining the specificity and sensitivity of cell culture without having to wait for the production of CPE as a diagnostic end-point (Griffiths *et al.*, 1984).

Following inoculation onto cell cultures, CMV is absorbed rapidly into the cell. CMV rapidly starts to produce α- and β-proteins but CMV DNA synthesis is delayed and protracted until several days after infection. This explains the long delay seen in conventional cell cultures, since CMV needs to replicate, produce daughter virions and infect neighbouring cells in order to produce the cytopathic effects shown in Figure 2C.11.

To speed up the diagnostic process, cells are inoculated with clinical specimens and stained after only 18 h incubation, using monoclonal antibodies directed against some of the α- and β-proteins of CMV (Figure 2C.12). This technique is termed 'shell vial assay' in the USA because of the vessels used for the sample processing (Gleaves *et al.*, 1984).

Enzyme Immunoassay (EIA)

The technique of DEAFF and antigenaemia provide results rapidly but still require subjective immunostaining and cell culture in the case of DEAFF. The technique of EIA could potentially overcome both of these problems by detecting soluble virus-specific proteins and by producing a colour change, visible to the naked eye, whenever CMV is present.

Some workers established EIA detection systems using polyclonal hyperimmune sera or monoclonal antibodies. The results indicated that EIA could detect small amounts of CMV complement-fixing (CF) antigen or of virus when added artificially to buffer systems. However, when clinical samples containing CMV were assayed, results of low sensitivity and/or specificity were obtained.

Detection of Viral DNA

Earlier reports of the detection of CMV by dot–blot methods have been completely superseded by PCR.

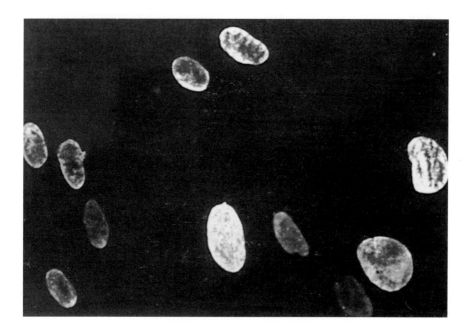

Figure 2C.12 Cytomegalovirus infection diagnosed by detection of early antigen fluorescent foci (DEAFF)

Different parts of the CMV genome have been chosen as targets by various authors, but there is no obvious advantage in any particular one. Ideally, one would wish to amplify a conserved region, but the degree of genetic variability found in clinical strains is only beginning to be defined. Potentially, PCR methods could be so sensitive that they detected low quantities, even latent virus, which would not necessarily be clinically relevant; accordingly, some authors have concluded that their nested PCR procedures do not provide prognostic information. We deliberately chose a non-nested procedure to avoid this problem, and find that PCR produces good prognostic information in both transplant patients (Kidd *et al.*, 1993) and HIV-positive individuals (Bowen *et al.*, 1997). Clearly, 'PCR' is not a single procedure and each laboratory should measure the clinical significance of its results through formal assessment (Kidd *et al.*, 1993; Einsele *et al.*, 1995; Bowen *et al.*, 1997; Shinkai *et al.*, 1997). The availability of fully quantitative PCR assays for CMV, especially in a real-time format, offers another approach for further refining prognostic values, as well as for understanding pathogenesis, as discussed previously.

Amniotic fluid should be tested in multiple replicates by PCR to avoid false negative results (Revello *et al.*, 1998).

Characteristics of the Various Assays Described

These are summarised in Table 2C.7. In the first three editions of this book, I described conventional cell culture as the 'gold standard' against which newer assays should be compared. In the fourth edition I proposed that this process is complete for PCR, so that it can be recommended as the new 'gold standard' for providing diagnostic information in a timely manner able to influence the management of individual patients. This conclusion is supported by a series of subsequent reports, so that any PCR assay which has had a published validation showing correlation with clinical end-points could be employed (Kidd *et al.*, 1993; Einsele *et al.*, 1995; Shinkai *et al.*, 1997). Note that the samples required, the sample extraction method and assay-specific details all differ among these validated assays, so colleagues should choose one system and follow the whole procedure exactly as described. We have always used whole blood because fractionation offers additional opportunities for sample contamination and mislabelling and so should only be performed if clear benefits can be shown. This choice is vindicated by a recent study which directly compared the utility of testing whole blood or blood fractions (Razonable *et al.*, 2002).

Advantages and Disadvantages of Virus Detection

1. The anatomical site of the infection can be documented (e.g. lung involvement in a patient with pneumonitis).
2. The patient's immune response is not required for diagnosis, so all infected immunocompromised patients, not just those able to mount an immune response, can be identified.
3. Rapid diagnostic methods have enabled infected patients to be recruited into therapeutic trials of potential antiviral agents so that patient management may be influenced.
4. PCR methods can quantify the amount of virus in clinical samples and allow quantitative virological assessment of antiviral agents.
5. If resistant virus emerges during a course of treatment, this may be detected by the assay and so provide an opportunity for prescription of an alternative drug.
6. A potential disadvantage is that the monoclonal antibodies or DNA probes used to detect CMV may be too specific and may identify only some strains of the virus, although this has not proved to be a problem to date.

Table 2C.7 CMV detection in body fluids

Method	Sensitivity	Specificity	Reliability	Rapidity	Proven prognostic value
Conventional cell culture	+ +	+ + +	+ +	+	+
Detection of early antigen fluorescent foci	+	+ + +	+ +	+ +	+
Antigenaemia	+ +	+ + +	+ +	+ + +	+
Polymerase chain reaction	+ + +	+ + +	+ +	+ +	+

Detection of Immune Response

IgG Antibody as a Marker of Past Infection

The detection of IgG antibodies against CMV is clearly indicative of infection sometime in the past. The individual is said to be seropositive and is liable to experience reactivations of his/her latent infection. The presence of IgG antibodies against CMV is thus a marker of potential infectivity; although a seropositive individual is 'immune' in the immunological sense, this term should not be used to imply protection from endogenous or exogenous infection.

Many assays have been described for the detection of CMV IgG antibodies. Those most frequently used are listed in Table 2C.8, together with estimates of their specificity, sensitivity, objectivity and rapidity. In patients with intact immunity, the CF test is perfectly adequate, provided that an efficient antigen is employed and that optimal incubation temperatures are used. Other tests (marked '+ +' in Table 2C.8) are more sensitive in that they produce higher antibody titres but they do not detect substantially more seropositive individuals in a population.

With immunocompromised patients, the CF test often gives false negative results by failing to detect low levels of IgG antibody. Thus, a more sensitive technique is required and any of those marked '+ +' in Table 2C.8 are satisfactory, with EIA being used most frequently. If an IF method is chosen, the IFA-LA assay should be avoided because all human sera bind to the IgG Fc receptor induced by CMV and this perinuclear fluorescence can be difficult to distinguish from the virus-specific nuclear fluorescence found with seropositive samples. ACIF is the IF method preferred, since it is unaffected by IgG binding to the Fc receptor.

Table 2C.8 Performance characteristics of several assays used to measure IgG antibodies against CMV

Method	Performance characteristics			
	Sensitivity	Specificity	Objectivity	Rapidity
Neutralisation	+	+ +	+	−
CF	+	+	+	+
IFA-LA	+ +	−	−	+ +
ACIF	+ +	+ +	+	+ +
Latex agglutination	+ +	+ +	+	+ + +
RIA	+ + +	+ +	+ +	+ +
EIA	+ + +	+ +	+ +	+ +

ACIF, anti-complement immunofluorescence; CF, complement fixing; EIA, enzyme immunoassay; IFA-LA, immunofluorescence assay for viral late antigens; RIA, radioimmunoassay.

IgG Antibody as a Marker of Acute Infection

Rising levels of IgG antibody were employed in the past but this approach has been completely superseded by assays for detecting virus itself. However, the detection of IgG antibodies of low avidity provides evidence of primary infection in the recent past, e.g. 16–20 weeks (Guerra et al., 2000).

Detection of IgM Antibodies

Attempts to detect CMV-specific IgM antibodies have been plagued by the use of methods of poor sensitivity and specificity and by interference from rheumatoid factor. Testing for IgM antibodies may be helpful in cases of suspected CMV mononucleosis. In all other cases of suspected active CMV replication, investigations using virus detection methods are recommended.

Problems Associated with Serological Diagnosis

1. Some immunocompromised patients fail to mount a typical immune response and die from disseminated CMV infection. If diagnoses are made solely by serology, these cases will not be identified.
2. The passive transfer of CMV IgG antibodies with blood products may produce 'seroconversions' if sensitive IgG assays are employed.
3. The major objection to detecting CMV infection serologically is that the diagnosis is delayed and so can have little effect on the management of an individual patient.

MANAGEMENT

Congenital Infection

The most important part of the management of these cases is to make an unequivocal diagnosis. This is usually accomplished in the case of those symptomatic at birth but is often impossible in those who are initially asymptomatic.

Babies born with symptoms are usually investigated using the appropriate tests; culture of urine or saliva for CMV. The presence of CMV in a neonate aged less than 3 weeks is clearly indicative of congenital infection.

Those born without symptoms are unlikely to have cultures performed and typically present from the age of 6 months onwards with sequelae such as hearing loss or mental retardation. These cases should be cultured for CMV but, if the virus is present, this does not guarantee that the infection was acquired congenitally rather than perinatally. Unfortunately, in each population which has been investigated, perinatal infection is at least 10 times more common than congenital infection, so that if the presence of CMV in a child aged, say 9 months, is taken as evidence of congenital infection, then such a diagnosis will be wrong in at least 90% of cases. The clinicians may be happy to accept the diagnosis when the clinical findings are reviewed but the child then has only a clinical diagnosis with compatible laboratory findings rather than a definitive virologically-proven diagnosis. Testing for specific IgM antibodies is of no help in this situation, since they should be present following congenital infection and will presumably be produced acutely in cases of perinatal infection, although this remains to be proven rigorously.

If CMV is found in a child who develops symptoms during infancy, it is worthwhile bleeding the mother and contacting the laboratory servicing her antenatal clinic to see if sera have been retained. Occasionally, a laboratory has kept a serum used to test for rubella status. If this serum has CMV IgG but not IgM antibodies, then it is unhelpful, since the mother may have had recurrent infection during pregnancy or, if she presented later than 16 weeks, primary infection early in pregnancy. If, however, the serum has low avidity antibodies or is IgM-positive, it will confirm that she had primary infection during pregnancy, which makes it more likely that her child's CMV was acquired congenitally. Similarly, if the mother seroconverts between early pregnancy and paediatric presentation, this supports a congenital transmission. Finally, the mother may remain seronegative, in which case the child cannot have had intrauterine infection and so the diagnosis of congenital infection can be excluded.

It will be evident from this discussion that the management of these cases would be greatly facilitated if it were possible to screen all new-borns for evidence of congenital infection, in a similar fashion to the established phenylketonuria screening programme. At present, cell culture is too cumbersome and expensive a technique to be used widely but it is hoped that one of the modern technologies described earlier will be able to fulfil this role reliably and, of course, cheaply.

Once the diagnosis of congenital infection has been established, an assessment should be made of the prognosis for the child and for a future pregnancy. An estimate of the child's prognosis can be given from the titre of neonatal viruria and the magnitude of the humoral immune reactivity present in the cord serum, but this can only divide cases crudely into high-, medium- and low-risk categories. More precise prognostic markers are required, especially of viral load. The prognosis for a future pregnancy is clear if the diagnosis has been definitely proven and the child was symptomatic at birth; since only one example of cytomegalic inclusion disease has been reported in consecutive siblings, the risk of an identical recurrence must be very low. If, however, the child developed symptoms during infancy, then the position is not so clear. No sibling cases have been reported but this might be because the correct diagnosis has not been made in the past. It remains possible, therefore, that a woman could have a future pregnancy damaged in a similar way. To be scientifically and legally correct, the risk cannot be given as zero but, on humanitarian grounds, the author usually emphasises that it must be very low. Before a definitive virological diagnosis is available, the differential diagnosis often includes a recessive gene for presentations with hearing loss, which has a recurrence risk of 25%. If the parents are prepared to gamble with their genes, then the virologist must not dissuade them from taking what must be a far lower risk with CMV. It is conventional to advise such women to wait 1 year between the estimated date of infection and trying to conceive, but there are no data to support this advice and no laboratory tests to determine whether it is 'safe' for an individual to proceed.

Having established the diagnosis and prognosis, treatment must be considered, including remedial therapy to compensate for hearing, speech or developmental defects. Ganciclovir has been studied in a dose-comparative trial (Whitley et al., 1997) which showed that the drug was relatively well tolerated over the 6 weeks' duration of therapy with no excess toxicity from the higher dose of 6 mg/kg b.d. As a result, this dose was compared against no treatment in a randomised controlled trial and significantly worse hearing was reported at 6 months among those who were not treated (Kimberlin et al., 2003). Thus, despite the toxicity of ganciclovir, which caused neutropenia and thrombocytopenia in substantial numbers of the neonates, this drug has become the standard of care for those born with CNS symptoms. Further controlled trials are required to determine the optimal duration of therapy and to determine whether the toxicity of ganciclovir can be justified in neonates born with symptoms outside the CNS, e.g. hepatosplenomegaly or thrombocytopenia purpura. Until such trials are conducted, this author concurs with the opinions of the investigators, that ganciclovir should not be used outside the setting of a controlled clinical trial (Whitley *et al.*, 1997; Kimberlin *et al.*, 2003). The toxicity profile of ganciclovir includes carcinogenesis in rodents and so possible therapeutic advantages must be balanced carefully against potential adverse consequences.

Finally, the parents should be informed about the nature of the child's illness and advised on its infectivity (see below).

Perinatal Infection

These cases produce few medical management difficulties. Most remain asymptomatic and undiagnosed. Cases of infantile pneumonitis should have samples of urine, saliva and nasopharyngeal aspirate cultured for CMV but, apart from bronchoscopy and/or lung biopsy, there is no way of proving that the pneumonitis is due to CMV in an individual case. The main medical importance of perinatal infection is the difficulty it produces for the diagnosis of congenital infection (see above) and the fear of contagion that it stimulates.

It is clear that children less than 18 months of age with perinatal infection can transmit CMV to their parents (Pass *et al.*, 1986). This presumably results from close contact with infected saliva during normal family life and so would be difficult to control completely. Control should be considered, however, if the mother is contemplating pregnancy, although care must be taken not to induce feelings of social isolation or rejection among the older sibling. There is no evidence that these children are contagious to adults outside the family but it seems prudent to advise the parents that the infants should avoid intimate contact with women who may be pregnant or with immunocompromised patients. Unfortunately, this advice, when ultimately passed to school teachers, can lead to the children being treated as lepers. The teaching staff may have to be reassured strongly to ensure that the children are not treated differently from any others. It usually suffices to emphasise that 10–20% of the children in the classroom are asymptomatically excreting CMV as a result of perinatal infection, so that routine hygienic precautions should be used by all staff for all children. The same advice should be given when the child has congenital CMV infection, irrespective of whether or not the virus has induced disease. It would be absurd to ostracise the occasional case of symptomatic congenital infection

knowing that literally hundreds of other children of the same age are excreting similar amounts of the same virus.

Postnatal Infection

Most cases of postnatal infection are asymptomatic and so do not require management. Exceptions are CMV mononucleosis or hepatitis, which may well be treated once a safe orally bioavailable anti-CMV drug becomes available.

When postnatal infection occurs in a pregnant woman, however, the possibility of termination of pregnancy requires consideration. Recurrent maternal infections are invariably asymptomatic and no laboratory test is currently available which can detect which immune women are transmitting the virus *in utero*. For these practical reasons, it is not possible to contemplate therapeutic intervention in these cases, even though some produce childhood damage (Fowler *et al.*, 1992), so discussion must be limited to primary maternal infections.

By analogy with rubella infection during pregnancy, it has been assumed that primary CMV infection will be most severe when it occurs during the first trimester, so therapeutic termination of such pregnancies would be justified if the diagnosis could be made sufficiently early. Studies have shown that asymptomatic primary CMV infection can be reliably diagnosed early in pregnancy by testing for IgG avidity and specific IgM antibodies. It has also been clearly shown that the vast majority of women in developed countries present early enough in pregnancy to allow the infection to be detected and for termination of pregnancy to be performed safely. Studies have confirmed the assumption that primary CMV infection is more severe at this stage of pregnancy, so severe that it produces a statistical excess of foetal losses. These results clearly suggest that some pregnancies involving the potentially most severely affected foetuses are terminated naturally, so that medical intervention directed towards the survivors may not be as beneficial as has been assumed.

Currently available data indicate that the risk that an individual foetus may survive to be born with cytomegalic inclusion disease following primary maternal infection before 28 weeks' gestation is about 4% (Griffiths and Baboonian, 1984; Stagno *et al.*, 1986). These results clearly demonstrate that, at present, there is no justification for recommending case finding of asymptomatic primary CMV infection by serological

Table 2C.9 Annual public health impact of congenital CMV

	USA	UK
Number of live births	4 000 000	700 000
Proportion congenitally infected	1%	0.3%
Number congenitally infected	40 000	2100
Number with cytomegalic inclusion disease (7%)	2800	147
Number fatal (12%)	336	18
Number with sequelae (90%)	2218	132
Number asymptomatic (93%)	37 200	1953
Number with sequelae (15%)	5580	293
Total number damaged	8134	443

After Stagno (1990).

screening during pregnancy, and no evidence that the offer of surgical termination of pregnancy in such cases would significantly reduce the incidence of disease attributable to congenital CMV infection (see Table 2C.9).

More subtle problems of an ethical or medico-legal nature are presented to a practising obstetrician when a woman develops symptoms due to primary CMV infection early in pregnancy. Two separate cases have been reported where mononucleosis was diagnosed at 22 and 18 weeks, respectively, and the pregnancies were surgically terminated. At first, the therapeutic intervention in these cases appears to be justified, since both foetuses showed signs of intrauterine infection. However, a selection bias is present because only successful reports have been published; where other pregnancies have been similarly interrupted, the cases have not been publicised following abortion of uninfected foetuses. Furthermore, the presence of intrauterine infection does not necessarily indicate that clinically evident disease would have presented itself in childhood, since the majority of congenitally infected infants develop normally.

In summary, there is no evidence to suggest that a symptomatic woman is more likely to deliver an affected baby than is an asymptomatic woman; therefore, whilst the final decision rests with the parents and their obstetrician, the same virological advice should be given to all. Amniocentesis with culture and PCR of the amniotic fluid has been performed in case series. Overall, these results show that, after 21 weeks' gestation, CMV can be detected in amniotic fluid in most cases. Amniocentesis frequently gives false negative results if performed before 21 weeks because foetal kidney function is required to excrete CMV into

the amniotic fluid. Given the need to make the diagnosis rapidly at this late stage of pregnancy, PCR has a distinct advantage over culture, but the parents must be counselled about the possibility of false negative results. In addition, quantitative PCR of amniotic fluid shows that high viral loads correlate with a high risk of disease. Coupled with the results of ultrasound scanning to assess foetal growth, amniotic fluid testing for CMV aids detection of some of the potentially most severely damaged cases, but the techniques are still restricted to specialised reference laboratories.

In two published independent cases, female members of paediatric medical or nursing staff requested termination after discovering that they had acquired asymptomatic primary CMV infection during pregnancy. Serological tests had been performed because they were caring for infants known to have congenital CMV infection. Virus isolates were obtained in each instance from the index case, the mother and the aborted foetus. In both cases, the maternal and foetal isolates were shown to be indistinguishable from each other by restriction enzyme analysis but were quite different from their respective index case. The conclusion is clear; primary CMV infection occurs commonly during pregnancy and will be found if women of childbearing age are investigated. Typing of strains in the published cases showed that the infections were not acquired from recognised occupational exposures, a finding which has important medical implications. There is little evidence that staff exposed professionally to infectious cases have an increased risk of contracting CMV infection, but it seems prudent to advise pregnant staff to avoid such contacts if possible by practising good hygiene precautions, such as handwashing after patient contact. This cautious approach is applied to female technical staff working with CMV in the laboratory, although we have never had a case of seroconversion among our predominantly seronegative staff. It should be emphasised that the same advice is given to female staff irrespective of their serological status; it should be clear that preconceptional humoral immunity in these women cannot be equated with a guarantee of protection for the foetus.

Immunocompromised Patients

The most important part of the management of these patients is to make the diagnosis of CMV infection rapidly. Once extensive damage to target tissues has occurred, as is shown in Figure 2C.13, then no

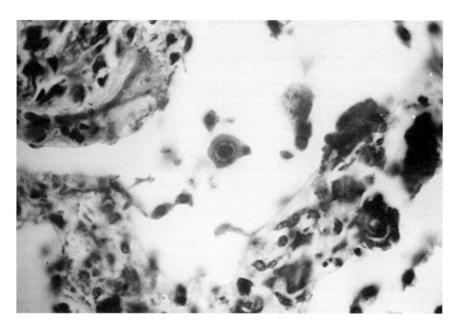

Figure 2C.13 The post mortem histological appearance of cytomegalovirus pneumonitis in a bone marrow allograft recipient. Reprinted from Griffiths. Diagnostic techniques for cytomegalovirus infection, **13**, 631–644 (1984) with permission from Elsevier

antiviral therapy can reasonably be expected to have a successful outcome. To provide advance warning of CMV disease, blood should be collected at least weekly from all allograft recipients and processed by one of the rapid diagnostic methods described in the previous paper.

If CMV is found in an allograft recipient, then the patient's condition should be reviewed with the clinicians. Many are asymptomatic but some may subsequently become unwell and the availability of rapid virological results may allow the clinicians to reduce immunosuppressive therapy before extensive dissemination of CMV has occurred. The importance of rapid diagnosis in the clinical management cannot be overemphasised, since the differential diagnosis of some illnesses requires an increase in immuno-suppressive therapy (e.g. renal allograft rejection episodes). Strategies for the use of antiviral drugs in asymptomatic patients found to have active infection with CMV will be discussed in the next section.

PREVENTION

Is Prevention Needed?

Prevention of an infection can be justified only if it leads to a reduction in ill-health, i.e. the infection itself need not necessarily be the target as long as the infectious process can be modified to prevent disease. Potential strategies by which this objective may be accomplished will be detailed, but first it is necessary to consider the magnitude of the problem in the two major populations: congenital and immunocompro-mised patients.

Congenital Infection

While it is well recognised that babies symptomatic at birth have a poor prognosis, the full effects on those babies who appear to be normal at birth are only now becoming apparent (Fowler *et al.*, 1992). However, the figures outlined in Table 2C.9 indicate that approxi-mately 8000 children/year in the USA and 400/year in the UK suffer overtly as a result of congenital CMV infection. If these figures are ultimately shown to be correct, then they will confirm congenital CMV infection as the second commonest known cause of mental retardation after Down's syndrome. Prevention of such a relatively common condition would be justifiable if this could be achieved safely and at low cost. A recent Institute of Medicine report estimates that $1 billion is spent annually in the USA providing care for these unfortunate children (Stratton, 2000).

Immunocompromised Patients

Infections form the commonest single cause of death in allograft patients. In bone marrow recipients, the single most important infection is CMV, responsible for approximately 15% of mortality before antiviral treatment became available. In recipients of solid organ transplants, several investigators report this virus to be a major cause of morbidity and mortality. In an analysis of hospital charges, CMV disease significantly increased costs, showing that if the expense of extra days spent in hospital is taken into account, then prevention of CMV disease should potentially be cost-effective (Kim *et al.*, 2000). Philosophically, also, it would seem sensible for health services to want to prevent CMV disease, if this can be done at reasonable cost, since its investment in high technology transplantation is wasted if the procedures are effective but the patients die from complications of the treatment.

Prevention of transmission. Knowledge of the potential routes of CMV transmission raises the possibility of prevention by interruption of infection. For example, seronegative renal allograft recipients could be matched to receive only kidneys from seronegative donors. Retrospective analysis by means of life-table survival curves has shown that CMV matching has a greater effect on the survival of cadaver kidney recipients than does matching the same patients for HLA class I status. However, CMV reinfection from the donor kidney has also been shown to cause disease, albeit at a rate lower than that found after primary infection (Grundy *et al.*, 1988). If seronegative kidneys were reserved for seronegative recipients, then more infected kidneys would be given to seropositive recipients and matching for other characteristics, such as HLA, might be prejudiced. Clearly, a controlled trial of the potential benefits of matching would be required before it could be justified as a clinical routine. While there is no doubt that matching could reduce morbidity and mortality due to CMV, there is equal concern that even greater morbidity and mortality due to graft rejection could result from a policy of matching for CMV. Put bluntly, patients and their relatives would not thank us for merely substituting one specific cause for another on the death certificate.

Likewise, seronegative recipients of all allografts could receive blood products only from seronegative donors, but infected blood might also lead to reinfection of seropositive recipients. A counsel of perfection would be to give only CMV seronegative blood or blood products to all pregnant women, all neonates or all immunocompromised patients, including those with AIDS. This would represent a major burden for the blood transfusion centres, all of which are hard-pressed to provide their current services without introducing further logistical and administrative problems. Alternatively, in-line filters could be used to remove leukocytes during blood transfusion, since this has been shown to reduce CMV transmission in a special care baby unit (Gilbert *et al.*, 1989).

Transmission could theoretically be reduced in the general population by advising women of child-bearing age to avoid salivary or sexual contact with seropositive consorts, but this clearly would be unpopular.

Pre-exposure immunisation. This strategy allows CMV exposure to occur but immunises the recipients beforehand, in the hope of preventing disease. Several vaccine candidates have undergone Phase I clinical testing (reviewed in Gonczol and Plotkin, 2001). These include recombinant soluble glycoprotein B, canarypox vectors expressing gB or pp65, as well as recombinant live attenuated Towne strains incorporating the novel genes from the Toledo strain. The recombinant soluble gB (with MF59 adjuvant) induced neutralising antibodies in seronegatives and boosted the neutralising titre in seropositives. The canarypox-gB did not induce neutralising antibodies, although it primed volunteers to respond to subsequent challenge with the Towne strain. The canarypox-pp65 induced CMI in seronegatives. It thus appears that we have several candidate vaccines which are immunogenic and safe and so should consider how they could be evaluated for efficacy.

In the past, vaccinologists assumed that efficacy would have to be proved by reducing the rate at which neonates were born with symptomatic congenital CMV to mothers given vaccine or placebo many years earlier. The practicalities, logistics and expense of conducting such studies are prohibitive. However, modern virology can now be employed in distinct patient populations to determine whether a vaccine protects against primary infection and can provide immunological control against high viral loads (see Table 2C.10). In the author's view, a vaccine which could protect one population of women and one population of transplant patients should be licensed for routine immunisation (e.g. of seronegative teenagers) with post-marketing active surveillance used to document the anticipated reduction in symptomatic congenital CMV infection. Certainly, there are no fears

Table 2C.10 Populations in whom efficacy of CMV vaccines could be evaluated using virological end-points

Populations given vaccine/placebo	Outcome
Seronegative workers at day-care primary centres Seronegative women with children at day-care centres Seronegative pregnant women immunised post-partum	Reduced CMV infection
Seronegative patients on waiting list for receipt of solid organs Seronegative donors of bone marrow to seropositive recipients	Reduced CMV viraemia/need for pre-emptive therapy

that widespread introduction of such a vaccine could affect herd immunity and so shift the incidence of primary infection into the child-bearing years, because the average age at which CMV is acquired in developed countries is already greater than the average age at pregnancy (Griffiths *et al.*, 2001). Furthermore, the Institute of Medicine report should provide a strong financial incentive for the necessary studies to be performed, because their economic analysis shows a cost-saving of $50 000 for each quality-adjusted life year gained by a hypothetical vaccine which costs $360 million to develop (Stratton, 2000).

Concern over the possible oncogenicity of CMV vaccines derives from theoretical considerations which are common to all live herpesvirus vaccines. The live-attenuated Towne strain of CMV vaccine reduced the severity of disease in seronegative recipients given seropositive kidneys (Plotkin *et al.*, 1991). It could not prevent reinfection of the recipients with a different strain of CMV but no evidence was found of reactivation of Towne vaccine virus when the patients were immunosuppressed. No excess of malignancies of any kind was found in the recipients of the vaccine.

Homosexual men are at greater risk of acquiring CMV infection than are heterosexual men and could be considered as candidates for the assessment of the efficacy of CMV vaccines. However, most are already seropositive and so studies would probably have to address the more difficult question of whether vaccination could prevent recurrent infection in this group (immunotherapy).

Vaccines could also be investigated for immunotherapy in patients receiving allografts. Clearly, there would be little point in attempting to present T cell epitopes at this time because the patients would be receiving drugs such as cyclosporin in order to suppress these responses. However, one could aim to present B cell epitopes with the hope of boosting the humoral immune response to keep the CMV load below that required to cause disease. In the case of bone marrow transplantation, immunisation of the donor prior to marrow harvest may potentially lead to adoptive transfer of immunity to the recipient.

Passive T cell immunotherapy has also been evaluated after bone marrow transplantation. Donor cells are expanded *in vitro* and passively administered to recipients. The clinical results show that the cells persist in recipients and a controlled trial to evaluate protective efficacy is currently under way.

TREATMENT

The drugs ganciclovir, foscarnet, cidofovir and fomivirsen (intravitreal only) have been licensed for serious or life-threatening CMV infections in immunocompromised patients, while valaciclovir is licensed only for prophylaxis. Ganciclovir is phosphorylated by the product of the *UL97* gene of CMV (Sullivan *et al.*, 1992) and then the triphosphate acts to inhibit virion DNA polymerase (*UL54*). Cidofovir is a phosphonate compound which is structurally analogous to a nucleoside monophosphate. It does not require activation by *UL97* but is converted to the diphosphate (structurally analogous to a nucleoside triphosphate) by cellular enzymes, and then inhibits *UL54*. Foscarnet is a low molecular weight analogue of the inorganic pyrophosphate product of DNA polymerase activity and so acts at a different site and does not require prior anabolism. Foscarnet and cidofovir must be administered by intravenous infusion; ganciclovir can now be given orally by means of the valganciclovir pro-drug, which is absorbed and cleaved in gastrointestinal cells to release ganciclovir. This pro-drug offers the potential of administering ganciclovir without the need for intravenous infusion (which is clinically important for a drug which causes neutropenia). However, clinical studies are required in each patient population to show that the drug is bioavailable. This has been done for liver transplant patients (Pescovitz *et al.*, 2000) but it remains to be proved that bone marrow transplant patients (who may have gastrointestinal graft-vs.-host disease) can also cleave the pro-drug ester. Ganciclovir produces neutropenia, which may be dose-limiting. In animal toxicology studies, ganciclovir has a cytostatic effect on the testis; the clinical significance of this for humans is unknown. Foscarnet is nephrotoxic, although this effect can be reduced by large volumes of normal saline. Foscarnet also affects ionised calcium levels and produces a fixed drug eruption on the skin of the genital area. Cidofovir is nephrotoxic and it is important that patients are hydrated and receive probenecid to decrease renal concentrations of drug.

Strategies for Deploying Antiviral Drugs

Based on the different stages of pathogenesis shown in Figure 2C.7, four distinct treatment strategies can be envisaged for CMV (see Table 2C.11). While these strategies have been evaluated formally in transplant patients, it is disappointing that they are only now being applied to the design of studies in AIDS patients. Recent results have, however, indicated that the same basic principles apply also to AIDS patients, so I will discuss the findings under the appropriate headings.

Prophylaxis

This approach is to give a drug active against CMV from the time of transplant, and Table 2C.12 lists the double-blind, randomised, placebo-controlled trials which have been conducted to date of such prophylaxis. Ganciclovir, the most potent drug *in vitro*, has been subjected to the rigours of several such trials but the other two licensed drugs, foscarnet and cidofovir, have not. In addition, Table 2C.12 shows that interferon-α (IFNα), aciclovir, valaciclovir and immunoglobulin have also been studied, although many physicians do not associate these therapies with anti-CMV activity.

The results summarised in Table 2C.12 show that ganciclovir has consistently demonstrated activity against CMV infection in all patient groups. It also reduced CMV disease in most groups, with some discrepancies which require discussion. After bone marrow transplant, ganciclovir had a strong trend towards protection which was significant in one study (Goodrich *et al.*, 1993) but failed to reach statistical significance in a second (Winston *et al.*, 1993). After heart transplant, ganciclovir had a significant effect in seropositive recipients (Merigan *et al.*, 1992) but not primary infections, while the opposite was seen in a second study (Macdonald *et al.*, 1995). Note that ganciclovir prophylaxis after bone marrow transplantation had no significant effect or even a trend in favour of survival; presumably, the drug-induced neutropenia facilitated bacterial and fungal infections, to which the patients succumbed (Goodrich *et al.*, 1993; Winston *et al.*, 1993). This illustrates the principle in Table 2C.11, that prophylaxis exposes all patients to the risk of side-effects and so should only be contemplated when a drug has no serious toxicity. In patients with AIDS, a trial of oral ganciclovir, 1 g t.d.s. vs. placebo, was termed 'prophylaxis' because patients did not have CMV disease at trial entry (Spector *et al.*, 1996). Note that this is not virological prophylaxis as defined in Table 2C.11. Nevertheless, PCR data show that the greatest effect of ganciclovir was seen when it was given prophylactically because the drug had less effect in those who were already PCR-positive at trial entry.

The results in Table 2C.12 also show that IFNα, aciclovir and valaciclovir each had anti-CMV effects *in vivo*, whereas there was no evidence of anti-CMV activity of immunoglobulin. This suggests that, if immunoglobulin does have clinical benefit against CMV disease, this is provided by interference with secondary phenomena rather than CMV itself. Note that the anti-CMV effect of aciclovir is clinically important; indeed, aciclovir is the only antiviral drug shown to improve survival when used for prophylaxis after bone marrow transplantation, presumably because its modest antiviral activity is not offset by bone marrow toxicity, as is the case with ganciclovir. A randomised comparison of prophylaxis with aciclovir or ganciclovir after liver transplant (not included in Table 2C.12) shows ganciclovir to be superior in

Table 2C.11 Strategies for deploying chemotherapy against CMV

Term used	When drug given	Risk of disease	Acceptable toxicity
Prophylaxis	Before active infection	Low	None
Suppression	After peripheral detection	Medium	Low
Pre-emptive therapy	After systemic detection	High	Medium
Treatment	Once disease apparent	Established	High

Table 2C.12 Double-blind, randomised, placebo-controlled trials of prophylaxis for CMV infection and disease after transplantation

Patient group	Study group	Dose	Planned duration of therapy (weeks)	No. of patients		Markers of efficacy in whole population					Reference
				Placebo	Drug	Reduced viraemia	Reduced excretion	Reduced disease	Increased survival	Reduced indirect	
RT$_x$	IFN	3×10^6 U 2/w	6	20	21	Yes	Yes	No	No	No	Cheeseman et al. (1979)
RT$_x$	IFN	3×10^6 U 3/w 6 w 3×10^6 U 2/w 8w	14	22	20	No	Yes	Yes	No	No	Hirsch et al. (1983)
RT$_x$	IFN	3×10^6 U 3/w 6w 3×10^6 U 2/w 8w	14	36	32	No	Yes	No	No	No	Lui et al. (1992)
RT$_x$	ACV	800–3200 mg/d	12	51	53	Yes	Yes	Yes	No	No	Balfour et al. (1989)
RT$_x$ with rejection	Ig	100 mg/kg	15	16	11	No	No	No	Yes	No	Metselaar et al. (1989)
RT$_x$	VACV	2 g q.d.s.	13	310	306	Yes	Yes	Yes	No	Yes	Lowance et al. (1999)
LT$_x$	Ig	150 mg/kg	16	72	69	No	No	No	No	No	Snydman et al. (1993)
LT$_x$	GCV	1 g t.d.s.	14	154	150	NG	NG	Yes	No	No	Gane et al. (1997)
HT$_x$	GCV	5 mg/kg b.d. 14 d 6 mg/kg o.d. 5/7 d until 28 d	4	73	76	No	Yes	Yes	No	Yes	Merigan et al. (1992)
HT$_x$	GCV	5 mg/kg o.d. 3/7 d until 42 d plus 14 d rejection	6 (+ rejection)	28	28	NG	Yes	No	NG	No	Macdonald et al. (1995)
BMT$_x$	GCV	2.5 mg/kg t.d.s. days −7 to −1 then 6mg/kg 5 d/w after engraftment	13.5 median	45	40	No	Yes	No	No	No	Winston et al. (1993)
BMT$_x$	GCV	After engraftment 5 mg/kg b.d. 5 d then o.d.	10.9 median	31	33	No	Yes	Yes	No	No	Goodrich et al. (1993)
BMT$_x$	ACV	500 mg/m^2 t.d.s. 1 m then 800 mg q.d.s. 6 m or placebo. Third arm 200–400 mg 1 m, then placebo	30	105	102*	Yes	Yes	Yes	Yes	No	Prentice et al. (1994)

BMT$_x$, bone marrow transplant; RT$_x$, renal transplant; HT$_x$, heart transplant; NG, not given; GCV, ganciclovir; ACV, aciclovir; IFN, interferon; Ig, immunoglobulin; VACV, valaciclovir; *third arm; d, days; w, weeks; m, months.

controlling CMV disease (Winston *et al.*, 1995), illustrating that the toxicity of ganciclovir is less prominent if bone marrow is not the organ being transplanted.

Early Treatment of Active Infection

Where allograft recipients are monitored closely to detect active CMV infection at the earliest possibility, trials have been conducted to determine whether early intervention with antiviral drugs can provide clinical benefit. There are two main approaches: *suppression*, where the drug is given after CMV has been detected at a peripheral site, such as in urine or in saliva; and *pre-emptive therapy*, where CMV is detected systemically, either from blood or the lung sampled by bronchoalveolar lavage. The collection of the latter sample is predicated on the immunopathological nature of CMV pneumonitis, so that therapy is directed at early virus replication before disease has become established. Both approaches have produced clinical benefit (see Table 2C.13). In particular, the study of ganciclovir in bone marrow transplants by Goodrich *et al.* (1991) showed this drug was literally life-saving when used in pre-emptive mode, in contrast to its lack of effect on mortality when used prophylactically (Goodrich *et al.*, 1993; Winston *et al.*, 1993). Again, the principles summarised in Table 2C.11 are prescient, showing that

Table 2C.13 Controlled clinical trials evaluating pre-emptive therapy

Patient group	Site sampled	Laboratory method	Patients randomised	Management allocation		Outcome compared to arm 1			Reference
				Arm 1	Arm 2	Duration viraemia	CMV disease	Survival	
BMT$_x$	BrW	Cytology DEAFF	40	Observation	GCV 5 mg/kg b.d. 14 d then o.d. until 120 d	NG	Reduced	Increased	Schmidt *et al.* (1991)
BMT$_x$	Urine Blood	DEAFF CCC	72	Placebo	GCV 5 mg/kg b.d. 7 d then o.d. until 100 d	NG	Reduced	Increased	Goodrich *et al.* (1991)
BMT$_x$	Blood Urine Throat	Culture (1 pos) PCR (2 pos)	37	Culture	PCR	NG	Reduced	Increased	Einsele *et al.* (1995)
BMT$_x$	Blood	Ag	226	GCV prophylaxis 5 mg/kg b.d. 5/7 d then 6 mg/kg o.d. 6/7 d until 100 d or placebo	GCV 5 mg/kg b.d. 7 d, o.d. 21 d	NG	Same	Same	Boeckh *et al.* (1996)
BMT$_x$	Blood	Ag	39	GCV 5 mg/kg b.d. 15 d	Fos 90 mg/kg b.d. 15 d	Same	Same	Same	Moretti *et al.* (1998)
BMT$_x$	Blood	Ag or PCR	213	GCV 5 mg/kg b.d. 14 d	Fos 60 mg/kg b.d. 14 d	Same	Same	Same	Reusser *et al.* (2002)
LT$_x$	Blood	Ag	22	GCV 5 mg/kg b.d. 7 d	oGCV 2 g t.d.s. 14 d then 1 g t.d.s. 28 d	NG	Same	Same	Singh *et al.* (2000)
LT$_x$	Blood	Ag	60	Observation	oGCV 1 g t.d.s. 14 d	Shorter	Same	Same	Rayes *et al.* (2001)
LT$_x$	Blood	PCR	69	Placebo	oGCV 1 g t.d.s. 8 w	Reduced	Reduced	Same	Paya *et al.* (2002)
LT$_x$ RT$_x$ BMT$_x$	Blood	PCR	48	GCV 5 mg/kg b.d. 14 d	GCV 5 mg/kg o.d. 14 d plus Fos 90 mg/kg o.d. 14 d	Same	Same	Same	Mattes *et al.* (2004)

BMT$_x$, bone marrow (or stem cell) transplant; LT$_x$, liver transplant; RT$_x$, renal transplant; GCV, ganciclovir; oGVC, oral ganciclovir; d, days; w, weeks; NG, not given; CCC, conventional cell culture; DEAFF, detection of early antigen fluorescent foci; PCR, polymerase chain reaction; Ag, antigenaemia; Fos, Foscarnet.

the toxicity of drugs for particular organs is as relevant as their antiviral potency, and that survival benefit can be achieved when the number of patients exposed to a toxic drug can be kept low by using laboratory markers to target therapy to individuals. The results in Table 2C.13 also show that where ganciclovir was compared to placebo or observation it usually produced less CMV disease, often accompanied by a survival benefit. In contrast, where ganciclovir was compared to another effective management, such as foscarnet or prophylaxis with ganciclovir, then no significant benefit was seen. The results in Table 2C.13 thus provide the evidence that ganciclovir and foscarnet are each effective anti-CMV compounds, that they can be given in combination (each at half dose) to minimise toxicity but do not show synergy *in vivo*, and that pre-emptive therapy and prophylaxis are each effective strategies for preventing CMV disease. Each of these strategies has its advantages and disadvantages (see Table 2C.14) and decisions about which to choose should be made locally and supported by continuing audit of what should now be a low incidence of CMV disease in transplant patients, e.g. 1–2% compared to approximately 15% before treatment became available.

In contrast, although pre-emptive therapy should be an effective strategy in AIDS patients, there is no evidence for this because controlled trials were not conducted to address the possibility. However, the PCR data at trial entry from a 'prophylaxis' trial in AIDS patients (Feinberg *et al.*, 1998) of valaciclovir vs. doses of aciclovir shown in two previous randomised, double-blind, placebo-controlled trials to be ineffective against CMV disease, can be interpreted to show that this drug worked best for pre-emptive therapy

(Griffiths *et al.*, 1998). This interpretation was initially controversial but is now supported by natural history studies from three separate research groups, showing that PCR viraemia identifies AIDS patients at high risk of imminent CMV disease. Although highly active antiretroviral therapy (HAART) has revolutionised the prognosis of AIDS patients, cases of CMV disease still occur in developed countries for two reasons. First, many individuals are unaware that they are infected with HIV and present with AIDS-defining conditions including CMV. Second, some patients have progressive HIV disease despite having tried all available antiretroviral compounds. In this latter group, a randomised placebo-controlled trial of pre-emptive therapy with valganciclovir is being conducted by the AIDS Clinical Trial Group (protocol 5030) triggered by the detection on a single occasion of CMV DNA in plasma. This is the first trial to apply the concepts of CMV pathogenesis learned from transplant patients to the parallel group of patients immunocompromised by HIV and the results are awaited with interest. In addition, it is known that the institution of HAART in a patient with asymptomatic CMV viraemia leads to prompt resolution of viraemia (Deayton *et al.*, 1999), so that HAART can be thought of as a form of pre-emptive therapy, analogous to reducing the dose of immunosuppressive drugs in a transplant patient with CMV infection.

Treatment of Established Disease

The treatment of an established disease is the most difficult strategy to pursue successfully, since the virus

Table 2C.14 Comparison of the proposed advantages of prophylaxis and pre-emptive therapy

Proposed advantages of prophylaxis	Proposed advantages of pre-emptive therapy
• Proven benefit in controlled clinical trials — CMV disease — Indirect effects	• Target resources on patients most at need (financial, skill)
• Avoids complicated logistical problems — Real-time laboratory assays — Organisation of sample collection — Geographical location	• Treat when viral load lower — Shorter treatment — Reduced recurrences — Reduced resistance?
• Protects against HSV, VZV	• Allows low level stimulation of immunity—reduces late-onset disease?
• Overall, may be more cost-effective — Cost of laboratory tests — Indirect effects of CMV — Other herpesviruses	• Protects patients non-compliant with prophylaxis
	• May also reduce indirect effects

Table 2C.15 Randomised controlled trials of therapy for established CMV disease

Patient group	Organ affected	Drug 1	Drug 2	Planned duration of therapy (days)	No. of patients		Significant markers of efficacy reported					Reference
					Drug 1	Drug 2	Reduced viraemia	Reduced excretion	Reduced disease	Reduced dissemination	Increased survival	
BMT$_x$	Upper GIT	GCV 2.5 mg/ kg t.d.s.	Placebo	14	18	19	No	Yes	No	No	No	Reed et al. (1990)
AIDS	Retina	GCV 5 mg/kg b.d. 14 d then o.d.	Foscarnet 60 mg/kg t.d.s. 14 d then 90 mg/kg o.d.	14 Induction then maintenance	127	107	ND	ND	No	No	Yes	Anonymous Studies of Ocular Complications of AIDS Research Group (1992)
AIDS	Lower GIT	GCV 5 mg/kg b.d. 14 d then o.d.	Placebo	14	32	30	No	Yes	No*	Yes	No	Dieterich et al. (1993)
AIDS	Retina (relapsed or active retinitis despite maintenance)	GCV 5 mg/kg b.d. 14 d then 10 mg/kg o.d. or foscarnet 90 mg/kg b.d. 14 d then 120 mg/kg o.d.	GCV plus foscarnet: continue existing maintenance dose, add induction dose of second drug for 14 d. For maintenance: GCV 5 mg/kg o.d. foscarnet 90 mg/kg o.d.	Life	183	96	ND	ND	Yes	ND	No	Anonymous Studies of Ocular Complications of AIDS Research Group (1996)

BMT$_x$, bone marrow transplant; GCV, ganciclovir; GIT, gastrointestinal tract; ND, not determined; * intention-to-treat analysis; Yes, subsidiary analysis.

may trigger pathological phenomena unresponsive to antiviral drugs and because extensive tissue damage is often followed by target organ failure and secondary opportunistic agents, which present their own management problems. It is thus salutary to note that, in contrast to the proven benefits of prophylaxis and pre-emptive therapy, no double-blind randomised placebo-controlled trial of anti-CMV therapy in established CMV disease has demonstrated that treatment at this late stage can provide a clinical benefit (see Table 2C.15).

One trial reported that ganciclovir and foscarnet are equipotent for the treatment of CMV retinitis in AIDS patients, but that foscarnet is associated with a significant survival benefit (Anonymous. Studies of Ocular Complications of AIDS Research Group, 1992). Although foscarnet should thus be considered the treatment of choice under these circumstances, the difficulties with intravenous administration, toxicity and cost of foscarnet usually lead clinicians to prescribe ganciclovir instead. This illustrates that the drugs available at present for the treatment of CMV are far from ideal, so the development of safe, orally bioavailable drugs is eagerly awaited. Note also that a randomised trial in AIDS patients showed that the combination of ganciclovir plus foscarnet was superior to either drug given alone (Anonymous. Studies of Ocular Complications of AIDS Research Group, 1996). In the absence of evidence for synergy between these two drugs *in vivo* against CMV (Mattes *et al.*, 2003), this outcome is best interpreted as the earliest example of combination antiretroviral therapy providing a transient clinical benefit against an opportunistic infection.

The management of established CMV retinitis is complex with multiple therapeutic options, including intravitreal injections of antiviral compounds as well as intraocular implantation of a device which slowly releases ganciclovir into the vitreous fluid (reviewed in Jacobson, 1997). These therapeutic options have frequently been evaluated by recruiting patients with peripheral retinitis which is not immediately sight-threatening and randomising them to immediate therapy vs. therapy with the same drug delayed until progression of retinitis has been observed (reviewed in Jacobson, 1997).

Note that CMV lung infection in AIDS patients is not routinely treated because of the theory that they do not mount the cell-mediated response required for immunopathology, and because cohort studies in the pre-HAART era showed no excess mortality among patients with *Pneumocystis carinii* pneumonia who were co-infected with CMV. CMV pneumonitis in allograft patients is treated with immunoglobulin in addition to ganciclovir because components of the preparation may possibly block the immunopathological response to target antigens in the lung.

CMV strains resistant to ganciclovir, ganciclovir plus foscarnet, or to ganciclovir plus foscarnet plus cidofovir, have been described in AIDS patients (Chou *et al.*, 1997). Genetic changes in *UL97* usually confer low-level resistance to ganciclovir. Continued selective pressure may select for *UL54* mutants, some of which are cross-resistant to cidofovir. Rare mutations in *UL54* can confer resistance to both ganciclovir and foscarnet (Chou *et al.*, 1997). Based on knowledge of the replication dynamics of CMV, it was predicted that CMV resistance was a greater problem than had been appreciated in the past and would be found in individuals with high-level replication receiving partially effective antiviral prophylaxis for a long time, e.g. more than 100 days (Emery and Griffiths, 2000). Recent clinical studies in transplant patients confirm this prediction and suggest that approximately 15–25% of patients with CMV disease in transplant (Limaye *et al.*, 2000) and AIDS patients (Bowen *et al.*, 1996; Hu *et al.*, 2002) have ganciclovir-resistant strains.

When HAART is introduced in a patient with established CMV retinitis, an inflammatory reaction may occur, leading to vitritis, which often impairs vision more than the underlying retinitis. This pathological interaction between CMV and the immune system might be avoided if CMV retinitis were prevented by using pre-emptive therapy. Interestingly, no exacerbation or reduction of any other CMV disease has been observed with HAART, whereas an increase in CMV pneumonitis might have been expected if the condition is immunopathologically mediated. In patients receiving ganciclovir maintenance therapy for CMV retinitis, this can be stopped once the CD4 count and HIV viral load have responded to HAART for more than 3 months.

Summary

Different strategies have been described, with advantages and disadvantages for different groups of patients. For transplant patients, several strategies are available and which is chosen by a particular unit will depend upon clinical preference and the laboratory support available (Bowen *et al.*, 1996; Emery, 2001; Hart and Paya, 2001) (Table 2C.14). However, such patients should clearly be managed by one of the proactive strategies (prophylaxis or pre-emptive therapy), since it would be unethical to continue to allow the natural history of CMV disease in these patients to proceed unchecked in the face of overwhelming benefit demonstrated in controlled clinical trials.

REFERENCES

Anonymous. Studies of Ocular Complications of AIDS Research Group (1992) Mortality in patients with the acquired immunodeficiency syndrome treated with either foscarnet or ganciclovir for cytomegalovirus retinitis. *N Engl J Med*, **326**, 213–220.

Anonymous. Studies of Ocular Complications of AIDS Research Group (1996) Combination of foscarnet and ganciclovir therapy vs. monotherapy for the treatment of relapsed cytomegalovirus retinitis in patients with AIDS. The Cytomegalovirus Retreatment Trial (abstr). *Arch Ophthalmol*, **114**, 23–33.

Balfour HH Jr, Chace BA, Stapleton JT *et al.* (1989) A randomized, placebo-controlled trial of oral acyclovir for the prevention of cytomegalovirus disease in recipients of renal allografts. *N Engl J Med*, **320**, 1381–1387.

Baskar JF, Smith PP, Ciment GS *et al.* (1996) Developmental analysis of the cytomegalovirus enhancer in transgenic animals. *J Virol*, **70**, 3215–3226.

Boeckh M, Gooley TA, Myerson D *et al.* (1996) Cytomegalovirus pp65 antigenemia-guided early treatment with ganciclovir versus ganciclovir at engraftment after allogeneic marrow transplantation: a randomized double-blind study. *Blood*, **88**, 4063–4071.

Boppana SB and Britt WJ (1995) Antiviral antibody responses and intrauterine transmission after primary maternal cytomegalovirus infection. *J Infect Dis*, **171**, 1115–1121.

Bowen EF, Sabin CA, Wilson P *et al.* (1997) Cytomegalovirus (CMV) viraemia detected by polymerase chain reaction identifies a group of HIV-positive patients at high risk of CMV disease. *AIDS*, **11**, 889–893.

Bowen EF, Wilson P, Cope A *et al.* (1996) Cytomegalovirus retinitis in AIDS patients: influence of cytomegaloviral load on response to ganciclovir, time to recurrence and survival. *AIDS*, **10**, 1515–1520.

Bresnahan WA and Shenk T (2000) A subset of viral transcripts packaged within human cytomegalovirus particles. *Science*, **288**, 2373–2376.

Britt WJ, Vugler L, Butfiloski E and Stephens EB (1990) Cell surface expression of human cytomegalovirus (HCMV) gp55-116 (gB): use of HCMV-recombinant vaccinia virus-infected cells in analysis of the human neutralizing antibody response. *J Virol*, **64**, 1079–1085.

Cha TA, Tom E, Kemble GW *et al.* (1996) Human cytomegalovirus clinical isolates carry at least 19 genes not found in laboratory strains. *J Virol*, **70**, 78–83.

Chee MS, Bankier AT, Beck S *et al.* (1990) Analysis of the protein-coding content of the sequence of human cytomegalovirus strain AD169. *Curr Top Microbiol Immunol*, **154**, 125–169.

Cheeseman SH, Rubin RH, Stewart A *et al.* (1979) Controlled clinical trial of prophylactic human-leukocyte interferon in renal transplantation. Effects on cytomegalovirus and herpes simplex virus infections. *N Engl J Med*, **300**, 1345–1349.

Chou S, Marousek G, Guentzel S *et al.* (1997) Evolution of mutations conferring multidrug resistance during prophylaxis and therapy for cytomegalovirus disease. *J Infect Dis*, **176**, 786–789.

Cope AV, Sabin C, Burroughs A *et al.* (1997a) Interrelationships among quantity of human cytomegalovirus (HCMV) DNA in blood, donor–recipient serostatus, and administration of methylprednisolone as risk factors for HCMV disease following liver transplantation. *J Infect Dis*, **176**, 1484–1490.

Cope AV, Sweny P, Sabin C *et al.* (1997b) Quantity of cytomegalovirus viruria is a major risk factor for cytomegalovirus disease after renal transplantation. *J Med Virol*, **52**, 200–205.

Deayton J, Mocroft A, Wilson P *et al.* (1999) Loss of cytomegalovirus (CMV) viraemia following highly active antiretroviral therapy in the absence of specific anti-CMV therapy. *AIDS*, **13**, 1203–1206.

Dieterich DT, Kotler DP, Busch DF *et al.* (1993) Ganciclovir treatment of cytomegalovirus colitis in AIDS: a randomized, double-blind, placebo-controlled multicenter study. *J Infect Dis*, **167**, 278–282.

Doniger J, Muralidhar S and Rosenthal LJ (1999) Human cytomegalovirus and human herpesvirus 6 genes that transform and transactivate. *Clin Microbiol Rev*, **12**, 367–382.

Einsele H, Ehninger G, Hebart H *et al.* (1995) Polymerase chain reaction monitoring reduces the incidence of cytomegalovirus disease and the duration and side effects of antiviral therapy after bone marrow transplantation. *Blood*, **86**, 2815–2820.

Emery VC (2001) Prophylaxis for CMV should not now replace pre-emptive therapy in solid organ transplantation. *Rev Med Virol*, **11**, 83–86.

Emery VC, Cope AV, Bowen EF *et al.* (1999) The dynamics of human cytomegalovirus replication *in vivo*. *J Exp Med*, **190**, 177–182.

Emery VC and Griffiths PD (2000) Prediction of cytomegalovirus load and resistance patterns after antiviral chemotherapy. *Proc Nat Acad Sci USA*, **97**, 8039–8044.

Feinberg JE, Hurwitz S, Cooper D *et al.* (1998) A randomized, double-blind trial of valaciclovir prophylaxis for cytomegalovirus disease in patients with advanced human immunodeficiency virus infection. AIDS Clinical Trials Group Protocol 204/Glaxo Wellcome 123-014 International CMV Prophylaxis Study Group. *J Infect Dis*, **177**, 48–56.

Fortunato EA and Spector DH (2002) Viral induction of site-specific chromosome damage (abstr). *Rev Med Virol* (in press).

Fowler KB, Stagno S, Pass RF *et al.* (1992) The outcome of congenital cytomegalovirus infection in relation to maternal antibody status. *N Engl J Med*, **326**, 663–667.

Gane E, Saliba F, Valdecasas GJ *et al.* (1997) Randomised trial of efficacy and safety of oral ganciclovir in the prevention of cytomegalovirus disease in liver-transplant recipients. The Oral Ganciclovir International Transplantation Study Group [corrected]. *Lancet*, **350**, 1729–1733.

Gerna G, Percivalle E, Sarasini A *et al.* (2002) The attenuated Towne strain of human cytomegalovirus may revert to both endothelial cell tropism and leuko- (neutrophil- and monocyte-) tropism *in vitro*. *J Gen Virol*, **83**, 1993–2000.

Ghazel P and Nelson JA (1993) Interactions between cytomegalovirus immediate-early proteins and the long terminal repeat of human immunodeficiency virus. *Rev Med Virol*, **3**, 47–56.

Gilbert GL, Hayes K, Hudson IL and James J (1989) Prevention of transfusion-acquired cytomegalovirus infection in infants by blood filtration to remove leucocytes. Neonatal Cytomegalovirus Infection Study Group. *Lancet*, **1**, 1228–1231.

Gleaves CA, Smith TF, Shuster EA and Pearson GR (1984) Rapid detection of cytomegalovirus in MRC-5 cells inoculated with urine specimens by using low-speed centrifugation and monoclonal antibody to an early antigen. *J Clin Microbiol*, **19**, 917–919.

Gonczol E and Plotkin S (2001) Development of a cytomegalovirus vaccine: lessons from recent clinical trials. *Exp Opin Biol Therap*, **1**, 401–412.

Goodrich JM, Bowden RA, Fisher L *et al.* (1993) Ganciclovir prophylaxis to prevent cytomegalovirus disease after allogeneic marrow transplant. *Ann Intern Med*, **118**, 173–178.

Goodrich JM, Mori M, Gleaves CA *et al.* (1991) Early treatment with ganciclovir to prevent cytomegalovirus disease after allogeneic bone marrow transplantation. *N Engl J Med*, **325**, 1601–1607.

Gor D, Sabin C, Prentice HG *et al.* (1998) Longitudinal fluctuations in cytomegalovirus load in bone marrow transplant patients: relationship between peak virus load, donor/recipient serostatus, acute GVDH and CMV disease. *Bone Marrow Transpl*, **21**, 597–605.

Gretch DR, Kari B, Rasmussen L *et al.* (1988) Identification and characterization of three distinct families of glycoprotein complexes in the envelopes of human cytomegalovirus. *J Virol*, **62**, 875–881.

Griffiths PD (1984) Diagnostic techniques for cytomegalovirus infection. *Clin Haematol*, **13**, 631–644.

Griffiths PD (1998) Studies of viral co-factors for human immunodeficiency virus *in vitro* and *in vivo*. *J Gen Virol*, **79**(2), 213–220.

Griffiths PD and Baboonian C (1984) A prospective study of primary cytomegalovirus infection during pregnancy: final report. *Br J Obstetr Gynaecol*, **91**, 307–315.

Griffiths PD, Feinberg JE, Fry J *et al.* (1998) The effect of valaciclovir on cytomegalovirus viremia and viruria detected by polymerase chain reaction in patients with advanced human immunodeficiency virus disease. AIDS Clinical Trials Group Protocol 204/Glaxo Wellcome 123-014. International CMV Prophylaxis Study Group. *J Infect Dis*, **177**, 57–64.

Griffiths PD, McLean A and Emery VC (2001) Encouraging prospects for immunisation against primary cytomegalovirus infection. *Vaccine*, **19**, 1356–1362.

Griffiths PD, Panjwani DD, Stirk P *et al.* (1984) Rapid diagnosis of cytomegalovirus infection in immunocompromised patients by detection of early antigen fluorescent foci. *Lancet*, **2**, 1242–1245.

Grob JP, Grundy JE, Prentice HG *et al.* (1987) Immune donors can protect marrow-transplant recipients from severe cytomegalovirus infections. *Lancet*, **1**, 774–776.

Grundy JE, Lui SF, Super M *et al.* (1988) Symptomatic cytomegalovirus infection in seropositive kidney recipients: reinfection with donor virus rather than reactivation of recipient virus. *Lancet*, **2**, 132–135.

Guerra B, Lazzarotto T, Quarta S *et al.* (2000) Prenatal diagnosis of symptomatic congenital cytomegalovirus infection. *Am J Obstetr Gynecol*, **183**, 476–482.

Hamprecht K, Maschmann J, Vochem M *et al.* (2001) Epidemiology of transmission of cytomegalovirus from mother to preterm infant by breastfeeding. *Lancet*, **357**, 513–518.

Hart GD and Paya CV (2001) Prophylaxis for CMV should now replace pre-emptive therapy in solid organ transplantation. *Rev Med Virol*, **11**, 73–81.

Hassan-Walker AF, Vargas Cuero AL, Mattes FM *et al.* (2001) CD8$^+$ cytotoxic lymphocyte responses against cytomegalovirus after liver transplantation: correlation with time from transplant to receipt of tacrolimus. *J Infect Dis*, **183**, 835–843.

Hirsch MS, Schooley RT, Cosimi AB, *et al.* (1983) Effects of interferon-alpha on cytomegalovirus reactivation syndromes in renal-transplant recipients. *N Engl J Med*, **308**, 1489–1493.

Hu H, Jabs DA, Forman MS *et al.* (2002) Comparison of cytomegalovirus (CMV) UL97 gene sequences in the blood and vitreous of patients with acquired immunodeficiency syndrome and CMV retinitis. *J Infect Dis*, **185**, 861–867.

Huang ES, Alford CA, Reynolds DW *et al.* (1980) Molecular epidemiology of cytomegalovirus infections in women and their infants. *N Engl J Med*, **303**, 958–962.

Jacobson MA (1997) Treatment of cytomegalovirus retinitis in patients with the acquired immunodeficiency syndrome. *N Engl J Med*, **337**, 105–114.

Keller R, Peitchel R, Goldman JN and Goldman M (1976) An IgG-Fc receptor induced in cytomegalovirus-infected human fibroblasts. *Immunol*, **116**, 772–777.

Kidd IM, Fox JC, Pillay D *et al.* (1993) Provision of prognostic information in immunocompromised patients by routine application of the polymerase chain reaction for cytomegalovirus. *Transplantation*, **56**, 867–871.

Kim WR, Badley AD, Wiesner RH *et al.* (2000) The economic impact of cytomegalovirus infection after liver transplantation. *Transplantation*, **69**, 357–361.

Kimberlin DW, Lin CY, Sanchez PJ *et al.* (2003) Effect of ganciclovir therapy on hearing in symptomatic congenital cytomegalovirus disease involving the central nervous system: a randomized, controlled trial. National Institute of Allergy and Infectious Disease Collaborative Antiviral Study Group. *J Pediatr*, **143**(1): 4–6.

Kondo K, Xu J and Mocarski ES (1996) Human cytomegalovirus latent gene expression in granulocyte-macrophage progenitors in culture and in seropositive individuals. *Proc Natl Acad Sci USA*, **93**, 11137–11142.

Kotenko SV, Saccani S, Izotova LS *et al.* (2000) Human cytomegalovirus harbors its own unique IL-10 homolog (cmvIL-10). *Proc Natl Acad Sci USA*, **97**, 1695–1700.

Limaye AP, Corey L, Koelle DM *et al.* (2000) Emergence of ganciclovir-resistant cytomegalovirus disease among recipients of solid-organ transplants. *Lancet*, **356**, 645–649.

Lowance D, Neumayer HH, Legendre CM *et al.* (1999) Valacyclovir for the prevention of cytomegalovirus disease after renal transplantation. International Valacyclovir Cytomegalovirus Prophylaxis Transplantation Study Group. *N Engl J Med*, **340**, 1462–1470.

Lui SF, Ali AA, Grundy JE *et al.* (1992) Double-blind, placebo-controlled trial of human lymphoblastoid interferon prophylaxis of cytomegalovirus infection in renal transplant recipients. *Nephrol Dialysis Transpl*, **7**, 1230–1237.

Macdonald PS, Keogh AM, Marshman D *et al.* (1995) A double-blind placebo-controlled trial of low-dose ganciclovir to prevent cytomegalovirus disease after heart transplantation. *J Heart Lung Transpl*, **14**, 32–38.

Mattes FM, Hainsworth E, Murdin-Geretti AM *et al.* (2004) A randomized, controlled trial comparing ganciclovir or ganciclovir plus foscarnet (each at half dose) for pre-emptive therapy of cytomegalovirus infection in transplant recipients *J Infect Dis* (in press).

Mattes FM, McLaughlin JE, Emery VC *et al.* (2000) Histopathological detection of owl's eye inclusions is still specific for cytomegalovirus in the era of herpesviruses 6 and 7. *J Clin Pathol*, **53**, 612–614.

Merigan TC, Renlund DG, Keay S *et al.* (1992) A controlled trial of ganciclovir to prevent cytomegalovirus disease after heart transplantation. *N Engl J Med*, **326**, 1182–1186.

Metselaar HJ, Rothbarth PH, Brouwer RM *et al.* (1989) Prevention of cytomegalovirus-related death by passive immunization. A double-blind placebo-controlled study in kidney transplant recipients treated for rejection. *Transplantation*, **48**, 264–266.

Meyers JD, Ljungman P and Fisher LD (1990) Cytomegalovirus excretion as a predictor of cytomegalovirus disease after marrow transplantation: importance of cytomegalovirus viremia. *J Infect Dis*, **162**, 373–380.

Moreno TN, Fortunato EA, Hsia K *et al.* (1997) A model system for human cytomegalovirus-mediated modulation of human immunodeficiency virus type 1 long terminal repeat activity in brain cells. *J Virol*, **71**, 3693–3701.

Moretti S, Zikos P, Van Lint MT *et al.* (1998) Foscarnet vs. ganciclovir for cytomegalovirus (CMV) antigenemia after allogeneic hemopoietic stem cell transplantation (HSCT): a randomised study. *Bone Marrow Transpl*, **22**, 175–180.

Muranyi W, Haas J, Wagner M *et al.* (2002) Cytomegalovirus recruitment of cellular kinases to dissolve the nuclear lamina. *Science*, **297**, 854–857.

Noyola DE, Demmler GJ, Nelson CT *et al.* (2001) Early predictors of neurodevelopmental outcome in symptomatic congenital cytomegalovirus infection. *J Paediatr*, **138**, 325–331.

Ott DE (2002) Potential roles of cellular proteins in HIV-1. *Rev Med Virol* (in press).

Pari GS, Kacica MA and Anders DG (1993) Open reading frames UL44, IRS1/TRS1, and UL36-38 are required for transient complementation of human cytomegalovirus oriLyt-dependent DNA synthesis. *J Virol*, **67**, 2575–2582.

Pass RF, Hutto C, Ricks R and Cloud GA (1986) Increased rate of cytomegalovirus infection among parents of children attending day-care centers. *N Engl J Med*, **314**, 1414–1418.

Pass RF, Stagno S, Britt WJ and Alford CA (1983) Specific cell-mediated immunity and the natural history of congenital infection with cytomegalovirus. *J Infect Dis*, **148**, 953–961.

Paya CV, Wilson JA, Espy MJ *et al.* (2002) Pre-emptive use of oral ganciclovir to prevent cytomegalovirus infection in liver transplant patients: a randomized, placebo-controlled trial. *J Infect Dis*, **185**, 854–860.

Pescovitz MD, Rabkin J, Merion RM *et al.* (2000) Valganciclovir results in improved oral absorption of ganciclovir in liver transplant recipients. *Antimicrob Agents Chemother*, **44**, 2811–2815.

Pleskoff O, Treboute C, Brelot A *et al.* (1997) Identification of a chemokine receptor encoded by human cytomegalovirus as a co-factor for HIV-1 entry. *Science*, **276**, 1874–1878.

Plotkin SA, Starr SE, Friedman HM *et al.* (1991) Effect of Towne live virus vaccine on cytomegalovirus disease after renal transplant. A controlled trial. *Ann Intern Med*, **114**, 525–531.

Prentice HG, Gluckman E, Powles RL *et al.* (1994) Impact of long-term acyclovir on cytomegalovirus infection and survival after allogeneic bone marrow transplantation. European Acyclovir for CMV Prophylaxis Study Group. *Lancet*, **343**, 749–753.

Rayes N, Seehofer D, Schmidt CA *et al.* (2001) Prospective randomized trial to assess the value of pre-emptive oral therapy for CMV infection following liver transplantation. *Transplantation*, **72**, 881–885.

Razonable RR, Brown RA, Wilson J *et al.* (2002) The clinical use of various blood compartments for cytomegalovirus (CMV) DNA quantitation in transplant recipients with CMV disease. *Transplantation*, **73**, 968–973.

Reed EC, Wolford JL, Kopecky KJ *et al.* (1990) Ganciclovir for the treatment of cytomegalovirus gastroenteritis in bone marrow transplant patients. A randomized, placebo-controlled trial. *Ann Intern Med*, **112**, 505–510.

Reusser P, Einsele H, Lee J *et al.* (2002) Randomized multicenter trial of foscarnet versus ganciclovir for pre-emptive therapy of cytomegalovirus infection after allogeneic stem cell transplantation. *Blood*, **99**, 1159–1164.

Revello MG, Sarasini A, Zavattoni M *et al.* (1998) Improved prenatal diagnosis of congenital human cytomegalovirus infection by a modified nested polymerase chain reaction. *J Med Virol*, **56**, 99–103.

Roback JD (2002) CMV and blood transfusions. *Rev Med Virol*, **12**, 211–219.

Schmidt GM, Horak DA, Niland JC *et al.* (1991) A randomized controlled trial of prophylactic ganciclovir for cytomegalovirus pulmonary infection in recipients of allogeneic bone marrow transplants; the City of Hope–Stanford–Syntex CMV Study Group. *N Engl J Med*, **324**, 1005–1011.

Shinkai M, Bozzette SA, Powderly W *et al.* (1997) Utility of urine and leukocyte cultures and plasma DNA polymerase chain reaction for identification of AIDS patients at risk for developing human cytomegalovirus disease. *J Infect Dis*, **175**, 302–308.

Singh N, Paterson DL, Gayowski T *et al.* (2000) Cytomegalovirus antigenemia directed pre-emptive prophylaxis with oral versus i.v. ganciclovir for the prevention of cytomegalovirus disease in liver transplant recipients: a randomized, controlled trial. *Transplantation*, **70**, 717–722.

Snydman DR, Werner BG, Dougherty NN *et al.* (1993) Cytomegalovirus immune globulin prophylaxis in liver transplantation. A randomized, double-blind, placebo-controlled trial. The Boston Center for Liver Transplantation CMVIG Study Group. *Ann Intern Med*, **119**, 984–991.

Soderberg-Naucler C, Fish KN and Nelson JA (1997) Reactivation of latent human cytomegalovirus by allogeneic stimulation of blood cells from healthy donors. *Cell*, **91**, 119–126.

Spector SA, McKinley GF, Lalezari JP *et al.* (1996) Oral ganciclovir for the prevention of cytomegalovirus disease in persons with AIDS. Roche Cooperative Oral Ganciclovir Study Group. *N Engl J Med*, **334**, 1491–1497.

Spiller OB, Hanna SM, Devine DV, Tufaro F (1997) Neutralization of cytomegalovirus virions: the role of complement. *J Infect Dis*, **176**, 339–347.

Stagno S (1990) Cytomegalovirus (abstr). *Infect Dis Fetus Newborn Infant*, 240–281.

Stagno S, Pass RF, Cloud G *et al.* (1986) Primary cytomegalovirus infection in pregnancy. Incidence, transmission to fetus, and clinical outcome. *J Am Med Assoc*, **256**, 1904–1908.

Stagno S, Reynolds D, Tsiantos A *et al.* (1975a) Cervical cytomegalovirus excretion in pregnant and nonpregnant women: suppression in early gestation. *J Infect Dis*, **131**, 522–527.

Stagno S, Reynolds DW, Pass RF and Alford CA (1980) Breast milk and the risk of cytomegalovirus infection. *N Engl J Med*, **302**, 1073–1076.

Stagno S, Reynolds DW, Tsiantos A *et al.* (1975b) Comparative serial virologic and serologic studies of symptomatic and subclinical congenitally and natally acquired cytomegalovirus infections. *J Infect Dis*, **132**, 568–577.

Stenberg RM and Stinski MF (1985) Autoregulation of the human cytomegalovirus major immediate-early gene. *J Virol*, **56**, 676–682.

Stratton KR (2000) *Vaccines for the 21st Century*, pp 1–460. National Academy Press, Washington.

Streblow DN, Soderberg-Naucler C, Vieira J *et al.* (1999) The human cytomegalovirus chemokine receptor US28 mediates vascular smooth muscle cell migration. *Cell*, **99**, 511–520.

Sullivan V, Talarico CL, Stanat SC, *et al.* (1992) A protein kinase homologue controls phosphorylation of ganciclovir in human cytomegalovirus-infected cells. *Nature*, **359**, 85.

van den Berg AP, Klompmaker LJ, Haagsma EB *et al.* (1991) Antigenemia in the diagnosis and monitoring of active cytomegalovirus infection after liver transplantation. *J Infect Dis*, **164**, 265–270.

Wertheim P, Buurman C, Geelen J *et al.* (1983) Transmission of cytomegalovirus by renal allograft demonstrated by restriction enzyme analysis. *Lancet*, **1**, 980–981.

Whitley RJ, Cloud G, Gruber W *et al.* (1997) Ganciclovir treatment of symptomatic congenital cytomegalovirus infection: results of a phase II study. National Institute of Allergy and Infectious Diseases Collaborative Antiviral Study Group. *J Infect Dis*, **175**, 1080–1086.

Winston DJ, Ho WG, Bartoni K *et al.* (1993) Ganciclovir prophylaxis of cytomegalovirus infection and disease in allogeneic bone marrow transplant recipients. Results of a placebo-controlled, double-blind trial. *Ann Intern Med*, **118**, 179–184.

Winston DJ, Huang ES, Miller M *et al.* (1985) Molecular epidemiology of cytomegalovirus infections associated with bone marrow transplantation. *Ann Intern Med*, **102**, 16–20.

Winston DJ, Wirin D, Shaked A and Busuttil RW (1995) Randomised comparison of ganciclovir and high-dose acyclovir for long-term cytomegalovirus prophylaxis in liver-transplant recipients. *Lancet*, **346**, 69–74.

Yeager AS, Palumbo PE, Malachowski N *et al.* (1983) Sequelae of maternally derived cytomegalovirus infections in premature infants. *J Paediatr*, **102**, 918–922.

Yurochko AD, Hwang ES, Rasmussen L *et al.* (1997) The human cytomegalovirus UL55 (gB) and UL75 (gH) glycoprotein ligands initiate the rapid activation of Sp1 and NF-κB during infection. *J Virol*, **71**, 5051–5059.

2D

Epstein–Barr Virus

Dorothy H. Crawford
University of Edinburgh, UK

INTRODUCTION

The discovery of Epstein–Barr virus (EBV) in 1964 resulted from the description by Denis Burkitt of a geographically restricted tumour occurring in African children (Burkitt, 1958). The tumour, which characteristically arises in the jaw, is now known to be of B lymphocyte origin and is called Burkitt's lymphoma (BL). Burkitt noticed that the geographical distribution of the tumour in Africa corresponded to that of holoendemic malaria, and was determined by the climatic conditions (high temperature and high rainfall) in which the malaria-carrying mosquito can breed. Because of this observation, Burkitt suggested that the tumour had an infectious aetiological agent for which the mosquito was the vector. This hypothesis led to electron microscopic studies on fresh tumour biopsy material, but this technique was unrewarding. Later, cell lines were grown in suspension culture from BL tumour material (Epstein and Barr, 1964) and in these cells virus particles were seen (Epstein *et al.*, 1964). Further studies showed this to be a new and distinct member of the herpesvirus group. Thus, Burkitt's initial postulate of an infectious agent being involved in the aetiology of the tumour proved to be correct and, although the mosquito does not play the role of vector for the virus, the association with hyperendemic malaria remains an important and constant finding.

Seroepidemiological studies have since shown that the virus is a ubiquitous agent; seropositivity increases with age in all communities studied, so that over 90% of adults worldwide are seropositive. When carrying out these studies Henle and Henle (1966) made the observation that a member of their staff seroconverted while undergoing an attack of acute infectious mononucleosis (IM). Further studies in collaboration with Yale University on college students proved that EBV is the sole aetiological agent in IM (Niederman *et al.*, 1970).

Early seroepidemiological and molecular studies also pinpointed an association between EBV infection and anaplastic nasopharyngeal carcinoma (NPC) (Old *et al.*, 1966; Wolf *et al.*, 1973), a geographically and genetically restricted tumour which is very common in southern China. However, for this tumour, as for BL, EBV does not act as the sole aetiological agent but is probably one of several necessary co-factors in the evolution of the tumour.

Since its discovery EBV has been associated with a variety of other lymphoid and epithelial tumours. These include lymphoproliferative lesions and lymphoma which develop in immunocompromised individuals (Crawford *et al.*, 1980), certain types of T cell lymphoma (Jones *et al.*, 1988), a subset of Hodgkin's lymphoma (Anagnostopoulos *et al.*, 1989) as well as a minority of gastric carcinomas (Tokunaga *et al.*, 1993). The benign epithelial lesion of oral hairy leukoplakia also contains replicating EBV (Greenspan *et al.*, 1985).

THE VIRUS

Structure

EBV is a DNA virus, which is a member of the family *Herpesviridae*, subfamily *Gammaherpesvirinae*, genus *Lymphocryptovirus*, showing a structure indistinguishable from other human herpesviruses by electron

Principles and Practice of Clinical Virology, Fifth Edition. Edited by A. J. Zuckerman, J. E. Banatvala, J. R. Pattison, P. D. Griffiths and B. D. Schoub
© 2004 John Wiley & Sons Ltd   ISBN 0 470 84338 1

microscopy. It is a large virus with a buoyant density in caesium chloride of 1.2–1.3 and a molecular weight of 100×10^6 Da. The central nucleic acid of the virion is surrounded by an icosahedral capsid consisting of 162 triangular capsomeres and measuring 100 nm in diameter (Figure 2D.1). This, in turn, is surrounded by an outer, irregularly shaped, lipid-containing envelope giving the mature particle a diameter of 150–200 nm. The viral envelope is derived from cellular membranes of infected cells and is acquired by budding of immature particles through the cell membrane. The envelope is essential for infectivity, and the sensitivity of the virus to ether and other lipid solvents results from its destruction.

The Viral Genome

The EBV genome is a linear double-stranded DNA molecule of 184 kb in length. Structurally the genome consists of alternating unique and internal tandem

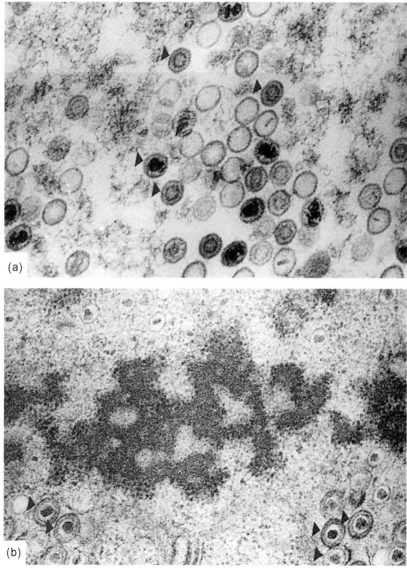

Figure 2D.1   Electron micrographs of the thin section of cells form an EB virus-immortalised lymphoblastoid cell line (M-ABA). Arrows indicate (a) immature virus particles and (b) enveloped virus-particles ($\times 39\,000$)

repeat regions flanked by terminal repeat (TR) sequences (Figure 2D.2). The genome sequence shows around 70 predicted open reading frames, which are designated by a four-letter and number acronym, e.g. BZLF1 refers to the first leftward open reading frame of the *Bam*HZ fragment of the genome (Baer *et al.*, 1984). Two strains of EBV have been defined—type 1 and type 2 (alternatively named A and B), which differ at the domains which code for the EB viral latent proteins. Although these types show no specific geographical restriction, in Western countries type 1 viruses are more commonly isolated than type 2. *In vitro* type 1 viruses are more efficient at immortalising B lymphocytes than type 2; however, neither type has a specific disease association. Variation within types occurs in the number of repeat sequences in each internal repeat, making it possible to define specific isolates by the size of their latent genes and/or their products. Analysis of these genes can therefore be used in epidemiological studies to monitor virus transmission within families or populations.

Following infection of B lymphocytes *in vitro*, EBV establishes a latent type of infection, with immortalisation of the cell and a restricted (latent) viral gene expression compatible with continued cell proliferation. The viral genome does not usually integrate into cellular DNA but forms a closed circular episome by covalent linkage of the terminal repeat elements. The episome replicates to give multiple copies shortly after infection and thereafter resides in the nucleus and replicates with cellular DNA, with equal partitioning to daughter cells allowing the copy number per clone to remain constant. These episomal forms can be activated to a lytic infection with the release of multiple viral progeny and cell death (Figure 2D.3).

Viral-coded Proteins

The viral genome is large enough to code for around 70 average-sized proteins, but not all of these have been identified and assigned to open reading frames on the viral genome. Nine viral-coded proteins are expressed in latently infected cells (Table 2D.1; Figure 2D.2) in addition to the classical herpesvirus immediate-early, early and late proteins associated with the lytic infection. The EBV genome also codes for two small RNA species (EBERS) which form abundant transcripts that are untranslated. Their function is unknown. In addition a complex series of spliced transcripts from the *Bam*A region of the genome is found in latently infected cells, but it is

uncertain whether any of these are translated into proteins.

Latent Proteins
(reviewed in detail in Bornkamm and Hammerschmidt, 2000)

The EB viral nuclear antigens (EBNAs) were first detected by anticomplementary immunofluorescence in the nuclei of latently infected EBV immortalised B cells (Reedman and Klein, 1973) (Figure 2D.4), and were subsequently identified as six separate proteins (EBNA1, EBNA2, EBNA3A, EBNA3B, EBNA3C; and leader protein (LP), also called EBNA1–6) which are translated from a long polycystronic mRNA by alternative splicing. EBNA1, EBNA2, EBNA3A and EBNA3C are required for *in vitro* B cell immortalisation, whereas EBNA3B and EBNALP are not (Table 2D.1).

EBNA 1 is coded by the *Bam*K open reading frame and characterised by a 20–45 kDa glycine–alanine (Gly–Ala) repeat sequence, which varies in length, causing the molecular weight of the protein to vary between viral isolates (65–85 kDa). The protein binds to the viral origin of replication and to metaphase chromosomes, thereby accounting for EBV episomal maintenance within the infected cell and equal partitioning into daughter cells at cell division. EBNA1 is essential for *in vitro* immortalisation of B cells and, although no oncogenic function has been attributed to the protein, mice expressing EBNA1 as a transgene in B cells have been reported to develop lymphoma (Wilson *et al.*, 1996).

The Gly–Ala repeat in EBNA1 renders the protein resistant to degradation in the proteosome. Thus, no EBNA1 peptides are displayed on the cell surface and cells expressing EBNA1 are not targets for cytotoxic T cells (Levitskaya *et al.*, 1995).

EBNA2 is an 86 kDa protein which is coded for by the *Bam*WYH open reading frames. Expression of EBNA2 is essential for immortalisation and the protein plays a pivotal role in this event by transactivating all the other latent viral genes. In addition, EBNA2 activates cellular genes, including the B cell activation antigens CD21 and CD23 and the oncogenes c-myc and c-fgr.

EBNA3A, EBNA3B, EBNA3C are a family of related proteins coded for by the BERF open reading frame, with molecular weights of 140–180 kDa. All three proteins inhibit transcriptional activation of EBNA2-responsive genes, thereby counterbalancing

Table 2D.1 EBV-coded latent proteins

Antigen complex	Molecular weight ($\times 10^{-3}$)	Expressed in:			
		BL	NPL	HD	PTLD
EB nuclear antigen (EBNA)					
1	65–97	+	+	+	+
2	75–105	−	−	−	+
3A	130–195	−	−	−	+
3B	145–160	−	−	−	+
3C	130–195	−	−	−	+
LP	20–130	−	−	−	+
Latent membrane protein (LMP)					
1	58–63	−	±	+	+
2A	54	−	+	+	+
2B	40	−	+	+	+

EBNA3A, EBNA3B, EBNA3C are also termed EBNA3, EBNA4 and EBNA6 respectively.
Leader protein (LP) is also termed EBNA5.
LMP2A and LMP2B are also termed terminal proteins 1 and 2.
BL, Burkitt's lymphoma; NPC, nasopharyngeal carcinoma; HD, Hodgkin's disease; PTLD, post-transplant lymphoproliferative disease.

the action of EBNA2. However, only EBNA3A and EBNA3C are essential for the immortalisation of B cells.

EBNA-LP is coded for by the BWRF1 open reading frame, which also forms the leader sequence of the EBNA RNAs. Because of multiple repeat regions in the DNA, EBNA-LP varies in size (20–130 kDa). The protein is not absolutely essential for immortalisation but enhances the immortalisation of infected B cells by complementing the growth-promoting effects of EBNA2.

Latent Membrane Proteins (LMPs)

LMP1 is coded for by the BNLF1 gene, and its expression is induced by EBNA2. BNLF1 is the most abundantly transcribed region of the genome in latently infected cells. The protein is mainly located in the plasma membrane of infected cells, where it associates with the cytoskeleton.

Structurally, LMP1 has six membrane-spanning domains with both the amino- and carboxy-termini in the cytoplasm. LMP1 is essential for the immortalisation and continued proliferation of B cells, and induces a tumourigenic phenotype on transfection into rodent fibroblasts. When transfected in B cells, LMP1 upregulates expression of the cell adhesion molecules, CD23 and CD40, inducing B cell activation and DNA synthesis. These changes mimic those seen following CD40-mediated B cell activation, many of which, in both cases are mediated by tumour necrosis factor receptor-associated factor (TRAF)-signalling molecules and the transcription factor NF-κB. The amino-terminus is essential for these effects, and a truncated form of LMP1 lacking this region, which is expressed in lytic infection and located in the viral envelope, lacks these properties. When transfected into squamous epithelial cell lines, LMP1 induces the membrane receptor molecules CD40 and the EGF receptor and inhibits terminal differentiation processes.

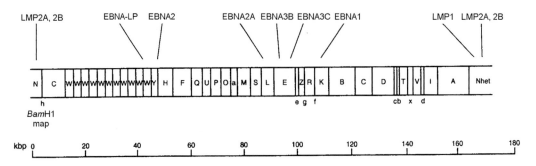

Figure 2D.2 Linear map of the EB virus genome, showing the open reading frames for the major latent proteins

Sequence analysis of the LMP1 gene in EBV isolates from different tumours and geographical locations has identified a common 30 bp deletion in the C-terminus as well as several point mutations when compared to the prototype genome. It has been suggested that this deletion increases the oncogenicity of the virus and is found at high frequency in EBV-associated malignancies (Chen *et al.*, 1992). However, other studies indicate that the incidence of the deletion in tumours does not exceed the level found in the healthy population in a particular geographical area (Khanim *et al.*, 1996).

LMP2A and LMP2B (also called terminal proteins 1 and 2) are formed by alternative splicing from an open reading frame which spans the terminal repeat sequences, and thus the intact gene is only formed and transcribed after the genome has circularised. Both are membrane proteins with 12 membrane-spanning segments, but whereas LMP2A has an amino-terminus of 119 amino acids, this is truncated in LMP2B. The amino-terminus of LMP2A associates with protein tyrosine kinases, and this interaction is thought to inhibit activation of infected B cells and thereby inhibit lytic viral replication and promote cell survival and maintenance of latency. The function of LMP2B is unknown.

Lytic Cycle Proteins

EBV lytic genes show extensive homology to those of other herpesviruses, and their expression similarly follows an orderly cascade, with the expression of each set being activated by the previous set and inhibited by the following set. They are divided into immediate-early, early and late, according to whether they are transcribed before (immediate-early and early) or after (late) viral DNA synthesis.

Immediate-early genes. EBV possesses two genes that can be classified as immediate-early genes, BZLF1 (Z) and BRLF1 (R), which together transactivate the early genes and thereby effect the switch from latent to lytic infection in B cells.

Early genes. First identified by the staining pattern of sera containing antibodies to EBV when applied to the Raji cell line, which lacks expression of the late genes, the early gene products (early antigens, EA) were characterised as diffuse (D) (nuclear and cytoplasmic staining) and restricted (R) (nuclear staining) (Henle *et al.*, 1971). It is now known that there are around 30 early proteins, most of which have enzyme functions required for viral DNA replication.

Late genes—viral capsid proteins. This antigen complex (VCA) consists of the non-glycosylated viral structural proteins but these have not yet been analysed in detail because of the lack of a fully lytic *in vitro* system for EBV. The major capsid protein is coded for by the BcLF1 open reading frame.

VCA can be detected by indirect immunofluorescence in around 10% of cells in a permissive cell line, such as P3HR1, using an EBV-positive human serum.

EBV glycoproteins. The EBV-coded glycoproteins are involved in viral infectivity and spread. Ten have been identified, most of which are inserted into membranes in an infected cell, and several of these become components of the viral envelope (membrane antigens, MA).

The major envelope glycoprotein gp340/220 is coded for by the BLLF1 open reading frame. The protein mediates virus attachment to the B cell surface by binding to the EBV receptor CR2 (also called CD21). Antibodies to gp340/220 prevent infection by blocking attachment, and the protein has therefore been developed as a vaccine candidate.

Gp110 is coded for by the BALF4 open reading frame and has homology with the herpes simplex virus (HSV) glycoprotein gB. It is localised in nuclear and cytoplasmic membranes of infected cells but is not detected in the viral envelope.

Gp85 is coded for by the BXLF2 open reading frame. It has homology to HSV glycoprotein gH and induces fusion between viral and cellular membranes. Gp85 requires another glycoprotein, gp25 (homologous to HSV gL), for its transport to the cell surface. Here it forms a trimolecular complex with gp42 and gp25, which is also present in the viral envelope. The complex mediates B cell infection by inducing fusion between viral and cellular membranes (gp85 and gp25) and viral penetration by binding to HLA class II molecules in the B cell surface (gp42). Gp42 is not required for infection of epithelial cells, which are HLA class II negative (Borza and Hutt-Fletcher 2002).

Human Homologues

EBV codes for homologues of human interleukin (IL)-10 (BCRF1, expressed late in the lytic cycle), and the cell survival gene bcl2 (BHRF1, coding for an early protein), which are thought to be important in immune evasion and cell survival respectively.

Host Range and Growth In Vitro

The host range of EBV is limited to man, its natural host, and some subhuman primates, including the gibbon, owl monkey, squirrel monkey and some species of tamarin, all of which can be infected experimentally.

In humans only B lymphocytes are regularly infected by the virus and this restriction of infection is probably accounted for by their expression of CR2 (the receptor for the C3d component of complement, also called CD21) the cell surface receptor used by EBV. A similar molecule found in a subpopulation of squamous epithelial cells may result in infection of these cells in the oropharyngeal cavity, although the extent and role of this infection in normal individuals is a controversial issue. Activated T cells and dendritic cells also express CR2 and may on rare occasions support EBV infection.

The classical method for demonstrating infectious virus in patient samples is the lymphocyte 'immortalisation' test, in which lymphocytes from EBV-negative donors are exposed to the filtered sample and then cultured. The presence of virus in the sample is indicated by the outgrowth of immortalised B cells into a lymphoblastoid cell line (see below). The technique is very time-consuming and slow to give results, and is therefore not recommended for routine use. A more rapid test enumerates the number of infected cells in an EBV negative B cell line 72 h after infection by staining for EBNA antigens. Polymerase chain reaction (PCR) detection of EBV DNA has virtually replaced these tests as a quicker and more sensitive assay; however, a positive PCR result does not necessarily denote infectivity.

EBV Immortalisation

When EBV is used to infect B lymphocytes *in vitro*, cell activation occurs within 24 h (Figure 2D.3). Initially, small resting B cells undergo blastogenesis, with an increase in HLA-DR expression, nuclear size and cytoplasmic volume, and the expression of B cell activation antigens on the cell surface. In particular, CD23 expression is reported to be essential for immortalisation. After 36 h DNA synthesis is initiated and cell division takes place at around 72 h. Around this time, immunoglobulin (Ig) can be detected in the cytoplasm of many infected B cells and it is subsequently secreted into the culture medium; IgM always predominates. This latter finding indicates that EBV is a potent polyclonal activator of Ig production by B cells. These early changes seen in B cells after infection with EBV are similar to those seen after stimulation with other B cell activators, such as the CD40 ligand. However, the polyclonal activa-

tion of B cells by EBV leads to immortalisation, which is a permanent rather than a transient event. Thus, once DNA synthesis is initiated, the cells will continue to proliferate in culture as EBV-positive B lymphoblastoid cell lines (LCLs).

EBNA2 and -LP are the first viral antigens to be detected in infected B cells, appearing as early as 12 h post-infection, and followed by the expression of all the other nuclear antigens by 24 h. LMP1 becomes detectable in these cells around 48 h post-infection; the kinetics of LMP2A and LMP2B expression is unknown. This viral gene expression (EBNA1, EBNA2, EBNA3A, EBNA3B, EBNA3C, EBNA-LP; LMP1, LMP2A and LMP2B) is seen in virtually all cells in an LCL and is termed 'full latent gene expression' or 'latency type 3' (Figure 2D.3). Two other forms of EBV latency exist; expression of EBNA1 only (latency 1) seen in BL cells, and EBNA1, LMP1, LMP2A (latency 2), seen in NPC and HD.

Only a minority ($< 1-10\%$) of cells in an LCL at any one time enter a productive phase resulting in viral progeny and cell death. LCL derived from different sources show varying degrees of permissiveness for viral replication. Tamarin-derived cell lines are the most permissive, with around 10% of lytically infected cells, and the tamarin B cell line B95-8, which was originally immortalised with IM-derived EBV, is used in most laboratories to obtain infectious virus for experimental purposes. Virus production into the culture supernanant medium can be induced by the addition of tetradecanoylphorbol-13-acetate (TPA) and sodium butyrate. Another cell line which can be induced to produce high levels of EBV, by the addition of antibodies to surface immunoglobulin, is BL-derived Akata.

Handling of EBV in the Laboratory

EBV is used as a tool for immortalising B lymphocytes *in vitro*, and EBV-positive cell lines, most of which produce small quantities of infectious virus, are grown in many laboratories for use in various assay systems. There is therefore general concern about the safety precautions necessary for handling this type of material. In this context it must be remembered that around 90% of the adult population have been infected by the virus and will continue to carry it as a lifelong infection of B lymphocytes and to excrete infectious virus particles into saliva. In addition, the virus is of low infectivity, and no authenticated cases of primary infection contracted in the laboratory have

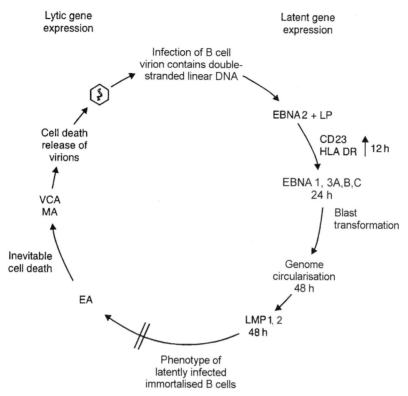

Figure 2D.3 EB virus gene expression and cellular events after infection of a resting B cell. EBNA, EB viral nuclear antigen; LMP, latent membrane protein; EA, early antigens; MA, membrane antigens; VCA, viral capsid antigens

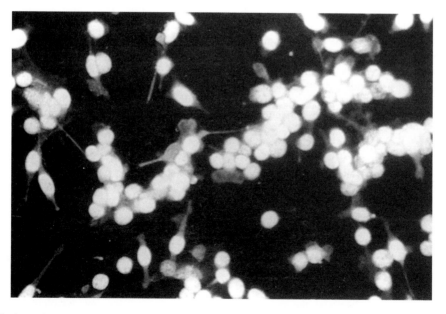

Figure 2D.4 A photomicrograph of cells from an EB virus immortalised adherent lymphoblastoid cell line (MABA) stained for EBNA. Bright nuclear fluorescence is seen in all cells. The cells are counterstained with Evans Blue ($\times$ 70)

been reported. EBV is classified as a hazard group 2 pathogen and therefore EBV-positive cell lines should be handled according to routine microbiological laboratory practice for this group.

EPIDEMIOLOGY

In seroepidemiological studies the presence or absence of IgG antibodies to VCA is generally used to screen sera, since these antibodies arise early in primary infection and thereafter persist for life. UK results show that seropositivity increases with age, reaching a level of around 90% in adults. Two peaks of seroconversion occur, one at 1–6 years and the other at 14–20 years (Figure 2D.5), with infection occurring later in high compared to low socioeconomic groups. These findings are very similar to those from other countries in the Western world. In developing countries seroconversion occurs early in life, with more than 90% of children over the age of 2 years being seropositive. Most seroconversions occur subclinically, but if primary infection is delayed until adolescence or early adult life, acute infectious mononucleosis may result.

EBV Infection in the Normal Seropositive Individual

In most individuals primary infection occurs subclinically during childhood, and thereafter a life-long carrier state exists in which a balance is maintained between the level of virus infection and the cellular and humoral immune mechanisms which keep the infection controlled. Continued low-grade virus shedding in the oropharynx can be found in most seropositive individuals and can be detected by the isolation of immortalising virus or the presence of viral DNA from saliva and throat washings. Furthermore, EBV DNA is present in circulating B cells and when large numbers of these are cultured from seropositive individuals, 'spontaneously immortalised' EBV-positive cell lines may arise, indicating the presence of a few cells capable of producing EBV in the culture. The origin and longevity of these circulating, infected B cells is much disputed; however, recent experimental evidence suggests that the virus establishes a stable, latent infection in a population of long-lived memory B cells. These cells evade immune surveillance mechanisms by expressing a very restricted number of genes; however, details of the exact gene expression have not been elucidated. Periodic reactivation of this latent B cell infection into lytic replication in

lymphoepithelial sites such as the tonsil, perhaps in association with B cell activation/maturation processes, would allow new virus production and replenishment of latently infected cells, and egress from the body.

EBV-specific, HLA class I-restricted, CD8-positive cytotoxic T cells are present in the circulation of all normal seropositive individuals. Many latent and lytic T cell epitopes have been identified, but the EBNA1 protein is not recognised due to a resistance to degradation by the proteosome. Thus, a life-long balance between virus infection and immune mechanisms is established which successfully controls the infection at subclinical levels in the healthy host. However, if this balance is altered by intercurrent disease or iatrogenic means which cause a decrease in the specific immune response, EBV-associated disease may occur.

EBV-ASSOCIATED DISEASES

EBV is an unusual virus in that it is associated with several disease states, in some of which it is the direct aetiological agent, whilst in others it acts as an essential co-factor in a complex series of events which lead to the disease. The EBV-associated tumours are shown in Table 2D.2. Infectious mononucleosis is the result of primary infection, whereas Burkitt's lymphoma and nasopharyngeal carcinoma occur in seropositive individuals as a result of a series of alterations in a cell type infected by EBV. Oral hairy leukoplakia and lymphoproliferative lesions occur in seropositive individuals in whom immunosuppression has allowed the cell populations naturally harbouring the virus to expand.

More recently, EBV has been associated with a variety of diseases, including subsets of T cell lymphomas (Jones *et al.*, 1988), Hodgkin's lymphoma (Anagnostopoulos *et al.*, 1989), and carcinoma of the stomach (Imai *et al.*, 1994). Here the tumour cells harbour viral DNA and express viral antigens; however, the exact role of the virus in these malignancies is still unclear. Further associations have been described with salivary gland tumours (Raab-Traub *et al.*, 1991), thymomas (Leywraz *et al.*, 1985) and leiomyosarcomas in immunodeficient children (Lee *et al.*, 1995).

Infectious Mononucleosis

Infectious mononucleosis (IM), or glandular fever, is an acute, self-limiting lymphoproliferative disease resulting from primary infection with EBV. It classically occurs in adolescents and young adults (15–25

Table 2D.2 EBV-associated tumours

Tumour	At risk population	EBV association
Lymphoid origin		
B lymphoproliferative disease (BLPD)	Post-transplant LPD	>90%
	HIV infection—primary central nervous system lymphoma	<100%
	—peripheral lymphoma	50%
Burkitt's lymphoma (BL)	African children—endemic BL	97%
	HIV infection—sporadic BL	25%
Hodgkin's disease (HD)	Children—developing countries	Overall 65%
	Young adults—high SE[1] groups	Mixed cellularity type 80%
	—history of IM	
T/NK cell lymphoma	Chronic active EBV	10–100% depending on histological type
	HIV infection	
Primary effusion lymphoma	HIV infection	70–80%; 100% contain HHV8 DNA
Non-lymphoid origin		
Nasopharyngeal carcinoma	S. Chinese and Inuit races—high incidence	Non-keratinised 100%
	Mayaks, Dyaks, Indonesians, Filipinos Vietnamese—moderate incidence	Keratinised 30–100%
Gastric carcinoma	Not identified	Adenocarcinoma 5–15%
Leiomyosarcoma	HIV infection / Immunodeficiency — mainly children	Not known

[1]SE, socio-economic.

years) in Western societies, where a susceptible seronegative population is present in this age group. Studies from the UK and USA in the 1970s showed that approximately 40% of school-leavers were EBV-seronegative (Figure 2D.5), and that clinical disease occurred in 50–74% of these individuals undergoing a primary infection, whereas the remainder (in common with most individuals before adolescence) seroconverted without overt clinical illness (University Health Physicians and Public Health Laboratory Service Laboratories, 1971). However, changing demography and life styles in the intervening 30 years is likely to have changed this pattern, and further studies are required to investigate this. Since the majority of those reaching the susceptible age for IM in the Western world are already seropositive, classical outbreaks of the disease are uncommon. The disease is more common in upper socioeconomic classes and in the Western world because these individuals have been relatively protected from infection during childhood.

Seroepidemiology

Following the original observation of a seroconversion in one individual at the time of an attack of IM (Henle and Henle, 1966) a large study was undertaken on serial serum samples from students at Yale University (Niederman *et al.*, 1970). The results of this study showed that: (a) no student having antibodies to EBV-associated antigens at entry to university later suffered from IM; (b) no student leaving the university without antibodies had suffered from IM during the years at university; and (c) about 50% of those who acquired EBV-specific antibodies during their years at university had clinical IM at the time of seroconversion. The other 50% seroconverted without significant illness. These data confirmed the causative role of EBV in IM.

Transmission

Detection of immortalising EBV in multiple samples of saliva and throat washings indicates that oral excretion of the virus occurs either continuously or intermittently in most seropositive individuals. It is therefore assumed that primary infection occurs by the oral route, by close contact with a virus-excreting individual. Childhood infection probably occurs through salivary contact with family members or other children, whereas the peak of seroconversion in late adolescence, which coincides with the age at which new social contacts are often made, is likely to occur during kissing. However, EBV has also been rescued from the uterine cervix of a few IM patients and normal seropositive women (Sixbey *et al.*, 1986), and from

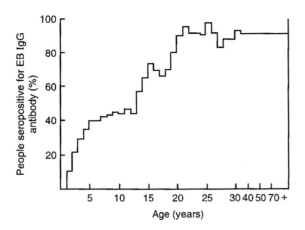

Figure 2D.5 Histogram analysis of IgG anti-VCA antibodies in sera from 1469 individuals. The percentage of seropositivity increases with age to a plateau of 92%

semen from healthy males (Israele *et al.*, 1991), suggesting that sexual intercourse is a possible route of spread. This is backed up by recent data from a large study in university students showing a strong correlation of previous sexual intercourse with EBV seropositivity and IM (Crawford *et al.*, 2002). IM can also be acquired by transfusion of fresh blood or organ transplantation from a seropositive to a seronegative individual.

Pathogenesis

EBV usually enters the body through the mouth, and a productive infection occurs in the oropharynx, from which site infectious virus particles are shed into the oral cavity and can be recovered from saliva and throat washings. Currently there is much debate regarding the cell type first infected by EBV. Extensive examination of IM tonsils reveals infected B cells expressing lytic antigens, but no infection of the overlying epithelium (Anagnostopoulos *et al.*, 1995). Thus, it is possible that EBV first infects B cells in tonsillar crypts, where the surface epithelium is incomplete and virus could access lymphocytes directly. This initial infection of B cells results in full latent gene expression (latency 3), cell activation and proliferation, thus amplifying the number of infected cells at the site of entry. These B lymphoblasts can be found in peripheral blood early in IM, and are thereby disseminated throughout the body. Their presence in the circulation stimulates a massive T cell response which is characteristic of IM. The symptoms of IM are

not caused directly by virus-infected B cells but are immunopathological in nature, resulting from massive cytokine production from CD8 T cells (Foss *et al.*, 1994), and to a lesser extent CD4 T cells and NK cells. Together, these cells are thought to control the infection by eliminating infected B lymphoblasts; however, some escape and establish life-long persistence.

Humoral Immunity

The antibody responses to EBV-associated antigens during primary infection form a characteristic pattern (Figure 2D.6). Classically, by the time of onset of clinical symptoms, IgM, IgA and IgG antibodies to VCA are present in the serum, as are IgG antibodies to components of the early antigen and membrane antigen complexes. Antibodies to the viral glycoproteins are neutralising and probably agglutinate virus particles, thus preventing further infection and spread of the virus. IgM and IgA antibodies to VCA and IgG anti-EA antibodies rise to a peak during the acute disease and decline to low or undetectable levels during convalescence. IgG antibodies to EBNA1 are not usually detectable in the serum until the convalescent period. Heterophil antibodies regularly appear in the serum early in IM, but their relationship to the virus and their role, if any, in controlling infection remain unclear. A variety of autoantibodies may be found in IM, which include cold agglutinins (anti-i), rheumatoid factors, anti-nuclear antibodies and antibodies to platelets and to smooth muscle. These antibodies, which may account for the raised total serum IgM level found in IM, are thought to be the result of the polyclonal activation of B cells caused by EBV infection. They are usually transient and harmless.

Cellular Immunity

One of the most distinctive features of IM is the presence, at the time of onset of clinical symptoms, of a lymphocytosis, and 'atypical' mononuclear cells in the peripheral blood (Figure 2D.7). The rise of lymphocyte count, which may be very marked (up to $15 \times 10^9/l$), is due to a vast increase in absolute numbers of T lymphocytes. These are highly activated CD8-positive, HLA class I-restricted, cytotoxic T cells specific for lytic (and to a lesser extent latent) antigens. During the acute phase of the disease, up to 40% of the total peripheral CD8[+] T cell numbers may be directed against a single EBV epitope. The lymphocytosis is

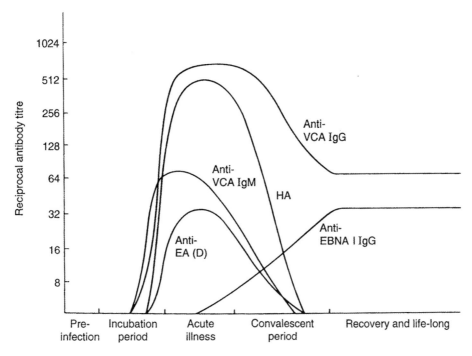

Figure 2D.6 Basic pattern of serum antibodies to EB virus-associated antigens before, during and after primary infection. HA, heterophil antibody; EA(D), diffuse form of early antigen; other abbreviations as in Figure 2D.3

accompanied by depression in most T lymphocyte functions, including those measured by delayed-type hypersensitivity testing and *in vitro* mitogen stimulation.

Histological Findings

Generally, tissue from IM patients is not available for study, but occasionally liver, bone marrow or lymph node biopsies are performed before the diagnosis is made. Also the histological findings on tissue from surgically removed tonsils and ruptured spleens, and post mortem specimens, have been described. In all cases the tissues are infiltrated with mononuclear cells, which are immunoblastic in appearance. These mainly consist of CD8$^+$ T cells with a minority population of EBERS-positive B cells. In the lymph node the pattern is generally described as 'reactive', with the infiltrate found in widely dilated sinuses and intersinusoidal cords extending into the interfollicular compartment, often obscuring the follicular centres. Virus-infected B cells are localised in the paracortical region, where occasional Hodgkin- or Reed–Sternberg-like cells may be present. In the liver the portal areas are

infiltrated and in the spleen the white pulp may be obscured by the extensive infiltrate, which extends throughout the parenchyma. Small aggregates of monocytoid cells and immunoblasts can be seen in the bone marrow. The histological findings are not diagnostic of IM in themselves, and may be difficult to distinguish from other causes of immunoblastic proliferations, e.g. Hodgkin's disease and non-Hodgkin lymphomas.

Clinical Features

Incubation period. As the source of infection is generally not determined, the incubation period is difficult to calculate; however, a period of 30–50 days is usual before symptoms occur.

Symptoms. Characteristically, IM begins abruptly with a sore throat and swelling of the neck, accompanied by non-specific symptoms such as malaise, fever, sweating, chills, headaches, stiff neck, anorexia and vague abdominal discomfort. A prodromal period characterised by lassitude and slight fever is described by some patients. The sore throat, which occurs in

80–90% of patients, is usually mild and clears after 7–14 days. It may, however, be severe enough to cause extreme pain and difficulty with swallowing, and occasionally gross tonsillar enlargement may lead to pharyngeal obstruction. In 25% of cases secondary infection of the pharynx occurs, commonly with a β-haemolytic streptococcus. Less commonly, patients present with jaundice, cough, myalgia or symptoms of one of the neurological complications of IM (see below).

Physical signs. Lymphadenopathy is present in the majority of cases at some time during the acute illness. The cervical nodes are most obviously involved, but generalised lymphadenopathy occurs, with the nodes often remaining palpable for several weeks. Glands are discrete and not severely tender. The additional presence of rubbery small glands in the axilla and groin indicates IM rather than a throat infection with involvement of cervical glands. Clinically detectable splenic enlargement occurs in 50–60% of patients and is usually accompanied by tenderness; however, ultrasound scanning detects splenomegaly in almost all cases. Mild hepatomegaly occurs in 15–25% of patients, and jaundice is clinically apparent in 5–10%. Fevers of 38–40°C are a regular feature during the first 1–2 weeks of IM, with the highest temperature often occurring at midday and being followed by drenching sweats.

Pharyngitis and palatal petechiae occur during the first week of the illness. These may be accompanied by a grey-white membrane which, when associated with pharyngeal oedema and tonsillar enlargement, can result in obstruction to the pharynx or trachea. Periorbital oedema is common early in this disease.

Two types of skin rashes can occur: a faint morbilliform eruption, which lasts 24–48 h, or a maculopapular rash, which occurs in almost all patients receiving ampicillin. The cause of the latter is unknown, but its presence is regarded by some as diagnostic of IM.

Other associated clinical conditions include encephalitis, meningitis, delirium, coma, psychosis, transverse myelitis, polyneuritis, mononeuritis, pericarditis, myocarditis, interstitial pneumonia and pleural effusions. None of these is common.

IM in children and the elderly. When IM occurs outside the classic age range of 15–25 years, it tends to present a less typical clinical picture. In children the disease is usually mild and does not require medical attention. Sore throat and cervical lymph node enlargement are usually present, but not invariably so. Occasionally children exhibit classic IM even as early as age 2 years.

The clinical onset of IM in the elderly is often insidious and occasionally bizarre. The disease can be severe, with hepatic, neurological and renal involvement.

IM in pregnancy. Infectious mononucleosis during pregnancy is uncommon, but where it has occurred there has rarely been deleterious effect on the foetus, and termination of pregnancy is not indicated.

IM in the immunosuppressed. When primary EBV infection occurs in immunocompromised patients, particularly after organ transplantation, it is often asymptomatic due to the inability to mount a T cell immune response. However, it may result in atypical disease, with gastrointestinal symptoms and/or signs of renal graft rejection and failure. Antibodies to EB viral antigens may be slow to develop, with neither IgM antibodies to VCA nor the heterophile antibody test being invariably positive. Some of these primary infections progress to lymphoproliferative disease and lymphoma (see below).

Course and convalescence. The illness usually resolves in 1–2 weeks but may last for several weeks, often with continued exhaustion on the slightest exertion and complaints of an inability to concentrate for several weeks after apparent recovery. Occasional patients, particularly those over 25 years of age, may experience intermittent fatigue over the following 2 years. Other patients suffer 'relapses' during the 6 months to 1 year following IM, with return of fever, sore throat and lymphadenopathy accompanied by a positive heterophil antibody test. The exact nature of these relapses is unclear, since the serological markers of primary infection may remain positive for up to a year, even in subclinical cases of seroconversion.

Complications. In the vast majority of cases IM is a benign and self-limiting disease from which complete recovery is the rule. However, certain morbid complications have been described in the literature, which account for around 30 deaths per year in the USA. The main causes of death are neurological complications, splenic rupture, hepatic failure and secondary infection. Approximately half the deaths are associated with X-linked lymphoproliferative syndrome (XLPS, see below).

Neurological complications. These include meningitis, encephalitis and the Guillain–Barré syndrome.

Each of these conditions may precede, accompany or postdate IM by several weeks. Recovery is usual.

Hepatic complications. Although many IM patients have biochemical evidence of hepatocellular damage, overt jaundice is uncommon (5–10%), and complete recovery occurs. However, more severe cases have been reported and these include massive hepatic necrosis, resulting in death if untreated by liver transplant.

Splenic rupture. This is a well-known but rare complication of IM, which may occur spontaneously or after mild trauma. The rupture gives rise to severe abdominal and shoulder pain and requires immediate surgical intervention.

Pharyngeal and tracheal obstruction. These may occur due to massive enlargement and oedema of the tonsils, adenoids, uvula and epiglottis, giving rise to an inability to swallow or to stridor with eventual cyanosis. A short course of corticosteroids usually gives a dramatic improvement, but intravenous hydration and feeding or tracheotomy may be necessary as emergency measures.

Immunological complications. These include haemolytic and aplastic anaemia, thrombocytopenia, hypogammaglobulinaemia, agranulocytosis and haemophagocytosis. These disorders may result from excess autoantibody production, such as to the blood group antigen i, due to B cell stimulation, or to abnormal suppression of haemopoiesis by T cells. Several of these conditions may be found in patients with X-linked lymphoproliferative disease (see below).

Chronic active EBV. Chronic active EBV infection, where symptoms of IM persist for more than a year, occurs rarely (around 1 in 2000 cases) and may result in death from hepatic failure, lymphoma, sepsis or haemophagocytic syndrome. In these cases there is a persistence of the acute IM-like serological profile, usually with grossly elevated titres of IgG antibody to VCA and EA-D, absence of IgG antibody to EBNA1, a positive monospot test and often detectable IgM antibodies to VCA. An atypical lymphocytosis is also present, which is mostly due to $CD8^+$ T cells. The viral load in saliva and peripheral blood is very high and in some cases EBNA-positive B cells can readily be detected in the circulation. These findings are likely to be due to inadequate immunological control of viral replication, and indeed in some cases a lack of EBV-specific memory T cells in the circulation has been demonstrated (Borysiewicz *et al.*, 1986).

Chronic active EBV has been treated with aciclovir and steroids, as well as a variety of agents such as interferons, but the results are disappointing. More recently, bone marrow transplant or adoptive immunotherapy have been used.

Chronic active IM can be distinguished from chronic fatigue syndrome (CFS) on clinical grounds and by an EB viral antibody screen. Around 10% of CFS patients have mildly elevated VCA and/or EA antibody titres, but no gross abnormalities can be found. These changes do not denote a specific aetiological association between EBV and CFS.

Laboratory findings. The classic finding in IM, after which the disease is named, is the 'atypical' mononuclear cells in the peripheral blood, which were first described by Downey and McKinlay (1923) (Figure 2D.7). Morphologically 'atypical' cells are large activated lymphocytes (10–20 μm in diameter) which, when stained with May–Grünwald–Giemsa stain, show abundant pale blue, vacuolated cytoplasm and an elongated or indented nucleus with coarse nuclear chromatin. These are mainly EBV-specific $CD8^+$ cytotoxic T cells (see above) and account for the leukocytosis regularly seen in the first 2 weeks of IM. A few atypical mononuclear cells occur in the peripheral blood in other acute virus infections, including cytomegalovirus, hepatitis B, influenza B and rubella, but they are most prominent in IM. Activated CD4 T cells and NK cells are also increased in numbers in acute IM. B lymphocytes are usually present in normal or slightly raised numbers and around 1 in 10^4–10^5 are infected with EBV and express all the latent viral proteins.

Abnormal liver function tests indicative of hepatocellular damage are found in 80–90% of patients. Liver enzymes are usually raised during the second and third week of the illness, and have returned to normal by the fifth week. In 30% of patients the bilirubin level is raised.

Diagnosis. The diagnosis of IM may be suspected on clinical grounds and substantiated by the haematological findings of 'atypical' lymphocytes, but a firm diagnosis of IM relies on the serological demonstration of antibodies to EBV-related antigens. A pre-illness specimen is rarely available to prove absence of antibody before the illness, and IgG antibodies to VCA are almost invariably present in the first serum sample received, having often already reached their peak. However, high levels of IgG anti-VCA antibodies are not of diagnostic significance, since variable levels are reached during the illness, and higher levels may occur in other conditions. The presence of IgM antibodies to VCA, with or without IgG antibodies to EA (D), and an absence of IgG anti EBNA1, are diagnostic. Commercial ELISA tests are available and reliable, although less sensitive than the traditional indirect immunofluorescence test. False-positive results in the IgM test may result from cross-linking between specific EB viral IgG and anti-IgM conjugate by rheumatoid factor, and therefore, if this factor is present in the serum, it should be absorbed out before testing. These days most laboratories rely on the heterophil antibody test, which has been simplified in a kit form as the Monospot test.

The heterophil antibody test. This classic test, variously called the Paul–Bunnell test, the Davidsohn–Henry test, or the Lee–Davidsohn test after the authors who described each variation (Davidsohn and Henry, 1969), detects an IgM heterophil antibody (HA) which causes haemagglutination of cells from species other than humans. The original test used a doubling dilution titration of serum and sheep red cells. The use of horse, rather than sheep, red cells was later found to increase the sensitivity of the test without loss of specificity. The test was modified to exclude Forssman antibody by absorption of the serum with guinea-pig kidney emulsion (GPK) before testing. A further refinement to confirm the specificity of the heterophil antibody titre was to compare the titres with and without absorption with ox cell stroma (OCS), which specifically removes the heterophil antibody of IM. Results were then usually expressed as three red cell agglutinin titres: (a) of unabsorbed serum; (b) of serum absorbed with GPK; and (c) of serum absorbed with OCS, and the diagnostic criterion commonly used was that the titre of (c) must be at least four-fold lower than the titre of (b), with the titre of (a) being 56 or higher.

The Monospot test. Slide tests are available which use absorption combined with agglutination and are quick and reliable. Drops of serum are placed on two squares on a slide; GPK is stirred into one drop and OCS into the other. Horse red cells are added to each square and stirred into the absorbed serum. Agglutination in the GPK square and not in the OCS square is indicative of IM.

The Monospot test is positive in around 85% of IM cases (as confirmed by positive anti-VCA IgM) and can persist for up to 6 months after recovery. Negative results are more common in sera from children with IM under 14 years than in those from older children or adults. This may be because HA arises due to the polyclonal stimulation of memory B cells, so if the priming exposure to the unknown 'heterophil' antigen has not yet occurred, no specific memory B cells would be present and no secondary rise could be induced. False-positive HA tests have been extensively recorded, particularly in association with pregnancy and autoimmune disease.

Treatment. This is largely supportive. High-dose aciclovir reduces virus production in the throat but does not shorten the duration of the illness, probably because the symptoms are immunopathological in nature and not caused directly by virus infection of B cells. The sore throat may be extremely painful and regular analgesics are then essential. Corticosteroids curtail the severity and duration of the symptoms, but are best reserved for severe cases of pharyngeal or tracheal obstruction, neurological and haematological complications.

Burkitt's Lymphoma

Burkitt's lymphoma (BL) is a tumour which occurs endemically in equatorial Africa and Papua New Guinea and sporadically worldwide. The African (endemic) form of the tumour is geographically restricted to those areas in which hyperendemic falciparum malaria occurs (Figure 2D.8). These are the low-lying areas of equatorial Africa and Papua New Guinea, with a rainfall of over 60 cm/year and a minimum temperature of 16°C.

The endemic and sporadic forms of BL are both monoclonal tumours of B lymphocytes which have indistinguishable histological appearances. However, whereas almost 100% of African BL are associated with EBV, only 12–25% of the sporadic cases are EBV-related.

Seroepidemiology

In the geographical areas where BL is endemic, almost all children over the age of 2 years have been infected by EBV and have IgG antibodies to VCA. However, in BL the pattern of antibodies to EBV antigens is altered when compared to normal matched controls. Sera from BL patients have IgG antibody titres to VCA with a geometric mean eight to ten times greater than

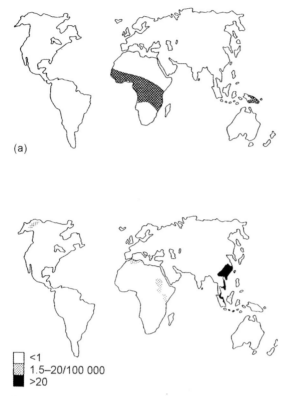

(a)

□ <1
▨ 1.5–20/100 000
■ >20

Figure 2D.8 Maps showing the worldwide distribution of (a) Burkitt's lymphoma and (b) nasopharyngeal carcinoma

matched control sera. IgG anti-EA (R) and anti-MA antibodies are also raised, and the levels of these serum antibodies vary with clinical events. Thus, after treatment, a drop in anti-EA (R) indicates a good prognosis, whereas a rise in anti-EA (R) and a fall in anti-MA may precede a recurrence of clinical disease. In a classic 7-year prospective epidemiological study carried out in Uganda by de Thé *et al.* (1978), 12 cases of BL developed in a cohort of 42 000 children. These 12 children had high titres of anti-VCA for months or years before the onset of the disease, indicating that BL does not result directly from primary infection. The study also showed a 30-fold increased risk of disease in those children with an anti-VCA titre of two doubling dilutions or more above the normal control population.

Pathogenesis

Association with EBV. Although it is very difficult to obtain absolute proof that a virus is involved in the aetiology of a human tumour, there is now much

evidence which points to the widely accepted view that EBV is involved in the aetiology of BL. In addition to the seroepidemiological evidence outlined above, multiple copies of the viral genome can be detected in the tumour cells of around 97% of African BL biopsy samples. The viral genome is clonal in the monoclonal BL B cell population, indicating that the infection event occurred before proliferation of the malignant cells. However, the viral gene expression is restricted to the latent antigen EBNA1, which is essential for maintenance of the viral genome in the cell, and EBERS and *Bam*A transcripts (latency 1) (Table 2D.1). No direct oncogenic role for these genes has been identified, although mice transgenic for EBNA1 develop lymphoma (Wilson *et al.*, 1996), and EBERS has been suggested to increase cell survival by inhibiting apoptosis (Komano *et al.*, 1999).

BL-derived cell lines. Lymphoid cell lines that are grown directly from BL biopsy material show the characteristic features of BL cells, with cellular markers consistent with a germinal centre B cell phenotype (CD10, CD77) and viral protein expression to restricted EBNA1 (latency 1). These differ from their *in vitro*, EBV-immortalised counterpart (see above) in several important respects, which indicate their increased malignant potential. Thus, BL-derived cell lines grow as colonies in soft agar and subcutaneously in nude mice whereas *in vitro* immortalised LCLs do not. BL cell lines are monoclonal, with all cells bearing surface immunoglobulin of one heavy chain isotype (usually M) and one light chain type, whereas *in vitro* immortalised cell lines are polyclonal in origin. There are also differences in growth characteristics, cellular gene expression and cytological appearances, reflecting their differing stages of B cell maturation (germinal centre cell vs. activated lymphoblast). However, with prolonged culture, the viral and cellular gene expression in BL cell lines may drift to resemble LCLs. Finally, BL cell lines consistently carry specific chromosomal translocations which are not present in *in vitro*-grown LCLs derived from normal individuals (see below).

Chromosomal abnormalities. It has been recognised for many years that fresh BL tumour cells and the derived cell lines (whether EBV-associated or not) show a reciprocal chromosomal translocation between the long arm of one chromosome 8 and chromosomes 14, 2 or 22. Each of these translocations results in the c-myc oncogene on chromosome 8 coming under the regulatory control of either the Ig heavy chain genes on chromosome 14 or, more rarely, the κ or λ light chain genes on chromosomes 2 and 22, respectively. The position of the chromosomal break points suggest that these translocations are the result of mistakes occurring during Ig gene rearrangements, Ig class switching, or during somatic hypermutation in a germinal centre cell. Furthermore, the translocated allele of c-myc frequently contains mutations. c-myc is a normal cellular gene which codes for a nuclear protein involved in the control of cell activation and proliferation. The BL translocations deregulate the gene, giving constitutive expression. In addition to this characteristic chromosomal translocation, BL cells often contain other genetic abnormalities, including a mutated p53 gene in about 30% of biopsy samples.

Co-factors in the pathogenesis of BL.

Since EBV is a ubiquitous agent, whereas EBV-associated BL occurs almost exclusively in those geographical areas of the world where malaria is hyperendemic, it is probable that malaria infection acts as one factor in the multifactorial aetiology of this disease. The association between BL and malaria is further substantiated by the finding that where malaria eradication has been successfully accomplished, the incidence of BL has dropped dramatically, and the incidence of BL in children with the sickle cell trait, which confers partial protection from malaria, is low.

Malaria infection acts as a chronic stimulator of germinal centre B cells and also as an immunosuppressant, causing a decreased EBV-specific cytotoxic T cell activity and increased numbers of EBV-infected B cells in the peripheral blood. It is postulated, therefore, that the combined lymphoid stimulation and immunosuppressive effects of malaria cause an increase in B cell turnover and a decrease in the elimination of EBV-positive B cells. However, at present it is unclear whether EBV acts to increase the population of cells susceptible to a chromosomal translocation, or to enhance the survival and proliferation of a cell population bearing the translocation. Whichever scenario is correct, it is assumed that the latent EBV growth-promoting genes (latency 3) must be expressed at this early stage of lymphomagenesis, but that a switch to the non-immunogenic EBNA1-only phenotype (latency1) occurs once their function is replaced by deregulated c-myc.

Clinical Features

African BL is a tumour that occurs in children aged 3–15 years, with a peak age incidence of 6–7 years. In those areas of Africa and Papua New Guinea where BL is endemic, it occurs with an incidence of 15 per 100 000 children aged 5–10 years, and is the commonest malignancy in this age range. It is more common in boys than girls and arises extranodally, typically in the area of the jaw, giving a characteristic presentation (Figure 2D.9). The tumour is usually found to be multifocal at presentation, the other sites commonly involved being the postorbital region, gastrointestinal tract, thyroid, liver, kidney, skeleton, testicles and ovaries, and the breast in adolescent girls. BL is a highly malignant tumour, with death supervening within a few months of clinical onset in untreated cases.

Diagnosis.

The diagnosis of BL in an endemic area is very often clear from the clinical features described above; however, histological evidence should be sought (Figure 2D.10). The tumour shows a characteristic histological picture of a poorly differentiated lymphocytic lymphoma with variable numbers of infiltrating histiocytes, giving the classic 'starry sky' appearance. BL is a monoclonal tumour of B cell origin, expressing the markers of a germinal centre B cell; CD10, CD77 and, in over 90% of cases, IgM.

Treatment.

Burkitt's lymphoma is very sensitive to chemotherapy, one dose of cyclophosphamide often being enough to cause complete regression of the tumour mass. Relapses do occur, however, and are progressively less responsive to therapy. For this reason, a full course of treatment should be given initially, in which case the prognosis is good.

Prevention.

The prevention of BL may theoretically be achieved by the eradication of malaria, which has already been achieved in small areas, such as some of the islands of Papua New Guinea, and the incidence of BL has fallen in these regions. Alternatively, prevention of BL development by a vaccine which prevents EBV infection has been suggested (see below).

Nasopharyngeal Carcinoma

Nasopharyngeal carcinoma (NPC) is a malignant tumour of the squamous epithelium of the nasopharynx, which is highly prevalent in southern China, where it is the commonest tumour in men and the second most common in women. In most other areas of the world the tumour is rare, but pockets of high incidence occur in North and Central Africa,

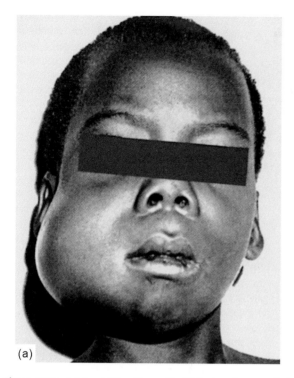
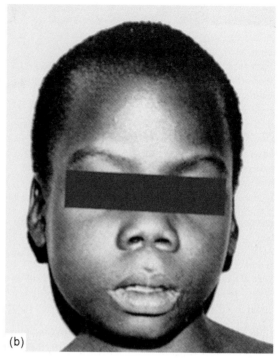

(a)

(b)

Figure 2D.9 Male child with a Burkitt's lymphoma of the jaw, (a) before treatment and (b) after treatment with cyclophosphamade (30 mg/kg body weight)

Malaysia, Indonesia, Vietnam, The Philippines and in the Inuit races of Alaska, Greenland and Iceland (see Figure 2D.8). The most undifferentiated form of the tumour, which is the most common, shows a 100% association with EBV regardless of the geographical location, whereas the association with the rarer, more differentiated, forms is controversial.

Seroepidemiology

The association between NPC and EBV was first demonstrated serologically (Old *et al.*, 1966) and later studies showed that sera from 100% of cases of undifferentiated NPC have high-titre antibodies to VCA. As in BL, the antibodies are present at a 10 times higher geometric mean titre than in matched controls, and show a unique reaction pattern. Thus, the anti-EA (D) component is the most frequently seen and is present at a higher titre than anti-EA (R). IgG and IgA Anti-EA (D) antibody titres rise as the disease progresses, fall in remissions, and may be undetectable in long-term survivors. Similarly, IgA antibodies to VCA are present in NPC sera and correlate with

disease progression. These IgA antibodies are also found uniquely in the saliva of NPC patients.

Pathogenesis

Association with EBV. The seroepidemiological data referred to above, and the finding of multiple clonal copies of the EBV genome in the malignant epithelial cells of 100% of undifferentiated NPC biopsy specimens, strongly suggest that the virus is involved in tumour aetiology. All the malignant epithelial cells express the EBV-coded antigen EBNA1, and LMP1 and LMP2 are expressed in around 50% of tumours (latency 2). Although the exact mechanisms involved in squamous epithelial cell transformation by EBV have not been resolved, the fact that LMP1 is a viral oncogene which can drive epithelial cell proliferation *in vitro* (Dawson *et al.*, 1990) and induce severe epithelial hyperplasia in transgenic mice (Wilson *et al.*, 1990), provides compelling evidence for an oncogenic role for EBV in NPC.

Co-factors in the pathogenesis of NPC. NPC is a genetically restricted tumour, being most common in

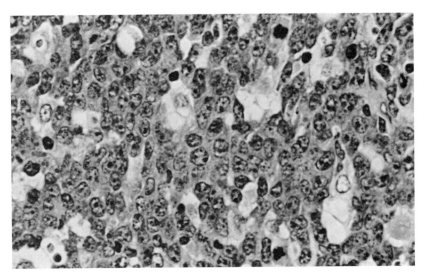

Figure 2D.10 Histological section of Burkitt's lymphoma, showing a uniform population of nucleolated lymphoid cells and scattered vacuolated macrophages (H & E × 800; courtesy of Professor P. Isaacson, University College Hospital)

southern Chinese and Inuits. It has an intermediate frequency in some negroid and mongoloid races and is rare in Caucasians. It has been noted that the first-generation immigrants from southern China to the USA retain the high frequency of the disease; although later generations show a declining incidence, which may be due to intermarriage with non-Chinese races. These data suggest a genetic factor in the aetiology of the disease, and this is backed up by family clustering and the finding of an association with certain HLA haplotypes (A2-BSin2, BW17-AW19, BW17-A blank). Environmental factors have also been suggested in the aetiology of NPC, particularly dietary components such as salted fish, which contain carcinogenic nitrosamines, and traditional herbal medicines containing phorbol esters, which are taken as snuff.

Clinical Features

NPC occurs at a rate of 98 per 100 000 of the population in southern China and is more common in men than in women. The age of onset of NPC varies with geographical distribution and histological type, the undifferentiated type being more common in high-risk areas in young patients, whereas the more differentiated types occur in older patients and constitute the bulk of sporadic cases. The tumour most commonly arises on the posterior wall of the nasopharynx in the fossa of Rosenmüller, where it

often remains silent, and rapidly metastasises to the draining lymph nodes. Thus, the most frequent presenting symptom of NPC is bilateral enlargement of lymph glands in the neck, which are firm, non-tender and fixed. The upper cervical chain of glands is most often involved in the initial spread. At this stage the primary tumour may be very small and difficult to locate. Less frequently, the presenting symptoms are associated with invasion by the primary tumour and include nasal obstruction, postnasal discharge, epistaxis, partial deafness and cranial nerve palsies. If untreated, the disease is rapidly fatal, with death being most often due to laryngeal and pharyngeal obstruction.

Diagnosis. The diagnosis of NPC is made on biopsy material from the primary tumour or an enlarged cervical lymph node. The cells are squamous epithelial in origin and three histological types are described in the World Health Organisation classification: (a) a well-differentiated squamous cell carcinoma with intercellular bridges and/or keratinisation; (b) a non-keratinising carcinoma; and (c) an undifferentiated carcinoma in which a heavy lymphocytic infiltration is often present, which may be so extensive as to lead to the mistaken diagnosis of lymphoma (Figure 2D.11). However, the lymphocytes, which are mainly T cells, are non-malignant. The term 'lymphoepithelioma' has been used to describe this third type, which occurs most commonly in the high-risk areas.

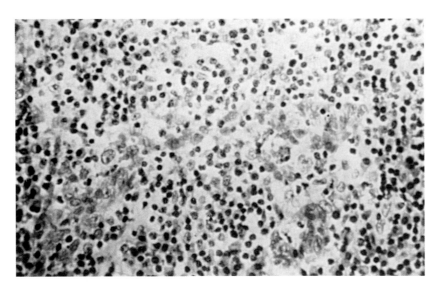

Figure 2D11. Histological section of undifferentiated nasopharyngeal carcinoma, showing scattered malignant epithelial cells and a heavy infiltrate of small lymphocytes (H & E × 400)

Serum antibody titres to EBV antigens can be used to confirm the diagnosis of NPC and to monitor the progress of the disease. Large-scale screening programmes in China have identified individuals with persistent IgA antibodies to VCA in serum and/or saliva, and follow-up of these cases has successfully detected 'precancerous' and early lesions.

Treatment. NPC is difficult to treat surgically because of the characteristic feature of early metastasis to regional lymph nodes. The tumour is resistant to chemotherapy, and therefore radiotherapy to the primary tumour and cervical lymph nodes is the treatment of choice. The overall prognosis is poor; however, the 5 year survival rate for early stage disease is around 60%.

Prevention. Although the precise role of EBV in the aetiology of NPC remains to be elucidated, it has been argued that prevention of primary infection by EBV using vaccination may be enough to break the chain of events which culminates in tumour formation. Vaccine preparations are discussed below.

Hodgkin's Disease

An association between EBV and Hodgkin's disease (HD) has long been suspected because HD is more common in people who have previously had IM than those who have not, and HD patients have high antibody titres to EBV lytic cycle antigens months or years before development of the disease. This association was firmly established when EBV DNA and expression of viral-coded proteins were demonstrated in malignant Hodgkin Reed–Sternberg (HR-S) cells in a proportion of cases. Multiple copies of clonal, circular EBV DNA can be detected in 40–60% of HD biopsies by Southern blotting, with confirmation of the HR-S cell location by detection of EBERS by *in situ* hybridisation (Anagnostopolous *et al.*, 1989). These cells also express EBNA1 and high levels of LMP1 and LMP2A, in the absence of other latent or lytic proteins (latency 2). The mixed cellularity type of HD is the most often associated with EBV.

The age distribution of HD is similar to that of EBV, showing a bimodal distribution, with one peak in childhood and another in adult life. Furthermore, the age of the early peak varies with geographical location, being later in Western societies (15–35 years) than in developing countries (5–10 years). This similarity initially suggested that HD may represent an atypical outcome to primary EBV infection; however, although most childhood HD in developing countries is EBV-associated, in Western societies non-EBV-associated HD predominates in the young, with EBV association increasing with age (reviewed in Jarrett, 2002).

The pathogenesis of EBV-associated HD is still unclear, although the presence of clonal viral DNA in

HR-S cells indicates infection at an early stage. In addition, expression of LMP1, which induces cell activation and proliferation while inhibiting apoptosis, and LMP2A, which enhances cell survival, is consistent with an oncogenic role for the virus. HR-S cells have now been definitively identified as germinal centre B cells, with functional immunoglobulin (Ig) gene rearrangements but defective Ig gene transcription (Marafioti et al., 2000), and it is therefore possible that EBV infection of these atypical cells allows the survival of a cell which would otherwise undergo apoptosis in the germinal centre.

EBV Infection in the Immunocompromised Host

EBV establishes a life-long persistent infection with latency in B lymphocytes and virus production into saliva in over 90% of the world's population (see above). This persistent infection is controlled mainly by EBV-specific cytotoxic T cells and it is not surprising, therefore, that when cell-mediated immunity is decreased there is often increased EBV production in saliva, high antibody titres to lytic cycle antigens (VCA and EA) and an increased viral load in peripheral blood lymphocytes. This pattern is sometimes called a 'reactivated infection', although generally no clinical symptoms ensue. In a few patients, however, EBV-associated lymphoproliferative lesions and lymphoma develop.

X-linked Lymphoproliferative Syndrome (X-LPS)
(reviewed by Gasper et al., 2002).

This rare syndrome (first called Duncan's syndrome) was recognised in 1974 by Purtilo and colleagues, who described a family in which six male kindred died of acute IM and/or malignant lymphoma (Purtilo et al., 1974). Since then, many such families have been reported, with affected members having an apparent inability to mount an effective immune response to primary EBV infection. X-LPS accounts for about half of the fatal IM cases reported, the other half being sporadic, with an equal sex distribution.

Clinically, the affected males are healthy until primary EBV infection occurs. The course of the disease is then fulminating and rapidly fatal in the majority of cases, with death commonly resulting from hepatic necrosis. A minority of patients progress to a chronic phase, often culminating in a fatal B cell lymphoma. These tumours

are mostly extranodal, commonly occurring in the central nervous system or gastrointestinal tract.

Histological studies on fatal cases show infiltration of tissues throughout the body with EBV-positive lymphoblastoid and plasmacytoid cells and T activated cells. These infiltrates are a particularly prominent feature in the liver, where dysregulated cytokine release from T cells leads to hepatic necrosis. Haemophagocytosis is seen in the tissues in almost all cases. There is no elective treatment for this disease, although etoposide may have some effect, and recently success has been reported with bone marrow transplantation.

Many abnormal immunological findings have been reported in X-LPS, although none is consistently found. These are more marked following EBV infection when combined T, B and NK cell abnormalities are reported.

The defective gene in X-LPS was identified in 1998 (Coffey et al., 1998; Sayos et al., 1998; Nichols et al., 1998) and the development of a diagnostic test rapidly followed. This identified a spectrum of clinical manifestations associated with the syndrome, including dysgammaglobulinaemia (incorporating some cases of common variable immunodeficiency), aplastic anaemia, lymphoid vasculitis with aneurysm formation and, rarely, non-EBV-associated lymphoma.

The X-LPS gene codes for a small src-homology 2 (SH2) domain containing cytoplasmic protein, alternatively called SH2D1A or SAP [signalling lymphocytic activation molecule (SLAM)-associated protein] which is expressed in T and NK cells. SAP appears to play a modulating role in T cell activation and is required for NK cell cytotoxicity; it is likely that the loss of these functions explains the X-LPS phenotype. However, this does not explain the link between EBV and X-LPS, since SAP expression is not specific to primary EBV infection. In this regard, the finding of rare X-LPS lymphoma in EBV-negative individuals indicates that the syndrome is not restricted to primary EBV infection, and it is now postulated that X-LPS is a more generalised immunodeficiency that can be triggered by a variety of virus infections. However, the exact nature of the immunological abnormality is still unclear.

Transplant Recipients
(reviewed by Hopwood and Crawford, 2000).

Iatrogenic immunosuppression following bone marrow or solid organ transplant results in an increased incidence of virus-associated tumours. B cell lymphomas are the second commonest tumours in this patient population (following skin tumours) and have a high morbidity and mortality. Termed 'post transplant lymphoproliferative disease' (PTLD), these tumours are mainly classified as large cell lymphoma, and develop in up to 10% of transplant recipients. Risk factors include high levels of immunosuppressive drugs (often in association with rejection episodes) and primary EBV infection following transplant. The latter is more common in children, who therefore have a higher incidence of PTLD than adults. Over 90% of PTLD patients are EBV-positive and the tumour cells generally express all the latent viral genes (latency 3) (Table 2D.1). Early lesions are often polyclonal B cell proliferations, but progression to a monoclonal lymphoma regularly occurs.

Clinically, PTLD may present as an IM-like syndrome, commonly in children undergoing primary infection (in which the virus may be acquired from the transplanted organ), and often within the first year of transplant. Alternatively, discrete tumours, frequently in the gastrointestinal tract, brain or transplanted organ, are seen in seropositive recipients, often several years after transplant. Because of the variable clinical presentation, diagnosis is often difficult and measurement of the viral load in peripheral blood has been used as an indicator of risk. However, although high viral load is found in the majority of PTLD patients, levels are very variable in healthy recipients, with some reaching those seen in PTLD. Therefore single estimations are not helpful and regular monitoring is required.

The pathogenesis of PTLD appears to be straightforward; immunosuppressive therapy following transplantation inhibits EBV-specific cytotoxic T cells, leading to uncontrolled proliferation of EBV-infected B cells. However, the lesions are often single and monoclonal, suggesting that, in addition to EBV, cellular factors are required for tumour outgrowth. The recent finding of non-functional Ig genes in a proportion of these tumours (Timms et al., 2003) suggests that EBV infection may have rescued an abnormal cell from apoptosis within the germinal centre.

Reduction of immunosuppressive therapy is now the first line of treatment for PTLD, and the antiviral drugs aciclovir or ganciclovir are sometimes added to this regimen, although their role in tumour regression is unproven. Complete tumour regression may be achieved by this treatment alone, particularly in early lesions, but relapses and recurrences are common and, despite additional chemotherapy and/or radiotherapy, the overall mortality is around 50%. Recent trials of immunotherapy for PTLD, including the humanised antibody to the B cell surface antigen CD20 (Kuehnle et al., 2000), as well as autologous (Rooney et al., 1998) or allogeneic (Haque et al., 2002) in vitro-grown EBV-specific cytotoxic T cells, have reported some success, although randomised controlled trials have not been performed.

Acquired Immunodeficiency Syndrome (AIDS)

The incidence of non-Hodgkin's lymphoma (NHL) in individuals infected with human immunodeficiency virus (HIV) is increased some 60-fold over the general population, and its development is an AIDS-defining illness. These tumours are not uniform in histological type or EBV association, and three principal types of HIV-associated NHL have been described:

1. Primary central nervous system lymphoma (PCNSL) is a rare tumour in the general population, which has 1000-fold increased incidence in HIV infection. It occurs at a late stage in the disease in the face of severe immunodeficiency, and is generally of the large cell lymphoblastoid type. PCNSL is invariably EBV-associated, showing full latent viral gene expression (latency 3). Definitive ante-mortem diagnosis may be difficult, but EBV DNA can be found in cerebrospinal fluid in most cases and detection is considered to be diagnostic.

2. Burkitt's lymphoma develops at a relatively early stage of HIV infection, when the immunodeficiency is mild. All AIDS BL tumours show the c-myc translocation typical of BL and around 25% show the cellular and viral gene expression described for African BL (see above), the other 75% being EBV-negative. The finding of BL in AIDS as well as in African children led to the suggestion that the polyclonal activation of B cells caused by both malaria and HIV infections may predispose to the development of BL by increasing B cell turnover, thereby increasing the likelihood of a c-myc gene translocation and EBV infection occurring in the same cell (Lenoir and Bornkamm, 1987).

3. Peripheral NHL occurs at a late stage of HIV infection and often presents at extranodal sites. Around 50% of these are EBV-associated, showing a lymphoblastoid phenotype with full latent viral gene expression (latency 3), similar to that of PTLD (see above).

Other types of lymphoma seen in HIV infection include HD, which shows a modestly raised incidence and a strong EBV association, and the human herpesvirus 8-associated primary infusion lymphoma, of which 70–80% show dual infection with EBV. All lymphomas associated with HIV infection respond poorly to treatment, due to the underlying disease; however, with the use of highly active antiretroviral therapy, their incidence is falling (Kirk et al., 2001).

Oral hairy leukoplakia (OHL) was first described in HIV-seropositive individuals, forming multiple characteristic corrugated white lesions on the lateral margin of the tongue. DNA hybridisation and immunocytochemical staining revealed EBV replicating in these lesions (Greenspan et al., 1985). OHL has now been recognised in other groups of immunocompromised patients. The lesion is painless and apparently harmless, but it can be successfully treated if required with continuous aciclovir therapy.

VACCINE DEVELOPMENT

Over the last two decades, work has been undertaken to develop a vaccine which would prevent primary infection by EBV. The antigen chosen for vaccine development is the MA antigen gp340/220 (see above), since it is this antigen to which neutralising antibodies are mainly directed. It was argued that this would prevent the development of BL and NPC by breaking a link in the chain of events which leads to the evolution of these diseases (Epstein, 1984). Such a vaccine preparation would have to be given very early in life to prevent natural infection in the BL- and NPC-susceptible populations. An effective vaccine preparation could also be useful in seronegative organ transplant recipients and those at risk of developing severe IM, such as the male offspring of XLPS carriers.

More recently, a peptide-based vaccine has been designed to induce cytotoxic T cell responses. To overcome the problem of the HLA class I restriction of the viral cytotoxic T cell response, a 'polytope' vaccine, containing multiple epitopes to which over 94% of the population should respond, has been formulated (Khanna et al., 1999). This vaccine is not designed to induce sterile immunity but to prevent disease. Both vaccines are in early clinical trials and, if satisfactory, are then expected to be tested for their ability to prevent or ameliorate the symptoms of IM.

REFERENCES

Anagnostopoulos I, Herbst H, Niedobitek G and Stein H (1989) Demonstration of monoclonal EBV genomes in Hodgkin's disease and ki-1-positive anaplastic large cell lymphoma by combined Southern blot and in situ hybridization. Blood, 74, 810–816.

Anagnostopoulos I, Hummel M, Kreschel C and Stein H (1995) Morphology, immunophenotype, and distribution of latently and/or productively Epstein–Barr virus-infected cells in acute infectious mononucleosis: implications for the interindividual infection route of Epstein–Barr virus. Blood, 85, 744–750.

Baer R, Bankier AT, Biggin MD et al. (1984) DNA sequence and expression of the B95-8 Epstein–Barr virus genome. Nature, 310, 207–211.

Bornkamm GW and Hammerschmidt W (2001) Molecular virology of Epstein–Barr virus. Phil Trans R Soc Lond Ser B, 356, 437–459.

Borysiewicz LK, Haworth SJ, Cohen J et al. (1986) Epstein–Barr virus-specific immune defects in patients with persistent symptoms following infectious mononucleosis. Qu J Med, 58, 111–121.

Borza CM and Hutt-Fletcher LM (2002) Alternate replication in B cells and epithelial cells switches tropism of Epstein–Barr virus. Nature Med, 8, 594–599.

Burkitt D (1958) A sarcoma involving the jaws in African children. Br J Surg, 46, 218–233.

Chen ML, Tsai CN, Liang CL et al. (1992) Cloning and characterization of the latent membrane protein (LMP) of a specific Epstein–Barr virus variant derived from the nasopharyngeal carcinoma in the Taiwanese population. Oncogene, 7, 2131–2140.

Coffey AJ, Brooksbank RA, Brandau O et al. (1998) Host response to EBV infection in X-linked lymphoproliferative disease results from mutations in an SH2-domain encoding gene. Nature Genet, 20, 129–135.

Crawford DH, Sweney P, Edwards JMB et al. (1981) Long term T cell-mediated immunity to Epstein–Barr virus in renal allograft recipients receiving cyclosporin A. Lancet, i, 10–12.

Crawford DH, Swerdlow AJ, Higgins C et al. (2002) Sexual history and Epstein–Barr virus infection. J Infect Dis, 186, 731–736.

Crawford DH, Thomas JA, Janossy G et al. (1980) Epstein–Barr virus nuclear antigen positive lymphoma after cyclosporin A treatment in patients with renal allograft. Lancet, i(8182), 1355–1356.

Davidsohn I and Henry JB (1969) Clinical Diagnosis by Laboratory Methods, 14th edn. (eds Todd and Sanford). Saunders, Philadelphia.

Dawson CW, Rickinson AB and Young LS. (1990) Epstein–Barr virus latent membrane protein inhibits human epithelial cell differentiation. Nature, 344, 777–780.

de Thé G, Geser A, Day NE et al. (1978) Epidemiological evidence for causal relationship between Epstein–Barr virus and Burkitt's lymphoma from Ugandan prospective study. Nature, 274, 756–761.

Downey H and McKinlay CA (1923) Acute lymphadenosis compared with acute lymphatic leukaemia. Arch Intern Med, 32, 82–112.

Epstein MA (1984) Leeuwenhoek lecture 1983. A prototype vaccine to prevent Epstein–Barr virus-associated tumours. Proc R Soc Ser B, 221, 1–20.

Epstein MA and Barr YM (1964) Cultivation in vitro of human lymphoblasts from Burkitt's lymphoma. Lancet, i, 702–703.

Epstein MA, Barr YM and Achong BG (1964) Virus particles in cultured lymphoblasts from Burkitt's lymphoma. *Lancet*, **i**, 702–703.

Foss H-D, Herbst H, Hummal M *et al.* (1994) Patterns of cytokine gene expression in infectious mononucleosis. *Blood*, **83**, 707–712.

Gaspar HB, Sharifi R and Thrasher AJ (2002) X-linked lymphoproliferative disease: clinical, diagnostic and molecular perspective. *Br J Haematol*, **119**, 585–596.

Greenspan JS, Greenspan D, Lennette ET *et al.* (1985) Replication of Epstein–Barr virus within the epithelial cells of oral hairy leukoplakia an AIDS-associated lesion. *N Engl J Med*, **313**, 1564–1571.

Haque T, Wilkie GM, Taylor C *et al.* (2002) Treatment of Epstein–Barr virus-positive post-transplantation lymphoproliferative disease with partly HLA-matched allogeneic cytotoxic T cells. *Lancet*, **360**, 436–442.

Henle G and Henle W (1966) Immunofluorescence in cells derived from Burkitt's lymphoma. *J Bacteriol*, **91**, 1248–1256.

Henle G, Henle W and Klein G (1971) Demonstration of two distinct components in the early antigen complex of Epstein–Barr virus-infected cells. *Int J Cancer*, **8**, 272–282.

Hopwood P and Crawford DH (2000) The role of EBV in post-transplant malignancies: a review. *J Clin Pathol*, **53**, 248–254.

Imai S, Koizumi S, Sugiura M *et al.* (1994) Gastric carcinoma: monoclonal epithelial malignant cells expressing Epstein–Barr virus latent infection protein. *Proc Natl Acad Sci USA*, **91**, 9131–9135.

Israele V, Shirlay P and Sixbey JW (1991) Excretion of the Epstein–Barr virus from the genital tract of men. *J Infect Dis*, **163**, 1341–1343.

Ito Y (1986) Vegetable activations of the viral genome and the causation of Burkitt's lymphoma and nasopharyngeal carcinoma. In *The Epstein–Barr Virus: Recent Advances* (eds MA Epstein and BG Achong), pp, 207–236. Heinemann, London.

Jarrett RF (2002) Viruses and Hodgkin's lymphoma. *Ann Oncol*, **13**, 23–29.

Jones JF, Shurin S, Abramowski C *et al.* (1988) T cell lymphomas containing Epstein–Barr viral DNA in patients with chronic Epstein–Barr virus infections. *N Engl J Med*, **318**, 733–741.

Khanim F, Yao Q-Y, Niedobitek G *et al.* (1996) Analysis of Epstein–Barr virus gene polymorphisms in normal donors and in virus-associated tumors from different geographic locations. *Blood*, **88**, 3491–3501.

Khanna R, Sherritt M and Burrows SR (1999) EBV structural antigens, gp350 and gp85, as targets for *ex vivo* virus-specific CTL during acute infectious mononucleosis: potential use of gh350/gp85 CTL epitopes for vaccine design. *J Immunol*, **162**, 3063–3069.

Kikuta H, Sakiyama Y, Matsumoto S *et al.* (1993) Fatal Epstein–Barr virus associated haemophagocytic syndrome. *Blood*, **82**, 3259–3264.

Kirk O, Pedersen C, Cozzi-Lepri A *et al.* (2001) Non-Hodgkin lymphoma in HIV-infected patients in the era of highly active antiretroviral therapy. *Blood*, **98**, 3406–3412.

Komano J, Maruo S, Kurozumi *et al.* (1999) Oncogenic role of Epstein–Barr virus-encoded RNAs in Burkitt's lymphoma cell line Akata. *J Virol*, **73**, 9827–9831.

Kuehnle I, Huls MH, Liu Z *et al.* (2000) CD20 monoclonal antibody (rituximab) for therapy of Epstein–Barr virus lymphoma after hemopoietic stem-cell transplantation. *Blood*, **95**, 1502–1505.

Lam KM-C, Syed N, Whittle H and Crawford DH (1991) Circulating Epstein–Barr virus-carrying B cells in acute malaria. *Lancet*, **337**, 876–878.

Lee ES, Locker J, Nalesnik M *et al.* (1995) The association of Epstein–Barr virus with smooth-muscle tumors occurring after organ transplantation. *N Engl J Med*, **332**, 19–25.

Lenoir G and Bornkamm G (1987) Burkitt's lymphoma: a human cancer model for the study of the multistep development of cancer. Proposal for a new scenario. In *Advances in Viral Oncology*, vol 6 (ed. G Klein), pp 173–206. Raven Press, New York.

Levitskaya J, Coram M, Levitsky V *et al.* (1995) Inhibition of antigen processing by the internal repeat region of the Epstein–Barr virus nuclear antigen-1. *Nature*, **375**, 685–688.

Leywraz S, Henle W, Chahinian AP *et al.* (1985) Association of Epstein–Barr virus with thymic carcinoma. *N Engl J Med*, **213**, 1296–1299.

Marafioti T, Hummel M, Foss H-D *et al.* (2000) Hodgkin and Reed–Sternberg cells represent an expansion of a single clone originating from a germinal centre B-cell with functional immunoglobulin gene rearrangements but defective immunoglobulin transcription. *Blood*, **95**, 1443–1450.

Nichols KE, Harkin DP, Levitz S *et al.* (1998) Inactivating mutations in an SH2 domain-encoding gene in X-linked lymphoproliferative syndrome. *Proc Natl Acad Sci USA*, **95**, 13765–13770.

Niederman JC, Evans AS, Subrahmanyan L and McCollum RW (1970) Prevalence, incidence and persistence of EB virus antibody in young adults. *N Engl J Med*, **282**, 361–365.

Old LJ, Boyse EA, Oettgen HF *et al.* (1966) Precipitating antibody in human serum to an antigen present in cultured Burkitt's lymphoma cells. *Proc Natl Acad Sci USA*, **45**, 1699–1704.

Purtilo DT, Cassel C and Yang JPS (1974) Fatal infectious mononucleosis. *N Engl J Med*, **291**, 736.

Raab-Traub N, Rajadurai P, Flynn K and Lanier AP (1991) Epstein–Barr virus infection in carcinoma of the salivary glands. *J Virol*, **65**, 7032–7036.

Reedman BM and Klein G (1973) Cellular localisation of an Epstein–Barr virus (EBV)-associated complement-fixing antigen in producer and non-producer lymphoblastoid cell lines. *Int J Cancer*, **11**, 499–520.

Rooney CM, Smith CA, Ng CYC *et al.* (1998) Infusion of cytotoxic T cells for the prevention and treatment of Epstein–Barr virus-induced lymphoma in allogeneic transplant recipients. *Blood*, **92**, 1549–1555.

Sayos J, Wu C, Morra M *et al.* (1998) The X-linked lymphoproliferative-disease gene product SAP regulates signals induced through the co-receptor SLAM. *Nature*, **395**, 462–469.

Sixbey JW, Nedrud JG, Raab-Traub N *et al.* (1984) Epstein–Barr virus replication in oropharyngeal epithelial cells. *N Engl J Med*, **310**, 1225–1230.

Tierney KJ, Steven N, Young LS and Rickinson AB (1994) Epstein–Barr virus latency in blood mononuclear cells: analysis of viral gene transcription during primary infection and in the carrier state. *J Virol*, **68**, 7374–7385.

Timms JM, Bell A, Flavell J *et al.* (2003) Epstein–Barr virus (EBV)-positive post-transplant lymphoproliferative disease frequently arises from B cells with randomly mutated or sterile immunoglobulin genes: a mechanistic link with EBV-positive Hodgkin's disease. *Lancet* (in press).

Tokunaga M, Land CE, Uemura Y *et al.* (1993) Epstein–Barr virus in gastric carcinoma. *Am J Pathol*, **143**, 1250–1254.

University Health Physicians and Public Health Laboratory Service Laboratories (1971) Infectious mononucleosis and its relationship to EB virus antibody. *Br Med J*, **5**, 643.

Wilson JB, Bell JL and Levine AJ (1996) Expression of Epstein–Barr virus nuclear antigen-1 induces B cell neoplasia in transgenic mice. *EMBO J*, **15**, 3117–3126.

Wilson JB, Weinberg W, Johnson R *et al.* (1990) Expression of the BJLF-1 oncogene of Epstein–Barr virus in the skin of transgenic mice induces hyperplasia and aberrant expression of keratin 6. *Cell*, **61**, 1315–1327.

Wolf HZW, Hansen H and Becker V (1973) EBV viral genomes in epithelial nasopharyngeal carcinoma cells. *Nature New Biol*, **244**, 245–247.

Roseoloviruses: Human Herpesviruses 6 and 7

Ursula A. Gompels

London School of Hygiene and Tropical Medicine, University of London, London, UK

INTRODUCTION

There is a group of viruses which infect almost all babies and persist for their lifetime. Lulled into complacency with their ubiquitous distribution, 'ignorance is not bliss', as these same viruses can be serious hazards during primary or reactivated infections, particularly in immunodeficient settings. When do these viruses cause pathology? How can they persist in cellular mediators of immunity, our own T lymphocytes and monocyte/macrophages? What can we learn from these well-adapted, persistent virus infections about our own immunity and can we use this knowledge to create new medicines for the future, which could also treat other conditions?

These are the roseoloviruses, *Human herpesvirus 6 and 7* (HHV-6, HHV-7). Fortunately, despite their widespread nature, these T lymphotropic and neurotropic viruses are generally regarded as benign infections; however, during some primary as well as secondary, reactivated infections in immunosuppressed patients severe complications have been recorded. In fact, in the last 15 or so years since their first identification there are at least 30 reports which have documented fatalities associated with these infections. This highlights the importance of their diagnosis and the role of better clinical care with available antiviral therapies, effective in some cases, plus the need for research and development of new therapeutic strategies plus better definition of *Roseolovirus* pathology and pathogenesis.

THE VIRUS

Biology

The general properties of HHV-6 and HHV-7 have been summarised in reviews, including the earlier version of this chapter (Gompels, 2000) and in descriptions of their complete genomic sequences (Table 2E.1). They are closely related, termed roseoloviruses, more distantly related to the cytomegaloviruses, and together forming the betaherpesvirus subgroup of human herpesviruses. There are two strain groups for HHV-6 (Ablashi *et al.*, 1993); the prototypes are strain U1102 for HHV-6 variant A (HHV-6A) and strain Z29 for variant B (HHV-6B); both genomes have been sequenced (Gompels *et al.*, 1995; Dominguez *et al.*, 1999). These show a closer relationship than many human cytomegalovirus (HCMV) strains. The HHV-6 variant strains differ by 5%, with increases primarily at the ends of the genomes overlapping repetitive sequences (Dominguez *et al.*, 1999; Gompels, 2000). There is also one hypervariable locus at the centre of the genome which also encodes a variable glycoprotein, U46 or gO, and marks a region of genomic reorganisation between herpesvirus subgroups (Gompels *et al.*, 1995; Kasolo *et al.*, 1997; Dominguez *et al.*, 1999; Gompels, 2000). Two strains of variant B genomic sequences are available and show less variation than between the variants (Dominguez *et al.*, 1999). The genomes of two strains of HHV-7, JI and RK, have also been sequenced and also show

Principles and Practice of Clinical Virology, Fifth Edition. Edited by A. J. Zuckerman, J. E. Banatvala, J. R. Pattison, P. D. Griffiths and B. D. Schoub
© 2004 John Wiley & Sons Ltd   ISBN 0 470 84338 1

Table 2E.1 Genomes of HHV-6 and HHV-7 strains

Virus NCBI http	Strain	Reference
HHV-6A	U1102	(Gompels *et al.*, 1995)
http://www.ncbi.nlm.nih.gov/entrez/query.fcgi?cmd = Retrieve&db = nucleotide&list_uids = 9628290&dopt = GenBank		
HHV-6B	Z29	(Dominguez *et al.*, 1999)
http://www.ncbi.nlm.nih.gov/entrez/query.fcgi?cmd = Retrieve&db = nucleotide&list_uids = 9633069&dopt = GenBank		
HHV-6B	HT	(Isegawa *et al.*, 1999)
http://www.ncbi.nlm.nih.gov/entrez/query.fcgi?cmd = Retrieve&db = nucleotide&list_uids = 4995977&dopt = GenBank		
HHV-7	JI	(Nicholas, 1996)
http://www.ncbi.nlm.nih.gov/entrez/query.fcgi?cmd = Retrieve&db = nucleotide&list_uids = 1236880&dopt = GenBank		
HHV-7	RK	(Megaw *et al.*, 1998)
http://www.ncbi.nlm.nih.gov/entrez/query.fcgi?cmd = Retrieve&db = nucleotide&list_uids = 9628718&dopt = GenBank		

less variation than beween the HHV-6A and B strain variant groupings (Nicholas, 1996; Megaw *et al.*, 1998).

Both HHV-6 and HHV-7 are T lymphotropic and neurotropic. *In vitro* HHV-6 can enter a wider variety of cell types, also sometimes confirmed in disseminated infections. A ubiquitous cellular receptor for HHV-6, CD46, has been identified, which is also a measles virus receptor, although HHV-6 interacts with a distinct site. CD46 interacts with the gH/gL/gQ complex of glycoproteins, which also mediate cellular fusion (Mori *et al.*, 2003; Santoro *et al.*, 2003). HHV-7 is more restricted and shares with HIV a cellular receptor, the CD4 antigen on helper T lymphocytes (Lusso *et al.*, 1994). As in other herpesviruses, there are likely to be multiple co-receptors and at least one other has been identified for HHV-7. These are the proteoglycan heparin or heparan sulphate, common virus receptors, which can bind to HHV-7 pp65 (ORF100) the homologue of HHV-6 glycoprotein gQ (U100), gp105 (Skrincosky *et al.*, 2000).

Both HHV-6 and HHV-7 have also been isolated from saliva and viral antigen has been identified in salivary epithelium, where the viruses may be secreted. Infection of the female genital tract has also been reported. HHV-7 appears to be more frequently shed in saliva or at higher detectable levels. This is likely to be the main route of host-to-host transmission. Other routes include iatrogenic transfer with blood products or organ transplants. Unlike the other human beta-herpesvirus, HCMV, HHV-6 and HHV-7 are not frequently shed in urine, although some virus can be detected.

Lytic Replication and Latency

Both HHV-6 and HHV-7 can be cultivated in activated cord blood lymphocytes or mononuclear cells (CBL, CBMC) or in peripheral blood lymphocytes or mononuclear cells (PBL, PBMC). Cord blood is used preferentially, as infection with laboratory strains can result in reactivation of resident latent virus from adult blood (Black *et al.*, 1989; Frenkel *et al.*, 1990; Katsafanas *et al.*, 1996). In routine culture both have been adapted to grow in CD4$^+$ T leukaemic cell lines, e.g. J-JHAN (Jurkat), HSB2, Molt-3 for HHV-6, and SupT-1 for HHV-7 (Cermelli *et al.*, 1997).

Both HHV-6 and HHV-7 have a cellular tropism for T lymphocytes. This has been shown *in vivo* during viraemia from acute infection as well as *in vitro*. The viruses infect and spread in these cells, showing a characteristic cytopathic effect of large cells (cytomegalia) and ballooning cells (Figure 2E.1). The cells are completely permissive for replication and virus production, where infection results in cell death by necrotic lysis. There is *in vitro* evidence that infection also causes cell death by apoptosis in uninfected or non-productively infected bystander cells (Inoue *et al.*, 1997; Secchiero *et al.*, 1997a). Both CD4$^+$, CD8$^+$ and γ/δ T lymphocytes can be infected, but the evidence suggests that activated CD4$^+$ T lymphocytes are the preferential target of fully permissive infection *in vivo* (Takahashi *et al.*, 1989; Lusso *et al.*, 1991). Antibody to CD3 (OKT3) has been shown to augment infection of HHV-6 in both primary (Roffman and Frenkel, 1991) and T leukaemic cell lines (H.A. Macaulay and U.A. Gompels, unpublished results).

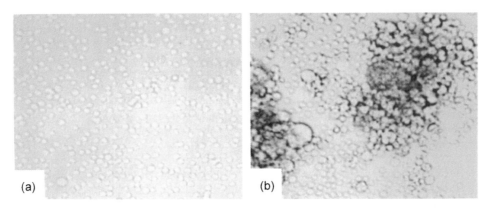

(a)   (b)

Figure 2E.1 The cytopathic effect of HHV-6 on CD4$^+$ T lymphocytes. This shows uninfected cells (JJhan T leukaemia cell line) in (a), and infected cells 5 days post-infection in (b). The cytopathic effect includes clumped, fused cells, cytomegalia (large cells, including multinucleated) and 'balloon cells' (cells which appear to have grossly enlarged cytoplasm). Infection and cell fusion can result subsequently in cell lysis

There is evidence for latency within monocytic/macrophage cells as well as bone marrow progenitor cells (Kondo *et al.*, 1991; Gompels *et al.*, 1993, 1994; Kempf *et al.*, 1997; Yasukawa *et al.*, 1997). A strong interaction has been recorded during primary infection and may also include a form of latency, with specific restricted transcripts (Kondo *et al.*, 2002, 2003). Latent infection of primary macrophages has also been observed for HHV-7 (Zhang *et al.*, 2002). HHV-7 can be detected by PCR in blood and saliva of asymptomatic adults in higher levels than HHV-6 (DiLuca *et al.*, 1995; Kidd *et al.*, 1996; Gautheret Dejean *et al.*, 1997). On this basis it has been suggested that HHV-7 may exist in a less controlled state of latency than HHV-6. Evidence has been presented that HHV-7 can reactivate HHV-6 (Katsafanas *et al.*, 1996). A latency gene has been identified for HHV-6, U94/Rep; it is highly conserved between strains but deleted in HHV-7 (Rapp *et al.*, 2001; Caselli *et al.*, 2002). U94/Rep has roles in gene expression and replication modulation, which may contribute to lower levels of HHV-6 identified during latency (Mori *et al.*, 2000; Rapp *et al.*, 2001; Caselli *et al.*, 2002; Dhepakson *et al.*, 2002; Turner *et al.*, 2002).

Molecular Biology

The genomes of HHV-6 and HHV-7 are, respectively, 153 kb and 145 kb in size. They are both bounded by terminal direct repeats of 8 kb and 6 kb, respectively, which themselves are bounded by repeated sequences similar to the telomeric repeats (GGGTTA) at the end of human chromosomes. Roles for these sequences in replication and latency have been proposed. The open reading frames in HHV-6 strain U1102 are designated U1–U100, with those in the direct repeats as DR1–DR7 (Gompels *et al.*, 1995). In HHV-7 similar nomenclature is used with homologous genes U2–U100 (Nicholas, 1996). A few genes are lacking in HHV-7 compared to HHV-6 but there are also a few HHV-7-specific genes, noted H1–H7 (Gompels *et al.*, 1995; Nicholas, 1996; Megaw *et al.*, 1998).

The genomes are most closely related to each other, with similarity between the encoded amino acid sequences in over 90% of the ORFs. Similarities to other vertebrate herpesviruses can be identified in only 20–30% of the ORFs, the 'conserved herpesvirus genes'. The organisation of these genes can be grouped into seven gene blocks (Gompels *et al.*, 1995; Nicholas, 1996; Megaw *et al.*, 1998). The arrangement of these gene blocks is subgroup-specific. HHV-6 and HHV-7 share with HCMV a betaherpesvirus organisation of these gene blocks.

Analyses of HHV-6 and HHV-7 coding sequences also place them within the betaherpesvirus subgroup of the *Herpesviridae*. They share the closest relation with human cytomegalovirus, the prototype betaherpesvirus, with approximately two-thirds of the genes encoding similar proteins. However, this relationship is distant and can only be determined by encoded amino acid sequences. Furthermore, HCMV is almost double the size, 230 kb, containing extended glycoprotein gene families absent from HHV-6 and HHV-7. HCMV is representative of beta-1 herpesviruses, the cytomegaloviruses, and HHV-6/-7 as beta-2 herpesviruses, the roseoloviruses.

The virus infects and spreads by cell fusion and candidate glycoproteins which mediate this process have been identified in each virus, the conserved gH and gL complex, encoded by HHV-6 and HHV-7 U48 and U82 (Liu et al., 1993a, 1993b; Gompels et al., 1995; Nicholas, 1996; Anderson and Gompels, 1999). These glycoproteins also form a complex with gQ (U100) in HHV-6 (Mori et al., 2003). Some functional interactions between betaherpesviruses have been observed, e.g. substitution of HCMV gH or gL glycoproteins can form complexes with HHV-6 gH/gL and may affect fusogenic spread of the viruses during reactivations (Anderson et al., 1996). Conserved replication and structural genes have been identified. An origin of lytic replication has been localised and characterised plus viral genes involved in replication, including enzyme targets of established antiviral drugs, such as a viral DNA polymerase, HHV-6 and HHV-7 U38, and phosphotransferase, HHV-6 and HHV-7 U69. Unlike HCMV, HHV-6 and HHV-7 encode an origin binding protein, 'OBP', homologue, HHV-6 and HHV-7 U73, which is found in alphaherpesviruses (Krug et al., 2001). This suggests a difference in replication strategy to HCMV, although HHV-6 and HHV-7 have more complicated origins then HSV and are more similar to other betaherpesviruses. These differences may affect replication strategies as well as the specificity of potential antivirals, which target replication. About one-third of HHV-6 and HHV-7 genes are specific to these two viruses and presumably reflect adaptations to their particular cellular tropism.

Both HHV-6 and HHV-7 also encode proteins with similarity to cellular products, chemokine receptors (U12 and U51), a chemokine (specific for HHV-6, U83) and members of the immunoglobulin superfamily, including an OX-2 homologue (HHV-6 and HHV-7 U85) (Gompels and Macaulay, 1995; Nicholas, 1996; Isegawa et al., 1998; Milne et al., 2000). Products of these genes may contribute an immunomodulatory role (see below).

Gene regulation appears to follow the same cascade as in other herpesviruses. There are 'immediate-early' (IE) or 'alpha' genes, which include regulators of virus gene expression, followed by 'early' (E) or 'beta' genes, including enzymes for DNA replication, then 'late' (L) or 'gamma' genes, which include structural genes for the virus particle. The IE genes are important in the switch between lytic replication and latency and include U86 and U89 sequence and positional homologues, respectively, of HCMV IE2 and IE1 as well as U16/17, also with HCMV positional homologues. In HHV-6 the IE1 gene also shows different organisation

between strain variants (Yamamoto et al., 1994). This IE region has a lower CG dinucleotide frequency then expected and this feature is a mark of regions in the host genome that are subject to DNA methylation, which can affect regulation of gene expression (Gompels et al., 1995). This is found in other betaherpesviruses and may reflect similarities in latency control in monocytic/macrophages or bone marrow progenitor cells.

Gene Therapy Applications

In gene therapy, virus vectors have been evaluated for tissue-specific gene delivery. Amplicon vectors have been constructed from both HHV-6 and HHV-7, which may have applications to delivery to stem cells or bone marrow progenitor cells (Deng and Dewhurst, 1998; Romi et al., 1999; Turner et al., 2002). These amplicons contain an origin of replication together with terminal sequences directing DNA packaging. The target gene in these vectors thus will be amplified to genome size, approximately 150 kb, before packaging into the capsid using helper virus. There are problems in that their efficiency appears much lower than similar amplicons derived from HSV-1 and, further, that cell lines expressing virus proteins for helper virus-free DNA packaging have not yet been described and would be necessary to minimise potential pathology.

Immunity

Neutralising antibodies are generated to both viruses after primary infections. Some of the antigens for this response have been defined and they include the conserved glycoproteins gB(U39), neutralising with complement, and the gH/gL complex (U48/U82), neutralising in the absence of complement (Liu et al., 1993a, 1993b; Anderson and Gompels, 1999). In HHV-6 there is a multiple spliced glycoprotein, gp 82/105, HHV-6 U100, gQ, which forms a complex with gH/gL, and this is also a target for neutralising antibodies. A homologue to this protein exists only in HHV-7 and not in other herpesviruses; HHV-7 gQ also induces neutralising antibodies (Skrincosky et al., 2000; Mori et al., 2003; Santoro et al., 2003). Monoclonal antibody reagents have been generated to both of these viruses and some of these have been developed into diagnostic assay systems. As yet none have 100% specificity but may be useful in characterising responses in patient groups. As with other human herpesviruses, many of the antibody responses generated are not relevant to a protective response but are useful in diagnostic systems. Thus, a high serological titre does not necessarily correspond to a high protective antibody response.

Cellular immunity has been demonstrated to both HHV-6 and HHV-7. The responses to HHV-6 and HHV-7 are largely specific, although some reactions show cross-reactivity, as would be predicted from sequence comparisons (Yasukawa *et al.*, 1993). Specific clones have been generated from both CD4$^+$ T lymphocytes and NK cells as well as antigen specific cell lines, e.g. to immunodominant p101. Thus, although HHV-6 and HHV-7 have the capacity to kill T lymphocytes, they can also generate a normal antiviral response, given antigen presentation to these cells.

Immunomodulation

Aside from direct cellular lysis of permissive T lymphocytes, HHV-6 and HHV-7 can also have effects which perturb the function of immune cells. The killing of T lymphocytes can also be mediated by T cell apoptosis in a bystander effect induced by HHV-6- or HHV-7-infected cells (Inoue *et al.*, 1997; Secchiero *et al.*, 1997a, 2001). Studies on HHV-7 show that it upregulates TNF-related apoptosis-inducing ligand (TRAIL) and induced cytotoxic responses in bystander cells through this pathway, while antigen-expressing cells become resistant through downregulation of TRAIL-R1, allowing persistence (Secchiero *et al.*, 2001). Direct virus effects on cellular proteins may also affect functions of immune cells. As mentioned above, HHV-6 and HHV-7 can affect surface expression of CD3 and CD4 antigens, thus affecting immune activation and signal transduction. HHV-6 downregulates CD3 and HHV-7 downregulates CD4 (Lusso *et al.*, 1991; Furukawa *et al.*, 1994; Secchiero *et al.*, 1997b). Multiple mechanisms involving both transcriptional and posttranscriptional events appear to be involved. HHV-6 can upregulate CD4 on a number of cell types, including NK and γδT cells *in vitro* and recently confirmed in a lymphoid tissue *ex vivo* system (Grivel *et al.*, 2003). This can affect the function of these cells, giving rise to abnormal signalling, and may reflect wider activation of the cell types. Interestingly, where CD4 expression is introduced in bone marrow progenitor cells, these are rendered sensitive to infection with HHV-7, so there may be a number of synergistic effects between these viruses (Yasukawa *et al.*, 1997). As in other herpesviruses, infection can lead to downregulation of major histocompatibility complex (MHC) class I molecules.

In HHV-7 the U21 gene product has been shown to downregulate class I, diverting it to lysosomes for breakdown. This immune escape mechanism can prevent detection of infected cells by cytotoxic T lymphocytes, thereby facilitating virus persistence (Hudson *et al.*, 2001).

A number of cytokines are abnormally regulated in HHV-6 infected cells. These include downregulation of IL-2 synthesis, leading to suppression of cellular proliferation (Flamand *et al.*, 1995). HHV-6 can inhibit the proliferative responses of PBMC (Horvat *et al.*, 1993), whereas levels of IL-2 can inhibit HHV-6 replication (Roffman and Frenkel, 1990). Other cytokines are upregulated by HHV-6 infection, including IL-10, IL-12, TNFα, and IL-1β (Flamand *et al.*, 1991; Li *et al.*, 1997). Although recent studies *in vitro* suggest suppression of IL-12, *in vivo* studies show upregulation of IL-12 during HHV-6 reactivation (Chapenko *et al.*, 2003; Smith *et al.*, 2003). These may be cell type- or gene-specific effects dependent on kinetics of expression and could affect generation of IL-12-dependent autoimmune T helper type (TH1) cells. Downregulation and upregulation of the chemokine RANTES has been observed in different epithelial or lymphoid cell types (Milne *et al.*, 1997; Grivel *et al.*, 2001), whereas IL-8 is upregulated in hepatic epithelial cells (Inagi *et al.*, 1996). In addition, HHV-6 can upregulate expression of monocyte cyclooxygenase-2 and prostaglandin E(2) (PGE2) synthesis, which is produced mainly in monocytic/macrophage cells; further PGE2 treatment of infected cells appeared to enhance virus replication (Janelle *et al.*, 2002). HHV-6 can enhance NK cell activity through IL-15, where it also has upregulated CD4 (Flamand *et al.*, 1996). HHV-6 virus infection can also upregulate TNF-κB receptors and chemokine receptors, EB1 or CCR7, which can further influence signalling in different cell types (Hasegawa *et al.*, 1994; Yoshida *et al.*, 1997). Interestingly, the ligand for CCR7, ELC/MIP3b, is most strongly expressed in thymus and lymph nodes, where these viruses can replicate (Yoshida *et al.*, 1997), and HHV-7 U12 is specific for this ligand (Nakano *et al.*, 2003).

HHV-6 infection has been shown *in vitro* to be associated with dysfunction of monocytes, as well as suppression of macrophage maturation in human bone marrow cultures. HHV-6 has also been shown to suppress *in vitro* cell differentiation and colony formation of haematopoietic progenitor cells (Knox and Carrigan, 1992; Isomura *et al.*, 1997), while HHV-7 infection has been shown to inhibit megakaryocyte survival or differentiation (Gonelli *et al.*, 2002). These findings correlate with some of the *in vivo* findings of HHV-6- and HHV-7-associated stem cell or bone marrow suppression. Recent data analysing cellular immune-specific gene expression after HHV-6 infection using microarrays suggest that infection leads to a TH1 phenotype (Mayne *et al.*, 2001). Interestingly, some similarities in immunomodulation have recently also been noted while characterising HHV-6-specific T cell lines from MS patients which were inefficient at virus clearance. These had decreased IL-4 and IL-10 (Tejada-Simon *et al.*, 2002).

Other direct effects on immunomodulation are possible by gene products which mimic the actions of immune regulatory molecules. These can have actions of either enhancing infection and/or modulating protective immunity. Both HHV-6 and HHV-7 encode a number of proteins which may affect immune recognition or activation. These include members of the immunoglobulin, chemokine receptor and chemokine protein families (Gompels *et al.*, 1995; Nicholas, 1996). Two chemokine receptor homologues are encoded by HHV-6 and HHV-7, U12 and U51. In HHV-6 both of these are functional CC chemokine receptors (Isegawa *et al.*, 1998; Milne *et al.*, 2000) and may play immunomodulatory roles (Murphy, 2001). U51 expression leads to downregulation of chemokine ligand RANTES transcription and secretion, a novel immunomodulatory mechanism, and has a unique specificity which overlaps cellular CCR1, 2, 3 and 5 chemokine receptors (Milne *et al.*, 2000). Recent results show these are ligand-inducible activities by calcium signalling similar to cellular receptors, although there may additionally be virus-specific constitutive pathways (Gompels and Dewin, 2003). U12 is regulated late and U51 early, thus they may play different roles in replication, affecting cellular spread, infected cell migration and cellular signalling. HHV-6, but not HHV-7, encodes a functional chemokine, U83, which has been shown specific for CCR2, to chemoattract monocytic cells, sites for latent infection, and may affect virus dissemination (Zou *et al.*, 1999, Littichau *et al.*, 2003). However, this gene is highly variable in different strains, and thus may encode a number of immunomodulatory specificities with different possible pathogenic effects (French *et al.*, 1999; D. Dewin and U. Gompels, unpublished results). Chemokines and their receptors are key mediators of an inflammatory response, therefore understanding the specificities of the HHV-6 and HHV-7 homologues may not only show new roles in modulating these virus infections but could also lead to novel immunotherapeutics for inflammatory disease in general.

HHV-6/-7 and HIV interactions. Both roseoloviruses and HIV can infect T lymphocytes and monocytic/macrophage cells; possible interactions of HHV-6 and HIV include control of gene expression and cellular receptor binding interference, competitive effects on cellular receptors for virus infection, as well as general immunomodulatory effects. Transactivation of the HIV LTR promoter of gene expression has been shown *in vitro* using reporter gene assays for HHV-6 proteins encoded by DR7, U16, U27, U89 and U94, as reviewed previously (Gompels *et al.*, 1995). It has also been shown *in vivo*, whereby HHV-6 gene expression (DR7) has been shown to reactivate a tat-deficient HIV provirus from latency (Kashanchi *et al.*, 1997). In addition HHV-6 can upregulate the HIV receptor CD4, whereas HHV-7 can compete for binding to this receptor and downregulate its expression (Lusso *et al.*, 1994). HHV-6 may also affect utilisation of the HIV co-receptors, the chemokine receptors CCR5 and CXCR4. Recent studies of ex-vivo lymphoid tissue HHV-6 infections show that HHV-6 upregulates CCR-5 ligand RANTES and that this can inhibit HIV infection by CCR5-utilising strains (Grivel *et al.*, 2001). Whereas *in vitro* studies in epithelial or infected endothelial cells already secreting or induced to express RANTES, show that HHV-6 can downregulate this RANTES secretion by expression of the HHV-6 chemokine receptor, U51, which can bind RANTES (Milne *et al.*, 2000; Caruso *et al.*, 2003). Thus, depending on cell type and stage of infection, HHV-6 could inhibit or enhance CCR5-utilising HIV strains, generally macrophage-tropic.

EPIDEMIOLOGY

HHV-6 and HHV-7 are common paediatric infections. Maternal antibodies are present at birth, then decrease to 6 months of age, when the seropositive rate increases (Yoshikawa *et al.*, 1989; Enders *et al.*, 1990; Hall *et al.*, 1994). With age, the serological titre appears to gradually decrease but persists, and the viruses establish lifelong infections characteristic of other herpesviruses. Up to 100% of adult populations are seropositive for these viruses (Enders *et al.*, 1990; Ward *et al.*, 1993; Yoshikawa *et al.*, 1993). A similar pattern exists for HHV-7, although infection appears to occur later during infancy and early childhood, with seropositivity increasing to adulthood (Yoshikawa *et al.*, 1993; Huang *et al.*, 1997; Yoshida *et al.*, 2002).

There is evidence for congenital and neonate infections (Hall *et al.*, 1994), although the majority of children appear to be infected during infancy by horizontal transmission, probably involving salivary fluid. There is no evidence for transmission by breast milk, but studies of strains in families show that the strain type is conserved and that either parent or closely related adults/siblings may transmit HHV-6 or HHV-7.

HHV-6B strains seem more prevalent in primary paediatric infections, where tested, primarily in 'Western' countries, with occasional HHV-6A infection (Van Loon *et al.*, 1995), but there appears to be geographic variation, as in an African country, Zambia, febrile paediatric infection with HHV-6A strains appears to have similar prevalence to HHV-6B (Kasolo *et al.*, 1997). Where both variant strain groups are prevalent, some sequences appear to be mixtures (Kasolo and Gompels, unpublished results). These studies have been done by DNA PCR followed by restriction enzyme digestions or nucleotide sequencing from PBMC during acute infections when there is sufficient viraemia, or 'DNAaemia', for assay. However, true distribution by strain-specific serology has yet to be performed, hampered by antibody cross-reactivity against whole virus antigen lysates and lack of single antigens with a combination of 100% specificity and immunodominance. Analyses of this distribution by strain-specific PCR on blood DNA is possible, from samples during acute primary infection, mostly in infants. There are problems collecting this information, however, as infant blood samples are not generally available and primary infection not routinely diagnosed.

Infection by HHV-6 or HHV-7 usually seems to give lifelong protective immunity. However, this may be largely dependent on the initial severity of the primary infection, route of infection and the nature of the specific response generated, as well as any later immune defects or modulation/suppression. Asymptomatic or symptomatic infections with multiple strains, both HHV-6A and HHV-6B or multiple HHV-6B strains, have been recorded even during infant primary infections (Van Loon *et al.*, 1995). Infection with HHV-6 does not appear to prevent subsequent infection with HHV-7, but it is possible, as it is with other related herpesviruses, that cross-reactive epitopes in some of the conserved proteins do generate cross-protective responses that may reduce the severity of symptoms or lead to asymptomatic infection.

CLINICAL FEATURES

Primary Infection

Fever and Rash (Exanthem Subitum, Roseola Infantum)

An extensive study of childhood infections with HHV-6, in a large USA paediatric population of 3000, has shown

that the primary characteristic of infant infections with HHV-6 is a high fever for 3–4 days (mean 39.4–39.7°C in different studies), with a small proportion of these (6–10%) additionally developing a rash, termed exanthem subitum (ES) (Hall *et al.*, 1994). HHV-6, primarily, and also HHV-7 cause ES (also known as roseola infantum or sixth disease), a mild skin rash in infants and young children which is accompanied by fever and can have rare but serious complications (Okada *et al.*, 1993; Hall *et al.*, 1994; Tanaka *et al.*, 1994). In infants diagnosed with ES, 80% had seroconversion or rise in HHV-6 antibodies, with a mean age of infection at 7.3 months (Pruksananonda *et al.*, 1992; Hall *et al.*, 1994). These are measles-like or rubella-like macular or papular rashes on the face, the trunk or both, which can confound measles and rubella surveillance and analyses of vaccine failures (Black *et al.*, 1996; Tait *et al.*, 1996; Kasolo *et al.*, 1997).

Febrile Seizure and Complications

Other symptoms previously only related to ES are also experienced in the febrile illness of primary paediatric infection with HHV-6, as it presents mostly without rash and thus is underdiagnosed (Hall *et al.*, 1994). These appear to be related to the level of virus replication, and include diarrhoea, respiratory symptoms, convulsions, cervical lymph node swelling and anterior fontanelle bulging (Okada *et al.*, 1993; Asano *et al.*, 1994; Hall *et al.*, 1994). HHV-6 diarrhoea appears to correlate with infection of the large intestine, as shown in children undergoing stem cell transplantation (Amo *et al.*, 2003). During primary infections there is a transient leukopenia observed, which is consistent with the ability of the virus to replicate in and kill lymphocytes. The relative complications observed in primary childhood infections with HHV-6 include skin rash (6–10%), febrile seizures (10%), hepatitis, bone marrow suppression, recurrent encephalitis, gastrointestinal (10%) and respiratory symptoms (sinusitis and pneumonitis, 10%) (Hall *et al.*, 1994). Some of these are serious and occasionally can lead to mortalities, as noted in the following sections.

Primary HHV-6 infection is a major paediatric infection and appears to be the first febrile episode in infants. Although generally a self-limiting illness, the USA study demonstrated that HHV-6 accounted for 20% of emergency ward visits from febrile illness for infants between 6–12 months (Hall *et al.*, 1994). In USA and Italy, in patients under the age of 2–3 years and admitted to hospital with acute febrile illnesses, 10–24% were due to primary HHV-6 infection (Hall *et al.*, 1994; Portolani *et al.*, 1993). In the Italian study, primary infections with this virus accounted for 40% of childhood hospitalisations for virus infections, higher by 10-fold than any other diagnosable agent (Portolani *et al.*, 1993). In a recent USA study of febrile infants under 90 days, evidence of active HHV-6 infection was found in 10% (Byington *et al.*, 2002).

The most common serious complication during primary HHV-6 infection is febrile seizure, which accounts for one-third of all febrile seizures under the age of 3 (Hall *et al.*, 1994). HHV-6 is also associated with recurrent seizures, meningoencephalitis, and other CNS complications which may have a fatal outcome, including occasional observations of epilepsy (Kondo *et al.*, 1993; Suga *et al.*, 1993; Hall *et al.*, 1994). A case-control study shows that the incidence of HHV-6 infection is similar in patients with febrile seizures and age-matched controls, suggesting that the febrile response to HHV-6 infection may be the main factor giving rise to seizures (Hukin *et al.*, 1998). However, there may also be a direct interaction of the virus with the CNS, as both HHV-6 and HHV-7 are commonly identified in brain autopsies and the DNA identified in CSF during associated neurological conditions. Occasional congenital infection with HHV-6B has been recorded, associated with seizures and poor neurological outcome (Lanari *et al.*, 2003). HHV-7 has also been associated with infant febrile convulsions during seroconversion (Clark *et al.*, 1997), as well as central nervous system (CNS) complications during exanthem subitum (Torigoe *et al.*, 1996).

Due to highly efficient infection during childhood, HHV-6 and HHV-7 primary infections in adults are rare, but where cases have been identified they appear more severe. For HHV-6, primary adult infection has been associated with fever and fits in a liver transplant patient. For HHV-7, primary infection in an immunocompetent adult was associated with encephalitis and flaccid paralysis, with active primary infection determined by antibody avidity and DNA PCR in serum and CSF (Ward *et al.*, 1989; Ward *et al.*, 2002b). The viruses have also been associated with infectious mononucleosis, where the patients are negative for main agents related with this disease, EBV and HCMV.

Secondary Reactivated Infections

In transplant patients receiving prophylactic immunosuppressive therapy, HHV-6 reactivation has been documented as one of the first human herpesviruses to reactivate, before HCMV and EBV infections (Wang et al., 1996). Complications due to HHV-6 and HHV-7 reactivations, as well as rare adult primary infections, can be seen in solid organ and stem cell or bone marrow transplant patients.

Solid Organ Transplantation

Most recent data for solid organ transplantation is disease associated with liver transplantation, with some also for renal. This has been reviewed recently (Razonable and Paya, 2002) and there are two areas, one of direct effects of HHV-6 reactivation, which includes anecdotal reports of fever, rash, pneumonitis, encephalitis, hepatitis and myelosuppression. The second area has the most current reports and is updated here; this is an indirect effect of virus replication through immunomodulation, leading to graft rejection or interactions amongst all three betaherpesviruses, in particular leading to HCMV disease (Dockrell *et al.*, 1997; DesJardin *et al.*, 1998, 2001; Emery, 2001; Humar *et al.*, 2002a, 2002b; Lautenschlager *et al.*, 2002b). In studies of 139 liver transplant patients by IgG/M antibodies, frequent HHV-6 reactivation (63%) was associated with severe CMV disease as well as older age and use of muromonab-CD3 as treatment for rejection. Similar results were found using quantitative PCR, where virus reactivation (at a viral load >2 log10 copies/µg input DNA) was common, 28% of 200 patients. There was symptomatic disease due to HHV-6 alone in 1%, but the main effect of HHV-6 reactivation was immunomodulatory, with a three- to four-fold increase in opportunistic infections and CMV disease with a subgroup of delayed rejections (>30 days) (Humar *et al.*, 2002a). Similar effects have been suggested for HHV-7, as well as HHV-6, reactivation in relation to HCMV disease in renal allograft patients (Osman *et al.*, 1996; DesJardin *et al.*, 1998; Kidd *et al.*, 2000). This indirect immunomodulatory effect has also been observed in liver transplant patients who were undergoing transplantation as a treatment for chronic hepatitis C (HCV) infection. In these patients, HHV-6 reactivation did not relate to increases in HCV viral load, but did correlate with more severe recurrence of HCV (biopsy-proven) in terms of hepatitis or fibrosis score, as well as fibrosis for patients with CMV disease (Humar *et al.*, 2002b). Investigations into mechanisms have suggested HHV-6 effects on increased adhesion molecule expression and lymphocyte infiltration in liver allografts and that this may also be a factor in rejection (Lautenschlager *et al.*, 2002a). In addition, in liver transplant patients, a prolonged suppression of HHV-6, but not HCMV, memory T cell response has been observed, correlating with HHV-6 viraemia (Singh *et al.*, 2002).

Stem Cell or Bone Marrow Transplantation

In cord blood, stem cell (PBSCT and CBSCT) and bone marrow (BMT) transplant patients a similar story is emerging, that of direct effects, in these cases primarily encephalitis, with also immunomodulatory effects leading to CMV infections or inhibiting graft outgrowth of specific lineages, also recently reviewed (Ljungman, 2002). Current reports identify HHV-6-associated encephalitis after virus reactivation in paediatric as well as adult unrelated cord blood and allogeneic bone marrow transplant patients (Zerr *et al.*, 2001; Chik *et al.*, 2002; MacLean and Douen, 2002; Rapaport *et al.*, 2002). Retrospective studies of allogeneic BMT patients identify HHV-6 as an independent risk factor for encephalitis, which can be paradoxically enhanced by CD3 antibody, often used for the prophylaxis of acute graft-vs.-host disease (Zerr *et al.*, 2001). Similar results were noted above in liver transplant patients using CD3 antibody. In this respect, it is of interest that CD3 antibody OKT3 *in vitro* can enhance HHV-6 cellular spread (Roffman and Frenkel, 1991; Macaulay and Gompels, unpublished results). Thus, differences in immunosuppressive regime may affect virus reactivation and sequelae.

Various neurological effects have been reported, including severe amnesia followed by HHV-6 encephalitis in an adult BMT patient (MacLean and Douen, 2002). HHV-6 DNA is identified in the CSF and there is viral DNAaemia prior to onset of disease (Chik *et al.*, 2002), with studies by quantitative PCR showing peaks at 2 weeks and 3 weeks post-transplantation in BMT and SCT patients, respectively (Ihira *et al.*, 2002; Tokimasa *et al.*, 2002). Real-time PCR has quantitated levels in BMT patients PBMC and CSF, range < 10–7500 EqCop/100 PBMCs and < 10–$415\,820$ EqCop/100 µl whole CSF, compared to healthy levels of 0.00015–0.0008 equivalent DNA copy number (EqCop)/100 only in PBMCs (Gautheret-Dejean *et al.*, 2002). The highest levels of DNAaemia during virus reactivation, greater than in exanthem subitum or BMT/PBSCT, were found in cord blood SCT (Sashihara *et al.*, 2002). This and the effect of certain CD3 antibodies appear to identify components that may enhance virus replication *in vivo*.

Cord blood is the best cell type to propagate virus *in vitro*.

HHV-6 skin rashes after 1 month post-transplantation may resemble GVHD (Yoshikawa *et al.*, 2001). Other direct effects in SCT patients include diarrhoea and HHV-6B was identified by PCR and *in situ* hybridisation in large intestinal cells (Amo *et al.*, 2003). Effects of immunomodulation by HHV-6 reactivation ($\geqslant 100$ copies/µg input DNA) have also been observed for allogeneic SCT, leading to CMV reactivation and correlating with an absence of CMV-specific lymphocyte proliferation post-transplantation (Wang *et al.*, 2002). Studies on treatment show some efficacy with ganciclovir (GCV), although aciclovir (ACV) is less potent (Chik *et al.*, 2002; Rapaport *et al.*, 2002; Tokimasa *et al.*, 2002). A case report of primary HHV-7, with neurological disease, acute myelitis, after unrelated BMT has been published (Ward *et al.*, 2002b). Prospective studies are required to further assess treatment options for and disease contributions by both these roseoloviruses in transplantation.

Associated Fatalities

Although usually a self-limiting infection, fatalities associated with HHV-6 and HHV-7 have also been recorded (Table 2E.2). These are primarily anecdotal reports, but a review of these point to potential risk factors which could indicate conditions for antiviral intervention. Potential risk factors include the higher viral load during primary infection or during reactivations following immunosuppression. In the paediatric group, fatalities are due to complications from ES or primary infections, other co-infections or underlying syndromes. Here the course can be rapid, with death between 15 days to 2 months. In infected adults, immunosuppressive conditions (e.g. in transplant recipients) or therapy can give rise to virus reactivation associated with mortalities, but also HHV-6 itself has an immunosuppressive effect which can underlie other fatal infections, notably fungal or other virus infections, such as HCMV. Table 2E.2 lists fatalities in both infected adults and children from either encephalitis or disseminated infections giving rise to heart disease, pneumonitis or hepatitis (one case). HHV-6 may be more pathogenic than HHV-7, as the fatalities reported are almost all for HHV-6, with only one exception for HHV-7, a paediatric case of fatal encephalitis in a peripheral blood stem cell transplant patient. Where variant strain group typing has been done for HHV-6 (Table 2E.2) (only eight cases), they

Table 2E.2   Fatal outcomes associated with HHV-6 or HHV-7 infections

Virus	Diagnosis	Fatal disease or complication	Reference
Paediatric			
HHV-6	Primary infection, ES	Encephalitis	Ahtiluoto *et al.* (2000)
HHV-6	Primary infection, ES	Encephalitis	Asano *et al.* (1992)
HHV-6	Primary complication	Griselli's syndrome	Wagner *et al.* (1997)
HHV-6B	Primary infection, Disseminated infection	Seizures, VZV co-infection	Ueda *et al.* (1996)
HHV-6B	Disseminated infection	Haemophagocytic syndrome	Portolani *et al.* (1997)
HHV-6	Disseminated infection	Pneumonia, T lymphocytopenia, thymic atrophy	Knox *et al.* (1995)
HHV-6	Disseminated infection	Interstitial pneumonitis, atypical lymphocyte infiltrates	Hoang *et al.* (1999)
HHV-6B	Disseminated infection after primary infection, ES	Acute myocarditis	Yoshikawa *et al.* (2002a)
HHV-6	Disseminated infection after primary infection, ES	Cardiac failure	Prezioso *et al.* (1992)
HHV-6	Disseminated infection	Severe myocarditis, B19 co-infection; no antiviral immunity	Rohayem *et al.* (2001)
HHV-6	Disseminated infection	Fulminant hepatitis	Asano *et al.* (1990)
HHV-7	Primary or reactivation	Encephalitis, stem cell transplant	Chan *et al.* (2002)
Adult			
HHV-6A	Primary infection	Multifocal meningoencephalitis	Beovic *et al.* (2001)
HHV-6	Primary infection	Demyelinating encephalomyelitis	Novoa *et al.* (1997)
HHV-6A	Reactivation	Encephalitis; after hormone treatment for prostate cancer, aged 85	Portolani *et al.* (2002)
HHV-6	Reactivation	Encephalitis; co-infection with HSV-1, 2/3 patients	Tang *et al.* (1997)
HHV-6	Reactivation	Encephalitis, then seizure in epilepsy patient	Wang *et al.* (1999)
HHV-6	Reactivation	Encephalitis, stem cell transplant	Tiacci *et al.* (2000)
HHV-6B	Reactivation	Encephalitis, bone marrow transplant	Drobyski *et al.* (1994)
HHV-6A	Reactivation	Encephalitis, bone marrow transplant	De Almeida Rodriguez *et al.* (1999)
HHV-6	Reactivation	Encephalitis, bone marrow transplant	Rapaport *et al.* (2002)
HHV-6	Reactivation	Fulminant myocarditis after steroid treatment hepatitis	Fukae *et al.* (2000)
HHV-6	Reactivation	Late mortality in liver transplant recipients; fungal infections predictor	Rogers *et al.* (2000)
HHV-6	Reactivation	Higher mortality rate, heart–lung transplant recipients, fungal disease	Jacobs *et al.* (2003)
HHV-6A	Primary, disseminated	Haemophagocytic syndrome, aplasia, then fulminant candidaemia in renal transplant recipient	Rogers *et al.* (2000)
HHV-6	Reactivation	Lymphocytopenia leading to CMV disease	Yoshikawa *et al.* (2002b)
HHV-6	Reactivation, dissemination	Pneumonitis, HIV co-infection	Knox and Carrigan (1994)

are equally divided between HHV-6A and HHV-6B, although HHV-6B was identified in the paediatric cases (3/3) and HHV-6A primarily in the adults (4/5).

Other Conditions

Vascular and Heart Disease

Like HCMV, HHV-6 and HHV-7 have been linked with vascular and heart disease, for both direct or indirect effects. Unusually severe infections with HHV-6 are associated with myocarditis, which occasionally

can be fatal (Table 2E.2), and HHV-6 reactivations in heart transplant patients are related to higher mortality (Jacobs *et al.*, 2003). Like HCMV, HHV-6 has also been shown *in vitro* to infect arterial endothelial cells and encodes proinflammatory chemokine and chemokine receptors. It can also modulate cellular chemokine expression in endothelial cells, all of which can affect the inflammatory response, an implicated co-factor in artherosclerosis (Isegawa *et al.*, 1998; Zou *et al.*, 1999; Milne *et al.*, 2000; Caruso *et al.*, 2003; Luttichau *et al.*, 2003). HHV-6 and HCMV have been implicated in vascular endothelial injury after bone marrow transplantation, with greater effects from reactivations with

HHV-6 alone or HHV-6 together with HCMV (Takatsuka *et al.*, 2003). Thus, all the betaherpesviruses may have distinct or synergistic effects on vascular/heart disease and further study is warranted.

Neurological Disease vs. 'Brain Commensal'

HHV-6 and HHV-7 have both been connected with neurological disease, but have also been identified as commensals in the brain. Thus, differential diagnoses, such as identifying active infection or higher viral loads in relevant tissue, are important. In the case of HHV-6 most data is for HHV-6 encephalitis, where detection of active infection by DNA in the CSF and serum combined with *in situ* hybridisation has been used. Cases of encephalitis have been primarily described in rare complications during primary infection or more frequently in immunosuppressed transplantation patients, as described above and previously (McCullers *et al.*, 1995; Kamei *et al.*, 1997; Novoa *et al.*, 1997; Gompels, 2000). Both viruses appear to be neurotropic in that they can be detected in brain autopsies of 'normal' immunocompetent adults, the exact proportion varying in different studies. In a Hong Kong study, HHV-6 was detected more frequently (43%) by PCR than HHV-7 (5%), with detection unrelated to age in 20–95 year-olds (Chan *et al.*, 1999, 2000). HHV-6 strain variant typing appeared to reflect the higher prevalence of HHV-6B in this population. Of the HHV-6 positives, 75% were HHV-6B and 25% HHV-6A. Out of the total brain autopsy sample size, 9/84 were HHV-6A (11%) and 27/84 HHV-6B (32%), similar to the prevalence found in a UK study (Lin *et al.*, 2002). Given the higher detection overall of HHV-6, compared to HHV-7, the former appears to present the greater hazard for potential CNS disease. Where comparative studies to other herpesviruses have been done in patients with neurological disease, the roseoloviruses presented in an equivalent proportion to HSV-1, a well-defined neurotropic virus. A study of CSF and serum DNA from 286 patients showed that 15% of these conditions were associated with active herpesvirus infections, with most of these due equally to HSV-1 or HHV-6/-7, which together accounted for most of the herpesvirus-linked clinically suspected encephalitis, meningitis or other disease of the CNS (Calvario *et al.*, 2002). Intriguingly, recent results show more frequent detection compared to 'normals' of HHV-6 in Alzheimer's disease brain autopsies (70% vs. 40%; Lin *et al.*, 2002).

Multiple Sclerosis Connection

Previous studies associated potential role for HHV-6 strain with MS by antigen staining in affected plaques and increased prevalence in serological studies, as well as detection of DNA in CSF and serum, as reviewed (Enbom, 2001). The association continues to be controversial, with conflicting studies reporting presence or absence of HHV-6 in CSF, serum or brain biopsies in relation to MS. Recent studies suggest increased exposure to HHV-6 and an inability to clear the infection, or immune abnormalities, which could also be from complications arising from MS.

Reports appear to discount a role for HHV-7 and point to a potential role for strain variants or infection with multiple strains. In a Latvian study, out of 113 neurological disorders and 150 blood donor controls, HHV-6 viraemia (DNA detected by PCR in both PBMC and plasma) was only detected in MS, predominantly in the active phase, while HHV-7 was detected with higher frequency in demyelinating diseases of the peripheral nervous system (Tomsone *et al.*, 2002). In a recent follow-up study from the same group, they examined the role of active HHV-6 infections/reactivations in relapsing remitting and secondary progressive MS by analysing HHV-6 plasma viraemia by DNA PCR, gene expression in PBMC by RT–PCR, and levels of IgM or IgG antibody. Their results showed that active HHV-6 was higher in MS than in other neurological conditions (Chapenko *et al.*, 2003). Similarly, in an American cohort, using a lymphoproliferation assay, more frequent responses to HHV-6 rather than HHV-7 were recorded in MS patients, although in this study differences were only seen for HHV-6A, 67% in MS compared to 33% healthy controls, while there were no differences between these groups in responses to HHV-6B and HHV-7, at approximately 75% and 25%, respectively (Soldan *et al.*, 2000). Studies using analyses of intrathecal antibodies also only identify HHV-6, not HHV-7, although in this case both HHV-6A and B antibodies (44% and 66% IgG, HHV-6B also IgM 44%, with none in controls) were implicated in MS patients in a Hungarian study (Ongradi *et al.*, 1999). However, other reports from Italy find equal prevalence of HHV-6 and HHV-7 in MS patients compared to controls in DNA PCR from PBMC, although in these cases serum or CSF were not analysed, nor strain variant typing; thus, although there may be regional differences, additional data would be required (Taus *et al.*, 2000). Further support for a role for HHV-6A is from Korea, where nested PCR identified HHV-6 in PBMC only in MS patients

(7/34; 21%) and none in healthy controls, and all strains were typed as HHV-6A (Kim *et al.*, 2000). Further, a Spanish study, also first by nested PCR on PBMC, showed in comparison to other herpesviruses that only HHV-6 was more prevalent in MS patients (2.3 times) (Alvarez-Lafuente *et al.*, 2002). In a follow-up using real-time quantitative PCR in PBMC, HHV-6B was found generally equivalent in 33 relapsing remitting MS patients compared to healthy controls, 33% and 26%, but HHV-6A was more prevalent, 20% compared to 4% in controls, and importantly only HHV-6A was detected in the serum, 15% of MS and none in controls (Alvarez-Lafuente *et al.*, 2002). Taken together, there does seem to be, in some regions, an active HHV-6A infection in a subgroup of MS patients which is distinct from controls.

Recent biopsy and autopsy studies of active lesions further identify HHV-6 in areas of demyelinating MS lesions. A biopsy study on patients who presented initially as having cerebral tumours later confirmed as MS, showed HHV-6 genome by *in situ* PCR in oligodendrocytes, lymphocytes and microglia, as well as antigen expression in astrocytes and microglia. This pattern may indicate mixtures of latent and lytic replication, although in some cells the significance of antigen expression in the absence of the viral genome is not clear, but might indicate phagocytic properties (Goodman *et al.*, 2003). A further autopsy study using laser microdissection found HHV-6 DNA by PCR in more samples from MS plaques than normal appearing white matter or control healthy brains or those with other neurological disease (Cermelli *et al.*, 2003). While this is important new data, it is difficult to differentiate causality from a bystander effect of HHV-6.

Preliminary indications of a connection between active HHV-6 replication and symptomatic MS suggest that HHV-6 may be a complicating factor in some MS patients. Interestingly, in studies investigating interferon-β (IFN-β) treatment of MS in USA, these patients also show decreased cell-free HHV-6 DNA in the serum and decreased HHV-6 IgM; *in vitro* virus replication is also sensitive to IFN-β (Hong *et al.*, 2002). In addition, using nested PCR of 215 samples from 59 MS patients in 5 months of follow-up, another study showed that HHV-6 could be detected in serum in more of those with clinical symptoms (22%, 4/18) than those in remission (6%, 11/197) (Berti *et al.*, 2002). The Latvian group also showed that reactivated HHV-6 infection was higher during periods of active MS disease (Chapenko *et al.*, 2003), while Knox *et al.* (2000), using virus isolation assay, had shown active viraemia in younger MS patients with shorter duration

of disease. In an Italian study, antibody responses to the HHV-6 latency gene U94/rep were studied and showed greater reactivity in MS sera than from patients with other neurological disease (87% vs. 44%), suggesting also differential exposure to HHV-6 (Caselli *et al.*, 2002). A recent study shows an association between HHV-6 IgM antibodies and early MS, as defined by clinically isolated syndromes at high risk for MS and short-duration active relapsing–remitting MS (Villoslada *et al.*, 2003). Are these examples of complications for rare adult primary infections with HHV-6?

One possible mechanism has been suggested to involve inefficient clearance of HHV-6 or immuno-modulation in MS patients (Tejada-Simon *et al.*, 2002). This USA study again detected HHV-6 in CSF and serum in greater prevalence in MS, and additionally showed that in these patients T cells specific for the immunodominant 101 kDa phospho-protein were less frequent than controls. Furthermore, derived T cell lines had decreased IL-4 and IL-10 with reduced IgG titres, but HHV-6 IgM was greater in MS patients than the controls. Another possible key is that soluble CD46 levels, the membrane-bound form of a receptor for HHV-6, are raised in serum from patients with MS and other inflammatory diseases (Soldan *et al.*, 2001).

Thus, in summary, the balance of the evidence points to a subgroup of MS patients who have active HHV-6 infections and difficulties in clearing the infection. Whether this is a cause or effect of MS is not clear. In many geographic regions, HHV-6A strains appear to be involved and future studies need to include this distinction. Controlled trials using valaciclovir showed no effect on MS, but HHV-6 is insensitive to this treatment *in vitro* (Bech *et al.*, 2002). Would specific antiviral interventions with more potent drugs, such as ganciclovir or foscarnet, help these patients clear HHV-6 and resolve symptoms, as appears to be the case in some bone marrow transplantation studies? Would such clinical trials further define a role for HHV-6 in MS?

HIV/AIDS Relationship

HHV-6/-7 appear among the first herpesviruses to reactivate in immunosuppressed HIV/AIDS patients in the absence of highly active retroviral therapy (HAART). By PCR, HHV-6 was detected at multiple sites with increased viral load in HIV/AIDS patients (Corbellino *et al.*, 1993; Knox and Carrigan, 1994;

Clark *et al.*, 1996). Studies of viral load detected by DNA PCR in saliva also showed increased secretion of HHV-7 in HIV/AIDS patients (DiLuca *et al.*, 1995). There may be a complicated relationship with HIV, because HHV-6 and HHV-7 can reactivate each other (Katsafanas *et al.*, 1996). These infections are difficult to monitor at the periphery in blood, since the level of the target cell for both HHV-6 and HHV-7, the CD4$^+$ cell, becomes very much reduced in late-stage AIDS patients. Accordingly, as detected by DNA PCR, levels of HHV-6 and HHV-7 decrease in PBMC in late-stage AIDS patients (Fairfax *et al.*, 1994; Fabio *et al.*, 1997), whereas the level increases in other tissues, due to disseminated infections, and virus can be detected in plasma, which is a marker for viraemia and virus reactivation (Secchiero *et al.*, 1995). In a longitudinal study of HHV-6 reactivation in two HIV-1-infected patients, the CD4$^+$ cell count decreased coincident with HHV-6 reactivation; one of the patients secreted both HHV-6A and -B variant strains, the other only HHV-6A (Iuliano *et al.*, 1997). In studies of HHV-6 disseminated infections in HIV/AIDS patients, increased HHV-6 DNA levels detected by quantitative PCR in various organs, correlated with higher levels of HIV, suggesting a role in AIDS progression (Emery *et al.*, 1999).

HHV-6 has been detected *in vivo* in AIDS retinitis. Usually it is detected in co-infections with HCMV, but it has also been identified on its own. HHV-6 and HCMV co-infections may affect their pathologies and interacting effects have been shown *in vitro*, where HHV-6 has been shown to infect retinal epithelium (Fillet *et al.*, 1996; Qavi *et al.*, 1996).

There are isolated reports of HHV-6 reactivations in AIDS patients associated with fatalities due to pneumonitis and encephalitis (Knox and Carrigan, 1994, 1995; Knox *et al.*, 1995a, 1995b). HHV-6 reactivations have also been associated in HIV-infected individuals with early phases of lymphadenopathy syndrome but not with malignant lymphoprolifera-tions (Dolcetti *et al.*, 1996). HHV-6 has been identified along with HIV in lymph node biopsies of AIDS patients in regions of hypocellularity using antigen specific markers for HHV-6 replication. It has been suggested that the HHV-6 reactivation at these sites is associated with cell damage in the lymph nodes, and *in vitro* studies show that the virus can reactivate HIV from latency in monocytes, identifying HHV-6A (Knox and Carrigan, 1996).

Presumably, since the advent of HAART treatment for HIV/AIDS, HHV-6/-7 reactivations and associated pathology are much reduced or negligible, but may be a risk in countries where HAART is unavailable.

Xenotransplantation

Roseoloviruses may be an important factor in xenotransplantion. In current applications of xeno-transplantation, porcine organs may be used in human transplantation. Much focus has been on the hazards from endogenous retroviruses, with possible patho-genic zoonoses. More recently, problems of endogenous herpesviruses have been aired, in particu-lar porcine cytomegalovirus, PCMV. Herds will need clearance of these viruses before applications in transplantation. Interestingly, genetic analyses of PCMV strains from a number of countries have shown that they are more closely related to the roseoloviruses, HHV-6 and HHV-7 (Goltz *et al.*, 2000; Widen *et al.*, 2001). Thus, potentially serious risks from porcine roseoloviruses during xenotrans-plantation include neurological disease from virus derived from infected donor organs, or possibly immunodeficiency due to infection of T lymphocytes. It is also possible that the porcine viruses may reactivate HHV-6, HHV-7 or HCMV, leading to associated pathologies described in the earlier sections. In a pig-to-primate (baboons) model, baboon CMV was reactivated together with PCMV, similar to that observed for HHV-6/-7 and HCMV during human transplantation, and there is some recent evidence for associated pathology (Mueller *et al.*, 2002). Generally, with natural routes of transmission, there is a host range barrier for zoonoses from animal herpesviruses, in particular for betaherpesviruses, which are usually species-specific. During transplantation, however, sys-temic infection may now be possible without barriers to infectivity, e.g. as presented during infectious entry to epithelial cells. There should be virtually no cross-protective immunity, given the genetic distances between the human and porcine viruses.

DIAGNOSIS

Infection with HHV-6 can be diagnosed by indirect immunofluorescence, virus isolation, PCR, RT-PCR, ELISA capture assays, and virus neutralisation assays. By electron microscopy (EM) the virus has the classic herpesvirus nucleocapsid morphology with irregular envelopment, including tegument proteins and a lipid bi-layer membrane containing surface projections com-posed of glycoproteins. EM is not sufficient to diagnose HHV-6 or HHV-7 from other herpesviruses. Indirect immunofluorescence using acetone-fixed whole infected cells in reaction with human sera and FITC conjugates is the main diagnostic tool. This is generally a sensitive assay but will not distinguish between HHV-6 strains or primary vs. reactivated infections. In addition, there is a large level of cross-reactivity between HHV-6- and HHV-7-positive sera. Some assays incorporate cross-blocking steps for both these viruses and claim specificity, others incorporate specific PCR-based assays (Black *et al.*, 1996; Tanaka-Taya *et al.*, 1996; Clark *et al.*, 1997; Ward *et al.*, 2002a). There are some antigens which can also cross-react with certain conserved proteins in HCMV but these are rare.

HHV-6 and HHV-7 serology are not sufficient to detect virus reactivation and associated pathology. Different assays have been used to distinguish primary vs. reactivated infections, including IgG avidity assays, levels of blood DNA, and differential detection of DNA in the blood vs. saliva (Ward *et al.*, 1993; Clark *et al.*, 1997). Primers for sensitive DNA PCR or cDNA RT–PCR have been described and most recently quantitative DNA PCR can be used to distinguish the almost universal latent compared to primary or secondary reactivated infections with viraemia, or 'DNAemia', associated with pathology. In latently infected adults the level of circulating cells harbouring latent HHV-6 or HHV-7 DNA has been estimated to be as little as 1–10 in a million, whereas during viraemia, levels can be a million times higher. Consequently, HHV-6 virus isolation from the blood is usually only observed during viraemia where there are high levels of circulating, actively replicating virus and correlates with DNAaemia, as well as detection of free virus in the serum as detected by DNA PCR (Secchiero *et al.*, 1995). However, there appears to be higher levels of HHV-7 circulating than HHV-6, due to differences in latency control, and this should be taken into account when only assaying PBMC (Cone *et al.*, 1993; Kidd *et al.*, 1996; Clark *et al.*, 1997). In exanthem subitum infants, DNA is detected in blood during the acute and convalescent stages (Tanaka-Taya *et al.*, 1996). Current markers for active HHV-6 and HHV-7 infection include virus isolation from blood, high levels of DNA in blood (DNAaemia), detection of DNA in the serum and, in the case of neurological disease, detection of DNA in the CSF. In addition, RT-PCR analyses of immediate-early, early and late gene expression are being developed to analyse virus reactivations (Chapenko *et al.*, 2003; Yoshikawa *et al.*, 2003).

In primary acute infections, viral load in PBMC is high, as detected by quantitative DNA PCR with 10 000 HHV-6 or a million HHV-7 genome equivalents/million PBMC in a study of febrile infants in the UK (Clark *et al.*, 1997), with similar or higher levels of HHV-6 estimated in the whole blood of febrile infants

in Zambia (Kasolo *et al.*, 1997). The virus DNA can be detected in plasma during childhood viraemia and adult reactivations, but not in healthy latently infected adults (Secchiero *et al.*, 1995). Using quantitative real-time PCR, diagnostic copy numbers associated with clinical symptoms can start to be applied for future treatment regimes. For example, recent retrospective studies on 78 stem cell transplant patients show median HHV-6 DNA levels of 1357 genome equivalent copies/million PBMC, most likely from virus reactivation, as 31 immunocompetent controls had levels below the quantitation threshold. Furthermore, higher patient loads were correlated with delayed neutrophil engraftment or severe graft-vs.-host disease and direct HHV-6-related symptoms (fever, rash, pneumonitis or myelosuppression) were related to a DNA load greater than 1000 copies/million PBMC (Boutolleau, 2003).

Specific tests for antigens which correlate with active infections or virus reactivation are being developed. In HHV-6 a 100 kDa phosphoprotein, p100 or p101, encoded by U11, is present in the tegument and has been identified as one of the immunodominant targets for antibody responses. Specific 101 kDa lymphoproliferative responses have also been measured between patient groups (Tejada-Simon *et al.*, 2002). In HHV-7 proteins with similar immunogenicity to p101, but lower molecular weight, 85/88 kDa, have been described and specific antibody reagents defined. The target for the 85 kDa protein is distinct, the HHV-7 U14 tegument protein (Stefan *et al.*, 1997). Specific antigen capture ELISA assays using the HHV-6 specific U94/rep latency gene have been used to discriminate patient groups in MS, and it will be interesting to compare to other patient groups, as this appears to be the only antigen latently expressed (Caselli *et al.*, 2002). Other strategies include antigen capture and antibody reagents as well as RT-PCR specific for late proteins and glycoproteins, such as U22 and U48/gH, which are markers for active infection (primary or reactivation), since their expression is dependent on virus DNA replication. Specific markers to distinguish between strains and HHV-6 or HHV-7 are being developed utilising HHV-6 or variant-specific genes, such as IE or the U83 chemokine genes (Schiewe *et al.*, 1994; Yamamoto *et al.*, 1994; French *et al.*, 1999).

TREATMENT

Given the genetic similarities between HHV-6 and HHV-7 with HCMV, many antiviral compounds active against HCMV may be expected to have similar effects on the replication of HHV-6 and HHV-7. In general this has been demonstrated *in vitro*. Ganciclovir (GCV) as well as related derivatives are effective inhibitors of HHV-6 and HHV-7 replication (Reymen *et al.*, 1995; Takahashi *et al.*, 1997), with some studies showing efficiency *in vivo*, although not completely effective (Rapaport *et al.*, 2002; Tokimasa *et al.*, 2002; Yoshida *et al.*, 2002). Both viruses encode homologues of proteins in HCMV which are targets for these agents' activity and sites for drug-resistant mutants. These are the homologues of the HCMV phosphotransferase, UL97, required for the phosphorylation of GCV, U69 in HHV-6 and HHV-7, as well as the virus-encoded DNA polymerase, HHV-6 and HHV-7 U38 (Gompels *et al.*, 1995; Nicholas, 1996). However, recent studies show that the HHV-6 phosphotransferase, U69, is 10-fold less active than HCMV UL97 in phosphorylating GCV, suggesting different sensitivities to this or related drugs with similar mechanisms of action (De Bolle *et al.*, 2002). Also active against these viruses are acyclic nucleoside phosphonate analogues, such as cidofovir (HMPC) (Takahashi *et al.*, 1997). Not all HCMV drugs are effective against HHV-6, and new benzimidazole ribonucleoside derivatives (i.e. BDCRB and maribavir, 1263W94) show significant activity *in vitro* to HCMV, but not HHV-6; thus, their potential application may discriminate between betaherpesvirus pathologies (Williams *et al.*, 2003).

Drugs which require thymidine kinase (TK) for activity are ineffective *in vitro*. This includes aciclovir (ACV) and its derivatives, brivudin (BVDU) and scrivudine (BVaraU) (Reymen *et al.*, 1995; Takahashi *et al.*, 1997). Like HCMV, this is consistent with the observation that both viruses do not encode the viral target for utilisation of the drug, thymidine kinase (Gompels *et al.*, 1995; Nicholas, 1996). However, there is some evidence from *in vivo* studies on HHV-6-associated inhibition of engraftment in bone marrow transplant patients, that high-dose aciclovir may have some therapeutic value, although the mechanism of action is unknown and preliminary comparative studies show that GCV is more effective (Wang *et al.*, 1996; Rapaport *et al.*, 2002).

Direct inhibitors of the virus DNA polymerase, such as foscarnet (phosphonoformic acid, PFA) or phosphonoacetic acid (PAA) and related compounds, have also been shown to be effective against these viruses *in vitro* (Reymen *et al.*, 1995; Takahashi *et al.*, 1997). As with treatment of other herpesvirus-associated pathologies, indiscriminate use of antiviral drugs could give rise to drug-resistant mutants. This has been shown after prolonged GCV usage and a common HHV-6 U69 point mutation identified (Manichanh *et al.*, 2001).

Some reports show efficacy of GCV *in vivo* against HHV-6 and HHV-7, but more prospective trials are required. However, where studied, GCV is not 100% effective, and thus other antivirals or combinations with immune therapeutic strategies are required, using, for example, DNA vaccines including targets for neutralising antibodies and cellular immunity or possibly passive immunity with humanised monoclonal antibodies. New targets for antiviral therapy are being evaluated and screening with existing drug compounds has shown other possible drugs with some activities, but mechanisms of action remain to be determined (Reymen *et al.*, 1995; Takahashi *et al.*, 1997; De Clercq *et al.*, 2001).

SUMMARY

In summary, HHV-6 and HHV-7 are widespread, T lymphotropic and neurotropic infant-fever viruses which form life-long persistent or latent infections which may reactivate to cause disease. Pathologies include encephalitis, disseminated infections, and immunomodulation leading to 'CMV' disease. These viruses can be particular threats, giving rise to occasional fatalities in some primary infections, usually paediatric cases, as well as in patient populations with immune suppression or disorders, such as bone marrow and solid organ transplant recipients or HIV/AIDS groups. There is also an association with neurological conditions and growing evidence of a connection with MS. In general, however, in the immunocompetent, HHV-6 and HHV-7 are well-adapted 'natural' vaccinations, and may provide a 'toolkit' for definition of novel immunomodulators. Better routine diagnosis (distinguishing latent from reactivated or *de novo* infections) using quantitative PCR or other methods, strain analyses, and more effective treatments with existing antivirals or new therapies are required.

ACKNOWLEDGEMENTS

The support of the Wellcome Trust, Royal Society, and UK Biological and Biochemical Sciences Research Council (BBSRC) are acknowledged.

REFERENCES

Ablashi D, Agut H, Berneman Z *et al.* (1993) Human herpesvirus-6 strain groups—a nomenclature. *Arch Virol*, **129**, 1–4.

Ahtiluoto S, Mannonen L, Paetau A et al. (2000) *In situ* hybridization detection of human herpesvirus 6 in brain tissue from fatal encephalitis. *Pediatrics*, **105**, 431–433.

Alvarez-Lafuente R, Martin-Estefania C, de las Heras V et al. (2002) Prevalence of herpesvirus DNA in MS patients and healthy blood donors. *Acta Neurol Scand*, **105**, 95–99.

Alvarez-Lafuente R, Martin-Estefania C, de Las Heras V et al. (2002) Active human herpesvirus 6 infection in patients with multiple sclerosis. *Arch Neurol*, **59**(6), 929–933.

Amo K, Tanaka-Taya K, Inagi R et al. (2003) Human herpesvirus 6B infection of the large intestine of patients with diarrhea. *Clin Infect Dis*, **36**, 120–123.

Anderson R and Gompels U (1999) N- and C-terminal external domains of human herpesvirus-6 glycoprotein H affect a fusion-associated conformation mediated by glycoprotein L binding the N terminus. *J Gen Virol*, **80**, 1485–1494.

Anderson RA, Liu DX and Gompels UA (1996) Definition of a human herpesvirus-6 betaherpesvirus-specific domain in glycoprotein gH that governs interaction with glycoprotein gL: substitution of human cytomegalovirus glycoproteins permits group-specific complex formation. *Virology*, **217**, 517–526.

Asano Y, Yoshikawa T, Kajita Y et al. (1992) Fatal encephalitis/encephalopathy in primary human herpesvirus-6 infection. *Arch Dis Childhood*, **67**, 1484–1485.

Asano Y, Yoshikawa T, Suga S et al. (1990) Fatal fulminant hepatitis in an infant with human herpesvirus-6 infection. *Lancet*, **335**, 862–863.

Asano Y, Yoshikawa T, Suga S et al. (1994) Clinical features of infants with primary human herpesvirus 6 infection (exanthem subitum, roseola infantum). *Pediatrics*, **93**, 104–108.

Bech E, Lycke J, Gadeberg P et al. (2002) A randomized, double-blind, placebo-controlled MRI study of anti-herpes virus therapy in MS. *Neurology*, **58**, 31–36.

Beovic B, Pecaric-Meglic N, Marin J et al. (2001) Fatal human herpesvirus 6-associated multifocal meningoencephalitis in an adult female patient. *Scand J Infect Dis*, **33**, 942–944.

Berti R, Brennan M, Soldan S et al. (2002) Increased detection of serum HHV-6 DNA sequences during multiple sclerosis (MS) exacerbations and correlation with parameters of MS disease progression. *J Neurovirol*, **8**, 250–256.

Black JB, Durigon E, KitePowell K et al. (1996) Seroconversion to human herpesvirus 6 and human herpesvirus 7 among Brazilian children with clinical diagnoses of measles or rubella. *Clin Infect Dis*, **23**, 1156–1158.

Black JB, Sanderlin KC, Goldsmith CS et al. (1989) Growth properties of human herpesvirus-6 strain Z29. *J Virol Methods*, **26**, 133–146.

Black JB, Schwarz TF, Patton JL et al. (1996) Evaluation of immunoassays for detection of antibodies to human herpesvirus 7. *Clin Diagn Lab Immunol*, **3**, 79–83.

Boutolleau D, Fernandez C, Andre E et al. (2003) Human herpesvirus (HHV)-6 and HHV-7: two closely related viruses with different infection profiles in stem cell transplantation recipients. *J Infect Dis*, **187**, 179–186.

Byington C, Zerr D, Taggart E et al. (2002) Human herpesvirus 6 infection in febrile infants ninety days of age and younger. *Pediatr Infect Dis J*, **21**, 996–999.

Calvario A, Bozzi A, Scarasciulli M et al. (2002) Herpes consensus PCR test: a useful diagnostic approach to the screening of viral diseases of the central nervous system. *J Clin Virol*, **25** (suppl), 71–78.

Caruso A, Favilli F, Rotola A et al. (2003) Human herpesvirus-6 modulates RANTES production in primary human endothelial cell cultures. *J Med Virol*, **70**, 451–458.

Caselli E, Boni M, Bracci A et al. (2002) Detection of antibodies directed against human herpesvirus 6 U94/REP in sera of patients affected by multiple sclerosis. *J Clin Microbiol*, **40**, 4131–4137.

Cermelli C, Berti R, Soldan SS et al. (2003) High frequency of human herpesvirus 6 DNA in multiple sclerosis plaques isolated by laser microdissection. *J Infect Dis*, **187**, 1377–1387.

Cermelli C, Pietrosemoli P, Meacci M et al. (1997) Supt-1: a cell system suitable for an efficient propagation of both HHV-7 and HHV-6 variants A and B. *Microbiologica*, **20**, 187–196.

Chan P, Chik K, To K et al. (2002) Case report: human herpesvirus 7 associated fatal encephalitis in a peripheral blood stem cell transplant recipient. *J Med Virol*, **66**, 493–496.

Chan P, Ng H, Cheung J et al. (2000) Prevalence and distribution of human herpesvirus 7 in normal brain. *J Med Virol*, **62**, 345–348.

Chan P, Ng H, Hui M et al. (1999) Presence of human herpesviruses 6, 7, and 8 DNA sequences in normal brain tissue. *J Med Virol*, **59**, 491–495.

Chapenko S, Millers A, Nora Z et al. (2003) Correlation between HHV-6 reactivation and multiple sclerosis disease activity. *J Med Virol*, **69**, 111–117.

Chik K, Chan P, Li C et al. (2002) Human herpesvirus-6 encephalitis after unrelated umbilical cord blood transplant in children. *Bone Marrow Transpl*, **29**, 991–994.

Clark DA, Ait-Khaled M, Wheeler AC et al. (1996) Quantification of human herpesvirus 6 in immunocompetent persons and post-mortem tissues from AIDS patients by PCR. *J Gen Virol*, **77**, 2271–2275.

Clark DA, Kidd IM, Collingham KE et al. (1997) Diagnosis of primary human herpesvirus 6 and 7 infections in febrile infants by polymerase chain reaction. *Arch Dis Childhood*, **77**, 42–45.

Cone RW, Huang M, Ashley R and Corey L (1993) Human herpesvirus 6 DNA in peripheral blood cells and saliva from immunocompetent individuals. *J Clin Microbiol*, **31**, 1262–1267.

Corbellino M, Lusso P, Gallo RC et al. (1993) Disseminated human herpesvirus 6 infection in AIDS (18). *Lancet*, **342**, 1242.

De Almeida Rodrigues G, Nagendra S, Lee C and De Magalhaes-Silverman M (1999) Human herpes virus 6 fatal encephalitis in a bone marrow recipient. *Scand J Infect Dis*, **31**, 313–315.

De Bolle L, Michel D, Mertens T et al. (2002) Role of the human herpesvirus 6 u69-encoded kinase in the phosphorylation of ganciclovir. *Mol Pharmacol*, **62**, 714–721.

De Clercq E, Andrei G, Snoeck R et al. (2001) Acyclic/carbocyclic guanosine analogues as anti-herpesvirus agents. *Nucleosides Nucleotides Nucleic Acids*, **20**, 271–285.

Deng H and Dewhurst S (1998) Functional identification and analysis of *cis*-acting sequences which mediate genome cleavage and packaging in human herpesvirus 6. *J Virol*, **72**, 320–329.

DesJardin JA, Cho E, Supran S et al. (2001) Association of human herpesvirus 6 reactivation with severe cytomegalovirus-associated disease in orthotopic liver transplant recipients. *Clin Infect Dis*, **33**, 1358–1362.

DesJardin JA, Gibbons L, Cho E *et al.* (1998) Human herpesvirus 6 reactivation is associated with cytomegalovirus infection and syndromes in kidney transplant recipients at risk for primary cytomegalovirus infection. *J Infect Dis*, **178**, 1783–1786.

Dhepakson P, Mori Y, Jiang Y *et al.* (2002) Human herpesvirus-6 rep/U94 gene product has single-stranded DNA-binding activity. *J Gen Virol*, **83**, 847–854.

DiLuca D, Mirandola P, Ragvaioli T *et al.* (1995) Human herpesviruses 6 and 7 in salivary glands and shedding in saliva of healthy and human immunodeficiency virus positive individuals. *J Med Virol*, **45**, 462–468.

Dockrell DH, Prada J, Jones MF *et al.* (1997) Seroconversion to human herpesvirus 6 following liver transplantation is a marker of cytomegalovirus disease. *J Infect Dis*, **176**, 1135–1140.

Dolcetti R, Di Luca D, Carbone A *et al.* (1996) Human herpesvirus 6 in human immmunodeficiency virus-infected individuals: association with early histologic phases of lymphadenopathy syndrome but not with malignant lymphoproliferative disorders. *J Med Virol*, **48**, 344–353.

Dominguez G, Dambaugh T, Stamey F *et al.* (1999) Human herpesvirus 6B genome sequence: coding content and comparison with human herpesvirus 6A. *J Virol*, **73**, 8040–8052.

Drobyski WR, Knox KK, Majewski D and Carrigan DR (1994) Brief report: Fatal encephalitis due to variant B human herpesvirus-6 infection in a bone marrow-transplant recipient. *N Engl J Med*, **330**, 1356–1360.

Emery V (2001) Human herpesviruses 6 and 7 in solid organ transplant recipients. *Clin Infect Dis*, **32**, 1357–1360.

Emery V, Atkins M, Bowen E *et al.* (1999) Interactions between beta-herpesviruses and human immunodeficiency virus in vivo: evidence for increased human immunodeficiency viral load in the presence of human herpesvirus 6. *J Med Virol*, **57**, 278–282.

Enbom M (2001) Multiple sclerosis and Kaposi's sarcoma—chronic diseases associated with new human herpesviruses? *Scand J Infect Dis*, **33**, 648–658.

Enders G, Biber M, Meyer G and Helftenbein E (1990) Prevalence of antibodies to human herpesvirus 6 in different age groups, in children with exanthema subitum, other acute exanthematous childhood diseases, Kawasaki syndrome, and acute infections with other herpesviruses and HIV. *Infection*, **18**, 12–15.

Fabio G, Knight SN, Kidd IM *et al.* (1997) Prospective study of human herpesvirus 6, human herpesvirus 7, and cytomegalovirus infections in human immunodeficiency virus-positive patients. *J Clin Microbiol*, **35**, 2657–2659.

Fairfax MR, Schacker T, Cone RW *et al.* (1994) Human herpesvirus 6 DNA in blood cells of human immunodeficiency virus-infected men: correlation of high levels with high CD4 cell counts. *J Infect Dis*, **169**, 1342–1345.

Fillet AM, Reux I, Joberty C *et al.* (1996) Detection of human herpes virus 6 in AIDS-associated retinitis by means of *in situ* hybridization, polymerase chain reaction and immunohistochemistry. *J Med Virol*, **49**, 289–295.

Flamand L, Gosselin J, DAddario M *et al.* (1991) Human herpesvirus 6 induces interleukin-1β and tumor necrosis factor α, but not interleukin-6, in peripheral blood mononuclear cell cultures. *J Virol*, **65**, 5105–5110.

Flamand L, Gosselin J, Stefanescu I *et al.* (1995) Immunosuppressive effect of human herpesvirus 6 on T-cell functions: suppression of interleukin-2 synthesis and cell proliferation. *Blood*, **85**, 1263–1271.

Flamand L, Stefanescu I and Menezes J (1996) Human herpesvirus-6 enhances natural killer cell cytotoxicity via IL-15. *J Clin Invest*, **97**, 1373–1381.

French C, Menegazzi P, Nicholson L *et al.* (1999) Novel, non-consensus cellular splicing regulates expression of a gene encoding a chemokine-like protein that shows high variation and is specific for human herpesvirus 6. *Virology*, **262**, 139–151.

Frenkel N, Roffman E, Schirmer EC *et al.* (1990) Cellular and growth-factor requirements for the replication of human herpesvirus 6 in primary lymphocyte cultures. *Adv Exp Med Biol*, **278**, 1–8.

Fukae S, Ashizawa N, Morikawa S and Yano K (2000) A fatal case of fulminant myocarditis with human herpesvirus-6 infection. *Intern Med*, **39**, 632–636.

Furukawa M, Yasukawa M, Yakushijin Y and Fujita S (1994) Distinct effects of human herpesvirus 6 and human herpesvirus 7 on surface molecule expression and function of CD4$^+$ T cells. *J Immunol*, **152**, 5768–5775.

Gautheret-Dejean A, Manichanh C, Thien-Ah-Koon F *et al.* (2002) Development of a real-time polymerase chain reaction assay for the diagnosis of human herpesvirus-6 infection and application to bone marrow transplant patients. *J Virol Methods*, **100**, 27–35.

Gautheret Dejean A, Aubin JT, Poirel L *et al.* (1997) Detection of human betaherpesvirinae in saliva and urine from immunocompromised and immunocompetent subjects. *J Clin Microbiol*, **35**, 1600–1603.

Goltz M, Widen F, Banks M *et al.* (2000) Characterization of the DNA polymerase loci of porcine cytomegaloviruses from diverse geographic origins. *Virus Genes*, **21**, 249–255.

Gompels U (2000) Human herpesviruses 6 and 7 (HHV-6 and HHV-7). *Principles and Practice of Clinical Virology*, 4th edn (eds A Zuckerman, JE Banatvala and J Pattison), pp 141–165. Wiley, Chichester.

Gompels UA, Carrigan DR, Carss AL and Arno J (1993) Two groups of human herpesvirus 6 identified by sequence analyses of laboratory strains and variants from Hodgkin's lymphoma and bone marrow transplant patients. *J Gen Virol*, **74**, 613–622.

Gompels U and Dewin D (2003) Chemokine receptor and chemokine ligand in human herpesvirus 6 (HHV-6), relationship to cellular receptors, inducible signalling and immunomodulation. *9th International Cytomegalovirus and Betaherpesvirus Workshop Abstract Book*, **103**, 77.

Gompels UA, Luxton J, Kehl KK and Carrigan DR (1994) Chronic bone marrow suppression in immunocompetent adult by human herpesvirus 6. *Lancet*, **343**, 735–736.

Gompels UA and Macaulay HA (1995) Characterization of human telomeric repeat sequences from human herpesvirus 6 and relationship to replication. *J Gen Virol*, **76**, 451–458.

Gompels UA, Nicholas N, Lawrence G *et al.* (1995) The DNA sequence of human herpesvirus-6: structure, coding content, and genome evolution. *Virology*, **209**, 29–51.

Gonelli A, Mirandola P, Grill V *et al.* (2002) Human herpesvirus 7 infection impairs the survival/differentiation of megakaryocytic cells. *Haematologica*, **87**, 1223–1225.

Goodman AD, Mock DJ, Powers JM *et al.* (2003) Human herpesvirus 6 genome and antigen in acute multiple sclerosis lesions. *J Infect Dis*, **187**, 1365–1376.

Grivel J, Ito Y, Faga G et al. (2001) Suppression of CCR5-but not CXCR4-tropic HIV-1 in lymphoid tissue by human herpesvirus 6. *Nature Med*, **7**, 1232–1235.

Grivel JC, Santoro F, Chen S et al. (2003) Pathogenic effects of human herpesvirus 6 in human lymphoid tissue *ex vivo*. *J Virol*, **77**, 8280–8289.

Hall CB, Long CE, Schnabel KC et al. (1994) Human herpesvirus-6 infection in children—a prospective study of complications and reactivation. *N England J Med*, **331**, 432–438.

Hasegawa H, Utsunomiya Y, Yasukawa M et al. (1994) Induction of G protein-coupled peptide receptor EBI 1 by human herpesvirus 6 and 7 infection in CD4$^+$ T cells. *J Virol*, **68**, 5326–5329.

Hoang M, Ross K, Dawson D et al. (1999) Human herpesvirus-6 and sudden death in infancy: report of a case and review of the literature. *J Forensic Sci*, **44**, 432–437.

Hong J, Tejada-Simon M, Rivera V et al. (2002) Anti-viral properties of interferon beta treatment in patients with multiple sclerosis. *Mult Scler*, **8**, 237–242.

Horvat RT, Parmely MJ and Chandran B (1993) Human herpesvirus 6 inhibits the proliferative responses of human peripheral blood mononuclear cells. *J Infect Dis*, **167**, 1274–1280.

Huang LM, Lee CY, Liu MY and Lee PI (1997) Primary infections of human herpesvirus-7 and herpesvirus-6: a comparative, longitudinal study up to 6 years of age. *Acta Paediatr*, **86**, 604–608.

Hudson A, Howley P and Ploegh H (2001) A human herpesvirus 7 glycoprotein, U21, diverts major histocompatibility complex class I molecules to lysosomes. *J Virol*, **75**, 12347–12358.

Hukin J, Farrell K, MacWilliam LM et al. (1998) Case-control study of primary human herpesvirus 6 infection in children with febrile seizures. *Pediatrics*, **101**, 1–7.

Humar A, Kumar D, Caliendo A et al. (2002a) Clinical impact of human herpesvirus 6 infection after liver transplantation. *Transplantation*, **73**, 599–604.

Humar A, Kumar D, Raboud J et al. (2002b) Interactions between cytomegalovirus, human herpesvirus-6, and the recurrence of hepatitis C after liver transplantation. *Am J Transplant*, **2**, 461–466.

Ihira M, Yoshikawa T, Suzuki K et al. (2002) Monitoring of active HHV-6 infection in bone marrow transplant recipients by real time PCR: comparison to detection of viral DNA in plasma by qualitative PCR. *Microbiol Immunol*, **46**, 701–705.

Inagi R, Guntapong R, Nakao M et al. (1996) Human herpesvirus 6 induces IL-8 gene expression in human hepatoma cell line, Hep G2. *J Med Virol*, **49**, 34–40.

Inoue Y, Yasukawa M and Fujita S (1997) Induction of T-cell apoptosis by human herpesvirus 6. *J Virol*, **71**, 3751–3759.

Isegawa Y, Mukai T, Nakano K et al. (1999) Comparisons of the complete DNA sequences of human herpesvirus 6 variants A and B. *J Virol*, **73**, 8053–63.

Isegawa Y, Ping Z, Nakano K et al. (1998) Human herpesvirus 6 open reading frame U12 encodes a functional β-chemokine receptor. *J Virol*, **72**, 6104–6112.

Isomura H, Yamada M, Yoshida M et al. (1997) Suppressive effects of human herpesvirus 6 on *in vitro* colony formation of hematopoietic progenitor cells. *J Med Virol*, **52**, 406–412.

Iuliano R, Trovato R, Lico S et al. (1997) Human herpesvirus-6 reactivation in a longitudinal study of two HIV-1 infected patients. *J Med Virol*, **51**, 259–264.

Jacobs F, Knoop C, Brancart F et al. (2003) Human herpesvirus-6 infection after lung and heart-lung transplantation: a prospective longitudinal study. *Transplantation*, **75**, 1996–2001.

Janelle M, Gravel A, Gosselin J et al. (2002) Activation of monocyte cyclooxygenase-2 gene expression by human herpesvirus 6. Role for cyclic AMP-responsive element-binding protein and activator protein-1. *J Biol Chem*, **277**, 30665–30674.

Kamei A, Ichinohe S, Onuma R et al. (1997) Acute disseminated demyelination due to primary human herpesvirus-6 infection. *Eur J Pediatr*, **156**, 709–712.

Kashanchi F, Araujo J, Doniger J et al. (1997) Human herpesvirus 6 (HHV-6) ORF-1 transactivating gene exhibits malignant transforming activity and its protein binds to p53. *Oncogene*, **14**, 359–367.

Kasolo FC, Mpabalwani E and Gompels UA (1997) Infection with AIDS-related herpesviruses in human immunodeficiency virus-negative infants and endemic childhood Kaposi's sarcoma in Africa. *J Gen Virol*, **78**, 847–856.

Katsafanas GC, Schirmer EC, Wyatt LS and Frenkel N (1996) *In vitro* activation of human herpesviruses 6 and 7 from latency. *Proc Natl Acad Sci USA*, **93**, 9788–9792.

Kempf W, Adams V, Wey N et al. (1997) CD68$^+$ cells of monocyte/macrophage lineage in the environment of AIDS-associated and classic-sporadic Kaposi sarcoma are singly or doubly infected with human herpesviruses 7 and 6B. *Proc Natl Acad Sci USA*, **94**, 7600–7605.

Kidd I, Clark D, Sabin C et al. (2000) Prospective study of human betaherpesviruses after renal transplantation: association of human herpesvirus 7 and cytomegalovirus co-infection with cytomegalovirus disease and increased rejection. *Transplantation*, **69**, 2400–2404.

Kidd IM, Clark DA, Ait-Khaled M et al. (1996) Measurement of human herpesvirus 7 load in peripheral blood and saliva of healthy subjects by quantitative polymerase chain reaction. *J Infect Dis*, **174**, 396–401.

Kim J, Lee K, Park J et al. (2000) Detection of human herpesvirus 6 variant A in peripheral blood mononuclear cells from multiple sclerosis patients. *Eur Neurol*, **43**, 170–173.

Knox K, Brewer J, Henry J et al. (2000) Human herpesvirus 6 and multiple sclerosis: systemic active infections in patients with early disease. *Clin Infect Dis*, **31**, 894–903.

Knox KK and Carrigan DR (1992) *In vitro* suppression of bone marrow progenitor cell differentiation by human herpesvirus 6 infection. *J Infect Dis*, **165**, 925–929.

Knox KK and Carrigan DR (1994) Disseminated active HHV-6 infections in patients with AIDS. *Lancet*, **343**, 577–578.

Knox KK and Carrigan DR (1995) Active human herpesvirus (HHV-6) infection of the central nervous system in patients with AIDS. *J Acqu Immun Defic Syndr Hum Retrovirol*, **9**, 69–73.

Knox KK and Carrigan DR (1996) Active HHV-6 infection in the lymph nodes of HIV-infected patients: *in vitro* evidence that HHV-6 can break HIV latency. *J Acqu Immun Defic Syndr Hum Retrovirol*, **11**, 370–378.

Knox KK, Harrington DP and Carrigan DR (1995a) Fulminant human herpesvirus-6 encephalitis in a human immunodeficiency virus-infected infant. *J Med Virol*, **45**, 288–292.

Knox KK, Pietryga D, Harrington DJ et al. (1995b) Progressive immunodeficiency and fatal pneumonitis associated with human herpesvirus 6 infection in an infant. *Clin Infect Dis*, **20**, 406–413.

Kondo K, Kondo T, Okuno T *et al.* (1991) Latent human herpesvirus 6 infection of human monocytes/macrophages. *J Gen Virol*, 72, 1401–1408.

Kondo K, Kondo T, Shimada K *et al.* (2002) Strong interaction between human herpesvirus 6 and peripheral blood monocytes/macrophages during acute infection. *J Med Virol*, 6, 364–369.

Kondo K, Nagafuji H, Hata A *et al.* (1993) Association of human herpesvirus 6 infection of the central nervous system with recurrence of febrile convulsions. *J Infect Dis*, 167, 1197–1200.

Kondo K, Sashihara J, Shimada K *et al.* (2003) Recognition of a novel stage of betaherpesvirus latency in human herpesvirus 6. *J Virol*, 77, 2258–2264.

Krug L, Inoue N and Pellett P (2001) Differences in DNA binding specificity among Roseolovirus origin binding proteins. *Virology*, 288, 145–153.

Lanari M, Papa I, Venturi V *et al.* (2003) Congenital infection with human herpesvirus 6 variant B associated with neonatal seizures and poor neurological outcome. *J Med Virol*, 70, 628–632.

Lautenschlager I, Harma M, Hockerstedt K *et al.* (2002a) Human herpesvirus-6 infection is associated with adhesion molecule induction and lymphocyte infiltration in liver allografts. *J Hepatol*, 37, 648–654.

Lautenschlager I, Lappalainen M, Linnavuori K *et al.* (2002b) CMV infection is usually associated with concurrent HHV-6 and HHV-7 antigenemia in liver transplant patients. *J Clin Virol*, 25 (suppl 2), S57–S61.

Li C, Goodrich JM and Yang X (1997) Interferon-γ (IFN-γ) regulates production of IL-10 and IL-12 in human herpesvirus-6 (HHV-6)-infected monocyte/macrophage lineage. *Clin Exp Immunol*, 109, 421–425.

Lin W-R, Wozniak M, Cooper R *et al.* (2002) Herpesviruses in brain and Alzheimer's disease. *J Pathol*, 197, 195–402.

Liu DX, Gompels UA, Foa-Tomasi L and Campadelli-Fiume G (1993a) Human herpesvirus-6 glycoprotein H and L homologs are components of the gp100 complex and the gH external domain is the target for neutralizing monoclonal antibodies. *Virology*, 197, 12–22.

Liu DX, Gompels UA, Nicholas J and Lelliott C (1993b) Identification and expression of the human herpesvirus 6 glycoprotein H and interaction with an accessory 40K glycoprotein. *J Gen Virol*, 74, 1847–1857.

Ljungman P (2002) β-Herpesvirus challenges in the transplant recipient. *J Infect Dis*, 186 (suppl 1), S99–S109.

Lusso P, De MA, Malnati M *et al.* (1991) Induction of CD4 and susceptibility to HIV-1 infection in human CD8[+] T lymphocytes by human herpesvirus 6. *Nature (Lond)*, 349, 533–535.

Lusso P, Malnati M, De MA *et al.* (1991) Productive infection of CD4[+] and CD8[+] mature human T cell populations and clones by human herpesvirus 6: transcriptional downregulation of CD3. *J Immunol*, 147, 685–691.

Lusso P, Secchiero P, Crowley RW *et al.* (1994) CD4 is a critical component of the receptor for human herpesvirus 7: interference with human immunodeficiency virus. *Proc Natl Acad Sci USA*, 91, 3872–3876.

Luttichau HR, Clark-Lewis I, Jensen PO *et al.* (2003) A highly selective CCR2 chemokine agonist encoded by human herpesvirus 6. *J Biol Chem*, 278, 10928–10933.

MacLean H and Douen A (2002) Severe amnesia associated with human herpesvirus 6 encephalitis after bone marrow transplantation. *Transplantation*, 73, 1086–1089.

Manichanh C, Olivier-Aubron C, Lagarde J *et al.* (2001) Selection of the same mutation in the U69 protein kinase gene of human herpesvirus-6 after prolonged exposure to ganciclovir *in vitro* and *in vivo*. *J Gen Virol*, 82, 2767–2776.

Mayne M, Cheadle C, Soldan S *et al.* (2001) Gene expression profile of herpesvirus-infected T cells obtained using immunomicroarrays: induction of proinflammatory mechanisms. *J Virol*, 75, 11641–11650.

McCullers J, Lakeman F and Whitley R (1995) Human herpesvirus 6 is associated with focal encephalitis. *Clin Infect Dis*, 21, 571–576.

Megaw AG, Rapaport D, Avidor B *et al.* (1998) The DNA sequence of the RK strain of human herpesvirus 7. *Virology*, 244, 119–132.

Milne R, Devaraj P, Nicholson N and Gompels U (1997) Characterisation of HHV-6 encoded G-protein coupled receptors. *Abstr Int Herpesvirus Workshop*, San Diego, CA.

Milne R, Mattick C, Nicholson L *et al.* (2000) RANTES binding and downregulation by a novel human herpesvirus-6 β chemokine receptor. *J Immunol*, 164, 2396–2404.

Mori Y, Akkapaiboon P, Yang X and Yamanishi K (2003) The human herpesvirus 6 U100 gene product is the third component of the gH-gL glycoprotein complex on the viral envelope. *J Virol*, 77, 2452–2458.

Mori Y, Dhepakson P, Shimamoto T *et al.* (2000) Expression of human herpesvirus 6B rep within infected cells and binding of its gene product to the TATA-binding protein *in vitro* and *in vivo*. *J Virol*, 74, 6096–6104.

Mori Y, Yang X, Akkapaiboon P *et al.* (2003) Human herpesvirus 6 variant A glycoprotein H-glycoprotein L-glycoprotein Q complex associates with human CD46. *J Virol*, 77, 4992–4999.

Mueller NJ, Barth RN, Yamamoto S *et al.* (2002) Activation of cytomegalovirus in pig-to-primate xenotransplantation. *J Virol*, 76, 4734–4740.

Murphy P (2001) Viral exploitation and subversion of the immune system through chemokine mimicry. *Nature Immunol*, 2, 116–122.

Nakano K, Tadagaki K, Isegawa Y *et al.* (2003) Human herpesvirus 7 open reading frame U12 encodes a functional β-chemokine receptor. *J Virol*, 77, 8108–8115.

Nicholas J (1996) Determination and analysis of the complete nucleotide sequence of human herpesvirus 7. *J Virol*, 70, 5975–5989.

Novoa LJ, Nagra RM, Nakawatase T *et al.* (1997) Fulminant demyelinating encephalomyelitis associated with productive HHV-6 infection in an immunocompetent adult. *J Med Virol*, 52, 301–308.

Okada K, Ueda K, Kusuhara K *et al.* (1993) Exanthema subitum and human herpesvirus 6 infection: clinical observations in fifty-seven cases. *Pediatr Infect Dis J*, 12, 204–208.

Ongradi J, Rajda C, Marodi C *et al.* (1999) A pilot study on the antibodies to HHV-6 variants and HHV-7 in CSF of MS patients. *J Neurovirol*, 5, 529–532.

Osman H, Peiris J, Taylor CE *et al.* (1996) Cytomegalovirus disease in renal allograft recipients: is human herpesvirus 7 a co-factor for disease progression? *J Med Virol*, 48, 295–301.

Portolani M, Cermelli C, Meacci M *et al.* (1997) Primary infection by HHV-6 variant B associated with a fatal case of hemophagocytic syndrome. *Microbiologica*, 20, 7–11.

Portolani M, Cermelli C, Moroni A *et al.* (1993) Human herpesvirus-6 infections in infants admitted to hospital. *J Med Virol*, **39**, 146–151.

Portolani M, Pecorari M, Tamassia M *et al.* (2002) Case of fatal encephalitis by HHV-6 variant A. *J Med Virol*, **65**, 133–137.

Prezioso PJ, Cangiarella J, Lee M *et al.* (1992) Fatal disseminated infection with human herpesvirus-6. *J Pediatr*, **120**, 921–923.

Pruksananonda P, Hall CB, Insel RA *et al.* (1992) Primary human herpesvirus 6 infection in young children. *N Engl J Med*, **326**, 1445–1450.

Qavi HB, Xu B, Green MT *et al.* (1996) Morphological and ultrastructural changes induced in corneal epithelial cells by HIV-1 and HHV-6 *in vitro*. *Curr Eye Res*, **15**, 597–604.

Rapaport D, Engelhard D, Tagger G *et al.* (2002) Antiviral prophylaxis may prevent human herpesvirus-6 reactivation in bone marrow transplant recipients. *Transpl Infect Dis*, **4**, 10–16.

Rapp J, Krug L, Inoue N *et al.* (2001) U94, the human herpesvirus 6 homolog of the parvovirus non-structural gene, is highly conserved among isolates and is expressed at low mRNA levels as a spliced transcript. *Virology*, **268**, 504–516.

Razonable R and Paya C (2002) The impact of human herpesvirus-6 and -7 infection on the outcome of liver transplantation. *Liver Transpl*, **8**, 651–658.

Reymen D, Naesens L, Balzarini J *et al.* (1995) Antiviral activity of selected acyclic nucleoside analogues against human herpesvirus 6. *Antiviral Res*, **28**, 343–357.

Roffman E and Frenkel N (1990) Interleukin-2 inhibits the replication of human herpesvirus-6 in mature thymocytes. *Virology*, **175**, 591–594.

Roffman E and Frenkel N (1991) Replication of human herpesvirus-6 in thymocytes activated by anti-CD3 antibody. *J Infect Dis*, **164**, 617–618.

Rogers J, Rohal S, Carrigan D *et al.* (2000) Human herpesvirus-6 in liver transplant recipients: role in pathogenesis of fungal infections, neurologic complications, and outcome. *Transplantation*, **69**, 2566–2573.

Rohayem J, Dinger J, Fischer R *et al.* (2001) Fatal myocarditis associated with acute parvovirus B19 and human herpesvirus 6 coinfection. *J Clin Microbiol*, **39**, 4585–4587.

Romi H, Singer O, Rapaport D and Frenkel N (1999) Tamplicon-7, a novel T-lymphotropic vector derived from human herpesvirus 7. *J Virol*, **73**, 7001–7007.

Rossi C, Delforge ML, Jacobs F *et al.* (2001) Fatal primary infection due to human herpesvirus 6 variant A in a renal transplant recipient. *Transplantation*, **27**, 288–292.

Santoro F, Greenstone HL, Insinga A *et al.* (2003) Interaction of glycoprotein H of human herpesvirus 6 with the cellular receptor CD46. *J Biol Chem*, **278**, 25964–25969.

Sashihara J, Tanaka-Taya K, Tanaka S *et al.* (2002) High incidence of human herpesvirus 6 infection with a high viral load in cord blood stem cell transplant recipients. *Blood*, **15**, 2005–2011.

Schiewe U, Neipel F, Schreiner D and Fleckenstein B (1994) Structure and transcription of an immediate-early region in the human herpesvirus 6 genome. *J Virol*, **68**, 2978–2985.

Secchiero P, Carrigan DR, Asano Y *et al.* (1995) Detection of human herpesvirus 6 in plasma of children with primary infection and immunosuppressed patients by polymerase chain reaction. *J Infect Dis*, **171**, 273–280.

Secchiero P, Flamand L, Gibellini D *et al.* (1997a) Human herpesvirus 7 induces CD4(+) T-cell death by two distinct mechanisms: necrotic lysis in productively infected cells and apoptosis in uninfected or nonproductively infected cells. *Blood*, **90**, 4502–4512.

Secchiero P, Gibellini D, Flamand L *et al.* (1997b) Human herpesvirus 7 induces the downregulation of CD4 antigen in lymphoid T cells without affecting p56(lck) levels. *J Immunol*, **159**, 3412–3423.

Secchiero P, Mirandola P, Zella D *et al.* (2001) Human herpesvirus 7 induces the functional up-regulation of tumor necrosis factor-related apoptosis-inducing ligand (TRAIL) coupled to TRAIL-R1 downmodulation in CD4(+) T cells. *Blood*, **98**, 2474–2481.

Singh N, Bentlejewski C, Carrigan D *et al.* (2002) Persistent lack of human herpesvirus-6 specific T-helper cell response in liver transplant recipients. *Transpl Infect Dis*, **4**(2), 59–63.

Skrincosky D, Hocknell P, Whetter L *et al.* (2000) Identification and analysis of a novel heparin-binding glycoprotein encoded by human herpesvirus 7. *J Virol*, **74**, 4530–4540.

Smith A, Santoro F, Di Lullo G *et al.* (2003) Selective suppression of IL-12 production by human herpesvirus 6. *Blood*, Jun 26 [Epub].

Soldan S, Fogdell-Hahn A, Brennan M *et al.* (2001) Elevated serum and cerebrospinal fluid levels of soluble human herpesvirus type 6 cellular receptor, membrane cofactor protein, in patients with multiplesclerosis. *Ann Neurol*, **50**, 486–493.

Soldan S, Leist T, Juhng K *et al.* (2000) Increased lymphoproliferative response to human herpesvirus type 6A variant in multiple sclerosis patients. *Ann Neurol*, **47**, 306–313.

Stefan A, Secchiero P, Baechi T *et al.* (1997) The 85 kDa phosphoprotein (pp85) of human herpesvirus 7 is encoded by open reading frame U14 and localizes to a tegument substructure in virion particles. *J Virol*, **71**, 5758–5763.

Suga S, Yoshikawa T, Asano Y *et al.* (1993) Clinical and virological analyses of 21 infants with exanthem subitum (roseola infantum) and central nervous system complications. *Ann Neurol*, **33**, 597–603.

Tait DR, Ward KN, Brown D and Miller E (1996) Measles and rubella misdiagnosed in infants as exanthem subitum (roseola infantum). *Br Med J*, **312**, 101–102.

Takahashi K, Sonoda S, Higashi K *et al.* (1989) Predominant CD4 T-lymphocyte tropism of human herpesvirus 6-related virus. *J Virol*, **63**, 3161–3163.

Takahashi K, Suzuki M, Iwata Y *et al.* (1997) Selective activity of various nucleoside and nucleotide analogues against human herpesvirus 6 and 7. *Antiviral Chem Chemother*, **8**, 24–31.

Takatsuka H, Wakae T, Mori A *et al.* (2003) Endothelial damage caused by cytomegalovirus and human herpesvirus-6. *Bone Marrow Transpl*, **31**, 475–479.

Tanaka K, Kondo T, Torigoe S *et al.* (1994) Human herpesvirus 7: another causal agent for roseola (exanthem subitum). *J Pediatr*, **125**, 1–5.

Tanaka-Taya K, Kondo T, Mukai T *et al.* (1996) Seroepidemiological study of human herpesvirus-6 and -7 in children of different ages and detection of these two viruses in throat swabs by polymerase chain reaction. *J Med Virol*, **48**, 88–94.

Tang YW, Espy MJ, Persing H and Smith TF (1997) Molecular evidence and clinical significance of herpesvirus co-infection in the central nervous system. *J Clin Microbiol*, **35**, 2869–2872.

Taus C, Pucci E, Cartechini E *et al*. (2000) Absence of HHV-6 and HHV-7 in cerebrospinal fluid in relapsing-remitting multiple sclerosis. *Acta Neurol Scand*, **101**, 224–228.

Tejada-Simon M, Zang Y, Hong J *et al*. (2002) Detection of viral DNA and immune responses to the human herpesvirus 6 101 kDa virion protein in patients with multiple sclerosis and in controls. *J Virol*, **76**, 6147–6154.

Tiacci E, Luppi M, Barozzi P *et al*. (2000) Fatal herpesvirus-6 encephalitis in a recipient of a T-cell-depleted peripheral blood stem cell transplant from a 3-loci mismatched related donor. *Haematologica*, **7**, 85–94.

Tokimasa S, Hara J, Osugi Y *et al*. (2002) Ganciclovir is effective for prophylaxis and treatment of human herpesvirus-6 in allogeneic stem cell transplantation. *Bone Marrow Transpl*, **29**, 595–598.

Tomsone V, Logina I, Millers A *et al*. (2002) Association of human herpesvirus 6 and human herpesvirus 7 with demyelinating diseases of the nervous system. *J Neurovirol*, **7**, 564–569.

Torigoe S, Koide W, Yamada M *et al*. (1996) Human herpesvirus 7 infection associated with central nervous system manifestations. *J Pediatr*, **129**, 301–305.

Turner S, DiLuca D and Gompels U (2002) Characterisation of a human herpesvirus variant A 'amplicon' and replication modulation by U94-Rep 'latency gene'. *J Virol Methods*, **105**, 331–341.

Ueda T, Miyake Y, Imoto K *et al*. (1996) Distribution of human herpesvirus 6 and varicella-zoster virus in organs of a fatal case with exanthem subitum and varicella. *Acta Paediatr Japon*, **38**, 590–595.

Van Loon NM, Gummuluru S, Sherwood DJ *et al*. (1995) Direct sequence analysis of human herpesvirus 6 (HHV-6) sequences from infants and comparison of HHV-6 from mother/infant pairs. *Clin Infect Dis*, **21**, 1017–1019.

Villoslada P, Juste C, Tintore M *et al*. (2003) The immune response against herpesvirus is more prominent in the early stages of MS. *Neurology*, **60**, 1944–1948.

Wagner M, Muller-Berghaus J, Schroeder R *et al*. (1997) Human herpesvirus-6 (HHV-6)-associated necrotizing encephalitis in Griscelli's syndrome. *J Med Virol*, **53**, 306–312.

Wang F, Larsson K, Linde A and Ljungman P (2002) Human herpesvirus 6 infection and cytomegalovirus-specific lymphoproliferative responses in allogeneic stem cell transplant recipients. *Bone Marrow Transplant*, **30**, 521–526.

Wang FZ, Dahl H, Linde A *et al*. (1996) Lymphotropic herpesviruses in allogeneic bone marrow transplantation. *Blood*, **88**, 3615–3620.

Wang J, Huff K, McMasters R and Cornford M (1999) Sudden unexpected death associated with HHV-6 in an adolescent with tuberous sclerosis. *Pediatr Neurol*, **21**, 488–491.

Ward K, Couto Parada X, Passas J and Thiruchelvam A (2002a) Evaluation of the specificity and sensitivity of indirect immunofluorescence tests for IgG to human herpesviruses-6 and -7. *J Virol Methods*, **106**, 107–113.

Ward K, White R, Mackinnon S and Hanna M (2002b) Human herpesvirus-7 infection of the CNS with acute myelitis in an adult bone marrow recipient. *Bone Marrow Transpl*, **30**, 983–985.

Ward KN, Gray JJ and Efstathiou S (1989) Brief report: Primary human herpesvirus 6 infection in a patient following liver transplantation from a seropositive donor. *J Med Virol*, **28**, 69–72.

Ward KN, Gray JJ, Fotheringham MW and Sheldon MJ (1993) IgG antibodies to human herpesvirus-6 in young children: changes in avidity of antibody correlate with time after infection. *J Med Virol*, **39**, 131–138.

Ward KN, Gray JJ, Joslin ME and Sheldon MJ (1993) Avidity of IgG antibodies to human herpesvirus-6 distinguishes primary from recurrent infection in organ transplant recipients and excludes cross-reactivity with other herpesviruses. *J Med Virol*, **39**, 44–49.

Widen F, Goltz M, Wittenbrink N *et al*. (2001) Identification and sequence analysis of the glycoprotein B gene of porcine cytomegalovirus. *Virus Genes*, **23**, 339–346.

Williams SL, Hartline CB, Kushner NL *et al*. (2003) *In vitro* activities of benzimadazole D- and L-ribonucleosides against herpesviruses. *Antimicrob Agents Chemother*, **47**, 2186–2192.

Yamamoto T, Mukai T, Kondo K and Yamanishi K (1994) Variation of DNA sequence in immediate-early gene of human herpesvirus 6 and variant identification by PCR. *J Clin Microbiol*, **32**, 473–476.

Yasukawa M, Inoue Y, Ohminami H *et al*. (1997) Human herpesvirus 7 infection of lymphoid and myeloid cell lines transduced with an adenovirus vector containing the CD4 gene. *J Virol*, **71**, 1708–1712.

Yasukawa M, Yakushijin Y, Furukawa M and Fujita S (1993) Specificity analysis of human $CD4^+$ T-cell clones directed against human herpesvirus 6 (HHV-6), HHV-7, and human cytomegalovirus. *J Virol*, **67**, 6259–6264.

Yoshida H, Matsunaga K, Ueda T *et al*. (2002) Human herpesvirus 6 meningoencephalitis successfully treated with ganciclovir in a patient who underwent allogeneic bone marrow transplantation from an HLA-identical sibling. *Int J Hematol*, **75**, 421–425.

Yoshida M, Torigoe S, Ikeue K and Yamada M (2002) Neutralizing antibody responses to human herpesviruses 6 and 7 do not cross-react with each other, and maternal neutralizing antibodies contribute to sequential infection with these viruses in childhood. *Clin Diagn Lab Immunol*, **9**, 388–393.

Yoshida R, Imai T, Hieshima K *et al*. (1997) Molecular cloning of a novel human CC chemokine EBI1-ligand chemokine that is a specific functional ligand for EBI1, CCR7. *J Biol Chem*, **272**, 13803–13809.

Yoshikawa T, Akimoto S, Nishimura N *et al*. (2003) Evaluation of active human herpesvirus 6 infection by reverse transcription-PCR. *J Med Virol*, **70**, 267–272.

Yoshikawa T, Asano Y, Kobayashi I *et al*. (1993) Seroepidemiology of human herpesvirus 7 in healthy children and adults in Japan. *J Med Virol*, **41**, 319–323.

Yoshikawa T, Ihira M, Asano Y *et al*. (2002) Fatal adult case of severe lymphocytopenia associated with reactivation of human herpesvirus 6. *J Med Virol*, **66**, 82–85.

Yoshikawa T, Ihira M, Ohashi M *et al*. (2001) Correlation between HHV-6 infection and skin rash after allogeneic bone marrow transplantation. *Bone Marrow Transpl*, **28**, 77–81.

Yoshikawa T, Ihira M, Suzuki K *et al*. (2002) Fatal acute myocarditis in an infant with human herpesvirus 6 infection. *J Clin Pathol*, **54**, 792–795.

Yoshikawa T, Suga S, Asano Y *et al.* (1989) Distribution of antibodies to a causative agent of exanthem subitum (human herpesvirus-6) in healthy individuals. *Pediatrics*, **84**, 675–677.

Zerr D, Gooley T, Yeung L *et al.* (2001) Human herpesvirus 6 reactivation and encephalitis in allogeneic bone marrow transplant recipients. *Clin Infect Dis*, **33**, 763–771.

Zhang Y, de Bolle L, Aquaro S *et al.* (2002) Productive infection of primary macrophages with human herpesvirus 7. *J Virol*, **75**, 10511–10514.

Zou P, Isegawa Y, Nakano K *et al.* (1999) Human herpesvirus 6 open reading frame U83 encodes a functional chemokine. *J Virol*, **73**, 5926–5933.

Kaposi's Sarcoma-associated Herpesvirus (Human Herpesvirus 8)

Abel Viejo-Borbolla, Cornelia Henke-Gendo and Thomas F. Schulz

Hannover Medical School, Germany

INTRODUCTION

The eighth human herpesvirus is associated with three forms of human neoplasia. It was first discovered in Kaposi's sarcoma (KS), with which it is strongly associated, hence the designation Kaposi's sarcoma-associated herpesvirus (KSHV) given to it by its discoverers (Chang *et al.*, 1994). It is also consistently found in a very rare form of B cell lymphoma, body cavity-associated lymphoma (BCBL) or primary effusion lymphoma (PEL). Finally, it is found in the plasma cell variant of multicentric Castleman's disease (MCD), particularly in HIV-infected individuals, and may also play a role in occasional cases of bone marrow failure in immunosuppressed individuals. To reflect its association with conditions other than KS, and to keep within the nomenclature adopted for other human herpesviruses, the term *Human herpesvirus 8* (HHV-8) is preferred by some authors.

The discovery of KSHV was initiated by careful epidemiological studies which had, for several decades, suggested the involvement of a transmissible agent in the pathogenesis of Kaposi's sarcoma. In spite of these leads, attempts by several groups to identify such an organism by conventional culture or morphological approaches had been unsuccessful. The development of molecular techniques combining PCR amplification with subtractive hybridisation (representational difference analysis, RDA), allowed Chang *et al.* (1994) to search for unknown DNA sequences present in Kaposi's sarcoma but not a control tissue. They initially identified two small DNA fragments with homologies to two oncogenic gammaherpesviruses, Epstein–Barr virus (EBV) and *Herpesvirus saimiri* (HVS) of squirrel monkeys. These were later shown to be part of a complete viral genome (Russo *et al.*, 1996) present in the endothelial tumour (spindle) cells of KS lesions (Boshoff *et al.*, 1995). After the discovery of KSHV in primary effusion lymphomas (PEL; Cesarman *et al.*, 1995a) several groups succeeded in establishing persistently infected cell lines from such lymphomas, and subsequently to visualise KSHV virions after chemical induction of the lytic replication cycle (Renne *et al.*, 1996; Said *et al.*, 1996). Ten years after its initial discovery, the available epidemiological and molecular evidence strongly suggests that KSHV is the cause of KS, PEL and the plasma cell variant of MCD, and thus a new human tumour virus.

VIRUS MORPHOLOGY AND CULTURE

KSHV has the characteristic morphological appearance of a herpesvirus (see Chapter 2A). An example of a KSHV virion, produced by the PEL-derived KS-1 cell line (Said *et al.*, 1996) after induction of the lytic cycle by treatment with phorbol esters, is shown in Figure 2F.1.

PEL-derived cell lines may be latently infected with KSHV only, or may be co-infected with EBV, if the original tumour also contained EBV (Said *et al.*, 1996; Renne *et al.*, 1996; further references in Schulz, 2001). In some cell lines (e.g. BCP-1, BCBL-1, KS-1) most

Principles and Practice of Clinical Virology, Fifth Edition. Edited by A. J. Zuckerman, J. E. Banatvala, J. R. Pattison, P. D. Griffiths and B. D. Schoub
© 2004 John Wiley & Sons Ltd ISBN 0 470 84338 1

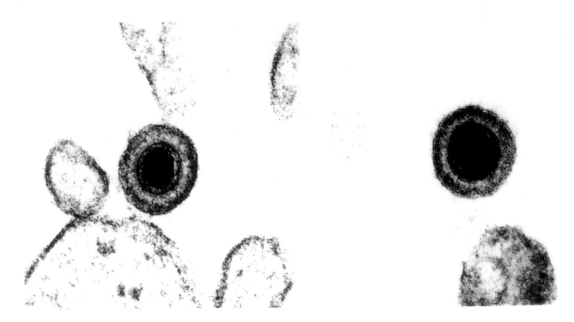

Figure 2F.1 Electron micrograph of KSHV in lytically induced KS-1 cells (Said *et al.*, 1996). The KSHV virion has the characteristic features of a herpesvirus. Courtesy of D. Ablashi, Advanced Biotechnologies

cells only express latent KSHV genes (see below), but some will spontaneously switch into lytic replication, whereas in others, e.g. the KSHV/EBV dually infected cell line HBL-6 (or BC-1), KSHV is much more strictly latent. The lytic replication programme can be switched on in all these cell lines by treatment with either phorbol esters (Renne *et al.*, 1996) or sodium butyrate (Miller *et al.*, 1996), but some cell lines are better virus producers (e.g. KS-1, BCBL-1, JSC-1, Cro-AP3) than others.

KSHV virus preparations obtained in this manner show only little infectivity *in vitro* when incubated with a number of permanent cell lines or primary cultures (Renne *et al.*, 1998; Flore *et al.*, 1998; Moses *et al.*, 1999; Ciufo *et al.*, 2001; Cerimele *et al.*, 2001; Lagunoff *et al.*, 2002). Early attempts showed that KSHV can be, albeit only inefficiently and transiently, propagated on the 293 embryonal kidney epithelial cell line (Renne *et al.*, 1998). More recently, primary endothelial cell cultures (Cannon *et al.*, 2000; Ciufo *et al.*, 2001) and endothelial cell lines immortalised by human papillomavirus E6/E7 (Moses *et al.*, 1999) or telomerase (Lagunoff *et al.*, 2002) have been found to be more efficiently infected. In these endothelial cell cultures most cells are infected in a latent form with minimal viral gene expression, expression of the viral latency-associated nuclear antigen 'LANA' (see below) in the majority, and evidence of lytic cycle

or structural viral proteins in only a few (Moses *et al.*, 1999; Cannon *et al.*, 2000; Ciufo *et al.*, 2001; Lagunoff *et al.*, 2002). Stable persistence of KSHV in endothelial cells *in vitro* may depend on the culture system used: in telomerase-immortalised endothelial cells KSHV appears not to be retained in infected cultures upon subsequent passage (Lagunoff *et al.*, 2002), whereas stable persistence has been found in the HPV-immortalised endothelial cell line (Moses *et al.*, 1999). Infection of endothelial cells results in morphological changes (spindle cell formation, piling up of infected cells) that vary with the cell culture system used (Moses *et al.*, 1999; Ciufo *et al.*, 2001; Lagunoff *et al.*, 2002).

It is also possible to isolate replicating KSHV on 293 cells from saliva (Vieira *et al.*, 1997), but this is very inefficient and requires detection of replicating KSHV by PCR. In these cells, KSHV replication can usually only be sustained for a few passages. Infection of keratinocyte cultures with KSHV has also been achieved (Cerimele *et al.*, 2001).

The inefficient persistence of KSHV in endothelial or epithelial cells is reminiscent of the rapid loss of KSHV from primary cultures of KS biopsies (Lebbé *et al.*, 1997) and contrasts with its stable long-term persistence in PEL-derived cell lines. It is therefore possible that cell lineage-specific factors affect the long-term latent persistence of KSHV *in vitro* as well as *in vivo*.

DIAGNOSTIC ASSAYS

Serological Assays

Several serological assays of varying sensitivity and specificity, such as immunofluorescence, enzyme-liked immunosorbent assays and immunoblotting, have been developed. Among the first KSHV antibody assays, latently infected PEL cell lines, such as BCP-1 or BCBL-1, were used as antigens for immunofluorescence assays (IFA) by incubating these cells, dried onto microscope slides, with patient sera and detecting specific antibody binding with fluorescein-conjugated secondary antibodies (Gao et al., 1996; Kedes et al., 1996; see Figure 2F.2). Positive cells show a typical speckled nuclear pattern which represents the main latent nuclear antigen of KSHV, the 225–234 kDa LANA-1 protein encoded by ORF73 (Rainbow et al., 1997). The sensitivity of this assay lies in the order of 80% or higher when suitable PEL cell lines (e.g. BCP-1) and sera from KS patients are used as standards. A 3% reactivity rate in this assay among healthy individuals from low-prevalence countries indicates a high specificity. In addition, an IFA performed on PEL cell lines, in which the lytic cycle can be efficiently induced by treatment with phorbol esters or sodium butyrate (e.g. BCBL-1; KS-1), detects antibodies to several viral structural proteins, in particular the ORF K8.1-encoded virion membrane glycoprotein (see below) (Lenette et al., 1996; Rezza et al., 1998). While thought to be more sensitive than the IFA for LANA-1 antibodies, the 'lytic' IFA suffers from a lower specificity in many laboratories. However, with some protocols good specificities for this assay have been reported (Schatz et al., 2001; Rezza et al., 1998), although the issue of interlaboratory comparability remains problematic with this assay.

Enzyme-linked immunosorbent assays (ELISAs) are based on either whole-virus lysates, recombinant viral proteins, in particular LANA-1, K8.1 glycoprotein, orf65/vSCIP (Simpson et al., 1996; Raab et al., 1998; see Schulz, 1998 for further references), or short chemically synthesised peptides derived from a combination of these three proteins (Tedeschi et al., 1999; Engels et al., 2000; Schatz et al., 2001; Lam et al., 2002). Sensitivity and specificity of these ELISAs are in the range 81–94% and 70–80%, respectively. Specificity of these assays can be increased by verifying a positive result in a more specific immunoblot. ELISAs based on the highly immunogenic K8.1 glycoprotein, which has no homologue in other herpesviruses, seem to perform with a comparatively high specificity (Engels et al., 2000; Schatz et al., 2001).

Combinations of different antigens or assays increase sensitivity and thus make it possible to detect even lower antibody titres, as in the early stages of asymptomatic infection or in the late stages of AIDS when KSHV-specific antibodies can vanish. Several serological testing algorithms have been evaluated, e.g. categorising individuals as seropositive if they had a high positive result on a K8.1-ELISA or an intermediate result in combination with a positive latent IFA (Engels et al., 2000). Others screen all samples by latent IFA and orf65/SCIP ELISA, confirming positive ELISA results by immunoblotting (Simpson et al., 1996). Recently, a multicentre study tested interassay concordance of 18 established as well as novel assays (Schatz et al., 2001). They advise combination of two IFAs against KSHV lytic and latent antigens, performed according to particular protocols. This combination gave a sensitivity of 89.1% and a specificity of 94.9%.

With the help of the assays mentioned in the previous paragraph it has been possible to gain some insight into the epidemiology of KSHV (see below). However, serological diagnosis of a KSHV infection in an individual, particularly from a low-risk population, may still be associated with a degree of uncertainty if antibodies to only one KSHV antigen or reactivity in only one assay are found. Simultaneous reactivity in several assays affords much higher certainty.

Molecular Biology Assays

By qualitative PCR, KSHV is easily detectable in fresh or frozen biopsies of KS, PEL or MCD, although the amount of KSHV DNA can be quite variable, particularly in KS biopsies. Detection in paraffin-embedded specimens generally may require the use of nested PCR, as does detection in peripheral blood, saliva or semen. Different primer combinations have been used successfully for this purpose (Chang et al., 1994; Whitby et al., 1995; further references in Schulz et al., 1999). To quantify the amount of KSHV DNA in peripheral blood or other specimen, several quantitative PCR assays, including competitive and real-time PCR, have recently been developed (Stamey et al., 2001; Boivin et al., 1999). Quantitative methods may become more important in clinical practice, since a measurable viral load of KSHV in patients' PBMCs has been reported to correlate with the presence of clinical symptoms and disease progression (Campbell et al., 2000). In particular, MCD (see below) seems to be associated with a high KSHV viral load (Boivin et

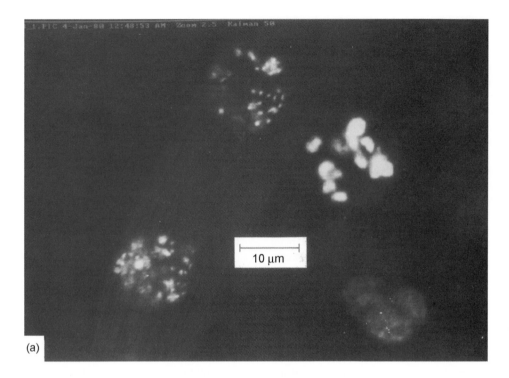

(a)

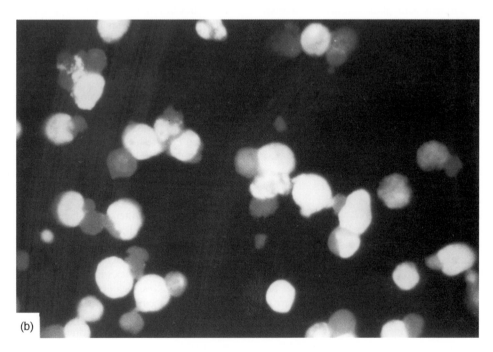

(b)

Figure 2F.2 Immunofluorescence pattern for latent (top) and lytic (bottom) KSHV antigens in PEL cells. The top panel shows the characteristic speckled nuclear pattern for the 'Latency associated nuclear antigen', LANA (Kedes *et al.*, 1996; Gao *et al.*, 1996), which is encoded by ORF73 (Rainbow *et al.*, 1997). The bottom panel shows the diffuse nuclear and cytoplasmic fluorescence seen on TPA- or sodium butyrate-induced PEL cells with patient sera

al., 2002; Oksenhendler et al., 2000). After transplantation, 11 of 12 patients with progressive KS disease have been shown to be positive by real-time PCR, whereas this was the case for only 6 of 31 with stable or remitting disease (Pellet et al., 2002). Detection of KSHV DNA in the peripheral blood of HIV-infected individuals has long been known to predict the onset of Kaposi's sarcoma (Whitby et al., 1995). Whether this is due to an increase in circulating KSHV-positive cells or to lytic (productive) viral replication needs to be resolved (Oksenhendler et al., 2000). KHSV viral load in PBMCs of seven out of eight patients suffering from AIDS-related progressive Kaposi's sarcoma became negative after complete or partial clinical response following initiation of a HIV triple therapy with protease inhibitors (Lebbé et al., 1998). Thus, quantitative PCR methods can serve as a diagnostic tool to monitor immunocompromised patients at high risk of KSHV-related diseases.

When dealing with the highly sensitive PCR methodology, the high risk of contamination and thus the possibility of false positive results always has to be kept in mind, especially when working with low concentrations of viral DNA, as is the case with KSHV. PCR contaminations might also be the reason for several reports on associations of KSHV with a number of diseases that have not been confirmed by others.

ORIGIN AND EVOLUTION OF KSHV

Phylogenetic analysis of its genomic sequence (Russo et al., 1996; Neipel et al., 1997) places KSHV with the gamma-2 subgroup of herpesviruses, the rhadinoviruses. This group includes several other animal herpesviruses, such as Herpesvirus saimiri (HVS), Equine herpesvirus 2 (EHV-2) and Murine herpesvirus 68 (MHV-68). Following the discovery of KSHV, attempts to understand its origin have resulted in the isolation or identification, by consensus PCR, of closely related rhadinoviruses in many non-human primates (reviewed in Greensill and Schulz, 2000). Thus, as shown in Figure 2F.3, fragments of viral DNA polymerase genes with close similarity to KSHV have been found in chimpanzees (PtRV-1 or PanRHV1), gorillas (GoRHV-1), mandrills (MnRHV1), African green monkeys (ChRV1) and macaques (RFHVMm, RFHVMn) (Rose et al., 1997; Greensill et al., 2000a, 2000b; Lacoste et al., 2000a, 2000b). In addition, a second group of gamma-2 herpesviral DNA polymerase fragments from chimpanzees (PanRHV2),

mandrills (MnRHV2), African green monkeys (ChRV2), and a virus isolate from macaques (RRV), appear to be slightly more distantly related to KSHV (Figure 2F.3; Desrosiers et al., 1997; Greensill et al., 2000a; Lacoste et al., 2000a, 2001). Although this is only based (in most cases) on relatively short DNA sequences, the fact that these two groups have now been found in many primate species suggests the existence of two distinct lineages of gamma-2 herpesviruses (rhadinoviruses), termed RV-1 and RV-2 (Figure 2F.3), in Old World primates. Despite attempts by several groups, only a representative of the RV-1 lineage, KSHV, has so far been found in humans. Whether a human RV-2 virus remains to be discovered, or whether it has died out during evolution, is not known at present.

The existence of closely related gamma-2 herpesviruses in non-human primates and the fact that their proximity reflects that of the host species (Figure 2F.3) would be in keeping with the accepted view of herpesvirus–host co-evolution (McGeoch et al., 2000). The study of genomic variation of KSHV isolates has also revealed the existence of particular KSHV variants in certain geographic regions, suggesting that KSHV has co-evolved with human populations. This is best illustrated by the pattern of variability found in the K1 gene at the left end of the KSHV genome (see Figures 2F.3, 2F.4 and 2F.5). K1 encodes a type I transmembrane protein with a cytoplasmic immunoreceptor tyrosine activation motif (ITAM)-containing signalling domain and an immunoglubulin superfamily-like extracellular domain which contains two highly variable regions, VR1 and VR2 (see Figure 2F.7) (Zong et al., 1999; Cook et al., 1999; Davidovici et al., 2001; Lacoste et al., 2000c; Biggar et al., 2000; Meng et al., 2001). Nucleotide substitutions that alter the protein sequence ('nonsynonymous' mutations) are more frequent in this region than those that do not ('synonymous' mutations), indicating that evolution of K1 is driven by some selective pressure. As illustrated in Figure 2F.4, K1 variants can be grouped into four or five major clades, A–E. The same clades can broadly be recognised in other genomic regions, where the variability between them is, however, much less than in the K1 gene. These five clades are all thought to be derived from one common ancestor, termed 'P' ('prototype'). Clade B is found exclusively in Africa or individuals descended from an African ancestor, while clade D is confined to old Asian populations, such as the Ainu, an old population on Hokkaido in the north of Japan (Zong et al., 1999; Meng et al., 2001). Clade E, which is closely related to clade D, was

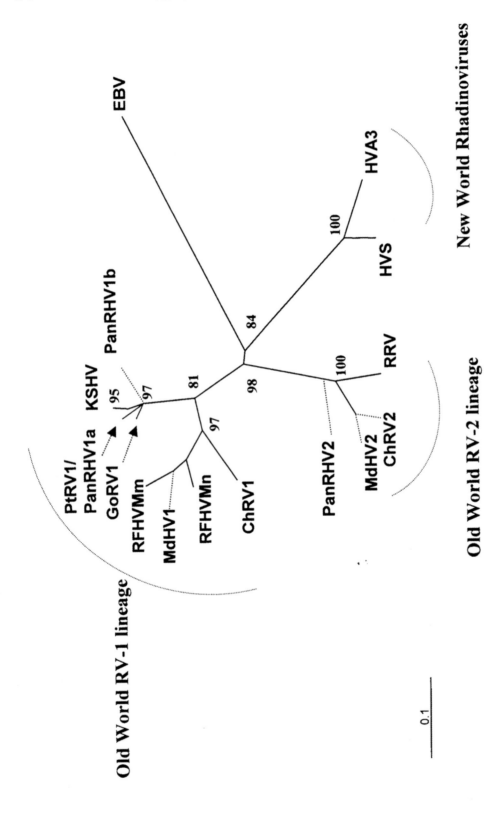

Figure 2F.3 Phylogenetic relationships among primate gamma-2 herpesviruses. The phylogenetic tree shown here was created by the neighbour-joining method of partial viral DNA polymerase sequences of the gamma-2 herpesviruses shown. Numbers at branchpoints denote bootstrap values to indicate the reliability of this analysis (values over 75% are generally taken to indicate a robust assignment to a branch). The figure shows that KSHV belongs to the RV-1 subgroup of gamma-2 herpesviruses with closely related viruses being found in many Old World primate species. In addition, a second group, RV-2, comprises slightly more distantly related gamma-2-herpesviruses in many primate species (see text). The 'New World' primate gamma-2-herpesviruses form a third branch (see text). The dotted lines indicate recently discovered family members for which the currently available sequences overlap only partially with the region of the DNA polymerase used to construct this tree

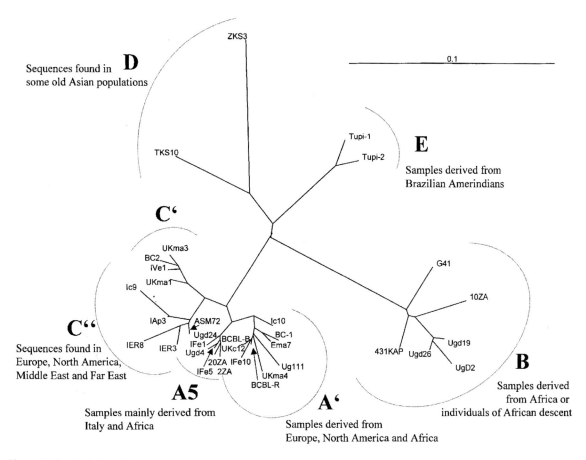

Figure 2F.4 Evolution of the K1 gene of KSHV: K1, located at the 'left' end of the KSHV genome (see Figure 2F.5), exists in five major variants. Some of these are associated with particular geographic regions or populations, indicating a possible co-evolution of K1 with human populations (see text)

found in Amerindian populations of Brazil (Biggar et al., 2000), an observation that would be compatible with the well-established migration of the original Amerindian people from Asia to the Americas. In contrast, KSHV clades A and C are now found in many parts of the world, most likely reflecting the mixing of populations over the last three millennia (Cook et al., 1999; Zong et al., 1999). However, geographic or ethnic associations can occasionally still be seen within individual clades: K1 sequences found in Ashkenazi and Sephardi Jews in Israel belonged to particular A and C subtypes (Davidovici et al., 2001) and a C subtype is found in Taiwan and Okinawa, reflecting the geographical proximity of these islands. In some cases the presence of particular subtypes in separate geographic locations, e.g. the wide distribution of the A5 subtype in Africa and its presence on the

east coast of Italy, could be hypothesised to be the result of old trading links (Cook et al., 1999; Lacoste et al., 2000c).

In addition to this pattern of evolution within human populations, recombination between different KSHV genomes and, in at least two cases, with related gamma-2 herpesviruses, appears to be another important factor in the evolution of KSHV. Evidence for multiple recombination events among 'P-type' sequences have been found in many KSHV sequences (Poole et al., 1999; Lacoste et al., 2000c; Kakoola et al., 2001; Zong, 2002). In addition, remnants of two so-far unidentified but more distantly related gamma-2 herpesviruses have been found in currently circulating KSHV variants. One, the 'M' type, has recombined into 'P-type' variants at the right end of the viral genome. Both the fact that this 'M' type has been seen in isolates from different parts of the world, and the observation of two separate lineages of the 'M' type indicate that this recombination event took place possibly in the order of 100 000 years ago (Poole *et al.*, 1999; Kakoola *et al.*, 2001; Lacoste *et al.*, 2000c; Zong, 2002). The other type ('Q' type) also originated from a recombination event with yet another gamma-2 herpesvirus at the right end of the KSHV genome, but has so far only been seen in South Africa (Alagiozoglou *et al.*, 2000; Zong *et al.*, 2002).

EPIDEMIOLOGY OF KSHV

Distribution in the General Population in Different Countries

The seroprevalence of KSHV in different geographic regions has been studied using immunofluorescence assays on PEL-derived cell lines, which detect antibodies to the latency-associated nuclear antigen (LANA), a hallmark of all KSHV-infected cells, or to structural proteins produced during lytic viral replication (Gao *et al.*, 1996; Kedes *et al.*, 1996; Simpson *et al.*, 1996; Lennette *et al.*, 1996). In addition, ELISAs or Western blot assays based on recombinant proteins [the ORF73-encoded LANA, the K8.1-encoded viral glycoprotein, the ORF65-encoded small capsid protein (SCIP) have been used; Simpson *et al.*, 1996; Raab *et al.*, 1998; Zhu *et al.*, 1999; Schatz *et al.*, 2001; further references in Schulz, 1999]. As outlined in the section on KSHV serology, none of these assays is 100% sensitive or specific. This means that exact seroprevalence rates, particularly in low-prevalence areas, have been difficult to determine. However, these assays have proved good enough to work out the distribution of KSHV in different countries and regions, and to define modes and risk factors of transmission in endemic countries as well as in population groups at high risk for sexually transmitted diseases.

The currently available seroepidemiology data indicate that KSHV is relatively rare in most northern, western and central European countries (data are available for the UK, Denmark, Sweden, France, Germany, The Netherlands and Hungary), with less than 5% of blood donors having antibodies to either KSHV LANA, the orf65-encoded SCIP protein, or the K8.1-encoded virion membrane glycoprotein (different antigens were used in the individual studies and the results are therefore difficult to compare) (Simpson *et al.*, 1996; Tedeschi *et al.*, 2000; further references in Schulz, 1999).

In comparison, infection with KSHV appears to be more widespread in some parts of Italy, Greece and, to a lesser extent, Spain (Gao *et al.*, 1996; Simpson *et al.*, 1996; Calabrò *et al.*, 1998; Whitby *et al.*, 1998; Andreoni *et al.*, 2001; Santarelli *et al.*, 2001; Perna *et al.*, 2000; Gambus *et al.*, 2001; further references in Schulz, 1999). In Italy, infection with KSHV appears to be more common among blood donors from regions previously reported to have a higher incidence of classic KS, such as Sicily or Sardinia, than in the centre or in prealpine regions (Calabrò *et al.*, 1998; Whitby *et al.*, 1998; Santarelli *et al.*, 2001; Perna, 2000; Rezza *et al.*, 1998; Serraino *et al.*, 2001; Andreoni *et al.*, 2001; further references in Schulz, 1999). Among Italian blood donors or hospital controls, KSHV seroprevalence increases with age, particularly in those over the age of 50, i.e the age group in which the incidence of classic KS is highest (Calabrò *et al.*, 1998; Serraino *et al.*, 2001).

In the USA, reported prevalence rates in blood donors vary; 0–3% for antibodies to LANA, 0–5 % for antibodies to orf65/SCIP, and 0–25% for antibodies measured by lytic IFA or an ELISA on purified virions (Kedes *et al.*, 1996; Gao *et al.*, 1996; Simpson *et al.*, 1996; Lennette *et al.*, 1996; Smith *et al.*, 1997; further references in Schulz, 1999). There may also exist regional or local variations in seroprevalence, since one study found a higher prevalence (15%) of antibodies to LANA or orf65/SCIP in Texas, particularly in individuals of less than high school education (Baillargeon *et al.*, 2001), and another study reported a higher prevalence rate in individuals of Black race and resident in particular parts of New York (Greenblatt *et al.*, 2001). In another study, the increased seroprevalence seen in Black or Hispanic individuals disappeared on multivariate analysis, which left only a history of syphilis and intravenous drug use as independent risk factors (Cannon *et al.*, 2001). These regional or local variations in seroprevalence may therefore reflect increased transmission in particular communities or risk groups (see below).

In contrast, all studies reported so far concur that antibodies to KSHV are frequently found in most African countries, particularly in sub-Saharan Africa. Antibodies to LANA, orf65/SCIP, K8.1 glycoprotein or undefined productive cycle antigens are found in approximately 40–60% of adults and adolescents in most parts of sub-Saharan Africa investigated so far, e.g. Uganda, Tanzania, The Gambia, Cameroon, South Africa, Eritrea, Malawi, Kenya and Egypt (Simpson *et al.*, 1996; Gao *et al.*, 1996; Lennette *et al.*, 1996; Ariyoshi *et al.*, 1998; Mayama *et al.*, 1998; Serraino *et al.*, 2001; Schatz *et al.*, 2001; Andreoni *et* al., 1999; Engels et al., 2000; Enbom, 1999; Rezza et al., 2000a; further references in Schulz, 1999). Occasional studies have even reported higher antibody prevalence rates by IFA for lytic KSHV antigens (Lennette et al., 1996). These high seroprevalence rates, obtained even with assays which detect antibodies to defined antigens, suggest that KSHV is widespread in Africa, and occurs not only in those regions (east and central Africa) where KS was known to exist before the arrival of HIV-1 (endemic KS) (see below). This could suggest an involvement of additional co-factors in the pathogenesis of endemic KS.

In Brazil, the prevalence of antibodies to LANA among blood donors was in the range 5–7% in two studies (Caterino-de-Araujo et al., 1999; Zago et al., 2000), while antibodies to purified virions were found in 16% of individuals belonging to low-income families in Belém, North Brazil (Freitas et al., 2002). In contrast, KSHV was found to be highly prevalent (LANA antibody prevalence rates >50%) in different Amerindian tribes and language groups in Brazil that had only little contact to the outside world (Biggar et al., 2000). As mentioned above, these individuals are infected with a KSHV variant that is related to those found in old Asian populations. Similarly, the Noirs Marron of French Guyana, a population of African descent living in remote villages, were also found by lytic immunofluorescence to have prevalence rates for KSHV antibodies of >15% among adults and reaching 27% in those above 40 years old (Plancoulaine et al., 2000). In Malaysia, India, Sri Lanka, Thailand and Japan KSHV prevalence was found to be low (Ablashi et al., 1999; Katano et al., 2000a; Satoh et al., 2001; Fujii et al., 1999).

In Saudi Arabia, KSHV infection was found to be infrequent (approximately 4–7%) in hospital controls used to assess KSHV prevalence in the general population (Almuneef et al., 2001; further references in Schulz, 1999).

A consistently observed feature of all these studies investigating the distribution of KSHV in the general population is the increase of KSHV prevalence with age. This is likely to reflect ongoing transmission throughout adult life, but may also be due to increased viral replication after reactivation of a latent KSHV infection in elderly individuals.

Thus, these studies conducted in different parts of the world indicate that, in spite of being an 'old' human virus that has co-evolved with human populations, KSHV has apparently become rare in many geographic regions, although in some of these it may have been retained in defined populations. It has, however, remained common in Africa.

Distribution in Homosexual Men

In accordance with the high incidence of AIDS KS in HIV-1 infected homo-bisexual men, KSHV is more common in this group than in the general population of the same country. This observation, which initially provided a strong argument for an association of KSHV with AIDS KS (Simpson et al., 1996; Melbye et al., 1998; Renwick et al., 1998; Martin et al., 1998; Rezza et al., 1998), has now been made consistently in many countries (Rezza et al., 2000b; Pauk et al., 2000; Perna et al., 2000; O'Brien et al., 1999). For example, about one-third of homosexual men participating in cohort studies in Denmark, the UK and Holland were infected with KSHV, as ascertained by the presence of antibodies to LANA-1 and the orf65-encoded capsid protein vSCIP (Melbye et al., 1998; Renwick et al., 1998; Simpson et al., 1996), although more recent studies in the USA have found lower prevalence rates (Casper et al., 2002). In some cohort studies, a decline of KSHV prevalence or incidence has been noted during the last two decades (Melbye et al., 1998; Renwick et al., 1998), but in other cohorts the rate of KSHV infection has remained stable (Osmond et al., 2002; Rezza et al., 2000b). KSHV is transmitted as a result of sexual contact in this group (see below) and it appears to have spread in this group as a separate epidemic independently of HIV-1 (Melbye et al., 1998; Dukers et al., 2000; O'Brien et al., 1999). Attempts have been made to back-calculate the beginning of this epidemic, but these are associated with some uncertainty and the answers may well differ for homosexual communities in different countries: thus, in Denmark KSHV may have been introduced into Danish homosexual men in the late 1970s through contact with US partners (Melbye et al., 1998), whereas in Holland the beginning of this epidemic was inferred to have occurred much earlier (Dukers et al., 2000) and KSHV was already highly prevalent in California in 1978–1979 (Osmond et al., 2002).

Transmission

Transmission in Childhood

In endemic countries or population groups (Africa, remote African or Amerindian populations in South America, African mothers in Europe; see above) the rapid increase of KSHV infection in children aged 1–12 years indicates that KSHV can be efficiently transmitted in childhood (Mayama et al., 1998; Andreoni et al., 1999, 2002; Gessain et al., 1999;

Plancoulaine *et al.*, 2000; Bourboulia *et al.*, 1998; Sitas *et al.*, 1999; Lyall *et al.*, 1999). In these situations young children are more likely to be infected if their mothers or siblings are infected, suggesting mother–child, or sibling–sibling transmission as a possible source of infection (Bourboulia *et al.*, 1998; Lyall *et al.*, 1999; Sitas *et al.*, 1999; Plancoulaine *et al.*, 2000). However, molecular analysis of KSHV strains found in Malawian families has suggested that both intra-familial and extrafamilial transmission of KSHV can occur (Cook *et al.*, 2002). In keeping with this, an epidemiological study among Egyptian children found that close contact with at least two other children in the community was a risk factor for KSHV infection (Andreoni *et al.*, 2002). Given the excretion of KSHV in saliva (see below), it is conceivable that saliva plays a role in transmitting KSHV from mother to child, sibling to sibling, or from other contact children (Andreoni *et al.*, 2002), although no direct evidence for this hypothesis currently exists. In addition, an association with hepatitis B virus (HBV) infection has been seen in one study, suggesting that in Africa KSHV may be transmitted along similar routes to HBV (Mayama *et al.*, 1998).

KSHV infection has also been noted in children in Italy (Calabrò *et al.*, 1998; Serraino *et al.*, 2001; Whitby *et al.*, 2000) but not in Spain (Gambus *et al.*, 2001).

Transmission in Adult Life

The gradual increase in seroprevalence during adult life, noted in many studies, would be compatible with the notion of continuing acquisition of KSHV infections. While in endemic countries or populations the majority of infections appear to occur before puberty, transmission during adulthood accounts for most infections in non-endemic countries.

In heterosexual adults of non-endemic countries, transmission during sexual contacts appears to represent one important route of infection. Thus, KSHV seroprevalence in Swedish women was found to be associated with an increased number of sexual partners and with a history of sexually transmitted diseases (STDs), particularly chlamydial infection and genital warts (Tedeschi *et al.*, 2000). A similar association of KSHV seroprevalence with *Human papillomavirus* infection (HPV) infection was seen in Spanish prostitutes, who are more frequently infected with KSHV than a control group (de Sanjose *et al.*, 2002). In Sicily, KSHV infection was more common in prostitutes, in men reporting contacts with prostitutes,

and in STD clinic attenders (Perna *et al.*, 2000), and contact with prostitutes was also seen as a risk factor for KSHV infection in men from Paris (Janier *et al.*, 2002).

Similarly, there is evidence from seroepidemiological studies pointing to a role for sexual transmission among heterosexual adults in KSHV endemic countries. Thus, an increased prevalence of KSHV among prostitutes in Africa has been seen in some studies but not in others (Lavreys *et al.*, 2003; Marcellin *et al.*, 2002; further references in Schulz, 1999). Similarly, there was no association between KSHV infection in husbands and wives in a population-based study among the Noir Marron of French Guyana (Plancoulaine *et al.*, 2000). Given the well-documented transmission of KSHV during sexual contact among gay men (see below), sexual transmission among heterosexual individuals would appear likely, and the reasons why this is seen in some but not in other studies are currently not clear.

The conditions facilitating sexual transmission of KSHV have been studied in most detail in homosexual men, among whom this virus is highly prevalent, even in non-endemic countries (see above). The high prevalence of KSHV in this group of men who, upon co-infection with HIV, also suffer from KS much more frequently than individuals who contracted HIV by another route, had provided one of the initial strong arguments in favour of an association of KSHV with KS (Simpson *et al.*, 1996; Kedes *et al.*, 1996; Gao *et al.*, 1996). Numerous studies conducted on this topic agree that KSHV infection among gay men is linked to behavioural patterns that predispose to infection with a sexually transmitted agent. Thus, KSHV infection is consistently seen to increase with the number of sexual partners (Melbye *et al.*, 1998; Martin *et al.*, 1998; O'Brien *et al.*, 1999; Dukers *et al.*, 2000). Epidemiological studies investigating the impact of detailed sexual behavioural variables on KSHV transmission have, however, arrived at different conclusions. While several early studies reported anal intercourse, either passive or active, as a risk factor (Melbye *et al.*, 1998; O'Brien *et al.*, 1999; Dukers *et al.*, 2000), others have identified oral–penile contact (Dukers *et al.*, 2000), deep kissing (Pauk *et al.*, 2000), as predisposing behavioural variables. The use of amyl nitrate ('poppers') has also emerged as a risk factor in some (Pauk *et al.*, 2000) but not other (Melbye *et al.*, 1998) studies.

Among body fluids that could transfer KSHV during sexual contacts, the highest copy numbers of KSHV DNA, as detected by PCR, are found in saliva (Blackbourn *et al.*, 1998; Pauk *et al.*, 2000; Vieira *et al.*, 1997; Stamey *et al.*, 2001; Biggar *et al.*, 2000). In contrast, KSHV is detected in semen only infrequently and at low copy number (Pauk *et al.*, 2000; further references in Schulz, 1999). It is thus likely that saliva may also represent an important vehicle for transmission of KSHV during sexual contact.

Another controversial issue is the importance of parenteral transmission. KSHV DNA can be detected in PBMCs, as well as in plasma or serum, of about 5–10% of infected individuals (Whitby *et al.*, 1995). Among transplant patients, KSHV transmission from donor to recipient has clearly been documented in individual cases (Regamey *et al.*, 1998; Luppi *et al.*, 2000a; Barozzi *et al.*, 2003). Whether parenteral transmission contributes significantly to the spread of KSHV among drug users is, however, controversial. While early studies (Simpson *et al.*, 1996; Gao *et al.*, 1996) found no evidence for an increased seroprevalence of KSHV among intravenous drug users, one recent study (Cannon *et al.*, 2001) observed intravenous drug use to be a risk factor for KSHV infection among US women with high-risk behaviour for HIV-infection, and another study noted an increase in KSHV among Italian HIV-infected intravenous drug users (Parisi *et al.*, 2002). However, no evidence for an association with intravenous drug use was found in a big prospective cohort study of more than a 1000 drug users in Amsterdam (Renwick *et al.*, 2002).

Although transmission of KSHV through organ or bone marrow transplantation may occur (Regamey *et al.*, 1998; Luppi *et al.*, 2000a), it appears that in endemic countries the majority of individuals who developed post-transplant KS were already infected with KSHV at the time of transplantation, rather than being infected through the transplanted organ (Parravicini *et al.*, 1997; Farge *et al.*, 1999). A recent report (Barozzi *et al.*, 2003) highlighted the possibility that KSHV-infected endothelial precursor cells may be transmitted from organ donor to recipient during transplantation and may develop into Kaposi's sarcoma.

To what extent this also applies in non-endemic countries and whether there is therefore a need, in non-endemic countries, to screen organ or bone marrow donors or blood to be transfused to immuno-suppressed individuals, is still under investigation.

THE ROLE OF KSHV IN NEOPLASTIC DISEASE

Kaposi's Sarcoma

Epidemiological Findings

Epidemiological studies allow the conclusion that Kaposi's sarcoma only develops in KSHV-infected individuals but that this remains a rare event, unless there is additional immune suppression, as a result of either organ transplantation or HIV infection. Other factors may also promote the emergence of Kaposi's sarcoma. Thus, KSHV DNA is nearly always detected in all epidemiological forms (HIV-associated, 'classic', endemic) and clinical stages (early patch/plaque, fully developed nodular) of KS (see Schulz, 1999, for detailed references). Detection of KSHV is possible in PBMC of 50–60% of patients with HIV-associated or 'classic' KS (e.g. Whitby *et al.*, 1995; for further references see Schulz, 1999). In addition, detection of KSHV in PBMC of HIV-infected individuals predicts the subsequent appearance of KS lesions (Whitby *et al.*, 1995). The presence of antibodies to KSHV in non-endemic areas is also strongly associated with having KS, or being at increased risk for KS, and, among HIV-1 infected individuals, is strongly predictive of the subsequent appearance of KS lesions (Gao *et al.*, 1996; Keddes *et al.*, 1996; Simpson *et al.*, 1996; Martin *et al.*, 1998; Renwick *et al.*, 1998). In Italy, there appears to be a correlation between regional seroprevalence rates and the incidence of classic KS (Calabrò *et al.*, 1998; Whitby *et al.*, 1998).

However, while classic KS remains a rare tumour in immunocompetent KSHV-infected individuals—the incidence rate range from 1–3 per 100 000 inhabitants, even in regions of Italy where KSHV seroprevalence rates are in the range 20–30% (Calabrò *et al.*, 1998; Whitby *et al.*, 1998)—it is much more common in immunosuppressed individuals. Among transplant recipients, KSHV infection increased the risk of post-transplant KS by a factor of 40–80 in different studies (Parravicini *et al.*, 1997; Farge *et al.*, 1999; Cattani *et al.*, 2000). Among HIV-infected homosexual men, approximately 40–50% of KSHV-infected individuals developed Kaposi's sarcoma within 5–10 years of primary infection with KSHV before the introduction of highly active retroviral therapy (HAART) (Renwick *et al.*, 1998; Martin *et al.*, 1998; O'Brien *et al.*, 1999; Jacobson *et al.*, 2000). Individuals who are already HIV-infected when they contract KSHV progress more rapidly towards disease than those who acquire HIV after KSHV (Renwick *et al.*, 1998; Jacobson *et al.*, 2000).

In The Gambia, West Africa, AIDS KS is markedly more common among HIV-1-infected than among HIV-2-infected individuals, although the KSHV prevalence appears to be comparable in these two groups (Ariyoshi *et al.*, 1998). Since KS in HIV-2 infected individuals is comparatively rare (Ariyoshi *et al.*, 1998), the co-factor role of HIV-1 may not be limited to immune suppression. An angiogenic role for the

HIV-1 Tat protein or inflammatory cytokines released during HIV infection has been suggested, and an induction of KSHV replication by HIV-1 Tat protein claimed (detailed references in Biberfeld *et al.*, 1998). However, it remains difficult to evaluate the importance of these possible pathogenic mechanisms at the epidemiological level.

In Africa, endemic KS (i.e. the clinically severe form of KS in HIV-negative individuals) is mainly found in East and Central Africa, in spite of a high KSHV prevalence in most of sub-Saharan Africa (Dedicoat and Newton, 2003). This observation strongly suggests the existence of other environmental co-factors that promote the development of KS in KSHV-infected individuals.

Pathology and Molecular Biology Findings

KSHV is present in the neoplastic component of KS lesions, the endothelial cell-derived spindle cell (Boshoff *et al.*, 1995; Rainbow *et al.*, 1997; further references in Schulz, 2001). Latent viral genes (orf K12/kaposin; orfK13/vFLIP; orf72/v-cyclin; orf73/LANA) are expressed in these cells (Rainbow *et al.*, 1997; Parravicini *et al.*, 2000; Katano *et al.*, 2000b; Staskus *et al.*, 1997; see Figure 2F.5; further references in Schulz, 2001). KS biopsies contain mainly circular episomal viral DNA, which is consistent with the latent infection (Judde *et al.*, 2000). However, some spindle cells in KS lesions can undergo lytic replication of KSHV (Staskus *et al.*, 1997; Katano *et al.*, 2000b) and, unlike many other oncogenic viruses, KSHV is therefore not strictly latent in neoplastic cells. Given the functional properties of some KSHV lytic cycle genes, e.g. induction of vascular endothelial growth factor (VEGF), angiogenic properties, etc. (see section on Pathogenesis, below), it is thought that some viral proteins expressed during the lytic cycle could contribute to the development of Kaposi's sarcoma. If this were the case, KSHV would differ from other human DNA tumour viruses which are thought to use viral proteins expressed during latent persistence to induce proliferation and tumourigenesis. Infection of primary endothelial cells with KSHV has been reported to result in an increased lifespan *in vitro* (Flore *et al.*, 1998), or in the adoption of a spindle cell-like phenotype by latently infected cells (Ciufo *et al.*, 2001).

The precise contribution of the viral genes highlighted in Figure 2F.5 to the pathogenesis of KS is not yet resolved. KSHV clearly has the capacity to interfere with the control of cellular proliferation, such as cell cycle control (v-cyc/orf72; LANA-1/orf73),

apoptosis (vFLIP/orf71; vbcl-2/orf16; survivin/orfK7) and intracellular signal transduction (vIL-6/orfK2; vIRF-1/orfK9; VIP/orfK1; vGCR/orf74; TMP/orfK15), and some of its proteins have chemotactic and/or angiogenic properties (vMIPs) or can protect virus-infected cells against attack by cytotoxic T lymphocytes or natural killer cells (MIR1,2/orfK3, orfK5) (see section on Pathogenesis, below, for a detailed discussion). Four viral proteins (vIRF, vGCR, VIP and 'kaposin') have transforming properties *in vitro*. It will be important to investigate the contribution of individual viral genes to the transformation of endothelial cells in the context of the whole viral genome, as has been possible for EBV. Studies of this kind are currently hampered by the lack of a suitable infectious molecular clone of KSHV or an animal model.

Primary Effusion Lymphoma (PEL)

Primary effusion lymphoma (PEL), also called body cavity-based lymphoma (BCBL), is a rare lymphoma in AIDS patients, characterised by its presentation as a malignant effusion in the peritoneal, pleural or pericardial space, most often in the absence of an obvious tumour mass. The lymphoma cells have pleomorphic or anaplastic features combining morphological aspects of large cell immunoblastic and anaplastic large cell lymphomas (references in Schulz, 2001). They are usually monoclonal and of B cell origin, as shown by a rearranged immunoglobulin locus and monotypic immunoglobulin light chain pattern, but express only few of the usual markers of B cell differentiation.

The majority of PEL cases described so far have been from AIDS patients, but there are also several reports of PEL in HIV-uninfected individuals (Cesarman *et al.* 1996; further references in Schulz, 2001). The presence of KSHV is now often considered an essential criterion for the diagnosis of PEL. However, rare cases of KSHV-negative effusion lymphomas of the B cell lineage, with an indeterminate surface marker phenotype and pleomorphic appearance, some of them CD30-positive, have been described (references in Schulz, 2001).

In most PEL cases the lymphoma cells are co-infected with Epstein–Barr virus (EBV) (Cesarman *et al.*, 1995a, 1995b; further detailed references in Schulz, 2001). However, several examples of PEL which contain only KSHV have now been reported and stable cell lines have been derived from some of them. Such 'KSHV-only' cell lines can induce lymphomas with malignant effusions in immunodeficient (SCID, BNX) mice, suggesting that, at least in this experimental model, the presence of EBV is not required for the induction of lymphoma (detailed references in Schulz, 2001).

During latency, EBV and KSHV genomes persist as covalently closed episomal circles of defined length, whereas lytic replication is associated with the presence of linear concatameric genomes of varying lengths. As judged by this criterion, different PEL cases have been shown to harbour either latent or lytically replicating KSHV genomes (Judde et al., 2000). Where latent (i.e. circular episomal) KSHV genomes were found, these can be present as either a single episome, or as multiple episomes with a varying number of terminal repeat units, indicating, respectively, a monoclonal or oligoclonal population (Judde et al., 2000).

Experiments on several PEL cell lines, as well as immunohistochemistry, immunofluorescence and in situ hybridisation studies on pathology specimens, indicate that four viral genes, LANA, v-cyc, v-FLIP and 'kaposin'/K12, may be expressed in a substantial proportion of lymphoma cells (Moore et al., 1996; Rainbow et al., 1997; Parravicini et al., 2000; Katano et al., 2000b; further references in Schulz, 1999, 2001). Where pathology samples have been studied by immunohistochemistry or immunofluorescence (Moore et al., 1996; Parravicini et al., 2000; Katano et al., 2000b), LANA has been found to be expressed in the vast majority, while vIL-6 protein expression is confined to a small proportion (2–5%) of tumour cells (Parravicini et al., 2000; Katano et al., 2000b). Other lytic proteins, e.g. K8 (a homologue of EBV Zta), K8.1 (a viral membrane glycoprotein), K9, K10 and K11 (proteins with sequence homology to interferon regulatory factors), orf59/PF-8 (a processivity factor) and orf65 (a minor capsid protein) have been detected in very few cells (<1%) or not at all (Katano et al., 2000b; Parravicini et al., 2000). This expression pattern is consistent with the notion that KSHV persists in most PEL tumour cells in a latent form, but that a small population of cells can switch into lytic viral replication. That vIL-6 is expressed in more lymphoma cells (2–5% by immunohistochemistry/immunofluorescence; significantly more by in situ hybridisation) than other lytic viral proteins (0–<1%) could be due to the fact that it is among the first 'early' genes to be expressed after induction of the lytic cycle in PEL cell lines in vitro (Sun et al., 1999). Its increased detection in uncultured PEL cells may therefore reflect higher protein levels in cells during the early stages of the lytic cycle. Alternatively, it has been suggested that there may be a particular latency programme for KSHV in PEL cells and that vIL-6 expression can occur independently from the activation of the lytic cascade, perhaps indicating a tissue-specific regulation of viral gene expression (Parravicini et al., 2000; Moore et al., 1996). Another example for preferential expression of a KSHV gene in B cells is the recently described homologue of interferon regulatory factors, vIRF 10.5/LANA-2 (Rivas et al., 2001).

Multicentric Castleman's Disease (MCD)

Castleman's disease is a localised lymphoproliferative condition, often found in the mediastinum or mesenterial or peripheral lymph nodes and characterised histologically by expanded germinal centres with B cell proliferation and vascular proliferation. Two histological types have been recognised: one is characterised by a pronounced plasma cell proliferation and persistence of the nodal architecture ('plasma cell variant'); and the other by abnormal germinal centres and abundant hyalinised vessels ('hyaline vascular variant'). Variants combining the features of these two types also occur.

Involvement of multiple lymph node sites occurs in multicentric Castleman's disease (MCD). MCD in AIDS patients is often associated with Kaposi's sarcoma and usually belongs to the plasma cell variant. KSHV can nearly always be detected by PCR in the lymph nodes or spleen affected by MCD in AIDS patients, but is much less common in MCD outside HIV infection (Soulier et al., 1995).

By immunohistochemistry or in situ hybridisation, KSHV is found in the B cells surrounding the follicular centres of MCD. As assessed by immunohistochemistry, KSHV-infected B cells express LANA, a hallmark of all KSHV-infected cells; 10–50% of follicular mantle cells have been found to express LANA in different studies (Parravicini et al., 1997, 2000; Katano et al., 2000b; further references in Schulz, 2001). About 5–25% of LANA-expressing follicular mantle B cells in MCD tissue also express vIL-6 and vIRF-1/K9 (Parravicini et al., 2000; Katano et al., 2000b; Figure 2F.6). Another viral vIRF homologue, vIRF-3/K10.5/LANA-2, is also expressed in a significant number of KSHV-infected B cells (Rivas et al., 2001), and a third vIRF homologue, encoded by orfK10, in about 5% of all mantle zone cells (Katano et al., 2000b). In addition, a small proportion of mantle zone cells also expresses other viral proteins that are associated with the early stages of lytic viral replication, such as PF-8 (processivity factor-8; encoded by orf59) and the K8 protein, a homologue of EBV BZLF-1, an activator of the lytic replication cycle (Parravicini *et al.*, 2000; Katano *et al.*, 2000b). Compared to PEL and KS tissue, KSHV thus appears to adopt a less restrictive pattern of gene expression in MCD tissue and this suggests that MCD may represent the result of active lytic viral replication in lymphoid tissue.

In keeping with this notion, the intensity of clinical symptoms in MCD patients, such as fever, or laboratory parameters reflecting disease activity, such as C-reactive protein, have been shown to correlate with the KSHV viral load in peripheral blood (Grandadam *et al.*, 1997; Oksenhendler *et al.*, 2000). Fluctuations of KSHV viral load in HIV-infected patients with MCD also mirror fluctuations in the plasma levels of human IL-6 and IL-10 and plasma HIV RNA copy numbers, indicating that active HIV infection can increase the severity of MCD by increasing KSHV viral load (Oksenhendler *et al.*, 2000). It is conceivable that, as postulated, the Tat protein of HIV-1 may be involved in this process, perhaps by inducing the expression of human IL-6 and IL-10 in lymphoid cells (detailed references in Oksenhendler *et al.*, 2000).

MCD can be a manifestation of a primary infection with KSHV in an HIV-infected individual (Oksenhendler *et al.*, 1998) or in transplant recipients (Parravicini *et al.*, 1997). This is in keeping with the idea that MCD may reflect active viral lytic replication in lymphoid tissue. It also highlights that co-infection with HIV-1, which can have a marked effect on KSHV replication (Oksenhendler *et al.*, 2000; Goudsmit *et al.*, 2000), may however not be required and that immunosuppression is sufficient to allow lytic replication in lymphoid tissue to an extent that produces clinically visible MCD lesions. Clinically visible MCD is, however, a rare outcome of primary KSHV infection, despite about 10% of HIV-1 infected individuals that seroconvert to KSHV having detectable KSHV viraemia in their peripheral blood (Goudsmit *et al.*, 2000).

Given the functional properties of vIL-6 (see below), it is likely that this viral protein plays a role in the pathogenesis of MCD. The plasmacytic phenotype of B cells in KSHV-associated cases of MCD may be the result of the activity of vIL-6 in this condition. Some authors prefer the term 'plasmablast' for these cells, to describe their large size and large vesicular nucleus with one or two prominent nucleoli (Dupin *et al.*, 2000). Interestingly, these KSHV-infected plasma cells always express IgM with λ-immunoglobulin light chains in all cases examined so far, indicating light chain restriction and the presence of a monotypic cell population (Dupin *et al.*, 2000). In some cases, these KSHV-infected plasmablasts are found in small clusters surrounding or replacing follicles, suggesting the emergence of microscopic plasmablastic lymphomas in MCD lesions (Dupin *et al.*, 2000).

Other Disease Associations

KSHV has been detected in occasional cases of HIV-negative angioimmunoblastic lymphadenopathy and germinal centre hyperplasia (detailed references in Schulz, 2001). Histologically, there may be prominent plasma cell proliferation and angiogenic changes in these cases, suggesting that viral proteins like vIL-6 and vMIP-I/II may have induced these transient changes.

In addition, a small number of case reports indicate that primary infection with KSHV, or KSHV reactivation, in transplant recipients may be associated with a transient thrombocytopenia, leukopenia and/or anaemia (Luppi *et al.*, 2000b; further references in Schulz, 2001).

PATHOGENESIS

This section focuses on the biochemical and cell biology features of individual KSHV genes. Understanding their contribution to pathogenesis is currently still hampered by the lack of an animal model. However, a broad understanding of the functional roles of individual KSHV proteins has been developed. Below, these are discussed in groups defined by their main functions, and these groups are illustrated in Figures 2F.5, 2F.7 and 2F.8.

The KSHV Genome

As explained above, KSHV is a gamma-2 herpesvirus (rhadinovirus), closely related to *Herpesvirus saimiri* (HVS) and *Rhesus rhadinovirus* (RRV). KSHV contains a long unique region (LUR) of 140.5 kb, with a GC content of 53.5%, flanked by 801 bp terminal tandem repeats (TR) rich in GC (84.5%) (Neipel *et al.*, 1997; Russo *et al.*, 1996) (Figure 2F.5). Within the LUR there are at least 90 putative open reading frames (ORFs). These ORFs are named and numbered following the nomenclature initially adopted for HVS. Genes lacking homology with other herpesviruses are designated by the letter K followed by a number.

Careful examination of the KHSV genome allows the identification of many genes with homology to cellular genes that are implicated in signalling transduction, cell cycle control and apoptosis. The same feature has also been found in all other known rhadinoviruses. It is believed that these genes were acquired by the virus from host cells in the distant past of herpesviral evolution, a process sometimes referred to as 'viral piracy'.

Cell Entry

Several groups have succeeded in infecting primary vascular endothelial cells, immortalised endothelial cells or keratinocytes. However, cell-free infection *in vitro* is inefficient and only low titres are achieved with virus produced from PEL cell lines (Cerimele *et al.*, 2001; Flore *et al.*, 1998; Lagunoff *et al.*, 2002; Moses *et al.*, 1999; Renne *et al.*, 1998). These virus stocks appear to have a particle:infectivity ratio in excess of 10^4, and there is some evidence that a significant proportion of virions in these stocks are defective (Nealon *et al.*, 2001).

Four structural glycoproteins, gB, gD, gH and the orfK8.1-encoded glycoprotein, have been documented in KSHV virions. These glycoproteins are candidates for promoting initial contact with KSHV receptor(s) and to initiate cell entry, since similar glycoproteins play such roles in other herpesviruses. Expression of gB, gH and gL on the surface of hamster cells and co-cultivation with human embryonic kidney cells or B lymphocytes resulted in cell-to-cell fusion (Pertel *et al.*, 2002), implying a role for these glycoproteins in fusion between the viral and cellular membranes.

KSHV has a wide tropism *in vitro* (Vieira *et al.*, 2001; Renne *et al.*, 1998; Cerimele *et al.*, 2001; Flore *et al.*, 1998; Lagunoff *et al.*, 2002; Moses *et al.*, 1999). This is probably due to the ability of KSHV to interact with ubiquitous host cell surface heparan sulphate and $\alpha3\beta1$ integrin molecules through gB (orf 8) and gpK8.1 (Akula *et al.*, 2002; Birkmann *et al.*, 2001) (see Figure 2F.7). The gB glycoprotein contains a RGD motif, known to be important for interaction with cell surface integrins. KSHV and its counterpart in macaques, RFHV (see section on Origin and Evolution, above, and Figure 2F.3), are the only herpesviruses known to date to have a gB protein containing a RGD motif. This may therefore be a feature of the RV-1 branch of primate rhadinoviruses (see section on Origin and Evolution, above). It has been shown that this motif plays a central role in KSHV entry at a post-adhesion step, suggesting the presence of more than one receptor for KSHV entry (Akula *et al.*, 2002). KSHV entry is inhibited by RGD peptides, by soluble $\alpha3\beta1$ integrin and by antibodies against $\alpha3$ and $\beta1$ (Akula *et al.*, 2002). All these observations point to $\alpha3\beta1$ integrin as one of the receptors for KSHV. Entry experiments using the human B cell line BJAB indicate that KSHV is endocytosed. KSHV infection induced the integrin-mediated activation of focal adhesion kinase (FAK), implicating a role for integrin and the associated signalling pathways in the entry of the virus, which result in morphological changes and cytoskeletal rearrangements (Naranatt *et al.*, 2003). Induction of intracellular signalling is due to binding and/or entry of virions, does not require cellular or viral gene expression, and seems to involve gB-mediated induction of FAK phosphorylation (Akula *et al.*, 2002; Naranatt *et al.*, 2003). Also, a role for phosphatidylinositol (PI) 3-kinase in early stages of the entry process and for PKC-ζ, MEK and ERK at later stages has been proposed (Naranatt *et al.*, 2003). It has been suggested that the interaction of KSHV with cell surfaces molecules, such as integrins, might generate a cellular state more prone to infection.

Latent Replication

KSHV persists in a latent form in the majority of the infected cells. During latency, the KSHV genome replicates and persists as extrachromosomal episomal DNA circles in the absence of virion production. Persistence is very efficient in rapidly dividing B cell lines obtained from PEL patients (PEL cell lines). Cell cultures established from KS tumours rapidly lose the KSHV genome after a few passages (Lebbe *et al.*, 1997). The reasons for this lack of long-term persistence of the episome in epithelial cells *in vitro* is currently unknown.

Latency is characterised by the presence of episomal viral DNA (Judde *et al.*, 2000; see section on Role of KSHV in Neoplastic Disease, above) and a restricted pattern of viral gene expression (see Figure 2F.5). Only five viral genes are currently known to be expressed during latency: the latency-associated nuclear antigen 1 (LANA-1/orf73); the viral homologue of a D-type cyclin (v-cyc/orf72); a homologue of the cellular inhibitor of the FLICE apoptosis complex (v-FLIP/orfK13); and a group of short membrane-associated proteins 'kaposin' A,B,C (orfK12) (see Figure 2F.5 and section on Role of KSHV in Neoplastic Disease, above; Jenner *et al.*, 2001). A considerable proportion of persistently infected B cells and B lymphoma cells in PEL and MCD, but not in KS endothelial cells, express K10.5/LANA-2, one of KSHV vIRF homologues (see above; Rivas et al., 2001). Among these five proteins, only LANA-1 has been detected in virtually all KSHV-infected cells by IF or IHC (Rainbow et al., 1997; Katano et al., 2000b).

LANA-1 is required for the persistence of the KSHV episomal genome (Ballestas et al., 1999; Garber et al., 2002; reviewed in Viejo-Borbolla et al., 2003a). LANA-1 binds to heterochromatin through its aminoterminal region and to the TR of KSHV genome through its C-terminal region (Piolot et al., 2001; Garber et al., 2002; Viejo-Borbolla et al., 2003b) (Figure 2F.5). The region responsible for binding to heterochromatin has been narrowed down to amino acids 5–22 (Piolot et al., 2001; Viejo-Borbolla et al., 2003b), but binding to heterochromatin seems to be modulated by a C-terminal domain of 15 amino acids (Viejo-Borbolla et al., 2003b). LANA-1 binds to two small motifs of 16 nucleotides within the KSHV terminal repeat (TR) subunit, termed LANA-binding sites 1 and 2 (LBS-1 and -2) (Garber et al., 2002). In this way, LANA-1 tethers viral episomes to host chromatin and thus ensures the distribution of KSHV genomes to daughter cells upon mitosis, in a manner similar to the EBNA-1 protein of Epstein–Barr virus (EBV) or the ORF73 protein of HVS (Collins and Medveczky, 2002). LANA-1 also mediates the replication of TR-containing plasmid DNA in transfected cells, thus illustrating its role in the replication of latent episomes (Garber et al., 2002; further references in Viejo-Borbolla et al., 2003a).

The functions of LANA-1 go beyond those of ensuring the replication, persistence and segregation to daughter cells of the KSHV genome. It has also been shown to bind to p53 and retinoblastoma protein (pRb) (Figure 2F.7) and, in this way, to inhibit the activation of p53-dependent promoters and to induce the activation of E2F-dependent genes (Friborg et al., 1999; Radkov et al., 2000). Moreover, LANA-1 can transform cells in co-transfection assays with a constitutively active Ha-ras (Radkov et al., 2000). LANA-1 has also been reported to act as a transcriptional activator and/or repressor and to associate with the mSin3 repressor complex through the N-terminal region (detailed references in Viejo-Borbolla et al., 2003a, 2003b). In addition, LANA-1 binds through the C-terminal region to several members of the female sterile homeotic (fsh) family of BET proteins, such as RING3, a cellular homeotic gene product and component of the 'mediator complex' which is involved in transcriptional regulation (Platt et al., 1999; Figure 2F.7). Recently, a role for LANA-1 in

promoting entry into S-phase has been described as a result of its interaction with GSK-3β, a kinase involved in phosphorylation and consequent degradation of β-catenin by the proteasome (Fujimuro et al., 2003). Association of GSK-3β with LANA-1 leads to its transfer to the nucleus, the stabilisation of β-catenin and increased β-catenin levels in infected cells, which allows activation of promoters containing Lef/Tcf-binding sites and entry into S-phase (Fujimuro et al., 2003).

Activation of the Viral Lytic Replication Cycle

Despite KSHV remaining latent in most of the infected cells (see section on Role of KSHV in Neoplastic Disease, above), a small population of virus-infected cells undergoes lytic (productive) viral replication, which allows the production and release of viral particles. This process, required for virus spread, normally results in cell death. It is thought that some lytic genes are involved in disease progression. This hypothesis is supported by two clinical observations: drugs that inhibit lytic KSHV replication prevent the development of clinical KS (see below); and an increase in KSHV replication is associated with the appearance of MCD lesions in immunocompromised patients (see above). Moreover, several observations (Bais et al., 1998; Montaner et al., 2003; Flore et al., 1998; further detailed references in Schulz, 2001, and Viejo-Borbolla et al., 2003a) indicate that lytic genes with autocrine and paracrine effects might play an important role in KSHV-related malignancies.

The switch between latent and lytic cycle is mediated by transcriptional activators of early and late lytic genes. In EBV two such proteins, E-RTA and ZTA, act synergistically to mediate activation of the EBV lytic cycle. A different scenario is observed in KSHV, where the product of orf50, RTA, is the key element in the activation cascade (Figure 2F.7). Ectopic expression of RTA in PEL cells triggers the lytic cycle, leading to the production of infectious virus (Sun et al., 1998; further references in Viejo-Borbolla, 2003a). RTA acts through binding to specific DNA sequences (Chang et al., 2002), and by interacting with cellular transcription factors (Gwack et al., 2002; Liang et al., 2002; Wang et al. 2003). RTA can also activate its own promoter (Deng et al., 2000) and cellular genes (Liang et al., 2002). The suppression of p53-mediated apoptosis and the interaction with signal transducer activator of transcription 3 (STAT3) leading to transcription of STAT-responsive genes suggest the implication of RTA in promoting cell proliferation

(Gwack et al., 2002). The product of KSHV orfK8 is K-bZIP, a homologue of EBV's ZTA (Gruffat et al., 1999). K-bZIP represses or enhances RTA-mediated gene activation (Izumiya et al., 2003; Wang et al. 2003). K-bZIP also binds to p53, and thereby represses p53-mediated apoptosis, presumably in order to create a favourable environment for viral replication (Park et al., 2000; Wu et al., 2002). K-bZIP can promote both CCAAT/enhancer binding protein alpha (C/EBPα) and p21^{CIP-1} expression and, through interaction with C/EBPα, is able to promote p21^{CIP-1}-mediated inhibition of entry into S phase (Wu et al., 2002). This probably creates a suitable environment for lytic viral replication by preventing competition with host-cell DNA synthesis for limited resources. C/EBPα, RTA and K-bZIP form a complex that associates with and activates the K-bZIP promoter (Wang et al., 2003). Therefore, both C/EBPα and K-bZIP can activate each other.

Regulation of the Cell Cycle

The product of orf72, v-cyc, has the functional properties of a D-type cyclin, i.e. it mediates phosphorylation, and thereby inactivation, of pRb through association with CDK6 (Chang et al., 1996; Swanton et al., 1997; Ellis et al., 1999; see Figure 2F.7). Other DNA tumour viruses, such as polyomaviruses, papillomaviruses and adenoviruses, also target the pRb pathway (for a review, see Helt and Galloway, 2003). Interestingly, PEL cell lines are defective for p16INK4a expression, a protein that promotes arrest in G$_1$ phase only upon the presence of pRb (Platt et al., 2002). Ectopic expression of p16INK4a induces a pRb-dependent G$_1$ cell cycle block in PEL cells, suggesting that pRb is functional in these KSHV-infected cells despite the presence of two proteins that target the pRb pathway, the v-cyc and LANA-1 (Platt et al., 2002).

V-cyc might play a role in KSHV oncogenicity, since it can promote the progression of resting cells into the S phase of the cell cycle (Swanton et al., 1997; Ellis et al., 1999; Lundquist et al., 2003). One mechanism of action of v-cyc seems to be the inactivation of STAT3, preventing growth-suppressive effects (Lundquist et al., 2003). Another mechanism might be the activation of the cyclin A promoter, a regulator of entry into S phase (Duro et al., 1999). Despite the homology with cellular D- and E-cyclins, KSHV v-cyc has some unique features. Thus, the CDK6/v-cyc complex required for phosphorylation of pRb is resistant to the cellular CDK inhibitors p16, p21 and p27 and to p16INK4a,

conferring resistance to the antiproliferative action of these inhibitors (Swanton et al., 1997; Platt et al., 2002). The CDK6/v-cyc complex can also phosphorylate and thereby inactivate Bcl-2, which leads to the activation of apoptotic pathways (Ojala et al., 2000). The action of vBcl-2 may counteract this (see section on Inhibition of Apoptosis, below).

The viral and cellular cyclins also differ in their ability to phosphorylate certain proteins. KSHV v-cyc does not induce phosphorylation of p107 (a pRb-related protein) and cannot thereby induce dissociation of p107 from E2F (Duro et al., 1999), but it is able to phosphorylate histone H1 and the cdk inhibitor p27^{kip} (Ellis et al., 1999). The cellular cyclin does not target these two proteins. These differences with respect to cellular D-type cyclins might explain why v-cyc avoids the CDK-inhibitor regulated checkpoints.

As mentioned above, LANA-1 is also able to promote the entry into S phase of transfected cells (Fujimoro et al., 2003).

Angiogenesis and B Cell Proliferation: vIL-6, vMIP-I-III, vGCR

KSHV-associated disorders express high levels of vascular endothelial growth factor (VEGF) and its receptor, kinase insert domain-containing receptor (KDR), which induces angiogenesis (for a review, see Hayward, 2003). In KS lesions, VEGF and other angiogenic factors stimulate the inflammatory and neovascular responses determining spindle cell proliferation, the predominant cell type within these lesions (Bais et al., 1998; detailed references in Hayward, 2003).

vIL-6

There is considerable evidence for a role of vIL-6 in the proliferation of infected B cells (reviewed in Schulz et al., 2001). Like its cellular counterpart, hIL-6, known to be important in B cell proliferation, vIL-6 is able to support the growth of IL-6-dependent B cells in vitro (Moore et al., 1996). However, there are differences between the two cytokines. Human IL-6 needs both subunits of the cell surface IL-6 receptor, IL-6Rα and gp130, to fulfil its stimulatory role, whereas vIL-6 only requires the latter (Molden et al., 1997; see Figure 2F.7). IL-6Rα and gp130 differ in expression patterns, with gp130 being more widely expressed. This may allow vIL-6 to stimulate a broader spectrum of cells.

In line with these predictions, vIL-6 has been shown to induce neurite outgrowth in the rat phaeochromocytoma cell line PC12 and to promote colony formation of human CD34$^+$ bone marrow progenitor cells. *In vivo*, vIL-6-transfected fibroblasts inoculated into nude mice induced hepatosplenomegaly, lymphadenopathy and polyclonal hypergammaglobulinaemia, accompanied by increased haematopoiesis of the myeloid, erythroid and megakaryocytic lineages and plasmacytosis in spleen and lymph nodes. Tumours developing in these animals were more extensively vascularised than those in control animals and expressed high levels of VEGF, which correlated with the amount of vIL-6 in these tumours. VEGF is also expressed in PEL-derived cell lines, and a neutralising antibody to VEGF blocked the formation of effusion lymphoma and bloody ascites in mice inoculated with PEL cell lines. VEGF can also be detected in the malignant effusions of PEL patients. VEGF-induced stimulation of vascular permeability may therefore be critical to the formation of the malignant ascites characteristic for this AIDS lymphoma. Finally, vIL-6 can also activate STAT3, Janus tyrosine kinase (JAK1) and the mitogen-activated protein kinase (MAPK) pathway (Molden *et al.*, 1997; detailed references for the effects of vIL-6 can be found in Schulz, 2001).

vGCR

Orf74 of KSHV has early lytic kinetics and encodes a G protein-coupled receptor (vGCR). KSHV and HVS vGCRs are homologues of the human IL-8 receptor. In contrast to its human homologue, KSHV vGCR shows ligand-independent, constitutive activity due to the presence of a point mutation in a sequence motif (DRY) that is highly conserved among GCRs (Arvanitakis *et al.*, 1997; Burger *et al.*, 1999). vGCR transfoms murine cells and induces VEGF-dependent angiogenesis, and KS-like lesions in transgenic mice, animals inoculated with transfected cells or transgenic animals following endothelial cell-specific infection by a retroviral vector expressing vGCR (Bais *et al.*, 1998; Montaner *et al.*, 2003; Yang *et al.*, 2000). Survival of vGCR-immortalised human umbilical endothelial cells (HUVEC) was dependent on autocrine signalling through KDR, a protein present in KS lesions, leading to the activation of the phosphatidyl-inositol 3′-kinase Akt/PI3K pathway and consequent NF-κB transcription factors (Montaner *et al.*, 2001; Bais *et al.*, 2003). The transcription of angiogenesis regulating genes, cytokines and pro-inflammatory genes was also found to be modulated upon vGCR expression (Polson *et al.*, 2002). vGCR activates the MAP kinases p38 and ERK-2, augments transcription of several KSHV lytic

genes (e.g. *orf*57) and increases production of vIL-6 and VEGF (Cannon *et al.*, 2003). Interestingly, despite its tumourigenic and angiogenic functions, vGCR is only expressed in approximately 10% of the KS cells (Chiou *et al.*, 2002). Similarly, infection of transgenic mice with a retroviral vector allowing endothelial cell-specific expression of vGCR resulted in the development of KS-like lesions, but expression of vGCR was confined to a small proportion of tumour cells. Expression of vGCR appeared to lead to the recruitment of other endothelial cells, suggesting that vGCR acts through paracrine mechanisms, probably by secreting angiogenic factors (Montaner *et al.*, 2003). The role of vGCR on disease progression in haematopoietic cells was analysed by using PEL cell lines expressing vGCR under the control of an inducible promoter (Cannon *et al.*, 2003). All these observations point to vGCR as a major player in the angiogenesis and thereby pathogenesis of KSHV.

vMIPs

Three chemokine homologues, vMIP-I-III, encoded by KSHV orfK6, orf4 and orf4.1, respectively, have been proposed to be important in promoting leukocyte chemotaxis, eosinophil migration and angiogenesis. They are members of the macrophage inflammatory protein (MIP) family, hence their name. Among them, vMIP-I has been reported to induce the expression of VEGF in PEL cell lines, in a similar way to vIL-6 (see above) (Liu *et al.*, 2001). Other viruses, such as mouse and human cytomegaloviruses, also encode functional chemokines (Alcami, 2003; Penfold, 1999). The vMIPs are also required for evading the immune response and inhibiting apoptosis (see below).

Inhibition of Apoptosis

Programmed cellular death, or apoptosis, is a complex process involving several cellular proteins (see Figure 2F.8). Viral infection triggers pathways resulting in apoptosis. To overcome this, viruses have developed mechanisms interfering with apoptotic pathways. This would allow them to increase the survival rate of virus-infected cells, thus increasing the time available for viral replication and spread within the host and to other individuals. Since inhibition of apoptotic pathways is one of the hallmarks of tumour cells, it is possible that viral proteins that interfere with apoptosis could also contribute to virus-mediated transformation. Figure 2F.8 summarises some of the ways by which KSHV inhibits programmed cellular death. Two different apoptotic pathways in mammalian cells result in the activation of effector caspases (Teodoro and Branton, 1997; see Figure 2F.8). The extrinsic pathway requires the activation of procaspases 8 and 10 by so-called 'death receptors', which belong to the TNF receptor gene superfamily, whereas in the intrinsic pathway mitochondria release caspase-activating proteins.

vFLIP

vFLIP [viral FLICE (Fas-associated death-domain-like IL-1β-converting enzyme)-inhibitory proteins], encoded by orfK13 is expressed on the same bicistronic transcript as v-cyc (Rainbow et al., 1997). It can block Fas-induced apoptosis and has been postulated to act as a tumour progression factor by interfering with apoptotic signals induced by virus-specific T killer cells (Djerbi et al., 1999; Thome et al., 1997; see Figure 2F.8). It has also been proposed to contribute to the continuous NF-κB activation observed in PEL cells (Liu et al., 2002).

K7/Survivin

K7 is the only currently known herpesviral inhibitor-of-apoptosis protein (IAP) homologue. Expressed during the lytic cycle in PEL cells, as shown by Northern blot using a K7-specific probe (Wang et al., 2002), K7 is a glycoprotein structurally related to survivin, as revealed by computational analysis (Wang et al., 2002). Human survivin, a member of the IAP family, protects cells from apoptosis by an unknown mechanism. K7 anchors to cellular membranes in the vicinity of Bcl-2 and binds to Bcl-2 (but not Bax), as shown by GST-pulldown assays, via its putative BH2 domain, and to caspase-3 via its BIR domain (Wang et al., 2002; see Figure 2F.8). Thus, K7 seems to be an adaptor molecule bringing together Bcl-2 and effector caspases, allowing the inhibition of the latter by Bcl-2 (Wang et al., 2002).

vBcl-2

Like all other gammaherpesviruses for which genomic sequences are available, KSHV expresses a viral homologue of human Bcl-2 (Cheng et al., 1997). The vBcl-2 mRNA is detected in PEL cell lines (Sarid et al., 1997) and protein expression could be shown for late stages of KS lesions (Widmer et al., 2002). vBcl-2 forms heterodimers with hBcl-2 (Sarid et al., 1997) and

it is believed that it may inhibit apoptosis in KSHV-infected cells (Cheng et al., 1997; Sarid et al., 1997). The mechanisms of action of vBcl-2 differ from those of the human Bcl-2 (Cheng et al., 1997). While human Bcl-2 forms heterodimers with members of the Bcl-2 family with pro-apoptotic roles (such as Bax and Bak), the viral homologue does not seem to do so (Cheng et al., 1997). Moreover, sequence comparison between the two proteins indicates a more restrictive regulation for human Bcl-2 than for vBcl-2 (Cheng et al., 1997). Finally, as mentioned above (see section on Regulation of the Cell Cycle), the CDK6–v-cyc complex phosphorylates and inactivates human Bcl-2, which results in apoptosis. However, vBcl-2 is not phosphorylated by the CDK6–v-cyc complex, allowing KSHV to overcome the v-cyc-induced apoptosis (Ojala et al., 2000). These differences seem to be due to variations in the protein structure between the two proteins (Huang et al., 2002). Thus, vBcl-2 lacks a non-structured loop where phosphorylation by the CDK6–v-cyc complex takes place (Huang et al., 2002).

vIRF-1, vIRF-2

Interferon regulatory factors (IRFs) are a family of interferon-responsive transcription factors that regulate expression of genes involved in pathogen response, cell proliferation and immune modulation through binding to interferon-stimulated response elements (ISREs) in the promoters of interferon-responsive genes. Among the members of the IRF family, IRF-3 and IRF-7 seem to be the key regulators for the induction of type I IFNs, the primary response against viral infection (for a review, see Stark et al., 1998). KSHV encodes four IRF homologues, named vIRFs (Moore et al., 1996; Russo et al., 1996). vIRF-1, encoded by orfK9, is a multifunctional protein that inhibits IFN signalling (Gao et al., 1997; Li et al., 2000; Moore et al., 1996). Expression of vIRF-1 inhibits IFN-signal transduction in reporter assays, downregulates expression of the cell cycle inhibitor p21[WAF-1CIP-1] and transforms NIH 3T3 cells (Gao et al., 1997). By Northern blot, vIRF-1 is weakly expressed in KSHV-infected B cells, while it is absent from spindle KS cells (Gao et al., 1997).

The ORF K11 encodes vIRF-2 (Burysek et al., 1999), another protein that also inhibits IFN-mediated cell death (Kirchhoff, 2002). The expression of CD95L, an apoptosis-inducing ligand of CD95/Apo-1/Fas, is upregulated by IFN-γ-activated IRF-1 (Kirchhoff et al., 2002). Both vIRF-1 and vIRF-2 inhibit IRF-1-induced expression of CD95L (Kirchhoff et al., 2002). The mechanism of action of vIRF-1 seems to involve the inhibition of IRF-1 binding to the CD95L promoter, whereas vIRF-2 might repress the induction of CD95L by interfering with NF-κB (Kirchhoff *et al.*, 2002).

It is conceivable that, by blocking interferon-induced signal transduction and/or apoptosis, vIRF-1 and vIRF-2 allow KSHV-infected cells to escape the effect of virus-specific T cells (see section on Escape from the Immune System, below).

LANA-2/orfK10.5

orfK10.5 is a latent gene whose product is another KSHV IRF homologue (vIRF-3) (Rivas *et al.*, 2001), which inhibits the activation of p53-dependent promoters and thereby restrains p53-mediated apoptosis (Rivas *et al.*, 2001). As it is a nuclear protein expressed in B cells during latency, it has also been referred to as LANA-2 (Rivas *et al.*, 2001).

vMIPs

A role for vMIP-I and -II (see above) in the inhibition of apoptosis has also been suggested (Liu *et al.*, 2001).

Induction of NF-κB as Protection Against Apoptosis

Several KSHV proteins (see above) can induce the NF-κB pathway which is known to have an anti-apoptotic effect. Inhibition of NF-κB in PEL cell lines promotes apoptosis (Keller *et al.*, 2000), thus highlighting the possibility that some of the NF-κB inducing KSHV proteins may also contribute to the protection against apoptosis.

KSHV Proteins with Transforming and Intracellular Signalling Activity

Kaposin

A group of transcripts originating in the K12/kaposin locus has been reported to encode several proteins (Sadler *et al.*, 1999). Among these, kaposin A, a type II transmembrane protein, is able to transform rodent fibroblasts to tumourigenicity (Kliche *et al.*, 2001; Muralidhar *et al.*, 1998). Recent data have shown that kaposin A induces lymphocyte aggregation and adhesion, probably through direct interaction with cytohesin-1 (Kliche *et al.*, 2001), a guanine nucleotide exchange factor for ARF GTPases and regulator of integrin-mediated cell adhesion (Figure 2F.7). The functions of kaposin B and C have not yet been established.

ORFs K1, K9 and 74

The products of three early and late genes, orfK1, orfK9 and orf74, (VIP, vIRF-1 and vGCR, respectively) have been shown to have transforming properties and to induce intracellular signalling pathways. VIP and vGCR cause tumours in transgenic mice, and activate several intracellular signal transduction pathways, including stress- and mitogen-induced kinases (Lee *et al.*, 1998a, 1998b; Lagunoff *et al.*, 1999, 2001; for references for vGCR, see above). VIP transforms rodent fibroblasts and is able to immortalise T lymphocytes when replacing the saimiri transforming protein (STP) in the HVS genome (Lee *et al.*, 1998a).

In spite of all these reports, no expression of K1/VIP or K9/vIRF-1 has so far been documented in the majority of tumour cells of KS, MCD or PEL. Although low-level expression cannot be excluded, the relevance of their *in vitro* transforming properties for the oncogenicity of KSHV is therefore not yet clear. The expression of vGCR in PEL and MCD tumours and in KS lesions has been observed by immunohistochemistry (Chiou *et al.*, 2002). Only a small proportion of the tumour cells expressed vGCR (Chiou *et al.*, 2002), in accordance with a proposed role for this membrane signalling protein in paracrine effects (see above; Bais *et al.*, 1998; Montaner *et al.*, 2003). In addition, LANA-1 has been found to transform rodent cells when co-transfected with activated Ha-ras (see above).

K15

A family of alternatively-spliced transcripts is transcribed late in the lytic replication cycle from eight exons located between orf75 and the TR. Proteins (terminal membrane protein; TMP) derived from these transcripts are predicted to contain up to 12 transmembrane domains and a common cytoplasmic domain containing a putative TRAF and Src kinase-binding motifs (Glenn *et al.*, 1999; Poole *et al.*, 1999; Choi *et al.*, 2000; Figure 2F.7). The largest K15-derived protein appears to have some functional similarities to LMP1 and LMP2A of EBV (Glenn *et al.*, 1999). Phosphorylation of the cytoplasmic domain of this protein by src kinases leads to the activation of NF-κB and of two MAPK (mitogen-acitvated kinase) pathways (Brinkmann *et al.*, 2003). The cytoplasmic domain of K15 proteins also interacts with several members of the TNF receptor-associated factors (TRAF) family, but the functional importance of this interaction is not yet understood (Glenn *et al.*, 1999;

Brinkmann *et al.*, 2003; see Figure 2F.7). Intracellular localisation studies have shown that TMP resides in the endoplasmic reticulum (ER) and mitochondria, where it interacts with HS1-associated protein X-1 (HAX-1), an inhibitor of Bax-induced apoptosis (Sharp *et al.*, 2002).

Escape from the Immune System

The interaction between viruses and their hosts during evolution has probably modelled the host immune system and has resulted in the development of viral strategies to evade the immune system. Many viruses encode proteins that target essential pathways of the immune system. KSHV has also acquired several mechanisms to protect infected cells from an attack by the immune system.

K3 and K5

The K3 and K5 proteins, unique to KSHV, are involved in protecting virus-infected cells against NK cells or cytotoxic T lymphocytes (Coscoy and Ganem, 2000). These membrane proteins, also termed modulator of immune recognition (MIR) 1 and 2, respectively, have been shown to downregulate MHC class I molecules (Coscoy and Ganem, 2000). MIR1 targets HLA-A, -B, -C and -E, whereas MIR2 does so primarily with HLA-A and -B. The synthesis or transport of MHC class I molecules (at least until the medial Golgi) is not affected but a higher rate of endocytosis and degradation of MHC class I molecules—possibly by an ubiquitin/proteasome-dependent mechanism—was observed (Means *et al.*, 2002; Lorenzo *et al.*, 2002; Figure 2F.7). Both MIR1 and -2 contain an amino terminal zinc finger belonging to the plant homeodomain (PHD) subfamily, involved in protein–protein interactions. This domain and the carboxy-terminal region are responsible for MIR-mediated endocytosis, whereas the transmembrane region is required for target specificity (Sanchez *et al.*, 2002).

Reports studying the expression of these proteins have shown that both MIR1 and MIR2 are expressed as early and late lytic genes following reactivation in PEL cell lines, whereas K3 transcripts were not detected in KS lesions (Sun *et al.*, 1999; Rimessi *et al.*, 2001; Jenner *et al.*, 2001).

Regulation of the Immune System by vIRFs

As explained above (see section on Inhibition of Apoptosis), the initial immune response against viral

infection is regulated by interferon regulatory factors (IRFs) through binding to interferon-stimulated response elements (ISREs) in the promoters of interferon-responsive genes. The mechanism by which vIRFs inhibit IFN-signal transduction seems to involve direct binding to IRFs p300/CREB binding protein (CBP) and other transcription factors impeding the formation of the transcriptional active complexes (Burysek *et al.*, 1999; Li *et al.*, 2000; Lin *et al.*, 2001; Seo *et al.*, 2000).

vIRF-1 is able to bind to the transcriptional co-activator CBP and inhibit its transcriptional activity (Seo *et al.*, 2000). It also interacts with the histone acetyl transferase p300 impeding its activity and modifying chromatin structure and blocking IRF3 recruitment of p300/CBP (Li *et al.*, 2000; Lin *et al.*, 2001) (see section on Inhibition of Apoptosis, above). As a consequence, cellular cytokine expression is affected, and this could be a mechanism to evade certain aspects of the immune response (Li *et al.*, 2000).

In a similar way to vIRF-1, vIRF-2 can also bind to IRFs and CBP/p300 and thereby inhibit virus-mediated induction of IFN type 1 gene transcription (Burysek *et al.*, 1999). Another mechanism of action of vIRF-2 involves the interaction with the IFN-induced, double-stranded RNA-activated serine-threonine kinase (PKR) (Burysek and Pitha, 2001), a main component of the host antiviral defence (for a review on PKR, see Levy and Garcia-Sastre, 2001). Such interaction blocks autophosphorylation of PKR and subsequent phosphorylation of PKR targets (Burysek and Pitha, 2001). Orf45 blocks phosphorylation and nuclear accumulation of IRF-7, and thereby virus-mediated induction of type I IFN-activated genes (Zhu *et al.*, 2002).

The Role of vMIPs in Blunting the Immune Response

The three viral β chemokines, viral macrophage inflammatory proteins (vMIP) I-III (see section on Angiogenesis and B Cell Proliferation, above) may also play a role in modulating the immune response. Other herpesviruses and poxviruses encode homologues of chemokines (see Alcami, 2003, and references cited therein). Little is known regarding the role of vMIP-III. vMIP-II binds to several chemokine receptors, either as an agonist or as an antagonist (Kledal *et al.*, 1997; Boshoff *et al.*, 1997), whereas vMIP-I is more selective, binding exclusively to and acting as an agonist of CCR8 (Dairaghi *et al.*, 1999; Endres *et al.*, 1999). The leukocyte infiltrate within KS lesions is composed mainly of mononuclear phagocytes and T cells, with the $CD4^+$ and $CD8^+$ cells having a marked type II cytokine profile (Sozzani *et al.*, 1998). This is probably due to the fact that both vMIP-I and -II act as chemoattractants for monocytes and Th2 cells and not Th1, NK or dendritic cells (Dairaghi *et al.*, 1999; Sozzani *et al.*, 1998; Weber *et al.*, 2001). This may allow the virus to skew the immune response from a type I, antiviral, response pattern towards a type II pattern (Weber *et al.*, 2001).

Orf4

The product of orf4, named KCP for KSHV complement control protein, has kinetics characteristic of a lytic protein which specifically increases the decay of classical C3-convertase (Spiller *et al.*, 2003; Jenner *et al.*, 2001). It is conceivable that KCP could enhance virus pathogenesis through evading complement attack, opsonisation and anaphylaxis (Spiller *et al.*, 2003).

ANTIVIRAL THERAPY

The introduction of highly active antiretroviral therapy (HAART) since 1996 has markedly reduced the incidence of AIDS KS in Western countries (Blum *et al.*, 1997; Conant *et al.*, 1997). This may be the consequence of an enhanced KSHV-specific immune response following HAART, but a direct effect of HIV proteinase inhibitors on KS has also been postulated (Sgadari *et al.*, 2002). Nevertheless, virus-specific therapy of KSHV-associated diseases still remains a problem, since antiherpesviral drugs known so far are only effective in combating lytic but not latent infection, which is common in KSHV infection. These drugs mainly act as inhibitors of viral replication by blocking the viral DNA polymerase. Latent episomal DNA is replicated by host DNA polymerases, implying that the latent stage of infection is not affected by these drugs (Medveczky *et al.*, 1997). *In vitro* assays have established that the replicative cycle of KSHV in PEL cell lines can be inhibited with cidofovir, ganciclovir and foscarnet, but not with aciclovir (Kedes and Ganem, 1997; Medveczky *et al.*, 1997). However, clinical studies with these classical antiviral drugs have produced controversial results. The use of intravenous ganciclovir or foscarnet therapy to treat cytomegalovirus disease did not affect the KSHV DNA load in PBMCs of seven patients analysed (Boivin *et al.*, 1999). Similar results have been

found in a pilot study by Little *et al.* (2003), in which no decrease of viral load of KSHV in PBMCs was observed after intravenous administration of cidofovir. In addition, all seven KS patients in this study showed disease progression. On the other hand, some retrospective studies and anecdotal reports do support the notion that these drugs are active against KSHV *in vivo*. Thus, both foscarnet and ganciclovir, but not aciclovir, had some activity in preventing the occurrence of Kaposi's sarcoma (Mocroft *et al.*, 1996; Glesby *et al.*, 1996). A randomised, placebo-controlled clinical trial originally performed to show the prevention of systemic cytomegalovirus diseases after CMV retinitis demonstrated a 75% risk reduction of KS among high-risk AIDS patients after high dose oral ganciclovir administration (Martin *et al.*, 1999). It therefore appears that ganciclovir and foscarnet can inhibit the replication and dissemination of KSHV prior to the emergence of Kaposi's sarcoma, but that they are of limited benefit in treating established disease.

There are some suggestions that other antiviral agents might be effective against KSHV infection. KSHV encodes a thymidine kinase homologue in orf21. This enzyme was shown to be competitively inhibited by zidovudine and stavudine *in vitro* and can also accept these antiretroviral compounds as substrates (Lock *et al.*, 2002). KSHV is also the first human virus known to encode for a dihydrofolate reductase, DHFR (ORF2). Although this early lytic enzyme has been shown to be nonessential for viral replication in cultured PEL cells and its activity was not detected in PBMCs, DHFR inhibitors, like methotrexate (MTX) or trimethoprim, might represent starting points for the design of new specific anti-KSHV agents (Cinquina *et al.*, 2000). MTX has already been shown to completely prevent TPA-induced viral DNA replication and to strongly decrease viral lytic transcript levels *in vitro* (Curreli *et al.*, 2002). Whether this is suitable for a therapeutic approach has to be further examined.

REFERENCES

Ablashi D, Chatlynne L, Cooper H *et al.* (1999) Seroprevalence of human herpesvirus-8 (HHV-8) in countries of Southeast Asia compared to the USA, the Caribbean and Africa. *Br J Cancer*, **81**, 893–897.

Akula SM, Pramod NP, Wang FZ and Chandran B (2002) Integrin α3β1 (CD 49c/29) is a cellular receptor for Kaposi's sarcoma-associated herpesvirus (KSHV/HHV-8) entry into the target cells. *Cell*, **108**, 407–419.

Alagiozoglou L, Sitas F and Morris L (2000) Phylogenetic analysis of human herpesvirus-8 in South Africa and identification of a novel subgroup. *J Gen Virol*, **81**, 2029–2038.

Alcami A (2003) Viral mimicry of cytokines, chemokines and their receptors. *Nature Rev Immunol*, **3**, 36–50.

Almuneef M, Nimjee S, Khoshnood K *et al.* (2001) Prevalence of antibodies to human herpesvirus 8 (HHV-8) in Saudi Arabian patients with and without renal failure. *Transplantation*, **71**, 1120–1124.

Andreoni M, El-Sawaf G, Rezza G *et al.* (1999) High seroprevalence of antibodies to human herpesvirus-8 in Egyptian children: evidence of nonsexual transmission. *J Natl Cancer Inst*, **91**, 465–469.

Andreoni M, Goletti D, Pezzotti P *et al.* (2001) Prevalence, incidence and correlates of HHV-8/KSHV infection and Kaposi's sarcoma in renal and liver transplant recipients. *J Infect*, **43**, 195–199.

Andreoni M, Sarmati L, Nicastri E *et al.* (2002) Primary human herpesvirus 8 infection in immunocompetent children. *J Am Med Assoc*, **287**, 1295–1300.

Ariyoshi K, Schim van der Loeff M, Corrah T *et al.* (1998) Kaposi's sarcoma and human herpesvirus 8 (HHV8) in HIV-1 and HIV-2 infection in The Gambia. *J Hum Virol*, **1**, 193–199.

Arvanitakis L, Geras RE, Varma A *et al.* (1997) Human herpesvirus KSHV encodes a constitutively active G-protein-coupled receptor linked to cell proliferation. *Nature*, **385**, 347–350.

Baillargeon J, Deng JH, Hettler E *et al.* (2001) Seroprevalence of Kaposi's sarcoma-associated herpesvirus infection among blood donors from Texas. *Ann Epidemiol*, **11**, 512–518.

Bais C, Santomasso B, Coso O *et al.* (1998) G-protein coupled receptor of Kaposi's sarcoma-associated herpesvirus is a viral oncogene and angiogenesis activator. *Nature*, **341**, 86–89.

Bais C, Van Geelen A, Eroles P *et al.* (2003) Kaposi's sarcoma associated herpesvirus G protein-coupled receptor immortalizes human endothelial cells by activation of the VEGF receptor-2/KDR. *Cancer Cell*, **3**, 131–143.

Ballestas ME, Chatis PA and Kaye KM (1999) Efficient persistence of extrachromosomal KSHV DNA mediated by latency-associated nuclear antigen. *Science*, **284**, 641–644.

Barozzi P, Luppi M, Facchetti F *et al.* (2003) Post-transplant Kaposi sarcoma originates from the seeding of donor-derived progenitors. *Nature Med*, **9**, 554–561.

Biberfeld P, Ensoli B, Stürzl M and Schulz TF (1998) Kaposi sarcoma-associated herpesvirus/human herpesvirus 8, cytokines, growth factors and HIV in the pathogenesis of Kaposi's sarcoma. *Curr Opin Infect Dis*, **11**, 97–105.

Biggar RJ, Whitby D, Marshall V *et al.* (2000) Human herpesvirus 8 in Brazilian Amerindians: a hyperendemic population with a new subtype. *J Infect Dis*, **181**, 1562–1568.

Birkmann A, Mahr K, Ensser A *et al.* (2001) Cell surface heparan sulfate is a receptor for human herpesvirus 8 and interacts with envelope glycoprotein K8.1. *J Virol*, **75**, 11583–11593.

Blackbourn DJ, Lennette ET, Ambroziak J *et al.* (1998) Human herpesvirus 8 detection in nasal secretions and saliva. *J Infect Dis*, **177**, 213–216.

Blackbourn DJ, Lennette E, Klencke B *et al.* (2000) The restricted cellular host range of human herpesvirus 8. *AIDS*, **14**, 1123–1133.

Blum L, Pellet C, Agbalika F *et al.* (1997) Complete remission of AIDS-related Kaposi's sarcoma associated with undetectable human herpesvirus-8 sequences during anti-HIV protease therapy. *AIDS*, **11**, 1653–1655.

Boivin G, Cote S, Cloutier N *et al.* (2002) Quantification of human herpesvirus 8 by real-time PCR in blood fractions of AIDS patients with Kaposi's sarcoma and multicentric Castleman's disease. *J Med Virol*, **68**, 399–403.

Boivin G, Gaudreau A, Toma E *et al.* (1999) Human herpesvirus 8 DNA load in leukocytes of human immunodeficiency virus-infected subjects: correlation with the presence of Kaposi's sarcoma and response to anticytomegalovirus therapy. *Antimicrob Agents Chemother*, **43**, 377–380.

Boshoff C, Endo Y, Collins PD *et al.* (1997) Angiogenic and HIV-inhibitory functions of KSHV-encoded chemokines. *Science*, **278**, 290–294.

Boshoff C, Schulz TF, Kennedy MM *et al.* (1995) Kaposi's sarcoma associated herpesvirus infects endothelial and spindle cells. *Nature Med*, **1**, 1274–1278.

Bourboulia D, Whitby D, Boshoff C *et al.* (1998) Serologic evidence for mother-to-child transmission of Kaposi sarcoma-associated herpesvirus infection. *J Am Med Assoc*, **280**, 31–32.

Brinkmann M, Glenn M, Rainbow L *et al.* (2003) Activation of mitogen-activated kinase and NF-κB pathways by a membrane protein encoded in the K15 gene of Kaposi sarcoma-associated herpesvirus (KSHV). *J Virol*, **77**, 9346–9358.

Burger M, Burger JA, Hoch RC *et al.* (1999) Point mutation causing constitutive signaling of CXCR2 leads to transforming activity similar to Kaposi's sarcoma herpesvirus-G protein-coupled receptor. *J Immunol*, **163**, 2017–2022.

Burysek L and Pitha PM (2001) Latently expressed human herpesvirus 8-encoded interferon regulatory factor 2 inhibits double-stranded RNA-activated protein kinase. *J Virol*, **75**, 2345–2352.

Burysek L, Yeow WS and Pitha PM (1999) Unique properties of a second human herpesvirus 8-encoded interferon regulatory factor (vIRF-2). *J Hum Virol*, **2**, 19–32.

Calabrò ML, Sheldon J, Favero A *et al.* (1998) Seroprevalence of Kaposi's sarcoma-associated herpesvirus (KSHV/HHV8) in different regions of Italy. *J Hum Virol*, **1**, 207–213.

Campbell TB, Borok M, Gwanzura L *et al.* (2000) Relationship of human herpesvirus 8 peripheral blood virus load and Kaposi's sarcoma clinical stage. *AIDS*, **14**, 2109–2116.

Cannon JS, Ciufo D, Hawkins AL *et al.* (2000) A new primary effusion lymphoma-derived cell line yields a highly infectious Kaposi's sarcoma herpesvirus-containing supernatant. *J Virol*, **74**, 10187–10193.

Cannon M, Philpott NJ and Cesarman E (2003) The Kaposi's sarcoma-associated herpesvirus G protein-coupled receptor has broad signaling effects in primary effusion lymphoma cells. *J Virol*, **77**, 57–67.

Cannon MJ, Dollard SC, Smith DK *et al.* (2001) Blood-borne and sexual transmission of human herpesvirus 8 in women with or at risk for human immunodeficiency virus infection. *N Engl J Med*, **344**, 637–643.

Casper C, Wald A, Pauk J *et al.* (2002) Correlates of prevalent and incident Kaposi's sarcoma-associated herpesvirus infection in men who have sex with men. *J Infect Dis*, **185**, 990–993.

Caterino-de-Araujo A, Calabro ML, de los Santos-Fortuna E *et al.* (1999) Searching for human herpesvirus 8 antibodies in serum samples from patients infected with human immunodeficiency virus type 1 and blood donors from Sao Paulo, Brazil. *J Infect Dis*, **179**, 1591–1592.

Cattani P, Nanni G, Graffeo R *et al.* (2000) Pretransplantation human herpes virus 8 seropositivity as a risk factor for Kaposi's sarcoma in kidney transplant recipients. *Transpl Proc*, **32**, 526–527.

Cerimele F, Curreli F, Ely S *et al.* (2001) Kaposi's sarcoma-associated herpesvirus can productively infect primary human keratinocytes and alter their growth properties. *J Virol*, **75**, 2435–2443.

Cesarman E, Chang Y, Moore PS *et al.* (1995a) Kaposi's sarcoma-associated herpesvirus-like DNA sequences in AIDS-related body-cavity-based lymphomas. *N Engl J Med*, **332**, 1186–1191.

Cesarman E, Moore PS, Rao P *et al.* (1995b) *In vitro* establishment and characterisation of two acquired immunodeficiency syndrome-related lymphoma cell lines (BC-1 and BC-2) containing Kaposi's sarcoma-associated herpesvirus-like (KSHV) DNA sequences. *Blood*, **86**, 2708–2714.

Cesarman E, Nador RG, Aozasa K *et al.* (1996) Kaposi's sarcoma-associated herpesvirus in non-AIDS-related lymphomas occurring in body cavities. *Am J Pathol*, **149**, 53–57.

Chang PJ, Shedd D, Gradoville L *et al.* (2002) Open reading frame 50 protein of Kaposi's sarcoma-associated herpesvirus directly activates the viral PAN and K12 genes by binding to related response elements. *J Virol*, **76**, 3168–3178.

Chang Y, Cesarman E, Pessin MS *et al.* (1994) Identification of herpesvirus-like DNA sequences in AIDS-associated Kaposi's sarcoma. *Science* **266**, 1865–1869.

Chang Y, Moore PS, Talbot SJ *et al.* (1996) Cyclin encoded by KS herpesvirus. *Nature*, **382**, 410.

Cheng EH, Nicholas J, Bellows DS *et al.* (1997) A Bcl-2 homolog encoded by Kaposi sarcoma-associated virus, human herpesvirus 8, inhibits apoptosis but does not heterodimerize with Bax or Bak. *Proc Natl Acad Sci USA*, **94**, 690–694.

Chiou CJ, Poole LJ, Kim PS *et al.* (2002) Patterns of gene expression and a transactivation function exhibited by the vGCR (ORF74) chemokine receptor protein of Kaposi's sarcoma-associated herpesvirus. *J Virol*, **76**, 3421–3439.

Choi JK, Lee BS, Shim SN, Li M and Jung JU (2000) Identification of the novel K15 gene at the rightmost end of the Kaposi's sarcoma-associated herpesvirus genome. *J Virol*, **74**, 436–446.

Cinquina CC, Grogan E, Sun R *et al.* (2000) Dihydrofolate reductase from Kaposi's sarcoma-associated herpesvirus. *Virology*, **268**, 201–217.

Ciufo DM, Cannon JS, Poole LJ *et al.* (2001) Spindle cell conversion by Kaposi's sarcoma-associated herpesvirus: formation of colonies and plaques with mixed lytic and latent gene expression in infected primary dermal microvascular endothelial cell cultures. *J Virol*, **75**, 5614–5626.

Collins CM and Medveczky PG (2002) Genetic requirements for the episomal maintenance of oncogenic herpesvirus genomes. *Adv Cancer Res*, **84**, 155–174.

Conant MA, Opp KM, Poretz D and Mills RG (1997) Reduction of Kaposi's sarcoma lesions following treatment of AIDS with ritonavir. *AIDS*, **11**, 1300–1301.

Cook PM, Whitby D, Calabro ML *et al.* (1999) Variability and evolution of Kaposi's sarcoma-associated herpesvirus in Europe and Africa. *AIDS*, **13**, 1165–1176.

Cook RD, Hodgson TA, Waugh AC *et al.* (2002) Mixed patterns of transmission of human herpesvirus-8 (Kaposi's sarcoma-associated herpesvirus) in Malawian families. *J Gen Virol*, **83**, 1613–1619.

Coscoy L and Ganem D (2000) Kaposi's sarcoma-associated herpesvirus encodes two proteins that block cell surface display of MHC class I chains by enhancing their endocytosis. *Proc Natl Acad Sci USA* **97**, 8051–8056.

Curreli F, Cerimele F, Muralidhar S *et al.* (2002) Transcriptional downregulation of ORF50/Rta by methotrexate inhibits the switch of Kaposi's sarcoma-associated herpesvirus/human herpesvirus 8 from latency to lytic replication. *J Virol*, **76**, 5208–5219.

Dairaghi DJ, Fan RA, McMaster BE *et al.* (1999) HHV8-encoded vMIP-I selectively engages chemokine receptor CCR8. Agonist and antagonist profiles of viral chemokines. *J Biol Chem*, **274**, 21569–21574.

Davidovici B, Karakis I, Bourboulia D *et al.* (2001) Seroepidemiology and molecular epidemiology of Kaposi's sarcoma-associated herpesvirus among Jewish population groups in Israel. *J Natl Cancer Inst*, **93**, 194–202.

Dedicoat M and Newton R (2003) Review of the distribution of Kaposi's sarcoma-associated herpesvirus (KSHV) in Africa in relation to the incidence of Kaposi's sarcoma. *Br J Cancer*, **88**, 1–3.

Deng H, Chu JT, Rettig MB *et al.* (2002) Rta of the human herpesvirus 8/Kaposi sarcoma-associated herpesvirus upregulates human interleukin-6 gene expression. *Blood*, **100**, 1919–1921.

Deng H, Young A and Sun R (2000) Auto-activation of the rta gene of human herpesvirus-8/Kaposi's sarcoma-associated herpesvirus. *J Gen Virol*, **81**, 3043–3048.

de Sanjose S, Marshall V, Sola J *et al.* (2002) Prevalence of Kaposi's sarcoma-associated herpesvirus infection in sex workers and women from the general population in Spain. *Int J Cancer*, **98**, 155–158.

Desrosiers RC, Sasseville VG, Czajak SC *et al.* (1997) A herpesvirus of rhesus monkeys related to the human Kaposi's sarcoma-associated herpesvirus. *J Virol*, **71**, 9764–9769.

Djerbi M, Screpanti V, Catrina AI *et al.* (1999) The inhibitor of death receptor signaling, FLICE-inhibitory protein defines a new class of tumor progression factors. *J Exp Med*, **190**, 1025–1032.

Dukers NH, Renwick N, Prins M *et al.* (2000) Risk factors for human herpesvirus 8 seropositivity and seroconversion in a cohort of homosexual men. *Am J Epidemiol*, **151**, 213–224.

Dupin N, Diss TL, Kellam P *et al.* (2000) HHV-8 is associated with a plasmablastic variant of Castleman's disease that is linked to HHV8-positive plasmablastic lymphoma. *Blood*, **95**, 1406–1412.

Duro D, Schulze A, Vogt B *et al.* (1999) Activation of cyclin A gene expression by the cyclin encoded by human herpesvirus-8. *J Gen Virol*, **80**, 549–555.

Ellis M, Chew YP, Fallis LS *et al.* (1999) Degradation of p27(Kip) cdk inhibitor triggered by Kaposi's sarcoma virus cyclin-cdk6 complex. *EMBO J*, **18**, 644–653.

Enbom M, Tolfvenstam T, Ghebrekidan H *et al.* (1999) Seroprevalence of *Human herpesvirus 8* in different Eritrean population groups. *J Clin Virol*, **14**, 167–172.

Endres MJ, Garlisi CG, Xiao H *et al.* (1999) The Kaposi's sarcoma-related herpesvirus (KSHV)-encoded chemokine vMIP-I is a specific agonist for the CC chemokine receptor (CCR)8. *J Exp Med*, **189**, 1993–1998.

Engels EA, Whitby D, Goebel PB *et al.* (2000) Identifying human herpesvirus 8 infection: performance characteristics of serologic assays. *J Acqu Immune Defic Syndr*, **23**, 346–354.

Farge D, Lebbe C, Marjanovic Z *et al.* (1999) Human herpesvirus 8 and other risk factors for Kaposi's sarcoma in kidney transplant recipients. Groupe Cooperatif de Transplantation d'Ile de France (GCIF). *Transplantation*, **67**, 1236–1242.

Flore O, Rafii S, Ely S *et al.* (1998) Transformation of primary endothelial cells by Kaposi's sarcoma-associated herpesvirus. *Nature*, **394**, 588–592.

Freitas RB, Freitas MR and Linhares AC (2002) Prevalence of human herpesvirus 8 antibodies in the population of Belem, Para, Brazil. *Rev Inst Med Trop Sao Paulo*, **44**, 309–313.

Friborg J Jr, Kong W, Hottiger MO and Nabel GJ (1999) p53 inhibition by the LANA protein of KSHV protects against cell death. *Nature*, **402**, 889–894.

Fujii T, Taguchi H, Katano H *et al.* (1999) Seroprevalence of human herpesvirus 8 in human immunodeficiency virus 1-positive and human immunodeficiency virus 1-negative populations in Japan. *J Med Virol*, **57**, 159–162.

Fujimuro M, Wu FY, ApRhys C *et al.* (2003) A novel viral mechanism for dysregulation of β-catenin in Kaposi's sarcoma-associated herpesvirus latency. *Nature Med*, **9**, 300–306.

Gambus G, Bourboulia D, Esteve A *et al.* (2001) Prevalence and distribution of HHV-8 in different subpopulations, with and without HIV infection, in Spain. *AIDS*, **15**, 1167–1174.

Gao SJ, Boshoff C, Jayachandra S *et al.* (1997) KSHV *orf K9* (vIRF) is an oncogene which inhibits the interferon signaling pathway. *Oncogene*, **15**, 1979–1985.

Gao SJ, Kingsley L, Li M *et al.* (1996) Seroprevalence of KSHV antibodies among North Americans, Italians, and Ugandans with and without Kaposi's sarcoma. *Nature Med*, **2**, 925–928.

Garber AC, Hu J and Renne R (2002) Latency-associated nuclear antigen (LANA) cooperatively binds to two sites within the terminal repeat, and both sites contribute to the ability of LANA to suppress transcription and to facilitate DNA replication. *J Biol Chem*, **277**, 27401–27411.

Gessain A, Mauclere P, van Beveren M *et al.* (1999) Human herpesvirus 8 primary infection occurs during childhood in Cameroon, Central Africa. *Int J Cancer*, **81**, 189–192.

Glenn M, Rainbow L, Aurad F *et al.* (1999) Identification of a spliced gene from Kaposi's sarcoma-associated herpesvirus encoding a protein with similarities to latent membrane proteins 1 and 2A of Epstein–Barr virus. *J Virol*, **73**, 6953–6963.

Glesby MJ, Hoover DR, Weng S *et al.* (1996) Use of antiherpes drug and the risk of Kaposi's sarcoma: data from the multicenter AIDS cohort study. *J Infect Dis*, **173**, 1477–1480.

Goudsmit J, Renwick N, Dukers NHTM *et al.* (2000) Natural history of HHV8 in the Amsterdam cohort studies (1984–

1997): analysis of seroconversions to orf65 and orf73. *Proc Natl Acad Sci USA*, **97**, 4838–4843.

Grandadam M, Dupin N, Calvez V *et al.* (1997) Exacerbations of clinical symptoms in human immunodeficiency virus type 1-infected patients with multicentric Castleman's disease are associated with a high increase in Kaposi's sarcoma herpesvirus DNA load in peripheral blood mononuclear cells. *J Infect Dis*, **175**, 1198–1201.

Greenblatt RM, Jacobson LP, Levine AM *et al.* (2001) Human herpesvirus 8 infection and Kaposi's sarcoma among human immunodeficiency virus-infected and -uninfected women. *J Infect Dis*, **183**, 1130–1134.

Greensill J, Sheldon JA, Renwick NM *et al.* (2000a) Two distinct γ-2 herpesviruses in African green monkeys: a second γ-2 herpesvirus lineage among old world primates? *J Virol*, **74**, 1572–1577.

Greensill J, Sheldon JA, Murthy KK *et al.* (2000b) A chimpanzee rhadinovirus sequence related to Kaposi's sarcoma-associated herpesvirus/human herpesvirus 8: increased detection after HIV-1 infection in the absence of disease. *AIDS*, **14**, F129–135.

Greensill J and Schulz TF (2000) Rhadinoviruses (gamma2-herpesviruses) of Old World primates: models for KSHV/HHV8-associated disease? *AIDS*, **14**(suppl 3), S11–S19.

Gruffat H, Portes-Sentis S, Sergeant A and Manet E (1999) Kaposi's sarcoma-associated herpesvirus (human herpesvirus-8) encodes a homologue of the Epstein-Barr virus bZip protein EB1. *J Gen Virol*, **80**(3), 557–561.

Gwack Y, Hwang S, Lim C *et al.* (2002) Kaposi's sarcoma-associated herpesvirus open reading frame 50 stimulates the transcriptional activity of STAT3. *J Biol Chem*, **277**, 6438–6442.

Hayward GS (2003) Initiation of angiogenic Kaposi's sarcoma lesions. *Cancer Cell*, **3**, 1–3.

Helt AM and Galloway DA (2003) Mechanisms by which DNA tumor virus oncoproteins target the Rb family of pocket proteins. *Carcinogenesis*, **24**, 159–169.

Huang Q, Petros AM, Virgin HW *et al.* (2002) Solution structure of a Bcl-2 homolog from Kaposi sarcoma virus. *Proc Natl Acad Sci USA*, **99**, 3428–3433.

Izumiya Y, Lin SF, Ellison T *et al.* (2003) Kaposi's sarcoma-associated herpesvirus K-bZIP is a coregulator of K-Rta: physical association and promoter-dependent transcriptional repression. *J Virol*, **77**, 1441–1451.

Jacobson LP, Jenkins FJ, Springer G *et al.* (2000) Interaction of human immunodeficiency virus type 1 and human herpesvirus type 8 infections on the incidence of Kaposi's sarcoma. *J Infect Dis*, **181**, 1940–1949.

Jaffe ES (1996) Primary body cavity-based AIDS-related lymphomas: evolution of a new disease entity. *Am J Clin Pathol*, **105**, 141–143.

Janier M, Agbalika F, de La Salmoniere P *et al.* (2002) Human herpesvirus 8 seroprevalence in an STD clinic in Paris: a study of 512 patients. *Sex Transm Dis*, **29**, 698–702.

Jansen-Durr P (1996) How viral oncogenes make the cell cycle. *Trends Genet*, **12**, 270–275.

Jenner RG, Alba MM, Boshoff C and Kellam P (2001) Kaposi's sarcoma-associated herpesvirus latent and lytic gene expression as revealed by DNA arrays. *J Virol*, **75**, 891–902.

Judde JG, Lacoste V, Briere J *et al.* (2000) Monoclonality or oligoclonality of human herpesvirus 8 terminal repeat sequences in Kaposi's sarcoma and other diseases. *J Natl Cancer Inst*, **92**, 729–736.

Kakoola DN, Sheldon J, Byabazaire N et al. (2001) Recombination in human herpesvirus-8 strains from Uganda and evolution of the K15 gene. J Gen Virol, 82, 2393–2404.

Katano H, Iwasaki T, Baba N et al. (2000a) Identification of antigenic proteins encoded by human herpesvirus 8 and seroprevalence in the general population and among patients with and without Kaposi's sarcoma. J Virol, 74, 3478–3485.

Katano H, Sato Y, Kurata T et al. (2000b) Expression and localization of human herpesvirus 8-encoded proteins in primary effusion lymphoma, Kaposi's sarcoma, and multicentric Castleman's disease. Virology, 269, 335–344.

Kedes DH and Ganem D (1997) Sensitivity of Kaposi's sarcoma-associated herpesvirus replication to antiviral drugs. J Clin Invest, 99, 2082–2086.

Kedes DH, Operskalski E, Busch M et al. (1996) The seroprevalence of human herpesvirus 8 (HHV 8): distribution of infection in Kaposi's sarcoma risk groups and evidence for sexual transmission. Nature Med, 2, 918–924.

Keller SA, Schattner EJ and Cesarman E (2000) Inhibition of NF-κB induces apoptosis of KSHV-infected primary effusion lymphoma cells. Blood, 96, 2537–2542.

Kirchhoff S, Sebens T, Baumann S et al. (2002) Viral IFN-regulatory factors inhibit activation-induced cell death via two positive regulatory IFN-regulatory factor 1-dependent domains in the CD95 ligand promoter. J Immunol, 168, 1226–1234.

Kledal TN, Rosenkilde MM, Coulin F et al. (1997) A broad-spectrum chemokine antagonist encoded by Kaposi's sarcoma-associated herpesvirus. Science, 277, 1656–1659.

Kliche S, Nagel W, Kremmer E et al. (2001) Signaling by human herpesvirus 8 kaposin A through direct membrane recruitment of cytohesin-1. Mol Cell, 7, 833–843.

Lacoste V, Judde JG, Briere J et al. (2000c) Molecular epidemiology of human herpesvirus 8 in africa: both B and A5 K1 genotypes, as well as the M and P genotypes of K14.1/K15 loci, are frequent and widespread. Virology, 278, 60–74.

Lacoste V, Mauclere P, Dubreuil G et al. (2000a) Simian homologues of human gamma-2 and betaherpesviruses in mandrill and drill monkeys. J Virol, 74, 11993–11999.

Lacoste V, Mauclere P, Dubreuil G et al. (2000b) KSHV-like herpesviruses in chimps and gorillas. Nature, 407, 151–152.

Lacoste V, Mauclere P, Dubreuil G et al. (2001) A novel gamma 2-herpesvirus of the Rhadinovirus 2 lineage in chimpanzees. Genome Res, 11, 1511–1519.

Lagunoff M, Bechtel J, Venetsanakos E et al. (2002) De novo infection and serial transmission of Kaposi's sarcoma-associated herpesvirus in cultured endothelial cells. J Virol, 76, 2440–2448.

Lagunoff M, Lukac DM and Ganem D (2001) Immuno-receptor tyrosine-based activation motif-dependent signaling by Kaposi's sarcoma-associated herpesvirus K1 protein: effects on lytic viral replication. J Virol, 75, 5891–5898.

Lagunoff M, Majeti R, Weiss A and Ganem D (1999) Deregulated signal transduction by the K1 gene product of Kaposi's sarcoma-associated herpesvirus. Proc Natl Acad Sci USA, 96, 5704–5709.

Lam LL, Pau CP, Dollard SC et al. (2002) Highly sensitive assay for human herpesvirus 8 antibodies that uses a multiple antigenic peptide derived from open reading frame K8.1. J Clin Microbiol, 40, 325–329.

Lavreys L, Chohan B, Ashley R et al. (2003) Human herpesvirus 8: seroprevalence and correlates in prostitutes in Mombasa, Kenya. J Infect Dis, 187, 359–363.

Lebbe C, de Cremoux P, Millot G et al. (1997) Characterization of in vitro culture of HIV-negative Kaposi's sarcoma-derived cells. In vitro responses to α-interferon. Arch Dermatol Res, 289, 421–428.

Lebbe C, Blum L, Pellet C et al. (1998) Clinical and biological impact of antiretroviral therapy with protease inhibitors on HIV-related Kaposi's sarcoma. AIDS, 12, F45–F49.

Lee H, Guo J, Li M et al. (1998b) Identification of an immunoreceptor tyrosine-based activation motif of K1 transforming protein of Kaposi's sarcoma-associated herpesvirus. Mol Cell Biol 18, 5219–5228.

Lee H, Veazy R, Williams K et al. (1998a) Deregulation of cell growth by the K1 gene of Kaposi's sarcoma-associated herpesvirus. Nature Med, 4, 435–440.

Lennette ET, Blackbourn DJ and Levy JA (1996) Antibodies to human herpesvirus type 8 in the general population and in Kaposi's sarcoma patients. Lancet, 348, 858–861.

Levy DE and Garcia-Sastre A (2001) The virus battles: IFN induction of the antiviral state and mechanisms of viral evasion. Cytokine Growth Factor Rev, 12, 143–156.

Li M, Damania B, Alvarez X et al. (2000) Inhibition of p300 histone acetyltransferase by viral interferon regulatory factor. Mol Cell Biol, 20, 8254–8263.

Liang Y, Chang J, Lynch SJ et al. (2002) The lytic switch protein of KSHV activates gene expression via functional interaction with RBP-Jκ (CSL), the target of the Notch signaling pathway. Genes Dev, 16, 1977–1989.

Lin R, Genin P, Mamane Y et al. (2001) HHV-8 encoded vIRF-1 represses the interferon antiviral response by blocking IRF-3 recruitment of the CBP/p300 coactivators. Oncogene, 20, 800–811.

Little RF, Mercad-Galindez F, Staskus K et al. (2003) A pilot study of cidofovir in patients with Kaposi sarcoma. J Infec Dis, 187, 149–153.

Liu C, Okruzhnov Y, Li H and Nicholas J (2001) Human herpesvirus 8 (HHV-8)-encoded cytokines induce expression of and autocrine signaling by vascular endothelial growth factor (VEGF) in HHV-8-infected primary-effusion lymphoma cell lines and mediate VEGF-independent antiapoptotic effects. J Virol, 75, 10933–10940.

Liu L, Eby MT, Rathore N et al. (2002) The human herpes virus 8-encoded viral FLICE inhibitory protein physically associates with and persistently activates the Iκ B kinase complex. J Biol Chem, 277, 13745–13751.

Lock MJ, Thorley N, Teo J and Emery VC (2002) Azidodeoxythymidine and didehydrodeoxythymidine as inhibitors and substrates of the human herpesvirus 8 thymidine kinase. J Antimicrob Chemother, 49, 359–366.

Lorenzo ME, Jung JU and Ploegh HL (2002) Kaposi's sarcoma-associated herpesvirus K3 utilizes the ubiquitin-proteasome system in routing class major histocompatibility complexes to late endocytic compartments. J Virol, 76, 5522–5531.

Lundquist A, Barre B, Bienvenu F et al. (2003) Kaposi's sarcoma-associated viral cyclin K overrides cell growth inhibition mediated by oncostatin M through STAT3 inhibition. Blood, 101, 4070–4077.

Luppi M, Barozzi P, Maiorana A et al. (1996) Human herpesvirus-8 DNA sequences in human immunodeficiency virus-negative angioimmunoblastic lymphadenopathy and benign lymphadenopathy with giant germinal center hyperplasia and increased vascularity. *Blood*, **87**, 3903–3909.

Luppi M, Barozzi P, Santagostino G *et al.* (2000a) Molecular evidence of organ-related transmission of Kaposi sarcoma-associated herpesvirus or human herpesvirus-8 in transplant patients. *Blood*, **96**, 3279–3281.

Luppi M, Barozzi P, Schulz TF *et al.* (2000b) Bone marrow failure associated with human herpesvirus 8 infection after transplantation. *N Engl J Med*, **343**, 1378–1385.

Lyall RG, Patton GS, Sheldon J *et al.* (1999) Evidence for horizontal and not vertical transmission of *Human herpesvirus 8* in children born to human immunodeficiency virus-infected mothers. *Pediatr Infect Dis J*, **18**, 795–799.

Marcelin AG, Grandadam M, Flandre P *et al.* (2002) Kaposi's sarcoma herpesvirus and HIV-1 seroprevalences in prostitutes in Djibouti. *J Med Virol*, **68**, 164–167.

Martin DF, Kuppermann BD, Wolitz RA *et al.* (1999) Oral ganciclovir for patients with cytomegalovirus retinitis treated with a ganciclovir implant. *N Engl J Med*, **340**, 1063–1070.

Martin JN, Ganem DE, Osmond DH *et al.* (1998) Sexual transmission and the natural history of human herpesvirus 8 infection. *N Engl J Med*, **338**, 948–954.

Mayama S, Cuevas L, Sheldon J *et al.* (1998) Prevalence of Kaposi's sarcoma associated herpesvirus (Human herpesvirus 8) in a young Ugandan population. *Int J Cancer*, **77**, 817–820.

McGeoch DJ, Dolan A and Ralph AC (2000) Toward a comprehensive phylogeny for mammalian and avian herpesviruses. *J Virol*, **74**, 10401–10406.

Means RE, Ishido S, Alvarez X and Jung JU (2002) Multiple endocytic trafficking pathways of MHC class I molecules induced by a Herpesvirus protein. *EMBO J*, **21**, 1638–1649.

Medveczky MM, Horvath E, Lund T and Medveczky PG (1997) *In vitro* antiviral drug sensitivity of the Kaposi's sarcoma-associated herpesvirus. *AIDS*, **11**, 1327–1332.

Melbye M, Cook PM, Hjalgrim H *et al.* (1998) Transmission of human herpesvirus 8 (HHV 8) among homosexual men follows the pattern of a 'Kaposi's sarcoma agent'. *Int J Cancer*, **77**, 543–548.

Meng YX, Sata T, Stamey FR *et al.* (2001) Molecular characterization of strains of Human herpesvirus 8 from Japan, Argentina and Kuwait. *J Gen Virol*, **82**, 499–506.

Miller G, Rigsby MO, Heston L *et al.* (1996) Antibodies to butyrate-inducible antigens of Kaposi's sarcoma-associated herpesvirus in patients with HIV-1 infection. *N Engl J Med*, **334**, 1292–1297.

Mocroft A, Youle M, Gazzard B *et al.* for the Royal Free/Chelsea and Westminster Hospitals Collaborative Group (1996) Anti-herpesvirus treatment and risk of Kaposi's sarcoma in HIV infection. *AIDS*, **10**, 1101–1105.

Molden J, Chang Y, You Y *et al.* (1997) A Kaposi's sarcoma-associated herpesvirus-encoded cytokine homolog (vIL-6) activates signaling through the shared gp130 receptor subunit. *J Biol Chem*, **272**, 19625–19631.

Montaner S, Sodhi A, Molinolo A *et al.* (2003) Endothelial infection with KSHV genes *in vivo* reveals that vGPCR initiates Kaposi's sarcomagenesis and can promote the tumorigenic potential of viral latent genes. *Cancer Cell*, **3**, 23–36.

Montaner S, Sodhi A, Pece S *et al.* (2001) The Kaposi's sarcoma-associated herpesvirus G protein-coupled receptor promotes endothelial cell survival through the activation of Akt/protein kinase B. *Cancer Res*, **61**, 2641–2648.

Moore PS, Boshoff C, Weiss RA and Chang Y (1996) Molecular mimicry of human cytokine and cytokine response pathway genes by KSHV. *Science*, **274**, 1739–1744.

Moses AV, Fish KN, Ruhl R *et al.* (1999) Long-term infection and transformation of dermal microvascular endothelial cells by human herpesvirus 8. *J Virol*, **73**, 6892–6902.

Moses AV, Jarvis MA, Raggo C *et al.* (2002) Kaposi's sarcoma-associated herpesvirus-induced upregulation of the c-kit protooncogene, as identified by gene expression profiling, is essential for the transformation of endothelial cells. *J Virol*, **76**, 8383–8399.

Muralidhar S, Pumfery AM, Hassani M *et al.* (1998) Identification of kaposin (open reading frame K12) as a human herpesvirus 8 (Kaposi's sarcoma-associated herpesvirus) transforming gene. *J Virol*, **72**, 4980–4988.

Naranatt PP, Akula SM, Zien CA *et al.* (2003) Kaposi's sarcoma-associated herpesvirus induces the phosphatidylinositol 3-kinase-PKC-zeta-MEK-ERK signaling pathway in target cells early during infection: implications for infectivity. *J Virol*, **77**, 1524–1539.

Nealon K, Newcomb WW, Pray TR *et al.* (2001) Lytic replication of Kaposi's sarcoma-associated herpesvirus results in the formation of multiple capsid species: isolation and molecular characterization of A, B, and C capsids from a gammaherpesvirus. *J Virol*, **75**, 2866–2878.

Neipel F, Albrecht JC and Fleckenstein B (1997) Cell-homologous genes in the Kaposi's sarcoma-associated rhadinovirus human herpesvirus 8: determinants of its pathogenicity? *J Virol*, **71**, 4187–4192.

O'Brien TR, Kedes D, Ganem D *et al.* (1999) Evidence for concurrent epidemics of human herpesvirus 8 and human immunodeficiency virus type 1 in US homosexual men: rates, risk factors, and relationship to Kaposi's sarcoma. *J Infect Dis*, **180**, 1010–1017.

Ojala PM, Yamamoto K, Castanos-Velez E *et al.* (2000) The apoptotic v-cyclin-CDK6 complex phosphorylates and inactivates Bcl-2. *Nature Cell Biol*, **2**, 819–825.

Oksenhendler E, Carcelain G, Aoki Y *et al.* (2000) High levels of human herpesvirus 8 viral load, human interleukin-6, interleukin-10, and C reactive protein correlate with exacerbation of multicentric castleman disease in HIV-infected patients. *Blood*, **96**, 2069–2073.

Oksenhendler E, Cazals-Hatem D, Schulz TF *et al.* (1998) Transient angiolymphoid hyperplasia and Kaposi's sarcoma after primary infection with human herpesvirus 8 in a patient with human immunodeficiency virus infection. *N Engl J Med*, **338**, 1585–1590.

Osmond DH, Buchbinder S, Cheng A *et al.* (2002) Prevalence of Kaposi sarcoma-associated herpesvirus infection in homosexual men at beginning of and during the HIV epidemic. *J Am Med Assoc*, **287**, 221–225.

Parisi SG, Sarmati L, Pappagallo M *et al.* (2002) Prevalence trend and correlates of HHV-8 infection in HIV-infected patients. *J Acqu Immune Defic Syndr*, **29**, 295–299.

Park J, Seo T, Hwang S *et al.* (2000) The K-bZIP protein from Kaposi's sarcoma-associated herpesvirus interacts with p53 and represses its transcriptional activity. *J Virol*, **74**, 11977–11982.

Parravicini C, Olsen SJ, Capra M *et al.* (1997) Risk of Kaposi's sarcoma-associated herpesvirus transmission from donor allografts among Italian posttransplant Kaposi's sarcoma patients. *Blood*, **90**, 2826–2829.

Parravicini C, Chandran B, Corbellino M *et al.* (2000) Differential viral protein expression in Kaposi's sarcoma-associated herpesvirus-infected diseases: Kaposi's sarcoma, primary effusion lymphoma, and multicentric Castleman's disease. *Am J Pathol*, **156**, 743–749.

Pauk J, Huang ML, Brodie SJ *et al.* (2000) Mucosal shedding of human herpesvirus 8 in men. *N Engl J Med*, **343**, 1369–1377.

Pellet C, Chevret S, Frances C *et al.* (2002) Prognostic value of quantitative Kaposi sarcoma-associated herpesvirus load in posttransplantation Kaposi sarcoma. *J Infect Dis*, **186**, 110–113.

Pellett PE, Spira TJ, Bagasra O *et al.* (1999) Multicenter comparison of PCR assays for detection of human herpesvirus 8 DNA in semen. *J Clin Microbiol* **37**, 1298–1301.

Penfold ME, Dairaghi DJ, Duke GM *et al.* (1999) Cytomegalovirus encodes a potent alpha chemokine. *Proc Natl Acad Sci USA*, **96**, 9839–9844.

Perna AM, Bonura F, Vitale F *et al.* (2000) Antibodies to human herpes virus type 8 (HHV8) in general population and in individuals at risk for sexually transmitted diseases in Western Sicily. *Int J Epidemiol*, **29**, 175–179.

Pertel PE (2002) Human herpesvirus 8 glycoprotein B (gB), gH, and gL can mediate cell fusion. *J Virol*, **76**, 4390–4400.

Piolot T, Tramier M, Coppey M *et al.* (2001) Close but distinct regions of human herpesvirus 8 latency-associated nuclear antigen 1 are responsible for nuclear targeting and binding to human mitotic chromosomes. *J Virol*, **75**, 3948–3959.

Plancoulaine S, Abel L, van Beveren M *et al.* (2000) Human herpesvirus 8 transmission from mother to child and between siblings in an endemic population. *Lancet*, **356**, 1062–1065.

Platt G, Carbone A and Mittnacht S (2002) p16INK4a loss and sensitivity in KSHV-associated primary effusion lymphoma. *Oncogene*, **21**, 1823–1831.

Platt GM, Simpson GR, Mittnacht S and Schulz TF (1999) Latent nuclear antigen of Kaposi's sarcoma-associated herpesvirus interacts with RING3, a homolog of the *Drosophila* female sterile homeotic (fsh) gene. *J Virol*, **73**, 9789–9795.

Polson AG, Wang D, DeRisi J and Ganem D (2002) Modulation of host gene expression by the constitutively active G protein-coupled receptor of Kaposi's sarcoma-associated herpesvirus. *Cancer Res*, **62**, 4525–4530.

Poole LJ, Zong JC, Ciufo DM *et al.* (1999) Comparison of genetic variability at multiple loci across the genomes of the major subtypes of Kaposi's sarcoma-associated herpesvirus reveals evidence for recombination and for two distinct types of open reading frame K15 alleles at the right-hand end. *J Virol*, **73**, 6646–6660.

Raab M-S, Albrecht J-C, Birkmann A *et al.* (1998) The immunogenic glycoprotein gp35-37 of human herpesvirus 8 is encoded by open reading frame K8.1. *J Virol*, **72**, 6725–6731.

Radkov SA, Kellam P and Boshoff C (2000) The latent nuclear antigen of Kaposi sarcoma-associated herpesvirus targets the retinoblastoma–E2F pathway and with the oncogene Hras transforms primary rat cells. *Nature Med*, **6**, 1121–1127.

Rainbow L, Platt GM, Simpson GR *et al.* (1997) The 222 to 234 kDa latent nuclear protein (LNA) of Kaposi's sarcoma-associated herpesvirus (human herpesvirus 8) is encoded by orf73 and is a component of the latency-associated nuclear antigen. *J Virol*, **71**, 5915–5921.

Regamey N, Tamm M, Wernli M *et al.* (1998) Transmission of human herpesvirus 8 inection from renal-transplant donors to recipients. *N Engl J Med*, **339**, 1358–1363.

Renne R, Blackbourn D, Whitby D *et al.* (1998) Limited transmission of Kaposi's sarcoma-associated herpesvirus in cultured cells. *J Virol*, **72**, 5182–5188.

Renne R, Zhong W, Herndier B *et al.* (1996) Lytic growth of Kaposi's sarcoma-associated herpesvirus (human herpesvirus 8) in culture. *Nature Med*, **2**, 342–346.

Renwick N, Dukers NH, Weverling GJ *et al.* (2002) Risk factors for human herpesvirus 8 infection in a cohort of drug users in The Netherlands, 1985–1996. *J Infect Dis*, **185**, 1808–1812.

Renwick N, Halaby T, Weverling GJ *et al.* (1998) Seroconversion for Kaposi's sarcoma-associated herpesvirus is highly predictive of KS development in HIV-1 infected individuals. *AIDS*, **12**, 2481–2488.

Rezza G, Dorrucci M, Serraino D *et al.* (2000b) Incidence of Kaposi's sarcoma and HHV-8 seroprevalence among homosexual men with known dates of HIV seroconversion. Italian Seroconversion Study. *AIDS*, **14**, 1647–1653.

Rezza G, Lennette ET, Giuliani M *et al.* (1998) Prevalence and determinants of anti-lytic and anti-latent antibodies to human herpesvirus-8 among Italian individuals at risk of sexually and parenterally transmitted infections. *Int J Cancer*, **77**, 361–365.

Rezza G, Tchangmena OB, Andreoni M *et al.* (2000a) Prevalence and risk factors for human herpesvirus 8 infection in northern Cameroon. *Sex Transm Dis*, **27**, 159–164.

Rimessi P, Bonaccorsi A, Sturzl M *et al.* (2001) Transcription pattern of human herpesvirus 8 open reading frame K3 in primary effusion lymphoma and Kaposi's sarcoma. *J Virol*, **75**, 7161–7174.

Rivas C, Thlick AE, Parravicini C *et al.* (2001) Kaposi's sarcoma-associated herpesvirus LANA2 is a B cell-specific latent viral protein that inhibits p53. *J Virol*, **75**, 429–438.

Rose TM, Strand KB, Schultz ER *et al.* (1997) Identification of two homologs of the Kaposi's sarcoma-associated herpesvirus (human herpesvirus 8) in retroperitoneal fibromatosis of different macaque species. *J Virol*, **71**, 4138–4144.

Russo JJ, Bohenzky RA, Chien M-C *et al.* (1996) Nucleotide sequence of Kaposi's sarcoma-associated herpesvirus (HHV 8). *Proc Natl Acad Sci USA*, **93**, 14862–14868.

Sadler R, Wu L, Forghani B *et al.* (1999) A complex translational program generates multiple novel proteins from the latently expressed kaposin (K12) locus of Kaposi's sarcoma-associated herpesvirus. *J Virol*, **73**, 5722–5730.

Said W, Chien K, Takeuchi S *et al.* (1996) Kaposi's sarcoma-associated herpesvirus (KSHV or HHV8) in primary effusion lymphoma: ultrastructural demonstration of herpesvirus in lymphoma cells. *Blood*, **87**, 4937–4943.

Sanchez DJ, Coscoy L and Ganem D (2002) Functional organization of MIR2, a novel viral regulator of selective endocytosis. *J Biol Chem*, **277**, 6124–6130.

Santarelli R, De Marco R, Masala MV *et al.* (2001) Direct correlation between human herpesvirus-8 seroprevalence and classic Kaposi's sarcoma incidence in Northern Sardinia. *J Med Virol*, **65**, 368–372.

Sarid R, Sato T, Bohenzky RA et al. (1997) Kaposi's sarcoma-associated herpesvirus encodes a functional Bcl-2 homologene. Nature Med, **3**, 293–298.

Satoh M, Toma H, Sato Y et al. (2001) Seroprevalence of Human herpesvirus 8 in Okinawa, Japan. Jpn J Infect Dis, **54**, 125–126.

Schatz O, Monini P, Bugarini R et al. (2001) Kaposi's sarcoma-associated herpesvirus serology in Europe and Uganda: multicentre study with multiple and novel assays. J Med Virol, **65**, 123–132.

Schulz TF (1998) Kaposi's sarcoma-associated herpesvirus (Human herpesvirus 8). J Gen Virol, **79**, 1573–1591.

Schulz TF (1999) Epidemiology of Kaposi's sarcoma-associated herpesvirus/human herpesvirus 8. Adv Cancer Res, **76**, 121–160.

Schulz TF (2001) KSHV/HHV8-associated lymphoprolifera-tions in the AIDS setting. Eur J Cancer, **37**, 1217–1226.

Schulz TF and Weiss RA (1995) A finger on the culprit. Nature, **373**, 17–18.

Seo T, Lee D, Lee B et al. (2000) Viral interferon regulatory factor 1 of Kaposi's sarcoma-associated herpesvirus (human herpesvirus 8) binds to, and inhibits transactivation of, CREB-binding protein. Biochem Biophys Res Commun, **270**, 23–27.

Serraino D, Toma L, Andreoni M et al. (2001) A seroprevalence study of human herpesvirus type 8 (HHV8) in eastern and Central Africa and in the Mediterranean area. Eur J Epidemiol, **17**, 871–876.

Sgadari C, Barillari G, Toschi E et al. (2002) HIV protease inhibitors are potent anti-angiogenic molecules and promote regression of Kaposi sarcoma. Nature Med, **8**, 225–232.

Sharp TV, Wang HW, Koumi A et al. (2002) K15 protein of Kaposi's sarcoma-associated herpesvirus is latently ex-pressed and binds to HAX-1, a protein with antiapoptotic function. J Virol, **76**, 802–816.

Simpson GR, Schulz TF, Whitby D et al. (1996) Prevalence of Kaposi's sarcoma-associated herpesvirus infection mea-sured by antibodies to recombinant capsid protein and latent immunofluorescence antigen. Lancet, **348**, 1133–1138.

Sitas F, Newton R and Boshoff C (1999) Increasing probability of mother-to-child transmission of HHV-8 with increasing maternal antibody titer for HHV-8. N Engl J Med, **340**, 1923.

Smith MS, Bloomer C, Horvat R et al. (1997) Detection of human herpesvirus 8 DNA in Kaposi's sarcoma lesions and peripheral blood of human immunodeficiency virus-positive patients and correlation with serologic measure-ments. J Infect Dis, **176**, 84–93.

Soulier J, Grollet L, Oksenhendler E et al. (1995) Kaposi's sarcoma-associated herpesvirus-like DNA sequences in multicentric Castleman's disease. Blood, **86**, 1276–1280.

Sozzani S, Luini W, Bianchi G et al. (1998) The viral chemokine macrophage inflammatory protein-II is a selective Th2 chemoattractant. Blood, **92**, 4036–4039.

Spiller OB, Blackbourn DJ, Mark L et al. (2003) Functional activity of the complement regulator encoded by Kaposi's sarcoma-associated herpesvirus. J Biol Chem, **278**, 9283–9289.

Stamey FR, Patel MM, Holloway BP and Pellett PE (2001) Quantitative, fluorogenic probe PCR assay for detection of human herpesvirus 8 DNA in clinical specimens. J Clin Microbiol, **39**, 3537–3540.

Stark GR, Kerr IM, Williams BR et al. (1998) How cells respond to interferons. Annu Rev Biochem, **67**, 227–264.

Staskus KA, Zhong W, Gebhard K et al. (1997) Kaposi's sarcoma-associated herpesvirus gene expression in endothe-lial (spindle) tumor cells. J Virol, **71**, 715–719.

Sun R, Lin SF, Gradoville L et al. (1998) A viral gene that activates lytic cycle expression of Kaposi's sarcoma-associated herpesvirus. Proc Natl Acad Sci USA, **95**, 10866–10871.

Sun R, Lin SF, Staskus K et al. (1999) Kinetics of Kaposi's sarcoma-associated herpesvirus gene expression. J Virol, **73**, 2232–2242.

Swanton C, Mann DJ, Fleckenstein B et al. (1997) Herpes viral cyclin/Cdk6 complexes evade inhibition by CDK inhibitor proteins. Nature, **390**, 184–187.

Tedeschi R, Caggiari L, Silins I et al. (2000) Seropositivity to human herpesvirus 8 in relation to sexual history and risk of sexually transmitted infections among women. Int J Cancer, **87**, 232–235.

Tedeschi R, De Paoli P, Schulz TF and Dillner J (1999) Human serum antibodies to a major defined epitope of human herpesvirus 8 small viral capsid antigen. J Infect Dis, **179**, 1016–1020.

Teodoro JG and Branton PE (1997) Regulation of apoptosis by viral gene products. J Virol, **71**, 1739–1746.

Thome M, Schneider P, Hofman K et al. (1997) Viral FLICE-inhibitory proteins (FLIPs) prevent apoptosis induced by death receptors. Nature, **386**, 517–521.

Vieira JD, Hunag L, Koelle DM and Corey L (1997) Transmissible Kaposi's-associated Herpesvirus (human herpesvirus 8) in saliva of men with a history of Kaposi's sarcoma. J Virol, **71**, 7083–7087.

Vieira J, O'Hearn P, Kimball L et al. (2001) Activation of Kaposi's sarcoma-associated herpesvirus (human herpes-virus 8) lytic replication by human cytomegalovirus. J Virol, **75**, 1378–1386.

Viejo-Borbolla A, Kati E, Sheldon J et al. (2003b) A domain in the C-terminal region of latency-associated nuclear antigen (LANA-1) of KSHV affects transcriptional activa-tion and binding to nuclear heterochromatin. J Virol, **77**, 7093–7100.

Viejo-Borbolla A, Ottinger M and Schulz TF (2003a) Human Herpesvirus 8: biology and role in the pathogenesis of Kaposi's sarcoma and other AIDS-related malignancies. Curr Infect Dis Rep, **5**, 169–175.

Wang HW, Sharp TV, Koumi A et al. (2002) Characteriza-tion of an anti-apoptotic glycoprotein encoded by Kaposi's sarcoma-associated herpesvirus which resembles a spliced variant of human survivin. EMBO J, **21**, 2602–2615.

Wang SE, Wu FY, Fujimuro M et al. (2003) Role of CCAAT/enhancer-binding protein alpha (C/EBPα) in activation of the Kaposi's sarcoma-associated herpesvirus (KSHV) lytic-cycle replication-associated protein (RAP) promoter in cooperation with the KSHV replication and transcription activator (RTA) and RAP. J Virol, **77**, 600–623.

Weber KS, Grone HJ, Rocken M et al. (2001) Selective recruitment of Th2-type cells and evasion from a cytotoxic immune response mediated by viral macrophage inhibitory protein-II. Eur J Immunol, **31**, 2458–2466.

Whitby D, Howard MR, Tenant-Flowers M et al. (1995) Detection of Kaposi sarcoma-associated herpesvirus (KSHV) in peripheral blood of HIV-infected individuals predicts progression to Kaposi's sarcoma. Lancet, **346**, 799–802.

Whitby D, Luppi M, Barozzi P *et al.* (1998) Human herpesvirus 8 seroprevalence in blood donors and patients with lymphoma from different regions of Italy. *J Natl Cancer Inst*, **90**, 395–397.

Whitby D, Luppi M, Sabin C *et al.* (2000) Detection of antibodies to human herpesvirus 8 in Italian children: evidence for horizontal transmission. *Br J Cancer*, **82**, 702–704.

Widmer I, Wernli M, Bachmann F *et al.* (2002) Differential expression of viral Bcl-2 encoded by Kaposi's sarcoma-associated herpesvirus and human Bcl-2 in primary effusion lymphoma cells and Kaposi's sarcoma lesions. *J Virol*, **76**, 2551–2556.

Wu FY, Tang QQ, Chen H *et al.* (2002) Lytic replication-associated protein (RAP) encoded by Kaposi sarcoma-associated herpesvirus causes p21CIP-1-mediated G_1 cell cycle arrest through CCAAT/enhancer-binding protein-α. *Proc Natl Acad Sci USA*, **99**, 10683–10688.

Yang TY, Chen SC, Leach MW *et al.* (2000) Transgenic expression of the chemokine receptor encoded by human herpesvirus 8 induces an angioproliferative disease resembling Kaposi's sarcoma. *J Exp Med*, **191**, 445–454.

Zago A, Bourboulia D, Viana MC *et al.* (2000) Seroprevalence of human herpesvirus 8 and its association with Kaposi sarcoma in Brazil. *Sex Transm Dis*, **27**, 468–472.

Zhong W and Ganem D (1997) Characterization of ribonucleoprotein complexes containing an abundant polyadenylated nuclear RNA encoded by Kaposi's sarcoma-associated herpesvirus (human herpesvirus 8). *J Virol*, **71**, 1207–1212.

Zhu FX, King SM, Smith EJ *et al.* (2002) A Kaposi's sarcoma-associated herpesviral protein inhibits virus-mediated induction of type I interferon by blocking IRF-7 phosphorylation and nuclear accumulation. *Proc Natl Acad Sci USA*, **99**, 5573–5578.

Zhu L, Wang R, Sweat A *et al.* (1999) Comparison of human sera reactivities in immunoblots with recombinant human herpesvirus (HHV)-8 proteins associated with the latent (ORF73) and lytic (ORFs 65, K8.1A, and K8.1B) replicative cycles and in immunofluorescence assays with HHV-8-infected BCBL-1 cells. *Virology*, **256**, 381–392.

Zong JC, Ciufo DM, Alcendor DJ *et al.* (1999) High-level variability in the ORF-K1 membrane protein gene at the left end of the Kaposi's sarcoma-associated herpesvirus genome defines four major virus subtypes and multiple variants or clades in different human populations. *J Virol*, **73**, 4156–4170.

Zong J, Ciufo DM, Viscidi R *et al.* (2002) Genotypic analysis at multiple loci across Kaposi's sarcoma herpesvirus (KSHV) DNA molecules: clustering patterns, novel variants and chimerism. *J Clin Virol*, **23**, 119–148.

3

Hepatitis Viruses

Tim J. Harrison, Geoffrey M. Dusheiko and Arie J. Zuckerman

Royal Free and University College Medical School, London, UK

INTRODUCTION

Hepatitis, characterised by necrosis and inflammation in the liver, may result from infection with a variety of viruses and is the main clinical outcome of infection with viruses from several different families. The predominantly hepatotropic viruses, which vary in prevalence throughout the world, may be considered together, although the biology of these viruses and the spectrum of diseases they cause differ considerably (see Table 3.1 for an overview).

The clinical spectrum of acute disease ranges from an asymptomatic or mild anicteric illness to acute disease with jaundice to severe prolonged jaundice or fulminant hepatitis (acute liver failure). Where the infection persists, chronic hepatitis may ensue and, here, the outcome is also variable. Inapparent or subclinical and anicteric infections are common. *Hepatitis A* and *E* viruses (HAV and HEV) do not persist in the liver and there is no evidence of direct progression to chronic liver damage. However, *Hepatitis B virus* (HBV), with or without its satellite, *Hepatitis D virus* (HDV, or the delta agent), and *Hepatitis C virus* (HCV), may be associated with persistent infection, a prolonged carrier state, and progression to chronic liver disease, which may be severe. In addition, there is substantial evidence of an aetiological association between infection with chronic hepatitis B and C and hepatocellular carcinoma (HCC), so that the hepatitis B vaccine can be considered to be the first vaccine against human cancer.

Pathology

Acute Hepatitis

The pathological features that are constant in all types of acute viral hepatitis consist of parenchymal cell necrosis and histiocytic periportal inflammation. The reticulin framework of the liver is usually well preserved, except in some cases of massive and submassive necrosis. The liver cells show necrotic changes that vary in form and intensity. The necrotic areas are usually multifocal, but necrosis frequently tends to be zonal, with the most severe changes occurring in the centrilobular areas. Individual hepatocytes are often swollen and may show ballooning but they can also shrink, giving rise to acidophilic bodies.

Dead or dying rounded liver cells are extruded into the perisinusoidal space. There are variations in the size and staining quality of the nuclei. Fatty changes in the liver are usually not marked, but some steatosis can be observed in chronic hepatitis C virus infection. A monocellular infiltration, which is particularly marked in the portal zones, is the characteristic mesenchymal reaction. This is also accompanied by some proliferation of bile ductules.

Kupffer cells and endothelial cells proliferate and the Kupffer cells often contain excess lipofuscin pigment. In the icteric phase of typical acute hepatitis, the walls of the hepatic vein tributaries may be thickened and frequently are infiltrated, with proliferation of the lining cells in the terminal hepatic veins. Cholestasis may occur in the early stages of viral hepatitis, and

Principles and Practice of Clinical Virology, Fifth Edition. Edited by A. J. Zuckerman, J. E. Banatvala, J. R. Pattison, P. D. Griffiths and B. D. Schoub
© 2004 John Wiley & Sons Ltd   ISBN 0 470 84338 1

Table 3.1   The principal agents of viral hepatitis

	HAV	HBV	HCV	HDV	HEV
Classification	*Picornaviridae,* Hepatovirus	*Hepadnaviridae*	*Flaviviridae,* Hepacivirus	Unclassified (viroid-like)	Calicivirus-like
Size (nm)	27	42	36	36–40	27–38
Genome	7.5 kb Linear ssRNA	3.2 kb Circular dsDNA*	9.4 kb Linear ssRNA	1.7 kb Circular ssRNA	7.5 kb Linear ssRNA
Structural proteins	VP1–4	HBcAg HBsAg	Nucleocapsid E1 (gp35) E2 (gp70)	HDAg (HBsAg)	ORF2 product
Transmission	Enteric	Parenteral	Parenteral	Parenteral	Enteric
Persistent infection	No	Yes	Yes	Yes	No
Vaccine	Yes	Yes	No	No	Under trial

*The HBV genome contains a single-stranded region.

plugs of bile thrombi may be found in the bile canaliculi; this is a more common feature in hepatitis E.

Spotty or focal necrosis with the associated mesenchymal reaction may also be found in anicteric hepatitis, but on the whole the lesions tend to be less severe than in the icteric type of illness. At the other extreme, there is rapid massive necrosis of the liver cells in fulminant hepatitis.

Repair of the liver lobules occurs by regeneration of hepatocytes; frequent mitoses, polyploidy, atypical cells and binucleated cells are found. There is gradual disappearance of the mononuclear cells from the portal tracts, but elongated histiocytes and fibroblasts may remain. The outcome of acute viral hepatitis may be complete resolution or fatal massive necrosis.

Chronic Hepatitis

The pathological features of chronic hepatitis B depend upon the stage of the disease, the host immune response and the degree of virus replication. In chronic hepatitis B with mild activity, only rare piecemeal necrosis is seen. Characteristic hepatocytes with eosinophilic 'ground-glass' cells are relatively common in anti-HBe positive patients with low levels of virus replication. Lobular hepatitis is more common in patients with active virus replication, and raised serum aminotransferases. CD8$^+$ cells predominate in areas of piecemeal necrosis. HBsAg and HBcAg can be detected by immunoperoxidase staining in routinely fixed liver biopsy sections. Patients with high levels of viraemia may have minimal hepatitis.

The pathological features of HCV infection are quite characteristic, albeit not pathognomonic. The presence

of HCV RNA in serum tends to correlate with some degree of hepatitis, so that disappearance of HCV RNA, e.g. following successful interferon-α (IFN-α) treatment, is followed by histological improvement. Typically, patients with chronic hepatitis C have mild portal tract inflammation with lymphoid aggregates or follicles and mild periportal piecemeal necrosis (Figure 3.1). Parenchymal steatosis, apoptosis and mild lobular inflammation are present and portal fibrosis or portal–central fibrosis may be present in later stages of disease. Bridging necrosis is not common. Rarely, granulomas can be observed. Although many of the lymphoid follicles are associated with bile ducts,

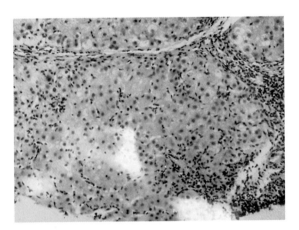

Figure 3.1   Section of a liver biopsy from a patient with chronic hepatitis C seen at low magnification. There is a moderate lymphocytic infiltrate in the portal tracts, with piecemeal necrosis. A scattered mild parenchymal inflammatory infiltrate is also present (H & E stain). Courtesy of Dr A. P. Dhillon, Department of Histopathology, Royal Free and University College Medical School

ductopaenia is not observed. Advanced disease, with cirrhosis or hepatocellular carcinoma, is not generally associated with distinguishing features.

HCV antigens have been detected in scattered groups of cells with granular cytoplasmic staining. The periportal lymphocytes around lymphoid follicles are mixed, but contain relatively large numbers of CD4 lymphocytes. A characteristic histological pattern of mild chronic hepatitis with portal lymphoid follicles and varying degrees of lobular activity is found in many patients with persistent hepatitis C infection.

Biochemical Tests of Liver Function

The serum levels of aspartic and alanine aminotransferase are elevated in acute hepatitis, as are levels of other enzymes released by the damaged liver cells. Usually, the levels of alanine aminotransferase (ALT) are higher than those of aspartic aminotransferase (AST), a difference particularly marked in hepatitis C. However, with progression of the disease to cirrhosis, the AST:ALT ratio may be reversed. Elevation of these enzymes may be the only abnormality to be found in individuals with asymptomatic and anicteric infections who are tested because of known exposure. Bilirubin is found in the urine and conjugated and total serum bilirubin levels are raised in most symptomatic infections. The leukocyte count is usually normal but some atypical lymphocytes are frequently found.

A progressive decline in serum albumin concentrations and prolongation of the prothrombin time are characteristically observed after decompensated cirrhosis has developed.

Clinical Manifestations of Acute Hepatitis

Differences between the clinical syndromes of acute hepatitis A, acute hepatitis B, and other forms of viral hepatitis become apparent on analysis of large numbers of well-documented cases, but these differences are not sufficiently reliable for the diagnosis of individual patients with icteric disease. Epidemiologic risk factors, e.g. travel, injections or sexual risk, can indicate a possible aetiology. Fever and headache are more frequent during the prodrome of acute hepatitis A. The late incubation period—early clinical phase is frequently heralded by a variety of non-specific symptoms, such as fatigue, anorexia, malaise and myalgias. A few days later, anorexia, nausea, vomiting and right upper quadrant abdominal pain can appear,

followed by passage of dark urine and clay-coloured stools and the development of jaundice of the sclera and skin. With the appearance of jaundice, there is usually a rapid subjective improvement in symptoms. The jaundice usually deepens during the first few days and persists for 1 or 2 weeks. The faeces then darken and the jaundice diminishes, at first rapidly and then more slowly, over an additional period of 2 weeks or so. The liver may be palpable in acute severe hepatitis, but only a minority of patients have palpable splenomegaly. Convalescence may be prolonged, although complete recovery in adults usually takes place within a few months. In children, the prodromal features may be mild or even absent, although anorexia, when present, tends to be severe. The icteric or post-icteric phase in children is short. The prodromal phase of hepatitis B and C is often prolonged and more insidious. Low-grade fever, arthralgias and skin rashes, particularly in hepatitis B, are not uncommon. The clinical features of the icteric phase are similar in all types of acute viral hepatitis. The mortality rate of acute hepatitis is low, approximately 0.1–3 deaths/1000 cases. Fulminant hepatitis can occur following acute hepatitis A–E; it is more common in hepatitis B. Hepatocellular failure develops rapidly; the patient may be deeply jaundiced or encephalopathy may occur before conspicuous jaundice is evident. Widespread haemorrhage occurs. The prothrombin time is prolonged; an altered prothrombin time is a more reliable indicator of prognosis, and of the need for liver transplantation, than the serum bilirubin or serum aminotransferases.

Fulminant hepatitis is unusual following hepatitis C infection but has been reported, particularly following chemotherapy or withdrawal of chemotherapy. High mortality rates for hepatitis occurring during pregnancy have been reported from India, the Middle East and North Africa in association with hepatitis E virus infection.

HEPATITIS A

Hepatitis A is endemic in all parts of the world, but the exact incidence is difficult to estimate because of the high proportion of asymptomatic and anicteric infections, differences in surveillance and differing patterns of disease. The degree of under-reporting is known to be very high. Serological surveys have shown that infection with hepatitis A virus is almost universal and, in developing countries, 80–90% of children have serological markers of past infection by the age of 5. In industrialised countries, improvements in sanitation have decreased the prevalence of antibodies in young adults to 5–20%.

Incubation Period

The incubation period of hepatitis A is 3–5 weeks, with a mean of 28 days. Subclinical and anicteric infections are common, particularly in children and, although the disease has, in general, a low mortality, adult patients may be incapacitated for many weeks. There is no evidence of persistence of the infection in the liver and progression to chronic liver damage does not occur. The virus replicates *in vivo* in the liver but it seems likely that the initial site of virus replication may be in the gut. This is not proven and the mechanism by which the virus reaches the liver is unknown, although a postulated transient viraemia is supported by occasional cases of HAV acquired from blood or blood products.

Mode of Spread

Hepatitis A virus is spread by the faecal–oral route, most commonly by person-to-person contact, and infection is particularly common in conditions of poor sanitation and overcrowding. Common source outbreaks result most frequently from faecal contamination of drinking water and food, but water-borne transmission is not a major factor in industrialised communities. On the other hand, many food-borne outbreaks have been reported in developed countries. This can be attributed to the shedding of large amounts of virus in the faeces (Figure 3.2) during the incubation period of the illness in infected foodhandlers, and the source of the outbreak can often be traced to uncooked food or food which has been handled after cooking. The consumption of raw or inadequately cooked shellfish cultivated in polluted water is associated with a high risk of HAV infection. For example, an epidemic with approximately 300 000 cases in Shanghai in 1988 was attributed to the ingestion of raw clams (Halliday *et al.*, 1991). However, although hepatitis A is common in developed countries, the infection occurs mainly in small clusters and often with only few identified cases. Hepatitis A is highly endemic in many tropical and subtropical areas with the occasional occurrence of large epidemics. The infection is acquired frequently by travellers from areas where the infection is of low prevalence to areas where hepatitis A is hyperendemic.

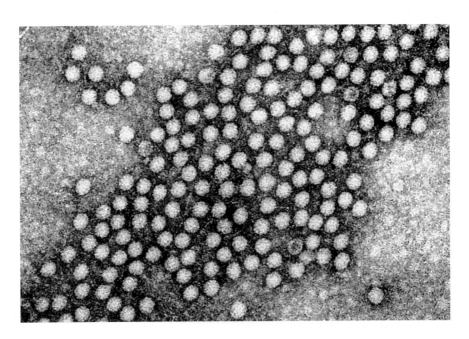

Figure 3.2 Electron micrograph showing HAV in faecal extracts obtained during the early acute phase of illness. The particles measure about 27 nm in diameter (× 170 000). From a series by Anthea Thornton and A. J. Zuckerman

Age Incidence

All age groups are susceptible to hepatitis A and disease severity increases with age. As noted above, most individuals in highly endemic areas are infected before 5 years of age but in many countries in northern Europe and in North America most clinical cases occur in adults. In countries where there has been improvement in socioeconomic conditions and sanitation, such as southern Europe and China, there has been an increase in the mean age of infection. In many developed countries, the prevalence of antibodies to hepatitis A has fallen to 5–10% of young adults and there is thus a large susceptible population. The diminishing incidence of hepatitis A is now matched by an increasing incidence of clinically apparent disease. This shift in age incidence is similar to that which occurred with poliomyelitis during and after World War II, reflecting improvement in socioeconomic and hygienic conditions and a consequent shift in herd immunity.

Seasonal Pattern

In temperate zones, the characteristic seasonal trend is for an increase in incidence in the autumn and early winter months, falling progressively to a minimum during the mid-summer. However, more recently the seasonal peak has been lost in some countries. In many tropical countries the peak of the infection tends to occur during the rainy season.

The Biology of Hepatitis A Virus

The hepatitis A virion is a non-enveloped particle measuring 25–28 nm in diameter (Figure 3.3) and containing a linear genome of single-stranded RNA, approximately 7500 nucleotides in length and coding for three major structural polypeptides with relative molecular mass (M_r) of 33 000, 29 000 and 27 000 (VP1, VP2 and VP3, respectively). A fourth, truncated VP4 polypeptide of only l7 amino acids has been predicted from the nucleotide sequence of the virus but has not been detected experimentally. X-ray crystallographic studies have not yet been reported but the basic structure of the capsid may be predicted from such studies of other picornaviruses; the antigenic structure has been defined further by analysis of neutralisation escape mutants selected by monoclonal antibodies. These studies suggest that the immunodominant

neutralisation site is a conformational epitope comprising residues of VP1 and VP3 (Ping and Lemon, 1992). It is believed that secondary or higher orders of protein structure may play essential roles in this antigenic site, because it has not been possible to detect this predominant antigen in virus preparations disrupted with detergent or following expression of recombinant protein (although expression of the entire HAV polyprotein may enable assembly of antigenic virus-like particles in cell culture, as noted below).

HAV is exceptionally stable; it is ether-resistant, stable at pH 3.0 and relatively resistant to inactivation by heat. HAV retains its physical integrity and biological activity at 60°C for 10 h but is inactivated after 5 min at 100°C. The virus also may be inactivated by ultraviolet irradiation and by treatment with a 1:4000 concentration of formaldehyde solution at 37°C for 72 h. There is also evidence that HAV is inactivated by chlorine at a concentration of 1 mg/l for 30 min.

Genetic Organisation

The organisation of the genome of HAV is similar to other picornaviruses and it was classified originally as Enterovirus type 72. However, there are substantial differences between HAV and the established four genera of the family *Picornaviridae*, e.g. an unusually low GC content of 38% and very limited sequence homology. Consequently, HAV has been reclassified in its own genus of the *Picornaviridae*, *Hepatovirus*.

Cloning and sequencing data (Cohen *et al.*, 1987) indicate that the genome of HAV consists of 7478 nucleotides with a 5' non-coding region of 733 nucleotides and a shorter non-coding region and poly(A) tract at the 3' terminus. A small protein (VPg) is bound covalently at the 5' terminus. A single open reading frame (ORF) extends from nucleotides 710–750 to about 60 nucleotides in advance of the 3' terminal poly(A) tract. This sequence can encode a polyprotein with a M_r of about 250 000. The predicted amino acid sequence compared with analogous regions of other picornaviruses suggests that the 5' region of the ORF codes for the three major structural proteins of the virus, along with the fourth, small VP4. The 3' region encodes a protease, which processes the polyprotein, a polymerase and other functions involved in genome replication. Dipeptide cleavage sites, which have been identified in a number of picornavirus polyproteins, are not conserved in hepatitis A virus but attempts have been made to predict the cleavage pattern and post-translational processing

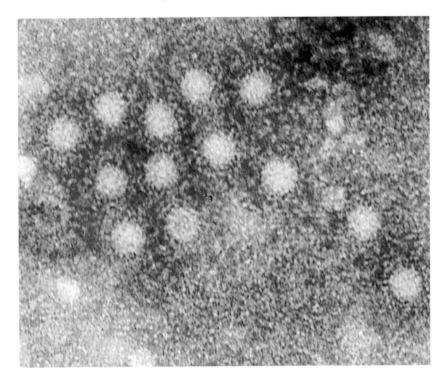

Figure 3.3 Electron micrograph showing a large aggregate of HAV particles heavily coated with antibody, giving the appearance of a 'halo'. 'Full' and 'empty' particles are shown (× 340 000). From a series by Anthea Thornton and A. J. Zuckerman

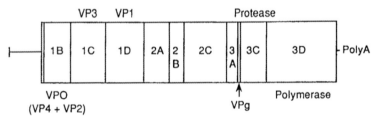

Figure 3.4 Organisation of the HAV genome. See text for details

of the polyprotein (Figure 3.4). The cellular receptor for HAV has been identified (Kaplan *et al.*, 1996).

Cell Culture

The successful propagation of hepatitis A virus in 1979 in primary monolayer and explant cell cultures and in continuous cell lines of primate origin was a major advance and opened the way to the preparation of hepatitis A vaccines. The viral capsid antigens are detectable by immunofluorescence and radioimmuno-assay, and the viral RNA by an indirect, quantitative autoradiographic plaque assay and by complementary DNA–RNA hybridisation and RT-PCR. HAV does not induce cytopathic changes in culture but tends to establish persistent infections and remain largely cell-associated. However, primary isolation of wild-type virus is difficult and several weeks elapse before antigen is detectable in the cytoplasm of infected cells. Thus, virus isolation is not a practical diagnostic technique in routine laboratories.

Adaptation to growth in cultured cells occurs with repeated passage, with more rapid production of intracellular antigen and with higher final yields. Virus adapted to growth in cell culture may become attenuated and the nucleotide sequences of wild-type

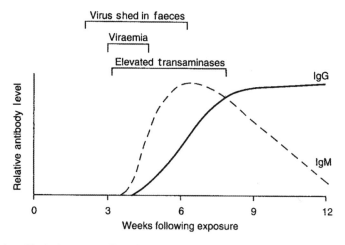

Figure 3.5 Serological profile during uncomplicated hepatitis A

and attenuated strains have been compared. There is evidence that changes in the 5′ non-coding region and the region encoding non-structural (2B/2C) polypeptides may be associated with attenuation and adaptation to cell culture.

Only one serotype of HAV has been identified in human volunteers infected experimentally, in patients from different outbreaks of hepatitis A and in naturally and experimentally infected chimpanzees and monkeys. This also has been confirmed by cross-neutralisation tests and by the protective efficacy of pooled human immunoglobulin obtained from different geographical regions. However, strain-specific differences exist, at least at the level of genomic nucleotide sequences from different isolates of HAV. A pairwise comparison of the nucleotide sequence of 168 bases from 152 strains of HAV revealed that these can be classified into seven genotypes, three of which were isolated from Old World monkeys.

Pathogenesis

The mechanisms underlying liver injury in hepatitis A are not understood. The initial non-cytopathic phase, during which virus replicates and is released, is followed by decreased virus multiplication and inflammatory cell infiltration, suggesting that immune mechanisms are involved in pathogenesis. Experimental evidence suggests that HLA-restricted, virus-specific T cells play a significant role in HAV-related hepatocellular injury. T cell clones have been derived from patients with acute hepatitis A and analysed for their phenotype. CD8+ clones isolated during the acute phase of the disease predominate over CD4+ clones; these CD8+ clones have cytotoxic activity and show specific cytotoxicity against autologous fibroblasts infected with HAV. These data support the hypothesis that liver cell injury in acute HAV infection is mediated by HAV-specific CD8+ T lymphocytes, and is not entirely due to an intrinsic cytopathic effect of the virus itself. The molecular targets of these cells are unknown.

Laboratory Diagnosis

Specific diagnosis of hepatitis A can be established by demonstrating the virus in faeces by enzyme immunoassay and radioimmunoassay or by immune electron microscopy and RT-PCR. Isolation of the virus in cell cultures is not appropriate for routine diagnosis.

Specific serological tests for hepatitis A antigen (HAAg) and antibodies include radioimmunoassay and enzyme immunoassays. Hepatitis A antibody (anti-HAV) is always demonstrable by such assays during the early phase of the illness and titres increase rapidly (Figure 3.5). Because antibody develops very early in the course of the infection, serological diagnosis of recent infection can be established by titrations of serial samples of serum or, more conveniently, by the demonstration of hepatitis A antibody of the IgM class, which is the simplest and most economical method of establishing the diagnosis. Hepatitis A IgM is detectable in serum for 45–60 days after the onset of symptoms. Liver biopsy is not usually required in acute hepatitis A. Titres of anti-HAV in IgG rise with convalescence and the antibody usually persists for many years. Recovery from infection is associated with lifelong immunity.

Clinical Course

Clinical disease with jaundice is uncommon in infants and young children and the infection may pass unnoticed in this group. Infection in adulthood results in acute icteric hepatitis in more than 70% of cases. The case fatality rate is 0.3–1.8%; the risk of serious complication increases significantly with age, and severe hepatitis is correspondingly more common in older persons. Recurrent hepatitis has been observed in patients (and experimentally inoculated Saimiri monkeys with acute disease) and may be associated with shedding of virus in stools. The relapses are generally benign, with eventual complete resolution. The absence of chronic infection indicates the effectiveness of the host immune response to HAV. In genetically susceptible individuals, it is possible that hepatitis A may trigger an autoimmune chronic hepatitis. Vento *et al.* (1991) identified individuals who possessed a defect in suppressor–inducer T lymphocytes controlling immune responses to the asialoglycoprotein receptor. These subjects developed a persistent response to the asialoglycoprotein receptor, and rarely autoimmune hepatitis after subclinical hepatitis A. Approximately 5% of patients with acute hepatitis A will develop cholestatic hepatitis, characterised by pruritis and steatorrhea.

Prevention and Control of Hepatitis A

Control of infection is difficult. Strict isolation of cases is not a useful control measure because faecal shedding of the virus is at its highest during the late incubation period and prodromal phase of the illness. Spread of hepatitis A is reduced by simple hygienic measures and the sanitary disposal of excreta.

Normal human immunoglobulin (NHIG), containing at least 100 IU/ml anti-HAV, will prevent or attenuate a clinical illness if given intramuscularly before exposure to the virus or early during the incubation period. The dosage should be at least 2 IU anti-HAV/kg body weight (Table 3.2), but in special cases, such as pregnancy or in patients with liver disease, the dosage may be doubled. Immunoglobulin does not always prevent infection and excretion of HAV, and inapparent or subclinical hepatitis may develop. The efficacy of passive immunisation is based on the presence of anti-HAV in the immunoglobulin, but the minimum titre of antibody required for protection has not yet been established. Immunoglobulin is used most commonly for close personal contacts of patients with hepatitis A and for those exposed to contaminated food. Immunoglobulin has also been used effectively for controlling outbreaks in institutions such as homes for the mentally handicapped and in nursery schools.

Prior to the availability of a vaccine, pre-exposure prophylaxis with immunoglobulin was recommended for persons without anti-HAV visiting highly endemic areas. After a period of 6 months the administration of immunoglobulin for travellers had to be repeated, unless it could be demonstrated that the recipient had developed his/her own anti-HAV. Because the shift in herd immunity led to reduced titres of anti-HAV in normal immunoglobulin in developed countries and a highly immunogenic vaccine has become available, a single dose of vaccine may be offered to travellers with the option of a booster dose 6–12 months later.

Hepatitis A Vaccines

There has been considerable interest in the development of both killed and attenuated hepatitis A vaccines and inactivated vaccines are now licensed in many countries. The virus grows poorly in cell culture but yields have been improved by adaptation and are sufficient to permit gradient purification. This virus is inactivated with formaldehyde and the antigen

Table 3.2 Passive immunisation with normal immunoglobulin for travellers to areas highly endemic for hepatitis A

Person's body weight (kg)	Period of stay <3 months	Period of stay >3 months
<25	50 IU anti-HAV (0.5 ml)	100 IU anti-HAV (1.0 ml)
25–30	100 IU anti-HAV (1.0 ml)	250 IU anti-HAV (2.5 ml)
>50	200 IU anti-HAV (2.0 ml)	500 IU anti-HAV (5.0 ml)

adsorbed to aluminium hydroxide and given intra-muscularly. These preparations are safe and immunogenic in man and have been shown to induce a protective immune response. Safety and immunogenicity studies and efficacy trials have been undertaken in volunteers (Flehmig *et al.*, 1989; Ellerbeck *et al.*, 1992; Werzberger *et al.*, 1992). The anti-HAV response includes neutralising antibodies. The currently licensed vaccines appear to be well-tolerated and immunogenic at doses of 720–1440 arbitrary 'ELISA' units (SKB) or l25–50 U (Merck). In the case of the SKB vaccine licensed in the UK, a single dose of 720 ELISA units of hepatitis A viral protein is sufficient for protection of adults of 16 years and over, with the option of a booster dose 6–12 months later. A juvenile formulation with 320 ELISA units/dose is available. Active immunisation induces higher levels of both total and neutralising antibodies than NHIG.

Inactivated vaccines of this type are useful for the protection of travellers from prosperous countries but are likely to be too costly for use in the developing world, where exposure usually occurs early in life. In developed countries, the vaccine should be given to travellers to countries where HAV is endemic, armed forces personnel, diplomats, staff of children's day care centres and of institutions for intellectually handicapped individuals, male homosexuals, intravenous drug abusers, haemophiliacs and sewage workers.

A combined hepatitis A and B vaccine is available and licensed for use in adults and children at risk of both infections; and a combined hepatitis A and typhoid vaccine is available and appropriate for use in travellers to areas where typhoid is endemic.

An economic appraisal of prophylactic measures against malaria, hepatitis A and typhoid in travellers deduced an unfavourable cost–benefit ratio for hepatitis A prophylaxis (Behrens and Roberts, 1994). However, this economic model is sensitive to the incidence of disease and suggests that hepatitis A immunisation can be made more cost-effective by targeting specific travellers. The addition of human immunoglobulin was recommended previously when travel is to occur within 4 weeks of receipt of vaccine, because of concern about the time taken to develop neutralising antibodies. However, a single dose of vaccine (1440 ELISA units) is effective. Ideally travellers should be given prophylaxis at least 4 weeks before, but should not be denied prophylaxis even when given up to the day of travel. After vaccination, anti-HAV antibodies may be detectable rapidly, although the minimum protective antibody level is uncertain. Data in chimpanzees suggest

protection against infection even if vaccine is administered shortly after exposure (Purcell *et al.*, 1992). The curtailment of Alaskan and Italian outbreaks by immunisation with a single dose without concurrent administration of immune globulin provides supportive evidence for at least some efficacy of one dose for post-exposure prophylaxis (McMahon *et al.*, 1996; Sagliocca *et al.*, 1999). The cost–benefit ratio of HAV vaccination probably is most beneficial when vaccine is given to frequent travellers to endemic areas. Where practical, testing for antibodies to hepatitis A prior to immunisation may be indicated in those aged 50 years or over, those born in areas of high endemicity and those with a history of jaundice. HAV vaccine is also recommended for individuals with significant chronic liver disease due to hepatitis B or C and who may have an increased risk of fulminant hepatic failure following HAV infection.

Attenuated strains of HAV have been developed and potentially may be useful as vaccines. This approach is attractive because live vaccines may be cheaper to produce (the attenuated virus grows more efficiently in cell culture), can be given orally and may induce a mucosal antibody response. As with vaccine strains of polioviruses, attenuation may be associated with mutations in the 5' non-coding region of the genome, which affect secondary structure. There is also evidence that mutations in the region of the genome encoding the non-structural polypeptides (region 2B/2C, Figure 3, Emerson *et al.*, 1992) may be important for adaptation to cell culture and attenuation. However, the markers of attenuation of HAV are not so well defined as those for the polioviruses and reversion to virulence may be a problem also. There is also concern that 'over-attenuated' viruses may not be sufficiently immunogenic.

Although there is some sequence variation between different isolates of HAV and evidence for different strains infecting non-human primates, there is only one serotype of the virus and immunity gives effective cross-protection against all strains. Considerable efforts have been made to define the epitope(s) involved. The immunodominant epitope may be highly conformational and involve alignment of domains from VP1 and VP3, posing problems for expression of immunogenic proteins using recombinant DNA technology. A recombinant vaccinia virus expressing most of the HAV capsid coding region has been shown to protect tamarin monkeys from subsequent challenge (Karayiannis *et al.*, 1993). Expression of the entire HAV polyprotein using a recombinant vaccinia virus led to assembly of virus-like particles in cells infected in culture.

HEPATITIS E

Epidemic hepatitis that resembled but was serologically distinct from hepatitis A was reported initially in the Indian subcontinent (Khuroo, 1980) and later in central and south-east Asia, the Middle East, North Africa and Central America. The disease also is a common cause of acute sporadic hepatitis in these countries. Sporadic cases have been observed in developed countries among migrant labourers and travellers returning from such areas. In contrast to prior epidemics of enterically-transmitted non-A, non-B hepatitis, HEV was found to be a common cause of acute hepatitis in a paediatric population in Egypt. Seroprevalence studies in Hong Kong suggest that hepatitis E accounts for one-third of non-A, non-B, non-C hepatitis, and that co-infection of hepatitis A and E can occur (Lok *et al.*, 1992). Recently, indigenous cases of hepatitis E have been reported in the USA and several European countries, including the UK. Rarely it could be transmitted by blood transfusion in countries where the disease is endemic (Arankalle and Chobe, 2000).

The average incubation period is slightly longer than for hepatitis A, with a mean of 6 weeks. The infection is acute and self-limiting. Clinical disease occurs predominantly in young adults and high mortality rates (up to 20%) have been reported in the third trimester of pregnancy. The infection is spread by the ingestion of contaminated water and probably by food, but secondary clinical cases seem to be uncommon.

Virus-like particles have been detected in the stools of infected individuals by immune electron microscopy using convalescent serum (Figure 3.6). However, such studies have often proved inconclusive and a large proportion of the excreted virus may be degraded during passage through the gut. The particles are slightly larger than those of hepatitis A, with a mean diameter of 32–34 nm. Cross-reaction studies between sera and virus in stools associated with a variety of epidemics in several different countries suggest a single viral serotype (Bradley, 1992).

Biology of HEV

Research into HEV advanced following the development of animal models (Bradley *et al.*, 1988). HEV was first transmitted to *Cynomolgus* macaques and subsequently a number of other species of monkeys and chimpanzees have been infected. The gallbladder bile

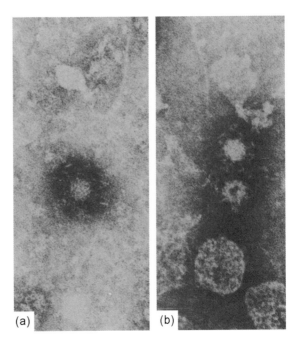

Figure 3.6 Immune electron microscopy of HEV from a faecal extract. (a) Particle coated with predominately IgG. (b) Particles coated with predominately IgM. Reproduced by permission from Purcell and Ticehurst (1988)

of infected monkeys was found to be a rich source of virus, enabling the molecular cloning of DNA complementary to the HEV (RNA) genome and elucidation of the entire 7.5 kb sequence (Tam *et al.*, 1991). The organisation of the genome is distinct from the picornaviruses; the non-structural polypeptides are encoded in the 5′ region and the structural polypeptides at the 3′ end. HEV resembles the caliciviruses in the size and organisation of its genome as well as the size and morphology of the virion, but remains unclassified.

Organisation of the HEV Genome

The HEV genome is a polyadenylated, positive-sense RNA of around 7500 nt and contains three ORFs (Figure 3.7). The first, of approximately 5 kb, begins 28 nt from the 5′ end of the genome and encodes motifs associated with NTP-binding, helicase and RNA-dependent RNA polymerase activities. A second ORF of around 2 kb begins 37 nt downstream of the

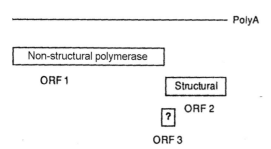

Figure 3.7 Organisation of the HEV genome. See text for details

first, terminates 68 nt from the poly(A) tail and is believed to encode the structural polypeptides. The third ORF is very short (369 nt) and overlaps the other two. The viral proteins may be subject to proteolytic processing and other post-translational modifications.

Pathogenesis

Macaque monkeys develop acute viral hepatitis associated with a rise in liver enzymes, the presence of HEV-specific viral particles in the stool and histological changes in the liver 21–45 days after HEV inoculation. Subclinical hepatitis E also may occur in experimental primates, and subclinical infections of humans may provide a reservoir for transmission. Ultrastructural changes in the livers of these experimental monkeys include infiltration of lymphocytes and polymorphonuclear lymphocytes around the necrotic area, swelling of mitochondria, dilation of smooth endoplasmic reticulum (ER), and presence of 27–34 nm virus particles during the acute phase of the disease. It is not known whether these changes reflect cytopathic liver injury or are immune-mediated. Negative-strand HEV RNA has been detected in small intestines, lymph nodes, colons and livers of pigs experimentally infected with swine and human HEV.

Diagnosis

Sequencing of the HEV genome has enabled the development of a number of specific diagnostic tests, e.g. HEV RNA was detected, using PCR, in stool samples obtained during an epidemic in Kanpur (northern India) and may also be detected in infected liver. Enzyme immunoassays, which detect IgG and

IgM anti-HEV, have been developed (Dawson et al., 1992). One assay employs four recombinant HEV antigens expressed in *Escherichia coli* as fusion proteins with glutathione-S-transferase, and another is based on synthetic peptides, representing antigens that were initially identified by blind immunoscreening using convalescent sera from infected individuals. Western blot assays are able to detect IgM anti-HEV. IgM is detected infrequently at initial presentation and disappears by 3 months after jaundice. IgG titres can be quite high, but tend to disappear over time. The diagnosis can be confirmed by PCR on faecal material from acutely infected patients. Bile from experimentally infected monkeys is also positive by PCR (Jameel et al., 1992). Attack rates have been higher in males than females and for adults rather than children. Evidence of secondary intrafamilial spread is uncommon.

Clinical Features

An early observation was the high mortality (10–20%) in pregnant women due to fulminant hepatitis. Fulminant hepatitis E has been reported in the UK, but appears to be a relatively infrequent cause elsewhere. In general, the disease is self-limited, with no evidence of chronic infection. Cholestatic disease can occur, which may be prolonged (Mechnik et al., 2001). Liver biopsies obtained during the acute illness show portal inflammation and cytoplasmic cholestasis. Stool specimens may reveal 27–32 nm virus-like particles when tested by immune electron microscopy (IEM) but RT-PCR is a more reliable assay for the virus. A recent observational study appears to confirm a high rate of severe or fulminant hepatitis in pregnant women. Babies born to women with acute disease are at risk of vertical transmission and may be at risk of perinatal morbidity. Liver transplantation is indicated for fulminant hepatitis E if survival otherwise seems unlikely.

Immunisation

Although individuals who recover from hepatitis E mount an antibody response, including to putative capsid antigens, it is not clear whether these antibodies protect against subsequent infection or, if so, how long that immunity lasts. Adult populations in endemic areas are susceptible to hepatitis E, with high attack rates in epidemics. Preliminary findings indicate that hyperimmune rabbit antisera against HEV antigens contain neutralising activity. However, the degree and longevity of protective immunity of macaque monkeys following recovery from experimental infection or immunisation with recombinant DNA or antigen preparations is controversial. The prospects for the development of hepatitis E vaccines have been reviewed (Panda and Nanda, 1997). Purdy *et al.* (1993) demonstrated that immunisation with a bacterially-expressed fusion protein, derived from the capsid region of the Burmese strain, protected *Cynomolgus* macaques from challenge with the homologous strain of virus. However, monkeys challenged with the Mexican strain excreted virus in their faeces, although there was no biochemical evidence (i.e. raised aminotransferases) of liver disease. In another study, an immunogen derived from the capsid region of the Pakistan strain was found to protect against infection with the Mexican strain (Tsarev *et al.*, 1997). Aside from the duration of a protective antibody response, other caveats are that animals are frequently challenged intravenously with HEV, rather than via the natural (oral) route, and that macaques do not suffer overt symptoms of hepatitis during infection—protection often is defined as the absence of elevated aminotransferases, despite evidence of virus replication (excretion in the faeces). A baculovirus-expressed candidate HEV vaccine (spanning amino acids (aa) 112–607 of the ORF 2 protein of the Pakistan strain) is undergoing a Phase II/III clinical trial in Nepal.

Sporadic Hepatitis E is Predominantly Zoonotic in Origin

The genomic sequences of HEV isolated initially from several Asian countries (Pakistan, China, India) were found to be similar to the Burmese prototype (now recognised as genotype 1) and less closely related to the strain isolated from Mexico (genotype 2). Genotype 1 viruses are associated with epidemic and sporadic hepatitis E throughout Asia and Africa and genotype 2 viruses also have been described from Nigeria. A third genotype of HEV was discovered in several herds of swine in the USA (Meng *et al.*, 1997) and has been implicated as the cause of rare cases of indigenous hepatitis E in individuals in the USA. Genotype 4 HEV, which has been described in China (Wang *et al.*, 2000) and Taiwan and seems to be the major cause of sporadic hepatitis E in that region, also has frequently been found infecting pigs. Thus, it seems that genotypes 3 and 4, and probably also the less well-

characterised hepatitis E viruses isolated in Europe and elsewhere, are responsible for sporadic cases of hepatitis E in humans that arise from zoonotic infection. In contrast, genotype 1 viruses, which have been implicated in all of the major Asian epidemics of hepatitis E, including in the Xinjiang Uighur autonomous region of China in 1988–1990, have not been isolated from pigs. Such epidemics typically result from massive faecal contamination of the water supply and the source of such contamination remains to be elucidated.

HEPATITIS B

Epidemiology

The discovery in 1965 of Australia antigen (now referred to as hepatitis B surface antigen, HBsAg), and the demonstration by Blumberg *et al.* (1965) and others of its association with type B hepatitis, led to rapid and unabated progress in the understanding of this complex infection. Hepatitis B remains a globally important disease. Low- (<2% of the population seropositive for HBsAg), intermediate- (2–8%) and high-prevalence (>8%) areas are recognised (Table 3.3). Several epidemiological studies indicate that the reported rates of hepatitis B infection have declined in western and northern Europe and the USA. Infection rates in children have declined in high prevalence areas where the universal immunisation of infants has been introduced.

In the past, hepatitis B was diagnosed on the basis of infection occurring approximately 60–180 days after the injection of human blood or plasma fractions or the use of inadequately sterilised syringes and needles. The development of specific laboratory tests for hepatitis B confirmed the importance of the parenteral routes of transmission, and infectivity appears to be especially related to blood. Transmission of the infection may result from accidental inoculation of minute amounts of blood or fluid contaminated with blood during medical, surgical and dental procedures; immunisation with inadequately sterilised syringes and needles; intravenous and percutaneous drug abuse; tattooing; body piercing; acupuncture; laboratory accidents; and accidental inoculation with razors and similar objects that have been contaminated with blood. However, several factors have altered the epidemiological concept that hepatitis B is spread exclusively by blood and blood products. These include the observations that under certain circumstances the virus is infective by mouth, that it is

Table 3.3 Prevalence of hepatitis B

	Northern Europe Western Europe Central Europe North America Australia	Eastern Europe Mediterranean Former USSR South-west Asia Central America South America	Parts of China South-east Asia Sub-Saharan Africa
HBsAg	0.2–0.5%	2–7%	8–20%
Anti-HBs	4–6%	20–55%	70–95%
Neonatal infection	Rare	Frequent	Very frequent
Childhood infection	Infrequent	Frequent	Very frequent

endemic in closed institutions and institutions for the mentally handicapped, that it is more prevalent in adults in urban communities and in poor socio-economic conditions, that there is a huge reservoir of carriers of markers of HBV in the human population, and that the carrier rate and age distribution of the surface antigen vary in different regions. There is much evidence for the transmission of hepatitis B by intimate contact and by the sexual route. Those with frequent changes of sexual partners, particularly male homo-sexuals, are at very high risk. HBsAg has been found in blood and in various body fluids such as saliva, menstrual and vaginal discharges, seminal fluid, colostrum, breast milk and serous exudates, and these have been implicated as vehicles of transmission of infection.

Perinatal Transmission

Viraemic mothers, especially those who are sero-positive for hepatitis B e Antigen (HBeAg), almost invariably transmit the infection to their infants. The mechanism of perinatal infection is uncertain, but it occurs probably during or shortly after birth as a result of a leak of maternal blood into the baby's circulation or of its ingestion or inadvertent inoculation. Such perinatal infections lead to a high rate of chronicity, estimated at around 90%, and individuals infected at such an early age may remain viraemic for decades. Perinatal transmission is an extremely important factor in maintaining the reservoir of the infection in some regions, particularly in China and south-east Asia. There is also a substantial risk of perinatal infection if the mother had acute hepatitis B in the second or third trimester of pregnancy or within 2 months of delivery. Although hepatitis B virus can infect the foetus *in utero*, this appears to be rare and is generally associated with ante-partum haemorrhage and tears

in the placenta. It has been suggested that the soluble HBeAg may cross the placenta and tolerise the foetus *in utero*.

However, mother-to-infant transmission does not account for at least 50% of infections in children, so that horizontal transmission, i.e. child-to-child trans-mission, must be equally important. The prevalence in children is quite low at 1 year of age but increases rapidly thereafter, and in many endemic regions the prevalence reaches a peak in children 7–14 years of age. Clustering of HBV also occurs within family groups, but does not appear to be related to genetic factors and does not reflect maternal or venereal transmission. The probability of a childhood infection becoming persistent declines with age, from around 90% in neonates to less than 5% in adolescence.

Chronic Hepatitis B

Chronic hepatitis B is defined as persistence of HBsAg in the circulation for more than 6 months. The 'carrier state' (the term may be inappropriate) may be lifelong and may be associated with liver damage, varying from mild chronic hepatitis to severe, active hepatitis, cirrhosis and primary liver cancer. Several risk factors have been identified in relation to its development. It is more frequent in males, more likely to follow infec-tions acquired in childhood than those acquired in adult life, and more likely to occur in patients with natural or acquired immune deficiencies. Chronic hepatitis B infection occurs in 90% of neonates or young infants, but in only 1–5% of immunocompetent adults. In countries where hepatitis B infection is common, the highest prevalence of HBsAg is found in young children, with steadily declining rates among older age groups. HBeAg has been reported to be more common in young than in adult carriers of hepatitis B, whereas the prevalence of anti-HBe seems to increase with age.

Survival of HBV is ensured by the reservoir of carriers, estimated to number over 350 million worldwide. The prevalence of carriers, particularly among blood donors, in northern Europe, North America and Australia is 0.1% or less; in central and Eastern Europe up to 5%; in southern Europe, the countries bordering the Mediterranean and parts of Central and South America the frequency is even higher; and in some parts of Africa, Asia and the Pacific region as many as 20% of the apparently healthy population may be HBsAg-positive (Table 3.3). There is an urgent need to introduce methods of interruption of transmission. The management of chronic hepatitis B is complex, with personal, social and economic implications.

Biology

In addition to the human HBV, a number of similar viruses that infect mammals and birds (but are not infectious for humans) have been described and the virus family has been named *Hepadnaviridae* (*hepa*totropic *DNA* viruses). The viruses have a similar genetic organisation and mode of replication and are characterised by a high degree of host specificity and tropism for the liver. Of the mammalian viruses, the *Woodchuck hepatitis virus* (WHV) and Beechey *Ground squirrel hepatitis virus* (GSHV) have been well characterised, the former being of interest as a model system for primary liver cancer because there is a high probability of progression to tumour for WHV-infected woodchucks. Of the avian viruses, the Pekin *Duck hepatitis B virus* (DHBV) has been well characterised and this animal model has been valuable in the elucidation of the hepadnavirus replication process.

Structure of Hepatitis B Virus

Electron microscopy of HBV-positive serum reveals three morphologically distinct forms of particle (Figure 3.8). The small, 22 nm spherical particles and tubular forms of roughly the same diameter are composed of the virus surface protein embedded in lipid and are synthesised in vast excess over the 42 nm, double-shelled virions. The latter comprise a 27 nm, electron-dense core surrounded by HBsAg that is distinct from the subviral particles in that there are

present pre-S1 epitopes (see below). The core or nucleocapsid consists of the genome surrounded by a second protein, hepatitis B core antigen (HBcAg). A third antigen, HBeAg, is found in soluble form in virus-positive sera and is related to the core antigen, as described below. The genome is DNA (Figure 3.9) and comprised of two strands held in a circular configuration by base-pairing at the 5′ ends (cohesive end region). One of the strands is incomplete (usually 50–80% full-length) and is associated with a polymerase which is able to fill in the single-stranded region when provided with suitable substrates.

The genomes of a variety of isolates of HBV have been cloned and the complete nucleotide sequences determined. There is some variation in sequence (up to 12% of nucleotides) between these isolates and up to eight genotypes (A–H) have been described on the basis of >8% nucleotide sequence divergence. However, the genetic organisation and other essential features are conserved. The genome is around 3200 base pairs in length and analysis of the protein coding potential reveals four conserved ORFs, the products of which are described below. These four ORFs are located on the same DNA strand and the strands of the genome have accordingly been designated + (incomplete strand) and − (complete strand), as shown in Figure 3.9. Other features include a motif of 11 base pairs, which is directly repeated near to the 5′ end of each strand of genomic DNA and plays an essential part in the replication strategy, two transcriptional enhancer elements, and binding sites for glucocorticoids and other cellular factors.

Hepatitis B Surface Antigen, HBsAg

The major (or small) surface protein is 226 amino acids long and found in non-glycosylated (p24) and glycosylated (gp27) forms. It is encoded in the 3′ half of the surface ORF and translated from the third of three in-phase initiation codons. Larger, pre-S proteins are translated utilising the two upstream initiation codons; translation from the second results in two intermediate-sized glycoproteins (gp33 and gp36) with a glycosylated 55 amino acid N-terminal extension, the pre-S2 domain. These middle surface proteins are minor components of virions and subviral particles. Translation of the entire ORF (pre-S1 + pre-S2 + S) gives rise to the large surface proteins (p39 and gp42) which are found predominantly in virions and perhaps also the tubular, 22 nm forms. A domain within the pre-S1 region seems to

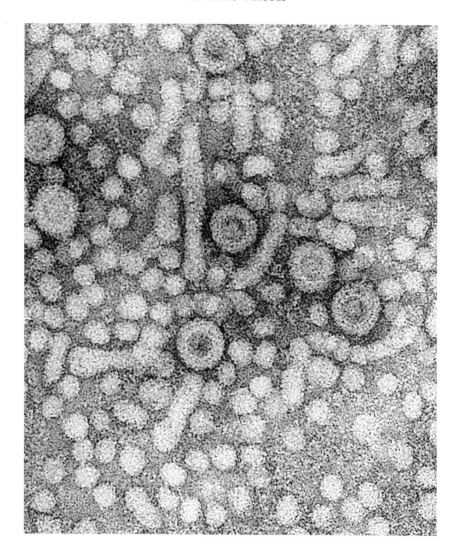

Figure 3.8 Electron micrograph of serum containing HBV after negative staining. The three morphological forms of the antigen are shown: (a) small pleomorphic spherical particles 20–22 nm in diameter (hepatitis B surface antigen); (b) tubular structures (a form of the surface antigen); (c) the 42 nm double-shelled virions, with a core surrounded by the surface antigen (× 300 000). Reproduced by permission from Zuckerman (1975)

be responsible for the attachment of the virus to a receptor on the hepatocyte. Synthesis of the pre-S1 protein also may act as a signal for virion assembly in the infected cell.

The subviral particles and the virion surface are composed of HBsAg anchored in a lipid bilayer derived from the endoplasmic reticulum of the host cell. The major antigenic determinant on the particles is the common, group-specific antigen, *a*, which is believed to form a 'double-loop' structure (aa 124–137 and aa 139–147) on the surfaces of the virions and

subviral particles. The formation of anti-*a* antibodies following vaccination seems to be sufficient to confer protective immunity. The major HBsAg protein also carries a pair of mutually exclusive subdeterminants, *d* or *y* and *w* or *r*, which in each case seem to correlate with variation at single amino acid positions (aa 122 and 160, respectively). Thus, four principal phenotypes of HBsAg are recognised—*adw*, *adr*, *ayw* and, more rarely, *ayr*—and these show differing geographical distribution. For example, in northern Europe the Americas and Australia subtype *adw* predominates,

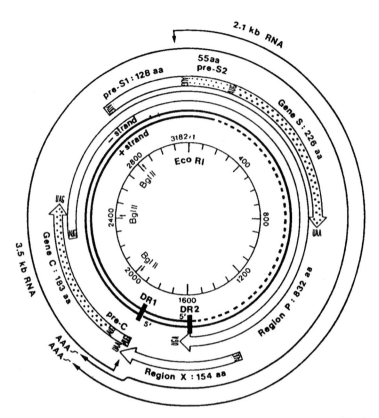

Figure 3.9 Structure and genetic organisation of the HBV genome. The broad arrows surrounding the genome represent the four large open reading frames of the L (−) strand transcript. The number of amino acids (aa) encoded are indicated in each case. The two thin arrows surrounding the broad arrows represent the two major HBV mRNAs. The partial restriction map and the numbering of the nucleotides indicated on the inner circle correspond to the ayw3 genome. DR1 and DR2 are the directly repeated sequences involved in the replication of the genome. Reproduced by permission from Tiollais *et al.* (1985) ©1985 Macmillan Magazines Limited

whilst *ayr* occurs in a broad zone that includes northern and western Africa, the eastern Mediterranean, Eastern Europe, northern and central Asia, and the Indian subcontinent. Both *adw* and *adr* are found in Malaysia, Thailand, Indonesia and Papua New Guinea, whereas subtype *adr* predominates in other parts of south-east Asia, including China, Japan and the Pacific Islands. The subtypes provide useful epidemiological markers of HBV.

Unusual variants which lack the group specific antigen, *a*, may be selected by antibody in immunised infants infected perinatally and in persistently infected individuals following treatment with hepatitis B immune globulin or a natural antibody response. Surface variants of HBV were first described in Italy, infecting children and adults in the presence of specific hepatitis B surface antibodies (anti-HBs) several months after successful immunisation with two generally licensed hepatitis B vaccines given with

and without hepatitis B immunoglobulin (Carman *et al.*, 1990). Epitope mapping of HBsAg in these patients revealed that monoclonal antibodies which normally bind to the *a* determinant failed to bind, suggesting that it was not present or that it was masked. Anti-core antibody was found in these patients. Further work established that, in at least one case, the infection was caused by a variant with a mutation leading to a substitution of arginine for glycine at aa position 145 in the immunodominant domain. This change, which seems to have been selected by antibody, has since been observed independently in the USA (McMahon *et al.*, 1992), Singapore (Harrison *et al.*, 1991) Japan and elsewhere. Other mutations have been described which lead to altered HBsAg, which escapes neutralisation by anti-HBs, but the arginine for glycine substitution at aa 145 seems to be the most common (Oon *et al.*, 1995; Nainan *et al.*, 2002).

Hepatitis B Core Antigen and Other Viral Proteins

The core protein (p22) is the major component of the nucleocapsid and has an arginine-rich domain at its carboxyl terminus, which presumably interacts with the viral nucleic acid. The importance of antibodies to this protein (anti-HBc) in the diagnosis of infection is discussed below. The core protein is translated from the second initiation codon in the core ORF (Figure 3.9). Translation from the upstream initiation codon yields a precursor protein (p25) which is processed to yield HBeAg. The precore region, between the two initiation codons, encodes a signal sequence which directs p25 to the endoplasmic reticulum, where it is cleaved by a cellular signal peptidase. HBeAg is secreted following further proteolysis, which removes the carboxyl-terminal domain. HBeAg is also expressed on the surface of the infected hepatocyte and is a major target for the cellular immune system. HBeAg is not an essential protein of the virus. Variants of HBV with mutations in the precore region (precore mutants), and which are defective for the synthesis of HBeAg, are discussed below.

The P open reading frame, which overlaps the other three, encodes the viral polymerase. This enzyme has both DNA- and RNA-dependent activities and the predicted aa sequence has been shown to have homology with retroviral reverse transcriptases. The polymerase protein also acts as the primer for minus strand DNA synthesis and has an 'RNase H' activity which degrades the RNA pregenome during minus strand synthesis. The fourth open reading frame has been termed X because the function of its product was originally obscure. It is now known that this protein acts as a transcriptional transactivator and may enhance the expression of the other viral proteins. Experiments using the woodchuck model (see above) confirm that a functional X gene is required for the establishment of infection *in vivo*.

Replication of the Virus

The essential elements of the replication strategy of the hepadnavirus genome were elucidated by Summers and Mason (1982) in an elegant series of experiments utilising subviral cores isolated from DHBV-infected duck hepatocytes. The hepadnaviruses are unique among animal DNA viruses in that they replicate through an RNA intermediate (Figure 3.10). On infection of the hepatocyte, the viral DNA is uncoated and converted to a covalently closed circular (super-coiled) form in the nucleus, and this is the template for transcription of the viral RNAs. There are at least four viral promoters and all of the RNAs are 3'-co-terminal, being polyadenylated in response to a signal in the core ORF. The largest RNAs are greater than genome length (ca. 3500 nucleotides) and, whilst some act as mRNAs for the synthesis of HBeAg, HBcAg and the viral polymerase, a subset are intermediates in the synthesis of progeny genomes. Binding of the polymerase to secondary structure at the 5' end (epsilon signal, ε) of the pregenome leads to packaging into immature viral cores in the cytoplasm (Figure 3.10, step 1). The amino-terminal domain of the viral polymerase acts as the primer for minus strand DNA synthesis and, following synthesis of a four nucleotide nascent strand, translocates to a complementary four-base sequence (τ) near to the 3' end of the RNA template (Figure 3.10, steps 2a and 2b) This protein remains covalently attached to the 5'-end of that strand in the mature virion. Minus strand synthesis proceeds by 'reverse transcription' of the pregenome by the viral polymerase, with concomitant degradation of the template (RNase H-like activity; Figure 3.10, step 3). The remaining oligoribonucleotide (which was the 5' end of the pregenome) is at the position of the direct repeat, DR1 (Figure 3.10, step 4), and is now believed to translocate to the other copy of the direct repeat, DR2, on the minus strand and to prime synthesis of the plus strand (Figure 3.10, step 5). The minus strand has a short terminal redundancy (approximately eight nucleotides) which permits the circularisation of the genome as the plus strand is synthesised (Figure 3.10, step 6). Completion of the core presumably starves the polymerase of precursor nucleoside triphosphates, leaving the plus strand incomplete. The cores are then coated with HBsAg to form mature virus particles.

HBV Infection and Chronic Hepatitis B

Following HBV infection, the first marker to appear in the circulation is HBsAg, which becomes detectable 2–8 weeks prior to biochemical evidence of liver damage or the onset of jaundice (Figure 3.11). Next to appear are the markers of the virion, such as the virus-specific DNA polymerase activity and the viral DNA, along with the soluble antigen, HBeAg. Two to four weeks after the appearance of the surface antigen, anti-HBc is detectable and persists throughout infection and after recovery. In acute infections, clearance of the virus is

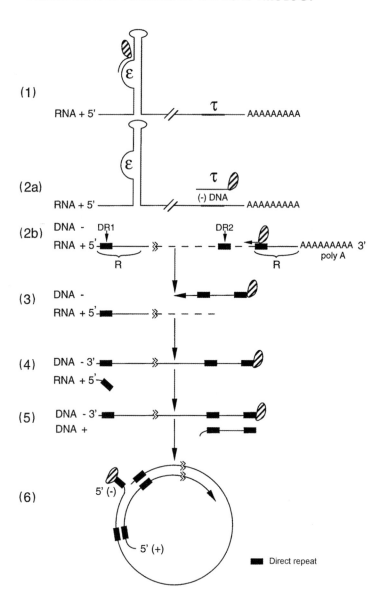

Figure 3.10 The replication strategy of the HBV genome. (1) Priming of minus (−) strand synthesis by the terminal protein (cross-hatched) on the bulge of the ε signal near the 5′ end of 3.5 kb pregenomic RNA. (2a) Translocation of the primer to a position (τ) near the 3′ end of the RNA template. (2b) The template shown as a linear structure; solid boxes indicate the direct repeat (DR) sequences and R the redundancy of the RNA. (3) Minus (−) strand DNA synthesis by reverse transcription with concomitant hydrolysis of the RNA template (RNase H-like activity). (4, 5) Translocation of the remaining 5′ oligoribonucleotide from DR1 to DR2 and priming of plus (+) strand DNA synthesis. (6) Circularisation of the genome through the redundancy in the minus strand and continuation of plus (+) strand synthesis. (Modified from Lien *et al.* (1986) *Journal of Virology*, **57**, 229–236. American Society of Microbiology, Washington)

marked by seroconversion, with the disappearance of HBeAg and the appearance of antibodies to it (anti-HBe). Later, during convalescence, HBsAg also disappears with the production of anti-HBs.

In 2–10% of infected adults and a much larger percentage of children infected perinatally, the immune system fails to clear virus replication and the infection persists. Chronic hepatitis B may be divided into two

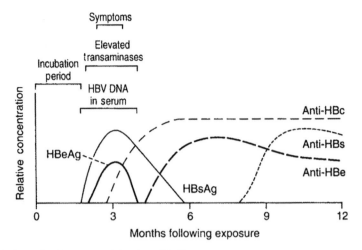

Figure 3.11 Serological profile of acute, resolving hepatitis B

phases (Figure 3.12). In the first, high levels of virus replication occur and the patient is seropositive for markers of the virion and for HBeAg. Although HBeAg correlates with the presence of the virus, in some cases when virus replication declines to very low levels, or when precore mutants are present, seroconversion to anti-HBe may occur without cessation of virus replication. Therefore, direct tests for the virus are more reliable for establishing infectivity, e.g. detection of viral DNA by hybridisation or PCR. During the first phase of chronicity, replicative forms of the HBV genome may be detected in the liver by Southern hybridisation of DNA extracted from biopsy material (Figure 3.13, lane A7). This replicative phase may persist for years, and even for life in individuals who were infected perinatally. More usually, levels of virus replication decline gradually until this is eliminated with seroconversion to anti-HBe. Rarely, there will be seroconversion also to anti-HBs, but in many cases, HBsAg will persist in the absence of virus replication. Examination of liver biopsies from patients in this second phase of chronicity often reveals that HBV DNA is now integrated chromosomally in the hepatocytes (Figure 3.13, lane B) and HBsAg seems to be produced following transcription of this integrated DNA. In fact, integration of virus DNA into the hepatocyte chromosomes seems to take place throughout the period of virus replication, and expansion of clones of such cells may be a stage in progression to neoplasia (see below). Integration of the viral genome is not believed to be required for replication of the virus and may, in fact, be the result of an abortive infection. Although replicative and integrated HBV DNA may sometimes be observed in

an individual biopsy specimen (Figure 3.13, lane C), it is not clear that both may be present in the same cell.

Occurrence of HBV in Extra-hepatic Tissues

As stated above, hepadnaviruses are essentially hepatotropic and it is not clear that they can replicate in other tissues. Sensitive hybridisation techniques have, however, enabled the detection of viral DNA at other sites, particularly in peripheral leukocytes, the bone marrow and spleen. Viral DNA in white blood cells usually occurs as monomeric or multimeric episomes or, rarely, may be integrated, and there have been reports that replicative forms also may be found. These findings have implications for virus transmission and for the possible recurrence of hepatitis B in individuals who have cleared virus replication from the liver.

Diagnostic Assays

Hepatitis B is usually diagnosed following the detection of HBsAg in serum. Current immunoassays for HBsAg detect 100–200 pg HBsAg/ml serum, corresponding to roughly 3×10^7 particles/ml. Most HBeAg-positive carriers have more than 10^5 genomes/ml serum. As noted above, HBeAg is a marker of viraemia but anti-HBe does not necessarily indicate clearance of virus replication. Immunity after infection with HBV is characterised by the presence of anti-HBs together with anti-HBc in serum. Immunity after

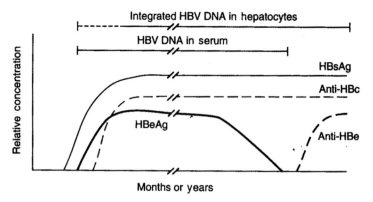

Figure 3.12 Serological profile of chronic hepatitis B with seroconversion

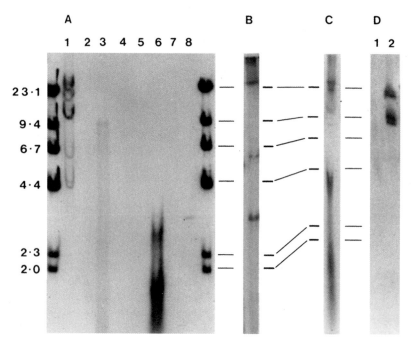

Figure 3.13 Analysis of the state of HBV DNA in the hepatocyte using the Southern blot hybridisation technique. Lane A1, integration of HBV DNA in the PLC/PRF/5 cell line; lane A6, HBV DNA replicative intermediates in the liver biopsy from an HBeAg-positive patient; lane B, integration of HBV DNA in an anti-HBe, HBsAg-positive patient without tumour; lane C, biopsy from an HBeAg-positive patient with both replicative forms and integrated HBV DNA; lanes D, biopsies from an anti-Be, HBsAg-positive patient with primary liver cancer. 1, biopsy from the non-tumourous part of the liver: 2, biopsy from the tumour showing integration of HBV DNA at three sites. All DNA samples were digested with the restriction enqyme *Hind*III. The leftmost lane shows radioactively labelled *Hind*III fragments of bacteriophage DNA as size markers, sizes are given in kilobase pairs alongside. (Modified from Harrison *et al.* (1986) *Journal of Hepatology*, **2**, 1–10. Elsevier Science Publishers BV, Amsterdam)

vaccination is characterised by the presence of anti-HBs alone. Anti-HBc of the IgM class is a valuable marker of acute infection (Table 3.4).

Detection of viral DNA is the optimal method of establishing hepatitis B viraemia and quantitative assays are valuable for monitoring virus loads during

antiviral therapy. Tests based on hybridisation of labelled probes or branched oligonucleotides are reliably quantitative but lack the sensitivity required to monitor the low virus levels achieved during successful therapy with nucleoside analogues. Currently, commercial assays based on real-time

Table 3.4 Interpretation of results of serological tests for hepatitis B

HBsAg	HBeAg	Anti-HBe	Anti-IgM	HBcIgG	Anti-HBs	Interpretation
+	+	−	−	−	−	Incubation period
+	+	−	+	+	−	Acute hepatitis B or persistent carrier state
+	+	−	−	+	−	Persistent carrier state
+	−	+	±	+	−	Persistent carrier state
−	−	+	±	+	+	Convalescence
−	−	−	−	+	−	Recovery
−	−	−	+	−	−	Infection with HBV without detectable HBsAg
−	−	−	−	+	−	Recovery with loss of detectable anti-HBs
−	−	−	−	−	+	Immunisation without infection. Repeated exposure to antigen without infection, or recovery from infection with loss of anti-HBc

PCR combine the requisite sensitivity with a wide dynamic range. Quantitative tests for HBV DNA are limited by a lack of standardisation of the assays and of widely accepted HBV DNA standards. Different assays vary in their sensitivities and linear ranges.

Acute Hepatitis B

The diagnosis of acute hepatitis B generally rests upon the finding of HBsAg and IgM anti-HBc in the serum of a patient with clinical and serum biochemical evidence of acute hepatitis. HBsAg is the first marker to appear in serum, followed by HBV DNA, HBeAg and DNA polymerase, and anti-HBc (Krogsgaard *et al.*, 1985). Levels of HBV DNA usually reach 10^5–10^8 genome equivalents/ml with the onset of symptoms, after which the levels decrease. In contrast, in patients who develop chronic hepatitis B, levels of HBV DNA remain high. A positive IgM anti-HBc test typically distinguishes acute from chronic hepatitis B, (but can be detected, usually at lower levels, in patients with severe chronic hepatitis B). By the time the patient consults a physician, HBV DNA and HBeAg often are no longer detectable in serum. The loss of HBeAg is a sign that the patient will clear HBsAg. HBsAg may be present only transiently in serum. The only evidence of infection may therefore be the presence of IgM anti-HBc or subsequent development of anti-HBc and anti-HBs.

Serum ALT concentrations typically rise in acute hepatitis B. Serum bilirubin concentrations increase in proportion to the severity of hepatic damage. During this phase, IgM anti-HBc in serum correlates with active hepatitis in patients. Antibodies to pre-S components appear early in the disease, and correlate with the disappearance of serological markers of HBV replication, suggesting a role in immunological clearance of HBV (Cupps *et al.*, 1990). Immune complexes may be responsible for some of the manifestations of the acute disease, such as a mild decrease in serum C3 and C4 concentrations. Autoantibodies, including abnormalities in rheumatoid factor, and anti-nuclear and anti-smooth muscle antibodies are also detectable in acute hepatitis.

In fulminant hepatitis B, extremely rapid clearance of HBeAg and HBsAg may occur. Fulminant hepatitis B is a life-threatening form of acute hepatitis B that is complicated by encephalopathy and bleeding due to liver failure. HBsAg may be negative at the time of presentation, and the diagnosis rests on the detection of IgM anti-HBc.

Chronic Hepatitis B

Many carriers are detected through routine screening for HBsAg or the presence of abnormal liver function tests. Older patients may present for the first time with complications of cirrhosis, or even hepatocellular carcinoma. Typically the levels of serum aminotransferases are elevated in patients with HBeAg, HBV DNA-positive chronic hepatitis, but some patients may have normal values. Many patients go on to develop moderate to severe HBeAg positive chronic hepatitis with raised serum ALT after several decades of infection, which can ultimately progress to cirrhosis. The levels of aminotransferases fluctuate with time.

Several phases of chronic hepatitis can be recognised. Typically in the immunotolerant phase, serum HBsAg and HBeAg are detectable; serum HBV DNA levels are high (usually $> 10^7$ copies/ml) serum aminotransferases are normal or minimally elevated. This phase is common in the young who are infected in the neonatal period, and may last 10–30 years after perinatal HBV infection. The immunotolerant phase is frequently followed by an 'immunoactive' phase, when symptoms of hepatitis may be present and serum aminotransferase levels are elevated. Exacerbations in serum aminotransferases may be observed, accompanied by a decrease in serum HBV DNA levels and ultimately followed by HBeAg seroconversion (i.e. HBeAg becomes undetectable, and anti-HBe detectable, in serum). Seroconversion rates are higher in those with raised serum ALT, and in patients with genotype D and (in Asia) genotype B infection. Seroconversion may occur following a sudden, asymptomatic exacerbation in serum aminotransferases. Once HBeAg is cleared, the disease remits temporarily and serum aminotransferases become normal.

Chronic hepatitis also may be observed in HBeAg-negative patients in whom HBsAg and anti-HBe are present in serum and serum HBV DNA is detectable using non-PCR-based methods; serum aminotransferase levels are elevated and liver biopsy shows necroinflammation. HBeAg is undetectable in these patients because of the predominance of mutant HBV genomes that cannot express HBeAg. Patients with HBeAg-negative (also called pre-core mutant) chronic hepatitis tend to be older, male, and to present with severe necro-inflammation and cirrhosis (Hadziyannis et al., 1983). HBeAg-negative chronic hepatitis has a variable course, often with fluctuating serum aminotransferases and serum HBV DNA levels. HBeAg may also become detectable transiently in these patients during acute flares. It is now known that such patients frequently are infected with variants of HBV with mutations in the precore region and which cannot synthesise HBeAg (Carman et al., 1989). In some cases, these patients may have been infected initially with a mixture of wild-type and variant virus, with clearance of the wild-type on seroconversion to anti-HBe. Precore variants may be selected during the process of seroconversion to anti-HBe, when hepatocytes expressing HBeAg are targeted for lysis by cytotoxic T cells. Different patterns of anti-HBe-positive disease can be discerned, but typically patients tend to have recurrent flares. Precore mutants can be detected in patients with fulminant hepatitis B but it is controversial whether infection with these variants ab initio, in the absence of wild-type virus, often leads to acute liver failure. Not all patients with fulminant hepatitis B are infected with precore mutants; other mutations, such as in the core promoter (Sterneck et al., 1996), as well as host factors, may be important. Hepatitis B viruses with double mutations in the core promoter have been associated with primary liver cancer in some regions of the world (Fang et al., 2002).

A spontaneous remission in disease activity may occur in approximately 10–15%/year of HBeAg positive carriers, characterised by the disappearance of detectable (by molecular hybridisation) HBV DNA from serum, followed by loss of HBeAg and seroconversion to anti-HBe. The inactive carrier state is characterised by very low serum HBV DNA levels in serum ($< 10^5$ copies/ml) and normal serum aminotransferases. Liver biopsies are not performed routinely in inactive HBsAg carriers but usually show little or no necroinflammation and mild or no fibrosis (although inactive cirrhosis may be present if transition to an inactive carrier state has occurred after many years). The prognosis of these patients, if stable without pre-existing advanced disease, is benign. However, a proportion of patients will develop active viral replication and raised ALT. Chronic hepatitis histologically is always associated with viral replication. If low levels of replication persist, serum HBsAg may become undetectable in serum and anti-HBs detectable. HBsAg may be lost in 1–2%/year of patients. However, a proportion of anti-HBe-positive individuals with low levels of HBV DNA may later develop higher levels of HBV replication and raised ALT and progress to HBeAg-negative chronic hepatitis.

Several genotypes (A–H) of HBV may be distinguished on the basis of DNA sequencing. HBV genotypes have been reported to correlate with spontaneous and interferon induced HBeAg seroconversion, activity of liver disease, and progression to cirrhosis and HCC, but further study is required. In China and Japan, where genotypes B and C circulate, there is evidence for increased pathogenicity, and likelihood of development of HCC, of genotype C over B.

Liver biopsy assessment by an experienced pathologist is considered to be an integral investigation by many hepatologists. The biopsy can be used to assess the progression of the disease and response to antiviral therapy. Normal concentrations of albumin, ALT and AST can be encountered in patients with established cirrhosis.

In HBeAg-positive patients, progression to cirrhosis occurs at an annual rate of 2–5.5%, with a cumulative

5 year incidence of progression of 8–20%. Progression to cirrhosis is generally faster in HBeAg-negative patients, at an annual rate of 8–20%. Recurrent exacerbations and bridging fibrosis with severe necroinflammatory change characterise patients more likely to progress. Recent retrospective studies have examined survival in compensated cirrhosis due to hepatitis B. The reported yearly incidence of hepatic decompensation is about 3%, with a 5 year cumulative incidence of 16%. In a European multicentre longitudinal study to assess the survival of 366 cases of HBsAg-positive compensated cirrhosis, death occurred in 23% of patients, mainly due to liver failure or hepatocellular carcinoma. The cumulative probability of survival in this cohort was 84% and 68% at 5 and 10 years, respectively. The worst survival was in HBeAg- and HBV DNA-positive subjects (Fattovich *et al.*, 1997). Chinese patients remaining HBeAg-positive were more likely to develop HCC.

Occult Hepatitis B

Occult hepatitis B (reviewed by Torbenson and Thomas, 2002) is defined as the presence of (usually low) levels of HBV DNA in serum in the absence of detectable HBsAg. Anti-HBc and/or anti-HBs may be present but are undetectable in a significant percentage of cases. Occult hepatitis B is of particular concern in individuals who are infected with HCV and in whom there is a high risk of development of advanced fibrosis and cirrhosis. The reported incidence in patients with hepatitis C varies from 0% in the UK to as high as 70–95% in Japan. There are several reports of HBV genomic sequences from such infections and a variety of mutations have been detected, including in the core promoter and surface open reading frame.

Pathogenesis of Hepatitis B Infection

HBV is not cytopathic to hepatocytes under most circumstances. Host immunity plays an important role in cellular injury and there is little correlation between the severity of the illness and the level of HBV replication. Patients with a poor T cell response may have high concentrations of virus in the liver, yet mild disease. The development of chronic infection is due to a failure of an adequate immune response, but the immune response is also responsible for disease pathogenesis during chronic infection. The subsequent expression of the disease involves a poorly understood interplay between viral and host factors. The nucleocapsid antigens (HBcAg and HBeAg) expressed on the cell membrane contain important targets of the immune response and cytotoxic T cells in acute hepatitis B.

Studies using transgenic mice and of acute hepatitis B in chimpanzees suggest that antiviral mechanisms of clearance of HBV may involve both targeted lysis of infected hepatocytes and inhibition of viral replication by non-cytolytic mechanisms (Guilhot *et al.*, 1993; Cavanaugh *et al.*, 1997; Guidotti and Chisari, 2001).

Intense hepatocyte lysis occurs in acute hepatitis B, apparently as a result of a polyclonal, multispecific cytotoxic lymphocyte immune response. The specific epitopes recognised by B as well as T cells are currently being mapped. However, experimental studies in the transgenic mouse model suggest that HBV replication also may be reduced by a complex interplay of cytotoxic T cell responses, apoptosis and downregulation of hepatitis B gene expression by several inflammatory cytokines. An association of MHC class II alleles (DRB*1302) with lack of persistent HBV infection has been reported (Thursz *et al.*, 1995).

The elimination of virus-infected hepatocytes is dependent on the recognition by cytotoxic T cells of viral determinants, in association with HLA proteins on the infected cells. Data derived from most experimental systems suggest that an acute, polyclonal and vigorous cytolytic T cell response usually occurs in acute symptomatic icteric hepatitis B, and that patients with acute self-limiting hepatitis B develop a polyclonal HLA class I restricted, cytotoxic T cell response against numerous epitopes in the HBV envelope, nucleocapsid and polymerase proteins. Several HLA-A2 restricted cytotoxic T cell epitopes have been defined.

Perinatal infection is almost always asymptomatic, and chronic infection ensues in 90% of cases. Rarely, infection acquired from an anti-HBe-positive mother may lead to severe hepatitis in the infant. The failure to eradicate HBV reflects an inadequate immune response to the virus, but the precise impairment of humoral and cellular immunity that determines the development and outcome of hepatitis B has not been characterised. Persistent infection is an unusual outcome in those patients with acute icteric hepatitis B and the mechanisms that lead to viral persistence are not well understood. In neonates, specific suppression of the cell-mediated immune response may favour infection, perhaps because of intrauterine exposure to HBeAg inducing tolerance to epitopes that are usually the target of the cytotoxic T cell response at a time when the immune system is immature. Clonal deletion of HBV-specific T cells may occur as a consequence of transplacental infection of the developing foetus or transplacental passage of viral antigens. In contrast to the vigorous polyclonal class I- and class II-restricted T cell response that can be identified in patients with acute icteric hepatitis B, in chronic disease the response in peripheral blood is relatively weak and focused, and insufficient to clear replicating virus.

Other mechanisms may also operate to prevent clearance of HBV: mutations abrogating the recognition of the wild-type hepatitis, including the natural variants of the HBcAg 18–27 core epitope that interfere with the recognition of the wild-type epitope and act as T cell receptor antagonists (Bertoletti et al., 1994). There is some evidence of a failure of interferon production in patients with chronic hepatitis B.

Prevention and Control of Hepatitis B

Passive Immunisation

Hepatitis B immunoglobulin (HBIG) is prepared from pools of plasma with high titres of anti-HBs and may confer temporary passive immunity under certain defined conditions. The major indication for the administration of HBIG is a single acute exposure to HBV, such as occurs when blood containing HBsAg is inoculated, ingested or splashed onto mucous membranes and the conjunctiva. The optimal dose has not been established but doses in the range of 250–600 IU have been used effectively. HBIG should be administered as early as possible after exposure and preferably within 48 h, usually 3 ml (containing 200 IU anti-HBs/ml) in adults. It should not be administered 7 days or more after exposure. It is generally recommended that two doses of HBIG should be given 30 days apart.

Results following the use of HBIG for prophylaxis in babies at risk of infection with HBV are encouraging if the immunoglobulin is given as soon as possible, and certainly within 12 h of birth. The dose of HBIG recommended in the newborn is 1–2 ml (200 IU anti-HBs/ml).

Active Immunisation

The major response of recipients of hepatitis B vaccine is to the common a determinant with consequent protection against all subtypes of the virus. First-generation vaccines were prepared from 22 nm HBsAg particles purified from plasma donations from asymptomatic (healthy) chronic carriers. These preparations are safe and immunogenic, but have been superseded in many countries by recombinant vaccines produced by the expression of HBsAg in yeast cells. The expression plasmid contains only the 3′ portion of the HBV surface ORF and only the major surface protein, without pre-S epitopes, is produced. Vaccines containing pre-S2 and pre-S1 as well as the major surface proteins expressed by recombinant DNA technology are available.

In many areas of the world with a high prevalence of HBsAg carriage, such as China and south-east Asia, the predominant route of transmission is perinatal. Administration of a course of vaccine, with the first dose immediately after birth, is effective in preventing transmission from an HBeAg-positive mother in approximately 70% of cases, and this protective efficacy rate may be increased to >90% if the vaccine is accompanied by the simultaneous administration of HBIG.

Immunisation against hepatitis B is now recognised as a high priority in preventive medicine in all countries and strategies for immunisation are being revised. Universal vaccination of infants and adolescents is recommended as a strategy to control the transmission of this infection. More than 150 countries now offer hepatitis B vaccine to all children, including the USA, Canada, Italy, France and most western European countries (Van Damme and Vorsters, 2002). Young infants, children, health care workers and susceptible persons (including travellers) living in certain tropical and sub-tropical areas where present socioeconomic conditions are poor and the prevalence of hepatitis B is high should also be immunised. It should be noted that in about 30% of patients with hepatitis B the mode of infection is not known and this is, therefore, a powerful argument for universal immunisation.

However, immunisation against hepatitis B is at present recommended in a number of countries with a low prevalence of hepatitis B only to groups which are at an increased risk of acquiring this infection. These groups include individuals requiring repeated transfusions of blood or blood products, prolonged in-patient treatment, patients who require frequent tissue penetration or need repeated circulatory access, patients with natural or acquired immune deficiency and patients with malignant diseases. Viral hepatitis is an occupational hazard among health care personnel and the staff of institutions for the mentally retarded and in some semi-closed institutions. High rates of infection with hepatitis B occur in narcotic drug addicts and intravenous drug abusers, sexually active male homosexuals and prostitutes.

Site of Injection for Vaccination and Antibody Response

Hepatitis B vaccination should be given in the upper arm or the anterolateral aspect of the thigh and not in the buttock. Many studies have shown that the antibody response rate was significantly higher in centres using deltoid injection than centres using the buttock. On the basis of antibody tests after vaccination, the Advisory Committee on Immunization Practices of the Centers of Disease Control, USA, recommended that the arm be used as the site for hepatitis B vaccination in adults, as have the Departments of Health in the UK.

Non-response to Current Hepatitis B Vaccines

Studies of the antibody response to the plasma-derived and recombinant DNA vaccines containing only the single antigen have shown that 5–10% or more of healthy immunocompetent subjects do not mount an anti-HBs antibody response to the surface antigen component present in these preparations (non-responders), or that they respond poorly (hyporesponders) (Zuckerman, 1996; Zuckerman *et al.*, 1997). Non-responders remain susceptible to infection with HBV.

While several factors are known to adversely affect the antibody response to HBsAg, including the site and route of injection, gender, advancing age, body mass (overweight), immunosuppression and immunodeficiency, evidence is accumulating that there is, at least in part, an association between immunogenetics and specific low responsiveness in different populations. Considerable experimental evidence is available suggesting that the ability to produce antibody in response to specific protein antigens is controlled by dominant autosomal class II genes of the major histocompatibility complex (MHC) in the murine model and in humans. Other mechanisms underlying non-responsiveness to current hepatitis single antigen vaccines remain largely unexplained.

The Kinetics of Anti-HBs Response to Immunisation and Booster Doses

The titre of vaccine-induced anti-HBs declines, often rapidly, during the months and years following a complete course of primary immunisation. The highest anti-HBs titres are generally observed 1 month after booster vaccination, followed by rapid decline during the next 12 months and thereafter more slowly. Mathematical models have been designed and an equation was derived consisting of several exponential terms with different half-life periods. It is considered by some researchers that the decline of anti-HBs concentration in an immunised subject can be predicted accurately by such antibody kinetics, with preliminary recommendations on whether or not booster vaccination is necessary (see review by Zuckerman, 1996).

If the minimum protection level is accepted at 10 IU/l, consideration should be given to the diversity of the individual immune response and the decrease in levels of anti-HBs, as well as to possible errors in quantitative anti-HBs determinations. It would then be reasonable to define a level of >10 IU/l and <100 IU/l as an indication for booster immunisation. It has been demonstrated that a booster inoculation results in a rapid increase in anti-HBs titres within 4 days. However, it should be noted that even this time delay might permit infection of hepatocytes.

Several options are therefore under consideration for maintaining protective immunity against hepatitis B infection:

- Relying upon immunological memory to protect against clinical infection and its complications, a view which is supported by *in vitro* studies showing immunological memory for HBsAg in B cells derived from vaccinated subjects who have lost their anti-HBs, but not in B cells from non-responders, and by post-vaccination surveys.
- Providing booster vaccination to all vaccinated subjects at regular intervals without determination of anti-HBs. This option is not supported by a number of investigators because non-responders must be detected. While an anti-HBs titre of about 10 IU/l may be protective, this level is not ideal from a laboratory point of view, since many serum samples may give non-specific reactions at this antibody level.
- Testing anti-HBs levels 1 month after the first booster and administering the next booster before the minimum protective level is reached.

No empirical data are available for the anti-HBs titre required for protection against particular routes of infection or the size of the infectious inoculum. The minimum protective level has been set at 10 IU/l against an international standard. However, the international standard is a preparation of immunoglobulin prepared from pooled plasma of individuals recovered from infection, rather than immunised subjects, and the antibody avidity is likely to be different. Furthermore, studies carried out in the 1980s indicated asymptomatic infection after immunisation in subjects and health care workers who had antibody titres below 50 IU/l.

There are studies showing that hepatitis B vaccine provides a high degree of protection against clinical symptomatic disease in immunocompetent persons, despite declining levels of anti-HBs (reviewed by Zuckerman and Zuckerman, 1998). These studies encouraged the Immunization Practices Advisory Committee of the United States, the National Advisory Committee on Immunisation of Canada and the European Consensus Group (2000) to recommend that routine booster immunisation against hepatitis B is not required. However, caution dictates that those at high risk of exposure, such as cardiothoracic surgeons and gynaecologists, would be prudent to maintain a titre of 100 IU/l of anti-HBs by booster inoculations, more so in the absence of an appropriate international antibody reference preparation. Breakthrough infections have been reported and, whereas long-term follow-up of children and adults indicated that protection is attained for at least 9 years after immunisation against chronic hepatitis B infection, even though anti-HBs levels may have become low or declined below detectable levels (reviewed by the European Consensus Group, 2000), brief periods of viraemia may not have been detected because of infrequent testing. Longer follow-up studies of immunised subjects are required to guide policy, as is well illustrated by a study carried out in Gambian children. Whittle *et al.* (2002) found, by a cross-sectional study in The Gambia, that the efficacy of hepatitis B vaccination against chronic carriage of HBV 14 years after immunisation was 94%, and the efficacy against infection was 80% and lower (65%) in those vaccinated at the age of 15–19 years. Further and longer follow-up studies of immunised subjects are therefore required to guide policy.

Hepatitis B Surface Antigen Variants

There is evidence that amino acid substitutions within the *a* determinant of the surface antigen can allow replication of HBV in vaccinated persons, since antibodies induced by the current vaccine do not recognise critical changes in the surface antigen domain. The emergence of variants of HBV, possibly due to selection pressure associated with extensive immunisation in an endemic area, was suggested by the findings of hepatitis B infection in individuals immu-

nised successfully (Zanetti *et al.*, 1988). These studies were extended subsequently by the finding of non-complexed HBsAg and anti-HBs and other markers of hepatitis B infection in 32 of 44 vaccinated subjects, and sequence analysis from one of these cases revealed a mutation in the nucleotide encoding the a determinant, the consequence of which was a substitution from glycine to arginine at amino acid position 145 (G145R) (Carman *et al.*, 1990).

Various mutations and variants of HBsAg have since been reported from many countries, including Italy, the UK, Holland, Germany, the USA, Brazil, Singapore, Taiwan, China, Japan, Thailand, India, West and South Africa (reviewed by Zuckerman and Zuckerman, 1999; Francois *et al.*, 2001). However, the most frequent and stable mutation was reported in the G145R variant. A large study in Singapore of 345 infants born to carrier mothers with HBsAg and HBeAg, who received HBIG at birth and plasma-derived hepatitis B vaccine within 24 h of birth and then 1 and 2 months later, revealed 41 breakthrough infections with HBV despite the presence of anti-HBs (Oon *et al.*, 1996). There was no evidence of infection among 670 immunised children born to carrier mothers with HBsAg and anti-HBe, nor in any of 107 immunised infants born to mothers without HBsAg. The most frequent variant was a virus with the G145R mutation in the *a* determinant. Another study in the USA of serum samples collected between 1981 and 1993 showed that 94 (8.6%) of 1092 infants born to carrier mothers became HBsAg-positive despite post-exposure prophylaxis with hepatitis B immunoglobulin and hepatitis B vaccine. Following amplification of HBV DNA, 22 children were found with mutations of the surface antigen, most being in aa 142–145; five had a mixture of wild-type HBV and variants and 17 had only the 145 variant (Nainan *et al.*, 1997).

A report from Taiwan (Hsu *et al.*, 1999) noted the increase in the prevalence of mutants of the *a* determinant of HBV over a period of 10 years in immunised children, from eight of 103 (7.8%) in 1984 to 10 of 51 (19.6%) in 1989, and 9 of 32 (28.1%) in 1994. This is of particular concern. The prevalence of HBsAg mutants among those fully immunised was higher than among those not vaccinated (12/33 vs. 15/153, $p = 0.0003$). In the 27 children with detectable mutants, the mean age of those vaccinated was lower than of those not vaccinated, and mutation occurred in a region with greatest hydrophilicity of the surface antigen (aa 140–149) and more frequently among those vaccinated than among those not vaccinated. More mutations to the neutralising epitopes were found in the 1994 survey in Taiwan (Hsu *et al.*, 1999).

Another important aspect is the evidence that HBsAg mutants may not be detected by all of the blood donor screening tests and by existing diagnostic reagents. Such variants may therefore enter the blood supply or spread by other means. This is emphasised by the finding in Singapore, between 1990 and 1992, of 0.8% of carriers of HBV variants in a random population survey of 2001 people (Oon et al., 1995, 1996). These findings add to the concern expressed in a study of mathematical models of HBV vaccination, which predict, on the assumption of no cross-immunity against the variant by current vaccines, that the variant will not become dominant over the wild-type virus for at least 50 years—but the G145R mutant may emerge as the common HBV in 100 (or more) years' time (Wilson et al., 1999).

It is important, therefore, to institute epidemiological monitoring of HBV surface mutants, employing test reagents which have been validated for detection of the predominant mutations, and consideration should be given to incorporating into current hepatitis B vaccines antigenic components which will confer protection against infection by the predominant mutant(s) (Zuckerman, 2000).

The Pre-S1 and Pre-S2 Domains and Third-generation Vaccines

There is evidence that the pre-S1 and pre-S2 domains of the surface antigen have an important immunogenic role in augmenting anti-HBs responses, preventing the attachment of the virus to hepatocytes and eliciting antibodies which are effective in viral clearance, stimulating cellular immune responses and circumventing genetic non-responsiveness to the S antigen.

These observations led to the development of a new triple antigen hepatitis B vaccine (Hepacare), a third-generation recombinant DNA vaccine containing pre-S1, pre-S2 and S antigenic components of hepatitis B virus surface antigen of both subtypes adw and ayw. All three antigenic components are glycosylated, closely mimicking the surface protein of the virus itself, produced in a continuous mammalian cell line, the mouse c127 clonal cell line, after transfection of the cells with recombinant HBsAg DNA. The vaccine is presented as an aluminium hydroxide adjuvant preparation of purified antigenic protein. Animal studies showed that the vaccine was well tolerated and a viral challenge study in chimpanzees demonstrated protective efficacy.

This vaccine was evaluated for reactogenicity and immunogenicity in a number of clinical trials (reviewed by Zuckerman and Zuckerman, 2002). The major conclusions from these studies were that the vaccine was safe and immunogenic and overcame the non-responsiveness to the single S antigen vaccines used widely in some 70% of non-responders, and that even a single dose of 20 μg of the triple antigen provided significant seroprotection levels of antibody.

However, the anticipated high costs of the triple antigen vaccine will limit the use of the triple antigen vaccine initially to the following groups:

- Vaccination of non-responders to the current single antigen(s) vaccines, who are at risk of exposure to HBV infection.
- Subjects with inadequate humoral immune response to single antigen hepatitis B vaccines, e.g. those over the age of 40 years, males, obese, smokers and other hyporesponders.
- Persons who require protection rapidly, e.g. health care employment involving potential exposure to parenteral procedures involving blood-to-blood contact (conventional schedules of immunisation with single antigen hepatitis B vaccines involve three doses at 0, 1 and 6 months, although accelerated schedules are also available).

Studies are required to determine the efficacy of the triple antigen vaccine in patients who are immunocompromised, and also to determine whether the inclusion of pre-S1 and pre-S2 antigenic components in this new vaccine will protect against the emergence of HBV surface antigen mutants.

Combined Immunoprophylaxis

Whenever immediate protection is required, e.g. for infants born to HBsAg-positive mothers (see above) or after accidental inoculation of non-immunised individuals, active immunisation with the vaccine should be combined with simultaneous administration of hepatitis B immunoglobulin at a different site. It has been shown that passive immunisation with up to 3 ml (200 IU of anti-HBs/ml) of HBIG does not interfere with an active immune response. A single dose of HBIG (usually 3 ml for adults; 1–2 ml for the newborn) is sufficient for healthy individuals. If infection has already occurred at the time of the first immunisation, virus multiplication is unlikely to be inhibited completely but severe illness and, most importantly, the development of the carrier state of HBV may be prevented in many individuals, particularly in infants born to carrier mothers.

Indications for Immunisation Against Hepatitis B

The current indications for the use of hepatitis B vaccines in the UK are given below. Many countries, including the USA and Italy, introduced universal immunisation for infants in 1992. The World Health Organisation recommended a decade ago that universal immunisation should be in place in areas with a prevalence of HBsAg greater than 8% by 1994 and in all countries by 1997, with integration of hepatitis B vaccine into the Expanded Programme of Immunization (EPI). These targets were not met and universal immunisation of infants worldwide remains a goal.

In 1996 the Department of Health and other government offices in the UK recommended immunisation for the following risk groups:

- Babies born to mothers who are chronic carriers of hepatitis B virus or to mothers who have had acute hepatitis B during pregnancy. In addition, babies born to mothers who are HBeAg-positive, who are HBsAg-positive without e markers (or where HBeAg/anti-HBe status has not been determined), or who have had acute hepatitis B during pregnancy should receive HBIG as well as active immunisation. Currently, vaccine without HBIG is recommended for babies born to mothers who are HBsAg-positive but known to be anti-HBe-positive.
- Parenteral drug misusers.
- Close family contacts of a case or carrier. Sexual contacts of patients with acute hepatitis B should also receive HBIG.
- Families adopting children from countries with a high prevalence of hepatitis B, particularly some countries in Eastern Europe, SE Asia and S America.
- Haemophiliacs (and others receiving regular blood transfusions or blood products), including carers responsible for the administration of such products.
- Patients with chronic renal failure. Higher doses of vaccine may be required in those who are immunocompromised.
- Health care workers, including students and trainees.
- Staff and students of residential accommodation for those with severe learning disabilities.
- Other occupational risk groups, including certain members of the emergency and prison services.
- Inmates of custodial institutions.
- Those travelling to areas of high prevalence.

Despite the availability of a vaccine, infection persists worldwide. In populous regions where mass immunisation has not started, there has not been a significant decline in HBsAg carrier rates, and therefore the carrier pool has increased with the increase in population. Nonetheless, notable successes through vaccination have emerged, particularly in Taiwan and Alaska. In Taiwan, the long-awaited impact of vaccination on the risk of hepatocellular carcinoma has been discernible (Chang et al., 1997).

Antiviral Therapy for Hepatitis B

Acute Hepatitis B

Most icteric patients with acute hepatitis B resolve their infection and do not require treatment. Fulminant hepatitis B is a severe form of acute infection complicated by encephalopathy and liver failure. Subgroups of fulminant hepatitis B, including hyperacute, acute and subacute, are defined by the interval between jaundice and encephalopathy. Subacute hepatic necrosis is characterised by a more protracted acute course and transition to chronic hepatitis with ongoing HBV replication. Patients with fulminant hepatitis (including acute and subacute forms) should be considered for liver transplantation, if appropriate. There are no controlled trials of lamivudine or adefovir for patients with acute fulminant or subacute fulminant hepatitis. Anecdotal reports suggest some efficacy of lamivudine in these patients, and carefully administered therapy could be tried, if administered early, and if there is evidence of ongoing HBV replication.

Chronic Hepatitis B

There is no established consensus as to which patients should be treated. Current treatments of chronic hepatitis B have limited long-term efficacy. In general, treatment of chronic hepatitis B should be targeted at patients with active disease and viral replication, preferably at a stage before signs and symptoms of cirrhosis or significant injury have occurred (Dusheiko et al., 1985). Eradication of the infection is possible in only a minority of patients. However, if HBV replication can be suppressed, the accompanying reduction in histological chronic active hepatitis lessens the risk of cirrhosis and hepatocellular carcinoma (Niederau et al., 1996).

Patients with mild chronic hepatitis should be monitored carefully at appropriate intervals. Therapy should be considered only if there is evidence of moderate to severe activity. HBeAg-positive patients should be followed for a few months to ascertain their status, and antiviral therapy should be considered if there is active HBV replication (HBV DNA above 10^5 copies/ml) and persistent elevation of aminotransferases after 3–6 months of observation. HBeAg-negative patients should be considered for antiviral therapy when the serum aminotransferases are raised and there is active viral replication (HBV DNA above 10^5 copies/ml). Many clinicians would consider a liver biopsy helpful for ascertaining the degree of necro-inflammation and fibrosis.

HIV and HBV co-infected patients whose immune status is preserved on highly active antiretroviral therapy (HAART) should be considered for anti-HBV therapy, with appropriate therapy for HIV infection to minimise resistance. If HAART is indicated for a patient co-infected with HIV, lamivudine can be utilised, as lamivudine is active against HIV and HBV. Adefovir also has activity against both viruses, although a lower dose is used for HBV. Tenofovir also is active against HBV and HIV; however, the efficacy of tenofovir in hepatitis B infection has not been elucidated in large controlled trials.

HBsAg-positive patients with extrahepatic manifestations and active HBV replication may respond to antiviral therapy. Patients with decompensated cirrhosis should be treated in specialist liver units, as the application of antiviral therapy is complex.

Prophylactic therapy is recommended for all patients undergoing liver transplantation for end-stage hepatitis B, to lower levels of HBV DNA to less than 10^5 copies/ml before transplantation. The optimal timing of transplantation has not been established, but selection of resistant strains before surgery should be avoided. Lamivudine and adefovir are suitable agents. Antiviral therapy for prophylaxis of recurrence post-transplantation probably requires lifelong continuation of treatment. The most promising prophylaxis, lamivudine together with lifelong HBIG treatment after transplantation, results in low rates of reinfection/reactivation after liver transplantation. Shorter courses of HBIG and other forms of prophylaxis, including adefovir in combination with lamivudine, are being studied. The optimal treatments for hepatitis B, including suitable combination therapies, are currently being evaluated. Response rates in HBeAg-positive patients are higher for all currently licensed agents for those patients with higher baseline ALT. Interferon remains a benchmark therapy for chronic hepatitis B. Approximately 35–40% of

HBeAg-positive patients are treated effectively by this agent, at a dose of 5–10 million IU/three times weekly (5 MIU daily in the USA) for 4–6 months. For HBeAg-positive patients, a 4–6 month course of interferon-α (IFN-α) can be considered. The subclinical exacerbation of the hepatitis and increases in serum aminotransferases frequently seen in responders suggests that IFN acts by augmenting the immune response to HBV, perhaps triggered by the inhibition of viral replication, the effects of IFN on cytotoxic T cells and the upregulation of MHC class I display. The rationale of first-line treatment with IFN-α is to achieve loss of HBeAg (and even subsequent loss of HBsAg) after a short, finite course of treatment. Sustained loss of HBeAg is generally associated with histological reduction in inflammation. Longer-term follow-up of responders shows that up to 65% of those who lose HBeAg become HBsAg-negative (Korenman et al., 1991; Lau et al., 1997). There are alternative options and strategies for treatment. Lamivudine can be given [100 mg daily for at least 1 year and maintained for 4–6 months after a virological response (loss of HBeAg) is achieved]. Loss of HBsAg has been observed. If a virological response is not achieved within 1 year, the likelihood that continuation of treatment will produce a response is offset by the cumulative risk of developing drug resistance over time. Therapy remains useful if HBV DNA is suppressed (histological improvement has been documented), but should be modified if a 1 log increase in HBV DNA is observed. Adefovir 10 mg daily is an effective alternative for lamivudine. As with lamivudine, the majority of patients do not show a virological response after 1 year. Adefovir can be given at a dose of 10 mg daily for at least 1 year, and maintained for 4–6 months after a virological response (loss of HBeAg) is achieved). Unlike lamivudine, the likelihood that continuation of treatment will produce a virological response is not apparently offset by the cumulative risk of developing drug resistance over time. Therapy remains useful if HBV DNA is suppressed (histological improvement has been documented). Long-term use of adefovir monotherapy (>2 years) will require monitoring for resistance and nephrotoxicity, because these data are not available.

For patients with HBeAg-negative moderate or severe chronic hepatitis, long-term treatment will be necessary for those treated with IFN-α, lamivudine or adefovir, because relapse rates are high when treatment is stopped. Approximately 10–25% of patients have long-term responses to treatment with IFN-α at doses of 9–10 MIU thrice weekly for 6–12 months (Brunetto et al., 1989).

Suppressive treatment aimed at reducing HBV DNA concentrations to delay histological progression may be the more realistic goal of treatment (these patients already are HBeAg-negative). Loss of HBsAg is highly unusual in these patients during or after treatment. Because most patients will require treatment for longer than 1 year, and perhaps for long periods to time, drug tolerance and resistance are important considerations. For young patients without advanced liver disease, a 12-month course of IFN-α, 5–6 or 9–10 MU thrice weekly, could be considered. The drug should be stopped at 1 year. Lamivudine or adefovir are alternatives, but it should be pointed out that long-term, rather than a finite course of treatment, will be required. Lamivudine can be given at a dose of 100 mg daily for at least 1 year. Suppression of HBV DNA is associated with histological improvement. The majority of anti-HBe-positive patients relapse if lamivudine is stopped after 1 year, despite suppression of HBV DNA, resistance being the major disadvantage of lamivudine monotherapy. Treatment should be continued until resistance occurs (greater than one log increase in DNA, or the hepatitis relapses on therapy). If resistance occurs, treatment with adefovir should be introduced. Similarly, Adefovir 10 mg daily is an effective substitute for either lamivudine or IFN monotherapy as a first-line therapy. Suppression of HBV DNA is associated with histological improvement. A high threshold of resistance is the major advantage of adefovir monotherapy in anti-HBe positive disease. Treatment should be continued while HBV DNA is suppressed. However, more information is needed on potential nephrotoxicity and drug resistance with long-term use.

Patients with decompensated cirrhosis are not candidates for IFN-α therapy because of the risk of side-effects. Patients with moderate to severe chronic hepatitis (HBeAg-positive or -negative) whether treated or not, and patients with advanced liver disease, should be monitored for the progression of liver disease and the development of complications, including hepatocellular carcinoma.

Interferon-α

IFN-αs are naturally occurring intercellular signalling proteins used therapeutically for their properties of inducing an antiviral state in cells, inhibiting cellular proliferation and immunomodulation. The IFNs have been classified into two types, based on receptor specificity. Type 1 IFNs (viral IFNs) include IFN-α (leukocyte) IFN-β (fibroblast) and IFN-ω. Type II IFN is also known as immune IFN, i.e. IFN-γ. The cellular activities of IFN-α are mediated by the products of the IFN-inducible genes. The natural IFN-α-producing cell is the precursor dendritic cell. IFN-γ is produced by cells of the immune system, including natural killer cells, CD4 Th1 cells and CD8 T cells following antigen-specific stimulation, and acts via a separate cell receptor. IFN-γ is critical for innate and adaptive immunity. Several IFN-αs, including HuIFN-α-n1 (Wellferon) rIFN-α2β (Intron A) and rIFN-α2α, (Roferon-A), have been licensed for the treatment of chronic hepatitis B. Recombinant methionyl human IFN consensus is a novel, non-naturally occurring type 1 IFN. These therapeutic preparations of type I IFNs consist of either a mixture of IFN species derived from virus-stimulated Namalwa cells (Wellferon) or recombinant DNA-produced, single-component IFN-α species. All are administered parenterally, either intramuscularly or subcutaneously, but can be given i.v. for patients with bleeding disorders. Wellferon is no longer in widespread use for the treatment of viral hepatitis.

Relative or absolute contraindications to IFN-α therapy include severe depression, Childs B/C cirrhosis, cirrhosis and hypersplenism, autoimmune hepatitis, hyperthyroidism, coronary artery disease, renal transplant, pregnancy, seizures, concomitant drugs, including several herbal remedies, diabetes/hypertension and retinopathy, thrombocytopenia, leukopenia, anaemia, high-titre autoantibodies and hyperthyroidism. The side-effects of IFN-α are relatively common, but are acceptable in most patients. Toxicity can be predicted in patients with low baseline white cell counts or thrombocytopenia, or pre-existing thyroid disease (Dusheiko, 1997). The risk of serious complications from IFN-α is rare. However, serious idiosyncratic complications, such as immune disorders, pneumonitis, retinal disease, renal disease or deafness can occur and the drug always must be prescribed with caution. Close monitoring is required throughout therapy, including regular clinical examinations, vital signs, urinalysis and usually monthly measurement of serum chemistries, complete blood counts and thyroid function tests, including thyroid stimulating hormone. A serum pregnancy test should be done to exclude pregnancy before starting treatment.

Interferons Linked to Polyethylene Glycol

The efficacy of IFN-α therapy is restricted by protein characteristics including poor stability, a short half-life and immunogenicity. The half-life varies from 4–16 h with peak concentrations of 3–8 h following i.m. or s.c. injection. By 24 h, little IFN-α remains in the circulation. Thus, frequent dosing is required to achieve effective therapeutic concentrations of drug in the plasma and large fluctuations in serum concentrations occur. Polyethylene glycol is an inert non-toxic polymer which can be used to modify the pharmacological properties of biologically active proteins without completely inactivating their intrinsic biological activity. Recent technology has enabled activation of the polyethylene glycol moiety through substitution of the hydroxyl group by an electrophilic functional group. The reactive functional group of activated PEG can be attached to a specific site, e.g. amine, sulphydryl group or other nucleophile on the protein. Until recently, mono-functional PEG derivatives used for protein pegylation were linear with M_rs of 12 000. New advances in pegylation technology have resulted in the development of branched PEGS of higher M_r (up to 60 000). The PEG polymer increases the half-life of the conjugated protein, protecting the protein from proteolysis and reducing renal clearance. This enables once-weekly dosing.

Reduced clearance of pegylated IFN results in increased circulation time and sustained systemic exposure of the pegylated compound. When the biological activity of a pegylated protein is measured *in vivo*, a direct relationship between the mass of the PEG conjugate and its biological activity is frequently observed. This is in contrast to the inverse relationship reported between PEG mass and biological activity of pegylated proteins *in vitro*, where the activity of pegylated compounds is decreased due to a reduction in their receptor-binding properties. The appropriate dose of pegylated IFN-α2β for body weight should be given.

M_r 12 000 and 40 000 pegylated IFN-αs have recently been licensed for the treatment of hepatitis C: the FDA has licensed pegylated IFN-α2β (PEG-Intron, Schering) and pegylated IFN-α2α (Pegasys, Roche) for the treatment of chronic hepatitis C, and studies are in progress in hepatitis B.

Nucleoside and Nucleotide Analogues

Lamivudine

Lamivudine (2′,3′-dideoxy-3′-thiacytidine [(±)-SddC], 3TC or Epivir) is a potent inhibitor of HBV, as well as HIV. The drug acts by inhibiting DNA synthesis through chain termination. The (−)-form [(−)-SddC], which is resistant to deoxycytidine deaminase, is the more active antiviral stereoisomer than the (+)-form. The negative enantiomer (−)-SddC does not appear to affect mitochondrial DNA synthesis. Metabolic studies have shown that the drug is converted to the monophosphate, diphosphate and triphosphate form. The drug is rapidly absorbed after oral administration, with a bioavailability of >80%. The majority of drug is excreted unchanged in the urine. Since 1990, lamivudine has been used in trials of treatment of HIV infection, and this compound has been licensed as a component of HAART. Lamivudine is active *in vitro* against human hepatitis B-transfected cell lines and in ducklings affected with DHBV, as well as in chimpanzees infected with HBV.

Large Phase III trials in patients with chronic hepatitis B have been completed. Doses above 25 mg reproducibly decrease HBV DNA levels in serum. HBV DNA generally became undetectable (by hybridisation assay) in more than 90% of patients who received 25–300 mg/day. In most patients, HBV DNA reappears after therapy is completed. In large trials in Asia and the West, approximately 15–20% of patients became HBeAg-negative after 12 months of treatment compared to 4% of placebo recipients. Histological improvement has been noted after 1 year of treatment. Lamivudine therapy has been consistently associated with a highly significant sustained reduction in levels of serum HBV DNA at the end of 1 year of therapy in up to 98%. Undetectable levels of HBV DNA were sustained in 44% of adults compared to 16% on placebo. Loss of HBe antigen with seroconversion to anti-HBe was observed in 17% after a year of treatment with lamivudine vs. 6% on placebo in adults. Histological improvement was the main outcome measure in the pivotal trial of lamivudine therapy in adults. Liver biopsies were scored according to the degree of necroinflammation and degree of fibrosis and an improvement in score of two or more HAI points was scored as improvement. Significant differences in the total HAI score were observed in those on lamivudine compared to those on placebo (Dienstag *et al.*, 1999). Lamivudine monotherapy reduces HBV DNA concentrations prior to liver transplant, but may be associated with subsequent resistance. Lamivudine and HBIG prophylaxis have proved effective for prevention of recurrent hepatitis B post-transplantation.

The drug seems to be well tolerated and relatively few serious side-effects have been reported. Serious side-effects have been observed in about 5% of patients; these include anaemia, neutropenia, an increase in liver enzymes, nausea and neuropathy. Increased lipases may occur, but uncommonly, and serious lactic acidosis has not been observed. Severe exacerbations of hepatitis accompanied by jaundice have been reported in patients whose HBV DNA became positive after stopping treatment, or after the development of resistance (Honkoop *et al.*, 1995). Reactivation of hepatitis was observed in patients who developed a methionine to valine or isoleucine substitution in the highly conserved YMDD motif of the HBV polymerase (Ling *et al.*, 1996). This motif is part of the active site of the polymerase, and this mutation parallels the M184 mutation seen in resistant HIV, where substitutions of valine and isoleucine for methionine also have been found. The major mutational patterns observed in patients with lamivudine resistance include L180M + M204V (previous notation L528M + M552V), V173L + L180M + M204V, M204I or L180M + M204I. These changes confer a marked decrease in sensitivity to lamivudine *in vitro*. The incidence of lamivudine resistance in chronic hepatitis rises from 24% after 1 year of treatment to 66% after 4 years. The incidence rises to 90% in HIV and HBV co-infected patients.

After lamivudine is stopped, HBV replication may reactivate and sometimes can be associated with severe 'flares' or exacerbation of hepatitis as HBV DNA increases in serum. The pathogenesis of this injury is not fully understood. Probably some of the injury is related to an immune response. The emergence of resistance could have a similar effect, as viral DNA increases. Combination studies with lamivudine and adefovir are in progress.

Adefovir Dipivoxil

Adefovir dipivoxil (bis-POM pMEA) 0-[2-[[bis[(pivaloyloxy)methyl]-phosphinyl]methoxy]ethyl]adenine) is an orally bioavailable prodrug of adefovir, a phosphonate nucleotide analogue of adenosine monophosphate. It requires cellular nucleoside kinases for activation to adefovir diphosphate and then acts as a competitive inhibitor and chain-terminator of HBV replication mediated by HBV DNA polymerase. The drug inhibits viral polymerases and terminates the growing DNA chain by acting as a competitive inhibitor of dATP. Because adefovir diphosphate lacks a 3' hydroxyl group, the compound causes premature termination of viral DNA synthesis upon its incorporation into the nascent DNA chain. Adefovir has activity against HBV, DHBV and WHV in cell culture models and against chronically infected animals. This agent also has some immunomodulatory activity and stimulates natural killer activity.

Adefovir is active *in vitro* against all known lamivudine-, emtricitabine-, famciclovir- and HBIG-resistant HBV, using both cell culture and enzyme assays. Resistance to adefovir is remarkably delayed in patients with chronic hepatitis B. Recently, a novel N236T mutation was reported in two anti-HBe-positive patients after 96 weeks of treatment, which was not detectable after 1 year of treatment. This mutant showed lowered susceptibility to adefovir. The mutation does not share cross-resistance with lamivudine. A low potential for resistance development with adefovir could be related to its close structural relationship with the natural substrate, which limits the potential for steric hindrance as a mechanism of resistance. In addition, adefovir contains a flexible acyclic linker that may allow adefovir to bind to HBV polymerase with different conformations, and thus further subvert steric hindrance. Adefovir also contains a phosphonate bond that is less susceptible to ATP-mediated chain terminator excision, which has been recognised as a mechanism of HIV resistance.

Following oral administration of single doses of adefovir dipivoxil 10 mg to patients with chronic hepatitis B or healthy subjects, maximum observed adefovir concentrations in plasma occur at a median 0.76–1.75 h following dosing, with mean values in the range 17.5–21.3 ng/ml. The mean adefovir area under the curve was 178–210 ng/h/ml. The long terminal elimination half-life allows for once-daily dosing. In preclinical studies, evidence for renal toxicity was noted in all species evaluated. This toxicity is characterised by a renal tubular nephropathy. The efficacy of adefovir dipivoxil has been investigated in patients with compensated liver disease and evidence of HBV replication, and in patients failing lamivudine therapy, including post-transplantation patients, patients with compensated and decompensated liver failure and patients co-infected with HIV. Two pivotal placebo-controlled clinical studies in patients with HBeAg- or anti-HBe-positive (pre-core mutant) chronic hepatitis B have been completed. An open-label study in liver transplantation patients with lamivudine-resistant HBV is continuing.

Doses of 5–125 mg/day have been assessed in the clinical development programme. In Phase I/II clinical studies in both HBeAg-positive and HBeAg-negative patients with chronic hepatitis B, statistically significant decreases in serum HBV DNA concentrations were demonstrated within the first week of treatment and were maintained for periods of treatment of up to 136 weeks. The antiviral response seen in Phase I/II studies indicated a suboptimal antiviral effect with 5 mg and maximal reductions in serum HBV DNA levels with doses of 30 mg and above. Data from previous studies indicated that dosing with 30 mg daily beyond 24 weeks is associated with the emergence of mild nephrotoxicity (seen at higher doses in HIV studies) that is reversible upon discontinuation of the drug. Multinational double-blind randomised placebo-controlled trials, in both HBeAg-positive and -negative patients with liver disease, have been completed. The primary endpoint of these studies was based on the quantitative assessment of histological improvement after 48 weeks of treatment using the Knodell HAI scoring score. Both necro-inflammatory activity and fibrosis showed greater improvement in adefovir dipivoxil 10 mg and 30 mg compared to placebo recipients ($p < 0.001$). Worsening of necro-inflammatory activity and fibrosis was seen in a greater proportion of the placebo groups ($p < 0.001$); HBV DNA concentration declined by 3.52 logs after 48 weeks in patients on 10 mg and 21% of patients were negative for HBV DNA by PCR. HBeAg seroconversion was observed in 12% of patients receiving 10 mg vs. 6% of placebo recipients. Improved responses were seen in patients with raised ALT (Marcellin et al., 2003). In anti-HBe-positive patients, a 3.9 log decline in HBV DNA concentration was observed in patients treated with 10 mg after 1 year, and improvements in ALT, hepatic necroinflammatory change and fibrosis were noted in treated patients (Hadziyannis et al., 2003). 51% of patients had undetectable HBV DNA by PCR vs. 0% of placebo recipients. The preferred treatment dose is 10 mg because of the favourable risk:benefit ratio.

Adefovir is effective in patients with lamivudine resistance, and has reduced the clinical consequences of lamivudine resistance in immunosuppressed patients, including HIV-positive patients and liver transplant patients, and patients with decompensated cirrhosis (Benhamou et al., 2001; Perrillo et al., 2000; Xiong et al., 1998). A 4–5 log change has been observed after adding adefovir salvage treatment in patients with lamivudine resistance. Caution will be required for patients with pre-existing renal damage, due to calcineurin inhibitors in liver transplant patients. An effect of adefovir on cccDNA has been observed in treated patients, but the significance of these findings requires further study.

New Nucleoside Analogues

Phase I and II trials with several new nucleoside analogues, including entecavir, emtricitabine, clevudine (L-FMAU) and L-dT are in progress.

Entecavir is a cyclopentyl guanine analogue, which is an inhibitor of all HBV polymerase functions. The drug is readily phosphorylated to the active triphosphate form. The drug is a potent inhibitor of WHV, and in humans with HBV at doses of 0.05–1 mg. In Phase II trials, 84% of patients were negative for HBV DNA by bDNA assay after 24 weeks of treatment. The drug is active against lamivudine-resistant variants and Phase III trials are in progress.

Emtricitabine (FTC) is a cytosine nucleoside analogue, with fluorine at the 5-position. Pilot studies have shown that the drug causes a 2–3 log reduction in HBV DNA at doses of 300 mg in patients treated for 8 weeks. In a Phase II study of 48 weeks duration, 61% of patients had undetectable HBV DNA. Drug-resistant mutants have been reported in 6% of treated patients (Lai et al., 2002).

Clevudine (L-FMAU) is a pyrimidine nucleoside analogue. Patients have been treated in Phase I dose escalating studies, and up to 3 log reductions in HBV DNA have been observed (Chong and Chu, 2002).

β-L thymidine (telbivudine), Val LdC and LdA are small molecule inhibitors of HBV DNA polymerase. These agents induce marked viral load reduction in the woodchuck infected with WHV. LdT is a specific and potent inhibitor of hepatitis B and is not active against HIV or other viruses. Clinical trials are in progress in HBeAg-positive patients at doses of 25–400 mg (Standring et al., 2001; Bryant et al., 2001). Phase I studies have shown a dose-dependent 2–4 log reduction in HBV DNA after 4 weeks of treatment. A Phase II trial testing doses of LdT 400 or 600 mg with or without lamivudine in HBeAg-positive patients is in progress. An interim analysis of the results at 24 weeks indicates that LdT 400 and LdT 600 mg result in 6 log declines in HBV DNA (compared to a 4 log decline in HBV DNA in lamivudine-treated patients).

At this time the long-term efficacy and safety of these new unlicensed drugs are unproven: chronic type B hepatitis disease will require relatively long courses of treatment, often in asymptomatic carriers, perhaps including children, and viral resistance may emerge. The end-points of treatment will require careful evaluation. Combination treatment may become necessary but may not be required for all patients.

Biological Response Modifiers

Interleukin-12 (IL-12) is a heterodimeric protein of M_r 75 000 and a member of the TNF receptor superfamily. This cytokine is a product of macrophages and dendritic cells. IL-12 promotes Th-1 and suppresses Th-2 cell development, suggesting that IL-12 may be useful therapeutically to promote a cellular immune response. The compound induces secretion of IFN-γ from T and NK cells, and increases the lytic activity of NK cells and facilitates specific CTL responses. The effect of systemic IL-12 treatment on autoantibody synthesis *in vivo* in HBeAg-expressing transgenic mice has been tested. Low-dose IL-12 significantly inhibited autoantibody (anti-HBe) production by shifting the Th-2-mediated response towards Th-1 predominance.

Additionally, previous studies suggest that a predominance of HBeAg-specific Th-2-type cells may contribute to chronicity in hepatitis B virus infection. Therefore, IL-12 may also prove beneficial in modulating the antibody and cellular immune response in acute hepatitis B to improve clearance of hepatitis B (Milich *et al.*, 1995). It has been shown that suppression of intrahepatic replication of HBV DNA in transgenic mice is mediated through cytokines such as IFN-γ and TNF. Fever, lethargy, anorexia, anaemia, thrombocytopaenia, stomatitis, pulmonary oedema and increased serum ALT have been observed in experimental animals. Pilot studies have begun in HBV-infected patients. IL-12 can also aggravate autoimmune processes, and deaths in patients with renal carcinoma have been observed. In two open label, multicentre, dose-escalation Phase I/II studies the efficacy of subcutaneously administered recombinant human IL-12 (rHuIL-12) was assessed in the treatment of chronic hepatitis B. At the end of treatment HBV DNA clearance was greater in patients treated with 0.50 µg/kg (25%) or with 0.25 µg/kg (13%) compared with those given 0.03 µg/kg, but the drug offers little advantage over existing treatments (Carreno *et al.*, 2000; Zeuzem and Carreno, 2001).

Thymosin is a synthetic 28 aa immune stimulant which is known to enhance suppressor T cell activity and B cell synthesis of IgG *in vitro*. Peptide preparations of thymosin have been evaluated in small controlled trials and HBV DNA has been noted to become negative in some of these patients and in chimpanzees with chronic hepatitis B. It is given parenterally by subcutaneous injection. This agent's possible therapeutic role was evaluated in a larger controlled trial, in which HBeAg seroconversion rates were not significantly different from recipients given placebo. Although approval for the treatment of hepatitis B has been granted in a few countries, the place of this drug is still being appraised. Few side-effects are observed with thymosin injected subcutaneously.

Immunotherapy

There has been a resurgence of interest in the possibility of therapeutic immunisation of chronically infected, HBV-positive patients to activate an immune response and eradicate viraemia. In a recent pilot study, 32 patients with HBeAg-positive, HBV DNA-positive chronic hepatitis B were immunised with three standard doses of GenHevac vaccine at monthly intervals. Six months after the first injection, 37% had undetectable DNA. Eight responders were given IFN-α to maintain virus inhibition (Pol *et al.*, 1994; Pol, 1995). More recent results have not suggested successful immunotherapy using HBV vaccine.

There is considerable interest in the possibility of provoking a cytotoxic immune response to HBV core epitopes, as the CTL response contributes to viral clearance in acute hepatitis B. A strong cytotoxic T cell response has been observed in HLA A2.1 individuals with acute hepatitis B against an epitope (FLPSDFFPSV) that contains an HLA A2 binding motif located between residues 18–27 of the hepatitis B nucleocapsid protein (Bertoletti *et al.*, 1993). This identification has led to development of a therapeutic vaccine (Theradigm HBV tm), in which this CTL epitope has been incorporated into a vaccine containing a T-helper cell epitope and two palmitic acid residues (CY-1899). In a pilot study, 90 patients with chronic hepatitis B infection received CY-1899. No significant changes in liver biochemistry or viral serology were observed during follow-up (Heathcote *et al.*, 1999).

Recently, DNA-based immunisation has been tested using purified plasmid DNA containing protein coding sequences and the regulatory elements required for their expression. The DNA is introduced into tissues by means of a parenteral injection and the number of cells transfected and the amount of protein produced is sufficient to produce a broad-based immune response to a wide variety of foreign proteins. A response to HBsAg has been achieved using this form of antigen presentation. A CD8$^+$ CTL response has been induced in BALB/C mice, suggesting a pathway for exogenous presentation of hepatitis B envelope protein via MHC class I expression (Davis *et al.*, 1995). The Pekin duck infected by DHBV has been immunised with a plasmid encoding the DHBV large (L) ORF, leading to a sustained decrease in viral replication and even to clearance of the intrahepatic viral cccDNA pool in some animals. Combination therapy data with lamivudine showed a pronounced antiviral effect (Thermet *et al.*, 2003). If the safety of DNA-mediated immunisation can be assured, this form of vaccination may also have therapeutic potential (Whalen and Davis, 1995).

Hepatitis B Virus and Primary Liver Cancer

Persistent infection with hepatitis B virus is associated with a high risk of developing hepatocellular carcinoma (HCC). However, the precise role played by the virus in causing this tumour remains to be elucidated.

Epidemiological Evidence

HCC is one of the 10 most common cancers in the world, with over 250 000 new cases each year. In areas where the tumour is particularly common, e.g. some regions of sub-Saharan Africa, China and South-east Asia, the age-adjusted incidence of HCC is over 30 new cases/100 000 population/year, whereas it is less than 5 cases/100 000/year in western Europe and North America. Primary liver cancer is more common among males than females and the incidence of the tumour increases with age, reaching a peak in the 30–50 age group.

When specific tests for the serological markers of HBV infection became available, it became clear that the geographical areas with a high incidence of primary liver cancer were coincident with those with a high prevalence of seropositivity for HBsAg. Furthermore, most patients from high-risk areas presenting with primary liver cancer proved to be HBsAg-positive or to have high titres of anti-HBc. There is often a considerable interval between the initial virus infection and development of HCC, although the tumour does occur in younger age groups in high-risk populations.

The relative risk of an HBsAg-carrier, compared to a matched non-carrier, developing primary liver cancer was estimated in an elegant prospective study carried out in Taiwan by Beasley and co-workers. Over 22 000 men, including more than 3000 HBsAg carriers, were followed for 75 000 man-years. The HBsAg carriers proved more than 200-fold more likely to develop HCC than members of the non-carrier group and more than 50% of the deaths in the former group were due to the tumour or to cirrhosis, another possible consequence of long-term HBV infection (Beasley and Hwang, 1991).

HBV DNA in Primary Liver Tumours

If HBV does indeed play a causal role in the development of primary liver cancer, then the tumours might be expected to contain virus-specific nucleic acid and perhaps also to express viral proteins. The first cell line to be established from a primary liver tumour from an HBsAg carrier (PLC/PRF/5) proved to secrete HBsAg in culture in the form of 22 nm particles with a morphology similar to those found in the plasma of persistently infected individuals. Some other HCC-derived cell lines are HBsAg-positive but many are negative. Similarly, immunohistochemistry of HBV-associated tumours shows that a minority produce HBsAg. Production of HBcAg by tumours seems to be rather less common.

Following the molecular cloning of the HBV genome, which made available hybridisation probes of high specific activity, the PLC/PRF/5 cell line was shown to contain HBV DNA integrated chromosomally at several sites (Figure 3.13, lane A1). Further analysis reveals considerable rearrangement of the viral DNA, although it is not clear whether these rearrangements were present in the original tumour or occurred during the establishment of the cell line (the genotype of the cultured cells appears to be stable with respect to the integrated HBV sequences). Other cell lines derived from HBV-associated primary liver tumours have also been shown to contain integrated HBV DNA.

Analysis by Southern hybridisation reveals integrated HBV DNA in approximately 80% of primary liver tumours from HBsAg carriers (Brechot et al., 1980; Chen et al., 1986). An example is illustrated in Figure 3.13, lane D2. It is possible that more sensitive techniques, such as PCR, may enable the detection of viral DNA sequences in tumours which test negative by hybridisation. In most cases, the tumours seem to be clonal with respect to the integrated viral DNA and seem to have arisen from a single cell. However, there is considerable variation between tumours in terms of the number of integrants and their location. Although HBV DNA is often found integrated into Alu or other satellite sequences, this is likely to reflect the size of such targets and it seems that the sites of integration in the cellular chromosomes are random.

Nucleic acid sequencing of the junctions between viral and cellular DNA shows that the direct repeats in the virus genome (see the account of the replication of the viral genome, above) are frequently located close to these junctions and may be 'hot spots' for recombination with host DNA. Because synthesis of progeny viral DNA in infected cells is cytoplasmic, it is likely that an intermediate(s) in the process of conversion of virion DNA to covalently closed circular DNA or progeny HBV DNA recycled from the cytoplasm to the nucleus is involved in the recombination.

Mechanisms of Oncogenesis

Because primary liver cancer most often develops in a liver which is affected by chronic hepatitis or cirrhosis (or both) it has been suggested that the involvement of HBV is mediated through these pathological changes and subsequent regeneration. However, it is clear that HCC is much more likely to develop in an HBV-infected cirrhotic liver than in the cirrhotic liver of an uninfected patient, and that tumours often develop in the livers of HBV-infected patients without an intermediate cirrhotic stage. The common finding of integrated viral DNA in tumours implies a more direct role of viral oncogenesis. However, the fact that up to 20% of tumours from HBsAg carriers may be negative for viral DNA suggests that other mechanisms sometimes may be involved.

Integrated viral DNA also may be detected in the livers of some HBsAg carriers without tumour, both in patients with ongoing virus replication and in those who have cleared replicating virus. The hybridisation techniques used are able to detect these integration events only if they occur at the same site in many cells and, because the sites of integration in the chromosomes appear to be random, this implies the clonal expansion of a cell with integrated viral DNA. The establishment of such clones in the liver may be the first step in a multistage process leading to carcinoma and there may be a role for other environmental factors (such as mycotoxins in the diet) in such a process. The long interval often seen between the initial virus infection and tumour development fits with this concept. Furthermore, because integration seems to occur repeatedly throughout the period of virus replication, the continuing accumulation of pre-neoplastic clones within the liver might increase the probability of progression to tumour for patients with long-term chronic infection.

Production of HBsAg in the livers of carriers who have cleared virus replication, as well as by some tumours, indicates that the surface mRNA may be actively transcribed from integrated viral DNA. The activity of this promoter makes attractive the promoter insertion hypothesis that aberrant transcription of cellular genes may result in loss of growth control. However, analysis of viral integration sites in tumours has only very rarely produced data supporting this hypothesis. In one tumour, the HBV genome has been found to be integrated into the gene for a retinoic acid receptor (Dejean et al., 1986), and in another a cyclin A gene was involved (Wang et al., 1990). However, these are isolated instances and it seems that a common mechanism of oncogenesis via insertional mutagenesis is extremely unlikely.

Another mechanism whereby viruses cause neoplastic transformation of cells is via the expression of a transforming gene introduced into the integrated viral genome. The HBV genome does not seem to contain such a gene and it has not been possible to transform cells in vitro using virus or viral DNA. The long interval between virus infection and tumour development also argues against such a direct mechanism. Nevertheless, the so-called X gene of HBV has been shown to encode a transcriptional transactivator and the possibility that this protein plays a role in disrupting the normal transcriptional control of the cell cannot be ruled out. Transactivation by the X protein seems to be through responsive elements such as the transcription factor AP-1 (jun/fos), AP-2, NF-κB and the CRE site. It has been shown that truncated pre-S proteins also may have transactivating properties. These may be produced in tumour cells by expression of integrated HBV DNA with virus–host junctions in the surface ORF.

HEPATITIS D

Delta hepatitis was first recognised following detection of a novel protein, delta antigen (HDAg), by immunofluorescent staining, in the nuclei of hepatocytes from patients with hepatitis B (Rizzetto et al., 1977). HDV is now known to be defective and require a helper function from HBV for its transmission. HDV is coated with HBsAg, which is needed for release from the host hepatocyte and for entry in the next round of infection. The agent is unique among human viruses, having an internal nucleocapsid comprising the genome surrounded by the delta antigen and enveloped by an outer protein coat of HBsAg. The genome consists of a single-stranded, circular RNA of around 1700 nucleotides, the delta antigen being encoded by antigenomic RNA (reviewed by Taylor, 1997).

Two major modes of HDV infection are known (Hadziannis, 1997). In the first, a susceptible individual is co-infected with HBV and HDV, often leading to a more severe form of acute hepatitis caused by HBV. Vaccination against HBV prevents such infections. In the second, an individual infected chronically with HBV becomes superinfected with HDV. This may accelerate the course of the chronic liver disease and cause overt disease in asymptomatic HBsAg carriers. HDV may be cytopathic, and HDAg directly cytotoxic. A less common type of infection has been seen in

HDAg-positive patients who have received liver transplants. Hepatocytes in the graft become infected with HDV circulating at the time of transplantation. In the absence of HBsAg, there is no cell-to-cell spread of the virus but HDV replication persists in isolated hepatocytes.

Epidemiology

Limited serological studies indicate a worldwide distribution of HDV in association with HBV. The infection is important epidemiologically in southern Europe, the Middle East (the Gulf States and Saudi Arabia), Japan and Taiwan, and parts of Africa and South America (Rizzetto, 1996). Three genotypes (I–III) of HDV are recognised on the basis of phylogenetic analysis and these are found, respectively, in southern Europe, Japan and Taiwan, and South America. There is evidence that the prevalence of δ infection is declining in southern Europe, particularly Italy (Gaeta *et al.*, 2000). It has been estimated that 5% of HBsAg carriers worldwide (approximately 15 million people) are infected with HDV. In areas of low prevalence of HBV, those at risk of hepatitis B, particularly intravenous drug users, are also at risk of HDV infection. Delta infection is associated with acute and chronic hepatitis, always in the presence of hepatitis B, and superinfection in a carrier of hepatitis B virus often leads to exacerbation of severe hepatitis. Epidemics with high mortality have been described in South America in association with severe hepatitis B.

The mode of transmission of HDV is similar to parenteral spread of HBV, so serological evidence of infection is found most frequently in western Europe and North America in multiply transfused individuals, such as patients with haemophilia, and in drug addicts, and is endemic in the Mediterranean Basin, the Middle East, West Africa, the Amazon Basin and some South Pacific Islands.

Structure and Replication of HDV

The HDV particle is approximately 36 nm in diameter and composed of an RNA genome associated with HDAg, surrounded by an envelope of HBsAg. The virus reaches higher concentrations in the circulation than HBV; up to 10^{12} particles/ml have been recorded. The HDV genome is a closed circular RNA molecule of 1679 nucleotides with extensive sequence complementarity that permits pairing of approximately 70% of the bases to form an unbranched rod structure. The genome thus resembles those of the satellite viroids and virusoids of plants and, similarly, seems to be replicated by the host RNA polymerase II, with autocatalytic cleavage and circularisation of the progeny genomes via *trans*-esterification reactions (ribozyme activity; Lazinski and Taylor, 1995; Lai, 1995). Consensus sequences of viroids, which are believed to be involved in these processes, also are conserved in HDV.

Unlike the plant viroids, HDV codes for a protein, HDAg, in an open reading frame in the antigenomic RNA. Around 600 copies of a polyadenylated mRNA, approximately 800 nt in length, may be detected in the cytoplasm of infected hepatocytes. The antigen, which contains a nuclear localisation signal, was originally detected in the nuclei of infected hepatocytes and may be detected in serum only after stripping off the outer envelope of the virion with detergent. The delta antigen is detectable in two forms in the infected hepatocyte. The 195 aa (small) form is required for HDV RNA replication and binds to the rod-like structures of the genome and genome complement. The larger (214 aa) form, which is structural and therefore required for virion assembly, seems to be synthesised following RNA editing. This process converts the termination codon at the end to the ORF for the short form to a tryptophan codon, resulting in a 19 aa carboxyl-terminal extension (Casey and Gerin, 1995).

Laboratory Diagnosis of HDV Infection

Specific serological tests are available to detect antibody to HDV; anti-HD IgM and anti-HD IgG, and for HDV RNA and HDAg. Co-infection and superinfection can be distinguished by correlation of the results of these tests with those for markers of HBV infection. Thus, in co-infection, HBsAg, HBeAg and HBV DNA become detectable in serum along with HDAg and HDV RNA. Co-existence of anti-HBc IgM with markers of HDV infection is a reliable indication of co-infection; anti-HD IgM becomes detectable, followed by anti-HD IgG. Markers of virus replication usually become undetectable during convalescence.

Superinfection of HBV carriers with HDV results frequently in persistent HDV infection. HD viraemia is followed by an anti-HD IgM, and then IgG, response. Markers of HBV replication may be suppressed during acute HDV infection. Anti-HD IgM persists with HDAg and HDV RNA in serum in chronic delta hepatitis.

Pathogenesis

The pathogenesis of the disease is uncertain. It has long been held that HDV is pathogenic and that the liver injury in hepatitis D is related to HDV itself. These data have been challenged recently with the observation that HDV re-occurs in liver-transplanted patients soon after grafting but without signs of HBV recurrence or evidence of liver damage. In these individuals, HDV may establish latent infection that is not dependent upon HBV for replication, and which is only associated with recrudescent liver injury after the acquisition of HBV. Hepatitis D virions cannot be released from the infected hepatocytes without an envelope supplied by HBV.

Fulminant hepatitis may occur in acute HDV and HBV infection, and outbreaks of severe hepatitis have been reported in Indians of the Amazon basin and in areas of Central Africa. Degenerative changes were observed in these patients, characterised by fine steatotic vacuolisation of hepatocytes, in keeping with a cytotoxic inflammatory lesion.

It is known that hepatitis D may interfere with HBV replication but the molecular mechanism has not been established. An increase in HDV replication has been noted in concurrent HDV and HIV replication, but this may not necessarily cause more severe hepatitis (Buti et al., 1991). There is also a large body of data to suggest that the pathogenesis of of HDV hepatitis is in part immunologically mediated.

Clinical Features

Hepatitis D causes acute, fulminant and chronic hepatitis, either as a co-infection with hepatitis B or as a superinfection in patients with chronic hepatitis B. Clinically there is a spectrum of disease and, in some co-infected or superinfected persons, HDV appears to be a pathogenic agent and to aggravate the underlying HBV infection. There is much interest in the study of pathogenicity caused by this agent.

Treatment

A number of investigators have evaluated interferon treatment of chronic type D hepatitis. HDV is sensitive to IFN-α, and doses of 3–10 mIU three times weekly for 6 months result in repression of hepatitis D and amelioration of biochemical signs of hepatitis, with a decrease in serum aminotransferases (Rizzetto et al.,

1986; Rosina et al., 1991; Saracco et al., 1989). Coincident with this decrease, HDV RNA disappears from serum in approximately 50% of cases. Unfortunately, many patients relapse when treatment is stopped. More recently, higher dose regimens have been employed, 9–10 mIU three times weekly for 12 months. Available antiviral drugs, including nucleoside analogues, are ineffective. Patients with decompensated liver disease should be considered for transplantation with prophylaxis against reinfection with HBV.

Immunisation

Immunisation against hepatitis B prevents HDV infection. Active immunisation with HDV synthetic or expressed gene products may modulate the infection in woodchuck models (Karayiannis et al., 1993).

HEPATITIS C

Hepatitis C Virus is Responsible for almost all Cases of Parenterally Transmitted Non-A, Non-B Hepatitis

The specific diagnosis of hepatitis types A, B and D revealed a previously unrecognised form of hepatitis which was clearly unrelated to any of these three types. Results obtained from several surveys of post-transfusion hepatitis in the USA and elsewhere provided strong epidemiological evidence of 'guilt by association' of an infection of the liver referred to as non-A, non-B hepatitis (Alter, 1988). This was the most common form of hepatitis occurring after blood transfusion in some areas of the world following the introduction of tests for HBsAg. Studies also showed that this infection was common in haemodialysis and other specialised units, that it occurs in a sporadic form in the general population and that it can be transmitted by therapeutic plasma components. There was also considerable evidence that the parenterally-transmitted infection, like hepatitis B, may become persistent and progress to chronic liver disease, cirrhosis and hepatocellular carcinoma. Transmission studies in chimpanzees helped establish that the main agent of parenterally acquired non-A, non-B hepatitis was likely to be an enveloped virus with a diameter of 30–60 nm (Bradley et al., 1985; He et al., 1987). These studies made available a pool of plasma known to contain a relatively high titre of the agent and enabled the molecular cloning of the genome of what we now know as *Hepatitis C virus* (HCV) (Choo *et al.*, 1989).

The Organisation of the HCV Genome

The genome of HCV (Figure 3.14) resembles those of the pestiviruses and flaviviruses. It comprises around 9400 nt of positive-sense RNA, lacks a 3' poly(A) tract and has a similar gene organisation (Choo *et al.*, 1991). It has been proposed that HCV should be designated the prototype of a third genus in the family *Flaviviridae*, *Hepacivirus*. All of the viral genomes from this family contain a single large ORF which is translated to yield a polyprotein (of around 3000 amino acids in the case of HCV) from which the viral proteins are derived by post-translational cleavage and other modifications.

There is a short, untranslated region at the 5' end of the genome of HCV and a further untranslated region at the 3' end, the large ORF accounting for over 95% of the sequence. The structural proteins are located towards the 5' end and the non-structural proteins towards the 3' end. The first product of the polyprotein is the non-glycosylated capsid protein, C, which complexes with the genomic RNA to form the nucleocapsid. A hydrophobic domain anchors the growing polypeptide in the endoplasmic reticulum and leads to cleavage by a cellular signal peptidase. The amino acid sequence of the nucleocapsid protein seems to be highly conserved among different isolates of HCV.

The next two domains in the polyprotein also have signal sequences at their carboxyl-termini and are processed in a similar fashion. The products are two glycoproteins, E1 (or gp35) and E2 (or gp70), which are found in the viral envelope. Alternative cleavage sites at the carboxyl-terminus of E2 may generate a small addition protein, p7. These glycoproteins have not been visualised *in vivo* and the molecular sizes are estimated from sequence data and expression studies *in vitro*. These envelope proteins are the focus of considerable interest as potential targets in tests for the direct detection of viral proteins and for anti-HCV vaccines.

As with many other RNA viruses, replication of the HCV genome is an error-prone process and the resulting mutations lead to the generation, within an infected individual, of a population of viruses with closely related, but different, nucleotide sequences. This has been termed the 'quasi-species effect'. The effect is particularly noticeable in the region of the genome (the hypervariable region, HVR-1), which encodes a domain at the amino-terminus of E2. Sequences within this region are highly variable within each individual, as well as between isolates of the virus, and divergence seems to be driven by the generation of neutralising antibodies which are targeted to that domain of E2. This hypothesis is supported by the observation that much less variability occurs in agammaglobulinaemic individuals. Thus, efforts to develop hepatitis C vaccines are hampered by variability of the most obvious target molecule and the efficacy of candidate vaccines is likely to be hampered by the rapid evolution of antibody escape mutants.

The non-structural region of the HCV genome is divided into regions NS2–NS5 (Figure 3.14). In the flaviviruses, NS3 has two functional domains, a protease which is involved in cleavage of the non-structural region of the polyprotein and a helicase which is assumed to be involved in RNA replication. Motifs within this region of the HCV genome have homology to the appropriate consensus sequences, suggesting similar functions. The HCV protease, which uses NS4a as a co-factor, is a major target of efforts to develop specific antiviral agents. Unlike the flaviviruses, HCV encodes a second protease activity—sequences at the NS2/NS3 junction are responsible for self-cleavage of that site. The HCV NS5, unlike that of the flaviviruses, is cleaved to yield NS5a and NS5b. NS5b contains the GDD motif common to viral RNA-dependent RNA polymerases and so is likely to be the HCV replicase and NS5a also may be involved in genome replication.

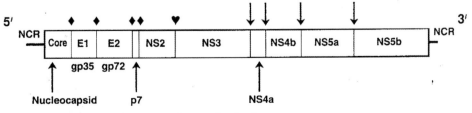

Figure 3.14   Organisation of the HCV genome. See text for details

Epidemiology of Hepatitis C

Infection with hepatitis C virus occurs throughout the world, with a current estimate of 170 million infected people. Much of the seroprevalence data are based on blood donors, who represent a carefully selected population in many countries. The prevalence of antibodies to HCV in blood donors varies from 0.02% in different countries. Almost 4 million Americans (1.8% of the population of the USA) have antibody to HCV, indicating ongoing or previous infection with this virus. Higher rates have been found in southern Italy, Spain, central Europe, Japan and parts of the Middle East, with as many as 19% in Egyptian blood donors. Until screening of blood donors was introduced, hepatitis C accounted for the vast majority of non-A, non-B post-transfusion hepatitis. However, it is clear that while blood transfusion and the transfusion of blood products are efficient routes of transmission of HCV, these represent a small proportion (about 15%) of cases of acute clinical hepatitis in the USA and a number of other countries (with the exception of patients with haemophilia). Current data indicate that in some 40–50% of patients in industrialised countries the source of infection cannot be identified; 35% or more of patients have a history of intravenous drug misuse; household contact and sexual exposure do not appear to be major factors in the epidemiology of this common infection, and occupational exposure in the health care setting accounts for about 2% of cases. Transmission of HCV from mother to infant occurs in about 10% of viraemic mothers and the risk appears to be related to the level of viraemia. The possibility of transmission *in utero* is also being investigated.

Diagnosis of HCV Infection

Cloning of the HCV genome made possible the development of specific diagnostic tests, including EIAs for antibody and RT-PCR for viraemia. Because expression of the original clone was detected by antibodies from the serum of an infected patient, it was an obvious candidate for development of an EIA to detect anti-HCV antibodies. A larger clone, C100, was assembled from a number of overlapping clones and expressed in yeast as a fusion protein, using human superoxide dismutase sequences to facilitate expression. This fusion protein formed the basis of first-generation tests for HCV infection (Kuo *et al.*, 1989). It is now known that antibodies to C100 are detected relatively late, following an acute infection. Furthermore, the first-generation assays were associated with a high rate of false positivity when applied to low-incidence populations and there were further problems with some retrospective studies on stored sera. Data based on this test alone should, therefore, be interpreted with caution.

Second and later generation tests include antigens from the nucleocapsid and further non-structural regions of the genome. The former (C22) is particularly useful because the sequence of the HCV core protein is relatively highly conserved, compared to other HCV proteins, and antibodies appear relatively early during infection. Supplementary tests involving several viral antigens bound to a solid substrate, recombinant immunoblot assays (RIBAs), are available and give a more detailed evaluation of the antibody profile of the patient. Antibody tests based on synthetic peptides also are available.

Routine testing of blood donations is now in place in most industrialised countries and prevalence rates vary from 0.2–0.5% in northern Europe to 1.2–1.5% in southern Europe and Japan. Many of those who are found to be antibody-positive have a history of parenteral risk, such as transfusion or administration of blood products or intravenous drug use. There is minimal evidence for sexual or perinatal transmission of HCV and it is not clear what the 'natural' routes of transmission are.

The availability of the nucleotide sequence of HCV made possible the use of the RT-PCR as a direct test for the genome of the virus itself. The first step is the synthesis of a complementary DNA copy of the target region of the RNA genome, using RT primed by the antigenomic PCR primer or random hexadeoxyribonucleotides. The product of this reaction is a suitable target for amplification. The concentration of virus in serum samples is often very low, so that the mass of product from the PCR reaction is insufficient for visualisation on a stained gel. Therefore, a second round of amplification (with nested primers) or detection of the primary product by Southern hybridisation is required. There is considerable variation in nucleotide sequences among different isolates of HCV and the 5' non-coding region, which seems to be highly conserved, is the preferred target for diagnostic PCR (Garson *et al.*, 1991). Hepatitis C viral load may be estimated by quantitative RT-PCR or by using a bDNA hybridisation assay. An immunoassay for the direct detection of the HCV core protein is currently under evaluation. This assay, based on a monoclonal antibody, provides an alternative means of quantifying viraemia in patients with relatively high viral loads.

Interpretation of Serological Tests for HCV

A negative EIA test is sufficient to rule out infection in individuals, such as blood donors, without risk factors for HCV infection. For those of low risk, a positive EIA requires confirmation and a supplementary assay for antibodies, such as RIBA, is valuable. Where the RIBA is negative, the EIA result is likely to have been a false positive. If the RIBA is positive, the patient is likely to have (or to have had) hepatitis C. RT-PCR may then be used to determine whether the patient is viraemic. Follow-up RT-PCR is also indicated where the result of the RIBA is indeterminate.

Individuals with even slightly raised serum aminotransferases should be tested for anti-HCV by EIA and any positive results confirmed by RIBA or assay for HCV RNA. In patients with biochemical or clinical evidence of liver disease, a positive EIA is sufficient to diagnose hepatitis C and testing for HCV RNA is valuable for confirmation. Quantitative assays for HCV RNA are valuable in monitoring the efficacy of antiviral therapy and may help predict long-term outcome.

Persistence of HCV Infection Is Common

Current data suggest that 60–80% of infections with HCV progress to chronicity. Thus, in contrast to HBV infection, where persistent infections of immunocompetent adults are rare, persistent HCV infection seems to be the norm. The morbidity of chronic hepatitis C is affected by many interactive factors, including age of acquisition, concomitant alcohol abuse, gender, co-existing viral disease and the host immune response.

Histological examinations of liver biopsies from 'healthy' HCV-carriers (blood donors) reveal that none has normal histology and that up to 70% have chronic active hepatitis and/or cirrhosis (Esteban *et al.*, 1991). It is not clear whether pathological changes result from direct cytopathology of the virus or are mediated by the immune response to infection. HCV infection also is associated with progression to HCC, e.g. in Japan, where the incidence of HCC has been increasing despite a decrease in the prevalence of HBsAg, HCV is the major risk factor. There is no DNA intermediate in the replication of the HCV genome or integration of viral nucleic acid and viral pathology may contribute to oncogenesis through cirrhosis and regeneration of liver cells. HCV infection rarely seems to cause acute liver failure.

In the USA, HCV accounts for 60–70% of chronic hepatitis, up to 50% of cirrhosis, end-stage liver disease and HCC. HCV causes an estimated 8000–10 000 deaths annually in the USA (Alter and Seeff, 2000).

Genotypes

The tremendous variation in the sequence of the genomes of various isolates of HCV has led to their classification into types and subtypes (Simmonds *et al.*, 1994) and up to 11 major genotypes are recognised. There is some evidence of variation between genotypes of viral pathogenicity and responsiveness to treatment (see below) but data are incomplete for most genotypes and other variables, such as the age of the patient and the duration of infection, confound interpretation.

Infections with types 1b and 1a are relatively common in Europe; infection with type 1b is frequent in southern Europe. Epidemiological differences in age distribution of major types, and the risk factors associated with particular genotypes, have become apparent. In Europe, types 3a and 1a are relatively more common in young individuals with a history of intravenous drug use. Type 1b accounts for most infections in those aged 50 or more. Type 4 infection is the most prevalent infection in Egypt, and many parts of the Middle East and Africa.

Although an inherently greater pathogenicity of type 1 HCV has been implied, these studies have not always been based on prospective follow-up or appropriately controlled to account for influences of several interdependent parameters and co-factors. Moreover, several clinical investigations have documented severe and progressive liver disease after infection with each of the well-characterised genotypes (1a, 1b, 2a, 2b, 3a, 4a, 5 and 6), so there is little evidence so far for variants of HCV that are completely non-pathogenic.

Treatment of Hepatitis C

Interferon-α

A considerable number of large, controlled therapeutic trials of IFN-α or IFN-α in combination with ribavirin, have been undertaken in acute and chronic hepatitis C infection.

Acute Hepatitis C

The mean incubation period of hepatitis C is 6–12 weeks. It is shorter with large inoculae (e.g. following administration of contaminated factor VIII). The acute course of HCV infection is clinically mild. Only 25% of cases are icteric, but patients with jaundice are more likely to clear the virus. Approximately 50–60% of patients will still have elevated serum aminotransferases 6 months after diagnosis (Alter *et al.*, 1992). Diagnosis may require testing for HCV RNA, because some patients may not have anti-HCV at the time that serum aminotransferases are elevated. Treatment is indicated for acute HCV infection because of the propensity of this virus to cause chronic disease; controlled trials indicate that treatment of the acute infection lessens the risk of chronic disease. It is not always clear whether treatment has benefited those patients who might have been convalescing spontaneously. The optimal form of treatment for acute hepatitis C is not yet determined. A trial of IFN-β in Japan, given intravenously for 1–3 months, did significantly reduce the risk of chronic hepatitis (Omata *et al.*, 1991). If a diagnosis of acute hepatitis C can be made, and the patient does not appear to be convalescing 2–4 months after the onset of the disease, IFN-α can be considered at a dose of 3–6 μg three times weekly for at least 6 months. Recent studies have made clear the fact that treatment benefits those patients who have been treated early, but it may be reasonable to allow 1–3 months to determine which patients might convalesce spontaneously (Jaeckel *et al.*, 2001). It is not yet clear whether pegylated IFN would offer an advantage, or whether combination treatment is essential (Hoofnagle, 2001).

Chronic Hepatitis C

There is evidence that alcohol and hepatitis C may synergistically aggravate hepatic injury, and the drinking of excess alcohol is discouraged because of this detrimental evidence (Sawada *et al.*, 1993; Miyakawa *et al.*, 1993). The patient should be advised not to donate blood. Patients can be told that the parenteral route is the most important route of transmission and that the virus is not easily transmitted except by this route.

IFN-α is indicated for the treatment of patients with chronic hepatitis C infection who are HCV RNA-positive and have elevated serum aminotransferases with histological moderate chronic hepatitis or more advanced lesions (Hoofnagle and Tralka, 1997; Anonymous, 1997). Thus, a liver biopsy generally is required. There is currently no substitute for liver biopsy to ascertain the grade (severity and extent of hepatic inflammation) or stage the disease (fibrosis).

Serum aminotransferases, bilirubin, alkaline phosphatase and prothrombin time should be measured. In patients whose lifestyle or geographic origin suggests that they are at risk of other viral infections, HBsAg and HIV infection need also be considered. It is not easy to chart the prognosis for patients seen at one point in time, however, as the disease progresses at variable rates in patients. It is not yet clear whether treating relatively mild, early disease in younger patients to prevent cirrhosis is a rational objective.

Four IFN-αs have been studied in large controlled trials of IFN-α. Several, including HuIFN-α-n1 (Wellferon) rIFN-α2β, (Intron A), and rIFN-α2α (Roferon-A) and Consensus interferon, have been evaluated for the treatment of chronic hepatitis C.

Ribavirin

Ribavirin is a synthetic guanosine nucleoside analogue, which possesses a broad spectrum of low-potency activity against both DNA and RNA viruses *in vitro* and *in vivo* (Fernandez *et al.*, 1986). Ribavirin shows only modest activity against hepatitis C virus but it increases the activity of IFN-α when the two agents are used in combination. The drug exerts its action after intracellular phosphorylation to mono-, di- and triphosphate nucleotides. The precise mode of action may include pertubation of intracellular nucleoside triphosphate pools, direct inhibition of the viral mRNA polymerase complex, mutagenesis of the viral genome and possibly enhancement of macrophage inhibition of viral replication. The combination of ribavirin and IFN-α has been shown to produce sustained virologic responses in about 40–50% of patients.

The major side-effects of the drug that have been reported include anaemia, a metallic taste, dry mouth, flatulence, dyspepsia, nausea, headaches, irritability, emotional lability, fatigue, insomnia, skin rashes and myalgia. Mild reversible anaemia is common. Modest increases in uric acid have been reported. Ribavirin is also teratogenic in animals and so is contraindicated in pregnancy; patients should not conceive for at least 6 months after stopping therapy.

Interferon plus Ribavirin

The recommended dosage of combination therapy is 3 million IU IFN-α injected subcutaneously three times weekly, and ribavirin 1000 mg administered orally in divided daily doses (1200 mg for patients weighing more than 70 kg).

Guidelines recommend antiviral therapy for those patients with chronic hepatitis C who are at highest risk of developing cirrhosis, i.e. patients with persistently increased serum ALT levels, detectable levels of HCV RNA and histological evidence of portal or bridging fibrosis or inflammation and necrosis. Recent clinical guidelines, including the EASL guidelines published in 1999, recommend that patients with moderate inflammation or moderate fibrosis should be considered for combination therapy with IFN-α plus ribavirin. The duration of therapy depends on the genotype and level of viraemia. Patients with genotypes 2 or 3 are treated for 6 months, as there is no advantage in prolonging treatment beyond this point. For patients with genotype 1, current data suggest that 6 months is sufficient, if the level of viraemia is low (less than 2 million copies/ml); 12 months of treatment is recommended if the level of viraemia is higher. Treatment should be continued only in patients with type 1 infection in whom HCV RNA has disappeared after 6 months of therapy. In naive patients in whom ribavirin is contraindicated, IFN monotherapy (3 million units or 9 µg, three times a week) should be administered for 12 months. It is important to manage the side-effects of therapy.

Careful clinical monitoring is suggested as an alternative to antiviral therapy for patients with less severe histological changes in whom cirrhosis may not develop. Studies have also shown that combination therapy with IFN-α plus ribavirin is beneficial in patients relapsing on IFN-α monotherapy.

Pegylated Interferons

The efficacy of pegylated IFN-α2a has been investigated in several controlled trials, and the outcome compared to standard IFN or IFN and ribavirin, based on virological, biochemical and histological responses. In these trials, sustained virologic responses were significantly higher in patients with chronic hepatitis C treated weekly with pegylated IFN-α than in those treated with IFN-α2a three million units thrice weekly (Reddy et al., 2001).

Pegylated IFN-α has proved significantly more effective in patients with hepatitis C than standard IFN. Recent studies have compared the efficacy of pegylated IFN-α2β plus ribavirin with standard IFN-α2β plus ribavirin for 48 weeks, or pegylated IFN-α2α and ribavirin. A high dose of pegylated IFN (1.5 µg/kg/week plus ribavirin 1–1.2 g daily) was more effective than standard IFN plus ribavirin for the treatment of HCV. Sustained virological responses were observed in 54% of those treated with high-dose pegylated IFN-α2β and ribavirin. Among patients with type 1 infection, the best response was observed in those treated with 1.5 µg/kg pegylated IFN (42%) vs. 33% for those treated with standard IFN and ribavirin (Manns et al., 2001).

A randomised Phase III trial of pegylated IFN-α2α and ribavirin has been published in abstract form. Pegylated IFN-α2α 180 µg/week plus ribavirin was superior to standard IFN-α2β plus ribavirin (1–2 g/day) for 48 weeks. Sustained virological responses for all genotypes were greater in recipients of pegylated IFN-α2α plus ribavirin (56%) compared to recipients of pegylated IFN-α2β plus ribavirin (45%). In recent studies, differences were observed in patients infected with genotypes 1 vs. non-1: e.g. 76% of patients with types 2 and 3 responded to pegylated IFN-α2α plus ribavirin, whereas 46% of patients with type 1 HCV responded to pegylated IFN-α2α plus ribavirin. Thus, these agents appear to be useful new treatment options that are more convenient for patients.

General Points about Treatment

Within genotypes, response rates may be higher for patients with lower virus concentrations and less advanced disease. Younger patients and patients without fibrosis or cirrhosis are also more responsive to therapy (Chemello et al., 1995). The mechanisms by which different genotypes might differ in responsiveness to treatment remain obscure. Patients with diverse circulating quasi-species may be less responsive to therapy than those with a single major species. Recent molecular evidence suggests that an IFN-sensitive region can be defined in the NS5a region in patients with genotype 1b infection. Patients with more amino acid substitutions in the NS5A gene (region 2209–2248) were more likely to have a complete response than patients with wild-type 1b (Enomoto et al., 1996).

Because autoimmune hepatitis is treated differently, and may be aggravated by IFN therapy, it is particularly advisable to exclude this diagnosis by measuring the titres of anti-smooth muscle and anti-liver kidney microsomal antibodies, even in those with a positive anti-HCV test, and to measure HCV RNA in anti-HCV-positive patients in whom IFN-α is contemplated.

Several small trials have suggested that IFN therapy improves liver function and reduces the incidence of HCC in patients with cirrhosis due to hepatitis B or C (Nishiguchi *et al.*, 1995). A recent, retrospective analysis of data for 913 patients with chronic viral hepatitis and cirrhosis from Italy and Argentina showed that IFN treatment lowered the rate of progression to hepatocellular carcinoma two-fold (International Interferon-α Hepatocellular Carcinoma Study Group, 1998). The risk reduction was apparently greater for patients with chronic hepatitis C and no evidence of infection with HBV. Treatment of hepatitis C may also reduce the indirect effects of this virus, including cryoglobulinaemia and lymphoma (reviewed in Zoulim *et al.*, 2003).

First reports of a new specific HCV serine protease inhibitor effective (BILN 2061) against hepatitis C are encouraging, as this new oral agent caused a dose-dependent 3–4 log drop in levels of viraemia in genotype 1 patients within 48 h (Lamarre *et al.*, 2003). Further developments in the field are anticipated.

Prevention of Hepatitis C

There are no vaccines available to protect contacts of individuals with hepatitis C. Difficulties in vaccine development include the sequence diversity between different viral groups and the substantial sequence heterogeneity among isolates in the N-terminal region of the E2 glycoprotein. However, secondary transmission should be relatively easy to prevent. The role of intrafamilial transmission requires clarification, but is relatively infrequent. Sexual transmission is possible and has been described, but fortunately this is a relatively inefficient and infrequent route. Young sexually active adults could be told of the advisability of condom use in general for casual sexual contact.

Mother-to-infant transmission has been observed, but appears to be unusual. Differences in the rates of maternal–infant transmission in different countries remain unexplained, and the importance of this route in perpetuating the reservoir of human infection is unknown, but could be relevant. Maternal–infant transmission is more likely in mothers with HCV RNA concentrations higher than 10^7 genomes/ml. Transmission from infected surgeons to their patients has been documented and verified by molecular epidemiological evidence (Esteban *et al.*, 1996). It is unknown whether higher levels of viraemia and particular forms of surgery are more likely to transmit infection.

Immunisation

There are currently no vaccines for the prevention of HCV infection. In the future, DNA vaccination may offer a suitable strategy. Physicians should consider vaccinating patients with chronic hepatitis C against HAV and HBV.

The GB Virus C and 'Hepatitis G' Virus

The discovery of HCV and HEV and their roles in causing parenterally-transmitted, epidemic and sporadic cases of non-A, non-B hepatitis does not rule out the possibility that there are other, unidentified human viruses which may cause hepatitis. Incubation times varied following transmission of non-A, non-B hepatitis to non-human primates, suggesting the involvement of more than one agent. The results of subsequent cross-challenge experiments seemed to support this conclusion, although retrospective analyses of samples from many of these studies implicate reinfection with HCV. Some sporadic cases of acute liver failure may be associated with a virus infection. Virus-like particles were detected by electron microscopy (Fagan *et al.*, 1992) but, although other viruses were excluded rigorously (Fagan and Harrison, 1994), a viral aetiology could not be confirmed by experimental transmission to potentially susceptible animals. Other viruses may exist which are spread by the faecal–oral route and have a tropism for the liver.

Application of molecular biological techniques led to the discovery, by two groups working independently, of a novel, parenterally-transmitted virus. This was given the provisional names GB virus C (GBV-C) (Simons *et al.*, 1995) and hepatitis G virus (HGV) (Linnen *et al.*, 1996). The structure of the genome GBV-C/HGV is typical of the *Flaviviridae* and, more specifically, is highly similar to HCV. Sequence variation among isolates of GBV-C/HGV, including in the region encoding the surface glycoproteins, seems to be rather less than for HCV but four genotypes, with varying geographical distribution, have been described.

The Clinical Significance of GBV-C/HGV Infection

Despite much effort, it has not been possible to identify recombinant antigens which react consistently in immunoassays with antibodies in the sera of infected individuals. Detection of the genome by RT-PCR remains the sole reliable method for diagnosing viraemia. Estimates of the prevalence of GBV-C/HGV infection in healthy individuals vary from 0.8% (blood donors with normal ALT levels in the USA) to 5.7% (Vietnam) and are much higher for those with parenteral risk factors, such as multiply transfused and HCV-positive individuals. Antibodies to the envelope (E2) glycoprotein seem to be a marker of recovery from past infection but their longevity remains to be established. GBV-C/HGV viraemia has been detected in patients with a variety of disorders, including chronic liver disease and acute liver failure, but a causative role remains unproved. Most individuals who become infected with GBV-C/HGV experience transient infections without symptoms, or have only mild elevations of serum aminotransferases as the sole evidence of liver involvement. Persistent infections of varying duration develop in around 5–10% of cases. Convincing evidence that the virus replicates in the liver has not been published in the peer-reviewed literature.

Whether GBV-C/HGV causes significant disease in a minority of those infected remains to be established. GBV-C/HGV may share a common pattern of transmission with HCV. Infection is common in risk groups such as intravenous drug users and the recipients of blood products, including haemophiliacs and patients with combined variable immunodeficiency. Instances of transmission through transfusion have been documented. Given their common mode of transmission, it is not surprising that co-infections may occur with HCV and GBV-C/HGV. However, it is not clear that co-infection worsens the course of chronic hepatitis C. Other co-infections also may occur and two papers (Xiang et al., 2001; Tillman et al., 2001) raise the intriguing possibility that co-infection with GBV-C/HGV may ameliorate HIV disease, although this finding has recently been challenged (Birk et al., 2002).

TTV and Related Viruses

Novel viral sequences were isolated in 1997 from a Japanese patient with post-transfusion hepatitis not associated with any of the conventional hepatitis viruses described above (Nishizawa et al., 1997). The agent was named TT virus after the initials of the patient and also has been referred to incorrectly as 'transfusion transmitted' virus. However, the presence of the virus in stool samples suggests that faecal–oral transmission may be a rather more common route. The virus also is found at high titres in saliva.

The TTV genome is a circular, single-stranded DNA molecule around 3.85 kb in size. TTV is now recognised as the prototype of a diverse group of viruses (including 'Yonban', 'Sanban', 'SENV' and others) with up to 30% divergence in sequence (unusually high for a DNA genome). Related viruses with smaller (around 2.9 kb) genomes have been dubbed 'TTV-like mini-viruses' (TLMV). TTV and TLMV belong to the family *Circoviridae* but are distinct from the circoviruses and a new genus, '*Anellovirus*', has been proposed (Hino, 2002). Eight genotypes of SENV have been described, SENV-A to SENV-H, each differing by at least 25% in nucleotide sequence. SENV-C, SENV-D and SENV-H are supposedly associated with transfusion hepatitis, and although the prevalence of these viruses is common in patients with non-A to non-E liver disease, a causal association has not been demonstrated and these should not be considered at present as candidate hepatitis viruses.

Sensitive PCR assays, targeted at conserved sequences in the untranslated region, are able to detect these viruses in more than 90% of the human population. Individuals may be infected with both TTV and TLMV, and with multiple genotypes of TTV. This extremely high prevalence in healthy individuals suggests that early reports associating TTV infection with acute liver failure and other disease states should be interpreted with caution. However, the formal possibility remains that a subset of TTV genotypes is pathogenic. The detection of (circular, double-stranded) replicative intermediates in liver and bone marrow (Okamoto et al., 2000a, 2000b) suggests that the virus replicates in these tissues, and perhaps also in other sites, and is shed into the blood and faeces. TTV DNA is found in saliva (78%), breast milk, semen (60%), cervical swabs and other body fluids of infected persons. TTV is also found in farm animals, including chickens (19%), cows (25%), pigs (20%), sheep (30%) and other mammals, including non-human primates.

REFERENCES

Alter HJ (1988) Transfusion-associated non-A, non-B hepatitis. The first decade. In *Viral Hepatitis and Liver Disease* (ed. Zuckerman AJ), pp 537–542. Alan R. Liss, New York.

Alter MJ, Margolis HS, Krawczynski K et al. (1992) The natural history of community-acquired hepatitis C in the United States. *N Engl J Med*, **327**, 1899–1905.

Alter HJ and Seeff LB (2000) Recovery, persistence and sequelae in hepatitis C infection: a perspective on long-term outcome. *Semin Liver Dis*, **20**, 17–35.

Anonymous (1997) *Management of Hepatitis C*. NIH Consensus Statement 1997 Mar 24–26, **15**, 1–41.

Arankalle VA and Chobe LP (2000) Retrospective analysis of blood transfusion recipients: evidence for post-transfusion hepatitis E. *Vox Sang*, **79**, 72–74.

Beasley RP and Hwang L-Y (1991) Overview on the epidemiology of hepatocellular carcinoma. In *Viral Hepatitis and Liver Disease* (eds Hollinger FB, Lemon SM, Margolis HS), pp 532–535. Williams and Wilkins, Baltimore.

Behrens RH and Roberts JA (1994) Is travel prophylaxis worth while? Economic appraisal of prophylactic measures against malaria, hepatitis A, and typhoid in travellers. *Br Med J*, **309**, 918–922.

Benhamou Y, Bochet M, Thibault V *et al.* (2001) Safety and efficacy of adefovir dipivoxil in patients co-infected with HIV-1 and lamivudine-resistant hepatitis B virus: an open-label pilot study. *Lancet*, **358**, 718–723.

Benhamou Y, Dohin E, Lunel-Fabiani F *et al.* (1995) Efficacy of lamivudine on replication of hepatitis B virus in HIV-infected patients. *Lancet*, **345**, 396–397.

Bertoletti A, Chisari FV, Penna A *et al.* (1993) Definition of a minimal optimal cytotoxic T-cell epitope within the hepatitis B virus nucleocapsid protein. *J Virol*, **67**, 2376–2380.

Bertoletti A, Costanzo A, Chisari FV *et al.* (1994) Cytotoxic T lymphocyte response to a wild-type hepatitis B virus epitope in patients chronically infected by variant viruses carrying substitutions within the epitope. *J Exp Med*, **180**, 933–943.

Birk M, Lindback S and Lidman C (2002) No influence of GB virus C replication on the prognosis in a cohort of HIV-1-infected patients. *AIDS*, **16**, 2482–2485.

Blumberg BS, Alter HJ and Visnich S (1965) A 'new' antigen in leukemia sera. *J Am Med Assoc*, **191**, 541–546.

Bradley DW (1992) Hepatitis E: epidemiology, aetiology and molecular biology. *Rev Med Virol*, **2**, 19–28.

Bradley DW, Krawczynski K, Cook EH Jr *et al.* (1988) Enterically transmitted non-A, non-B hepatitis: etiology of disease and laboratory studies in non-human primates. In *Viral Hepatitis and Liver Disease* (ed. Zuckerman AJ), pp 138–147. Alan R. Liss, New York.

Bradley DW, McCaustland KA, Cook EH *et al.* (1985) Posttransfusion non-A, non-B hepatitis in chimpanzees. Physicochemical evidence that the tubule-forming agent is a small, enveloped virus. *Gastroenterology*, **88**, 773–779.

Brechot C, Pourcel C, Louise A *et al.* (1980) Presence of integrated hepatitis B virus DNA sequences in cellular DNA of human hepatocellular carcinoma. *Nature*, **286**, 533–535.

Brunetto MR, Oliveri F, Rocca G *et al.* (1989) Natural course and response to interferon of chronic hepatitis B accompanied by antibody to hepatitis B e antigen. *Hepatology*, **10**, 198–202.

Bryant ML, Bridges EG, Placidi L *et al.* (2001) Anti-HBV specific β-L-2′-deoxynucleosides. *Nucleosides Nucleotides Nucleic Acids*, **20**, 597–607.

Buti M, Esteban R, Español MT *et al.* (1991) Influence of human immunodeficiency virus infection on cell-mediated immunity in chronic D hepatitis. *J Infect Dis*, **163**, 1351–1353.

Carman WF, Jacyna MR, Hadziyannis S *et al.* (1989) Mutation preventing formation of hepatitis B e antigen in patients with chronic hepatitis B infection. *Lancet*, **2**, 588–591.

Carman WF, Zanetti AR, Karayiannis P *et al.* (1990) Vaccine-induced escape mutant of hepatitis B virus. *Lancet*, **336**, 325–329.

Carreno V, Zeuzem S, Hopf U *et al.* (2000) A phase I/II study of recombinant human interleukin-12 in patients with chronic hepatitis B. *J Hepatol*, **32**, 317–324.

Casey JL and Gerin JL (1995) Hepatitis D virus RNA editing: specific modification of adenosine in the antigenomic RNA. *J Virol*, **69**, 7593–7600.

Cavanaugh VJ, Guidotti LG and Chisari FV (1997) Interleukin-12 inhibits hepatitis B virus replication in transgenic mice. *J Virol*, **71**, 3236–3243.

Chang MH, Chen CJ, Lai MS *et al.* (1997) Universal hepatitis B vaccination in Taiwan and the incidence of hepatocellular carcinoma in children. *N Engl J Med*, **336**, 1855–1859.

Chemello L, Bonetti P, Cavalletto L *et al.* (1995) Randomized trial comparing three different regimens of α2a-interferon in chronic hepatitis C. *Hepatology*, **22**, 700–706.

Chen J-Y, Harrison TJ, Lee C-S *et al.* (1986) Detection of hepatitis B virus DNA in hepatocellular carcinoma. *Br J Exp Pathol*, **67**, 279–288.

Chong Y and Chu CK (2002) Understanding the unique mechanism of L-FMAU (Clevudine) against hepatitis B virus: molecular dynamics studies. *Bioorg Med Chem Lett*, **12**, 3459–3462.

Choo QL, Kuo G, Weiner AJ *et al.* (1989) Isolation of a cDNA clone derived from a blood-borne non-A, non-B viral hepatitis genome. *Science*, **244**, 359–362.

Choo QL, Richman KH, Han JH *et al.* (1991) Genetic organization and diversity of the hepatitis-C virus. *Proc Natl Acad Sci USA*, **88**, 2451–2455.

Cohen JI, Ticehurst JR, Purcell RH *et al.* (1987) Complete nucleotide sequence of wild-type hepatitis A virus: comparison with different strains of hepatitis A virus and other picornaviruses. *J Virol*, **61**, 5–59.

Cupps TR, Hoofnagle JH, Ellis RW *et al.* (1990) *In vitro* immune responses to hepatitis B surface antigens S and preS2 during acute infection by hepatitis B virus in humans. *J Infect Dis*, **161**, 412–419.

Davis HL, Schirmbeck R, Reimann J *et al.* (1995) DNA-mediated immunization in mice induces a potent MHC class I-restricted cytotoxic T lymphocyte response to the hepatitis B envelope protein. *Hum Gene Ther*, **6**, 1447–1456.

Dawson GJ, Chau KH, Cabal CM *et al.* (1992) Solid-phase enzyme-linked immunosorbent assay for hepatitis-E virus IgG and IgM antibodies utilizing recombinant antigens and synthetic peptides. *J Virol Methods*, **38**, 175–186.

Dejean A, Bougueleset L, Grzeschik K-H *et al.* (1986) Hepatitis B virus DNA integration in a sequence homologous to v-erb-A and steroid receptor genes in a hepatocellular carcinoma. *Nature*, **322**, 70–72.

Dienstag JL, Schiff ER, Wright TL *et al.* (1999) Lamivudine as initial treatment for chronic hepatitis B in the United States. *N Engl J Med*, **341**, 1256–1263.

Dusheiko G (1997) Side-effects of α-interferon in chronic hepatitis C. *Hepatology*, **26**, 112S–121S.

Dusheiko G, Dibisceglie A, Bowyer S *et al.* (1985) Recombinant leukocyte interferon treatment of chronic hepatitis B. *Hepatology*, **5**, 556–560.

Ellerbeck EF, Lewis JA, Nalin D *et al.* (1992) Safety profile and immunogenicity of an inactivated vaccine derived from an attenuated strain of hepatitis A. *Vaccine*, **10**, 668–672.

Emerson SU, Huang YK, McRill C *et al.* (1992) Mutations in both the 2B-gene and 2C-gene of hepatitis A virus are involved in adaptation to growth in cell culture. *J Virol*, **66**, 650–654.

Enomoto N, Sakuma K, Asahina Y *et al.* (1996) Mutations in the non-structural protein 5a gene and response to interferon in patients with chronic hepatitis B 1b infection. *N Engl J Med*, **334**, 77–81.

Esteban JI, Gomez J, Martell M *et al.* (1996) Transmission of hepatitis C virus by a cardiac surgeon. *N Engl J Med*, **334**, 555–560.

Esteban JI, Lopez-Talavera JC, Genesca J *et al.* (1991) High rate of infectivity and liver disease in blood donors with antibodies to hepatitis-C virus. *Ann Intern Med*, **115**, 443–449.

European Consensus Group on Hepatitis B Immunity (2002) Are booster immunisations needed for lifelong hepatitis B immunity? *Lancet*, **355**, 561–565.

Fagan EA, Ellis DS, Tovey GM *et al.* (1992) Toga virus-like particles in acute liver failure attributed to sporadic non-A, non-B hepatitis and recurrence after liver transplantation. *J Med Virol*, **38**, 71–77.

Fagan EA and Harrison TJ (1994) Exclusion in liver by polymerase chain reaction of hepatitis B and C viruses in acute liver failure attributed to sporadic non-A, non-B hepatitis. *J Hepatol*, **21**, 587–591.

Fang ZL, Yang JY, Ge XM *et al.* (2002) Core promoter mutations (A(1762)T and G(1764)A) and viral genotype in chronic hepatitis B and hepatocellular carcinoma in Guangxi, China. *J Med Virol*, **68**, 33–40.

Fattovich G, Giustina G, Degos F *et al.* (1997) Morbidity and mortality in compensated cirrhosis type C: a retrospective follow-up study of 384 patients. *Gastroenterology*, **112**, 463–472.

Fernandez H, Banks G and Smith R (1986) Ribavirin: a clinical overview. *Eur J Epidemiol*, **2**, 1–14.

Flehmig B, Heinricy U and Pfisterer M (1989) Immunogenicity of a killed hepatitis A vaccine in seronegative volunteers. *Lancet*, **I**, 1039–1041.

Francois G, Kew M, Van Damme P *et al.* (2001) Mutant hepatitis B viruses: a matter of academic interest only or a problem with far-reaching implications? *Vaccine*, **19**, 3799–3815.

Gaeta GB, Stroffolini T, Chiaramonte M *et al.* (2000) Chronic hepatitis D: a vanishing disease? An Italian multicenter study. *Hepatology*, **32**, 824–827.

Garson JA, Ring CJA and Tuke PW (1991) Improvement of HCV genome detection with 'short' PCR products. *Lancet*, **338**, 1466–1467.

Guidotti LG and Chisari FV (2001) Non-cytolytic control of viral infections by the innate and adaptive immune response. *Annu Rev Immunol*, **19**, 65–91.

Guilhot SL, Guidotti G and Chisari FV (1993) Interleukin-2 downregulates hepatitis-B virus gene expression in transgenic mice by a posttranscriptional mechanism. *J Virol*, **67**, 7444–7449.

Hadziyannis SJ (1997) Hepatitis delta—review. *J Gastroenterol Hepatol*, **12**, 289–298.

Hadziyannis SJ, Lieberman HM, Karvountzis GG *et al.* (1983) Analysis of liver disease, nuclear HBcAg, viral replication, and hepatitis B virus DNA in liver and serum of HBeAg vs. anti-HBe positive carriers of hepatitis B virus. *Hepatology*, **3**, 656–662.

Hadziyannis SJ, Tassopoulos NC, Heathcote EJ *et al.* (2003) Adefovir dipivoxil for the treatment of hepatitis B e antigen-negative chronic hepatitis B. *N Engl J Med*, **348**, 800–807.

Halliday ML, Kang L-Y, Zhou T-K *et al.* (1991) An epidemic of hepatitis A attributable to the ingestion of raw clams in Shanghai, China. *J Infect Dis*, **164**, 852–859.

Harrison TJ, Anderson MG, Murray-Lyon IM *et al.* (1986) Hepatitis B virus DNA in the hepatocyte. A series of 160 biopsies. *J Hepatol*, **2**, 1–10.

Harrison TJ, Hopes EA, Oon CJ *et al.* (1991) Independent emergence of a vaccine-induced escape mutant of hepatitis B virus. *J Hepatol*, **13**(suppl 4), S105–S107.

He LF, Alling D, Popkin T *et al.* (1987) Determining the size of non-A, non-B hepatitis virus by filtration. *J Infect Dis*, **156**, 636–640.

Heathcote J, McHutchison J, Lee S *et al.* (1999) A pilot study of the CY-1899 T-cell vaccine in subjects chronically infected with hepatitis B virus. *Hepatology*, **30**, 531–536.

Hino S (2002) TTV, a new human virus with a single stranded circular DNA genome. *Rev Med Virol*, **12**, 151–158.

Honkoop P, De Man RA, Heijtink RA *et al.* (1995) Hepatitis B reactivation after lamivudine. *Lancet*, **346**, 1156–1157.

Hoofnagle JH (2001) Therapy for acute hepatitis C. *N Engl J Med*, **345**, 1495–1497.

Hoofnagle JH and Tralka TS (1997) The National Institutes of Health consensus development conference: management of hepatitis C—Introduction. *Hepatology*, **26**, 1S; and The National Institutes of Health consensus development conference panel statement: management of hepatitis C. *Hepatology*, **26**, 2S–10S.

Hsu HY, Chang MH, Liaw SH, Ni YH and Chen HL (1999) Changes of hepatitis B surface antigen variants in carrier children before and after universal vaccination in Taiwan. *Hepatology*, **30**, 1312–1317.

International Interferon-α Hepatocellular Carcinoma Study Group (1998) Effect of interferon-α on progression of cirrhosis to hepatocellular carcinoma: a retrospective cohort study. *Lancet*, **351**, 1535–1539.

Jaeckel E, Cornberg M, Wedemeyer H *et al.* (2001) Treatment of acute hepatitis C with interferon-α2β. *N Engl J Med*, **345**, 1452–1457.

Jameel S, Durgapal H, Habibullah CM *et al.* (1992) Enteric non-A, non-B hepatitis: epidemics, animal transmission, and hepatitis E virus detection by the polymerase chain reaction. *J Med Virol*, **37**, 263–270.

Kaplan G, Totsuka A, Thompson P *et al.* (1996) Identification of a surface glycoprotein on African green monkey kidney cells as a receptor for hepatitis A virus. *EMBO J*, **15**, 4282–4296.

Karayiannis P, Saldanha J, Monjardino J *et al.* (1993) Immunisation of woodchucks with hepatitis δ antigen expressed by recombinant vaccinia and baculoviruses, controls HDV superinfection. *Prog Clin Biol Res*, **382**, 193–199.

Khuroo MS (1980) Study of and epidemic of non-A, non-B hepatitis. Possibility of another human hepatitis virus distinct from post-transfusion non-A, non-B type. *Am J Med*, **68**, 818–824.

Korenman J, Baker B, Waggoner J *et al.* (1991) Long-term remission of chronic hepatitis B after α-interferon therapy. *Ann Intern Med*, **114**, 629–634.

Krogsgaard K, Kryger P, Aldershvile J *et al.* (1985) Hepatitis B virus DNA in serum from patients with acute hepatitis B. *Hepatology*, **5**, 10–13.

Kuo G, Choo Q-L, Alter HJ *et al.* (1989) An assay for circulating antibodies to a major etiologic virus of human non-A, non-B hepatitis. *Science*, **244**, 362–364.

Lai CL, Rosmawati M, Lao J *et al.* (2002) Entecavir is superior to lamivudine in reducing hepatitis B virus DNA in patients with chronic hepatitis B infection. *Gastroenterology*, **123**, 1831–1838.

Lai MMC (1995) Molecular biologic and pathogenetic analysis of hepatitis δ virus. *J Hepatol*, **22**, 127–131.

Lamarre D, Anderson PC, Bailey M *et al.* (2003) An NS3 protease inhibitor with antiviral effects in humans infected with hepatitis C virus. *Nature*, **426**, 186–189.

Lau DT, Everhart J, Kleiner DE *et al.* (1997) Long-term follow-up of patients with chronic hepatitis B treated with interferon-α. *Gastroenterology*, **113**, 1660–1667.

Lazinski DW and Taylor JM (1995) Intracellular cleavage and ligation of hepatitis δ virus genomic RNA: regulation of ribozyme activity by *cis*-acting sequences and host factors. *J Virol*, **69**, 1190–1200.

Ling R, Mutimer D, Ahmed N *et al.* (1996) Selection of mutations in the hepatitis B virus polymerase during therapy of transplant recipients with lamivudine. *Hepatology*, **24**, 711–713.

Linnen J, Wages J, ZhangKeck ZY *et al.* (1996) Molecular cloning and disease association of hepatitis G virus: a transfusion-transmissible agent. *Science*, **271**, 505–508.

Lok ASF, Kwan W, Moeckli R *et al.* (1992) Seroepidemiological survey of hepatitis E in Hong Kong by recombinant-based enzyme immunoassays. *Lancet*, **340**, 1205–1208.

McMahon BJ, Beller M, Williams J *et al.* (1996) A program to control an outbreak of hepatitis A in Alaska by using an inactivated hepatitis A vaccine. *Arch Pediatr Adolesc Med*, **150**, 733–739.

McMahon G, Ehrlich PH, Moustafa ZA *et al.* (1992) Genetic alterations in the gene encoding the major HBsAg-DNA and immunological analysis of recurrent HBsAg derived from monoclonal antibody-treated liver transplant patients. *Hepatology*, **15**, 757–766.

Manns MP, McHutchinson JG, Gordon SC *et al.* (2001) Peginterferon-α2β plus ribavirin compared with interferon-α2β plus ribavirin for initial treatment of chronic hepatitis C: a randomised trial. *Lancet*, **358**, 958–965.

Marcellin P, Chang TT, Lim SG *et al.*; Adefovir Dipivoxil 437 Study Group (2003) Adefovir dipivoxil for the treatment of hepatitis B. *N Engl J Med*, **348**, 808–816.

Mechnik L, Bergman N, Attali M *et al.* (2001) Acute hepatitis E virus infection presenting as a prolonged cholestatic jaundice. *J Clin Gastroenterol*, **33**, 421–422.

Meng XJ, Purcell RH, Halbur PG *et al.* (1997) A novel virus in swine is closely related to the human hepatitis E virus. *Proc Natl Acad Sci USA*, **94**, 9860–9865.

Milich DR, Wolf SF, Hughes JL *et al.* (1995) Interleukin 12 suppresses autoantibody production by reversing helper T-cell phenotype in hepatitis B e antigen transgenic mice. *Proc Natl Acad Sci USA*, **92**, 6847–6851.

Miyakawa H, Sato C, Izumi N *et al.* (1993) Hepatitis C virus infection in alcoholic liver cirrhosis in Japan: its contribution to the development of hepatocellular carcinoma. *Alcohol Alcoholism*, **1A**(suppl), 85–90.

Nainan OV, Khristova ML, Bytm K *et al* (2002) Genetic variation of hepatitis B surface antigen coding region among infants with chronic hepatitis B virus infection. *J Med Virol*, **68**, 319–327.

Nainan OV, Stevens CE, Taylor PE *et al.* (1997) Hepatitis B virus (HBV) antibody resistant mutants among mothers and infants with chronic HBV infection. In *Viral Hepatitis and Liver Disease* (eds Rizzetto M, Purcell RH, Gerin JL and Verme G), pp 132–134. Edizioni Minerva Medica, Turin.

Niederau C, Heintges T, Lange S *et al.* (1996) Long-term follow-up of HBeAg-positive patients treated with interferon-α for chronic hepatitis B. *N Engl J Med*, **334**, 1422–1427.

Nishiguchi S, Kuroki T, Nakatani S *et al.* (1995) Randomised trial of effects of interferon-α on incidence of hepatocellular carcinoma in chronic active hepatitis C with cirrhosis. *Lancet*, **346**, 1051–1055.

Nishizawa T, Okamoto H, Konishi K *et al.* (1997) A novel DNA virus (TTV) associated with elevated transaminase levels in posttransfusion hepatitis of unknown etiology. *Biochem Biophys Res Commun*, **241**, 92–97.

Okamoto H *et al.* (2000a) Replicative forms of TT virus DNA in bone marrow cells. *Biochemistry*, **270**, 657–662.

Okamoto H, Takahashi M, Nishizawa T *et al.* (2000b) Replicative forms of TT virus DNA in the liver. *J Virol*, **74**, 5161–5167.

Omata M, Yokosuka O, Takano S *et al.* (1991) Resolution of acute hepatitis C after therapy with natural interferon-β. *Lancet*, **338**, 914–915.

Oon CJ, Lim GK, Ye Z *et al.* (1995) Molecular epidemiology of hepatitis B virus vaccine variants in Singapore. *Vaccine*, **13**, 699–702.

Oon C-J, Tan K-L, Harrison TJ and Zuckerman AJ (1996) Natural history of hepatitis B surface antigen mutants in children. *Lancet*, **348**, 1524.

Panda SK and Nanda SK (1997) Development of vaccines against hepatitis E virus infection. In *The Molecular Medicine of Viral Hepatitis* (eds Harrison TJ and Zuckerman AJ), pp 45–62. Wiley, Chichester.

Perrillo R, Schiff E, Yoshida E *et al.* (2000). Adefovir dipivoxil for the treatment of lamivudine-resistant hepatitis B mutants. *Hepatology*, **32**, 129–134.

Ping LH and Lemon SM (1992) Antigenic structure of human hepatitis A virus defined by analysis of escape mutants selected against murine monoclonal antibodies. *J Virol*, **66**, 2208–2216.

Pol S (1995) Immunotherapy of chronic hepatitis B by anti HBV vaccine. *Biomed Pharmacother*, **49**, 105–109.

Pol S, Driss F, Michel M-L *et al.* (1994) Specific vaccine therapy in chronic hepatitis B infection. *Lancet*, **344**, 342.

Purcell RH, D'Hondt E, Bradbury R *et al.* (1992) Inactivated hepatitis A vaccine: active and passive immunoprophylaxis in chimpanzees. *Vaccine*, **10**(suppl 1), S148–S151.

Purcell RH and Ticehurst JR (1988) Enterically transmitted non-A, non-B hepatitis: epidemiology and clinical characteristics. In *Viral Hepatitis and Liver Disease* (ed. Zuckerman AJ), pp 131–137. Alan R. Liss, New York.

Purdy MA, McCaustland KA, Krawczynski K *et al.* (1993) Preliminary evidence that a trpE-HEV fusion protein protects cynomolgus macaques against challenge with wild-type hepatitis E virus (HEV). *J Med Virol*, **41**, 90–94.

Reddy KR, Wright TL, Pockros PJ *et al.* (2001) Efficacy and safety of pegylated (40 kDa) interferon-α2α compared with interferon-α2α in non-cirrhotic patients with chronic hepatitis C. *Hepatology*, **33**, 433–438.

Rizzetto M (1996) Changing epidemiology of viral hepatitis worldwide. Implications for prevention and therapy. *Med Microbiol Lett*, **5**, 455–457.

Rizzetto M, Canese MG, Arico S *et al.* (1977) Immuno-fluorescence detection of new antigen-antibody system (delta/anti-delta) associated to hepatitis B virus in liver and in serum of HBsAg carriers. *Gut*, **18**, 997–1003.

Rizzetto M, Rosina F, Saracco G *et al.* (1986) Treatment of chronic δ hepatitis with α-2 recombinant interferon. *J Hepatol*, **2**, S229–S233.

Rosina F, Pintus C, Meschievitz C *et al.* (1991) Long-term interferon treatment of chronic δ hepatitis: a multicenter Italian study. *Prog Clin Biol Res*, **364**, 385–391.

Sagliocca L, Amoroso P, Stroffolini T *et al.* (1999) Efficacy of hepatitis A vaccine in prevention of secondary hepatitis A infection: a randomised trial. *Lancet*, **353**, 1136–1139.

Saracco G, Mazzella G, Rosina F *et al.* (1989) A controlled trial of human lymphoblastoid interferon in chronic hepatitis B in Italy. *Hepatology*, **10**, 336–341.

Sawada H, Takada A, Takase S *et al.* (1993) Effects of alcohol on the replication of hepatitis C virus. *Alcohol Alcoholism*, **1**(suppl), 85–90.

Simmonds P, Alberti A, Alter HJ *et al.* (1994) A proposed system for the nomenclature of hepatitis C viral genotypes. *Hepatology*, **19**, 1321–1324.

Simons JN, Leary TP, Dawson GJ *et al.* (1995) Isolation of novel virus-like sequences associated with human hepatitis. *Nature Med*, **1**, 564–569.

Standring DN, Bridges EG, Placidi L *et al.* (2001). Antiviral β-L-nucleosides specific for hepatitis B virus infection. *Antivir Chem Chemother*, **12**(suppl 1), 119–129.

Sterneck M, Gunther S, Santantonio T *et al.* (1996) Hepatitis B virus genomes of patients with fulminant hepatitis do not share a specific mutation. *Hepatology*, **24**, 300–306.

Summers J and Mason WS (1982) Replication of the genome of a hepatitis B-like virus by reverse transcription of an RNA intermediate. *Cell*, **29**, 403–415.

Tam AW, Smith MM, Guerra ME *et al.* (1991) Hepatitis E virus (HEV)—molecular cloning and sequencing of the full-length viral genome. *Virology*, **185**, 120–131.

Taylor J (1997) Replication of hepatitis D virus. In *The Molecular Medicine of Viral Hepatitis* (eds Harrison TH, Zuckerman AJ), pp 1331–1140. Wiley, Chichester.

Thermet A, Rollier C, Zoulim F *et al.* (2003) Progress in DNA vaccine for prophylaxis and therapy of hepatitis B. *Vaccine*, **21**, 659–662.

Thursz MR, Kwiatkowski D, Allsopp CEM *et al.* (1995) Association between an MHC class II allele and clearance of hepatitis B virus in the Gambia. *N Engl J Med*, **332**, 1065–1069.

Tillmann HL, Heiken H, KnapikBotor A *et al.* (2001) Infection with GB virus C and reduced mortality among HIV-infected patients. *N Engl J Med*, **345**, 715–724.

Tiollais ● *et al.* (1985) The hepatitis B virus. *Nature*, **317**, 389–495.

Torbenson M and Thomas DL (2002) Occult hepatitis B. *Lancet Inf Dis*, **2**, 479–486.

Tsarev SA, Tsareva TS, Emerson SU *et al.* (1997) Recombinant vaccine against hepatitis E: dose response and protection against heterologous challenge. *Vaccine*, **15**, 1834–1838.

Van Damme P and Vorsters A (2002) Hepatitis B control in Europe by universal vaccination programmes: the situation in 2001. *J Med Virol*, **67**, 433–439.

Vento S, Garofano T, Di Perri G *et al.* (1991) Identification of hepatitis A virus as a trigger for autoimmune chronic hepatitis type 1 in susceptible individuals. *Lancet*, **337**, 1183.

Wang J, Chenivesse X, Henglein B *et al.* (1990) Hepatitis B virus integration in a cyclin A gene in a hepatocellular carcinoma, *Nature*, **343**, 555–557.

Wang YC, Zhang HY, Ling R *et al.* (2000) The complete sequence of hepatitis E virus genotype 4 reveals an alternative strategy for translation of open reading frames 2 and 3. *J Gen Virol*, **81**, 1675–1686.

Werzberger A, Mensch B, Kuter B *et al.* (1992) A controlled trial of a formalin-inactivated hepatitis A vaccine in healthy children. *N Engl J Med*, **327**, 453–457.

Whalen RG and Davis HL (1995) DNA-mediated immunization and the energetic immune response to hepatitis B surface antigen. *Clin Immunol Immunopathol*, **75**, 1–12.

Whittle H, Jaffar S, Wansborough M *et al.* (2002) Observational study of vaccine efficacy 14 years after trial of hepatitis B vaccination in Gambian children. *Br Med J*, **325**, 569–572.

Wilson JN, Nokes DJ and Carman WF (1999) The predicted pattern of emergence of vaccine-resistant hepatitis B: a cause for concern? *Vaccine*, **17**, 973–978.

Xiang JH, Wunschmann S, Diekema DJ *et al.* (2001) Effect of coinfection with GB virus C on survival among patients with HIV infection. *N Engl J Med*, **345**, 707–714.

Xiong XF, Flores C, Yang H *et al.* (1998) Mutations in hepatitis B DNA polymerase associated with resistance to lamivudine do not confer resistance to adefovir *in vitro*. *Hepatology*, **28**, 1669–1673.

Zanetti AR, Tanzi E, Manzillo G *et al.* (1988) Hepatitis B variant in Europe. *Lancet*, **2**, 1132–1133.

Zeuzem S and Carreno V (2001) Interleukin-12 in the treatment of chronic hepatitis B and C. *Antiviral Res*, **52**, 181–188.

Zoulim F, Chevallier M, Maynard M *et al.* (2003) Clinical consequences of hepatitis C virus infection. *Rev Med Virol*, **13**, 57–68.

Zuckerman AJ (1975) *Human Viral Hepatitis*. Elsevier/North Holland, Amsterdam.

Zuckerman AJ (2000) Effect of hepatitis B virus mutants on efficacy of vaccination. *Lancet*, **355**, 1382–1384.

Zuckerman AJ and Zuckerman JN (1999) Molecular epidemiology of hepatitis B virus mutants. *J Med Virol*, **58**, 193–195.

Zuckerman JN (1996) Nonresponse to hepatitis B vaccines and the kinetics of anti-HBs production. *J Med Virol*, **50**, 283–288.

Zuckerman JN, Sabin C, Craig FM *et al.* (1997) Immune response to a new hepatitis B vaccine in healthcare workers who had not responded to standard vaccine: randomised double blind dose–response study. *Br Med J*, **314**, 329–333.

Zuckerman JN and Zuckerman AJ (1998) Is there a need for boosters of hepatitis B vaccines? *Viral Hepatitis Rev*, **4**, 43–46.

Zuckerman JN and Zuckerman AJ (2002) Recombinant hepatitis B triple antigen vaccine. *Expert Rev Vaccine*, **1**, 141–144.

4

Viruses Associated with Acute Diarrhoeal Disease

Ulrich Desselberger* and Jim Gray**

Addenbrooke's Hospital, Cambridge, UK

INTRODUCTION

Gastroenteritis in humans can be caused by viruses, bacteria and parasites. The pathogenesis differs considerably, depending on the infectious agent. Clinical symptoms, however, are similar and range from mainly upper gastrointestinal symptoms including vomiting to acute watery or bloody diarrhoea without any vomiting, or combinations thereof. Viral gastroenteritis is a global problem in infants and young children (Bern *et al.*, 1992).

Viruses which are known to cause human gastroenteritis (Figure 4.1) belong to genera of different virus families (Blacklow and Greenberg, 1991; van Regenmortel *et al.*, 2000):

- Rotaviruses (a genus of the *Reoviridae*).
- Noroviruses (previously termed 'Norwalk-like viruses' or 'small round structured viruses'; SRSVs) and Sapoviruses (previously termed 'Sapporo-like viruses' or 'classical caliciviruses'; two genera of the *Caliciviridae*).
- Astroviruses (*Astroviridae*).
- Enteric adenoviruses (group F of the *Adenoviridae*).

*Present address: Virologie Moléculaire et Structurale, UMR 2472, CNRS, 1 Avenue de la Terrasse, Bât. 14B, 91198 Gif-sur-Yvette Cedex, France. E-mail: ulrich.desselberger@gv.cnrs-gif.fr
**Present address: Enteric Virus Unit, Enteric, Respiratory and Neurological Virus Laboratory, Central Public Health Laboratory, Health Protection Agency, 61 Colindale Avenue, London NW9 5DF, UK. E-mail: jim.gray@hpa.org.uk

In terms of relative frequency of incidence in children, rotaviruses were found to account for 30–60%, caliciviruses for 8–30%, astroviruses for 6–9% and enteric adenoviruses for 3–6% of all cases of viral gastroenteritides (Bon *et al.*, 1999; Pang *et al.*, 2000). In adults, caliciviruses are the most frequent viral cause of diarrhoea. Thus, recently the significance of caliciviruses for gastroenteric disease has been increasingly recognised.

Other viruses found in the gastrointestinal tract that are not regularly associated with diarrhoea are:

- Enteroviruses (*Picornaviridae*).
- Reoviruses (*Reoviridae*).
- Toroviruses (*Coronaviridae*).
- Coronaviruses (*Coronaviridae*).
- Parvoviruses (*Parvoviridae*).

Human immunodeficiency virus (HIV; a member of the family *Retroviridae*) can infect the gut directly. Under conditions of immunosuppression, the following viruses were also found to infect the gut and cause disease:

- Herpes simplex viruses (*Herpesviridae*).
- Cytomegalovirus (*Herpesviridae*).
- Picobirnaviruses (*Birnaviridae*).

Many of the obligatory human gastroenteritis viruses do not grow at all, or not very well, in cell culture, and therefore virus isolation is not the diagnostic method of choice. By contrast, electron microscopy (EM) permits the differentiation of viruses on the basis of their characteristic morphology (Figure

Principles and Practice of Clinical Virology, Fifth Edition. Edited by A. J. Zuckerman, J. E. Banatvala, J. R. Pattison, P. D. Griffiths and B. D. Schoub
© 2004 John Wiley & Sons Ltd ISBN 0 470 84338 1

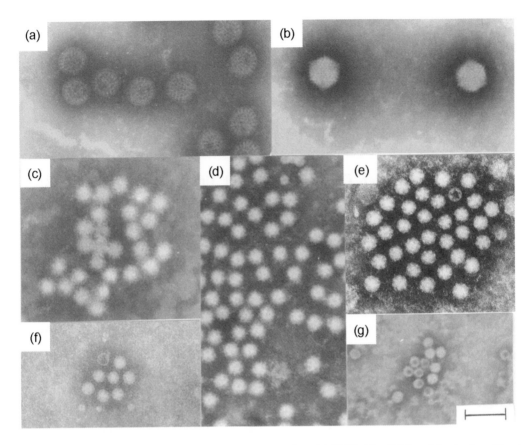

Figure 4.1 Electron micrographs of (a) rotavirus, (b) enteric adenovirus, (c) SRSV, (d) calicivirus, (e) astrovirus, (f) enterovirus and (g) parvovirus. Negative staining with 3% phosphotungstate, pH 6.3; bar = 100 nm. Astroviruses: courtesy of Mr T. Lee and Dr J. Kurtz, Oxford Public Health Laboratory; all other viruses: courtesy of Dr J. Gray, Clinical Microbiology and Public Health Laboratory, Cambridge

4.1); however, the sensitivity of detection (approximately 10^6 particles/ml) is low. In general, detection of rotaviruses is easy, as these viruses are shed in very large numbers (up to 10^{11} particles/ml faeces) during the peak of the illness. Astroviruses also occur in large numbers and are readily detected. Other viruses, particularly caliciviruses, are often only produced in relatively low numbers (i.e. below the detection level of EM) and only very early into the clinically apparent disease. The method of reverse transcription (RT)-polymerase chain reaction (PCR), which has much greater sensitivity (20–100 RNA molecules are detectable per reaction) is increasingly being used in diagnostic laboratories. RT-PCR and serological techniques using recombinant antigens have helped to recognise the true extent of human infections with caliciviruses and astroviruses, which has been found to be much higher than previously thought.

Most viral gastroenteritis infections follow two distinct epidemiological patterns. In childhood, diarrhoea occurs as endemic disease, mainly caused by rotaviruses of group A, caliciviruses, astroviruses and adenoviruses of subgroup F. By the age of 5 years many children have been infected with all these agents, often without apparent symptoms. The main mode of transmission seems to be oro-faecal, but possibly also by droplets and close contact. By contrast, epidemics are mainly caused by caliciviruses and sometimes by astroviruses and group B and C rotaviruses. All ages can be affected, and viruses are quite often transmitted by infected food (e.g. shellfish) or water (Hedberg and Osterholm, 1993; Gray et al., 1997).

Treatment largely follows guidelines established in 1985, mainly using oral rehydration fluids containing electrolytes and sugar (reviewed by Desselberger, 1999). Bismuth subsalicylate has been found to be

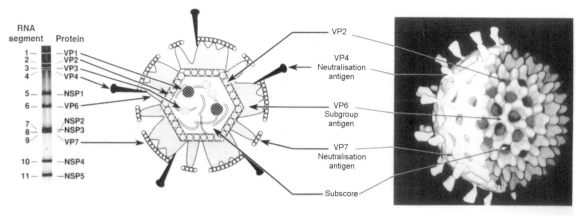

Figure 4.2 RNA profile (10% SDS polyacrylamide gel, silver-stained), protein products (gene protein assignment) and particle structure (reconstruction from cryoelectron micrographs) of rotavirus. From Mattion *et al.* (1994), published by Marcel Dekker, New York

beneficial in children with acute watery diarrhoea (Figueroa-Quintanilla *et al.*, 1993). Agents such as diphenoxylate or loperamide against abdominal cramping should be avoided, as they can have serious side-effects. In severe cases of diarrhoea, rapid fluid replacement by parenteral administration may be required. In developing countries where children are often malnourished as well, supplementary nutrition is an important component of the therapy. Public health measures to confine outbreaks include frequent hand-washing, proper disinfection, removal of infected faeces and contaminated food or water, and taking infected individuals out of work. Outbreaks in clinical wards may require temporary closure to new admissions and restrictions on placements of staff.

Viruses regularly and irregularly causing acute gastroenteritis will be briefly described below (for concise reviews, see Hart and Cunliffe, 1997; Desselberger, 1998b; for more extensive information, see Kapikian, 1994a; Chiba *et al.*, 1997; Chadwick and Goode, 2002; Cohen *et al.*, 2002; Desselberger and Gray, 2003). According to the relative degree of importance of different viruses for clinical human disease, rotaviruses and caliciviruses are presented more extensively than the other viruses.

ROTAVIRUSES

Structure, Genome and Gene–Protein Assignment

Rotaviruses are the major cause of severe gastroenteritis among children of <5 years of age worldwide and also of acute diarrhoea in the young of many mammalian species (calves, piglets, lambs, fowls, etc.) causing 500 000–600 000 deaths each year. They were discovered as the cause of human disease in 1973 (Bishop *et al.*, 1973; Flewett *et al.*, 1973). Rotaviruses possess a genome consisting of 11 segments of double-stranded (ds) RNA encoding six structural proteins (VP1, VP2, VP3, VP4, VP6 and VP7) and six non-structural proteins (NSP1–NSP6). The wheel-like structure of the particle (Latin *rota* = wheel) as seen by EM is pathognomonic (Figure 4.1). The structural proteins of the particle constitute an inner layer (VP1–VP3; 'the core'), an intermediate layer (VP6; 'the inner capsid'), and an outer layer (VP4, VP7; 'the outer capsid') of the particle (Figure 4.2). Details of the three-dimensional structure have been elucidated in a number of excellent studies by several groups (e.g. Prasad *et al.*, 1988, 1990, 1996; Lawton *et al.*, 1997a,b; Prasad and Estes, 1997; Lawton *et al.*, 1999, 2000; Pesavento *et al.*, 2001; Yeager *et al.*, 1990, 1994; Petitpas *et al.*, 1998; Lepault *et al.*, 2001). According to their findings, the triple-layered capsid is ordered in five-, three- and two-fold symmetry axes and is perforated by 132 aqueous channels (classes I–III, in three symmetry positions). The class I channels are necessary components to allow transcription in sub-viral particles (see below).

Complete gene–protein assignments have been established for several strains; the protein–function correlations are only partially known. Details describing sizes of RNA segments and their products, as well as post-translational modification and possible function(s) of the virus-encoded proteins, are summarised in Table 4.1. Functions are reviewed in more detail below.

Classification

A classification scheme for rotaviruses has been derived from immunological reactivities of three of its components as well as from genomic sequence comparisons and has been established as follows (Estes, 2001):

1. According to the serological cross-reactivity of the inner capsid protein VP6, five groups (A–E) have been firmly established, and two more groups (F,G) are likely to exist. Within group A rotaviruses, there are subgroups (I; II; I + II; non-I; non-II) according to their exclusive reactivities with two VP6-specific monoclonal antibodies.

2. Both surface proteins, VP4 and VP7, elicit antibodies which neutralise in vitro and in vivo (Offit et al., 1986) and are therefore considered to be involved in protection. In order to characterise strains, a dual classification scheme distinguishing types, similar to that developed for influenza viruses, has been established (so far only for group A rotaviruses). The system differentiates G types (VP7-specific, G for glycoprotein) and P types (VP4-specific, P for protease-sensitive protein). So far, 14 different G types and more than 20 P types have been detected, indicating extensive genomic diversity within group A rotaviruses. Whereas the correlation of G serotypes and their genotypes is practically complete, for many P genotypes no serotype has yet been established. Thus, it has been agreed to designate the P serotype and genotype separately but jointly, the latter in square brackets: for example, the human Wa strain is classified as G1P1A[8], the human DS-1 strain as G2P1B[4], etc. (Desselberger, 1998a; Estes, 2001).

As VP4 and VP7 are coded for by different RNA segments (segments 4 and 7, 8 or 9, depending on strain, respectively; see Table 4.1) and as rotaviruses were found to reassort readily in doubly-infected cells in vitro and in vivo, various combinations of VP4 and VP7 types have been observed in natural rotavirus isolates (Estes, 2001; Desselberger et al., 2001).

Replication

Rotaviruses spread via the oro-faecal route and infect the small intestine after oral ingestion. Multiplication occurs in the mature epithelial cells at the tips of the villi of the small intestine. Rotaviruses grow well in secondary monkey kidney cells and in immortalised monkey kidney cell lines (MA104, BS-C1) in the presence of trypsin, and therefore their replication in vitro could be studied in detail (Estes, 2001). Triple-layered particles (i.e. the infectious virions) attach to the host cells via the outer layer protein VP4. Virus entry is by receptor-mediated endocytosis or direct penetration. The cellular receptor(s) have not yet been fully characterised, but some animal strains use sialic acid on glycolipids (Ciarlet et al., 2002). Other strains seem to recognise galactose (Jolly et al., 2001). In addition to glycolipids, several integrins have been proposed to mediate intake, possibly in a post-attachment step, acting as co-receptors (Coulson et al., 1997; Hewish et al., 2000; Guerrero et al., 2000). The heat shock cognate protein (hsc70) may also be involved as a co-receptor (Guerrero et al., 2002). Replication is exclusively in the cytoplasm. After removal of the outer capsid by lysosomal enzymes, the viral RNA-dependent RNA polymerase (coded for by RNA 1) is activated in double-layered particles, and by use of the VP1/VP2/VP3 transcription complex (Lawton et al., 2000) large numbers of positive-stranded RNA molecules are transcribed and exit the double-layered particle via its 12 aqueous channels, located on the edges of the five-fold axes of symmetry. This process is ATP-dependent. The new RNA molecules act as mRNAs, and their translation products start to accumulate in the cytoplasm. NSP3 is intimately involved in translation by binding to the 3′ end of mRNA and the eukaryotic translation factor eIF4G (Vende et al., 2000). Molecules of mRNA seem to be pulled through VP2 oligomers (the nascent 'core') by means of a complex formation with NSP2, which has NTPase activity and acts as a molecular motor (Taraporewala et al., 1999; Taraporewala and Patton, 2001; Schuck et al., 2001; Patton, 2001). NSP5 is also involved at this stage (Berois et al., 2003). Double-layered particles form, consisting of VP1, VP2, VP3 and VP6 and several of the nonstructural proteins, and containing one genome-equivalent of packaged single-stranded RNA (which is then replicated to form dsRNA). They accumulate and form pseudocrystalline aggregates termed 'viroplasm' (intracytoplasmic inclusion bodies). By budding through the rough endoplasmic reticulum (RER), double-layered particles incorporate VP7 and VP4 to form the third, outer layer (a transient, RER-derived envelope is shed before complete maturation). Triple-layered infectious virions are released by cell lysis. The non-structural proteins have been implicated as supporting various stages of morphogenesis; e.g. NSP2, probably complexed with NSP5, is involved in ssRNA packaging and NSP4 was

Table 4.1 Genes, gene protein assignments and functions of proteins of group A rotavirus

RNA segment			Protein product				Functions
No.	Size (bp)	Description	Deduced MW (kDa)	Location	No. of molecules per virion	Post-translational modification	
1	3302	VP1	125.0	Inner core	12	–	RNA-dependent RNA polymerase; ss RNA binding; complex with VP3
2	2690	VP2	94.0	Core	120	Myristoylation	RNA binding; required for replicase activity of VP1
3	2591	VP3	88.0	Inner core	12	–	Guanylyl transferase; methyl transferase; complex with VP1
4	2362	VP4	86.8	Outer capsid (dimer)	120	Proteolytic cleavage to VP5* and VP8*	Haemagglutinin; cell attachment; neutralisation antigen (ab protective); fusogenic; protease-enhanced infectivity; virulence (mice, piglets)
5	1611	VP5 (NSP1)	58.7	Non-structural	NA	–	RNA binding; virulence (mice); nonessential for replication (some strains)
6	1356	VP6	44.8	Inner capsid (trimer)	780	Myristoylation	Group- and subgroup-specific antigen; protection (by intra-cellular neutralisation)?
7[a]	1059	VP9 (NSP3)	34.6	Non-structural (dimer)	NA	–	RNA binding (3′ end); competing with cellular PABP for interaction with EIF4G1 (translation); inhibiting host cell translation
8[a]	1104	VP8 (NSP2)	36.7	Non-structural (octamer)	NA	–	RNA binding; NTPase; helicase; + strand RNA packaging; virulence (mice)
9[a]	1062	VP7	37.4[b]	Outer capsid (trimer)	780	Cleavage of signal sequence; glycosylation	Neutralisation antigen (ab protective); Ca^{2+} binding
10	751	VP12 (NSP4)	20.3	Non-structural	NA	Glycosylation (→VP10, NS28); trimming	Intracellular receptor for VP6 (morphogenesis); viral enterotoxin (secreted cleavage product); protection by spec.ab; virulence (mice, piglets)
11	667	VP11 (NSP5)	21.7	Non-structural	NA	0-glycosylation, phosphorylation	RNA binding; protein kinase; interacting with NSP2 and NSP6
		NSP6	12.0	Non-structural	NA	–	Interacting with NSP5

[a]This gene protein assignment is of the SA11 rotavirus strain.
[b]Second in-frame initiation codon located 30 codons downstream (deduced MW33.9 kDa).
Modified from Estes (2001).

proposed to act as intracellular receptor in the RER to attract single-shelled particles for maturation to double-shelled particles (for details of structure–function correlations and replication, see Estes, 2001; Prasad and Estes, 1997; Lawton et al., 2000). In immunodeficient hosts and under certain experimental conditions, rotaviruses undergo genome rearrangements (for review, see Desselberger, 1996).

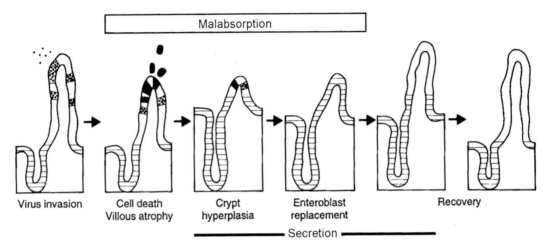

Figure 4.3 Rotavirus pathogenesis. Development of damage to gut mucosa, diarrhoea and repair. From Phillips (1989) published by Elsevier

Pathogenesis

Extensive cellular necrosis of the gut epithelium leads to villous atrophy, loss of digestive enzymes, a reduction of absorption and increased osmotic pressure in the gut lumen, resulting in the onset of diarrhoea. This is followed by a reactive crypt cell hyperplasia accompanied by increased fluid secretion, which also contributes to the severity of diarrhoea. Local pathogenesis is shown diagrammatically in Figure 4.3.

Viral factors determining the pathogenicity of rotaviruses have been investigated in several animal models (piglets, mice, rabbits; for review, see Burke and Desselberger, 1996). The protein product of RNA segment 4, VP4, has been found to be a major determinant of pathogenicity in several systems, but products of other structural genes (VP3, VP7) and of non-structural genes (NSP1, NSP2, NSP4) have also been implicated.

The recent discovery of NSP4 as an enterotoxin (Ball et al., 1996) has provided an explanation of the old observation that rotavirus-infected animals exhibit profuse diarrhoea *prior to* the detection of histologic lesions. NSP4 or a peptide thereof [amino acids (aa) 114–135] induce dose- and age-dependent diarrhoea in laboratory animals (mice, rats) *in the absence of histological changes* (Ball et al., 1996). NSP4 produces an increase in intracellular Ca^{2+} concentration, disturbing the cellular electrolyte homeostasis (Tian et al., 1994, 1995). Recently it was found that a peptide of NSP4, which is active as an enterotoxin, is secreted from infected cells (Zhang et al., 2000) and is able to

induce intracellular Ca^{2+} elevation and diarrhoea in mice. It is thought that the secreted protein binds to a (still hypothetical) receptor and thus affects uninfected cells (Zhang et al., 2000; Tafazoli et al., 2001). Antibody to NSP4 has been shown to reduce the severity of diarrhoeal disease in suckling mice.

Immune Responses and Correlates of Protection

After neonatal or primary rotavirus infection, a mainly serotype-specific humoral immune response is elicited, providing homotypic immunity, but there is also partial protection developing against subsequent rotavirus infections by other serotypes (Velasquez et al., 1996). The exact correlates of protection remain to be determined (Offit, 1994) but levels of rotavirus-specific coproantibodies of the IgA subclass seem to correlate best with protection (Coulson et al., 1992; Feng et al., 1994, 1997; Yuan et al., 1996), although not in all cases (O'Neal et al., 2000). Humoral antibodies might be directed towards the type-specifying antigens VP7 and VP4, but also towards the inner capsid protein VP6 (Burns et al., 1996; Herrmann et al., 1996; Feng et al., 1997). There is a rotavirus-specific cytotoxic T cell response, but its exact role in overcoming the infection or in protection against subsequent infections is not known (Offit, 1994; Franco and Greenberg, 1995). Natural infection or appropriate vaccination (see below) seem to protect from severe disease in subsequent infections (Coulson et al., 1992; Velasquez et al., 1996), even if the serotype of the challenging virus differs from that of the previous infections or those contained in a vaccine.

Illness, Diagnosis and Treatment

After a short incubation period of 1–2 days the onset of the illness is sudden, with watery diarrhoea lasting 4–7 days, vomiting and rapid dehydration. All degrees of severity of disease are seen, including inapparent infections by so-called 'nursery strains', central nervous system infections (Iturriza-Gomara et al., 2002a) and chronic infections and hepatitis in children with immunodeficiencies (Gilger et al., 1992).

Diagnosis of a rotavirus infection is relatively easy, as large numbers of virus particles (up to 10^{11} particles/ml faeces) are shed. The main techniques used to detect them are enzyme-linked immunoassays (ELISAs), passive particle agglutination tests (PPATs) and, when searching comprehensively for diarrhoeogenic viruses, EM (Table 4.2). Serological assays have been used to establish G and P types of rotavirus isolates, but application of this technology depends on the presence of double-shelled virus particles in the clinical specimen. Molecular techniques are therefore increasingly being applied for the purpose of typing, and also detection. Rotavirus-specific oligonucleotide primers complementary to common and type-specific regions of the VP6, VP7 and VP4 genes allow sensitive detection, subgroup determination and typing for both G and P types, respectively, by RT-PCR (Gouvea et al., 1990; Gentsch et al., 1992; Iturriza-Gómara et al., 2002c, 2003).

Treatment is by oral, subcutaneous or intravenous rehydration and sometimes pain relief, as indicated above. The formulae of oral rehydration salt (ORS) solutions and reduced osmolarity 'light ORS', recommended by WHO, are widely used (Desselberger, 1999; Table 4.3). Oral immunoglobulins seem to have an effect on the duration of diarrhoea and virus shedding but are not routinely used (Desselberger, 1999; Bass, 2003).

Epidemiology

The epidemiology of group A rotavirus infections is complex, as, at any one time within a geographical location, rotaviruses of different G types co-circulate (for review, see Desselberger et al., 2001). The relative incidence of G types also changes over time in the same location. Approximately 95% of co-circulating strains are types G1–G4 in most places, typically G1P1A[8], G2P1B[4], G3P1A[8] and G4P1A[8] (Iturriza-Gomara et al., 2000), but other G types may be represented at high frequencies, particularly in tropical areas (Desselberger et al., 2001). Recently, G9 rotaviruses have been isolated as one of the predominant outbreak strains in several locations in the USA (Ramachandran et al., 1998) and in the UK (Iturriza-Gómara et al., 2002b). Group B rotaviruses have caused outbreaks of diarrhoea in children and adults in China (Hung, 1988) and have been isolated from sporadic cases of gastroenteritis in Calcutta, India (Krishnan et al., 1999; Kobayashi et al., 2001). Group C rotaviruses are associated with small outbreaks in humans (e.g. Caul et al., 1990). Besides the accumulation of point mutations (genomic drift; Iturriza-Gómara et al., 2002c), gene reassortment (genomic shift; Iturrizza-Gómara et al., 2001, 2002c) seems to play a major role in generating the increasing diversity of rotaviruses.

Vaccine Development

Rotavirus infections have been recognised as a major cause of infection and diarrhoea, associated with approximately 600 000 annual cases of death worldwide (Bern et al., 1992), and therefore development of vaccine candidates has been a major goal and has been

Table 4.2 Diagnostic tests for the main causes of viral gastroenteritis

Virus	EM, IEM	ELISA	PPAT	PCR
Rotavirus	+	+ +	+	+ + + (RT)
Enteric adenovirus	+[a]	+ +	−	+ + +
Calicivirus	±	+ +	−	+ + + (RT)
Astrovirus	+	+	−	+ + + (RT)

[a]Only 30–40% are of types 40 and 41.
Sensitivity: EM, 10^6 particles/ml; IEM, 10^5; ELISA, 10^5 (and soluble antigen); PPAT, 10^5 (and soluble antigen); PCR/RT-PCR, 10^1–10^2.
The scale − to + + + indicates relative levels of sensitivities and relevant diagnostic usefulness.

Table 4.3 Oral rehydration salt (ORS) solutions for the treatment of rotavirus-related diarrhoea

Component	Osmolarity (mmol/l)		
	WHO ORS	'ORS light'	'ORS reduced' 2002
Sodium	90	60	75
Potassium	20	20	20
Chloride	80	50	65
Citrate	10	10	10
Glucose	111	84	75
Total osmolarity	**311**	**224**	**245**

Modified from Desselberger (1999) and WHO (2002; http://www.who.int).

in progress since the early 1980s. Results have been mixed for some time, owing to the enormous genomic and antigenic diversity of rotaviruses (for review, see Kapikian, 1994b; Desselberger, 1998c). Mainly animal rotaviruses (of simian or bovine origin) have been used as live attenuated vaccines. In many cases protection from *infection and/or mild disease* was only modest (40–50%). By contrast, 70–80% protection from *severe disease including dehydration* was recently achieved (Rennels *et al.*, 1996; Joensuu *et al.*, 1997; Pérez-Schael *et al.*, 1997), particularly when applying a cocktail of viruses, e.g. as a tetravalent vaccine containing a rhesus monkey rotavirus (RRV) of G3 type and monoreassortants individually carrying the VP7 gene of human serotypes G1, G2 and G4 in the RRV genetic background. A tetravalent RRV-based reassortant vaccine (Rotashield®) received Food and Drug Administration (FDA) approval as a universal vaccine in the USA in August 1998, and recommendations for its usage have been issued (CDC, 1999a). More than 1.5 million doses were administered in the following 10 months. During that time cases of intussusception were observed in vaccinees, particularly within 3–7 days after the first dose, with a relative risk of 27.9 (95% confidence interval 10.8–72.1; Murphy *et al.*, 2001), and an attributable risk of one case of intussusception for every 4700–9500 children vaccinated (Murphy *et al.*, 2001) or one case in 11 000 children vaccinated (Kramarz *et al.*, 2001) was calculated. These observations led the CDC and the American Academy of Pediatrics to withdraw the recommendation for use in infants (CDC, 1999b,c). Recent ecological studies have failed to demonstrate an increase in the incidence of intussusception during the time of usage of the Rotashield vaccine (Chang *et al.*, 2001; Simonsen *et al.*, 2001), suggesting that the attributable risk may be much smaller. There are currently no plans to reintroduce the Rotashield vaccine in either developed or developing countries (for review see Offit *et al.*, 2003).

Other approaches to immunisation are under investigation at present. There are several other live attenuated candidate vaccine strains under investigation: the bovine WC3 virus (G6P7[5]) and G1 and P1A[8] reassortants thereof (Clark *et al.*, 1996) and the human strain 89-12 (G1P1A[8], Bernstein *et al.*, 1998, 1999). The application of virus-like particles (VLPs) originating from baculovirus recombinants expressing structural proteins (VP2, VP6, VP4, VP7) (Conner *et al.*, 1996), enhancement of rotavirus immunogenicity by microencapsidation (Offit *et al.*, 1994) and DNA-based vaccines (Herrmann *et al.*, 1996; Chen *et al.*, 1997, 1998) are also under further investigation.

ENTERIC ADENOVIRUSES

Genome and Structure

Adenoviruses are non-enveloped icosahedral viruses of 70–80 nm diameter, possessing a genome of linear dsDNA of approximately 35 000 bp and a capsid with 240 hexons and 12 pentons at the vertices which carry projecting fibres (Shenk, 1996). Their three-dimensional structure has been elucidated (Stewart *et al.*, 1991).

Classification

Human adenoviruses occur in 51 distinct serotypes ordered into six different subgroups (A–F). The classification is based on immunological, biochemical and biological differences. Within subgroups, serotypes are differentiated by the reactivity of the two major capsid proteins, hexon and fibre. Within each subgroup DNA sequence homology is greater than 85%. Adenoviruses regularly associated with gastroenteritis are classified in subgroup F, as serotypes 40 and 41.

Replication and Pathogenesis

All adenoviruses grow well in human epithelial cells, with the exception of the enteric adenoviruses types 40 and 41. Those can be grown in Graham 293 cells (a human embryonic kidney cell line transformed by adenovirus type 5 DNA). Replication has been studied in detail, mainly with adenovirus types 2 and 5 of subgroup C. Cell attachment is facilitated by the fibre protein, and uptake is via receptor-mediated endocytosis. Members of the immunoglobulin superfamily have been implicated as receptors, and integrins possibly as co-receptors. Following uncoating, viral DNA moves to the nucleus and a phased early and late gene expression is initiated. The early protein E1A acts as a transcriptional activator and is a potent blocker of apoptosis and interferon (IFN)-α and -β expression. Late gene expression is at the onset of viral DNA replication and is accompanied by blockage of cellular mRNA expression. Virus assembly is in the cytoplasm. Virus particles are released after cell death, mediated by disruption of the cytoskeleton. Some adenovirus proteins seem to decrease the expression of MHC class I antigens on the surface of infected cells, thus hindering susceptibility to adenovirus-specific cytotoxic T lymphocytes, and also to counteract tumour necrosis factor alpha (TNF-α) expression (for details, see Shenk, 1996).

Adenoviruses replicate in the epithelia of the human respiratory and gastrointestinal tracts as well as in the conjunctiva and in lymphocytes. Various viral factors contribute to the pathogenesis. Whilst the pentons are directly cytotoxic, early viral proteins counteract TNF and apoptosis, and downregulate the expression of MHC class I molecules, thus preventing recognition by cytotoxic T cells. There is persistence of adenovirus infection in lymphoid cells, the mechanism of which is poorly understood (Horwitz, 2001).

Diagnosis

Detection of enteric adenoviruses in faecal specimens is mainly by ELISAs using subgroup F-specific monoclonal antibodies. EM followed by immune EM (IEM) can also be used to identify these agents. Adenoviruses are detected in 4–15% of stools from children with gastroenteritis in many hospitals, outpatients clinics and day care centres (Krajden et al., 1990). PCR techniques have also been applied to the diagnosis of adenovirus infection (e.g. Xu et al., 2000; Allard et al., 2001). However, of all the adenoviruses detected in faeces, only 30–50% belong to subgroup F, comprising types 40 and 41, the others being mainly members of subgroups B and D, primarily infecting the respiratory tract. Of 2 and 5 year-old children, 14% and 50%, respectively, possess neutralising antibodies to adenoviruses types 40 and 41, suggesting that there are likely to be many inapparent infections.

Clinical Symptoms and Treatment

Clinically, adenovirus-associated diarrhoea does not differ from those caused by other viruses, although the duration of symptoms may last slightly longer (3–11 days). The stools are watery and non-bloody (in contrast to bacterial diarrhoeas). Fever and vomiting are common. Usually adenovirus gastroenteritis is a mild disease, and treatment is symptomatic. Ribavirin has been used in a few cases (Kapelushnik et al., 1995). Cidofovir is active against adenovirus in vitro and has been used to treat diarrhoea complicated by disseminated adenovirus infections in children after bone marrow transplantation (de Clercq, 1996; Legrand et al., 2001). In those cases the diarrhoeogenic adenovirus was of type 31.

Epidemiology

Adenovirus infections occur worldwide as epidemic, endemic or sporadic infections. Enteric adenoviruses are mainly endemic, but outbreaks in hospitals and boarding schools have been reported. Most infections are in infancy and early childhood. The incidence of enteric adenovirus infections is 4–7/100 person years in small children without a seasonal preference. In immunocompromised persons, adenoviruses can cause severe systemic disease. Different genomic subtypes within types 40 and 41 have been observed (de Jong et al., 1993).

Prevention and Control

At present there is no vaccine candidate for enteric adenoviruses. Control of hospital outbreaks is by cohort nursing of patients, use of gloves, gowns and goggles, and disinfection with sodium hypochlorite.

NOROVIRUSES AND SAPOVIRUSES
(HUMAN CALICIVIRUSES)

Introduction

This group of viruses was first recognised from an outbreak of gastroenteritis in an elementary school in Norwalk, Ohio, USA in 1968, affecting half of the students and teachers (Kapikian *et al.*, 1972). The outbreak was not due to a bacterial pathogen, and, finally, using IEM, the causative agent *Norwalk virus* (NV) was visualised as a 27–35 nm virus particle. Upon cloning and sequencing of the genome, NV has been classified unequivocally as a member of the family *Caliciviridae* (Cubitt, 1994; Kapikian *et al.*, 1996). With the advent of molecular diagnostic techniques, it has become apparent that noroviruses (previously termed Norwalk-like viruses or 'SRSVs') and sapoviruses (previously termed Sapporo-like viruses or 'classical caliciviruses') are major causes of outbreaks of diarrhoea and vomiting in various population groups and are now recognised as the second most important cause of viral gastroenteritis (Fankhauser *et al.*, 1998; Koopmans, 2001).

Structure and Genome

Typically, the surface of the particle carries cup-shaped depressions (Fig. 1d), which have given the name to this viral family (Latin *calix* = goblet, cup). The morphology of caliciviruses has been analysed in more detail using cryoelectron microscopy and image reconstruction, when it was possible to produce norovirus particles from insect cells which were infected with a baculovirus recombinant expressing the capsid protein (e.g. Prasad *et al.*, 1994a,b, 1999). The capsid consists of 90 dimers of a single capsid protein of 58 kDa molecular weight (monomer), which are arranged in such a way that large hollows are seen at the five-fold and three-fold axes and represent what appears to be the cup-like structures of caliciviruses. Each dimer forms a basal shell (S) domain. This is joined by a flexible hinge to a protruding (P) domain which is further subdivided into subunits P1 and P2.

The genome consists of single-stranded RNA of positive polarity and approximately 7.7 kb in size. Full-length sequences of cDNAs from three different caliciviruses (NV, *Southampton virus* and *Manchester virus*) have been obtained (Jiang *et al.*, 1993; Lambden *et al.*, 1993; Liu *et al.*, 1995). The single-stranded RNAs of positive polarity are polyadenylated and have a length of 7.3–7.7 kb (Figure 4.4). The genome composition of the sapoviruses bears a greater similarity to that of several animal caliciviruses than to human noroviruses (Matson *et al.*, 1995; Liu *et al.*, 1995, 1999). All calicivirus genomes have three open reading frames (ORFs), ORF1 encoding non-structural proteins with helicase, protease and RNA-dependent RNA polymerase (RdRr) functions, ORF2 the viral capsid protein, and ORF3 at the 3' end of the genome encoding a small protein of as-yet unknown function (Figure 4.4). There is a major difference between the genomes of noroviruses and sapoviruses in that for sapoviruses ORF2 is in the same reading frame as ORF1 and is thus contiguous with the RdRr gene. For noroviruses, ORF1 and ORF2 overlap by a few nucleotides with a -2 frameshift for ORF2 (Liu *et al.*, 1995; Clarke and Lambden, 2001).

Classification

Noroviruses and sapoviruses constitute two of the four genera of the family *Caliciviridae* (Mayo, 2002; the other two being *Vesivirus* and *Lagovirus*, infecting animals). Sequence comparison has allowed division of the noroviruses into two, possibly three, genogroups (see Table 4.4), genogroups I and II containing at least seven or eight different human type species (Koopmans, 2001; Koopmans *et al.*, 2003). A bovine calicivirus (*Jena virus*) is closely related to genogroup I noroviruses (Liu *et al.*, 1999), whilst a porcine enteric calicivirus (PEC) is related to sapoviruses (Vinjé *et al.*, 2000a).

Replication

As there is no *in vitro* cell culture system available for human caliciviruses, their replication can at present be deduced only from that of animal caliciviruses that have a similar genome organisation and can be propagated in cell cultures; e.g. feline calicivirus grows in CRFK cells, and an infectious cDNA clone has been constructed (Sosnovtsev and Green, 1995). From this it appears that viruses interact with species-specific receptors. Proteins deduced from ORF1 may arise from appropriate co- and post-translational cleavage of a polyprotein precursor, in a way similar to the cleavage cascade identified for picornaviruses (for further details, see Estes *et al.*, 1997).

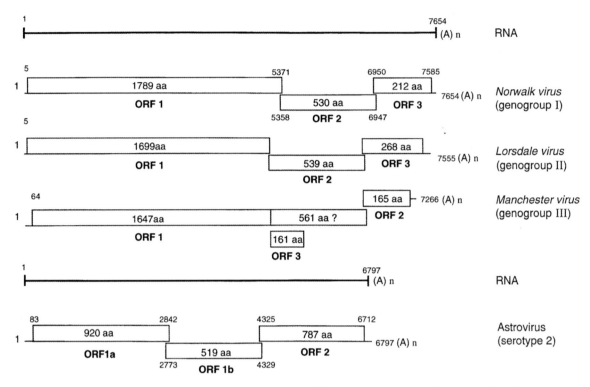

Figure 4.4 Genomic organisation of Norwalk virus (a norovirus of genogroup I), Lorsdale virus (a norovirus of genogroup II), Manchester virus (a sapovirus) and of astrovirus (serotype 2). For nomenclature of noroviruses, see Table 4.2. ORF, open reading frame; aa, amino acids; (A)$_n$, poly(A) tail of RNA. From Estes *et al.* (1997) and Matsui and Greenberg (2001); slightly modified

Pathogenesis

The incubation period ranges from 10 to 50 h, and diarrhoea lasts 24–48 h. Ileum biopsies from ill volunteers showed that a symptomatic illness correlated with broadening and blunting of intestinal villi, crypt hyperplasia, cytoplasmic vacuolisation and lymphocytic infiltration of the lamina propria (Guo and Saif, 2003). Small intestinal brush border enzymes are decreased, and malabsorption and diarrhoea with abdominal cramps, nausea and vomiting result.

Laboratory Diagnosis

This is mainly by direct EM or IEM, by ELISA (Herrmann *et al.*, 1995) or, more recently, by RT-PCR assays (e.g. Ando *et al.*, 1995). For the latter to be successful, broadly reactive primers must be available in order to detect most of the human caliciviruses. Initial use of such primers looked promising (Green *et al.*, 1995). Vinjé *et al.* (2000a) have developed primers

with which 90% of outbreaks initially diagnosed by EM could be detected. These techniques have also been applied to detecting caliciviruses in shellfish and other foodstuffs (Lees *et al.*, 1995; Atmar *et al.*, 1996) from which human infections frequently originate.

Immune Responses

The immune responses against human calicivirus infections have been examined in adult volunteer studies, using IEM and more recently ELISAs with recombinant antigens. However, there is the problem that most volunteers have been infected with such viruses some time before experimental exposure, and proper neutralisation assays are not available. Interestingly, more than 50% of adult volunteers appear to be susceptible (Graham *et al.*, 1994; Gray *et al.*, 1994).

Volunteer studies have shown that pre-existing calicivirus-reactive antibodies do not protect from reinfection in the longer run; on the contrary, higher pre-existing antibody levels seem to condition for more

Table 4.4 Classification of current genogroups and genotypes of human noroviruses

Genogroup	Genotype	Type species
I	1	Norwalk/1968/USA
	2	Southampton/1991/UK
	3	Desert Shield/395/1990/Saudi Arabia
	4	Chiba 407/1987/Japan
	5	Musgrove/1989/UK
	6	Hesse 3/1997/Germany
	7	Winchester/1994/UK
II	1	Hawaii/1971/USA
	2	Melksham/1994/UK
	3	Toronto 24/1994/Canada
	4	Bristol/1993/UK
	5	Hillingdon/1990/UK
	6	Seacroft 1990/UK
	7	Leeds/1990/UK
	8	Amsterdam/1998/The Netherlands
III?	1	Alphatron/1998/The Netherlands

Modified from Green *et al.* (2001) and Koopmans *et al.* (2003).

severe illness upon reinfection (Gray *et al.*, 1994). Some volunteers who fell ill after initial NV challenge remained immune when rechallenged 6–14 weeks later.

Clinical Course

The clinical symptoms were studied in 50 volunteers and were as follows: 41 (82%) became infected and of those 68% were symptomatic and 32% asymptomatic. The most common symptoms were nausea, headache and abdominal cramps followed by diarrhoea and vomiting. Severe symptoms lasted for only 12–48 h (Graham *et al.*, 1994). Persistent infection with caliciviruses and other viruses associated with chronic diarrhoea has been found in children with severe combined immunodeficiency (SCID) and in patients with the acquired immune deficiency syndrome (AIDS) (Grohmann *et al.*, 1993).

Epidemiology

The availability of recombinant proteins expressed from cloned cDNAs has allowed the study of age-dependent antibody prevalence in both developed and developing countries. Epidemic gastroenteritis produced by caliciviruses is relatively mild. There is likely to be a large number of inapparent infections in early childhood, as it has been shown that 50% of 3 year-old children in the UK already have NV-specific antibodies, a number that increases to 80% in early adulthood (Figure 4.5; Gray *et al.*, 1993). In other countries, NV-specific antibodies are produced after primary infection even earlier (China) or later (Japan) in life (Figure 4.5). In general, children appear to be infected with caliciviruses much more frequently than was previously recognised (Gray *et al.*, 1993; Numata *et al.*, 1994).

Outbreaks of acute gastroenteritis, which can be related to food or water-borne sources, occur frequently in recreational camps, hospitals, schools, cruise ships, nursing homes, etc. (Nakata *et al.*, 2000; Koopmans, 2001) and are associated with the ingestion of contaminated drinking or recreational water, uncooked shellfish, eggs, salads and cold foods. Mixed infections with caliciviruses of different genogroups have been observed (Gray *et al.*, 1997), and, as a consequence of this, genome recombination was found to occur (Jiang *et al.*, 1999; Vinjé *et al.*, 2000b). Worldwide, outbreaks occur year round, and nosocomial infections with caliciviruses are common. The viruses are highly infectious and have been found to spread rapidly in volunteer studies. The primary and secondary attack rates are high (above 50%). Transmission is by the faecal–oral route and by projectile vomiting producing an aerosol which scatters these viruses in the environment. Viral shedding does not normally persist beyond 100 h after the initial infection, but can be prolonged for up to 2 weeks. Shedding has also been observed in volunteers who remained well.

Prevention

The most efficient methods of prevention are measures of good hygiene (handwashing, disinfection and disposal of contaminated faeces and material, hygienic processing of food, withdrawal from work of ill food handlers, hospital staff, etc.) and sometimes closure of facilities (hospitals, nurseries, etc.). A vaccine seems possible, e.g. derived from VLPs (Jiang *et al.*, 1992) or from transgenic plants ('edible vaccines'; Mason *et al.*, 1996, 2002; Yu and Langridge, 2001), but better understanding of the significance of antibody responses for protective immunity is required. Prophylactic surveillance of key personnel in hospitals or food production (including keeping people with vomiting

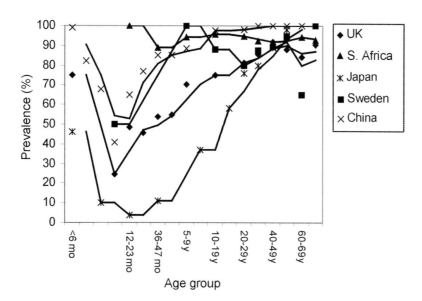

Figure 4.5 Age-related seroprevalence of antibody to Norwalk virus in different countries. UK, Gray *et al.* (1993); Sweden, Hinkula *et al.* (1995); South Africa, Smit *et al.* (1999); China, Jing *et al.* (2000); Japan, Numata *et al.* (1994)

and loose stools off work) and of water sources helps to reduce calicivirus-induced outbreaks.

ASTROVIRUSES

Astroviruses are members of the family *Astroviridae* (van Regenmortel *et al.*, 2000). Virions possess a genome of single-stranded RNA of positive polarity and no envelope, like the *Picornaviridae* and *Caliciviridae* (Matsui and Greenberg, 2001).

Structure and Genome

Morphologically, astroviruses are 28–30 nm particles with typical five- or six-pointed star patterns on their surface, and sometimes also knob-like structures. Studies by cryo-EM revealed a rippled solid capsid shell decorated with 30 dimeric spikes (Matsui and Greenberg, 2001).

The astrovirus genome (Figure 4.4) of approximately 6.8 kb comprises three ORFs (1a, 1b and 2), coding for a viral protease (ORF1a), an RNA-dependent RNA polymerase (ORF1b) and structural proteins (ORF2) (Willcocks *et al.*, 1994). There is a 70 base overlap in ORF1a and ORF1b containing sequences directing ribosomal frameshifting (to a -1

frame) for the reading of ORF1b (Lewis and Matsui, 1994, 1996; Marczinke *et al.*, 1994; Brierley and Vidakovic, 2003).

Classification

By 1995, seven serotypes had been distinguished by solid phase IEM and had been confirmed as different genotypes (Noel *et al.*, 1995). Recently, a genotype 8 has been identified which, although rare overall, had relatively high incidences in Egypt and Spain (Naficy *et al.*, 1999, 2000; Guix *et al.*, 2002).

Replication

Astroviruses grow well in some cell cultures (human embryonic kidney, monkey kidney or human colon carcinoma cells) in the presence of trypsin (Lee and Kurtz, 1981). After adsorption to and uncoating in cells (a receptor has so far not been identified), astroviruses produce full-length and subgenomic RNAs, the former leading to translation of ORF1a and ORF1a–ORF1b fusion proteins and the latter directing the production of the ORF2 protein precursor (Geigenmüller *et al.*, 2002, 2003). As mentioned above, the viral RNA polymerase is made from ORF1b by −1 ribosomal frameshifting (efficiency approximately 5%).

Transfection of naked full-length genome RNA was shown to lead to the production of infectious virus, allowing a reverse genetics system from cDNA to be set up (Geigenmüller et al., 1997).

Pathogenesis

This is mainly deduced from studies of in vitro infected cells and of experimental animals. Adsorption occurs through a cellular receptor likely to contain sialic acid, and replication takes place in the cytoplasm. Animals infected with species-specific astroviruses (lambs, calves) show infection of mature enterocytes (at the tip of the villi) of the small intestine at 14–38 h post-infection, and diarrhoea is observed on days 2–4.

Clinical Course, Diagnosis, Treatment and Prevention

Clinically, astrovirus disease is similar to that caused by rotaviruses, although often milder. Diagnosis is by EM, IEM (typing), astrovirus-specific ELISA (detecting seven types; Herrmann et al., 1990) and generic and type-specific RT-PCR (Noel et al., 1995). Treatment is symptomatic, and prevention in outbreaks consists of measures to interrupt person-to-person spread (good hygiene, disinfection, surveillance of food sources, etc.). At present, there is no specific antiviral treatment and no vaccine.

Epidemiology

Astroviruses are found in humans, lambs, calves, deer, piglets, mice, dogs and ducks, causing diarrhoea in most cases except for ducks, in which they cause acute hepatitis. Astroviruses are very species-specific. Human astrovirus infections are seen in infants and the elderly as endemic infections and occasionally as the cause of food-borne outbreaks of diarrhoea. The seasonal incidence peak is in the winter. Transmission is via the faecal–oral route, person-to-person contact and possibly fomites. The incidence of astrovirus infections in hospital-based studies has mostly been ≤5% of viral causes of diarrhoea, but much higher incidence figures (>10%) were recorded in Guatemala and Thailand. The incidence of different serotypes was determined from a collection of isolates in Oxford, UK (Lee and

Kurtz, 1994) and has been complemented recently by an age-stratified study of the prevalence of neutralising astrovirus antibodies in Utrecht, The Netherlands (Koopmans et al., 1998; Table 4.5). According to this, serotype 1 is most frequently found, followed by serotypes 2–4 at medium and serotypes 5–7 at the lowest frequency. The seroprevalence figures suggest that individuals can become infected by more than one serotype. Astrovirus infection is frequent in childhood (often inapparent), and 75% of 10 year-old children have astrovirus antibodies (Koopmans et al., 1998). A high percentage (15%) of cases of diarrhoea in HIV-infected individuals is due to astrovirus infection (Grohmann et al., 1993). Large food-borne outbreaks of astrovirus gastroenteritis have been recorded (e.g. Oishi et al., 1994).

Co-circulation of multiple astrovirus serotypes was shown by several groups in different locations (e.g. Noel et al., 1995; Mustafa et al., 2000; Monroe et al., 2001). The different types cluster in two genogroups (A: types 1–5, B: types 6 and 7; Belliot et al., 1997). The assignment of genotype 8 to a genogroup seems to depend on the genome area used for comparison and therefore the possibility has been raised that RNA recombination might have occurred (Belliot et al., 1997; Monroe et al., 2001).

Although enteric astroviruses have been isolated from animals, e.g. turkeys (Koci et al., 2000), there is so far no firm indication that human astroviruses may have arisen from an animal reservoir.

GASTROINTESTINAL VIRUSES NOT REGULARLY ASSOCIATED WITH ACUTE DIARRHOEAL DISEASE

Details of the virology, immunology, diagnosis, clinical symptoms and epidemiology of these viruses are found in other chapters.

Enteroviruses and Parechoviruses

Enteroviruses (polioviruses, coxsackieviruses and echo-viruses) and parechoviruses, all members of two genera of the *Picornaviridae*, infect humans via the alimentary tract, where they have their first site of replication (lymphoid tissues of the pharynx and the gut). Virus is usually excreted in the stool for several to many weeks and can also be isolated with ease from the pharynx during the first 2 weeks of infection. Most infections are asymptomatic. The main disease foci are the central

Table 4.5 Incidence of astrovirus serotypes in Oxford, UK, 1976–1992, and prevalence of astrovirus type-specific neutralising antibodies in Utrecht, The Netherlands, 1994–1996

Astrovirus type	Astrovirus isolates Oxford, UK[a] (n = 291) (% type)	Astrovirus neutralising antibody Utrecht, The Netherlands[b] (n = 242) (% type-specific antibody)
1	64.9	91
2	11.3	31
3	9.3	69
4	11.3	56
5	2.1	36
6	0.3	16
7	0.7	10

[a]From Lee and Kurtz (1994).
[b]From Koopmans et al. (1998).
For astrovirus type 8, see text.

nervous system (spinal cord, brain, meninges), heart (myocardium and pericardium), skeletal muscles and skin, which are reached after a viraemic step originating from the gut (Melnick, 1996).

Diarrhoea is not a regular symptom of primary infection. Some echoviruses (notably types 4, 11, 14, 18, 19 and 22) as well as *Coxsackie virus A1* have been documented as associated with outbreaks of diarrhoea (Townsend *et al.*, 1982; Patel *et al.*, 1985; Melnick, 1996), but a consistent association has not been established.

Aichivirus, proposed as a new genus of the *Picornaviridae* (Yamashita *et al.*, 1998), has been found to be a consistent cause of sporadic cases and outbreaks of human gastroenteritis in Japan (Yamashita *et al.*, 1991, 1993) and also to be the cause of traveller's diarrhoea in SE Asia (Yamashita *et al.*, 1995).

Reoviruses

Orthoreovirus, another genus of the family *Reoviridae*, also primarily infects the gut via M cells and the first round of replication occurs in the Peyer's patches. From there they are carried in a viraemic step (or by retrograde transport along the autonomous nerves) to the central nervous system, where they have their main disease targets in neuronal or ependymal cells. Reovirus pathogenesis has been studied in detail in mice, and particular pathogenetic factors have been associated with particular gene products (Tyler and Fields, 1996).

At the end of human childhood, antibodies against all three serotypes of reovirus are found, suggesting past infection. No firm association of reovirus

infection with any distinct human disease has so far been established, although reoviruses are not infrequently seen in the gut; an association with mild diarrhoea has been suggested (Tyler and Fields, 1996).

Coronaviruses and Toroviruses

These two genera of the family *Coronaviridae* (Enjuanes *et al.*, 2000) cause respiratory and gastrointestinal infections in humans. Toroviruses, a well-established cause of diarrhoea in calves and of asymptomatic infection in horses (Koopmans and Horzinck, 1994), were recently found to be associated with acute and possibly persistent diarrhoea in children (Koopmans *et al.*, 1997; Waters *et al.*, 2000).

Coronaviruses are a recognised major cause of the common cold in man (McIntosh, 1996) and were discovered very recently (March, 2003) as the cause of the severe acute respiratory syndrome (SARS). They cause gastroenteritis in animals (Kim *et al.*, 2001) and were found to be associated with cases of human diarrhoea, but coronavirus-like particles were also seen in symptomless healthy subjects. The true significance of coronavirus infection for human enteric disease remains to be established (Siddell and Snijder, 1998; Holmes, 2001).

Parvoviruses

These viruses are well-known pathogens of diarrhoea in animals. However, in humans no firm association with diarrhoea has been made, although parvovirus-like particles are not infrequently observed by EM as 'small round viruses' in human faeces (Fig. 4.1g).

Human Immunodeficiency Virus

The clinical virology of this member of the family *Retroviridae* (subfamily *Lentivirinae*) is extensively discussed elsewhere in this book. Here it should be mentioned that there is evidence for primary HIV infection in gut-associated lymphoid tissue and in enterocytes, which may contribute to an enteropathy with chronic diarrhoea in AIDS patients (e.g. Nelson *et al.*, 1988; Kotler *et al.*, 1991; Heise *et al.*, 1991; Rabeneck, 1994).

Cytomegalovirus and Herpes Simplex Virus

These two members of the family *Herpesviridae* are frequent co-infectants/superinfectants in the gut of HIV-infected individuals, causing mainly chronic colitis (Dieterich and Rahmin, 1991; Montec *et al.*, 1994), but also oesophagitis, gastritis and cholangitis (Theise *et al.*, 1991). There may be interaction between HIV and cytomegalovirus infections in causing gut disease (Skolnik *et al.*, 1988). With the introduction of highly active antiretroviral therapy (HAART) in 1996, it has become less urgent to initiate or maintain a specific anti-CMV therapy with ganciclovir (Whitcup *et al.*, 1999; Pollok, 2001).

Picobirnaviruses

This recently established family, *Birnaviridae* (Leong *et al.*, 2000), consists of bisegmented RNA viruses of approximately 60 nm in diameter and icosahedral structure. They were found in the gut of rats, guinea-pigs, pigs and calves and to be associated with cases of diarrhoea, although not regularly. Recently, besides astroviruses, caliciviruses and adenoviruses, picobirnaviruses were found to be significantly associated with diarrhoea in AIDS patients in a case–control study (Grohmann *et al.*, 1993; Giordano *et al.*, 1999). Similar bisegmented dsRNA viruses have been demonstrated to infect *Cryptosporidium* spp. but they are much smaller (30 nm in diameter), and there is little sequence identity between them and the typical picobirnaviruses (Wang and Wang, 1991; Khramtsov and Upton, 2000; Xiao *et al.*, 2001). Reagents derived from the genomic sequence (Rosen *et al.*, 2000) will allow the epidemiology of human and related picobirnaviruses to be unravelled.

ACKNOWLEDGEMENTS

The authors gratefully acknowledge fruitful discussions with Dr John Kurtz (Oxford) and Dr Marion Koopmans (Amsterdam), and the excellent secretarial support of Lynne Bastow and Narguesse Stevens.

REFERENCES

A complete list of references is available from the authors upon request.

Allard A, Albinson B and Wadell G (2001) Rapid typing of human adenoviruses by a general PCR combined with restriction endonuclease analysis. *J Clin Microbiol*, **39**, 498–505.

Ando T, Monroe SS, Gentsch JR *et al.* (1995) Detection and differentiation of antigenically distinct small round-structured viruses (Norwalk-like viruses) by reverse transcription-PCR and Southern hybridization. *J Clin Microbiol*, **33**, 64–71.

Atmar RL, Neill FH, Woodley CM *et al.* (1996) A collaborative evaluation of a method for the detection of Norwalk virus in shellfish tissue using the polymerase chain reaction. *Appl Environm Microbiol*, **62**, 254–258.

Ball JM, Tian P, Zeng CQY *et al.* (1996) Age-dependent diarrhea induced by a rotaviral non-structural glycoprotein. *Science*, **272**, 101–104.

Bass D (2003) Treatment of viral gastroenteritis. In *Viral Gastroenteritis* (eds Desselberger U, Gray J), pp 93–104. Elsevier Science, Amsterdam.

Belliot G, Laveran H and Monroe SS (1997) Detection and genetic differentiation of human astroviruses: phylogenetic grouping varies by coding region. *Arch Virol*, **142**, 1323–1334.

Bern C, Martines J, de Zoysa I *et al.* (1992) The magnitude of the global problem of diarrhoeal disease: a ten year update. *Bull WHO*, **70**, 705–714.

Bernstein DI, Smith VE, Sherwood JR *et al.* (1998) Safety and immunogenicity of live, attenuated human rotavirus vaccine 89–12. *Vaccine*, **16**, 381–387.

Bernstein DJ, Sack DA, Rothstein E *et al.* (1999) Efficacy of live, attenuated human rotavirus vaccine 89-12 in infants: a randomized placebo-controlled trial. *Lancet*, **354**, 287–290.

Berois M, Sapin C, Erle I *et al.* (2003) Rotavirus non-structural protein NSP5 interacts with major core protein VP2. *J Virol*, **77**, 1757–1763.

Bishop RF, Davidson GP, Holmes IH and Ruck BJ (1973) Virus particles in epithelial cells of duodenal mucosa from children with viral gastroenteritis. *Lancet*, **ii**, 1281–1283.

Blacklow NR and Greenberg HB (1991) Viral gastroenteritis. *N Engl J Med*, **325**, 252–264.

Bon F, Fascia P, Dauvergne M *et al.* (1999) Prevalence of group A rotavirus, human calicivirus, astrovirus and adenovirus type 40 and 41 infections among children with acute gastroenteritis in Dijon, France. *J Clin Microbiol*, **37**, 3055–3058.

Brierley D and Vidakovic M (2003) Ribosomal frameshifting in astroviruses. In *Viral Gastroenteritis* (eds Desselberger U, Gray J), pp 587–606. Elsevier Science, Amsterdam.

Burke B and Desselberger U (1996) Rotavirus pathogenicity. *Virology*, **218**, 299–305.

Burns JW, Siadat-Pajouh M, Krishnaney AA *et al.* (1996) Protective effect of rotavirus VP-specific IgA monoclonal antibodies that lack neutralizing activity. *Science*, **272**, 104–107.

Caul EO, Ashley CR, Darville JM *et al.* (1990) Group C rotavirus associated with fatal enteritis in a family outbreak. *J Med Virol*, **30**, 201–205.

Centers for Disease Control and Prevention. Advisory Committee on Immunization Practices (ACIP) (1999a) Rotavirus vaccine for the prevention of rotavirus gastroenteritis among children. *Morbid Mortal Weekly Rep*, **48** (RR-2), 1–22.

Centers for Disease Control and Prevention. Advisory Committee on Immunization Practices (ACIP) (1999b) Intussusception among recipients of rotavirus vaccine—United States, 1998–1999. *Morbid Mortal Weekly Rep*, **48**, 577–581.

Centers for Disease Control and Prevention, Advisory Committee on Immunization Practices (ACIP) (1999c) Withdrawal of rotavirus vaccine recommendation. *Morbid Mortal Weekly Rep*, **48**, 1007.

Chadwick D and Goode JA (eds) (2002) *Gastroenteritis Viruses*. Ciba Foundation Symposium No. 238, 323 pp Wiley, Chichester.

Chang HH, Smith PF, Ackelsberg J *et al.* (2001) Intussusception, rotavirus diarrhoea, and rotavirus vaccine among children in New York State. *Pediatrics*, **108**, 54–60.

Chen SC, Fynan EF, Robinson HL *et al.* (1997) Protective immunity induced by rotavirus DNA vaccines. *Vaccine*, **15**, 899–902.

Chen SC, Jones DH, Fynan EF *et al.* (1998) Protective immunity induced by oral immunization with a rotavirus DNA vaccine encapsulated in microparticles. *J Virol*, **72**, 5757–5761.

Chiba S, Estes MK, Nakata S and Calisher CH (eds) (1997) Viral gastroenteritis. *Arch Virol*, **142** (suppl 12), p. 311.

Ciarlet M, Ludert JE, Iturriza-Gómara M *et al.* (2002) Initial interaction of rotavirus strains with N-acetylneuraminic (sialic) acid residues on the cell surface correlates with VP4 genotype, not species of origin. *J Virol* **76**, 4087–4095.

Clark HF, Offit PA, Ellis RW *et al.* (1996) WC3 reassortant vaccines in children. *Arch Virol*, **12** (suppl): 187–198.

Clarke IN and Lambden PR (2001) The Molecular Biology of Human Caliciviruses. *Novartis Found Symp*, **238**, 180–191 (Discussion pp 191–196).

Cohen J, Garbarg-Chenon A and Pothier CH (eds) (2002) *Les Gastroentérites Virales*, pp 325. Elsevier SAS, Paris.

Conner ME, Zarley CD, Hu B *et al.* (1996) Virus-like particles as a rotavirus subunit vaccine. *J Infect Dis*, **174** (suppl 1), S88–S92.

Coulson BS, Grimwood K, Hudson IL *et al.* (1992) Role of antibody in clinical protection of children during reaction with rotavirus. *J Clin Microbiol*, **30**, 1678–1684.

Coulson BS, Londrigan SH and Lee DJ (1997) Rotavirus contains integrin ligand sequences and a disintegrin-like domain implicated in virus entry into cells. *Proc Natl Acad Sci USA*, **94**, 5389–5394.

Crawford SE, Mukherjee SK, Estes MK *et al.* (2001) Trypsin cleavage stabilizes the rotavirus VP4 spike. *J Virol*, **75**, 6052–6061.

Cubitt WD (1994) Caliciviruses. In *Viral Infections of the Gastrointestinal Tract* (ed. Kapikian AZ), pp 549–568. Marcel Dekker, New York.

De Clercq E (1996) Therapeutic potential of cidofovir (HPMPC, Vistide) for the treatment of DNA virus (i.e. herpes-, parvo- pox- and adenovirus) infections. *Verhandelingen—Koninklijke Academie Voor Geneeskunde Van Belgie*, **58**, 19–47.

de Jong JC, Bijlsma K, Wermenbol AG *et al.* (1993) Detection, typing and subtyping of enteric adenoviruses 40 and 41 from fecal samples and observation of changing incidences of infection with these types and subtypes. *J Clin Microbiol*, **31**, 1562–1569.

Desselberger U (1996) Genome rearrangements of rotaviruses. *Adv Virus Res*, **46**, 69–95.

Desselberger U (1998a) Reoviruses. In *Topley and Wilson's Microbiology and Microbial Infections, vol I, Virology* (eds Collier L and Mahy B), pp 537–550. Edward Arnold, London.

Desselberger U (1998b) Viral gastroenteritis. *Curr Opin Infect Dis*, **11**, 565–575.

Desselberger U (1998c) Prospects for vaccines against rotaviruses. *Rev Med Virol*, **8**, 43–52.

Desselberger U (1999) Rotavirus infections: guidelines for treatment and prevention. *Drugs*, **58**, 447–452.

Desselberger U and Gray J (eds) (2003) *Viral Gastroenteritis*. Series Perspectives in Medical Virology. Elsevier Science, Amsterdam.

Desselberger U, Iturriza-Gómara M and Gray J (2001) Rotavirus Epidemiology and Surveillance. *Novartis Found Symp*, **238**, 125–147.

Dieterich DT and Rahmin M (1991) Cytomegalovirus colitis in AIDS: presentation in 44 patients and a review of the literature. *J AIDS* **4** (suppl), S29–S35.

Enjuanes L, Brian D, Cavanagh D *et al.* (2000) *Coronaviridae*. In *Virus Taxonomy* (eds van Regenmortel MHV *et al.*) Seventh Report of the International Committee on Taxonomy of Viruses, pp 835–849. Academic Press, San Diego.

Estes MK (2001) Rotaviruses and their replication. In *Fields Virology* (eds Knipe DM, Howley PM *et al.*), 4th edn, pp 1747–1785. Lippincott Williams and Wilkins, Philadelphia.

Estes MK, Atmar RL and Hardy ME (1997) Norwalk and related diarrhea viruses. In *Clinical Virology* (eds Richman DD, Whitley RJ and Hayden FG), pp 1073–1095. Churchill Livingstone, New York.

Fankhauser RL, Noel JS, Monroe SS, Ando T, Glass RI (1998) Molecular epidemiology of 'Norwalk-like viruses' in outbreaks of gastroenteritis in the United States. *J Infect Dis*, **178**, 1571–1578.

Feng N, Burns JW, Bracy L *et al.* (1994) Comparison of mucosal and systemic humoral immune responses and subsequent protection in mice orally inoculated with a homologous or a heterologous rotavirus. *J Virol*, **68**, 7766–7773.

Feng N, Vo PT, Chung D *et al.* (1997) Heterotypic protection following oral immunization with live heterologous rotavirus in a mouse model. *J Infect Dis*, **175**, 330–341.

Figueroa-Quintanilla D, Salazar-Lindo E, Sack RB *et al.* (1993) A controlled trial of bismuth subsalicylate in infants with acute watery diarrheal disease. *N Engl J Med*, **328**, 1653–1658.

Flewett TH, Bryden AS and Davies H (1973) Virus particles in gastroenteritis. *Lancet*, **ii**, 1497.

Franco MA and Greenberg HB (1995) Role of B cells and cytotoxic T lymphocytes in clearance and immunity to rotavirus infection in mice. *J Virol*, **69**, 7800–7806.

Geigenmüller U, Grinzton NH and Matsui SM (1997) Construction of a genome-length cDNA clone for human astrovirus serotype 1 and synthesis of infectious RNA transcripts. *J Virol*, **71**, 1713–1717.

Geigenmüller U, Ginzton NH and Matsui SM (2002) Studies on intracellular processing of the capsid protein of human astrovirus serotype 1 in infected cells. *J Gen Virol*, **83**, 1691–1695.

Geigenmüller U, Méndez E and Matsui SM (2003) Studies on the molecular biology of human astrovirus. In *Viral Gastroenteritis* (eds Desselberger U and Gray J), pp 573–586. Elsevier Science, Amsterdam.

Gentsch JR, Glass RI, Woods P et al. (1992) Identification of group A rotavirus gene 4 types of polymerase chain reaction. *J Clin Microbiol*, **30**, 1365–1373.

Gilger MA, Matson DO, Conner ME et al. (1992) Extraintestinal rotavirus infections in children with immunodeficiency. *J Pediatr*, **120**, 912–917.

Giordano MO, Martinez LC, Rinaldi D et al. (1999) Diarrhea and enteric emerging viruses in HIV-infected patients. *AIDS Res Hum Retrovir*, **15**, 1427–1432.

Gouvea V, Glass RI, Woods P et al. (1990) Polymerase chain reaction amplification and typing of rotavirus nucleic acid from stool specimens. *J Clin Microbiol*, **28**, 276–282.

Graham DY, Jiang X, Tanaka T et al. (1994) Norwalk virus infection of volunteers: new insights based on improved assays. *J Infect Dis*, **170**, 34–43.

Gray JJ, Cunliffe C, Ball J et al. (1994) Detection of immunoglobulin M (IgM), IgA, and IgG Norwalk virus-specific antibodies by indirect enzyme-linked immunosorbent assay with baculovirus-expressed Norwalk virus capsid antigen in adult volunteers challenged with Norwalk virus. *J Clin Microbiol*, **32**, 3059–3063.

Gray JJ, Green J, Cunliffe C et al. (1997) Mixed genogroup SRSV infections among a party of canoeists exposed to contaminated recreational water. *J Med Virol*, **52**, 425–429.

Gray JJ, Jiang X, Morgan-Capner P et al. (1993) Prevalence of antibodies to Norwalk virus in England: detection by enzyme-linked immunosorbent assay using baculovirus-expressed Norwalk virus capsid antigen. *J Clin Microbiol*, **31**, 1022–1025.

Green J, Gallimore CI, Norcott JP et al. (1995) Broadly reactive reverse transcriptase polymerase chain reaction in the diagnosis of SRSV-associated gastroenteritis. *J Med Virol*, **47**, 392–398.

Green K, Chanock R and Kapikian A (2001) Human caliciviruses. In: *Field's Virology* (eds Knipe DM, Howley PM et al.) 4th edn, pp 841–874. Lippincott Williams & Wilkins, Philadelphia.

Grohmann GS, Glass RI, Pereira HG et al. (1993) Enteric viruses and diarrhea in HIV-infected patients. *N Engl J Med*, **329**, 14–20.

Guerrero CA, Bouyssounade D, Zárate S et al. (2002) The heat shock cognate protein 70 is involved in rotavirus cell entry. *J Virol*, **76**, 4096–4102.

Guerrero CA, Méndez E, Zárate S et al. (2000) Integrin β3 mediates rotavirus entry. *Proc Nat Acad Sci USA*, **97**, 14644–14649.

Guix S, Caballero S, Villena C et al. (2002) Molecular epidemiology of astroviruses in Spain. *J. Clin Microbiol*, **40**, 133–139.

Guo MZ and Saif LJ (2003) Pathogenesis of enteric calicivirus infections. In *Viral Gastroenteritis* (eds Desselberger U, Gray J), pp. 489–503. Elsevier Science, Amsterdam.

Hart CA and Cunliffe NA (1997) Viral gastroenteritis. *Curr Opin Infect Dis*, **10**, 408–413.

Hedberg CW and Osterholm MT (1993) Outbreaks of foodborne and waterborne viral gastroenteritis. *Clin Microbiol Rev*, **6**, 199–210.

Heise C, Daudekar S, Kumar P et al. (1991) Human immunodeficiency virus infection of enterocytes and mononuclear cells in human jejunal mucosa. *Gastroenterology*, **100**, 1521–1527.

Herrmann JE, Chen SC, Fynan EF et al. (1996) Protection against rotavirus infections by DNA vaccination. *J Infect Dis*, **174** (suppl 1), S93–S97.

Herrmann JE, Novak NA, Perron-Henry DM et al. (1990) Diagnosis of astrovirus gastroenteritis by antigen detection with monoclonal antibodies. *J Infect Dis*, **161**, 226–229.

Hewish MJ, Takada Y and Coulson BS (2000) Integrins a2b1 and a4b1 can mediate SA11 rotavirus attachment and entry into cells. *J Virol*, **74**, 228–236.

Hinkula J, Ball JM, Lofgren S et al. (1995) Antibody prevalence and immunoglobulin IgG subclass pattern to Norwalk virus in Sweden. *J Med Virol*, **47**, 52–57.

Holmes KV (2001) Coronaviruses. In *Fields Virology* (eds Knipe DM, Howley PM, Griffin D et al.), 4th edn, pp 1187–1203. Lippincott Williams & Wilkins, Philadelphia.

Horwitz MS (2001) Adenoviruses. In *Fields Virology* (eds Knipe DM, Howley PM, Griffin D et al.), 4th edn, pp 2301–2326. Lippincott Williams & Wilkins, Philadelphia.

Hung T (1988) Rotavirus and adult diarrhoea. *Adv Virus Res*, **35**, 193–218.

Iturriza-Gómara M, Auchterlonie IA, Zaw W et al. (2002a) Rotavirus gastroenteritis and CNS infection: characterisation of the VP7 and VP4 genes of rotavirus strains isolated from paired faecal and CSF samples of a child with CNS disease. *J Clin Microbiol*, **40**, 4797–4799.

Iturriza-Gómara M, Cubitt D, Steele D et al. (2002b) Characterization of rotavirus G9 strains isolated in the UK between 1995 and 1998. *J Med Virol*, **61**, 510–517.

Iturriza-Gómara M, Desselberger U and Gray J (2003) Molecular epidemiology of rotaviruses: genetic mechanisms associated with diversity. In *Viral Gastroenteritis* (eds Desselberger U and Gray J), pp. 317–344. Elsevier Science, Amsterdam.

Iturriza-Gómara M, Green J, Brown D et al. (2000) Molecular epidemiology of human group A rotavirus infections in the UK between 1995 and 1998. *J Clin Microbiol*, **38**, 4394–4401.

Iturriza-Gómara M, Isherwood B, Desselberger U and Gray J (2001) Reassortment *in vivo*: driving force for diversity of human rotavirus strains isolated in the United Kingdom between 1995 and 1999. *J Virol*, **75**, 3696–3705.

Iturriza-Gómara M, Wong C, Blome C et al. (2002c) Molecular characterisation of VP6 genes of human rotavirus isolates: correlation of genogroups with subgroups and evidence of independent segregation. *J Virol*, **76**, 6596–6601.

Jiang X, Espul C, Zhong WM et al. (1999) Characterization of a novel human calicivirus that may be a natural recombinant. *Arch Virol*, **144**, 2377–2387.

Jiang X, Wang M, Graham DY *et al.* (1992) Expression, self-assembly, and antigenicity of the Norwalk virus capsid protein. *J Virol*, **66**, 6527–6532.

Jiang X, Wang M, Wang K *et al.* (1993) Sequence and genomic organization of Norwalk virus. *Virology*, **195**, 51–61.

Jing Y, Qian Y, Huo Y *et al.* (2000) Seroprevalence against Norwalk-like human caliciviruses in Beijing, China. *J Med Virol*, **60**, 97–101.

Joensuu J, Koskenniemi E, Pang XL *et al.* (1997) Randomized placebo controlled trial of rhesus–human reassortant rotavirus vaccine for prevention of severe rotavirus gastroenteritis. *Lancet*, **350**, 1205–1209.

Jolly CJ, Beisner B, Ozser E and Holmes IH (2001) Non-lytic extraction and characterization for receptors for multiple strains of rotavirus. *Arch Virol*, **146**, 1307–1323.

Kapelushnik OR, Delukina M, Nagler A *et al.* (1995) Intravenous ribavirin therapy for adenovirus gastroenteritis after bone marrow transplantation. *J Pediatr Gastroenterol Nutrit*, **21**, 110–112.

Kapikian AZ (ed.) (1994a) *Viral Infections of the Gastrointestinal Tract*, 2nd edn, pp 785. Marcel Dekker, New York.

Kapikian AZ (1994b) Jennerian and modified Jennerian approach to vaccination against rotavirus diarrhea in infants and young children: an introduction. In *Viral Infections of the Gastrointestinal Tract* (ed. Kapikian AZ), 2nd edn, pp 409–517. Marcel Dekker, New York.

Kapikian AZ, Estes MK and Chanock RM (1996) Norwalk group of viruses. In *Fields Virology* (eds Fields BN, Knipe DM, Howley PM *et al.*), pp 783–810. Lippincott-Raven, Philadelphia.

Kapikian AZ, Wyatt RG, Dolin R *et al.* (1972) Visualisation by immune electron microscopy of a 27 nm particle associated with acute infectious non-bacterial gastroenteritis. *J Virol*, **10**, 1075–1081.

Khramtsov NV and Upton SJ (2000) Association of RNA polymerase complexes of the parasitic protozoan *Cryptosporidium parvum* with virus-like particles: heterogeneous system. *J Virol*, **74**, 5788–5795.

Kim SY, Song DS and Park BK (2001) Differential detection of transmissible gastroenteritis virus and porcine epidemic diarrhea virus by duplex RT-PCR. *J Vet Diagn Invest*, **13**, 516–520.

Kobayashi N, Naik TN, Kusuhara Y *et al.* (2001) Sequence analysis of genes encoding structural and non-structural proteins of a human group B rotavirus detected in Calcutta, India. *J Med Virol*, **64**, 583–588.

Koci MD, Seall BS and Schultz-Cherry S (2000) Molecular characterisation of an avian astrovirus. *J Virol*, **74**, 6173–6177.

Koopmans M (2001) Molecular Epidemiology of Human Enteric Caliciviruses in The Netherlands. *Novartis Found Symp*, **238**, 197–214 (Discussion, pp 214–218).

Koopmans M and Horzinek M (1994) Toroviruses of animal and humans: a review. *Adv Virus Res*, **43**, 233–273.

Koopmans MP, Bijen MHL, Monroe SS and Vinje J (1998) Age-stratified seroprevalence of neutralising antibodies to astrovirus types 1 to 7 in humans in The Netherlands. *Clin Diagn Lab Immunol*, **5**, 33–37.

Koopmans MP, Goosen ES, Lima AA *et al.* (1997) Association of torovirus with acute and persistent diarrhoea in children. *Pediatr Infect Dis J*, **16**, 504–507.

Koopmans M, van Strien E and Vennema H (2003) Molecular epidemiology of human caliciviruses. In *Viral Gastroenteritis* (eds Desselberger U and Gray J), pp 523–554. Elsevier Science, Amsterdam.

Kotler DP, Reka SA, Borcich A *et al.* (1991) Detection, localization and quantitation of HIV-associated antigens in intestinal biopsies from patients with AIDS. *Am J Pathol*, **139**, 823–830.

Krajden M, Brown M, Petrasek A *et al.* (1990) Clinical features of adenovirus enteritis: a review of 127 cases. *Pediatr Infect Dis J*, **9**, 636–641.

Kramarz P, France EK, Destefano F *et al.* (2001) Population-based study of rotavirus vaccination and intussusception. *Pediatr Infect Dis J*, **20**, 410–416.

Krishnan T, Sen A, Choudhury JS *et al.* (1999) Emergence of adult diarrhoea rotavirus in Calcutta, India. *Lancet*, **353**, 380–381.

Lambden PR, Caul EO, Ashley CR *et al.* (1993) Sequence and genome organization of a human small round-structured (Norwalk-like) virus. *Science*, **259**, 516–518.

Lawton JA, Estes MK and Prasad BV (1997a) Three-dimensional visualization of mRNA release from actively transcribing rotavirus particles. *Nature Struct Biol*, **4**, 118–121.

Lawton JA, Estes MK and Prasad BV (1999) Comparative structural analysis of transcriptionally competent and incompetent rotavirus-antibody complexes. *Proc Natl Acad Sci USA*, **96**, 5428–5433.

Lawton JA, Estes MK and Prasad BV (2000) Mechanism of genome transcription in segmented dsRNA viruses. *Adv Virus Res*, **55**, 185–229.

Lawton JA, Zwng CQ, Mukherjee SK *et al.* (1997b) Three-dimensional structural analysis of recombinant rotavirus-like particles with intact and amino-terminal-deleted VP2: implications for the architecture of VP2 capsid layer. *J Virol*, **71**, 7353–7369.

Lee T and Kurtz JB (1981) Serial propagation of astrovirus in tissue culture with the aid of trypsin. *J Gen Virol*, **57**, 421–424.

Lee TW and Kurtz JB (1994) Prevalence of astrovirus serotypes in the Oxford region 1976–92, with evidence for 2 new serotypes. *Epidemiol Infect*, **112**, 187–193.

Lees DN, Henshilwood K, Green J *et al.* (1995) Detection of small round structured viruses in shellfish by reverse transcription-PCR. *Appl Environm Microbiol*, **61**, 4418–4424.

Legrand F, Berrebi D, Houhou N *et al.* (2001) Early diagnosis of adenovirus infection and treatment with cidofovir after bone marrow transplantation in children. *Bone Marrow Transpl*, **27**, 621–626.

Leong JC, Brown D, Dobos P *et al.* (2000) Birnaviridae. In *Virus Taxonomy* (eds Van Regenmortel MHV *et al.*). Seventh Report of the International Committee on Taxonomy of Viruses, pp 481–490. Academic Press, San Diego.

Lepault J, Petitpas I, Erk I *et al.* (2001) Structural polymorphism of the major capsid protein of rotavirus. *EMBO J*, **20**, 1498–1507.

Lewis TL and Matsui SM (1994) An astrovirus frameshift signal induces ribosomal frameshifting *in vitro*. *Arch Virol*, **140**, 1127–1135.

Lewis TL and Matsui SM (1996) Astrovirus ribosomal frameshifting in an infection–transfection transient expression system. *J Virol*, **70**, 2869–2875.

Liu BL, Clarke IN, Caul EO *et al.* (1995) Human enteric caliciviruses have a unique genome structure and are distinct from the Norwalk-like viruses. *Arch Virol*, **140**, 1345–1356.

Liu BL, Lambden PR, Günther H *et al.* (1999) Molecular characterization of a bovine enteric calicivirus: relationship to the Norwalk-like virus. *J Virol*, **73**, 819–825.

Marczinke B, Bloys AJ, Brown TDK *et al.* (1994) The human astrovirus RNA-dependent RNA polymerase coding region is expressed by ribosomal frameshifting. *J Virol*, **68**, 5588–5595.

Mason HS, Ball JM, Shi JJ *et al.* (1996) Expression of Norwalk virus capsid protein in transgenic tobacco and potato and its immunogenicity in mice. *Proc Natl Acad Sci USA*, **93**, 5335–5340.

Mason HS, Warzecha H, Mor T and Arntzen CJ (2002) Edible plant vaccines: applications for prophylactic and therapeutic molecular medicine. *Trends Mol Med*, **8**, 324–329.

Matson DO, Zhong W, Nakata S *et al.* (1995) Molecular characterization of a human calicivirus with closer sequence relatedness to animal caliciviruses than other known human caliciviruses. *J Med Virol*, **45**, 215–222.

Matsui SM and Greenberg HB (2001) Astroviruses. In *Fields Virology* (eds Knipe DM, Howley PM *et al.*), 4th edn, pp 875–893. Lippincott, Williams & Wilkins, Philadelphia.

Mattion NM, Cohen J and Estes MK (1994) The rotavirus proteins. In *Viral Infections of the Gastrointestinal Tract* (ed. Kapikian AZ), 2nd edn, pp 169–249. Marcel Dekker, New York.

Mayo MA (2002) Virus taxonomy—Houston 2002. *Arch Virol*, **147**, 1071–1076.

McIntosh K (1996) Coronaviruses. In *Fields Virology* (eds Fields BN, Knipe DM, Howley DM *et al.*), 3rd edn, pp 1095–1103. Lippincott-Raven, Philadelphia.

Melnick JL (1996) Enteroviruses: polioviruses, coxsackie-viruses, echoviruses, and newer enteroviruses. In *Fields Virology* (eds Fields BN, Knipe DM, Howley PM *et al.*), 3rd edn, pp 655–712. Lippincott-Raven, Philadelphia.

Mentec H, Laport C, Laport J *et al.* (1994) Cytomegalovirus colitis in HIV-1 infected patients: a prospective research in 55 patients. *AIDS*, **8**, 461–467.

Monroe SS, Holmes JL and Belliot GM (2001) Molecular Epidemiology of Human Astroviruses. *Novartis Found Symp*, **238**, 237–245 (Discussion pp 245–249).

Murphy TV, Garguillo PM, Massoudi MS *et al.* (2001). Intussusception among infants given an oral rotavirus vaccine. *N Engl J Med*, **344**, 564–572.

Mustafa H, Palombo EA and Bishop RF (2000) Epidemiology of astrovirus infection in young children hospitalized with acute gastroenteritis in Melbourne, Australia, over a period of four consecutive years, 1995–1998. *J Clin Microbiol*, **38**, 1058–1062.

Naficy AB, Abu-Elyazeed R, Holmes JL *et al.* (1999) Epidemiology of rotavirus diarrhoea in Egyptian children and implications for disease control. *Am J Epidemiol*, **150**, 770–777.

Naficy AB, Rao MR, Savarino SJ *et al.* (2000) Astrovirus diarrhea in Egyptian children. *J Infect Dis*, **182**, 685–690.

Nakata S, Honma S, Namata KK *et al.* (2000) Members of the family *Caliciviridae* (NV and SV) are the most prevalent causes of gastroenteritis outbreaks among infants in Japan. *J Infect Dis*, **181**, 2029–2032.

Nelson JA, Reynolds-Kohler C, Margaretten W *et al.* (1988) Human immunodeficiency virus detected in bowel epithelium from patients with gastrointestinal symptoms. *Lancet*, **i**, 259–262.

Noel JS, Lee TW, Kurtz JB *et al.* (1995) Typing of human astroviruses from clinical isolates by enzyme immunoassay and nucleotide sequencing. *J Clin Microbiol*, **33**, 797–801.

Numata K, Nakata S, Jiang E *et al.* (1994) Epidemiological study of Norwalk virus infections in Japan and Southeast Asia by enzyme-linked immunosorbent assays with Norwalk virus capsid protein produced by the baculovirus expression system. *J Clin Microbiol*, **32**, 121–126.

Offit PA (1994) Rotaviruses. Immunological determinants of protection against infection and disease. *Adv Virus Res*, **44**, 161–202.

Offit PA, Clark HF, Blavat G *et al.* (1986) Reassortant rotaviruses containing structural proteins VP3 and VP7 from different parents induce antibodies protective against each parental serotype. *J Virol*, **60**, 491–496.

Offit PA, Clark HF and Ward RL (2003) Current state of development of rotavirus vaccines. In *Viral Gastroenteritis* (eds Desselberger U, Gray JS), pp 345–356. Elsevier Science, Amsterdam.

Offit PA, Khoury CA, Moser CA *et al.* (1994) Enhancement of rotavirus immunogenicity by microencapsulation. *Virology*, **203**, 134–143.

Oishi I, Yamazaki K, Kimoto T *et al.* (1994) A large outbreak of acute gastroenteritis associated with astrovirus among students and teachers in Osaka, Japan. *J Infect Dis*, **170**, 439–443.

O'Neal CM, Harriman GR and Conner ME (2000). Protection of the villus epithelial cells of the small intestine from rotavirus infections does not require IgA. *J Virol*, **74**, 4102–4109.

Pang X-L, Honma S, Nakata S and Vesikari T (2000) Human caliciviruses in acute gastroenteritis of young children in the community. *J Infect Dis*, **181** (suppl 2), S288–S294.

Patel JR, Daniel J and Mathan VI (1985) An epidemic of acute diarrhoea in rural Southern India associated with echovirus type 11 infection. *J Hyg (Camb)*, **95**, 483–492.

Patton JT (2001) Rotavirus RNA Replication and Gene Expression. *Novartis Found Symp*, **238**, 64–77.

Pérez-Schael I, Guntiñas MJ, Pérez M *et al.* (1997) Efficacy of the rhesus rotavirus-based quadrivalent vaccine in infants and young children in Venezuela. *N Engl J Med*, **337**, 1181–1187.

Pesavento JB, Lawton JA, Estes MK and Prasad BVV (2001) The reversible condensation and expansion of the rotavirus genome. *Proc Natl Acad Sci USA*, **98**, 1381–1388.

Petitpas I, Lepault J, Vachette P *et al.* (1998) Crystallization and preliminary x-ray analysis of rotavirus protein VP6. *J Virol*, **72**, 7615–7619.

Phillips AD (1989) Mechanisms of mucosal injury: human studies. In *Virus and the Gut* (ed. Farthing MJG), pp 30–40. Swan, London.

Pollok RCG (2001) Viruses causing diarrhoea in AIDS. *Novartis Found Symp*, **238**, 276–282 (Discussion, pp 282–288).

Prasad BVV, Burns JW, Marietta E *et al.* (1990) Localization of VP4 neutralization sites in rotavirus by three-dimensional cryo-electron microscopy. *Nature*, **343**, 476–479.

Prasad BVV and Estes MK (1997) Molecular basis of rotavirus replication: structure–function correlations. In *Structural Biology of Viruses* (eds Chiu A, Burnett RM and

Garcia RL), pp 239–268. Oxford University Press, New York.

Prasad BVV, Hardy ME, Dokland T *et al.* (1999) X-ray crystallographic structure of the Norwalk virus capsid. *Science*, **286**, 287–290.

Prasad BVV, Matson DO and Smith AJ (1994a) Three-dimensional structure of calicivirus. *J Mol Biol*, **240**, 256–264.

Prasad BVV, Rothnagel R, Jiang X *et al.* (1994b) Three-dimensional structure of baculovirus-expressed Norwalk virus capsids. *J Virol*, **68**, 5117–5125.

Prasad BVV, Rothnagel K, Zeng CQ *et al.* (1996) Visualization of ordered genomic RNA and localization of transcriptional complexes in rotaviruses. *Nature*, **382**, 471–473.

Prasad BVV, Wang GJ, Clerx JP *et al.* (1988) Three-dimensional structure of rotavirus. *J Mol Biol*, **199**, 269–275.

Rabeneck L (1994) AIDS enteropathy: what's in a name? *J Clin Gastroenterol*, **19**, 154–157.

Ramachandran M, Gentsch JR, Parashar UD *et al.* (1998) Detection and characterization of novel rotavirus strains in the United States. *J Clin Microbiol*, **36**, 3223–3229.

Rennels MB, Glass RI, Dennehy PH *et al.* (1996) Safety and efficacy of high-dose rhesus–human reassortant rotavirus vaccines—report of the multicenter trial US rotavirus vaccine efficacy group. *Pediatrics*, **97**, 7–13.

Rosen BI, Fang ZY, Glass RI and Monroe SS (2000) Cloning of human picobirnavirus genomic segments and development of a RT-PCR detection assay. *Virology*, **277**, 316–329.

Schuck P, Taraporewala Z, McPhie P and Patton JT (2001) Rotavirus non-structural protein NSP2 self-assembles into octamers that undergo ligand-induced conformational changes. *J Biol Chem*, **276**, 9679–9687.

Shenk T (1996) Adenoviridae: the viruses and their replication. In *Fields Virology* (eds Fields BN, Knipe DM, Howley PM *et al.*), 3rd edn, pp 2111–2148. Lippincott-Raven, Philadelphia.

Siddell SG and Snijder EJ (1998) Coronaviruses, toroviruses and arteriviruses. In *Topley and Wilson's Microbiology and Microbial Infections, vol 1, Virology*, 9th edn (eds Collier L and Mahy BWJ), pp 463–484. Edward Arnold, London.

Simonsen L, Morens DM, Elixhauser A *et al.* (2001) Incidence trends in infant hospitalization for intussusception: impact of the 1998–1999 rotavirus vaccination program in 10 US States. *Lancet*, **358**, 1224–1229.

Skolnik PR, Kosloff BR and Hirsch MS (1988) Bidirectional interactions between human immunodeficiency virus type 1 and cytomegalovirus. *J Infect Dis*, **157**, 508–513.

Smit TK, Bos P, Peenze I *et al.* (1999) Seroepidemiological study of genogroup I and II calicivirus infections in South and Southern Africa. *J Med Virol*, **59**, 227–231.

Sosnovtsev SV and Green K (1995) RNA transcripts derived from a cloned full-length copy of the feline caliciviruses genome do not require VP6 for infectivity. *Virology*, **210**, 383–390.

Stewart PL, Burnett RM, Cyrklaff M *et al.* (1991) Image reconstruction reveals the complex molecular nature of adenoviruses. *Cell*, **67**, 145–154.

Tafazoli F, Zeng CQY, Estes MK *et al.* (2001) The NSP4 enterotoxin of rotavirus induces paracellular leakage in polarized epithelial cells. *J Virol*, **75**, 1540–1546.

Taraporewala TF, Chen D and Patton JT (1999) Multimers formed by the rotavirus nonstructural protein NSP2 bind to RNA and have nucleoside triphosphatase activity. *J Virol*, **73**, 9934–9943.

Taraporewala TF and Patton JT (2001) Identification and characterization of the helix-destabilizing activity of rotavirus non-structural protein NSP2. *J Virol*, **75**, 4519–4527.

Theise ND, Rotterdam H and Dieterich D (1991) Cytomegalovirus esophagites in AIDS diagnosis by endoscopic biopsy. *Am J Gastroenterol*, **86**, 1123–1126.

Tian P, Estes MK, Hu Y *et al* (1995) The rotavirus nonstructural glycoprotein NSP4 mobilizes Ca^{2+} from the endoplasmic reticulum. *J Virol*, **69**, 5763–5772.

Tian P, Hu Y, Schilling WP *et al.* (1994) The nonstructural glycoprotein of rotavirus affects intracellular calcium levels. *J Virol*, **68**, 251–257.

Townsend TR, Bolyard EA, Yolken RH *et al.* (1982) Outbreak of Coxsackie A1 gastroenteritis: a complication of bone marrow transplantation. *Lancet*, **i**, 820–823.

Tyler KL and Fields BN (1996) Reoviruses. In *Fields Virology*, (eds Fields BN, Knipe DM, Howley PM *et al.*), 3rd edn, pp 1597–1623. Lippincott-Raven, Philadelphia.

Van Regenmortel M, Fauquet CM, Bishop DHL *et al.* (2000) *Virus Taxonomy. Classification and Nomenclature of Viruses.* Seventh Report of the International Committee on Taxonomy of Viruses. Academic Press, San Diego.

Velasquez FR, Matson DO, Calva JJ *et al.* (1996) Rotavirus infection in infants as protection against subsequent infection. *N Engl J Med*, **355**, 1022–1028.

Vende P, Piron M, Castagne N and Poncet D (2000) Efficient translation of rotavirus mRNA requires simultaneous interaction of NSP3 with the eukaryotic translation initiation factor eIF4G and the mRNA 3′ end. *J Virol*, **74**, 7064–7071.

Vinjé J, Deijl H, van der Heide R *et al.* (2000a) Molecular detection and epidemiology of Sapporo-like viruses. *J Clin Microbiol*, **38**, 530–536.

Vinjé J, Green LD, Gallimore CI *et al.* (2000b) Genetic polymorphism across the three open reading frames of Norwalk-like caliciviruses. *Arch Virol*, **145**, 223–243.

Wang AL and Wang CC (1991) Viruses of the protozoa. *Ann Rev Microbiol*, **45**, 251–263.

Waters V, Ford-Jones RL, Petric M *et al.* (2000) Etiology of community-acquired pediatric viral diarrhea: a prospective longitudinal study in hospitals, emergency departments, pediatric practices and child care centres during the winter rotavirus outbreak, 1997–1998. The Pediatric Rotavirus Epidemiology Study for Immunization Study Group. *Pediatr Infect Dis J*, **19**, 843–848.

Whitcup SM, Fortin E, Lindblad AS *et al.* (1999) Discontinuation of anticytomegalovirus therapy in patients with HIV infection and cytomegalovirus retinitis. *J Am Med Assoc*, **282**, 1633–1637.

Willcocks MM, Brown TDK, Madeley CR *et al.* (1994) The complete sequence of a human astrovirus. *J Gen Virol*, **75**, 1785–1788.

Xiao L, Limor J, Bern C and Lal AA (2001) Tracking *Cryptosporidium parvum* by sequence analysis of small double stranded RNA. *Emerg Infect Dis*, **7**, 141–145.

Xu W, McDonough MC and Erdman DD (2000) Species-specific identification of human adenoviruses by a multiplex PCR. *J Clin Microbiol*, **38**, 4114–4120.

Yamashita T, Kobayashi S, Sakae K *et al.* (1991) Isolation of cytopathic small round viruses with BSC-1 cells from patients with gastroenteritis. *J Infect Dis*, **164**, 954–957.

Yamashita T, Sakae K, Ishihara Y *et al.* (1993) Prevalence of newly isolated cytopathic small round virus (*Aichi* strain) in Japan. *J Clin Microbiol*, **31**, 2938–2943.

Yamashita T, Sakae K, Kobayashi S *et al.* (1995) Isolation of cytopathic small round virus (*Aichi* virus) from Pakistani children and Japanese travellers from South-East Asia. *Microbiol Immunology*, **39**, 433–435.

Yamashita T, Sakae K, Tsuzuki H *et al.* (1998) Complete nucleotide sequence and genetic organization of *Aichi* virus, a distinct member of the *Picornaviridae* associated with acute gastroenteritis in humans. *J Virol*, **72**, 8408–8412.

Yeager M, Berriman JA, Baker TS *et al.* (1994) Three-dimensional structure of the rotavirus haemagglutinin VP4 by cryo-electron microscopy and difference map analysis. *EMBO J*, **13**, 1011–1018.

Yeager M, Dryden KA, Olson NH *et al.* (1990) Three-dimensional structure of rhesus rotavirus by cryoelectron microscopy and image reconstruction. *J Cell Biol*, **110**, 2133–2144.

Yu J, Langridge WH (2001) A plant-based multicomponent vaccine protects mice from enteric diseases. *Nature Biotechnol*, **19**, 548–552.

Yuan LZ, Ward LA and Rosen BI (1996) Systemic and intestinal antibody secreting cell responses and correlates of protective immunity to human rotavirus in a gnotobiotic pig model of disease. *J Virol*, **70**, 3075–3083.

Zhang M, Zeng CQY, Morris PA and Estes MK (2000) A functional NSP4 enterotoxin peptide secreted from rotavirus-infected cells. *J Virol*, **74**, 11663–11670.

5

Influenza

Chris W. Potter

University of Sheffield, Sheffield, UK

INTRODUCTION

Although occasionally occurring as sporadic infections, influenza is more commonly and dramatically seen as local outbreaks or widespread epidemics: these occur in most parts of the world, and in some countries in most years. Epidemics can arise at any time but are usually concentrated in months of high relative humidity: they occur explosively, often with little or no warning, and the number of people infected can vary from a few hundred to hundreds of thousands. In addition, history records some nine occasions since AD 1700 when influenza has caused pandemics, and at these times millions were infected. In many cases epidemics are short-lived, lasting days or weeks; however, those occurring in large groupings can continue in successive waves for months. It is the large number of persons infected during an outbreak of influenza, together with our proven inability to prevent or to contain these outbreaks, which has focused so much study and research on this disease.

Influenza is a short-lived but relatively severe respiratory infection in healthy adults, and the large number of patients involved in an epidemic can include a significant number of deaths. Epidemics can be disruptive to industry, with loss of productivity, and to services such as medical, postal, power, police and education; can cause depressed immunity to other infectious diseases; can cause depression and behavioural complications which may continue for months after the acute phase of illness has passed; and infection is life-threatening to the elderly and to patients with predisposing heart, chest or metabolic disease. Epidemics can be traced anecdotally from the fifth century BC, the Hundred Years War and

the court of Mary Tudor, to the more exact records of the last 100 years; nevertheless, knowledge gained during this latter period, including the past 70 years when the virus could be isolated and studied in the laboratory, has done little to prevent epidemics or help treat patients: it is not surprising, therefore, that influenza has been referred to as the 'last plague'.

Such has been the impact of epidemic influenza on communities that it is easy to understand the interest of researchers, physicians, diagnostic laboratories, health authorities and pharmaceutical companies in this infection, and the large investment of both time and money into the study of this disease. Thus, since the first isolation of an influenza virus in ferrets in 1933, research into the nature and control of the disease has led to the setting up of many research laboratories devoted to the study of influenza viruses, and to the commissioning of an international network of communicating laboratories by the World Health Organisation (WHO) to monitor the antigenic changes in the infecting viruses and the incidence and spread of infection. As a result of these activities, a large volume of information is available concerning influenza viruses: whether application of this knowledge can be ordered to diminish the impact of influenza on individuals or to prevent the epidemics and pandemics which will inevitably occur in the future remains to be seen (Kitler *et al.*, 2002). Although many questions concerning influenza and influenza viruses remain unanswered, much of the scientific information necessary to achieve the above aims is available; but an enormous number of resources are necessary for their implementation, and this must be considered in competition with other priorities.

Principles and Practice of Clinical Virology, Fifth Edition. Edited by A. J. Zuckerman, J. E. Banatvala, J. R. Pattison, P. D. Griffiths and B. D. Schoub
© 2004 John Wiley & Sons Ltd   ISBN 0 470 84338 1

THE VIRUSES

Structure

The influenza viruses belong to the genera *Influenza virus A*, *B* and *C* in the family *Orthomyxoviridae*. Studies on the structure of influenza viruses carried out during the past years have brought knowledge of this subject to a point far in advance of that for other viruses, with the possible exception of human immunodeficiency virus. Influenza viruses grown in embryonated eggs and examined in the electron microscope show particles, approximately spherical and with a diameter of 80–120 nm: after serial passage in the laboratory, some strains produce filamentous particles, and pleomorphic forms are not uncommon (Stuart-Harris *et al.*, 1985). The electron microscopic appearance of influenza virus particles is shown in Figure 5.1a, and a diagram showing the components that make up the particles is shown in Figure 5.1b.

The chemical composition of the virus particles has been determined. Each particle is composed of approximately 1% RNA, 70–75% protein, 20–24% lipid and 5–8% carbohydrate. Structurally, the virus consists of a single strand of RNA of negative polarity (Lamb and Krug, 1996) and molecular weight $4–6 \times 10^6$ segmented into eight fragments: the molecular weights of the fragments range from 3×10^5 to 1×10^6. The RNA is closely associated with the nucleoprotein (NP) to form the ribonuclear protein (RNP), a helical structure termed the nucleocapsid; the NP has a molecular weight of approximately 60 kDa, and there are approximately 1000 molecules in each virus particle. The NP is a type-specific antigen, occurs in one of three antigenic forms, and these different forms provide the basis for the classification of influenza viruses into types A, B and C.

Surrounding the nucleocapsid is a second protein referred to as the matrix or membrane protein (M1); this protein is a major protein of the virus particle, contributing 35–45% of the particle mass. The molecular weight of the M1 protein is 23 kDa, and there are approximately 3000 molecules in each virus particle. A second M protein, termed M2 and coded by the same gene segment as the M1 protein, is important in virus replication (see below); there are 14–68 molecules of M2 present in each virus particle. External to the M1 protein the particles have a viral membrane; this is a lipid bilayer which constitutes approximately 20–24% of the virus particle.

Two virus glycoproteins are inserted into the membrane; these are rod-shaped structures radiating out from the virus particles to give the spiky appearance of the surface (Figure 5.1). The first of these glycoproteins is the haemagglutinin (HA), which is composed of two separate molecules, termed HA1 and HA2, joined together by a disulphide bond (Skehel *et al.*, 1984). The complete HA molecule is composed of three of these subunits, each of molecular weight 75–80 kDa and 20% carbohydrate to give a total molecular weight of approximately 225 kDa. There are approximately 1000 HA molecules on each virus particle: each HA particle is 14–16 nm in length and 4 nm in diameter, and is attached to the lipid membrane by a hydrophobic tip. The HA forms 25–30% of the protein of the virus. The function of the HA is the attachment of the virus to receptors on the

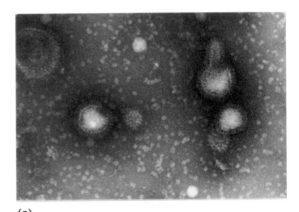

(a)

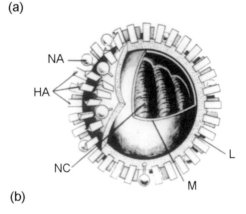

(b)

Figure 5.1 Structure of influenza virus particle: (a) electron microscopic appearance; (b) diagram of structural components. HA, haemagglutinin; L, lipid bilayer in which the HA and NA subunits are inserted; M, matrix protein; NA, neuraminidase; NC, nucleocapsid consisting of nucleoprotein (NP) subunits closely associated with the viral RNA

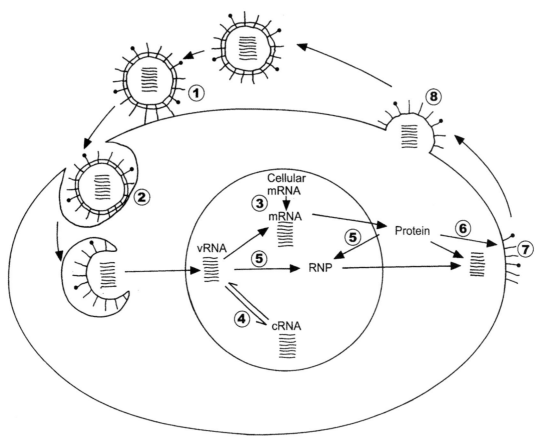

Figure 5.2 Replication of influenza virus. 1, binding of HA to cell receptors; 2, fusion of viral and endosomal membranes; 3, cap snatching; 4, replication; 5, encapsidation of vRNA by NP to form RNP; 6, glycosylation of HA and NA; 7, lipid rafts; 8, budding

surface of host cells during the initial stages of virus infection: the HA also attaches to receptors on erythrocytes causing haemagglutination, a property which forms the basis of *in vitro* tests for virus and virus antibody (see Serology). The subtype classification of influenza viruses is based on the different antigenic forms of the HA molecule.

The second glycoprotein radiating from the surface of the virus particle is the neuraminidase (NA). There are 100–200 NA molecules on the surface of each virus particle: they are 10 nm long and 4 nm in diameter and composed of four identical subunits, each of molecular weight approximately 60 kDa, and an unknown amount of carbohydrate; these structures account for some 7% of the total viral protein. The NA molecules are attached to the viral membrane by a stalk terminated by a hydrophobic tip; the complete structure has a mushroom appearance (Laver *et al.*, 1984) and a total molecular weight of approximately

200–250 kDa. The function of the NA is not fully understood; suggested functions include the removal of sialic acid residues from cell surfaces to promote virus absorption, and the removal of virus receptors on the infected cell surface to mediate in the release of newly formed virus particles (Colman, 1998). The NA does not appear to have a function in virus entry, replication or assembly. Again, the NA glycoprotein is antigenically variable, and these differences are used in the subtype classification of the viruses.

Influenza virus particles also contain an RNA-dependent RNA polymerase complex; this consists of three proteins, termed polymerase basic protein 1 (PB1), polymerase basic protein 2 (PB2) and polymerase acidic protein (PA): the molecular weights vary (range 80–90 kDa) and there are approximately 50 molecules of each species in each virus particle, which are closely associated with the nucleocapsid. These P-proteins have a complex role in virus-specific RNA synthesis during virus replication. Finally, the virus RNA codes for two non-structural proteins, termed NS1 and NS2: NS1 is synthesised early after infection, while NS2, now termed nuclear export protein (NEP), appears late and is found in virus particles (Paragas *et al.*, 2001). The function of these molecules remains an important subject of current research (see below) and mutant viruses with defects in the RNA fragment coding for these proteins are unable to synthesise sufficient viral RNA or M1 proteins.

Most studies on the structure of influenza virus particles have been carried out on influenza A viruses; however, sufficient work has been done with influenza B viruses to suggest general similarity in size, composition and structure. Some differences have been found, but the significance of these to virus natural history and epidemiology is not known. The influenza B viruses differ from influenza A viruses by the presence of an antigenically distinct NP, and this, together with the antigenic specificity of other virus proteins and glycoproteins, characterises a virus type with marked differences in epidemiological behaviour. The size, composition and structure of influenza C viruses are similar to those of influenza A: the main difference is an antigenically distinct NP, and the absence of the NA glycoprotein. These differences again characterise a virus which has epidemiological properties distinct from those of both influenza viruses A and B.

Replication

Most studies on the replication of influenza viruses have been carried out using influenza A strains, but the limited number of studies with influenza B viruses have not indicated major differences in the mechanism of replication of this virus type. When an influenza A virus is inoculated onto cell cultures, there are three possible outcomes. First, the virus may fail to initiate infection, commonly because the cells do not possess the receptors essential for virus absorption. Second, the virus may undergo an incomplete growth cycle, known as abortive infection; this occurs in a variety of cell lines, including HeLa cells, L cells and human diploid fibroblast cells. There is at present no accepted explanation for abortive infection, but because of a block at some stage of the normal replication cycle large numbers of virus particles are produced which are deficient in RNA content and are non-infective. Abortive infection is also seen when excessive amounts of virus are inoculated onto permissive cells, such as the cells of the amniotic membrane of the embryonated

hen's egg, where the effect is described as the Von Magnus phenomenon. Third, infection may be permissive and result in the production of infectious virus; the various stages of replication are shown in Figure 5.2.

Permissive infection by influenza virus occurs in human, baboon and monkey kidney cells and in the cells lining the amniotic and allantoic cavities of the embryonated hen's egg. Infection is initiated by adsorption of the virus to the cell surface. In addition, infection can occur in other cells, provided that trypsin is added to the medium, since cleavage of the HA into HA1 and HA2 is essential for virus replication. Adsorption requires the interaction of two molecules: these are sialic acid-containing receptors on the surface of the cell, and the virus haemagglutinin. Some 28 species of sialic acid receptors, together with sugar chains, are known (Suzuki *et al.*, 2001), and the specificity is important, since avian influenza viruses bind to some receptors while human influenza viruses bind to others; thus, receptor characteristics are important in determining virus-host range (Matrosovich *et al.*, 1997). However, this is not absolute, since pathogenicity is affected by genetic determinants and some viruses can cross species barriers via other receptors (Stray *et al.*, 2000). The binding function of the HA is shown in studies which indicate that specific antibody to the HA prevents virus adsorption. Adsorption provokes receptor-mediated endocytosis of the virus particles via clathrin-coated pits which can be seen by electron microscopy to appear approximately 20 min after infection. This in turn is followed by fusion of the viral envelope to endosomal membranes, a procedure which requires the acidic environment at pH 5.0–6.0 in the endosomes, and the cleavage of the HA into HA1 and HA2. The low pH also frees the M1 protein from RNP, thus allowing the RNA protease complex to migrate to the cell nucleus. The acidic environment within the virus particle that allows this is achieved via the M2 protein in the virus membrane, which acts as a channel to allow H+ ions into the virion, and is brought about by lysosomal proteases and lipase enzyme and mediated by the NP (Wang *et al.*, 1997).

The events of virus replication in the cell nucleus are complex and remain to be fully understood (Lamb and Krug, 1996). Our information to date suggests that transcription of the messenger RNA (mRNA) from all RNA fragments takes place immediately after entry into the cell nucleus. Initially, similar amounts of each mRNA are produced; however, this is followed by a regulatory phase in which the synthesis of mRNA coding for the NP and the NS1 predominate: it is clear that mRNA synthesis is regulated at all stages, and that this regulation is controlled by virus proteins, such as the P proteins, NP and NS1 (Portela *et al.*, 1999). Synthesis of mRNA involves, sequentially, cap recognition and binding, endonuclease activity, initiation and then elongation to produce a functional mRNA. First, the polymerase complex binds to a methylated cap structure present on heterologous, cellular RNA; this cap recognition is a function of PB2 protein. Second, a nucleotide sequence of 10–30 bases is cleaved from the cap structure by endonuclease activity, termed 'cap snatching'. This structure forms the starter molecule for mRNA synthesis: it has been suggested that this cleavage is one of the functions of PB1 or PB2 proteins (Blok *et al.*, 1996). The cap sequence incorporates a G complementary to the penultimate C of the vRNA to complete the initiation step, and this is a function of the PB1 protein. Finally, elongation takes place in the normal manner to produce complete mRNAs; this step requires binding to NP, and elongation is thought to be controlled by the PA protein. Cap snatching from the host RNA requires host RNA synthesis, and virus replication is dependent on this process; for this reason inhibitors such as α-amanitin inhibit influenza virus replication. Finally, it is evident that interactions occur between PB1 and PB2 and PB1 and PA but none has been demonstrated between PB2 and PA to date; the place of these interactions in viral replication remains to be determined. The mRNAs leave the cell nucleus and bind to ribosomes, and translation of viral proteins is initiated; again, we are not fully informed of the details.

The synthesis of cRNA, and subsequently vRNA, occurs after the time of peak production of mRNA and protein synthesis. Full-length vRNAs are produced and exist in approximately equimolar amounts of each throughout infection, and they are all synthesised in the infected cell nucleus. The process clearly requires the RNA polymerase to switch to a replicase mode; however, the process is poorly understood. In addition, the switch requires NP but again the exact function of this in replication remains to be determined. In contrast to the production of mRNA, cRNA is a full-length copy of RNA; it is neither capped nor polyadenylated and does not require a primer.

The time sequence for the appearance of the various viral proteins has been studied extensively: the presence of NP can be detected approximately 2 h after virus infection, and the concentration rises to a maximum at 5–6 h; the NP1 protein appears 5 h after infection, and has been identified in the cytoplasm and, to a lesser extent, the nucleus of infected cells; the HA and NA appear approximately 3 h after infection.

It is apparent that the processes described above interfere with the normal host cell functions; specifically, there is a preferential synthesis of viral components at the expense of host cell components. One of the chief mediators of the above is the NS1 protein, which is one of the most abundantly produced proteins synthesised in infected cells (Liu *et al.*, 1997). The NS1 protein inhibits the processing of cellular RNA by a number of mechanisms: the result of this is the cessation of cellular gene expression, and in particular their nuclear export. An important consequence of this activity of NS1 is to antagonise interferon production and thus interfere with the cellular response to virus infection (Garcia-Sastre, 2001): indeed, this may be the most important role of NS1, since it is not essential for viral replication, as seen in studies in which NS1 mutants replicate in interferon-negative cells.

Assembly of new virions within infected cells begins with the binding of NP to newly synthesised vRNAs to form RNP (Elton *et al.*, 1999). RNPs exit the nucleus in association with M1 and NEP proteins, and at the cell membrane they are enclosed by an envelope which contains HA, NA and M2 proteins; it is proposed that the M1 protein is the major driving force in this process (Gomez-Puertas *et al.*, 2000). Virus escapes by budding from lipid rafts in the plasma membrane: the process of virus release is detectable 5–6 h after infection, and is maximal 7–8 h after infection. The mechanism for viral release from the host cell is not completely understood, but an important element in this process is believed to be the NA, which prevents limitation of virus release through aggregation by the removal of sialic acid residues from the viral envelope and at the cell membrane.

VIRAL VARIATION

Historical Aspects

The explosive nature of epidemic influenza, together with a large number of patients involved and the specific clinical features of this disease, has given credibility to records of this infection from the beginning of the eighteenth century: improved and more precise data, and the laboratory isolation and study of influenza viruses since 1933 have given accurate records for the past 100 years. The incidence of outbreaks and the numbers of patients involved have not decreased during this period. History records frequent, almost annual, epidemics of influenza in some countries in most years; these are associated with

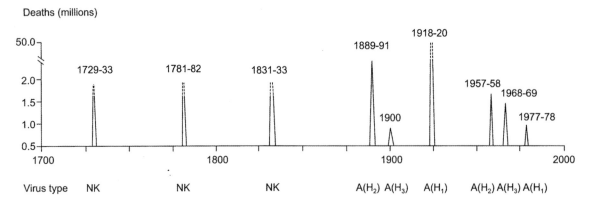

Figure 5.3 Incidence and extent of influenza pandemics since AD 1700. Gives years of pandemics, estimated number of influenza deaths in each pandemic and haemagglutinin type (HA1, HA2 or HA3) of causal virus. NK not known

attack rates of 5–30% of the population, a significant increase in rates of hospitalisation and deaths, predominantly among the elderly and the very young, and the disruption of services and social life (Potter, 2001). In addition to the above, history records nine pandemics since 1700, which began at a focal point and spread rapidly through the world to infect hundreds of millions of individuals; these are shown in Figure 5.3. Accurate documentation of pandemics is first seen in the pandemic which spread from Russia, into Europe and the USA in the years 1889–1892: infection presented as an upper respiratory tract infection of sudden onset and short duration; the total number of cases was high; and deaths were most numerous amongst infants and the elderly, but were recorded in a relatively small percentage of approximately 0.05% of the 25–30% of the world population infected. The pandemic of 1918–1920 originated in China or the USA, and is known as the Spanish influenza. This pandemic spread worldwide for some 6–8 months, and then gave rise to an infection of unusual virulence which commonly caused a severe and new form of pneumonia; some 40–50 million deaths occurred, principally among young adults (Potter, 1998). The effects of the pandemic caused international panic. The number of deaths recorded is probably only a fraction of the true number: many countries did not record figures; India was said to have lost a generation, and 1.5 million deaths occurred in sub-Saharan Africa. The propaganda surrounding the World War of 1914–1918 undermined the accuracy of data from Europe; and the Bolshevik revolution in Russia resulted in ignorance of the effects of the pandemic in that country (Crosby, 1976).

The definition of a pandemic of influenza is an outbreak of infection arising in a specific geographical region, spreading worldwide and infecting a high percentage of people, and caused by a strain of influenza virus which could not have arisen by mutation from strains previously circulating. Thus, the influenza outbreaks of 1932–1933 and 1947–1948 were caused by viruses related to each other and to the virus that caused the pandemic of 1918–1920; by the above definition, the widespread outbreaks of 1932 and 1947 were not pandemics. However, a pandemic did occur in 1957, which originated in China, spread through the world, infecting 40–50% of people and causing over 1 million deaths, mainly in the elderly population; however, fatalities among younger victims were more conspicuous in the early months of the pandemic than later, and this is noted in other pandemics (Simonsen et al., 1998). Pandemic infection occurred again in 1968 and the event was similar to that of 1957 (Figure 5.3). Pandemic infection broke out in 1976 and was due to an influenza virus very closely related to a virus strain which disappeared in 1947. This pandemic was therefore limited to the young, since many persons born before 1947 had seen this virus previously and had retained immunity to infection. Prior to 1976 the appearance of a new pandemic virus had been accompanied by the disappearance of the virus subtype previously causing infections in man; however, from 1976 the old and new subtypes co-circulated, and this behaviour continues to this day (2004).

No discernible pattern for pandemics can be seen in the times between pandemics that would allow prediction of future pandemics; however, the largest gap between pandemics over the last 150 years is 40 years, which suggests that the next pandemic will occur before the year 2017. In conclusion, the historical record of influenza indicates almost annual occurrences of epidemics punctuated at intervals of 10–40 years by pandemics: nothing has been introduced over the last 100 years to suggest that this situation will not continue into the future (Potter, 2001).

Antigenic Shift

Since 1933, the viruses which cause the two types of outbreak, pandemic and epidemic, have been isolated and compared in the laboratory. Viruses isolated from patients infected in the years 1933–1946 and 1947–1956 show wide variations, and cross-haemagglutination inhibition (HI) tests using antiserum from virus-infected ferrets show no serological cross-reactivity (Table 5.1); however, sequence data indicate that the two groups of virus, represented by A/PR/8/34 and A/FM/1/47, are related and are included in the subtype H1. In addition, RNA sequences recovered and amplified by the polymerase chain reaction (PCR) from post mortem lung tissue from two US soldiers who died in September 1918, and a third sample from an Alaskan Inuit woman who had been interred in permafrost since her death from influenza in November 1918, indicated that the 1918–1920 pandemic was also caused by an influenza A (H1) virus (Taubenberger et al., 1997). In contrast, the pandemic subtypes which emerged to cause the pandemics of 1957 and 1968 are unrelated to each other and to the H1N1 subtype, and could not have arisen by mutation from the preceding subtypes. This absolute specificity for the HA of the different subtypes indicates that in the years when pandemic infections are recorded, new influenza virus subtypes have emerged in a population that has no immunity; this is known as antigenic shift. Since it is principally antibody to the virus HA which is

equated with immunity (see later), infection by influenza viruses in the previous years does not induce HI antibody to the newly emerged virus strain. The historical pattern for pandemic influenza is for a new virus subtype to emerge and spread rapidly, causing explosive outbreaks in many countries. As a result of infection, immunity to the new subtype is built up over a period of years, and further outbreaks are more limited. However, after 10–40 years, a new virus subtype emerges with an HA which does not cross-react with antibody to the HA of the previous virus subtype, and to which the population is therefore largely susceptible, to initiate a new cycle of influenza pandemic and epidemics. These sudden changes in antigenicity can also occur in the virus NA molecule.

Although the HA antigens of influenza A virus subtypes show no cross-reactivity in HI tests (Table 5.1), some expressions of relatedness are seen in the phenomenon known as 'original antigenic sin', first reported by Francis et al. (1953). This term describes the observation that infection by influenza virus induces antibody to the infecting virus and recalls antibody to the other virus subtypes that the individual has experienced previously; indeed, the titre of antibody to the earlier infecting subtypes can be several-fold greater than that to the current infecting virus. This is probably due to stimulation of B memory cells, which persist after infection, being stimulated by new virus serotype, and suggests a relatedness in the HA antigens of different virus serotypes not detected in HI and other serological tests.

The importance of antigenic shift in producing new antigenic subtypes which spread to cause pandemic infection is evident; but despite some 100 years of intensive research, the origin of these new viruses is uncertain. The problem has been of great interest to a large number of virologists; and experiments, epidemological studies and imagination have produced a number of theories. For example, new virus subtypes

Table 5.1 Antigenic shift in the haemagglutinin of influenza A viruses

Virus subtype	Virus strain	Serum HI antibody titre to influenza virus[a]			
		A/PR/8/34	A/FM/1/47	A/Sing/1/57	A/HK/1/68
H1N1	A/South Carolina/1/18	NK	NK	NK	NK
	A/PR/8/34	1280	<10	<10	<10
	A/FM/1/47	<10	640	<10	<10
H2N2	A/Sing/1/57	<10	<10	1280	<10
H3N2	A/HK/1/68	<10	<10	<10	1280

NK = not known.
[a]Influenza A viruses grown in eggs were tested in HI tests with antisera from ferrets infected intranasally with live virus and bled 3–4 weeks later. The serum HI antibody titre against 8 HA units of virus is listed.

may arise by spontaneous mutation or be introduced from cosmic sources: although both these views are present in the literature, only a minority of scientists consider them valid explanations, and convincing evidence to support either of these theories is lacking. Thus, random mutations would be expected to produce intermediary strains and such strains have not been identified; detailed analysis has shown that new virus subtypes have multiple sequence differences, and it is difficult to imagine these all occurring simultaneously. The most widely-held theory for the origin of new influenza viruses is that new virus subtypes are reassortant viruses resulting from double infection of a single cell. The appearance of a new influenza virus subtype is paralleled usually by the disappearance of the old subtype, with the one exception of 1976, and it would therefore seem unlikely that the dual infection was by two subtypes of human influenza viruses. However, influenza A viruses infect other species, including horses and particularly birds: dual infection with the human and animal or bird viruses in a species which could support the replication of both could result in the production of a reassortant virus with a surface antigen(s) from the non-human virus and infectivity from the human virus. This theory is scientifically tenable: reassortant viruses can be produced in the laboratory from human and animal parents; reassortants can be identified following mixed infection of animals or birds; influenza viruses can cross species barriers; and antigenic analysis of two human virus subtypes has revealed similarities between HA in these viruses and known avian viruses. In contrast, although animals have been infected with human influenza viruses following human infection, no epidemiological evidence has been found to suggest that the HA of an animal or avian influenza virus has subsequently occurred in a novel human influenza subtype which then caused pandemic infection. Influenza B viruses do not occur in animals and do not exhibit antigenic shift: this has been put forward as indirect evidence for reassortment as the mechanism for the emergence of new influenza A virus subtypes. It has been suggested that reassortment of the whole HA molecule from an avian influenza virus into the new pandemic strain is not essential, and that only some of the sequences from the avian virus may be necessary to produce an HA of radically different antigenic form.

Finally, it has been suggested that there are a limited number of influenza virus subtypes which are recycled in the human population. Evidence for this theory comes from seroepidemiological studies of antibody to influenza viruses in sera taken at different times from subjects of different ages. By this means, antibody can be detected over a period of 100 years, since the presence of antibody to a particular virus subtype in persons of known age can indicate dates when the viruses circulated in the population, even before virus isolation was possible. Analysis of the results indicate when pandemics occurred and which virus serotype was responsible. Thus, the pandemics beginning in the years 1889, 1900, 1918, 1957, 1968 and 1976 are shown to be due to influenza A virus subtypes H2, H3, H1, H2, H3 and H1, respectively (Figure 5.3). Thus, of the 15 HA types identified in nature, only influenza viruses A (H1, H2 and H3) have caused pandemics; and over the observation period, they have occurred sequentially. From these observations it has been suggested that only these subtypes can cause pandemics and that these three exist cryptically in nature, and can emerge when the antibody state of the population has fallen to levels which allow pandemics to occur. A cycle of approximately 70 years involving the three subtypes mentioned above would satisfy this requirement. The evidence supporting this theory remains fragile. Although serological studies have detected the presence of antibody to influenza virus A (H3), which was first seen in 1968, in serum from aged persons collected before the pandemic, no reservoir for the virus in humans or animals before this date has been found. Again, it can be argued that no reservoir is necessary to support this theory: reassortants may be appearing all the time and only when a reassortant emerges which is capable of spreading rapidly in human populations, and when the immune status of the population has waned by the death of the older generations, can pandemic infection occur due to a virus similar to that which has occurred in years past. It is clear from the above that the origin of new virus serotypes is not proven; but the advances made in recent years in influenza surveillance, diagnosis and antigen analysis will be applied to the virus which causes the next pandemic, and this may prove the mechanism for antigenic shift.

More recent concern for the next pandemic has been demonstrated by the outbreak of influenza A (H5N1) virus infection in chickens in South China and later in Hong Kong, which caused extensive mortality (March 1997): from these infections, known as the Hong Kong Incident, 17 cases occurred in humans, five of which were fatal (de Jong et al., 1997). Following these events the Hong Kong authorities barred further importation and slaughtered 1.7 million chickens (December 1997); since this time no further human cases have been reported. The episode has underlined a number of points. First, avian viruses have little infectivity for humans (see above), and in spite of massive exposure only a small number of human cases occurred: in the

Table 5.2 Antigenic drift in the haemagglutinin of influenza A (H3N2)

Virus subtype	Virus strain	Serum HI antibody titre to influenza virus[a]				
		A/HK/1/68	A/Eng/42/72	A/PC/1/73	A/Vic/3/75	A/Bang/79
H3N2	A/Hong Kong/1/68	1280	320	40	40	<10
	A/England/42/72	240	2560	80	120	40
	A/Port Chalmers/1/73	40	120	5120	320	160
	A/Victoria/3/75	<10	40	640	1280	160
	A/Bangkok/1/79	<10	<10	80	160	640

[a]See footnote to Table 5.1.

same time period in 1968, influenza virus A (H3) virus emerged to cause half a million cases of influenza. Second, the episode evoked a rapid and intense response by virologists and others and the strategy of slaughtering vast numbers of chickens emphasised the international concern of pandemic influenza, based on the history of the massive epidemics and great mortality in the past, and the will to take rapid and dramatic action in the face of a possible pandemic. Third, although the avian virus A(H5) had little infectivity for humans, recombination of this strain with the human influenza A virus could have produced a recombinant and the start of a pandemic. Finally, influenza A (H5 and H9) viruses still persist in parts of China and have been responsible for some human infection. This is receiving very close monitoring at present, since it may provide the seeds for a new pandemic virus in the future.

Antigenic Drift

In addition to the large pandemics of influenza virus infections seen every 10–40 years due to the occurrence of new influenza virus subtypes showing antigenic shift, there are also epidemics of a smaller nature occurring in the intervening years. When the viruses from the various epidemics between pandemics are compared in cross-haemagglutination tests, they exhibit strain differences. Thus, although all the viruses belong to the same subtype they do not cross-react completely; these changes are termed antigenic drift. Table 5.2 shows the HA variants found in some influenza viruses isolated in 1968–1979; all belong to the same subtype but were associated with the epidemics of 1968, 1972, 1973, 1975 and 1979. The virus of 1968 (A/HK/1/68) reacts most strongly with homologous antiserum, and cross-reactions are seen with other viruses in the series; the degree of cross-reactivity decreases as the time difference increases. The same is true for the other virus strains in the series;

and similar drift can be seen in the strains isolated from 1979 to the present day (not shown). The practical effects of antigenic drift are that infection by one strain may induce some cross-reacting antibody and partial immunity to infection by other viruses of the same subtype, and the degree of cross-immunity is directly related to the degree of cross-reactivity. In this way viruses may alter from year to year, giving rise to the new strains that cause fresh epidemics.

A theory for the mechanism of antigenic drift is generally agreed amongst scientific workers. This theory proposes that virus variants occurring naturally by mutation are selected by antibody pressure in an immune or partially immune population; since these new viruses are not neutralised completely by antibody to pre-existing virus strains, they are capable of causing new epidemics. Selection based on the relatively small changes in the antigenicity of the virus HA that characterises antigenic drift can be achieved in the laboratory and in animal models; thus, virus strains with antigenic changes detected by serological and biochemical techniques can be recovered by growth in low concentrations of antibody. Antigenic drift also occurs in the NA antigen. Epidemics due to new virus strains exhibiting antigenic drift are not as great as those showing antigenic shift, since partial immunity is present in persons with cross-reacting antibody due to previous infection. Finally, antigenic drift has been shown for influenza A subtypes H1, H2 and H3, and also for influenza B, and probably accounts for all the interpandemic outbreaks seen in the past.

VIRUS CLASSIFICATION

The influenza viruses are classified into types A, B and C, principally on the basis of possessing distinct NP antigens. Influenza A viruses affect humans, pigs, birds, horses and other species; however, only humans are infected by influenza types B and C. The antigenic differences of the HA and NA antigens of influenza A viruses provide the basis of their classification into subtypes. This classification is of practical importance, since cross-immunity between viruses of different subtypes does not occur, and the antigenic differences are critical for the understanding of virus epidemiology and for vaccine production. Many schemata for the classification of influenza viruses have been proposed in the past, but at the present time the agreed classification is shown in Table 5.3. Previously, the results of serological studies suggested that the HA of the influenza virus strain which affects swine, termed H_{SW}, is similar to that which caused the pandemic of 1918–1920, and this has been confirmed by comparisons of the sequence data from the two viruses. Strains occurring in the years 1933–1948 were classified as subtype HO; and those occurring in 1947–1957 were termed H1. Recent studies have shown that the HA of all these viruses are related, and the classification shown in Table 5.3 groups these viruses into a single subtype, termed H1. The H2 subtypes caused infections in humans in 1957–1968, and the H3 from 1968 to the present time (2004); the H1 serotype reappeared in 1976 and has also caused infection since that time. The HA of human subtype H3 cross-reacts with the HA of equine influenza virus Heq2 and avian influenza virus Hav7, and these three are now grouped together into a single subtype, H3. Further subtype classification is dependent on evidence of cross-reactivity between the various viruses, and the classification shown in Table 5.3 gives the new and old designations. To date, a total of 15 distinct HAs have been recognised among the human influenza A viruses: the

most recently recognised subtypes are H14, identified in 1990 in a virus infecting wild ducks in Russia, and H15, identified in viruses affecting birds in Australia and reported in 1996. In spite of intensive investigation, no further subtypes have been recognised in any of the many species tested.

Antigenic differences also occur in the NA antigen of the influenza A viruses. The antigenic form designated N1 is found in all human influenza A viruses isolated prior to 1957, and the form N2 has been found in all human isolates recovered since that time; a recurrence of infection by strains having the N1 neuraminidase occurred in 1976, and these strains have been regularly recovered from patients since that date. The other antigenic variants of the NA occur in viruses isolated from birds and horses (Table 5.3).

Using the above classification it is possible to describe any influenza virus in terms of its subtype specification. Every influenza virus is referred to as A or B, followed consecutively by the place of isolation, the laboratory number and the year of isolation: following this designation, the subtype designation is given in parentheses. Thus, influenza virus A/Hong Kong/1/68 (H3N2) signifies an influenza A virus isolated from a patient in Hong Kong in 1968, and of subtype H3N2. Within any subtype as described above, a number of strains can occur as a result of antigenic drift, and these are important in epidemiology and in vaccine design, since antibody against one strain does not completely neutralise viruses of other strains: thus, minor variations need to be identified and, where necessary, alterations to vaccine composition made according to these observations. Viruses of different subtype strains can be distinguished by a variety of tests, including HI tests using homologous and heterologous sera, reactions with monoclonal antibody rather than polyclonal convalescent sera from infected ferrets, and sequence studies on the RNA coding for viral HA and NA. In this way, large numbers of differing strains are identified within any one influenza A subtype, and tracking the antigenic drift which gives rise to these is of crucial importance in influenza research. However, these studies of strain differences are not a routine procedure; they remain an important function of influenza virus research centres collaborating closely with the WHO.

PATHOGENESIS

Influenza has been described as an unchanging disease caused by a constantly changing virus; however, history suggests that clinical disease does vary in

Table 5.3 Nomenclature of influenza A viruses

Haemagglutinin		Neuraminidase	
Subtype	(Previous designation)	Subtype	(Previous designation)
H1	(HO, H1, H_{Sw})	N1	(N1)
H2	(H2)	N2	(N2)
H3	(H3, Heq2, Hav7)	N3	(Nav2, Nav3)
H4	(Hav4)	N4	(Nav4)
H5	(Hav5)	N5	(Nav5)
H6	(Hav6)	N6	(Nav6)
H7	(Heq1, Hav1)	N7	(Neq1)
H8	(Hav8)	N8	(Neq2)
H9	(Hav9)	N9	(Nav6)
H10	(Hav2)		
H11	(Hav3)		
H12	(Hav10)		
H13	(–)		
H14	(–)		
H15	(–)		

severity at times, particularly in 1918 and again in 1997 during the Hong Kong Incident, and in an outbreak in Liverpool in 1951. Studies of the influenza viruses which affect birds and man suggest that pathogenicity is related to: the cleavability of the HA into HA1 and HA2; interactions between the HA and NA molecules, evident from studies of strains resistant to neuraminidase inhibitors; the independent structure of the NA; the role of the PB2 protein; and the host interferon response. These various factors could act singularly or in combinations, and the strategy for virus virulence may not have a single explanation. Although an area of intense research, no explanation(s) for the differing virulence among human influenza viruses has emerged to date (reviewed by Zambon, 2001), and the reason for the extreme virulence of the 1918 pandemic virus remains unknown.

There is no agreed explanation for the pathogenesis of human influenza, and reasons for some features of disease are not known. However, histological and virological investigations by a number of workers have broadly delineated the effects of virus infection. Infection is the result of inhaling respiratory droplets from infected persons; these droplets containing virus are deposited on the mucous blanket lining the respiratory tract. Much virus is destroyed by non-specific immune barriers, such as mucous binding, which is functional at this site or inactivated by natural inhibitors containing sialic acid present in serum or mucosal fluids, which can bind to virus haemagglutinins and competetively inhibit virus binding to cells (Matrosovich and Klenk, 2002); however, some virus escapes these inhibitors and is released from mucus by the action of virus neuraminidase and attaches by the virus HA to receptors on the cells of the respiratory epithelium: epithelial cells of both the upper and lower respiratory airways are rich in these receptors. The receptors are rich in sialic acid, and it is specifically the human receptors on these cells of the respiratory epithelium that human influenza viruses attach to (see above). Following viral attachment, replication proceeds: virus can be isolated following acute infection from 1–7 days, with peak titres usually occurring at 48–72 h after the onset of symptoms. Histological studies on nasal exudate cells and tracheal biopsies have indicated that the major site of virus infection is the ciliated columnar epithelial cells. Following infection these cells become progressively rounded and swollen, and the nucleus appears shrunken and pyknotic; the cytoplasm becomes vacuolated, the nucleus degenerates and ciliation is lost. Immunofluorescence studies have shown these cells to contain much virus-specific protein.

The progression of changes in the cells of the respiratory epithelium suggests that they begin in the tracheal bronchial epithelium and then ascend. Thus, early lesions in the tracheobronchial mucosa have been described in uncomplicated influenza, as evidenced by clinical bronchitis and tracheitis; the tissues show increased permeability of vascular capillary walls, oedema, polymorphonuclear infiltration and phagocytosis of degenerate epithelial cells. The basement membrane is not affected.

Because of the generalised symptoms present in uncomplicated influenza, viraemic spread from the respiratory tract has been suggested and virus can replicate in other cells, such as macrophages. Influenza has been associated with ECG and EEG changes; some unconfirmed reports of virus antigen in brain and heart have been recorded; and influenza has been temporally associated with cases of virus encephalitis, particularly among children. However, demonstration of viraemia has not been conclusive; blood samples from children infected with influenza were not found to contain virus when tested by the very sensitive PCR technique (Mori et al., 1997). In addition, the failure to prove viraemia at least in some cases leaves unexplained the myalgia and degree of prostration which are commonly seen in influenza, and the sudden and the marked temperature rise which occurs following infection. The virus has been shown to have strong pyrogenic properties when inoculated intravenously into animals, but the quantities of virus needed to demonstrate this effect are unnaturally high. It has been postulated that the mononuclear cell infiltration of infected tissue which occurs during infection may result in the release of pyrogens, and that infection results in the induction of cytokines which may be relevant to the systemic symptoms, but these hypotheses remain unproven.

CLINICAL FEATURES

Uncomplicated Infection

Influenza has been described as an unchanging disease due to a changing virus, and this description underlines the relative constancy of the clinical presentation of the infection. Detailed analysis of the symptoms seen in the groups of patients studied in the years 1937–1941, 1947 and 1957 indicate some differences in the relative incidence of some symptoms; however, these are probably due to the variable opinions of different observers. Although the clinical presentation of uncomplicated influenza in any one age group is generally agreed, variations in the incidence of certain symptoms does occur for different ages; thus, croup is more a feature of infection in young children; sore throats are seen more commonly in adults; vomiting and convulsions are rarely seen except in infants; and myalgia is more common in adults.

Following droplet infection from infected individuals, the incubation period is 48 h, but may vary from 24 to 96 h; the variation is probably dependent on the size of the infecting dose. The onset of the illness is usually abrupt, and many patients can pinpoint the hour of onset. The symptoms in adults commonly include a marked fever, headache, photophobia, shivering, a dry cough, malaise, aching of muscles and a dry tickling throat which can lead to the voice becoming husky and even lost. The fever is usually continuous and classically lasts 3 days, at which point the temperature falls and the symptoms abate; in a percentage of cases, a second spike may occur after this time which is smaller than the first but gives the common biphasic fever curve. Of the acute symptoms listed, the cough may persist for several days; the eyes are often watery, burning and painful in movement; the nose can be blocked or may have a purulent discharge; cervical adenopathy is unusual but has been described; and myalgia is most severe in the leg muscles, but also may involve the extremities. Although the infection usually resolves within 7 days, patients commonly complain of feeling listless and unwell for weeks after acute infection, and depression is a common residual complaint.

Studies of the clinical illness resulting from infection by influenza B virus show close similarity to those caused by influenza A virus. Thus, infection is commonly a 3 day illness with predominant systemic symptoms. Some authors have suggested that influenza B infections are milder than those caused by influenza A, with less myalgia and a higher incidence of nasal symptoms, and differences have been reported for the incidence of sweating and other symptoms; however, these differences are small. In contrast, influenza C infection is usually a relatively mild respiratory infection of young children and a mild upper respiratory tract infection of adults, which is rarely diagnosed.

Tracheobronchitis and Bronchitis

All series of patients studied have included a small proportion in whom the respiratory symptoms were more severe. These patients have a productive cough, chest tightness and substernal soreness. Rales and rhonchi are commonly heard but the lungs are radiologically clear. These symptoms are most commonly seen in patients with chronic obstructive bronchitis and in older persons, and it is evident that age and chronic pulmonary disease predispose to bronchitis, which can result in death from influenza in some patients.

Pneumonia

Pneumonia in patients with influenza virus infection can be a primary viral pneumonia or secondary bacterial infection. In viral pneumonia, patients develop persistent fever with leukocytosis, dyspnoea, hypoxia and cyanosis following the acute symptoms described above. Sputum specimens will show no clear bacteriological cause, and a proportion of these patients will die of diffuse haemorrhagic pneumonia as a direct result of infection. Autopsies show congested, dark red lungs, and the mucosa of the trachea and bronchi will be hyperaemic; microscopic examination of lung sections has consistently revealed tracheitis and bronchiolitis with haemorrhage, hyperaemia, a small cellular infiltrate and loss of ciliated epithelium. An alveolar exudate containing both neutrophils and mononuclear cells in haemorrhage is common. Influenza viral pneumonia is relatively uncommon, but cases have been demonstrated in many influenza epidemics: pneumonia can occur in previously young and healthy persons, but it is more commonly associated with patients with pre-existing cardiovascular disease, such as rheumatic heart disease. The pathology of the viral pneumonia which killed many relatively young and previously healthy people during 1918–1920 was unique to that epidemic, and contained pathological features not described before or since (Crosby, 1976). Thus, following the acute symptoms of influenza described above, some patients showed increasing tracheobronchitis and bronchiolitis, shortage of breath, and the appearance of mahogany spots around the mouth which would extend and coalesce into a violaceous cyanosis until 'a white man could not be distinguished from a coloured'. With increasing cyanosis, blood-stained fluid would froth from the mouth and death would follow from suffocation. The time from onset of infection to death varied from a few hours to 2–3 days. Post mortem examination would not show the signs of secondary bacterial pneumonia: rather, the lungs contained up to a litre of blood-stained, frothy and fibrin-free fluid; petechial and confluent haemorrhages were seen in the lining of the trachea and bronchi; and the lung tissue exhibited intense inflammatory changes with marked adenopathy.

The pneumonia following influenza virus infection can be a secondary bacterial pneumonia; this is more common than primary viral pneumonia, and usually occurs late in the course of the disease. It usually ensues after a period of improvement from the acute symptoms of infection. The symptoms and signs are those of a typical bacterial pneumonia and of the organisms involved. *Staphyloccocus aureus* is the most common, but *Streptococcus pneumoniae*, *Haemophilus influenzae* and other bacteria may also be found. The association of *S. aureus* with secondary bacterial pneumonia following influenza is much more common than might be anticipated, and there appears to be a good reason for this: infection of cells by influenza A virus requires cleavage of the virus HA by proteases, and some strains of *S. aureus* produce such enzymes; thus, in secondary bacterial pneumonia *S. aureus* and influenza viruses may each promote infection by the other (Tashiro *et al.*, 1987). The incidence of secondary bacterial pneumonia is most common in the elderly and those with underlying disease, such as congestive heart failure and chronic bronchitis; in addition, patients with diabetes mellitus, renal disease, alcoholism and those who are pregnant may also have increased susceptibility to secondary bacterial infection.

Myositis and Myoglobinuria

In addition to myalgia, which is a characteristic feature of acute influenza infection, clinical myositis and myoglobinuria can occur. Symptoms usually develop soon after the subsidence of the acute upper respiratory tract symptoms: the muscles are painful and tender to touch, but neurological symptoms are not evident. Laboratory studies have shown changes in serum transaminases and creatinine phosphokinase levels in many of these patients, and histological examination of muscle biopsies has revealed necrosis of the muscle fibres and a mononuclear cell infiltration.

Reye's Syndrome

A syndrome characterised by encephalopathy and fatty liver degeneration was originally described in 1929, and more fully characterised by Reye *et al.* (1963). Later observers noted an association of recent viral infection with this syndrome, now termed Reye's syndrome, and the aetiology of the condition has been intensely researched. Originally thought to be a rare condition, it is now recognised as more common; cases have been reported from many countries, and analyses of series of patients have been published in the UK and USA (Corey *et al.*, 1976). Typically, a previously normal child has a virus-type prodromal illness followed in a few days by vomiting, altered consciousness and occasionally, convulsions; the liver may be enlarged, and there is evidence of hepatic dysfunction, with raised transaminases and blood ammonia levels. 40–50% of patients admitted to hospital for Reye's syndrome die. At autopsy an enlarged, pale and fatty liver is usually seen, and histological examination shows diffuse panlobar microvesicular fatty infiltration. The brain shows evidence of encephalitis with cerebral oedema.

The association of Reye's syndrome with a preceding viral infection was noted in early studies of this disease. An association with prior infection with influenza B virus was first reported; however, subsequent studies associated Reye's syndrome with prior infections of other viruses, including influenza A virus, varicella zoster virus, herpes simplex virus, coxsackie virus B5, echovirus, adenoviruses and cytomegalovirus. The incidence of Reye's syndrome by age and the nature of preceding infection is seen in the results of a series of 367 cases studied in the USA between 1973 and 1974 (see Figure 5.4). The modal age was 11–14 years; although a significant number of cases occurred in younger children, the syndrome was rarely seen in patients aged 18 years or older. A prior respiratory tract infection was recorded for the majority of patients; in some patients this was identified as influenza B infection, seen mainly in children aged 11–15 years, while varicella was identified in other cases, mainly in children aged 3–8 years (Figure 5.4b). Outbreaks of Reye's syndrome have been recorded in conjunction with influenza A and influenza B epidemics, and the clustering of cases in the winter months is illustrated in Figure 5.4a. Finally, the mortality rate for the series illustrated in Figure 5.4 was 41%.

An experimental disease similar to Reye's syndrome can be induced in mice by intravenous inoculation with influenza B virus; and other studies have suggested that acute viral infection in conjunction with co-factors may be responsible for initiating the pathology of the disease. In particular, the use of high concentrations of aspirin in conjunction with acute virus infection has been suggested as a possible precondition for the development of Reye's syndrome. There is epidemiological data to support this association and Reye's

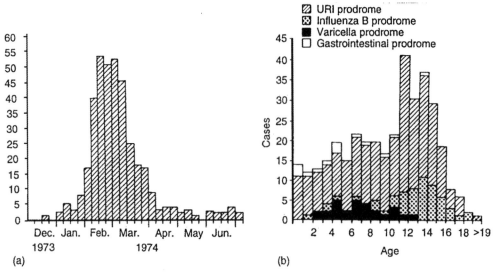

Figure 5.4   Seasonal occurrence (a) and age and associated infection (b) in 367 cases of Reye's syndrome. URI, upper respiratory infection. Data from Corey *et al.* (1976)

syndrome is now rare, following widespread advice to give paracetamol, not aspirin, to febrile children.

Otitis Media

Although considered by many to be a bacterial infection, or a bacterial infection secondary to viral disease, it has been increasingly recognised that otitis media could be the result of influenza infection. Diagnosis of this in young children is associated with influenza epidemics, and in many cases bacterial causes of infection cannot be demonstrated. Association of influenza with otitis media is now sufficiently recognised epidemiologically, but there is a need for detailed virological examination of patients presenting with otitis media, particularly in the age group 0–4 years (Fleming, 2000); this has not been published at the time of writing (2004).

Congenital Malformations

The literature contains a number of reports of an increased incidence of congenital malformations (Conover and Roessmann, 1990) and neural tube defects (Lynberg *et al.*, 1994) following influenza virus infection during pregnancy. In contrast, transplacental passage of the virus has not been demonstrated

satisfactorily (Irvine *et al.*, 2000), and prospective studies of congenital abnormalities following epidemics of influenza have failed to establish a relationship between influenza virus infection and these abnormalities. Follow-up studies of influenza during pregnancy have indicated increased severity of influenza among pregnant women, but no evidence of increased medical problems among the offspring. No conclusions are justified from our present knowledge: the recommendation for immunisation of pregnant women in the USA is a recognition of the severity of this infection in this group, in which, during the pandemics of 1898 and 1918, the death rate was considerable; and for the fetus a precaution of what might happen, rather than one based on evidence for what has been demonstrated.

Other Complications

Although influenza in healthy adults is normally severe but of short duration, resolving in 3–5 days, complications can occur, particularly in elderly patients and in those with predisposing conditions, as outlined above. In addition, virus infection can result in a number of other less well-understood complications. Influenza can cause ketoacidosis in diabetic patients, even in relatively mild cases of infection. Infection has been implicated in acute viral encephalitis and in Guillain–Barré syndrome, and deaths have been reported in both these groups. Histological examination of brain tissue has shown no gross abnormalities but small changes consistent with virus encephalitis have been shown, and virus has been isolated at autopsy from the lungs of fatal cases of encephalitis. The pathogenesis of the neurological complication is unknown, since virus recovery from the brain has been infrequently documented.

Epidemiological studies have associated some sub-types of influenza A with sudden unexplained death and sudden infant death syndrome, sometimes called 'cot death syndrome' (Zink *et al.*, 1987). Firm data associating acute influenza infection with sudden infant death syndrome have been sought by many workers in the past, but have been difficult to obtain; and the association is made on circumstantial evidence and remains speculative. Influenza virus infection, and the association of this infection with secondary *S. aureus* infection (see above), can result in toxic shock syndrome; this complication of influenza infection has been reported by a number of observers. Finally, reports of the association of maternal influenza with schizophrenia and Parkinson's disease in the offspring are in the literature, but the evidence of association is both fragile and contradictory. Thus, the earlier, retrospective studies of small groups of patients infected during influenza epidemics suggest an increased risk of schizophrenia where infection took place in the second trimester of pregnancy (O'Callaghan, 1991); however, other similar studies have failed to confirm these results. A review of these studies, while offering some support for an association, has pointed out methodological difficulties, particularly in the earlier studies, which relied on small numbers of patients asked to recall events of 20 or more years past and questionable evidence for past influenza infection (Bradbury and Miller, 2000). Three larger studies published in 1999 found no evidence of an association between influenza virus infection in pregnancy and later schizophrenia in the offspring: these results would appear to end the debate, but research continues.

DIAGNOSIS OF INFECTION

During epidemics of influenza, large numbers of patients are seen with similar influenza symptoms: if it has been established that influenza virus is circulating in the community, an association of patients with contacts diagnosed as having influenza may suggest that the diagnosis is self-evident. However, influenza A and B can co-circulate, and mixed infections of influenza and other viruses have been reported; under these circumstances presumptive diagnosis can be misleading. Again, the symptoms of influenza in any group of patients are clearly different from those caused by other virus infections; however, the symptoms and signs for any one patient may vary, such that a diagnosis on clinical grounds cannot be confidently made. In contrast, concordance between clinical diagnosis and labora-tory-proved cases of influenza are held to be good, with correlations of 70% being reported. It may be held that clinical diagnoses in the time of epidemics are relatively easy and possibly of limited value; however, laboratory diagnosis of isolated cases of suspected influenza should be carried out, since clinical assessment is more difficult, and infection may represent the first case of an impending epidemic or infection by a new virus strain; diagnosis of these cases may not be of benefit to the individual patient, but is an important signal of what may happen subsequently in the community. The recognition of index cases activates preventative mea-sures to protect subjects for whom influenza is a life-threatening condition.

Traditionally, the laboratory diagnosis of influenza is based upon the isolation and identification of virus from pathological specimens, and/or a demonstration of a significant increase in specific antibody titre between serum specimens collected at the onset of disease and 2–3 weeks later. The isolation of virus can be achieved in a limited number of cases, since virus may have disappeared by the time the specimens are taken, and the methods used for virus isolation may lack sensitivity; however, direct methods of detecting viral nucleic acid by PCR, and viral protein by ELISA tests or with fluorescein-labelled antibody are increas-ingly available, refined and rapid. Serological tests provide the most sensitive and practical alternative for diagnosis in the absence of virus isolation; but, since they require a convalescent serum specimen, the diagnosis is retrospective. However, a diagnosis may be made on a single serum sample by demonstrating the presence of a virus-specific IgM response; such responses may be present for about 8 weeks, occasion-ally longer, following influenza infection.

Virus Isolation and Identification

Pathological Specimens

Influenza viruses replicate in the upper respiratory tract, and are present in these tissues and in respiratory secretions; virus is not found in other tissues, although occasional reports of virus isolation from brain, heart tissue and blood are documented. Serial specimens of respiratory secretions from patients with influenza indicate that the maximum titre of virus is present on days 2 and 3 after the onset of symptoms, but virus is detectable from days 1 to 5. Throat or nasopharyngeal swabs can be taken into a suitable transport medium, or nasal washings can be collected: comparative studies have shown that virus can more commonly be isolated from nasal washings than from other specimens. In all cases, the rapid transfer of specimens, or proper maintenance of specimens where delay may occur, is important for virus isolation.

Culture in Embryonated Hens' Eggs

Influenza viruses A and B, present in pathological specimens and collected into transport medium, can be cultured by amniotic inoculation of 10–12 day embryonated hens' eggs. The virus is adsorbed from the fluid of the amniotic cavity onto the cells of the amniotic membrane where multiplication occurs, releasing newly formed virus back into the amniotic fluids. After 2–3 days of incubation, virus can be present in high titres in the amniotic fluid and can be detected by adding aliquots of harvested amniotic fluid to chick, turkey, guinea-pig or human erythrocytes and observing haemagglutination. Egg fluids negative for virus can be passed to further embryonated eggs and retested: experience has shown that additional passage is unwarranted, and specimens which do not reveal virus after two egg passages are recorded as negative.

Cell Culture

Pathological specimens can be inoculated onto cultures of kidney cells from rhesus monkeys, baboons, chicks or a variety of other species; in addition, the cells of other tissues or transformed cells can be used but may require the addition of trypsin to ensure the cleavage of virus HA into HA1 and HA2 necessary for virus replication. Experience has shown that rhesus monkey and baboon kidney cells are probably the most sensitive. After adsorption and incubation of virus-infected cells, newly produced virus can be detected by a number of methods. First, free virus released into the maintenance medium of the cell culture can be detected by haemagglutination with erythrocytes, as described for amniotic fluid (see above). Second, since virus is released slowly from the cell surface of infected cells, erythrocytes will adhere directly to these infected cells; this phenomenon is termed haemadsorption, and can be observed under the microscope. Finally, and more

rapidly, virus can be detected in infected cells by fixation and staining with specific fluorescein-labelled antibody (Brumbeck and Wade, 1996).

Virus Recognition

Influenza viruses isolated from embryonated hens' eggs or cell culture can be identified by serological methods. First, influenza virus can be recognised as A, B or C by complement fixation (CF) tests using extracts of infected cells or embryonic membranes, which contain high titres of NP antigen, and standard antisera against influenza A, B or C viruses. The NP antigen is found for all influenza A, B or C virus types, and antibody against one type does not react with soluble antigen of another type: thus, the influenza type can be unequivocally identified in this manner.

Further classification of influenza isolates into sub-types and strains is a highly specialised responsibility of WHO reference laboratories; these determinations are carried out on virus isolates forwarded from laboratories to these centres. Each virus isolate is tested by HI tests against antisera raised in experimental animals against a range of virus subtypes and strains: the titre of each serum against homologous virus is known from prior testing. The submitted virus strains are standardised to contain a fixed amount of HA activity by titration against erythrocytes, and then reacted against a range of dilutions of each antiserum. By observing the patterns of HI against the various antisera, the virus subtype and strain is identified. Should the virus isolate not be inhibited by any of the sera to the same titre as known for homologous virus, then the strain may be a new subtype or strain: homologous serum against the strain is then prepared in animals, and more extensive cross-HI tests performed. These tests require the constant addition of new antisera to the battery used, and experience in interpreting the results.

In addition, to identify the HA of a virus isolate, the NA is also typed. This is done by identifying which antisera prepared against the various influenza NAs inhibit the NA of unknown virus to the same titre as against homologous virus; the indicator system in this test is an NA substrate, such as fetuin.

Rapid Diagnosis

Immunoreactions

Since influenza virus is very rarely isolated from symptom-free persons, the isolation of virus from patients may be taken as proof of infection without the need for diagnostic serology; however, using conventional egg and cell cultures (see above), this procedure takes at least 2–3 days, and in practice probably a week, to complete. Since clinicians have antiviral agents for the treatment of influenza to hand, and may confidently expect additions to this armoury in the near future, more rapid methods of diagnosis are needed if these compounds are to be used rationally. In addition, more rapid diagnostic methods would allow the earlier initiation of measures to limit the spread of infection. One procedure for rapid diagnosis relies on the direct identification of virus or virus antigens present in the respiratory secretions in the early days of illness: virus and virus-infected cells can be removed either in throat washings or scraped from the tissue surface with a metal spoon. In the laboratory, the cells are placed on a glass slide, fixed and stained by an indirect immunofluorescence or an ELISA technique using antisera against influenza virus; the immunofluorescence can be accelerated by treatment with microwave irradiation for a few seconds (Hite and Huang, 1996). The procedure can be completed within 1–2 h of specimens arriving in the laboratory, and offers obvious advantages. Many workers have investigated methods using this principle; some are convinced of the value of the technique, while others have been disappointed with the specificity of antisera available and the level of background reaction, particularly fluorescence, which makes the test difficult to interpret; however, better reagents are becoming available and the method offers a considerable advance over existing methods for the future. In one comparative study of virus identification made by a traditional culture method and direct fluorescent antigen test, and using a reverse transcriptase PCR procedure to resolve discrepancies, a 90% correlation was reported for influenza A and B infections (Chan et al., 2002).

Molecular Biology

Developments in molecular biology have provided reagents and techniques for the diagnosis of many infectious agents and these have been applied to the detection of influenza viruses. Thus, influenza virus RNA can be detected by molecular hybridisation using DNA probes labelled with either isotopes or biotin (Uryvaev et al., 1990). Viruses can be detected by PCR: virus RNA sequences are transcribed into cDNA by reverse transcriptase, and then amplified using specific DNA primers (RT-PCR); the amplified sequence is then detected by polyacrylamide gel electrophoresis as a molecule of predicted molecular weight. The sensitivity of the RT-PCR technique is unsurpassable, since theoretically one RNA sequence can be amplified to several million DNA sequences; thus, the technique offers exquisite sensitivity, but great care must be taken to avoid cross-contamination (Zhang and Evans, 1991). Again, RT-PCR shows a high concordance with results obtained from slower culture and serological methods (Zambon and Ellis, 2001); and enzyme digestion of the PCR product can be used to differentiate virus strains and rapidly record antigenic drift (Ellis et al., 1997; Cooper and Subbarao, 2000). Finally, a quantitative RT-PCR, now being devised, could be used to determine viral load. Details of the methodology of these techniques, together with comparisons of sensitivity and lists of other procedures mentioned above, have recently been fully reviewed (Ellis and Zambon, 2002).

Serology

Although isolation and identification of virus from respiratory secretions is recommended to establish a diagnosis for all suspected cases of influenza, virus cannot be isolated from all cases of infection. More commonly the diagnosis is made retrospectively by the demonstration of a rise in serum antibody to the infecting virus. For this, blood samples are taken as early after the onset of symptoms as possible (acute specimen), and 14–21 days later (convalescent specimen): these sera are each titrated for virus antibody, and the demonstration of a four-fold or greater increase in antibody titre in the convalescent serum as compared to the acute serum is diagnostic of infection. A common method of measuring antibody titre is by CF: soluble antigen is extracted from embryonic membranes of infected cells, and is reacted against a range of dilutions of the acute and convalescent sera. This test is often positive for patients from whom virus could not be isolated.

A more specific test for antibody to influenza virus is the HI test. For this, paired sera from patients with suspected influenza infection are treated to remove non-specific inhibitors, and a series of dilutions made: to each dilution is then added a standard quantity of intact virus, and after incubation chick cells are added. The presence of antibody is indicated by inhibition of haemagglutination, and the highest serum dilution that inhibits haemagglutination is recorded as the titre of HI antibody in the serum specimen. A further technique for detecting serum antibody is the haemadsorption inhibition test. In this test, mixtures of standard virus and serum dilution are inoculated on to appropriate cells, such as monkey kidney cells, and incubated: after 2–3 days the cultures are washed, guinea-pig erythrocytes are added, and the cultures viewed under a microscope. The presence of haemadsorption indicates virus replication and the absence of antibody, whilst no haemadsorption indicates neutralisation by antibody in the serum. Again, by testing each serum over a range of dilutions the titre of antibody can be determined, and a four-fold or greater rise in titre is diagnostic of infection.

Infection by influenza virus results in a rise of serum antibody titre, but the requirements for equal or greater than four-fold rise in titre of HI or CF antibody reflects the inaccuracy of these tests for detecting increases in antibody. A more precise method of measuring antibody is by the single radial haemolysis technique. Here, influenza virus is coated onto sheep red cells, and suspended in melted agar with complement: the agar is poured into dishes or onto glass slides and, after setting, wells are cut in the agar and inoculated with dilutions of test sera. The presence of antibody in the sera is detected by lysis of the red cells as antibody combines with complement and antigen on the red cell surface. This lysis can be seen with the naked eye, and the amount of antibody present is directly related to the area of haemolysis. The procedure is more sensitive than CF or HI antibody and has a greater degree of precision: a 50% increase in zone area of haemolysis reflects a rise in antibody and is evidence of recent infection. Sera do not require pre-treatment to remove the non-specific inhibitors which plague the HI test. Lastly, antibody can be measured by ELISA, and reagents and appropriate protocols are on the market; studies have shown that ELISA readings correlate with HI titres, and the procedure is becoming increasingly popular.

TREATMENT AND PREVENTION

The clinical severity of influenza, with high temperatures, respiratory symptoms, myalgia and severe prostration, requires most patients to seek bed rest during the acute phase of illness; the exhaustion and depression which follow may require further rest and convalescence. During epidemics, symptoms can affect tens of thousands of individuals, causing disruption to industry, services and social life; causing a significant number of deaths; and resulting in complications such as pneumonia and Reye's syndrome, which are life-threatening to both old and young. From these observations, it is clearly desirable that adequate means of treatment and prevention should be developed; but despite the need,

which has been recognised throughout the past century, progress has been relatively slow, and the impact of epidemic influenza has changed little. Some progress has been made, and this can be summarised under the separate headings of treatment and prevention.

Treatment

General

At the present time the treatment of influenza is usually symptomatic. Patients are advised to remain in bed for 2–3 days until the acute symptoms have subsided. The symptoms of headache and fever were commonly treated with salicylates, but in view of the evidence that a combination of salicylates and acute influenza infection underlies the pathogenesis of Reye's syndrome in children, paracetamol is given in place of salicylates. Codeine linctus may relieve the cough; insomnia may be treated with barbiturates or promethazine (an antihistamine with hypnotic side-effects); and antibiotics are indicated where chest complications are present or suspected. The use of prophylactic antibiotics in patients with chronic chest disease who thus have a higher risk of developing postinfluenzal pneumonia is contentious: some advocate this practice, but the incidence of secondary bacterial pneumonia is not reduced and infection may be by antibiotic-resistant organisms.

Since the earliest conception of antiviral chemotherapy, influenza has been one of the target diseases against which suitable antiviral compounds should be developed. The search for such compounds has used three methods. First there is the rational approach, which predicts a potentially valuable substance that would interfere with virus replication: this requires an exact knowledge of the molecular events of virus infection and multiplication, and such information is not complete; however, this approach identified ribavirin. The second method is the serendipity approach, which requires the random screening of chemical compounds in the hope that an active compound will be found by chance; this method identified amantadine. Lastly, there is the structural approach: the three-dimensional structures of the HA and NA of influenza virus have been elucidated and the identification of the active sites in these structures in virus replication predicts the structure of compounds which may interfere with their function; this strategy led to the development of the neuraminidase inhibitors.

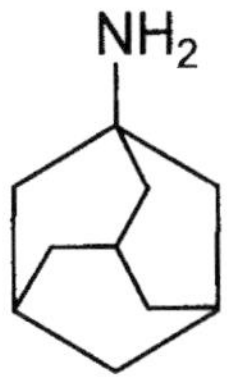

L - Amantadine

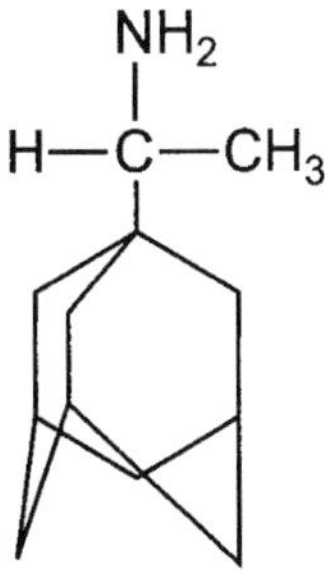

Rimantadine

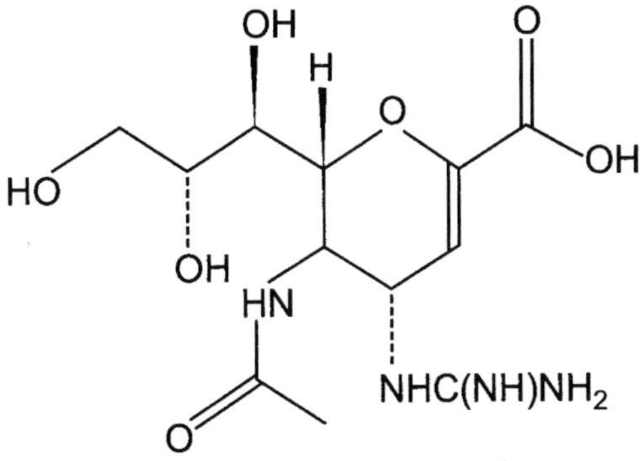

Zanamivir (Relenza)

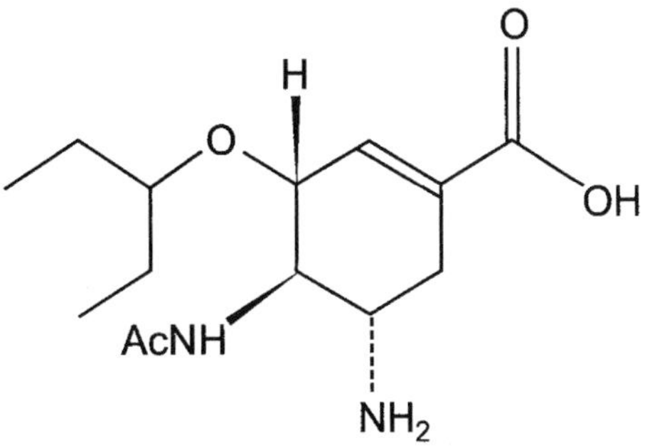

Oseltamivir (Tamiflu)

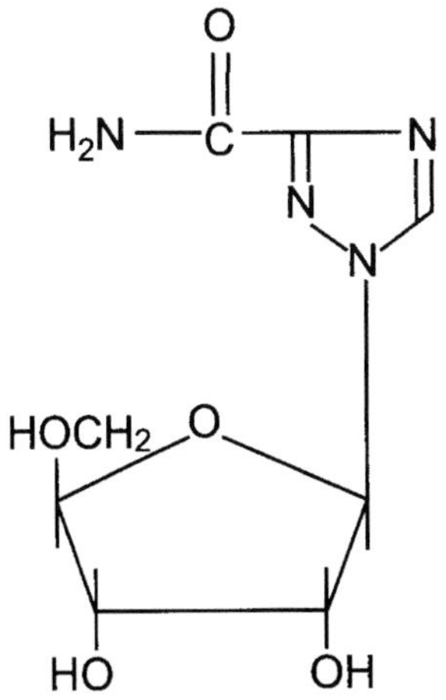

Ribavirin

Figure 5.5 Structure of some antiviral compounds active against influenza virus infection

Amantadine, Rimantadine

Amantadine and rimantadine are synthetic, water-soluble primary amines with a symmetrical structure; basically, they consist of a stable base with an active amino group (Figure 5.5). In experimental studies, the compounds have been shown to inhibit the growth of influenza virus in cell culture; to limit virus replication in mice, ferrets and other experimental animals; to reduce tissue damage by influenza virus in infant rats; and to protect hamsters from infection from virus-infected animals placed in the same cage (Potter and Oxford, 1977). On the other hand, the compounds are not equally active against all influenza virus strains; resistant strains arise during treatment; naturally occurring resistant strains have been isolated; and the compounds are not active against influenza B viruses. Studies on the mode of action of amantadine have indicated two features of antiviral activity. First, the compound acts at the level of virus uncoating by lysosomal enzymes: this process requires the ion channel formed by the M2 protein and a fall in pH (see above) for optimal enzyme activity, but amantadine blocks this channel and thus uncoating and subsequent virus replication is limited. Second, the action of amantadine on the M2 ion channel actively inhibits the transport of HA and other viral subunits at the cell surface, which in turn limits virus assembly (Lin et al., 1997).

Clinical studies with amantadine have shown that the compound can occasionally induce mild neurological symptoms; these include insomnia, loss of concentration and mental disorientation. The symptoms are quickly shown by susceptible individuals, and cease when treatment is stopped. If these symptoms do not occur within 24 h of initiation of amantadine treatment, they are unlikely to occur at all. With these reservations in mind, amantadine has been subjected to clinical trials, and satisfies the basic requirements of non-toxicity. Both prophylactic and therapeutic studies have been carried out. In the most convincing prophylactic studies, index cases of influenza were identified in closed groups of subjects in schools or universities, and unaffected volunteers from among the contacts were given either amantadine or a placebo: these studies indicate an approximate 70% protection for those taking amantadine prophylactically (Dolin et al., 1982). In a therapeutic study carried out among patients attending general practitioners, volunteers with symptoms of influenza were treated with either amantadine or placebo in a double-blind study. The diagnosis of influenza was confirmed by demonstrating a significant rise in serum HI antibody, and only patients in whom the diagnosis was confirmed were included in the subsequent analysis. Amantadine significantly reduced the duration of fever (51 h as opposed to 74 h in the placebo group), and illness (2.5 days as opposed to 3.5 days). The study inadvertently included patients shown subsequently to be suffering from influenza B infection; this provided an added control to the study, since no therapeutic effect was demonstrable against this infection, and amantadine is known to have no antiviral activity against influenza B virus. It is suggested that rimantadine is the preferred compound, since, although not as effective as amantadine, it is less toxic (Arruda and Hayden, 1996).

Ribavirin

The structure of the synthetic nucleoside analogue 1-β-D-ribofuranosyl-1, 2,4-triazole carboxymide (ribavirin) is shown in Figure 5.5. The compound has been shown to inhibit the replication of a wide range of RNA and DNA viruses in vitro, including both influenza A and influenza B, and to limit influenza virus replication in mice and ferrets. The compound probably acts by inhibition of virus nucleic acid synthesis, through alterations to cell metabolism: antiviral compounds which act in this way, through alteration to cell metabolism, have broad antiviral activity and do not generate resistant forms; these two properties are true for ribavirin. Ribavirin is well-tolerated in concentrations 200-fold greater than those necessary to inhibit virus replication; however, the compounds have been reported to have immunosuppressive effects, although these are completely reversible once treatment is stopped. Clinical studies have demonstrated a significant therapeutic effect on symptoms of both influenza A and B (Stein et al., 1987); and the compound is very effective in animal studies when given by aerosol combined with rimantadine or amantadine (Hayden, 1996).

Neuraminidase Inhibitors

The activity of the neuraminidase enzyme, situated on the outer surface of the influenza virus particle, is important in the replication of both influenza A and B viruses. The three-dimensional crystalline structure of this glycoprotein has been established (Laver et al., 1984), and although the structure can vary between influenza strains, X-ray crystallography and site-directed mutagenesis indicate that the active site is conserved (Laver et al., 1999). It is apparent, therefore, that drugs that combine with the active site would have antiviral activity. The first active antineuraminidase compound, 4-guanidino-Neu5Ac2en, (zanamivir, Relenza), was shown to have a good antiviral activity against influenza A and B *in vitro* and, given as an aerosol, was safe and effective in animal models and in clinical studies (Monto *et al.*, 1999). The structure of this compound is shown in Figure 5.5. The second compound with similar structure and properties (3R, 4R,55)-4-acetoamido-5-amino-3-(1 ethylopropoxy)-1 cyclohexane-1 carbozylic acid (oseltamivir, Tamiflu), given orally as a prodrug, shows similar antiviral activity in volunteer studies (Nicholson *et al.*, 2000) and is also licensed for treatment; and early reports in the literature suggest that several other similar compounds are in development.

Treatment of young adults with these compounds is demonstrably effective: the incidence, severity and duration of illness can be reduced significantly, and resistant strains are unusual and are compromised in the ability to replicate (Blick *et al.*, 1995). Licence for both these neuraminidase inhibitors has been given in many countries as a result of convincing clinical results. Controlled trials also show that neuraminidase inhibitors can be given prophylactically to family members of an index case and so interrupt transmission of influenza.

Prevention

It is clear from our knowledge of the epidemics and pandemics due to influenza, and morbidity, mortality and disruptive effects associated with these outbreaks, that both individuals and communities would benefit greatly from the use of effective vaccines. To this end, various forms of vaccines have been developed during the last 50 years: despite this, the efficacy of influenza vaccines is still questioned, and the ability of vaccines to limit epidemic infection has not been proven.

Immunity to Influenza

The antigens of the influenza virus particle which stimulate immunity to subsequent infections have been identified. The virus proteins have been purified and separately inoculated into groups of experimental animals; the results of challenge studies indicate that immunity is induced by the host responses to the virus HA and, to a lesser extent, to the NA. Some evidence suggests that the immune response to the M2 and NP proteins may contribute to immunity, but there is little evidence to suggest that these are major factors.

Studies to determine which immune responses correlate with protection against infection indicate that the serum antibody titre against the HA is the most important; thus, susceptibility to influenza virus infection is inversely related to the titre of serum HI antibody. This is true for both experimental challenge with attenuated virus and natural infection with virulent virus; and a serum HI antibody titre of approximately 30–40 and 20–30 represents a 50% protective level of antibody against infection by homologous influenza A and B virus, respectively (Potter and Oxford, 1979). Further, the degree of cross-immunity for viruses of different subtype or strain is directly related to the degree of cross-reactivity of the HA antigens: immunisation with an influenza virus vaccine confers no protection against challenge with virus of different subtype, since there is no cross-reactivity of the HA of the two viruses. In addition to conferring relative protection against infection, the serum HI antibody is reported to both reduce the severity of infection and decrease virus

Table 5.4 Response of volunteers to immunisation with whole or ether-split influenza virus vaccine and results of subsequent challenge infection

Vaccine (A/Scotland/74 + B/Hong Kong/73)[a]	Number (%) with HI titre $\geqslant 40$		Total number (%) infected by challenge virus[b]
	Preimmunisation	Postimmunisation	
Whole virus	7/24 (29)	18/24 (75)	3/24 (12.5)
Split virus	7/24 (29)	22/24 (92)	0/24
Saline control	6/27 (22)	6/27 (22)	11/27 (41)

[a]Vaccine given subcutaneously in 0.5 ml volume, and containing equivalent concentration of virus HA; control group given 0.5 ml saline only.
[b]$10^{7.4}$ egg infectious dose (EID) of live virus 1 month after immunisation.

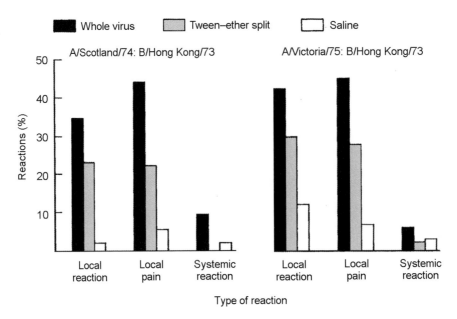

Figure 5.6   Reactions of volunteers to immunisation with influenza virus vaccines (see also Table 5.4)

spreading from infected persons. Similar studies have shown that serum neuraminidase inhibiting (NI) antibody also confers protection against influenza virus infection: this has been shown in studies with experimental animals and in observations of natural infection in humans. Thus, antineuraminidase antibody has been shown to confer protection against the clinical effects of influenza virus infection, not infection *per se*, and in the presence of a NI antibody, infection will induce protective HI antibody whilst clinical symptoms are considerably reduced and may not occur. A generally held view is that the serum HI antibody is more important in determining immunity than the serum NI antibody. Local IgA antibody against virus antigens contributes to immunity, as indicated by several studies. The importance of cellular immune responses in immunity to infection remains to be established (McMichael *et al.*, 1983); however, cellular immunity is an important prerequisite for humoral antibody production in response to vaccines and in the resolution of clinical disease.

From the above it is clear that an influenza vaccine must contain the surface HA and NA antigens of the virus in a form which will stimulate serum HI and NI antibody, local IgA antibody and possibly cellular immunity. It is essential that the vaccine contains the antigens of recently isolated virus strains: although some cross-reactivity and corresponding cross-immunity are seen between viruses of the same

subtype, the most solid immunity is found following immunisation with virus homologous to the infecting strain. Thus, whatever the type of vaccine used, the virus contents should be reviewed annually and changed to match new variants as they occur.

Whole Virus Vaccines

Whole, inactivated virus vaccines are prepared by inoculating the currently circulating strain of influenza virus into embryonated hens' eggs: at the present time and for the last two decades, strains of influenza A(H3N2) and (H1N1) and influenza B have been circulating in any one year; thus, the currently infecting strains of each of the three viruses are grown in parallel. Allantoic fluids are harvested after 2–3 days of incubation, centrifuged by zonal centrifugation to concentrate and purify the particles, inactivated with formalin or β-propiolactone and standardised by haemagglutinin content for intramuscular inoculation. The three viruses are mixed to contain 15 μg HA of each virus in each dose. Clinical studies with vaccines prepared in this manner have recorded some local pain in approximately 20–30% of vaccinees and symptomatic reactions, such as fever, headache and muscle pain, in about 5% of persons; however, these responses are usually mild and ephemeral. The vaccine induces serum HI and NI

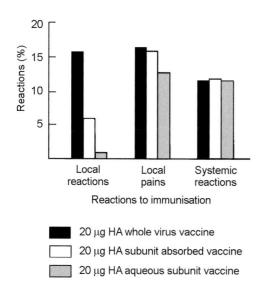

Figure 5.7 Reactions of volunteers to immunisation with influenza virus vaccines

a vaccine containing virus of the new subtype against which the vaccinees have had no past experience is relatively short-lived, and 60–80% of the antibody may have disappeared by 12 months after immunisation.

Split Virus Vaccines

Because of the relatively high incidence of reactions seen in vaccinees given whole, inactivated virus vaccine, attempts have been made to produce a product which is less reactogenic, while preserving the ability to induce satisfactory titres of serum antibody. For this, virus pools grown, purified and inactivated as described in the previous section are treated with detergents to disrupt the virus particles: inoculation of virus manufactured in this way induces fewer reactions in volunteers than whole virus vaccines (Figure 5.6), and the serum antibody responses and protection afforded against subsequent challenge are similar (Table 5.4). For these reasons, many prefer split vaccines to whole virus vaccines.

Subunit Virus Vaccines

Since only virus HA and NA antigens are required to induce immunity, vaccines containing purified surface antigens and free of virus RNA and core proteins have been investigated; these are conventionally given as aqueous suspension, but may be administered with carrier compounds to enhance the immune response (Podda, 2001). Volunteers given aqueous subunit vaccines intramuscularly experience fewer reactions than those given whole virus vaccines (Figure 5.7). In years of antigenic drift when the population is primed, serum HI antibody responses to whole and subunit

antibody responses which confer protection on 60–90% of volunteers against challenge virus infection (an example is shown in Table 5.4) and significant prevention of hospitalisation and deaths in the elderly. The vaccine may be given annually to the young or elderly and higher doses may be given to the elderly, who give relatively poor immune responses to conventional vaccine (Keital et al., 1996). The serum antibody response persists at a protective level for 1–5 years, depending on the vaccine virus strain and the age of the vaccinees; however, subsequent infecting virus strains may show antigenic drift and the vaccine-induced antibody will be less effective in protecting against these new strains. In contrast, the antibody response to

Table 5.5 Response of volunteers to immunisation with inactivated influenza vaccines

Previous experience[a]	Nature of influenza A (H1N1) vaccine given	Percentage with serum HI titres ⩾40 and geometric mean titre (in parentheses)		
			Postimmunisation	
		Preimmunisation	1 dose	2 doses
Primed	Whole virus	20 (13)	95 (465)	–
	Subunit—absorbed	32 (19)	100 (578)	–
	Subunit—aqueous	33 (10)	100 (622)	–
Unprimed	Whole virus	0	77 (70)	96 (259)
	Subunit—absorbed	0	50 (27)	88 (176)
	Subunit—aqueous	0	25 (14)	94 (99)

[a]Older subjects who had been exposed to influenza A (H1N1) viruses in 1933–1957 (primed) and subjects born after 1957 (unprimed). Number of subjects in each group varied from 12 to 30.

saline vaccines are similar, and since aqueous vaccines are less reactogenic, these are preferred (Table 5.5). However, when vaccinees are not primed by previous exposure to viruses of the same subtype, the serum HI antibody response to whole vaccine is significantly greater than for subunit vaccine; in order to achieve protective levels of antibody, two doses of subunit vaccine may be necessary, and the search for an acceptable adjuvant to overcome this need is an important research activity. However, the response to whole virus vaccine is not as good in times of antigenic shift as in a primed population, and again two doses of vaccine are needed. Thus, two doses of either vaccine are required when priming is not present and, as whole vaccines are more reactogenic, subunit vaccines are again preferred.

As mentioned above, subunit vaccines remain short of ideal in protecting the population against influenza, and experimental studies to find a suitable carrier/ adjuvant to enhance antibody reproduction has been pursued vigorously for some years. A large number of adjuvants are known but few are suitable for intramuscular injection: ISCOMS and M57 enhance serum antibody responses, but there is an increase in the incidence of reactions; and immune modulators such as IL-2 enhance antibody responses in mice but have not been investigated in volunteers. At this time of writing (2004), attempts to increase the immunogenicity of subunit virus vaccines by incorporating adjuvants have not identified an agreed safe, suitable and acceptable carrier. The best vaccines available at the moment are aqueous subunit vaccines, but many authorities hold that these are not sufficiently potent for completely successful immunisation, and we anxiously await further developments.

Live Virus Vaccines

Inactivated influenza vaccines induce serum HI and NI antibodies to protective levels in the majority of vaccinees; however, the local IgA antibody and cellular immune responses are disappointing. In contrast, there is evidence that immunisation with live, attenuated influenza vaccine induces a full range of immune responses and a more solid immunity than inactivated vaccines. These findings, the known shortcomings of inactivated vaccines, the resistance of general practitioners and the public to immunisation against influenza by injection, and the reactogenicity to inactivated vaccine have continued to encourage the development of live vaccines against this infection. Influenza viruses can be attenuated by serial passage in

embryonated hens' eggs, chemical mutation or by laboratory passage at reduced temperatures; using these techniques, viruses can be produced which infect and immunise volunteers without producing appreciable clinical illness. Unfortunately, these methods require a long and unpredictable time to complete— probably too long for vaccine to be available for immunisation against current influenza variants. To circumvent this problem, attenuated viruses produced by one of the above methods have been mixed with wild-type viruses causing current infections to produce reassortants, which contain the RNA fragments coding for the wild-type HA and NA and all the other genetic material from the attenuated strain. These reassortants can be produced relatively quickly in the laboratory and, when inoculated intranasally into volunteers, produce few and mild symptoms, induce both serum and local HI and NI antibody against the wild-type virus and immunity to challenge virus infection (Beare, 1982). Two strains, A/Ann Arbor/6/60 (H2N2) and B/ Ann Arbor/1/66, have been used to produce attenuated influenza A and B vaccine reassortants for over three decades (Maassab and De Borde, 1985); in all studies, the selected reassortants have been shown to be safe and effective, easily administered and suitable for all ages (Potter, 1994).

Some problems of live, attenuated influenza virus vaccines have not been overcome. The development of a suitable influenza virus vaccine initially requires the production and purification of a suitable reassortant from an established, suitable and attenuated virus and the wild-type virus. Then, under strictly controlled conditions, the virus must be shown to be attenuated for humans and to be genetically stable, since there is a possibility that the virus may revert to a virulent variant when inoculated into volunteers. In a series of developmental tests the vaccine virus must be shown to be attenuated for various groups of volunteers of different ages and susceptibility, to induce antibody responses, and to protect against challenge virus infection: only after these satisfactory tests can a licence be given for general use. At the present time, these studies are estimated to take 2 years to complete: this makes their development impractical, because by the time the vaccine can be made available, the epidemic strain against which it has been prepared will probably have disappeared, to be replaced by new strains requiring a new vaccine. Despite these setbacks, studies have continued to find methods for the more rapid development of live vaccine; should a method be found that reduces the development to 6–8 months, live vaccine strains, with all the attendant advantages, will become practical. Alternatively, should the long history of efficacy and safety of reassortant vaccines based on the A/Ann Arbor/6/60 (H2N2) and B/Ann Arbor/1/66 viruses be accepted, and this appears to be the case for many licensing authorities, then many of the protracted studies on safety listed above may be considered unnecessary and the development of these vaccines accelerated. No live influenza virus vaccines are available for general use in Western countries at the present time, and vaccines against influenza viruses are limited to one of the forms of inactivated vaccines given intramuscularly, as discussed above. Licence for a live influenza vaccine was expected recently, but a live vaccine against another disease was shown to produce a few unwarranted reactions, which has forced licensing authorities to re-evaluate live influenza vaccines once again.

Other Approaches to Vaccine Development

In addition to the above influenza vaccines, several other approaches are possible and are being researched at the present time. Large quantities of influenza virus antigens can be made by cloning the relevant genes into a variety of vehicles for expression, or by growing viruses in cell cultures; this would make vaccines more available, since quantity would not be limited by the availability of embryonated hens' eggs. Again, cDNA derived from virus RNA can be selectively mutated and then rescued when transferred into helper cells (Parkin et al., 1997): these deletion mutants cannot revert to virulent virus and are therefore safe, and could be developed as attenuated vaccines. A more practical technique has been developed which allows virus to be produced from susceptible cells transfected with plasmids coding for each of the eight gene segments of the virus RNA (Fodor et al., 1999); this opens the possibility of laboratory-designed live influenza vaccines (Hoffman et al., 2002; Neumann and Kawaoka, 2002).

One of the limitations of influenza vaccine usage is the requirement to inoculate intramuscularly; to obviate this, inactivated vaccines have been tested intranasally. Saline, inactivated vaccines given intranasally are poor immunogens: these vaccines need to be combined with adjuvant/carrier to be effective, but none has received general approval for human use at the present time (Potter and Jennings, 1999), although a limited licence has been given for the adjvuant MF59 (Podda, 2001). Intramuscular immunisation with the NA antigen has been proposed: antibody to the NA permits subsequent infection by wild-type virus; however, this infection would not cause clinical illness,

but would induce immunity comparable to that following natural infection. This strategy has proved successful in experimental influenza. Finally, DNA vaccines coding for virus HA have been used successfully in animal models, and represent an exciting development for the future (Wong et al., 2001).

Recommendations

At the present time, no live attenuated influenza virus vaccine is available for general use, and the new and novel methods of producing vaccine outlined above remain a hope for the future. The currently available vaccines are inactivated vaccines produced from virus grown in hens' eggs: of these, the most popular are the aqueous subunit vaccines, which have replaced the earlier whole and split virus vaccines in many countries. These vaccines produce relatively few reactions, and such reactions are usually mild and of relatively short duration; they produce serum antibody in the large majority of subjects, and immunity to infection in 60–90% of vaccinees. Early fears that these vaccines may be unsuitable in certain patient groups, such as those with multiple sclerosis, AIDS or diabetes, have been largely discounted by more recent and larger studies.

A large literature assembled over the past three decades attests to the safety and the efficacy of inactivated influenza vaccine: these studies were carried out in children, in healthy adults and in the elderly. Meta-analysis of collected studies from the literature in both healthy young and elderly people indicates that immunisation is both safe and effective in producing immunity; and in the elderly can prevent approximately one in five cases of influenza illness, one in four hospitalisations from pneumonia and influenza, and one in four deaths, where there is a good match between the influenza strains in the vaccine and those in circulation (Vu et al., 2002). With this information to hand, it is difficult to understand the reluctance of some patients, and indeed some practitioners, to use immunisation more widely; immunisation rates for vulnerable people in many Western countries are less than 20%. Finally, although inactivated influenza vaccines are effective in the elderly population, they are less effective than in younger people, since the immune response is impaired by age; however, recent clinical studies suggest that a combination of inactivated vaccine given intramuscularly and live vaccine given intranasally can be more effective than killed vaccine on its own. The anticipated licensing of live vaccines could result in this strategy being used to further protect the vulnerable and aged population.

Vaccine is recommended in most Western countries for all aged over 65 years, patients with chronic lung or heart disease, patients with metabolic disorders such as diabetes, renal disease or immunodeficiencies, including children, for whom influenza is life-threatening, and residents of institutions for the elderly or disabled; other groups, such as household contacts of high-risk persons and health care workers, should be considered for immunisation, together with pregnant women after the first trimester. Recently, researchers have recommended that the use of vaccine should be extended to young children for whom influenza is a more serious clinical disease, and in whom the virus replicates to higher titres, thus identifying them as a focus of infection for others. For the remainder of the population, immunisation against influenza is a debatable subject; some authorities hold that vaccines should be available for all and used according to the wishes of doctors and patients, while others protest that the further widespread use of vaccine is not justified.

REFERENCES

Arruda E and Hayden FG (1996) Update on therapy of influenza and rhinovirus infections. *Antiviral Chemother*, **4**, 175–187.

Beare AS (ed.) (1982) Research into immunization of humans against influenza by means of living viruses. In *Basic and Applied Influenza Research*, pp 211–234. CRC Press, Boca Raton FL.

Blick TJ, Tiong T, Sahasrabudhe A *et al.* (1995) Generation and characterization of an influenza virus neuraminidase variant with decreased sensitivity to the neuraminidase inhibitor 4-guanidine-neu 5 AC 2 en. *Virology*, **214**, 475–484.

Blok V, Cianci C, Tibbles KW *et al.* (1996) Inhibition of the influenza virus RNA-dependent RNA polymerase by antisera directed against the carboxy-terminal region of the PB2 subunit. *J Gen Virol*, **77**, 1025–1033.

Bradbury TN and Miller GA (2000) Season of birth in schizophrenia: a review of evidence, methodology and aetiology. *Psychol Bull*, **98**, 569–594.

Brumback BG and Wade CD (1996) Simultaneous rapid culture for four respiratory viruses in the same cell monolayer using a differential multicoloured fluorescent confirmatory stain. *J Clin Microbiol*, **34**, 798–801.

Chan KH, Maldeis N, Pope W *et al.* (2002) Evaluation of the Directigen flu A and B test for rapid diagnosis of influenza type A and B infections. *J Clin Microbiol*, **40**(5), 1675–1680.

Colman P (1998) Structure and function of the neuraminidase. In *Textbook of Virology* (eds Nicholson KG, Webster RG and Hay AJ), pp 65–73. Blackwell, London.

Conover RT and Roessmann U (1990) Malformation complex in an infant with intrauterine influenza viral infection. *Arch Pathol Lab Med*, **114**, 535.

Cooper LA and Subbarao K (2000) A simple restriction fragment length polymorphism-based strategy that can distinguish the internal genes of human H1N1, H3N2 and H5N1 influenza A viruses. *J Clin Microbiol*, **38**(7), 2579–2583.

Corey L, Rubin RJ, Hattwick MAW *et al.* (1976) A nationwide outbreak of Reye's syndrome. *Am J Med*, **61**, 615–625.

Crosby AW (1976) *Epidemic and Peace, 1918*. Greenwood Press, Westford, CT.

de Jong JC, Claas ECJ and Osterhaus ADME (1997) A pandemic warning. *Nature*, **389**, 534.

Dolin R, Reichman RC, Madore P *et al.* (1982) A controlled trial of amantadine and rimantadine in the prophylaxis of influenza A infection. *N Engl J Med*, **307**, 580–584.

Ellis JS, Sadler CJ, Laidler H *et al.* (1997) Analysis of influenza A (H3N2) strains isolated in England during 1995–1996 using polymerase chain reaction. *J Med Virol*, **51**, 234–241.

Ellis JS and Zambon MC (2002) Molecular diagnosis of influenza. *Rev Med Virol*, **12**, 1–5.

Elton D, Medcalf E, Bishop K *et al.* (1999) Identification of amino acid residues of influenza virus nucleoprotein essential for RNA binding. *J Virol*, **73**, 7357–7367.

Fleming DM (2000) The contribution of influenza to combined acute respiratory infections, hospital admissions and deaths in winter. *Commun Dis Public Health*, **3**, 32–38.

Fodor E, Devenish L, Engelhardt P *et al.* (1999) Rescue of influenza A virus from recombinant DNA. *J Virol*, **73**, 9679–9682.

Francis T Jr, Davenport FM and Hennessy AV (1953) A serological recapitulation of human infection with different strains of influenza virus. *Trans Assoc Am Physic*, **66**, 231–239.

Garcia-Sastre A (2001) Inhibition of interferon-mediated antiviral responses by influenza A viruses and other negative-strand RNA viruses. *Virology*, **279**, 375–384.

Gomez-Puertas P, Albo C, Perez-Pastrana E *et al.* (2000) Influenza virus matrix protein is a major driving force in virus budding. *J Virol*, **75**, 11538–11547.

Hayden FG (1996) Combination antiviral therapy for respiratory virus infections. *Antiviral Res*, **29**, 45–48.

Hite SA and Huang YT (1996) Microwave-accelerated direct immunofluorescent staining for respiratory syncytial virus and influenza A virus. *J Clin Microbiol*, **34**, 1819–1820.

Hoffman E, Krauss S, Perez D *et al.* (2002) Eight-plasmid system for rapid generation of influenza virus vaccines. *Vaccine*, **20**, 3165–3170.

Irvine WL, James DK, Stephenson T *et al.* (2000) Influenza virus infection in the second and third trimester of pregnancy: a clinical and socioepidemiological study. *Br J Obstet Gynaecol*, **107**, 1289–1290.

Keital WA, Cate TR, Atmar RL *et al.* (1996) Increasing doses of purified influenza virus haemagglutinin and sub-virus vaccines enhance antibody responses in the elderly. *Clin Diagn Lab Immunol*, **3**, 507–510.

Kitler ME, Gavinio P and Lavanchy D (2002) Influenza and the work of the World Health Organization. *Vaccine*, **20**(S2), 5–14.

Lamb RA and Krug RM (1996) Orthomyxoviridae: the viruses and their replication. In *Field's Virology*, 3rd edn (eds Fields BN, Knipe DM and Howley PM), pp 1353–1395. Lippincott-Raven, Philadelphia, PA.

Laver WG, Colman PM, Ward CW *et al.* (1984) Influenza virus neuraminidase: structure and variation. In *The Molecular Biology and Epidemiology of Influenza* (eds Stuart-Harris CH and Potter CW), pp 77–89, Academic Press, London.

Laver WG, Bischofberger N and Webster RG (1999) Disarming flu viruses. *Sci Am*, **280**, 78–87.

Lin T-I, Heider J and Schroeder C (1997) Different modes of inhibition by amantane amine derivatives and natural polyamines of the functionally reconstituted influenza M2 proton channel protein. *J Gen Virol*, **78**, 767–774.

Liu J, Lynch PA, Chien C-Y *et al.* (1997) Crystal structure of the unique structural multifunctional RNA-binding domain of the influenza virus NS1 protein. *Nature Struct Biol*, **4**, 891–899.

Lynberg MC, Khovry MJ, Lu X *et al.* (1994) Maternal 'flu, and the risk of neural tube defects: a population-based case-control study. *Am J Epidemiol*, **140**, 244–255.

Maassab HF and DeBorde DC (1985) Development and characterization of cold-adapted viruses for use as live virus vaccines. *Vaccine*, **3**, 355–369.

Matrosovich MN, Gambaryan AS, Teneberg S *et al.* (1997) Avian influenza viruses differ from human viruses by recognition of sialoligo-saccharides and gangliosides and by a higher concentration of the HA receptor-binding site. *Virology*, **233**, 224–234.

Matrosovich M and Klenk H-D (2002) Natural and synthetic sialic acid-containing inhibitors of influenza virus receptor binding. *Rev Med Virol*, **12**, 1–13.

McMichael AJ, Gotch FM, Noble GR *et al.* (1983) Cytotoxic T-cell immunity to influenza. *N Engl J Med*, **309**, 13–17.

Monto AS, Fleming DM, Henry D *et al.* (1999) Efficacy and safety of the neuraminidase inhibitor zanamivir in the treatment of influenza A and B virus infections. *J Infect Dis*, **180**, 254–261.

Mori I, Nagafuji H, Matsumoto K *et al.* (1997) Use of the polymerase chain reaction for demonstration of influenza virus dissemination in children. *Clin Infect Dis*, **24**, 736–737.

Neumann G and Kawaoka Y (2002) Generation of influenza A virus from cloned cDNAs—historical perspective and outlook for the new millennium. *Rev Med Virol*, **12**, 13–30.

Nicholson KG, Aoki FY and Osterhaus ADME (2000) Efficacy and safety of oseltamivir in treatment of acute influenza: a randomised controlled trial. *Lancet*, **355**, 1845–1850.

O'Callaghan E (1991) Schizophrenia after post-prenatal exposure to 1957 H2-influenza epidemic. *Lancet*, **337**, 1248–1250.

Paragas J, Talon J, O'Neill RE *et al.* (2001) Influenza B and C virus NEP (NS2) proteins possess nuclear export activities. *J Virol*, **75**(16), 7375–7383.

Parkin NT, Chiu P and Coelingh K (1997) Genetically engineered live attenuated influenza A virus vaccine candidates. *J Virol*, **71**(4), 2772–2778.

Podda A (2001) The adjuvanted influenza vaccines with novel adjuvants: experience with the MF59-adjuvanted vaccine. *Vaccine*, **19**(17–19), 2673–2680.

Portela A, Zurcher T, Nieto A *et al.* (1999) Replication of orthomyxoviruses. *Adv Virus Res*, **54**, 319–348.

Potter CW (1994) Attenuated influenza virus vaccines. *Rev Med Virol*, **4**, 279–292.

Potter CW and Oxford JS (1977) Animal models of influenza virus infection as applied to the investigation of antiviral compounds. In *Chemoprophylaxis and Virus Infection of the Respiratory Tract*, vol 2. (ed. Oxford JS), pp 1–26. CRC Press, Boca Raton, FL.

Potter CW and Oxford JS (1979) Determinants of immunity to influenza infection in man. *Br Med Bull*, **35**, 69–75.

Potter CW (1998) Chronicle of influenza pandemics. In *Textbook of Influenza* (eds Nicholson KG, Webster RG and Hay AJ), pp 3–18. Oxford: Blackwell Science.

Potter CW and Jennings R (1999) Intranasal immunization with inactivated influenza vaccines. *Pharmaceut Sci Technol Today*, **2**(10), 402–408.

Potter CW (2001) A history of influenza. *J Appl Microbiol*, **91**, 1–8.

Reye RDK, Morgan C and Baral J (1963) Encephalopathy and fatty degeneration of the viscera: a disease entity in childhood. *Lancet*, **ii**, 749–752.

Simonsen L, Clark MJ, Schonberger LB *et al.* (1998) Pandemic versus epidemic influenza mortality: a pattern of changing age distribution. *J Infect Dis*, **178**, 53–60.

Skehel JJ, Daniels RS, Douglas AR *et al.* (1984) Studies on the haemagglutinin. In *The Molecular Biology and Epidemiology of Influenza* (eds Stuart-Harris CH and Potter CW), pp 61–68. Academic Press, London.

Stein DS, Creticos CM, Jackson GG *et al.* (1987) Oral ribavirin treatment of influenza A and B. *Antimicrob Ag Chemother*, **31**, 1285–1287.

Stray SJ, Cummings RD and Air GM (2000) Influenza virus infections of desialylated cells. *Glycobiology*, **10**, 649–658.

Stuart-Harris CH, Schild GC and Oxford JS (1985) *Influenza: The Viruses and the Disease*, pp 22–40. Edward Arnold, London.

Suzuki Y, Ito T, Suzuki T *et al.* (2001) Sialyl sugar chains as receptors and determinants of host range of influenza A viruses. In *Options for the Control of Influenza*, vol IV (eds Osterhaus A, Cox N and Hampson A), pp 521–525. Excerpta Medica, Amsterdam.

Tashiro M, Ciborowski P, Klenk H-D *et al.* (1987) Role of *Staphylococcus aureus* in the development of influenza pneumonia. *Nature (Lond)*, **325**, 536–537.

Taubenberger JK, Reid AH, Krafft AE *et al.* (1997) Initial genetic characterisation of the 1918 'Spanish influenza virus'. *Science*, **275**, 1793–1796.

Uryvaev LV, Rusavskaia EA, Sinagutullina NM *et al.* (1990) Detection of influenza A virus RNA by molecular hybridisation of nucleic acids using biotin treated probes. *Voprosy Virusologii*, **35**, 464–466.

Vu T, Farish S, Jenkins M *et al.* (2002) A meta-analysis of effectiveness of influenza vaccine in persons aged 65 years and over living in the community. *Vaccine*, **20**, 1831–1836.

Wang P, Palese P and O'Neill RE (1997) The NP1-1/NP1-3 (karyopherin α) binding site on the influenza A virus nucleoprotein NP is a nonconventional nuclear location signal. *J Virol*, **83**, 337–355.

Wong JP, Zabielski MA, Schmaltz FL *et al.* (2001) DNA vaccination against respiratory influenza virus infection. *Vaccine*, **19**, 2461–2467.

Zambon MC (2001) The pathogenesis of influenza in humans. *Rev Med Virol*, **11**, 227–241.

Zambon MC and Ellis JS (2001) Molecular methods for diagnosis of influenza. In *Options for the Control of Influenza*, vol IV (eds Osterhaus A, Cox N and Hampson A), pp 267–273. Excerpta Medica, Amsterdam.

Zhang WD and Evans DH (1991) Detection and identification of human influenza virus by the polymerase chain reaction. *J Virol Methods*, **33**, 165–189.

Zink P, Drescher J, Verhagen W *et al.* (1987) Serological evidence of recent influenza A (H3N2) infections in forensic cases of sudden infant death syndrome (SIDS). *Arch Virol*, **93**, 223–232.

6

Parainfluenza Viruses

Stelios Psarras[1], Nikolaos G. Papadopoulos[1] and Sebastian L. Johnston[2]

[1]*University of Athens, Greece, and* [2]*Wright–Fleming Institute of Infection and Immunity, Imperial College London, UK*

INTRODUCTION

Human parainfluenza viruses (HPIV) are the second leading cause after respiratory syncytial virus (RSV) of hospitalisation for respiratory tract illness (RTI) in young children. Although the characteristic HPIV-mediated illness is laryngotracheobronchitis (croup), the repertoire of the virus in the paediatric population also includes upper respiratory tract infection and the development of bronchiolitis and pneumonia. Parainfluenza viruses are also able to trigger community-acquired RTI requiring hospitalisation in adults, as well as morbidity and mortality in immunocompromised patients.

Vaccination against these important respiratory pathogens is not, as yet, available for clinical use. However, recently established reverse genetics systems have allowed for the recovery of infectious HPIV cDNAs and their manipulation has led to the development of promising vaccine candidates. Results from reverse genetics-based genome modification studies have also shed light on the complex pattern replication of, and immunity against, HPIVs. Further unravelling of the molecular and epidemiological aspects of HPIV infection, as well as efficient nucleic acid-based detection methods, would be of much benefit in the battle against these pathogens. For instance, improvement of our understanding of the mechanisms used by HPIVs to escape interferon-driven antiviral immune surveillance should assist the development of effective intervening strategies in the future. To that end, antiviral agents targeting particular events in the viral life-cycle,

e.g. attachment to and replication in target cells, are under development.

TAXONOMY

Parainfluenza viruses are single-stranded negative-sense enveloped RNA viruses belonging to the order *Mononegavirales*. Human parainfluenza viruses comprise five members; HPIV1, HPIV2, HPIV3, HPIV4A and HPIV4B. They are all members of the large family *Paramyxoviridae* and of its subfamily *Paramyxovirinae*, but they are classified into different genera (Figure 6.1). Thus, human and animal PIV1s and PIV3s belong to the genus *Respirovirus* (formerly *Paramyxovirus*), whereas PIV2s and PIV4s are members of the genus *Rubulavirus*. The human pathogen mumps virus is also a member of the genus *Rubulavirus*. These two genera, together with the genus *Morbillivirus* (to which measles virus belongs), form part of the subfamily *Paramyxovirinae*, whereas the subfamily *Pneumovirinae* contains the genus *Pneumovirus*, with the most important member being human RSV, as well as the genus *Metapneumovirus*, to which belongs the recently isolated human metapneumovirus (hMPV) (van den Hoogen *et al.*, 2002).

Sendai virus (SeV), simian virus 5 (SV5) and bovine PIV3 (BPIV3) are well-studied animal counterparts of HPIV1, HPIV2 and HPIV3, respectively. SeV was originally isolated from the lung of a fatal case of pneumonitis in a newborn in Sendai, Japan, in 1953, but it is considered to be a murine virus; it is also referred to as murine PIV1 (MPIV1), since it readily

Principles and Practice of Clinical Virology, Fifth Edition. Edited by A. J. Zuckerman, J. E. Banatvala, J. R. Pattison, P. D. Griffiths and B. D. Schoub
© 2004 John Wiley & Sons Ltd   ISBN 0 470 84338 1

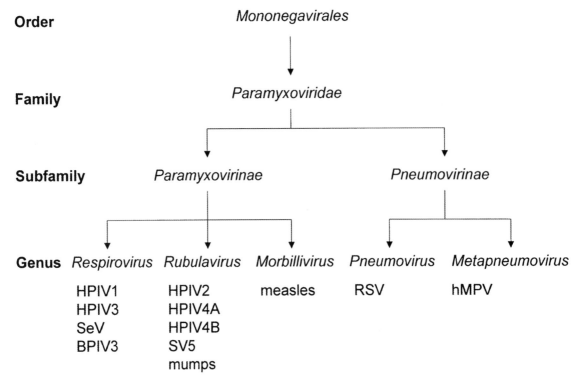

Figure 6.1 Classification of parainfluenza and related viruses. For abbreviations see text

infects and causes disease in mice and no further cases of the human disease have been reported. The related avian Newcastle disease virus (NDV) belongs to the genus *Avulavirus* of the subfamily *Paramyxovirinae*.

STRUCTURE AND PHYSICAL PROPERTIES

The non-segmented, negative-stranded RNA species of PIVs form genomes approx. 15–16 kb long, encoding at least six mRNAs. They also contain short (less than 100 nt long) untranslated regions at their 3' and 5' ends, named 'leader' and 'trailer', respectively, which contain important replication and transcription promoter elements (see Replication). The gene order starting from the 3' end is: N–P–M–F–HN–L. The coding proteins have molecular weights of 40–250 kDa, and consist of the nucleocapsid [nucleocapsid protein (N or NP); phosphoprotein (P); polymerase (L)] and the envelope [haemagglutinin neuraminidase (HN); fusion protein (F); matrix protein (M)] of the virion.

Viral RNA is encapsidated within multiple copies of the N protein, resulting in nuclease-resistant helical nucleocapsids. These are further associated with P and L proteins to form the ribonucleoprotein (RNP) complex. Accordingly, N is present in abundance in the RNP of the virion to perform its encapsidation function (2600 molecules), whereas the proportion of the L and P proteins is lower (30 and 300 molecules, respectively) (Lamb *et al.*, 1976). Shifts in reading frame, as well as readthrough and RNA-editing events, allow for the encoding of additional protein species by the P, M and F parts of the genome (see Replication). These species, designated V, C and D, are characteristic of each HPIV subtype, playing important roles in replication, assembly, maturation and virulence of these viruses.

The resulting virions are pleomorphic, roughly spherical, lipid-containing enveloped particles, 120–300 nm in total diameter. The nucleocapsid strands are 12–17 nm in diameter, with cross-striations at intervals of 4 nm to give a herringbone appearance. Lipids comprise 20–25% and carbohydrates 6% by weight of virus particles. Their total molecular weight is at least 500×10^6 Da and their density in sucrose is 1.18–1.20 g/ml. The virions are sensitive to lipid solvents, non-ionic detergents, formaldehyde and oxidising agents.

RECEPTORS, VIRUS ENTRY AND HOST RANGE

Infection of target cells by PIVs is initiated by attachment of virus to the host cell through interaction of the HN glycoprotein with a sialic acid-containing cell surface receptor. F and HN envelope proteins then regulate the process that allows the fusion of the virus envelope with the plasma membrane. Following penetration, the virion becomes uncoated and the viral nucleocapsid material is released into the cytoplasm.

PIVs may show preferences for the side from which they enter a particular cell type. HPIV3, for instance, can enter type II alveolar polarised epithelial cells from both the apical and basolateral domains, but preferentially enter and are released from the apical surface (Bose *et al.*, 2001). Microtubules seem to actively regulate the release process.

Both sialoglycoproteins (e.g. glucophorin) (Suzuki *et al.*, 1984; Wybenga *et al.*, 1996) and gangliosides can serve as specific viral receptors for PIVs (Holmgren *et al.*, 1980; Suzuki *et al.*, 1985; Umeda *et al.*, 1984). It has been shown that SeV is able to bind to both ganglio-series and neolacto-series gangliosides, with a terminal *N*-acetylneuraminic acid (NeuAc) linked to galactose (Gal) by an α2-3 linkage (NeuAcα2-3Gal) as isoreceptor (Holmgren *et al.*, 1980; Suzuki *et al.*, 1985; Umeda *et al.*, 1984). In contrast, HPIV1 and HPIV3 subtypes bind only to neolacto-series gangliosides and with different binding specificity (Suzuki *et al.*, 2001). In particular, HPIV1 binds only to gangliosides containing *N*-acetylactosamine α2-3 linked to NeuAc, whereas HPIV3 binds in addition to gangliosides of identical composition but with an α2-6 linkage or containing a different terminal sialic acid (*N*-glyconyl-neuraminic acid; NeuGc). Thus, HPIVs seem to differentially recognise the oligosaccharide core structure of their cognate receptors, a feature consistent with the different infection patterns of the target cells. Moreover, according to a recent report, additional molecules, such as heparan sulphate, may regulate binding and entry of HPIV3 (Bose and Banerjee, 2002).

A current hypothesis suggests that upon binding to its sialic acid-containing receptor, HN undergoes a conformational change which triggers other conformational changes in the F protein (Lamb, 1993). Heptad repeats contained within the latter confer a trimeric core coiled-coil formation and proteolytic cleavage into two subunits (membrane distal F_2 and membrane proximal F_1) is required for the exposure of the hydrophobic fusion peptide contained in the new N-terminus of the F_1 subunit. The fusion peptide contains 25 hydrophobic residues, highly conserved among the paramyxovirus species.

Indeed, for HPIV1, -2 and -3 efficient membrane fusion by the F protein also requires the participation of HN (Hu *et al.*, 1992; Moscona and Peluso, 1991). However, this is not true for SV5, since its F protein can mediate membrane fusion in the absence of HN (Bagai and Lamb, 1995), in a unique manner that probably differs even from those exhibited by other similarly structured viral fusion proteins (Baker *et al.*, 1999).

HN not only mediates the attachment of the virus to cell surface receptors but also possesses neuraminidase activity, i.e. the ability to cleave the sialic acid moiety of those receptors. Evidence from studies with NDV HN suggests that both the attachment and the hydrolytic activity of PIV HNs are co-localised in a single site with two conformationally switched states. In this way HN can promote the release of newly formed virions from the cell surface, allowing them to penetrate additional cells (Huberman *et al.*, 1995). However, this is not the only way of PIV propagation. PIV envelope proteins accumulating in the cell surface of the infected cells can fuse with neighbouring cells, leading to syncytium formation. Again, neuraminidase activity of HN controls the process by modulating the number of available receptors on the adjacent cells (Moscona and Peluso, 1992). In particular, it has been reported that syncytium formation by HPIV3 is reduced when the target cells are infected at high multiplicity of infection (MOI). The absence of cytopathic effect (CPE) from these 'persistently infected' cells is due to sialic acid cleavage by the HN neuraminidase in a manner proportional to viral loading (Moscona and Peluso, 1993). This phenomenon can be reproduced at low MOI by addition of exogenous (bacterial or viral) neuraminidase. On the other hand, high MOI HPIV-1 and -2 infection fails to inhibit syncytial formation *in vitro*. Interestingly, the observed CPE cannot be blocked by bacterial or NDV neuraminidase treatment, but it is significantly reduced by HPIV3 neuraminidase, suggesting different cleavage specificities of PIVs neuraminidases (Ah-Tye *et al.*, 1999). Nevertheless, these data show that in addition to the above-mentioned differences in binding specificities, CPE formation also seems to be differentially

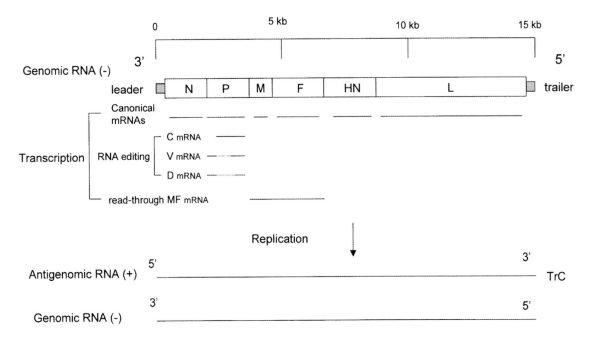

Figure 6.2 Genomic organisation and main transcriptional and replication events of parainfluenza viruses. The genomic organisation of the PIV genome (3′ to 5′ direction), as found in the RNP complex of the virion is shown in the upper part of the scheme. Cistron sizes were designed to roughly correspond to the original sequence length, thus depicting relative sizes (in thousands of RNA bases; kb). Upon RNP release into the cytoplasm of a target cell, canonical as well as alternative transcriptional events produce the six main mRNAs and additional species (for their role in virus life, see text). Dashed lines within V and D products represent sequences not included in the fusion mRNAs and indicate inclusion of the second ORF. Promoter sequences found in the 3′ (leader) end of the genome drive not only the transcription but also a round of replication ignoring gene initiation and stop signals, thus producing the antigenomic RNA (depicted in the 5′ to 3′ direction). Promoter elements (TrC) found in the 3′ of the latter trigger a second round of replication, generating negative-sense original PIV RNA

regulated by the individual HPIV serotypes, a fact that might have particular impact on their pathogenesis pattern.

Viral interference, a state whereby cells infected by a specific virus are refractory to subsequent infections by a challenge virus, is induced by several mechanisms including attachment interference. Accordingly, expression of NDV HN inhibits infection of the target cells by NDV (Morrison and McGinnes, 1989). Furthermore, it seems that the neuraminidase activity of HPIV3 depletes the cells of the available appropriate receptors and protects them from reinfection, not only by HPIV3 but also by HPIV2 (Horga *et al.*, 2000). This heterologous interference pattern suggests additional regulatory mechanisms of PIV infection and propagation.

It is plausible to assume that the binding specificities of parainfluenza viruses would determine the host range of particular subtypes. Indeed, sialoglycoproteins

localised on erythrocyte membranes mediate the well-studied PIV-mediated agglutination of these cells (haemadsorption activity). In addition, blood group I-type gangliosides able to bind HPIVs have been detected in the cell surface from human and bovine, but not equine, erythrocytes. Accordingly, HPIV1 and HPIV3 are unable to induce agglutination of equine erythrocytes, but succeed in agglutinating human and bovine-derived ones (Suzuki *et al.*, 2001).

However, receptor specificity is not the only determinant of PIVs' host range. Cell-specific replication patterns, as well as cell-specific escape from immune regulatory mechanisms of the virus, seem to play a more important role, as described in the following sections.

Finally, it should be noted here that the host range for some PIV species has not been conclusively defined, e.g. SV5, originally isolated from monkey tissue, seems to be a canine virus. Similarly, SeV, considered to be mainly a murine virus, has recently been reported to propagate equally well as its homologue HPIV1 in the respiratory tract of primates (Skiadopoulos et al., 2002a).

REPLICATION

Upon release of the viral RNP into the cytoplasm, transcription is the first event initiating the viral replication cycle. Transcription is thought to start at the 3′ end of viral RNA and generates the six essential mRNAs by a sequential start–stop mechanism. Conserved sequences flanking the 3′ and 5′ termini of each PIV gene, termed gene start (GS) and gene end (GE), mediate transcription initiation and termination/polyadenylation, respectively.

Following this initial transcription phase, sequences located in the leader of the 3′ end of PIV RNA promote the replication of the nascent RNA, so that the entire genome is copied into a positive-sense replica called the antigenome. A prerequisite for this synthesis is the ability for read-through transcription, ignoring the gene start and gene stop signals of each particular mRNA through mechanisms yet to be defined. Subsequently, promoter sequences found in the 3′ end (trailer) of the PIV antigenome drive the synthesis of genomic RNA, leading to the replication of the entire PIV genetic material (Figure 6.2).

The whole transcription and replication procedure is thought to be mediated by the RNA-dependent RNA polymerase complex of P and L proteins, and the nucleocapsid N protein. Indeed, efficient HPIV3 transcription and replication has been demonstrated by a minireplicon (i.e. an otherwise 'empty' recombinant viral genome containing only the promoter elements for transcription and replication) when these three proteins were provided in-trans by co-transfection (Durbin et al., 1997). When these three proteins were provided in-trans, infectious HPIV2 could be rescued from the full-length HPIV2 cDNA (Kawano et al., 2001). It seems that P acts as transactivator of L, which is the catalytic subunit of the polymerase complex. Moreover, the L protein is not able to bind by itself to the N-RNA complex to initiate RNA synthesis, but requires the formation of the L–P complex. Interestingly, N–P and P–P complexes have also been observed in the infected cells. The N–P complex seems to play an important role in encapsidation of the nascent RNA chains during genome replication. Genetic analysis of HPIV3 revealed that the N-terminus of the P protein is responsible for the formation of the soluble N–P complex, whereas the C-terminus mediates P binding

to the N-RNA template, as well as the formation of the stable L–P complex (De et al., 2000). In addition to the role of viral proteins, cellular actin microfilaments seem to play an important role in HPIV3 RNA synthesis and replication (Gupta et al., 1998).

The promoter elements for SeV and HPIV3 replication have been mapped (Hoffman and Banerjee, 2000; Tapparel and Roux, 1996). The first 12 nucleotides of the 3′ leader are essential for HPIV3 replication driven by the leader (Le) promoter. Similarly, the first 12 nucleotides of the 3′ terminus of the antigenome are critical for the synthesis of genomic DNA driven by the so-called trailer complementary (TrC) promoter (Hoffman and Banerjee, 2000). Interestingly, mutations in the leader of SeV have been recently shown to affect viral replication and pathogenesis in a mouse model (Fujii et al., 2002).

Analysis of paramyxovirus minireplicons as well as infectious recombinant viruses revealed that many members of the family, with the remarkable exception of RSV (Samal and Collins, 1996), obey the so-called 'rule of six' (Calain and Roux, 1993): replication of their RNA is efficient only if the nucleotide length of the genome is a multiple of six. This special feature, thought to reflect an association of the NP protein strictly with six nucleotides in the nucleocapsid, is indeed dominant in HPIV3 replication; however, it is not an absolute prerequisite, as in SeV for instance, since HPIV3 replication in minireplicons is efficient even when the genome length cannot be divided by six (Durbin et al., 1997). Similar findings have been reported for HPIV2 (Kawano et al., 2001).

Apart from the 'canonical' N, P, M, F, HN and L proteins, a number of alternative transcriptional and translational events generated additional gene products by PIVs (Figure 6.2). Many of these proteins modulate the transcription and/or replication processes of these viruses.

In particular, an overlapping open reading frame (ORF) located within the P region encodes the non-structural C protein (Spriggs and Collins, 1986b). The C protein of SeV has been reported to inhibit RNA replication by downregulating the promoter of genomic RNA (Cadd et al., 1996). It also contributes to the SeV pathogenicity for mice (Kurotani et al., 1998).

A polymerase slippage on a cis-acting sequence motif in the template P gene leads to the addition of non-templated nucleotides during mRNA synthesis. Transcription of these elements leads to reading frame shifts and internal ORFs are expressed as chimeras fused to the amino-terminus of the P protein. This RNA editing leads to the translation of an additional V protein by the HPIV3 genome. In HPIV2, however, which lacks the above-mentioned C ORF, it is actually the insertion of two G residues that produces the mRNA encoding the P protein, whereas the unedited mRNA (which is actually the exact copy of the P gene) encodes the V protein (Kawano *et al.*, 2001). The differences between the PIV subtypes do not stop here: the V protein is a structural protein detected in the HPIV2 virion (Ohgimoto *et al.*, 2001), but is a non-structural component of SeV (Lamb and Choppin, 1977), whereas the HPIV1 genome does not encode V protein at all (Matsuoka *et al.*, 1991). The V protein seems to play an important role in generation and maturation of HPIV2 virions. In particular, recovery of infectious virions from a HPIV2 cDNA modified to lack V protein expression [HPIV2V(−)] was successful by the usual reverse genetics protocols, but the titres obtained were 10–100 times lower than those of unmodified HPIV2, although RNA synthesis was not impaired in the former. Furthermore, HPIV2V(−) virions were anomalous in size, consisting of heterogenous populations and larger mean diameter (220 nm vs. 165 nm) (Kawano *et al.*, 2001).

Finally, RNA editing of the P region in HPIV3 and BPIV3 results in the generation of a unique protein named D, not encountered in other paramyxoviruses, which is the fusion product of the N-terminus of P protein and a second internal ORF (Galinski *et al.*, 1992; Pelet *et al.*, 1991).

In addition to synthesising monocistronic mRNA, the viral polymerase in some cases ignores the termination GE and initiation GS signals. Accordingly, bicistronic M–F readthrough transcripts are abundant in cells infected by HPIV1 or HPIV3, but not by SeV (Bousse *et al.*, 1997; Spriggs and Collins, 1986a). This capacity to read through was due to *cis*-elements contained in the long non-coding region of the HPIV1 F gene and, when these sequences were introduced in the SeV M–F boundary, they conferred M–F read-through transcription in the modified *Respirovirus* (Bousse *et al.*, 2002). This modification was further shown to reduce the levels of F protein and virus propagation in the infected cells, resulting in reduced pathogenicity of the virus for mice. Thus, failure of transcriptional termination in specific gene boundaries of the PIV genome may form an additional regulatory mechanism of replication and pathogenesis associated with the parainfluenza viruses.

The mechanisms regulating PIV replication may also contribute to determination of tissue tropism by these viruses. Although MDBK cells are refractory to HPIV1, the virus is able to infect them and its genetic material is transcriptionally active in this environment. However, replication seems to be severely impaired,

since only trace amounts of genomic RNA and no nucleocapsid formation is detectable following infection, rendering these cells non-permissive for HPIV1 infection (Tao and Ryan, 1996). Amino acid differences observed at given positions in the otherwise highly homologous BPIV3 and HPIV3 proteins are host range-specific and consistent with the ability of each strain to preferentially propagate in either bovine or primate tissues (Bailly *et al.*, 2000).

During PIV replication the nascent RNA associates with the N–P complex to form the helical nucleocapsid. For HPIV1 it has been reported that the matrix protein M plays a central role in this encapsidation procedure (Coronel *et al.*, 2001). At the end of the whole process the nucleocapsids associate with the viral envelope proteins (M, HN and F) at the plasma membrane. This leads finally to the budding and release of the new infectious virions from the cell surface.

VIRAL TRANSMISSION, INCUBATION AND SHEDDING

Parainfluenza viruses are transmitted by inhalation of virus-laden droplets expelled into the air from lower respiratory or nasal secretions of infected individuals. In an isolated population of an Antarctic station, HPIV1 and HPIV3 were the main pathogens detected after a respiratory tract illness (RTI) outbreak, probably transmitted by newly arriving personnel from abroad (Parkinson *et al.*, 1979). No RTI was recorded in periods of no arrivals.

After an incubation period of 2–8 days, viral replication occurs in the nasopharyngeal epithelium and 1–3 days later it is spread throughout the tracheobronchial tree. The virus normally does not multiply outside the respiratory tract.

Recurrent infection is a common event and seems to occur more than once, even during adulthood (Marx *et al.*, 1999). However, symptomatology becomes progressively more restricted to the upper respiratory tract.

In the remote community model mentioned above, HPIVs could be isolated throughout a period of complete social isolation of greater than 8 months, suggesting prolonged viral shedding in humans (Muchmore *et al.*, 1981). In another study, shedding of HPIV3 at 4–6 weeks after onset of RTI was observed in a paediatric population (Frank *et al.*, 1981). Increased shedding has been also correlated with more severe RTI symptoms in HPIV1-infected children (Hall *et al.*, 1977). In addition, persistent infection has been demonstrated *in vitro*, where the level of viral neuraminidase activity has been shown to play an important role in the process (Moscona and Peluso, 1992). Finally, it should be noted that, similar to RSV, HPIVs survive for long periods on skin, cloth and other material (Brady *et al.*, 1990), a fact that emphasises the importance of prophylaxis (such as hand washing) particularly within the hospitals and clinics.

PATHOGENESIS

HPIV infection and illness is associated with both upper and lower respiratory tract symptoms. Furthermore, HPIVs have been clearly associated with the development of croup, pneumonia and bronchiolitis in susceptible individuals, mainly children (see Epidemiology and Clinical Features). Pathological features of these conditions, such as airway inflammation, necrosis and sloughing of the epithelium, oedema, excessive mucus production, alveolar filling and interstitial infiltration of the lungs should therefore be considered consequences of HPIV-associated airway lesions, as has been shown in some reports (Marx *et al.*, 1999). In the case of croup, the vocal cords, larynx, trachea and bronchi become swollen, leading to obstruction to the inflow of air. This is clinically manifested by stridor and in drawing of the soft tissues around the rib cage.

Cytopathic effects, caused mainly by syncytium formation, are thought to be of crucial importance for HPIV pathogenesis. Thus, HPIV1 and HPIV2 have been shown to readily infect and propagate in cultured human tracheal epithelial cells (Stark *et al.*, 1991). CPE, including early syncytium formation, has also been demonstrated in this system. The role of HN–receptor interaction in the process has been demonstrated in experiments using variants of HPIV3 that contain single amino acid changes in HN. These altered HN molecules show increased avidity for sialic acid receptors and, as a result, the respective variants are highly fusogenic and destroy a cell monolayer more rapidly than wild-type (wt) HPIV3. More importantly, they cause more severe alveolitis and interstitial pneumonitis than wt HPIV3 in a reliable cotton rat model for PIV infection (Prince *et al.*, 2001).

The main body of evidence concerning HPIV-mediated airway inflammation comes from animal studies, as early experimental infection studies of human volunteers (Kapikian *et al.*, 1961; Smith *et al.*, 1967; Tremonti *et al.*, 1968; Lefkowitz and Jackson, 1966) have not been continued and HPIV

inoculation was found to be poorly infectious (Clements *et al.*, 1991b).

In particular, several rat and mice strains develop bronchiolitis and pneumonia following PIV infection, with characteristics similar to the human pathology (Porter *et al.*, 1991; Mo *et al.*, 1995; Sorden and Castleman, 1991). C57BL/6J mice inoculated with non-fatal doses of SeV secreted high levels of inflammatory cytokines (IFN-γ, IL-2, IL-6, TNFα) in their bronchoalveolar (BAL) fluid, peaking between day 7 and day 10, the time point at which the virus was cleared from the lungs (Mo *et al.*, 1995). Infiltration of BAL fluid and bronchioles by inflammatory cells (neutrophils, lymphocytes, macrophages and mast cells) has been reported in a SeV-infected rat strain (Sorden and Castleman, 1991). In addition, the expression of chemokines, such as monocyte chemotactic protein-1 (MCP-1), regulated on activation normal T cell expressed and secreted protein (RANTES), growth-related oncogene-α (GRO-α) and IL-8 are induced by SeV in human cells (Hua *et al.*, 1996; Le Goffic *et al.*, 2002). Moreover, the chemokines RANTES and macrophage inflammatory protein-1α (MIP-1α) have been also found elevated in nasal secretions of paediatric patients with acute upper respiratory illness attributed to a number of respiratory viruses, including HPIV (Bonville *et al.*, 1999).

Airway inflammation and hyperresponsiveness are also induced by HPIV3 in guinea-pigs, characterised by increased release of and response to histamine and BAL enrichment with eosinophils, neutrophils and monocytes (Folkerts *et al.*, 1993; Graziano *et al.*, 1989; van Oosterhout *et al.*, 1995). Eosinophil accumulation is well correlated with the degree of airway responsiveness, as well as with the significantly elevated eotaxin levels following HPIV3 inoculation (Scheerens *et al.*, 1999). Interestingly, the viral content detected in the lungs of inoculated animals pre-sensitised with ovalbumin (i.e eosinophil-enriched) was considerably reduced (80%) as compared to the non-sensitised ones (Adamko *et al.*, 1999). Treatment with an antibody to IL-5, a known eosinophil chemoattractant, reversed the ovalbumin effect and inhibited viral clearance. Thus, similarly to what has been previously reported for RSV (Domachowske *et al.*, 1998), eosinophils, when activated by the HPIV virus, apart from mediating inflammatory activity, may also exert antiviral activity.

Finally, both HPIV2 and HPIV3 have been reported to induce expression of intercellular adhesion molecule-1 (ICAM-1) in tracheal and other human epithelial cells (Tosi *et al.*, 1992a; Gao *et al.*, 2000).

Notably, ICAM-1 also serves as receptor for the majority of rhinoviruses, another important group of respiratory pathogens. This increase may induce adhesion of inflammatory cells in airway epithelium, further augmenting local inflammation, as has been shown for neutrophils in *in vitro* systems (Tosi *et al.* 1992a, 1992b). Indeed, from the limited human studies available, HPIV3 infection has been associated with BAL neutrophilia in a patient experiencing unilateral bronchiolitis obliterans (Peramaki *et al.*, 1991), whereas bronchial neutrophils and total eosinophils were found to be significantly increased in otherwise healthy individuals during common cold caused by respiratory viruses including HPIV (Trigg *et al.*, 1996).

The above data clearly indicate the inflammatory influence of PIV infection, consistent with an early report showing increased nasal secretion of interferon in children infected by PIVs (Hall *et al.*, 1978); however, further human studies would be required to establish this notion and its clinical impact.

ANTIGENICITY AND IMMUNITY

Sera obtained from subjects 1–2 weeks following HPIV infection contain antibodies able to inhibit HPIV-induced adsorption of erythrocytes to cultured cells. To detect these so-called 'haemagglutination inhibition' (HI) antibodies (see Diagnosis), sera should be heated at 56°C for 30 min and treated with potassium periodate to inactivate specific heat-labile and stable inhibitors of the process (McLean, 1982). HI antibodies persist in the host for several years, whereas complement-fixing antibodies against the whole virion (V-CF) appear 1–2 weeks later and tend to persist only for around 1 year. Neutralising antibodies are detected at the same time as HI antibodies. Antibody production in children aged less than 2 years may be delayed until recurrent infections occur.

Antibodies can be elicited against the HN, N, P, F and M proteins (Komada *et al.*, 1989, 1992; Rydbeck *et al.*, 1987). However, HN seems to possess the greatest antigenic capacity. Its antigenic sites lie within coiled-coil regions of the molecule (van Wyke Coelingh *et al.*, 1987). Henrickson and Savatski (1997) mapped 21 epitopes in HPIV1 HN. They are organised in five non-overlapping antigenic sites (I–V) and a sixth site connecting sites I, II and III. By examining clinical isolates collected during a period of 35 years and from different geographic regions, these authors provided evidence showing that only 33% of these epitopes were conserved among isolates. Two sites were found in all

isolates, but another one was missing from isolates collected in the last 15 years. Similarly, some mono-clonal antibodies against HN and N of HPIV1 strains generated in the 1990s did not react with isolates obtained in the 1970s and 1980s (Komada *et al.*, 1992). By contrast, an earlier report found a single change in the HPIV1 HN antigenic pattern in a limited number of isolates obtained between 1981 and 1989, suggesting HN homogeneity (Hetherington *et al.*, 1994). Mono-clonal antibodies raised against HPIV3 allowed the mapping of five, two, six and six epitopes in HN, F, N and M proteins, respectively (Rydbeck *et al.*, 1987); this analysis revealed a limited antigenic variation among isolates obtained throughout a 6 year period.

At least 20 epitopes have been located in the F protein of HPIV3 (van Wyke Coelingh and Tierney, 1989). From those, only 14, organised in three non-overlapping antigenic sites, induce the production of neutralising antibodies. In addition, HPIV3 frequently accumulates mutations producing F epitopes that efficiently bind to antibodies but are resistant to neutralisation. Similarly, antibodies against HPIV4 (of both subtypes) can be divided into three groups: those showing high neutralis-ing, HI and haemolysis inhibition activities; those neutralising the virus but unable to inhibit haemagglu-tination; and those exhibiting low neutralising and HI activity (Komada *et al.*, 1989). The F protein appears to possess neutralisation epitopes; many of the antibodies generated against the F protein neutralise the virus via mechanisms not including inhibition of fusion (van Wyke Coelingh and Tierney, 1989).

The HN glycoproteins of related PIV subtypes may be antigenically dissimilar, even if they share common epitopes. This is the case, for instance, for HPIV3 and BPIV3 (Ray and Compans, 1986). However, even when the amino acid identity between HN proteins of closely related viruses is high (e.g. between HPIV1 and SeV), there may be a limited conservation of epitopes and high antigenic diversity (Komada *et al.*, 1992). In the case of the HPIV4 couple (4A and 4B), antigenicity of N protein is highly conserved between the species, but monoclonal antibodies raised against F or HN proteins show low cross-reactivity with the hetero-logous subtype viruses, although there is a high degree of amino acid identity between the respective glyco-proteins (Komada *et al.*, 1989). By constructing HPIV4B cDNAs with putative N-glycosylation sites identical to those of 4A, Komada *et al.* (2000) were able to show that the mutant 4B subtype was antigenically closer to 4A than to the wt HPIV4B, suggesting that N-glycosylation pattern determines, at least partially, the limited cross-reactivity observed between PIV species.

The severity of respiratory illness and the duration of virus shedding seem to be reduced in the presence of high titres of neutralising antibodies (Chanock *et al.*, 1961). However, the fact that HPIV3, for instance, can reinfect an individual within a short time interval and even in the presence of neutralising antibodies (Glezen *et al.*, 1984; Welliver *et al.*, 1982; Bloom *et al.*, 1961) and may cause infection of a persistent nature (Gross *et al.*, 1973; Muchmore *et al.*, 1981), suggests that the virus fails to induce a state of long-lasting immunity. These events cannot be explained by the relatively stable antigenic determinants. On the other hand, the fact that the most severe symptoms develop in subjects with defects in cell-mediated immunity or severe immunodeficiency syndromes (Dorman *et al.*, 1999; Taylor *et al.*, 1998) indicates that the interaction of PIVs with the T cell compartment of the host's immune response may be of crucial importance for the fate of both the virus and the infected host.

Cytokine induction in response to HPIV3 has been shown to inhibit both T cell proliferation and cytotoxicity *in vitro* (Sieg *et al.*, 1994, 1995). In particular, HPIV3-induced IL-10 inhibited proliferation of CD3$^+$ peripheral blood mononuclear cells (PBMCs) derived from healthy human donors and infected *in vitro* by the virus (Sieg *et al.*, 1996). In addition, the HPIV3-infected lymphocytes failed to respond to IL-2, suggesting that IL-10 mediates an inhibition of T cell function which may support enhanced virus survival. HPIV3 infects and replicates poorly in human monocytes, simultaneously increasing their survival by induction of granulocyte macrophage colony forming factor (GM-CSF) expression (Plotnicky-Gilquin *et al.*, 2001). In the same set of experiments it was shown that the virus replicates extensively in human dendritic cells (DCs), accelerating their apoptosis. The surviving DCs seem to undergo maturation via increased production of IL-12 following HPIV3 treatment, but mature DCs were poor stimulators of allogeneic T cell proliferation (Plotnicky-Gilquin *et al.*, 2001). Thus, HPIV3 infects and differentially regulates growth and response of these two professional antigen presenting cell populations. Infected DCs may actually contribute to the active dissemination of the virus, whereas only small numbers of surviving pulmonary DCs should be able to reach the draining lymph nodes; however, these cells would have low stimulatory properties, thus aiding survival of the virus. The infected monocytes might also constitute a reservoir for HPIV3.

HPIV3 induces the expression of major histocompatibility complex (MHC) class I and class II molecules in human alveolar epithelial cells (Gao *et al.*, 1999). Although IFN-β is also induced and acts as an intermediate in this process, viral antigens contribute also to MHC induction. MHC class I induction is virus replication-independent, whereas infectious virions are required for induced expression of MHC class II molecules. Such an induction pattern could contribute to HPIV3 infection immunopathology by increasing CTL-mediated lysis of respiratory epithelium. Indeed, cell-mediated immune response to HPIV3 viral antigens has been reported to be increased among young children developing bronchiolitis (i.e. increased lysis of airway epithelial cells) compared to those experiencing only upper RTI (Collins *et al.*, 1995).

PIVs also show the ability to escape IFN-mediated antiviral immune responses. Type I IFN (IFN-α and IFN-β) responses are mediated by both STAT1 and STAT2 transcription factors, whereas type II (IFN-γ) uses only STAT1 as intermediate. It has been shown that the V protein of SV5 is responsible for blocking IFN antiviral responses in human cells by targeting STAT1 for degradation by the proteasome (Didcock *et al.*, 1999). Although practically all PIVs seem to resist interferon responses (Young *et al.*, 2000), there are differences in the mechanisms used by the individual members of the subfamily to achieve this. In particular, HPIV3, SeV and SV5 have been shown to block both type I and II IFN pathways, whereas HPIV2 is able to block only type I, by downregulating STAT2 (Young *et al.*, 2000). Accordingly, HPIV2 replication is severely impaired in IFN-γ pretreated cells (Andrejeva *et al.*, 2002). The inability of HPIV2 to block IFN-γ-mediated defence can give us a clue as to why HPIV2 infections are generally less severe than HPIV3-mediated ones (see Clinical Features). In addition, STAT2 seems to form an intracellular determinant of PIV host range, being an accessory to STAT1 degradation by certain PIVs in human cells. When human STAT2 was transfected into mouse cells it conferred STAT1 degradation ability and escape from type I response to SV5 in an otherwise refractory environment (Parisien *et al.*, 2002).

Finally, HPIV3 has been shown to induce type I IFN expression in human epithelial cells (Gao *et al.*, 2001), consistent with the reported elevated IFN levels following parainfluenza infection in children (Hall *et al.*, 1978). HPIV3-induced IFN-α/β inhibits signals downstream of CIITA mRNA accumulation, a transcription factor regulating the IFN-γ-induced MHC class II expression. On the other hand, HPIV3 antigens directly inhibit CIITA mRNA accumulation (Gao *et al.*, 2001), the overall effect being an inhibition of the IFN-γ-induced MHC class II expression in epithelial

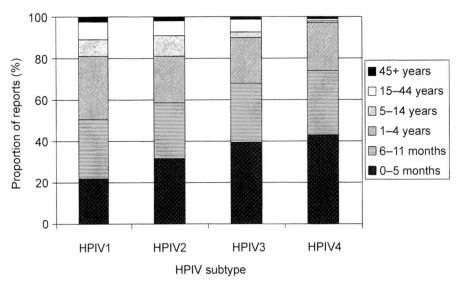

Figure 6.3 Age distribution of HPIV laboratory reports in England and Wales, 1985–1987. Adapted from Laurichesse *et al.*
(1999)

cells, i.e. the primary target of respiratory virus
replication (Gao *et al.*, 2001). This may result in
regulation of CD4$^+$ cell activation, in addition to PIV-
mediated regulation of macrophages, B cells and
dendritic cells.

EPIDEMIOLOGY

Parainfluenza viruses are second only to RSV as
leading causes of hospitalisation for RTI in young
children. It has been estimated that they account for
40% of acute paediatric LRTIs in cases where a viral
agent has been isolated (Glezen *et al.*, 1971) and for
20% of hospitalisations for paediatric respiratory
illnesses (Murphy *et al.*, 1988).

Of the human pathogens, HPIV1 and HPIV2 are
generally more associated with croup, upper RTI and
pharyngitis (Knott *et al.*, 1994), whereas HPIV3 is in
addition a major cause of infant bronchiolitis and is
also associated with the development of pneumonia in
susceptible subjects (Hall, 2001). HPIV4 subtypes
cause a rather mild illness, but lower respiratory tract
symptoms have been documented (Lindquist *et al.*,
1997).

HPIVs affect mainly the paediatric population.
Thus, HPIV infection was determined to be the cause
of 9% of paediatric admissions for acute RTIs over a
2 year period in England (Downham *et al.*, 1974).
Serological evidence suggests that almost 50% of

infants have been infected by HPIV3 by the time
they reach their first birthday (Parrot *et al.*, 1962). In
contrast, HPIV1 and HPIV2 are encountered more
frequently in toddlers and preschool children. By
collecting data from England and Wales for the period
1975–1997, Laurichesse *et al.* (1999) were able to
illustrate the different age distribution patterns of all
four HPIV subtypes (Figure 6.3). In contrast, they
could not find any significant differences in sex
distribution.

HPIV1 outbreaks are the most intense and well
defined of all human PIV species. They are well
correlated with sharp biennial rises in croup outbreaks
usually recorded in the autumn (Hall, 2001). HPIV2
outbreaks follow those of type 1, usually in a biennial
manner, and are generally less predictable; however, a
similar incidence has been recorded (Hall, 2001).
HPIV3 infections seem to be more frequent (Laurichesse *et al.*, 1999) and to occur yearly, with peaks of
isolates recorded during spring and summer. Outbreaks of this virus last longer than those of the other
members of the family (Hall, 2001). HPIV4 isolates are
rare and, accordingly, their seasonal pattern is less well
characterised. The patterns of isolations of HPIV1–
HPIV4 in England and Wales are illustrated in Figure
6.4 for the period 1975–1997 (Laurichesse *et al.*, 1999).

Croup incidence is associated more with HPIV1
epidemiology than with the other HPIV subtypes. In a
study conducted between winter and spring of 3
consecutive years in Canadian patients with croup,

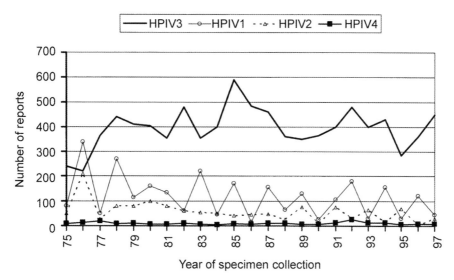

Figure 6.4 Distribution of HPIV1-3 isolates in England and Wales for the period 1975–1997. Adapted from Laurichesse *et al.* (1999)

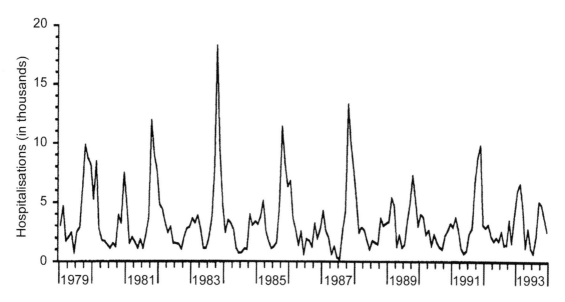

Figure 6.5 Collective data from croup hospitalisations (children aged <15 years) in the USA, 1979–1993. 22.5% of all croup hospitalisations per biennium and 36.7% in odd-numbered years can be attributed to HPIV1. Reproduced from Marx *et al.* (1997)

HPIV1 was isolated in 30.3% of the cases and HPIV3 in 3.5%. Peak monthly HPIV1 isolation occurred in November in this study and in January in another study of similar design (McLean, 2000).

By analysing croup hospitalisation collective data from the USA, Marx *et al.* (1997) confirmed the unique pattern of HPIV1 epidemics: HPIV1 has produced national epidemics of acute RTI in the USA in the odd-numbered years between 1979 and 1993, whereas it was rarely isolated in between the peaks. Notably, HPIV-1 was calculated to be responsible for ~18% of all cases in croup recorded and ~37% of all cases with

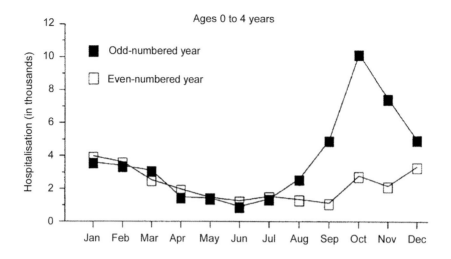

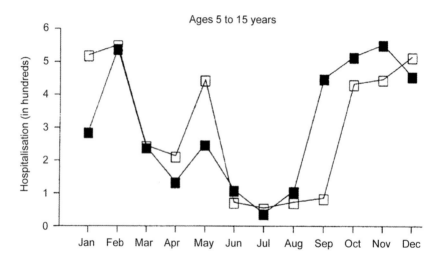

Figure 6.6 Seasonal distribution of croup during odd- and even-numbered years in US pediatric populations, 1979–1993. Reproduced from Marx *et al.* (1997)

determined aetiology, indicating the leading role of this HPIV subtype in the disease. While the major peaks of croup occurred biennially during October in odd-numbered years, minor peaks were produced annually around February (Figure 6.5). Interestingly, these trends were also age-dependent, with epidemics in children under 5 years closely following the biennial pattern, whereas in older individuals the annual winter peaks were equal in height to those of the autumn. In addition, there were no apparent differences between odd- and even-numbered years in the magnitude of the

autumn peaks (Figure 6.6). The pattern of the autumn peaks coincided well with peaks of HPIV1 isolation across the USA (Marx *et al.*, 1997). Accordingly, croup hospitalisations in years when HPIV1 was present were 18 000 more than in the 'inactive' years (annual mean 41 000). A study that included successive cohorts, followed over a period of 20 years (1974–1993) in Nashville, of 1429 otherwise healthy infants and young children less than 5 years of age, revealed that HPIV3 was the most common HPIV pathogen isolated from LRTI specimens (Reed *et al.*, 1997). In particular, HPIV3 accounted for 59%, whereas HPIV1 and HPIV2 accounted for 29% and 12%, respectively, of the parainfluenza isolates. In all, HPIV isolates represented 17.4% of all viral cultures that yielded a virus in this study, with 10% of the children having a symptomatic HPIV3 LRT infection. The higher incidence of HPIV3 infections was consistent with the annual epidemic pattern of HPIV3 isolation during this period, in contrast to the biennial outbreaks of HPIV1 and HPIV2 (see also Figure 6.4). In addition, in accordance with the data of Laurichesse et al. (1999; see Figure 6.3), HPIV3 was more frequently isolated from children aged 3–12 months, whereas the other two species were more common in the second year of life.

Another population-based prospective study suggested that during their respective epidemic seasons, HPIV1 and HPIV3, but not HPIV2, were among the most commonly detected infectious agents in adult patients hospitalised for lower RTI (together with RSV and influenza A and B) (Marx et al., 1999). Importantly, no HPIV1 and very few HPIV3 infections could be documented in between the epidemic seasons. Although similar rates of incidence were observed for HPIV1 and HPIV3 in this adult population in the epidemic seasons (2.5% and 3.2% of hospitalised patients, respectively), the likelihood of clinically serious disease was greater for HPIV3 infection. In contrast, the role of HPIV2 was emphasised in a study among hospitalised children with middle and lower RTIs, where it was suggested that HPIV2 is predominantly associated with inspiratory difficulty, as compared with HPIV1 and HPIV3 (Korppi et al., 1988).

Thus, epidemiological data have provided strong evidence documenting the association of parainfluenza virus with upper and lower LTI. However, they are all based on viral isolation and serological assays. Future studies thus might reveal a greater contribution of these viruses by using the efficient polymerase chain reaction (PCR)-based assays recently established (see Diagnosis).

CLINICAL FEATURES

As stated above, acute laryngotracheobronchitis (croup) is the major clinical manifestation and a hallmark feature of HPIV (especially HPIV1) infection in children. The syndrome is characterised by croupy cough, inspiratory stridor, cry or hoarse voice, difficulty during inspiration and indrawing of the chest wall in the subcostal, intercostal or supraclavicular areas (McLean, 2000). The majority of patients experience cough and runny nose a couple of days

before the onset of the disease but they do not develop marked fever. There are frequent rhonchi in the lungs, but no rales and, since the air entrance into the chest is inhibited, the breath sounds are generally reduced. Accordingly, diminished inflation of the lungs is revealed in some cases by radiology. In some cases there is also severe airway obstruction due to gross swelling of the epiglottis or the aryepiglottic folds of the larynx, that may require emergency tracheotomy to re-establish inspiration. Upon hospitalisation (usually 3–24 h after the onset of the clinical syndrome) the symptoms usually subside relatively quickly (1–2 days). Influenza, measles and chickenpox may also induce croup in paediatric patients.

Parainfluenza viruses have also been involved in lower RTIs and other complications of upper RTIs. 30–50% of the patients developing upper RTI due to parainfluenza infection may experience otitis media (Knott et al., 1994). 15% of HPIV infections also involve the lower respiratory tract, with some 2.8% of the patients requiring hospitalisation (Reed et al., 1997). A study analysing the prevalence of HPIV1 and HPIV2 in US children under 6 years of age, receiving emergency treatment and/or requiring admission due to lower RTIs during the fall of 1991, reported that PIVs were associated with croup (48%), bronchiolitis (10%), pneumonia (12%), cough with fever (29%) and wheeze with fever (19%) (Henrickson et al., 1994). HPIV association with bronchiolitis has also been clearly documented (Welliver et al., 1986; Hall, 2001). Pneumonia and bronchiolitis due to HPIV3 infection occur mainly in the first 6 months of life, as is also the case for RSV (Reed et al., 1997).

A report examining data collected over a period of 20 years, concerning immunocompetent children aged under 5 years with clinically significant RTI, revealed the absence of significant differences in clinical signs and symptoms between the three main HPIV serotypes. The most common symptoms were coryza and cough, with fewer than 10% of cases experiencing high body temperatures (Reed et al., 1997). The authors also could not find significant differences between upper and lower RTI among the subtypes, with lower RTIs being more rare than expected. In contrast, HPIV3 was more often associated with acute otitis than HPIV1 and HPIV2 combined (Reed et al., 1997).

Although HPIV infection is thought to concern mainly paediatric patients, it has been also associated with lower RTI in adults. Association of HPIV3 with adult croup has been recently documented, providing evidence suggesting that the disease may be severe in adults as well as in the paediatric population (Woo et al., 2000). Furthermore, in a prospective study among adults hospitalised during 1991–1992, HPIV1-mediated symptoms and disease included wheezing, rhonchi and one case of lobar pneumonia (Marx *et al.*, 1999). Wheezing and rhonchi were also recorded among HPIV3-infected patients and at rates significantly higher than those reported among patients experiencing a bacterial pneumonia (*C. pneumoniae*, *M. pneumoniae*, etc.). 27% of HPIV3-infected hospitalised patients developed lobar pneumonia.

Nosocomial spread of community-acquired parainfluenza viruses, introduced into transplantation units by staff or visitors, may cause severe infection of patients receiving immunosuppressive treatment following bone marrow transplantation. The severity depends on the degree of immunosuppression, the virus subtype, the presence of other infections and the timing of the infection (before or after transplantation, etc.) (Wendt and Hertz, 1995). A high mortality rate due to pneumonia has been reported for HPIV infections in cases of children and adults receiving bone marrow transplantation as well as in infants with combined immunodeficiency (Frank *et al.*, 1983; Wendt *et al.*, 1992). IFN-γ-deficient patients are also more susceptible to HPIV3 infection (Dorman *et al.*, 1999).

Although rare, parainfluenza infection has been also shown to affect tissues other than the respiratory tract, such as the central nervous system and brain. Thus, PIV has been isolated from children or adults with meningitis (Arguedas *et al.*, 1990; Arisoy *et al.*, 1993; Vreede *et al.*, 1992). Furthermore, the presence of PIV has also been documented in conditions such as Guillain–Barré and Reye's syndromes (Roman *et al.*, 1978; Powell *et al.* 1973).

DIAGNOSIS

Identification of parainfluenza viruses in clinical specimens can be achieved by detecting whole virus, viral proteins and viral RNA in clinical samples, as well as by investigating host antibody responses. Methods include: identification of the virion or viral proteins with the use of electronic microcopy or immunofluorescence, respectively; virus culture and identification based on cytopathic effects exerted on cultured cells; a variety of serology techniques to detect antibody responses; and detection of PIV genetic material by reverse transcriptase PCR (RT-PCR).

Nasopharyngeal secretions or throat swabs constitute the preferred specimens for all PIV detection methods, with the latter generally giving less satisfactory results (McLean, 2000). For children under 5 years of age a fine-bore catheter is passed through a nostril into the nasopharynx. Suction by a syringe externally attached to the catheter is then used for the collection of the sample. Older children and adults can undergo nasal aspiration or lavage, or can gargle 5–10 ml 0.15 mol/l saline and expel the fluid into appropriate containers.

Whole Virus Detection

For electron microscopic detection, microdrops of secretion or garglings are placed on carbon-coated electron microscope grids (300 mesh), dried in air and stained for 30 s in 2% phosphotungstic acid (McLean, 2000). Immediately after negative staining, electron microscopic examination can be performed and virions morphologically identified as paramyxoviruses (~140 nm total diameter, roughly spherical; see Structure) can be observed within 5–15 min. Although quick, this method requires, in addition, immunofluorescence for HPIV subtyping, and requires expert personnel.

Protein-based Methods

Immunofluorescence-based subtyping requires the centrifugation of nasopharyngeal secretions or garglings to precipitate material onto the cups of 12-cup Teflon-coated slides (McLean, 1982). Throat swabs can also be directly smeared onto cups that are then dried at 40°C and fixed for 10 min in acetone. Rabbit antisera or purified antibodies raised against HPIV (and if desired other viruses) can then be added as soluble minidrops to wells in the fixed slides. Following incubation at 37°C for 30 min, the slides are exposed to a secondary, fluoroscein-labelled antibody and counterstained with 0.01% naphthalene black in PBS. After extensive washing with PBS, the slides can be examined under a fluorescence microscope. Immunofluorescent foci in the cytoplasm of cells exposed to subtype specific antibody, which are absent when the specimen is incubated with heterologous antisera, documents serotype-specific HPIV infection of the patient. This method, when used in combination with electron microscopy, allows same-day confirmation of parainfluenza infection. However, the timing of sampling is of crucial importance, since acute infection, during which viral shedding is greatest, may have occurred before hospitalisation. In addition, the detection of antigen in nasal specimens of immunocompromised and elderly patients has been claimed to be a rather insensitive method (Sable and Hayden,

1995; Whimbley and Ghosh, 2000; Englund *et al.*, 1997).

In addition to conventional immunofluorescence microscopy, flow cytometry analysis has also been used for the detection of PIVs (Henrickson, 1995). Enzyme-linked, radio- and fluoroimmunoassay (EIA, RIA, FIA) techniques have been applied to PIV detection, showing sensitivities 75–95% with polyclonal sera (Henrickson, 1995). Optical immunoassay (OIA), a method applied for the detection of other viruses, has not been developed for the HPIVs to date.

Virus Culture

For the virus to be recovered by tissue culture techniques, nasopharyngeal secretions or throat swabs are resuspended in 2 ml cell culture medium containing 10% fetal bovine serum (FBS). Viral suspensions retain viability in this medium and can be kept, if necessary, for 24 h at 4°C before being transferred to tissue culture. For longer delays, freezing at −70°C is recommended. Centrifugation at 2000 × g for 10 min allows precipitation of bacteria and desquamated cells; supernatants containing the viral population can then be inoculated onto human fibroblast or primary monkey kidney (PMK) cell cultures. A good alternative to PMK cells, although less sensitive for primary isolation of HPIV1 and -2, is the monkey kidney-derived LLC-MK$_2$ continuous cell line. (Henrickson, 1995) Inoculation should be performed at both 37°C and 33°C, since some strains seem to prefer the lower temperature conditions prevailing in the upper respiratory tract. Most HPIV clinical isolates can be detected 10 days after initial inoculation.

Haemagglutinin containing viruses such as HPIVs and influenza viruses can then be identified by their ability to induce erythrocyte haemadsorption by infected cells. For the haemadsorption test, the supernatants should be removed and the monolayer exposed to 0.1% guinea-pig or avian erythrocytes suspended in 0.15 mol/l saline. Haemadsorption is then observed under a light microscope. By then adding 0.5% suspensions of guinea-pig or avian erythrocytes in saline to cells plated in 96-well plates and inoculated by two-fold serial dilution of viral preparations, the titre of specimens can be determined with precision (McLean, 2000).

Since all HPIVs and influenza viruses haemadsorb, serotyping (haemadsorption inhibition test; HAdI) is necessary for confirmation of the patient's virus type or subtype. To that end 250 μl suspensions containing 10 antibody units of antisera raised against each PIV and influenza serotype are mixed with the fresh, titrated viral isolate, diluted so that the latter contains four haemagglutinating doses. Since even in normal sera PIV-mediated haemagglutination-inhibiting activities are present, an inactivation step should be performed before the haemadsorption test. Such nonspecific activities are sensitive to heat or periodate treatment or incubation with receptor-destroying enzyme (RDE); the latter binds to and inactivates serum-derived PIV-binding activities (Canchola *et al.*, 1965; Smith *et al.*, 1975). After a 10 min incubation at room temperature, 0.5% suspensions of erythrocytes are added and the serotype against which the specific antiserum inhibits haemadsorption corresponds with the serotype of the viral isolate.

Alternatively, cells inoculated with specimen and showing haemadsorption can be removed from the plastic surface by pipetting and placing on Teflon-coated slides. Acetone fixed slides are incubated with anti-PIV antibodies for immunofluorescent detection as described above. The latter determination of PIV serotype can be completed within 3 h, whereas the haemadsorption inhibition assay requires 2 h. However, the rate-limiting step for both final procedures is prior tissue culture isolation, which usually needs 10 days to be completed, making this method complex and time-consuming.

Serological Techniques

The prerequisite for serological identification of PIV infection is collection of both acute phase and convalescent blood samples. The former should be collected as soon as possible after onset of the symptoms, whereas the latter is obtained, usually after 1–3 weeks, provided that any fever and all other associated symptoms have resolved. Sera should be separated from clots after collection and stored at −20°C for further processing. The paired sera should then be treated with heat and periodate or receptor-destroying enzyme to inactivate inhibitory substances and are applied as serial two-fold dilutions in haemagglutination inhibition (HI) tests against four haemagglutinating doses of each parainfluenza serotype (McLean, 2000). Virus infection is considered to be confirmed if antibody conversion from negative to positive can be documented. Alternatively, if both sera are positive, a four-fold difference in antibody titre is considered confirmation of serological evidence of infection with the respective PIV serotype. Although the final step of this method is quick (2 h), the requirement for a specimen during convalescence limits the usefulness of this method to retrospective diagnosis. Furthermore, this method is not that sensitive for young infants, where antibody may be detected only after recurrent infections in some cases (McLean, 2000).

Apart from HI antibodies, neutralising and complement-fixing antibodies can also be detected in patients' paired sera, although the latter method is thought not to be such a useful test for clinical diagnosis (McLean, 2000). For neutralisation tests, cultured cells should be inoculated with 100-tissue culture infective doses of PIV subtypes mixed with two-fold serial dilutions of patients' sera; 3 days later, haemadsorption assays should be inhibited by positive sera.

RIA and ELISA tests are also available for detection of antibody responses to detect HPIV infection, although they are not widely used.

RNA-based Diagnosis

Recently established RT-PCR protocols allow the specific detection of PIV genetic material from clinical specimens (Karron et al., 1994). PIVs are RNA viruses, therefore total RNA should first be extracted from nasopharyngeal secretions or throat swabs by standard molecular biology techniques. The specimens should be kept at $-70°C$ to avoid deterioration of the genomic material. A good practice is to store samples at $-70°C$ in appropriate virus transport medium (VTM) (e.g. Hanks' balanced salt solution enriched with 0.5% bovine serum albumin; Corne et al., 1999). If throat swabs are taken they can be broken directly into a denaturing solution to inactivate all RNAse enzyme activity and then stored or transported at room temperature (Carman et al., 2000). Extracted RNA is reverse-transcribed into cDNA and amplified by PCR, using serotype-specific primers that have been designed with the aid of computer software, usually against the HN or P coding regions of HPIVs 1–4, to exploit differences in nucleotide sequence occurring between species (Corne et al., 1999; Aguilar et al., 2000). Nucleotide diversity observed within each serotype (e.g. van Wyke Coelingh et al., 1988; Henrickson and Savatski, 1992) should also be taken into account, and areas of high homology are selected for serotype-specific primer pairs design. (Corne et al., 1999). The products (amplicons) have different sizes, usually within the range 100–1000 base pairs, depending on the serotype, and can be easily visualised under a UV transilluminator, following electrophoresis in a 1.5–2% agarose gel in the presence of the DNA dye ethidium bromide. This test can be readily accomplished within 1 working day, which is of importance for the effective treatment of patients. Multiplex RT-PCRs are also available that allow the simultaneous determination of HPIV1–HPIV3 (Corne et al., 1999) or all HPIV serotypes (Aguilar et al., 2000) from clinical samples.

In order to improve specificity and sensitivity, the amplicons can be hybridised with labelled synthesised DNA probes directed against regions of the amplicon. Alternatively, RT-PCR can be combined with enzyme immunoassay techniques (RT-PCR–EIA), consisting of hybridisation of the HPIV amplicon with biotinylated RNA probes generated against amplicon internal sequences (Karron et al., 1994). Moreover, PCR amplicons may be used as templates for a second PCR round, with primers designed against internal (nested) oligonucleotides located within the already amplified region. Nested RT-PCR protocols are usually characterised by increased sensitivity and are also required for subtyping in cases where first-round products do not discriminate between serotypes (Echevarria et al., 1998).

Amplified DNA species can also be sequenced and the diversity of individual serotypes within characteristic genes, such as HN, can be studied, providing valuable epidemiological information concerning particular outbreaks (Echevarria et al., 2000).

Finally, PIV RT-PCRs can be part of more extended multiplex protocols, allowing the simultaneous detection of additional respiratory pathogens (Fan et al., 1998; Hindiyeh et al., 2001; Kehl et al., 2001; Liolios et al., 2001; Freymuth et al., 1997; Grondahl et al., 1999). Such a multiplex method allowing the simultaneous detection of HPIV1–HPIV3 and other respiratory viruses (e.g. influenzas A and B, as well as RSVs A and B) has been recently developed and has achieved high sensitivity and specificity scores when tested in clinical samples (Hexaplex; Kehl et al., 2001). Thus, in addition to being quick and easy, it allows for the simultaneous detection of multiple pathogens. This highly sensitive test also permits the detection of PIVs in samples with low virus copy numbers, or viral RNA without live virus, both of which may be missed by conventional cell culture techniques (Fan et al., 1998). The detection limits of multiplex RT-PCR protocols can go down to one (1) $TCID_{50}$ for cultured PIV viruses (Corne et al., 1999) or 100–140 copies/ml, depending on the serotype (Fan et al., 1998). The sensitivity of this highly specific and rapid method is generally at least as high as combined tissue culture and immunofluorescence (Corne et al., 1999) and is sometimes even more sensitive (Aguilar et al., 2000;

Fan *et al.*, 1998). The ability to simultaneously detect additional respiratory pathogens renders thus multiplex RT-PCR a beneficial tool for PIV detection in clinical samples.

PREVENTION

There are no established HPIV vaccines available for clinical use at present. BPIV3 is a promising vaccine candidate against HPIV3, with which it shares sequence and antigenic similarities (Clements *et al.*, 1991a). The bovine subtype is characterised by attenuated replication in the respiratory tract of primates; however, it is immunogenic and protective against HPIV3 challenge and antibody responses are under investigation in Phase II clinical trials in infants (Lee *et al.*, 2001). The bovine attenuated PIV3 induced antibodies in seronegative children (Karron *et al.*, 1995a), while another attenuated, serially passaged, cold-adapted human PIV3 (Hall *et al.*, 1992) gave promising results in both seronegative and seropositive children and in infants aged 6 months–10 years (Karron *et al.*, 1995b).

In contrast to attenuated type 3 viruses, the type 1 SeV, although considered as a murine subtype, has been recently shown to replicate efficiently in the upper and lower respiratory tract of primates as well as human PIV1 (Skiadopoulos *et al.*, 2002a). This, together with the fact that this serotype was originally isolated from humans, has so far excluded its use as a vaccine in humans.

Recently, using reverse genetics, a recombinant infectious PIV virus was produced expressing the HN and F proteins of HPIV1 on the cold-adapted HPIV3 backbone mentioned above (Skiadopoulos *et al.*, 1999). This construct was shown to protect against HPIV1 challenge in primates (Skiadopoulos *et al.*, 2002b), while retaining its attenuated phenotype. In addition, by replacing the HPIV3 HN and F sequences with chimaeric open reading frames, encoding the HPIV2 ectodomains fused with the transmembrane and cytoplasmic domains of HPIV2, Skiadopoulos *et al.* (2002b) succeeded in generating a vaccine candidate against HPIV2.

This methodology allows inclusion of more than one antigenic viral glycoprotein in the attenuated backbone. Thus, a recombinant HPIV3 was generated that additionally expressed HN of HPIV1 and HPIV2; the resultant infectious virions conferred immunity against all three HPIVs in hamsters, while retaining the attenuated pattern of infection (Skiadopoulos *et al.*, 2002b). Further extension of the repertoire could include vaccination against other respiratory pathogens, such as RSV types A and B (Schmidt *et al.*, 2002). Clinical studies evaluating the clinical efficacy of such elegant recombinant vaccine candidates in humans are awaited with particular interest.

TREATMENT

A major problem limiting development and use of efficient therapeutic treatments is the lack of availability of a rapid and reliable diagnostic test. An additional obstacle seems to be that many clinicians do not recognise HPIV infections among the common pathogens in adult respiratory infections (Hall, 2001). The major clinical need is in young children with croup. Current therapy includes supportive care; children are usually placed in plastic tents supplied with cool, moist oxygen (croupette), and recovery usually occurs after 1–2 days (McLean, 2000). Intranosocomial prophylaxis is also important for the inhibition of further spread of the virus.

Studies investigating the action of steroids in mild to severe croup have been recently systematically reviewed and analysed (Moss *et al.*, 2002). Although smaller studies may bias results to show larger effects, it has been shown that nebulised steroids are effective in significantly reducing the severe manifestations of croup (e.g. improvement of croup scores by 5 h) in children attending the emergency departments of hospitals.

As stated above (e.g. Clinical Features), croup is not the only manifestation of HPIV-mediated disease. Some patients may develop tracheobronchitis, bronchiolitis or pneumonia, each one requiring specific treatment. Thus, excessive secretions may require emergency removal by bronchoscopic aspiration, whereas antibiotics are administered in bacterially complicated HPIV-triggered pneumonia.

HPIV replication and pathology are currently a target of potential drug inhibitors, synthetically generated or even derived from natural sources (Jiang *et al.*, 2001). The broad-spectrum antiviral agent ribavirin and its analogues are known to bind and inhibit HPIVs (Gabrielsen *et al.*, 1992; Ghose *et al.*, 1989). Aerosolised ribavirin, a synthetic guanosine analogue, has been used in immunocompromised patients for parainfluenza virus infections (Elizaga *et al.*, 2001; Englund *et al.*, 1997; Nichols *et al.*, 2001), however, the results were not impressive and further clinical trials are needed (Bowden, 1997). Sialic acid analogues, such as the 4-guanidino-Neu5Ac2en (GU-DANA; zanamivir) used for the treatment of influenza infections (Greengard *et al.*, 2000), also inhibit HN neuraminidase action and syncytial formation by HPIV3 (Porotto *et al.*, 2001) and are thus potential candidates as inhibitory agents of viral entry and cytopathology. However, PIV variants (HN mutants) with increased receptor binding avidity can escape the inhibitory effect of this agent (Murrell *et al.*, 2003). Recently, synthetically modified pyrimidine bases of uracil have been shown to specifically inhibit SeV replication (Saladino *et al.*, 2001). Whether this ability also holds for HPIV1 and other members of the family, as well as its clinical significance, remains to be elucidated.

REFERENCES

Adamko DJ, Yost BL, Gleich GJ *et al.* (1999) Ovalbumin sensitization changes the inflammatory response to subsequent parainfluenza infection. Eosinophils mediate airway hyperresponsiveness, m(2) muscarinic receptor dysfunction, and antiviral effects. *J Exp Med*, **190**, 1465–1478.

Aguilar JC, Perez-Brena MP, Garcia ML *et al.* (2000) Detection and identification of human parainfluenza viruses 1, 2, 3, and 4 in clinical samples of pediatric patients by multiplex reverse transcription-PCR. *J Clin Microbiol*, **38**, 1191–1195.

Ah-Tye C, Schwartz S, Huberman K *et al.* (1999) Virus-receptor interactions of human parainfluenza viruses types 1, 2 and 3. *Microb Pathog*, **27**, 329–336.

Andrejeva J, Young DF, Goodbourn S and Randall RE (2002) Degradation of STAT1 and STAT2 by the V proteins of simian virus 5 and human parainfluenza virus type 2, respectively: consequences for virus replication in the presence of α/β and γ interferons. *J Virol*, **76**, 2159–2167.

Arguedas A, Stutman HR and Blanding JG (1990) Parainfluenza type 3 meningitis. Report of two cases and review of the literature. *Clin Pediatr*, **29**, 175–178.

Arisoy ES, Demmler GJ, Thakar S and Doerr C (1993) Meningitis due to parainfluenza virus type 3: report of two cases and review. *Clin Infect Dis*, **17**, 995–997.

Bagai S and Lamb RA (1995) Quantitative measurement of paramyxovirus fusion: differences in requirements of glycoproteins between simian virus 5 and human parainfluenza virus 3 or Newcastle disease virus. *J Virol*, **69**, 6712–6719.

Bailly JE, McAuliffe JM, Skiadopoulos MH *et al.* (2000) Sequence determination and molecular analysis of two strains of bovine parainfluenza virus type 3 that are attenuated for primates. *Virus Genes*, **20**, 173–182.

Baker KA, Dutch RE, Lamb RA and Jardetzky TS (1999) Structural basis for paramyxovirus-mediated membrane fusion. *Mol Cell*, **3**, 309–319.

Bloom HH, Johnson KM, Jacobsen R and Chanock RM (1961) Recovery of parainfluenza viruses from adults with upper respiratory illness. *Am J Hyg*, **74**, 50–59.

Bonville CA, Rosenberg HF and Domachowske JB (1999) Macrophage inflammatory protein-1α and RANTES are present in nasal secretions during ongoing upper respiratory tract infection. *Pediatr Allerg Immunol*, **10**, 39–44.

Bose S and Banerjee AK (2002) Role of heparan sulfate in human parainfluenza virus type 3 infection. *Virology*, **298**, 73–83.

Bose S, Malur A and Banerjee AK (2001) Polarity of human parainfluenza virus type 3 infection in polarized human lung epithelial A549 cells: role of microfilament and microtubule. *J Virol*, **75**, 1984–1989.

Bousse T, Matrosovich T, Portner A *et al.* (2002) The long non-coding region of the human parainfluenza virus type 1 f gene contributes to the read-through transcription at the m–f gene junction. *J Virol*, **76**, 8244–8251.

Bousse T, Takimoto T, Murti KG and Portner A (1997) Elevated expression of the human parainfluenza virus type 1 F gene downregulates HN expression. *Virology*, **232**, 44–52.

Bowden RA (1997) Respiratory virus infections after marrow transplant: the Fred Hutchinson Cancer Research Center experience. *Am J Med*, **102**, 27–30; discussion 42–43.

Brady MT, Evans J and Cuartas J (1990) Survival and disinfection of parainfluenza viruses on environmental surfaces. *Am J Infect Control*, **18**, 18–23.

Cadd T, Garcin D, Tapparel C *et al.* (1996) The Sendai paramyxovirus accessory C proteins inhibit viral genome amplification in a promoter-specific fashion. *J Virol*, **70**, 5067–5074.

Calain P and Roux L (1993) The rule of six, a basic feature for efficient replication of Sendai virus defective interfering RNA. *J Virol*, **67**, 4822–4830.

Canchola JG, Chanock RM, Jeffries BC *et al.* (1965) Recovery and identification of human myxoviruses. *Bacteriol Rev*, **29**, 496–503.

Carman WF, Wallace LA, Walker J *et al.* (2000) Rapid virological surveillance of community influenza infection in general practice. *Br Med J*, **321**, 736–737.

Chanock RM, Bell JA and Parott RH (1961) Natural history of parainfluenza infection. In *Perspectives in Biology*, vol 2 (ed. Pollard M), pp 126–139. Burgess, Minneapolis, MN.

Clements ML, Belshe RB, King J *et al.* (1991a) Evaluation of bovine, cold-adapted human, and wild-type human parainfluenza type 3 viruses in adult volunteers and in chimpanzees. *J Clin Microbiol*, **29**, 1175–1182.

Clements ML, Belshe RB, King J *et al.* (1991b) Evaluation of bovine, cold-adapted human, and wild-type human parainfluenza type 3 viruses in adult volunteers and in chimpanzees. *J Clin Microbiol*, **29**, 1175–1182.

Collins PL, Chanock RM and McIntosh K (1995) Parainfluenza viruses. In *Field's Virology*, 3rd edn, vol 1 (eds Fields BN, Knipe DM and Howley PM), pp 1205–1241. Lippincott-Raven, Philadelphia, PA.

Corne JM, Green S, Sanderson G *et al* (1999) A multiplex RT-PCR for the detection of parainfluenza viruses 1-3 in clinical samples. *J Virol Methods*, **82**, 9–18.

Coronel EC, Takimoto T, Murti KG *et al.* (2001) Nucleocapsid incorporation into parainfluenza virus is regulated by specific interaction with matrix protein. *J Virol*, **75**, 1117–1123.

De BP, Hoffman MA, Choudhary S *et al.* (2000) Role of NH(2)- and COOH-terminal domains of the P protein of human parainfluenza virus type 3 in transcription and replication. *J Virol*, **74**, 5886–5895.

Didcock L, Young DF, Goodbourn S and Randall RE (1999) The V protein of simian virus 5 inhibits interferon signalling by targeting STAT1 for proteasome-mediated degradation. *J Virol*, **73**, 9928–9933.

Domachowske JB, Dyer KD, Bonville CA and Rosenberg HF (1998) Recombinant human eosinophil-derived neurotoxin/RNase 2 functions as an effective antiviral agent against respiratory syncytial virus. *J Infect Dis*, **177**, 1458–1464.

Dorman SE, Uzel G, Roesler J *et al.* (1999) Viral infections in interferon-γ receptor deficiency. *J Pediatr*, **135**, 640–643.

Downham MA, McQuillin J and Gardner PS (1974) Diagnosis and clinical significance of parainfluenza virus infections in children. *Arch Dis Child*, **49**, 8–15.

Durbin AP, Siew JW, Murphy BR and Collins PL (1997) Minimum protein requirements for transcription and RNA replication of a minigenome of human parainfluenza virus type 3 and evaluation of the rule of six. *Virology*, **234**, 74–83.

Echevarria JE, Erdman DD, Meissner HC and Anderson L (2000) Rapid molecular epidemiologic studies of human parainfluenza viruses based on direct sequencing of amplified DNA from a multiplex RT-PCR assay. *J Virol Methods*, **88**, 105–109.

Echevarria JE, Erdman DD, Swierkosz EM *et al.* (1998) Simultaneous detection and identification of human parainfluenza viruses 1, 2, and 3 from clinical samples by multiplex PCR. *J Clin Microbiol*, **36**, 1388–1391.

Elizaga J, Olavarria E, Apperley J *et al.* (2001) Parainfluenza virus 3 infection after stem cell transplant: relevance to outcome of rapid diagnosis and ribavirin treatment. *Clin Infect Dis*, **32**, 413–418.

Englund JA, Piedra PA and Whimbey E (1997) Prevention and treatment of respiratory syncytial virus and parainfluenza viruses in immunocompromised patients. *Am J Med*, **102**, 61–70; discussion 75–76.

Fan J, Henrickson KJ and Savatski LL (1998) Rapid simultaneous diagnosis of infections with respiratory syncytial viruses A and B, influenza viruses A and B, and human parainfluenza virus types 1, 2, and 3 by multiplex quantitative reverse transcription–polymerase chain reaction–enzyme hybridization assay (Hexaplex). *Clin Infect Dis*, **26**, 1397–1402.

Folkerts G, Verheyen AK, Geuens GM *et al.* (1993) Virus-induced changes in airway responsiveness, morphology, and histamine levels in guinea-pigs. *Am Rev Respir Dis*, **147**, 1569–1577.

Frank AL, Taber LH, Wells CR *et al.* (1981) Patterns of shedding of myxoviruses and paramyxoviruses in children. *J Infect Dis*, **144**, 433–441.

Frank JA Jr, Warren RW, Tucker JA *et al.* (1983) Disseminated parainfluenza infection in a child with severe combined immunodeficiency. *Am J Dis Child*, **137**, 1172–1174.

Freymuth F, Vabret A, Galateau-Salle F *et al.* (1997) Detection of respiratory syncytial virus, parainfluenzavirus 3, adenovirus and rhinovirus sequences in respiratory tract of infants by polymerase chain reaction and hybridization. *Clin Diagn Virol*, **8**, 31–40.

Fujii Y, Sakaguchi T, Kiyotani K *et al.* (2002) Involvement of the leader sequence in sendai virus pathogenesis revealed by recovery of a pathogenic field isolate from cDNA. *J Virol*, **76**, 8540–8547.

Gabrielsen B, Phelan MJ, Barthel-Rosa L *et al.* (1992) Synthesis and antiviral evaluation of N-carboxamidine-substituted analogues of 1-β-D-ribofuranosyl-1,2,4-tria-zole-3-carboxamidine hydrochloride. *J Med Chem*, **35**, 3231–3238.

Galinski MS, Troy RM and Banerjee AK (1992) RNA editing in the phosphoprotein gene of the human parainfluenza virus type 3. *Virology*, **186**, 543–550.

Gao J, Choudhary S, Banerjee AK and De BP (2000) Human parainfluenza virus type 3 upregulates ICAM-1 (CD54) expression in a cytokine-independent manner. *Gene Expr*, **9**, 115–121.

Gao J, De BP and Banerjee AK (1999) Human parainfluenza virus type 3 upregulates major histocompatibility complex class I and II expression on respiratory epithelial cells: involvement of a STAT1- and CIITA-independent pathway. *J Virol*, **73**, 1411–1418.

Gao J, De BP, Han Y *et al.* (2001) Human parainfluenza virus type 3 inhibits γ-interferon-induced major histocompatibility complex class II expression directly and by inducing α/β interferon. *J Virol*, **75**, 1124–1131.

Ghose AK, Crippen GM, Revankar GR *et al.* (1989) Analysis of the *in vitro* antiviral activity of certain ribonucleosides against parainfluenza virus using a novel computer-aided receptor modeling procedure. *J Med Chem*, **32**, 746–756.

Glezen WP, Frank AL, Taber LH and Kasel JA (1984) Parainfluenza virus type 3: seasonality and risk of infection and reinfection in young children. *J Infect Dis*, **150**, 851–857.

Glezen WP, Loda FA, Clyde WA Jr *et al.* (1971) Epidemiologic patterns of acute lower respiratory disease of children in a pediatric group practice. *J Pediatr*, **78**, 397–406.

Graziano FM, Tilton R, Hirth T *et al.* (1989) The effect of parainfluenza 3 infection on guinea pig basophil and lung mast cell histamine release. *Am Rev Respir Dis*, **139**, 715–720.

Greengard O, Poltoratskaia N, Leikina E *et al.* (2000) The anti-influenza virus agent 4-GU-DANA (zanamivir) inhibits cell fusion mediated by human parainfluenza virus and influenza virus HA. *J Virol*, **74**, 11108–11114.

Grondahl B, Puppe W, Hoppe A *et al.* (1999) Rapid identification of nine microorganisms causing acute respiratory tract infections by single-tube multiplex reverse transcription-PCR: feasibility study. *J Clin Microbiol*, **37**, 1–7.

Gross PA, Green RH and Curnen MG (1973) Persistent infection with parainfluenza type 3 virus in man. *Am Rev Respir Dis*, **108**, 894–898.

Gupta S, De BP, Drazba JA and Banerjee AK (1998) Involvement of actin microfilaments in the replication of human parainfluenza virus type 3. *J Virol*, **72**, 2655–2662.

Hall CB (2001) Respiratory syncytial virus and parainfluenza virus. *N Engl J Med*, **344**, 1917–1928.

Hall CB, Douglas RG Jr, Simons RL and Geiman JM (1978) Interferon production in children with respiratory syncytial, influenza, and parainfluenza virus infections. *J Pediatr*, **93**, 28–32.

Hall CB, Geiman JM, Breese BB and Douglas RG Jr (1977) Parainfluenza viral infections in children: correlation of shedding with clinical manifestations. *J Pediatr*, **91**, 194–198.

Hall SL, Stokes A, Tierney EL *et al.* (1992) Cold-passaged human parainfluenza type 3 viruses contain ts and non-ts mutations leading to attenuation in rhesus monkeys. *Virus Res*, **22**, 173–184.

Henrickson KJ (1995) Human parainfluenza viruses. In *Diagnostic Procedures for Viral, Rickettsial and Chlamydial Infections*, 7th edn (eds Lennette EH, Lennette DA and Lennette ET), pp 481–494. American Public Health Association, Washington, DC.

Henrickson KJ, Kuhn SM and Savatski LL (1994) Epidemiology and cost of infection with human parainfluenza virus types 1 and 2 in young children. *Clin Infect Dis*, **18**, 770–779.

Henrickson KJ and Savatski LL (1992) Genetic variation and evolution of human parainfluenza virus type 1 hemagglutinin neuraminidase: analysis of 12 clinical isolates. *J Infect Dis*, **166**, 995–1005.

Henrickson KJ and Savatski LL (1997) Antigenic structure, function, and evolution of the hemagglutinin-neuraminidase protein of human parainfluenza virus type 1. *J Infect Dis*, **176**, 867–875.

Hetherington SV, Watson AS, Scroggs RA and Portner A (1994) Human parainfluenza virus type 1 evolution combines co-circulation of strains and development of geographically restricted lineages. *J Infect Dis*, **169**, 248–252.

Hindiyeh M, Hillyard DR and Carroll KC (2001) Evaluation of the Prodesse Hexaplex multiplex PCR assay for direct detection of seven respiratory viruses in clinical specimens. *Am J Clin Pathol*, **116**, 218–224.

Hoffman MA and Banerjee AK (2000) Precise mapping of the replication and transcription promoters of human parainfluenza virus type 3. *Virology*, **269**, 201–211.

Holmgren J, Svennerholm L, Elwing H *et al.* (1980) Sendai virus receptor: proposed recognition structure based on binding to plastic-adsorbed gangliosides. *Proc Natl Acad Sci USA*, **77**, 1947–1950.

Horga MA, Gusella GL, Greengard O *et al.* (2000) Mechanism of interference mediated by human parainfluenza virus type 3 infection. *J Virol*, **74**, 11792–11799.

Hu XL, Ray R and Compans RW (1992) Functional interactions between the fusion protein and hemagglutinin-neuraminidase of human parainfluenza viruses. *J Virol*, **66**, 1528–1534.

Hua J, Liao MJ and Rashidbaigi A (1996) Cytokines induced by Sendai virus in human peripheral blood leukocytes. *J Leukoc Biol*, **60**, 125–128.

Huberman K, Peluso RW and Moscona A (1995) Hemagglutinin-neuraminidase of human parainfluenza 3: role of the neuraminidase in the viral life cycle. *Virology*, **214**, 294–300.

Jiang RW, Ma SC, But PP and Mak TC (2001) New antiviral cassane furanoditerpenes from *Caesalpinia minax*. *J Nat Prod*, **64**, 1266–1272.

Kapikian AZ, Chanock RM, Reichelderfer TE *et al.* (1961) Inoculation of human volunteers with parainfluenza virus type 3. *J Am Med Assoc*, **178**, 537–541.

Karron RA, Froehlich JL, Bobo L *et al.* (1994) Rapid detection of parainfluenza virus type 3 RNA in respiratory specimens: use of reverse transcription-PCR-enzyme immunoassay. *J Clin Microbiol*, **32**, 484–488.

Karron RA, Wright PF, Hall SL *et al.* (1995a) A live attenuated bovine parainfluenza virus type 3 vaccine is safe, infectious, immunogenic, and phenotypically stable in infants and children. *J Infect Dis*, **171**, 1107–1114.

Karron RA, Wright PF, Newman FK *et al.* (1995b) A live human parainfluenza type 3 virus vaccine is attenuated and immunogenic in healthy infants and children. *J Infect Dis*, **172**, 1445–1450.

Kawano M, Kaito M, Kozuka Y *et al.* (2001) Recovery of infectious human parainfluenza type 2 virus from cDNA clones and properties of the defective virus without V-specific cysteine-rich domain. *Virology*, **284**, 99–112.

Kehl SC, Henrickson KJ, Hua W and Fan J (2001) Evaluation of the Hexaplex assay for detection of respiratory viruses in children. *J Clin Microbiol*, **39**, 1696–1701.

Knott AM, Long CE and Hall CB (1994) Parainfluenza viral infections in pediatric outpatients: seasonal patterns and clinical characteristics. *Pediatr Infect Dis J*, **13**, 269–273.

Komada H, Ito M, Nishio M *et al.* (2000) N-glycosylation contributes to the limited cross-reactivity between hemagglutinin neuraminidase proteins of human parainfluenza virus type 4A and 4B. *Med Microbiol Immunol (Berl)*, **189**, 1–6.

Komada H, Kusagawa S, Orvell C *et al.* (1992) Antigenic diversity of human parainfluenza virus type 1 isolates and their immunological relationship with Sendai virus revealed by using monoclonal antibodies. *J Gen Virol*, **73**, 875–884.

Komada H, Tsurudome M, Ueda M *et al.* (1989) Isolation and characterization of monoclonal antibodies to human parainfluenza virus type 4 and their use in revealing antigenic relation between subtypes 4A and 4B. *Virology*, **171**, 28–37.

Korppi M, Halonen P, Kleemola M and Launiala K (1988) The role of parainfluenza viruses in inspiratory difficulties in children. *Acta Paediatr Scand*, **77**, 105–111.

Kurotani A, Kiyotani K, Kato A *et al.* (1998) Sendai virus C proteins are categorically non-essential gene products but silencing their expression severely impairs viral replication and pathogenesis. *Genes Cells*, **3**, 111–124.

Lamb RA (1993) Paramyxovirus fusion: a hypothesis for changes. *Virology*, **197**, 1–11.

Lamb RA and Choppin PW (1977) The synthesis of Sendai virus polypeptides in infected cells. II. Intracellular distribution of polypeptides. *Virology*, **81**, 371–381.

Lamb RA, Mahy BW and Choppin PW (1976) The synthesis of sendai virus polypeptides in infected cells. *Virology*, **69**, 116–131.

Laurichesse H, Dedman D, Watson JM and Zambon MC (1999) Epidemiological features of parainfluenza virus infections: laboratory surveillance in England and Wales, 1975–1997. *Eur J Epidemiol*, **15**, 475–484.

Lee MS, Greenberg DP, Yeh SH *et al.* (2001) Antibody responses to bovine parainfluenza virus type 3 (PIV3) vaccination and human PIV3 infection in young infants. *J Infect Dis*, **184**, 909–913.

Lefkowitz LB and Jackson GG (1966) Dual respiratory infection with parainfluenza and rhinovirus. The pathogenesis of transmitted infection in volunteers. *Am Rev Resp Dis*, **93**, 519–528.

Le Goffic R, Mouchel T, Aubry F *et al.* (2002) Production of the chemokines monocyte chemotactic protein-1, regulated on activation normal T cell expressed and secreted protein, growth-related oncogene, and interferon-γ-inducible protein-10 is induced by the Sendai virus in human and rat testicular cells *Endocrinology*, **143**, 1434–1440.

Lindquist SW, Darnule A, Istas A and Demmler GJ (1997) Parainfluenza virus type 4 infections in pediatric patients. *Pediatr Infect Dis J*, **16**, 34–38.

Liolios L, Jenney A, Spelman D *et al.* (2001) Comparison of a multiplex reverse transcription-PCR-enzyme hybridization assay with conventional viral culture and immunofluorescence techniques for the detection of seven viral respiratory pathogens. *J Clin Microbiol*, **39**, 2779–2783.

Marx A, Gary HE Jr, Marston BJ *et al.* (1999) Parainfluenza virus infection among adults hospitalized for lower respiratory tract infection. *Clin Infect Dis*, **29**, 134–140.

Marx A, Torok TJ, Holman RC *et al.* (1997) Pediatric hospitalizations for croup (laryngotracheobronchitis): biennial increases associated with human parainfluenza virus 1 epidemics. *J Infect Dis*, **176**, 1423–1427.

Matsuoka Y, Curran J, Pelet T *et al.* (1991) The P gene of human parainfluenza virus type 1 encodes P and C proteins but not a cysteine-rich V protein. *J Virol*, **65**, 3406–3410.

McLean DM (1982) *Immunological Investigation of Human Virus Diseases*. Churchill Livingstone, Edinburgh.

McLean DM (2000) Parainfluenza viruses. In *Principles and Practice of Clinical Virology*, 4th edn (eds Zuckerman AJ, Banatvala JE and Pattison JR), pp 279–291. Wiley, Chichester.

Mo XY, Sarawar SR and Doherty PC (1995) Induction of cytokines in mice with parainfluenza pneumonia. *J Virol*, **69**, 1288–1291.

Morrison TG and McGinnes LW (1989) Avian cells expressing the Newcastle disease virus hemagglutinin-neuraminidase protein are resistant to Newcastle disease virus infection. *Virology*, **171**, 10–17.

Moscona A and Peluso RW (1991) Fusion properties of cells persistently infected with human parainfluenza virus type 3: participation of hemagglutinin- neuraminidase in membrane fusion. *J Virol*, **65**, 2773–2777.

Moscona A and Peluso RW (1992) Fusion properties of cells infected with human parainfluenza virus type 3: receptor requirements for viral spread and virus-mediated membrane fusion. *J Virol*, **66**, 6280–6287.

Moscona A and Peluso RW (1993) Persistent infection with human parainfluenza virus 3 in CV-1 cells: analysis of the role of defective interfering particles. *Virology*, **194**, 399–402.

Moss WJ, Ryon JJ, Monze M *et al.* (2002) Suppression of human immunodeficiency virus replication during acute measles. *J Infect Dis*, **185**, 1035–1042.

Muchmore HG, Parkinson AJ, Humphries JE *et al.* (1981) Persistent parainfluenza virus shedding during isolation at the South Pole. *Nature*, **289**, 187–189.

Murphy BR, Prince GA, Collins PL *et al.* (1988) Current approaches to the development of vaccines effective against parainfluenza and respiratory syncytial viruses. *Virus Res*, **11**, 1–15.

Murrell M, Porotto M, Weber T *et al.* (2003) Mutations in human parainfluenza virus type 3 hemagglutinin-neuraminidase causing increased receptor binding activity and resistance to the transition state sialic acid analog 4-GU-DANA (Zanamivir). *J Virol*, **77**, 309–317.

Nichols WG, Corey L, Gooley T *et al.* (2001) Parainfluenza virus infections after hematopoietic stem cell transplantation: risk factors, response to antiviral therapy, and effect on transplant outcome. *Blood*, **98**, 573–578.

Ohgimoto S, Ohgimoto K, Niewiesk S *et al.* (2001) The haemagglutinin protein is an important determinant of measles virus tropism for dendritic cells *in vitro*. *J Gen Virol*, **82**, 1835–1844.

Parisien JP, Lau JF and Horvath CM (2002) STAT2 acts as a host range determinant for species-specific paramyxovirus interferon antagonism and simian virus 5 replication. *J Virol*, **76**, 6435–6441.

Parkinson AJ, Muchmore HG, Scott LV *et al.* (1979) Parainfluenzavirus upper respiratory tract illnesses in partially immune adult human subjects: a study at an Antarctic station. *Am J Epidemiol*, **110**, 753–763.

Parrot RH, Vargosko AJ, Kim HW *et al.* (1962) Acute respiratory diseases of viral etiology. III. Myxoviruses: parainfluenza. *Am J Publ Health*, **52**, 907–917.

Pelet T, Curran J and Kolakofsky D (1991) The P gene of bovine parainfluenza virus 3 expresses all three reading frames from a single mRNA editing site. *EMBO J*, **10**, 443–448.

Peramaki E, Salmi I, Kava T *et al.* (1991) Unilateral bronchiolitis obliterans organizing pneumonia and bronchoalveolar lavage neutrophilia in a patient with parainfluenza 3 virus infection. *Resp Med* **85**, 159–161.

Plotnicky-Gilquin H, Cyblat D, Aubry JP *et al.* (2001) Differential effects of parainfluenza virus type 3 on human monocytes and dendritic cells. *Virology*, **285**, 82–90.

Porotto M, Greengard O, Poltoratskaia N *et al.* (2001) Human parainfluenza virus type 3 HN-receptor interaction: effect of 4-guanidino-Neu5Ac2en on a neuraminidase-deficient variant. *J Virol*, **75**, 7481–7488.

Porter DD, Prince GA, Hemming VG and Porter HG (1991) Pathogenesis of human parainfluenza virus 3 infection in two species of cotton rats: *Sigmodon hispidus* develops bronchiolitis, while *Sigmodon fulviventer* develops interstitial pneumonia. *J Virol*, **65**, 103–111.

Powell HC, Rosenberg RN and McKellar B (1973) Reye's syndrome: isolation of parainfluenza virus. Report of three cases. *Arch Neurol*, **29**, 135–139.

Prince GA, Ottolini MG and Moscona A (2001) Contribution of the human parainfluenza virus type 3 HN-receptor interaction to pathogenesis *in vivo*. *J Virol*, **75**, 12446–12451.

Ray R and Compans RW (1986) Monoclonal antibodies reveal extensive antigenic differences between the hemagglutinin-neuraminidase glycoproteins of human and bovine parainfluenza 3 viruses. *Virology*, **148**, 232–236.

Reed G, Jewett PH, Thompson J *et al.* (1997) Epidemiology and clinical impact of parainfluenza virus infections in otherwise healthy infants and young children <5 years old. *J Infect Dis*, **175**, 807–813.

Roman G, Phillips CA and Poser CM (1978) Parainfluenza virus type 3: isolation from CSF of a patient with Guillain–Barré syndrome. *J Am Med Assoc*, **240**, 1613–1615.

Rydbeck R, Love A, Orvell C and Norrby E (1987) Antigenic analysis of human and bovine parainfluenza virus type 3 strains with monoclonal antibodies. *J Gen Virol*, **68**, 2153–2160.

Sable CA and Hayden FG (1995) Orthomyxoviral and paramyxoviral infections in transplant patients. *Infect Dis Clin North Am*, **9**, 987–1003.

Saladino R, Crestini C, Palamara AT *et al.* (2001) Synthesis, biological evaluation, and pharmacophore generation of uracil, 4(3*H*)-pyrimidinone, and uridine derivatives as potent and selective inhibitors of parainfluenza 1 (Sendai) virus. *J Med Chem*, **44**, 4554–4562.

Samal SK and Collins PL (1996) RNA replication by a respiratory syncytial virus RNA analog does not obey the rule of six and retains a non-viral trinucleotide extension at the leader end. *J Virol*, **70**, 5075–5082.

Scheerens J, Folkerts G, Van Der Linde H *et al.* (1999) Eotaxin levels and eosinophils in guinea pig bronchoalveolar lavage fluid are increased at the onset of a viral respiratory infection. *Clin Exp Allerg*, **29** (suppl 2), 74–77.

Schmidt AC, Wenzke DR, McAuliffe JM *et al.* (2002) Mucosal immunization of rhesus monkeys against respiratory syncytial virus subgroups A and B and human parainfluenza virus type 3 by using a live cDNA-derived vaccine based on a host range-attenuated bovine parainfluenza virus type 3 vector backbone. *J Virol*, **76**, 1089–1099.

Sieg S, King C, Huang Y and Kaplan D (1996) The role of interleukin-10 in the inhibition of T-cell proliferation and apoptosis mediated by parainfluenza virus type 3. *J Virol*, **70**, 4845–4848.

Sieg S, Muro-Cacho C, Robertson S *et al.* (1994) Infection and immunoregulation of T lymphocytes by parainfluenza virus type 3. *Proc Natl Acad Sci USA*, **91**, 6293–6297.

Sieg S, Xia L, Huang Y and Kaplan D (1995) Specific inhibition of granzyme B by parainfluenza virus type 3. *J Virol*, **69**, 3538–3541.

Skiadopoulos MH, Surman SR, Riggs JM *et al.* (2002a) Sendai virus, a murine parainfluenza virus type 1, replicates to a level similar to human PIV1 in the upper and lower respiratory tract of African green monkeys and chimpanzees. *Virology*, **297**, 153–160.

Skiadopoulos MH, Tao T, Surman SR *et al.* (1999) Generation of a parainfluenza virus type 1 vaccine candidate by replacing the HN and F glycoproteins of the live-attenuated PIV3 cp45 vaccine virus with their PIV1 counterparts. *Vaccine*, **18**, 503–510.

Skiadopoulos MH, Tatem JM, Surman SR *et al.* (2002b) The recombinant chimeric human parainfluenza virus type 1 vaccine candidate, rHPIV3-1cp45, is attenuated, immunogenic, and protective in African green monkeys. *Vaccine*, **20**, 1846–1852.

Smith GB, Purcell RH and Chanock RM (1967) Effect of amantadine hydrochloride on parainfluenza type 1 virus infections in adult volunteers. *Am Rev Resp Dis*, **95**, 689–690.

Smith WD, Wells PW, Burrells C and Dawson AM (1975) Immunoglobulins, antibodies and inhibitors of parainfluenza 3 virus in respiratory secretions of sheep. *Arch Virol*, **49**, 329–337.

Sorden SD and Castleman WL (1991) Brown Norway rats are high responders to bronchiolitis, pneumonia, and bronchiolar mastocytosis induced by parainfluenza virus. *Exp Lung Res*, **17**, 1025–1045.

Spriggs MK and Collins PL (1986a) Human parainfluenza virus type 3: messenger RNAs, polypeptide coding assignments, intergenic sequences, and genetic map. *J Virol*, **59**, 646–654.

Spriggs MK and Collins PL (1986b) Sequence analysis of the P and C protein genes of human parainfluenza virus type 3: patterns of amino acid sequence homology among paramyxovirus proteins. *J Gen Virol*, **67**, 2705–2719.

Stark JM, Huang YT, Carl J and Davis PB (1991) Infection of cultured human tracheal epithelial cells by human parainfluenza virus types 2 and 3. *J Virol Methods*, **31**, 31–45.

Suzuki T, Harada M, Suzuki Y and Matsumoto M (1984) Incorporation of sialoglycoprotein containing lacto-series oligosaccharides into chicken asialoerythrocyte membranes and restoration of receptor activity toward hemagglutinating virus of Japan (Sendai virus). *J Biochem (Tokyo)*, **95**, 1193–1200.

Suzuki T, Portner A, Scroggs RA *et al.* (2001) Receptor specificities of human respiroviruses. *J Virol*, **75**, 4604–4613.

Suzuki Y, Suzuki T, Matsunaga M and Matsumoto M (1985) Gangliosides as paramyxovirus receptor. Structural requirement of sialo-oligosaccharides in receptors for hemagglutinating virus of Japan (Sendai virus) and Newcastle disease virus. *J Biochem (Tokyo)*, **97**, 1189–1199.

Tao T and Ryan KW (1996) Host range restriction of parainfluenza virus growth occurs at the level of virus genome replication. *Virology*, **220**, 69–77.

Tapparel C and Roux L (1996) The efficiency of Sendai virus genome replication: the importance of the RNA primary sequence independent of terminal complementarity. *Virology*, **225**, 163–171.

Taylor CE, Osman HK, Turner AJ *et al.* (1998) Parainfluenza virus and respiratory syncytial virus infection in infants undergoing bone marrow transplantation for severe combined immunodeficiency. *Commun Dis Publ Health*, **1**, 202–209.

Tosi MF, Stark JM, Hamedani A *et al.* (1992a) Intercellular adhesion molecule-1 (ICAM-1)-dependent and ICAM-1-independent adhesive interactions between polymorphonuclear leukocytes and human airway epithelial cells infected with parainfluenza virus type 2. *J Immunol*, **149**, 3345–3349.

Tosi MF, Stark JM, Smith CW *et al.* (1992b) Induction of ICAM-1 expression on human airway epithelial cells by inflammatory cytokines: effects on neutrophil-epithelial cell adhesion. *Am J Respir Cell Mol Biol*, **7**, 214–221.

Tremonti LP, Lin JS and Jackson GG (1968) Neutralizing activity in nasal secretions and serum in resistance of volunteers to parainfluenza virus type 2. *J Immunol*, **101**, 572–577.

Trigg CJ, Nicholson KG, Wang JH *et al.* (1996) Bronchial inflammation and the common cold: a comparison of atopic and non-atopic individuals. *Clin Exp Allergy J Br Soc Allerg Clin Immunol*, **26**, 665–676.

Umeda M, Nojima S and Inoue K (1984) Activity of human erythrocyte gangliosides as a receptor to HVJ. *Virology*, **133**, 172–182.

van den Hoogen BG, Bestebroer TM, Osterhaus AD and Fouchier RA (2002) Analysis of the genomic sequence of a human metapneumovirus. *Virology*, **295**, 119–132.

van Oosterhout AJ, van Ark I, Folkerts G *et al.* (1995) Antibody to interleukin-5 inhibits virus-induced airway hyperresponsiveness to histamine in guinea-pigs. *Am J Respir Crit Care Med*, **151**, 177–183.

van Wyke Coelingh K and Tierney EL (1989) Antigenic and functional organization of human parainfluenza virus type 3 fusion glycoprotein. *J Virol*, **63**, 375–382.

van Wyke Coelingh KL, Winter CC, Jorgensen ED and Murphy BR (1987) Antigenic and structural properties of the hemagglutinin-neuraminidase glycoprotein of human parainfluenza virus type 3: sequence analysis of variants selected with monoclonal antibodies which inhibit infectivity, hemagglutination, and neuraminidase activities. *J Virol*, **61**, 1473–1477.

van Wyke Coelingh KL, Winter CC and Murphy BR (1988) Nucleotide and deduced amino acid sequence of hemagglutinin-neuraminidase genes of human type 3 parainfluenza viruses isolated from 1957 to 1983. *Virology*, **162**, 137–143.

Vreede RW, Schellekens H and Zuijderwijk M (1992) Isolation of parainfluenza virus type 3 from cerebrospinal fluid. *J Infect Dis*, **165**, 1166.

Welliver R, Wong DT, Choi TS and Ogra PL (1982) Natural history of parainfluenza virus infection in childhood. *J Pediatr*, **101**, 180–187.

Welliver RC, Wong DT, Sun M and McCarthy N (1986) Parainfluenza virus bronchiolitis. Epidemiology and pathogenesis. *Am J Dis Child*, **140**, 34–40.

Wendt CH and Hertz MI (1995) Respiratory syncytial virus and parainfluenza virus infections in the immunocompromised host. *Semin Respir Infect*, **10**, 224–231.

Wendt CH, Weisdorf DJ, Jordan MC *et al.* (1992) Parainfluenza virus respiratory infection after bone marrow transplantation. *N Engl J Med*, **326**, 921–926.

Whimbley E and Ghosh S (2000) Respiratory syncytial virus infections in immunocompromised adults. *Curr Clin Top Infect Dis*, **20**, 232–255.

Woo PC, Young K, Tsang KW *et al.* (2000) Adult croup: a rare but more severe condition. *Respiration*, **67**, 684–688.

Wybenga LE, Epand RF, Nir S *et al.* (1996) Glycophorin as a receptor for Sendai virus. *Biochemistry*, **35**, 9513–9518.

Young DF, Didcock L, Goodbourn S and Randall RE (2000) Paramyxoviridae use distinct virus-specific mechanisms to circumvent the interferon response. *Virology*, **269**, 383–390.

7

Respiratory Syncytial Virus

Caroline Breese Hall

University of Rochester School of Medicine, Rochester, NY, USA

INTRODUCTION

On the barely born
the Gods bestow
the most potential,
the greatest woe.
CBH

Respiratory syncytial virus (RSV) infections are a common and concerning conundrum. This ubiquitous agent is the major respiratory pathogen of young children, with life-threatening illness occurring most frequently in the first few months of life, and is commonly followed by the sequelae of recurrent wheezing. Worldwide acute respiratory disease is the leading cause of morbidity and mortality in young children, causing an estimated 4 million deaths each year in children within the first 5 years of life (Selwyn, 1990). Viruses are the most frequent cause, and RSV is the leading viral agent. Much about this virus, however, we do not understand—its immunity, its 'inner soul' and its control.

The initial name bestowed upon RSV was chimpanzee coryza agent (CCA), since it was first isolated in 1956 from a colony of chimpanzees suffering from the common cold. The human source of the pathogen was subsequently recognised by an identical agent being recovered from the respiratory secretions of an infant with pneumonia (Long strain) and from a child with laryngotracheobronchitis (Chanock *et al.*, 1957).

The virus has now been recognised throughout the world as causing widespread outbreaks of pneumonia and bronchiolitis in infants, and tracheobronchitis and upper respiratory tract infections in older children and adults. In temperate climates the virus produces yearly outbreaks in the winter to early spring. The predictability of its pattern of activity is singular among respiratory viruses.

THE VIRUS

RSV belongs to the family *Paramyxoviridae* and is classified in the genus *Pneumovirus*. In size, RSV lies between the larger paramyxoviruses and the smaller influenza viruses. RSV is an enveloped RNA virus with non-segmented, single-stranded, negative-sense genome. The two large envelope glycoproteins, which are integral to the immunity and pathogenesis, project from the surface, giving the envelope a thistle-like appearance (Figure 7.1) (Collins *et al.*, 1996).

The RSV genome encodes 11 proteins; eight are structural (L, G, F, N, P, M, M2-1 and SH) and two are non-structural (NS1 and NS2). The function of the 11th protein, M2-2, is not yet defined. The glycosylated F (fusion) and G (attachment) proteins and the small non-glycosylated hydrophobic protein, SH (or 1A), are transmembrane surface proteins. The viral capsid proteins associated with the mRNA of the genome are the nucleoprotein (N), the phosphoprotein (P) and the polymerase (L). The matrix proteins present in RSV are the non-glycosylated, M, M2-1 and M2-2 (membrane-associated proteins). The genome of the A2 strain of RSV is composed of 15 222 nucleotides, and the complete sequence of the A2 strain gene has now been delineated.

The roles of these proteins in eliciting an immune response and in protection still require further study. F and G are the major protective antigens and evoke

Principles and Practice of Clinical Virology, Fifth Edition. Edited by A. J. Zuckerman, J. E. Banatvala, J. R. Pattison, P. D. Griffiths and B. D. Schoub
© 2004 John Wiley & Sons Ltd   ISBN 0 470 84338 1

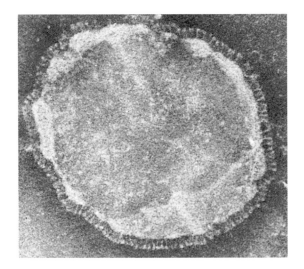

Figure 7.1 Negative contrast electron micrograph of RSV. The fringed envelope is variable in shape. The surface projections are about 15 nm long and the envelope contains a helical nucleocapsid which may occasionally be visible (negative contrast, 3% potassium phosphotungstate, pH 7.0; ×200 000). Courtesy of Professor C.R. Madeley

after initial RSV infection, but the response to the G protein is more variable. In young infants, the heavily glycosylated G protein is a poorer immunogen, and pre-existing maternal antibody results in a greater degree of dampening of the infant's own antibody response.

Antigenic variation among strains of RSV has resulted in the two major strain groups, designated A and B, which have been delineated on the basis of their reactions with monoclonal and polyclonal antisera. The major antigenic differences between these two strain groups have been linked to the G protein (Johnson *et al.*, 1987). The amino acid homology between G proteins of the two strain groups is ∼55%, and the antigenic relatedness is only 3–7%. The F protein, on the other hand, is relatively conserved, as are the N, P, M2, NS1 and NS2 proteins. The prototype A and B strains exhibit greater than 90% amino acid homology. Intra-group variations also occur, with an amino acid diversity for the G protein within the group varying from about 12% for group B to about 20% for group A (Cane and Pringle, 1995, 2001).

In tissue culture, RSV produces a characteristic syncytial appearance with eosinophilic cytoplasmic inclusions. RSV has a growth cycle which, after inoculation, consists of a period of adsorption of 2 h, followed by an eclipse period of 12 h. The subsequent log phase of replication of the new virus lasts for approximately 10 h. At the time when maximal quantities of virus are obtained, about half of the virus remains cell-associated on the surface of the cell.

neutralising antibodies (Table 7.1). The F protein also evokes fusion inhibiting antibodies, probably independent of the neutralisation activity (West *et al.*, 1994). Antibody to the F protein also provides heterologous immunity to both strain groups, whereas antibody to G affords little protection against heterologous strains. Infants are able to produce both F and G antibody

Table 7.1 Respiratory syncytial virus (RSV)

Viral proteins		Functions
Structural		
Surface		
F	Fusion	Penetration; major protection antigen
G	Attachment	Viral attachment; major protective antigen
SH (1A)	Small hydrophobic	Unknown
Matrix		
M	Matrix	? Mediates nucleocapsid to envelope
M2-1	Small envelope	Transcriptional regulation; unique to pneumoviruses
M2-2	Small envelope	Unknown
Nucleocapsid-associated		
N, NP	Nucleoprotein	Major RNA-binding nucleocapsid protein
P	Phosphoprotein	Major phosphorylated protein, RNA-dependent RNA polymerase activity
L	Large polymerase complex	Large nucleocapsid-associated protein; major polymerase subunit; RNA-dependent RNA polymerase activity
Non-structural		
NS1(1C)	Non-structural	Function unknown, unique to pneumoviruses
NS2(1B)	Non-structural	Function unknown, unique to pneumoviruses

Reproduced by permission from Hall (2001b).

Under certain conditions, such as repeated high passage, continuous infection may develop, which is associated with a diminished amount of cell-free virus and a loss of the characteristic cytopathic effect.

EPIDEMIOLOGY

RSV has a global distribution and an epidemic personality. Its seasonal pattern (Figure 7.2) is distinctive in that it predictably produces a sizeable outbreak of infections each year (Kim *et al.*, 1973). However, the timing and length of the outbreaks of RSV vary according to the geography. Warmer climates tend to have more prolonged outbreaks with less pronounced peaks of activity. In the UK and the temperate parts of the USA, the peak period of RSV activity generally has occurred from January to March, and in the USA RSV activity usually lasts for 20 or more weeks, stretching from November to May (CDC, 2002b).

The role of strain variation in the epidemiology, severity and clinical impact of an RSV outbreak remains unclear. Strains from both groups appear to circulate concurrently, although the proportion from each group may vary by year and locale (Hall *et al.*, 1990; Cane, 2001). In most areas in which it has been examined, A strains tend to dominate and outbreaks composed almost entirely of B strains are uncommon. Studies of strains from cities across the USA have shown substantial annual differences suggesting that the more influencing factors may be local rather than national (Anderson *et al.*, 1991). Homotypic immunity to previous strains may also play a role, as several

distinct, but varying, genotypes within a strain group appear to predominate each year in a community (Peret *et al.*, 1998; Cane, 2001). Some, but not all, evidence has suggested that the magnitude of an outbreak and the severity of the clinical illness are greater with A strain infections (Hall *et al.*, 1990; McConnochie *et al.*, 1990; Toms, 1990).

In most places the size of the annual RSV outbreak will fluctuate, with alternating years being more severe in some areas. Nevertheless, over 11 consecutive years the number of hospital admissions for children with RSV lower respiratory tract disease in Washington, DC, did not vary more than 2.7-fold, demonstrating the consistent and persistent impact of this virus (Kim *et al.*, 1973). Furthermore, when RSV attains its peak activity in a community, it is usually the solo actor among the company of major respiratory viruses. Other epidemic pathogens, such as influenza and parainfluenza viruses, tend to precede or follow the RSV outbreak, but may coincide occasionally.

Several generalisations may be made about the clinical epidemiology of RSV: (a) RSV is highly contagious; (b) lower respiratory tract disease associated with primary infection is almost entirely confined to the child under 3 years of age; (c) lower respiratory tract disease during the first couple of weeks of life is relatively uncommon compared to the subsequent 6–9 months; and (d) reinfections are frequent throughout life (Henderson *et al.*, 1979; Glezen *et al.*, 1986; Hall *et al.*, 1991).

Fifty per cent or more of infants have been estimated to acquire RSV infection during their first year of exposure to RSV, and approximately 40% of these infections will result in lower respiratory tract disease.

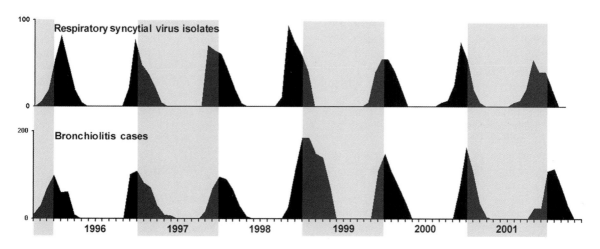

Figure 7.2.

Essentially, all children have been infected with RSV during the first 3 years of life. In a prospective longitudinal study of families in Houston, Texas, Glezen *et al.* (1986) showed that 69% of infants in the first year of life were infected with RSV, and one-third of those infections were associated with lower respiratory tract disease. In the second year of life, 83% of the infants acquired RSV infection and 16% had lower respiratory tract disease. Even during the third and fourth years of life, one-third to one-half of the children were infected with RSV, with lower respiratory tract disease occurring in about one-quarter (Glezen *et al.*, 1986). The attack rate in day care centres is even higher, with 65–98% of the children becoming infected during each of the first 3 years of life and up to one-half of the infections being manifest as lower respiratory tract disease (Henderson *et al.*, 1979). Recurrent infections, therefore, are not only common but may occur within a year.

RSV appears to spread with equal facility and alacrity on hospital wards housing young children (Hall *et al.*, 1979; Hall, 2000a; Berner *et al.*, 2001; Goldmann, 2001). The properties of RSV explain why it has been a major nosocomial hazard on paediatric wards. Epidemics occur yearly, resulting in the admission of a large number of young infants with primary infection who tend to shed virus in high titres and sometimes for prolonged periods. Those in contact with these infants admitted with RSV lower respiratory tract disease, no matter what their age, compose a large susceptible population, as immunity is not durable. Most of these cross-infections result in symptomatic illness, and about half will involve the lower respiratory tract. The morbidity, cost, and mortality may be high, particularly in young children with underlying prematurity, cardiopulmonary, and immunodeficiency diseases (Hall *et al.*, 1979, 1986; Hall, 2000a; Isaacs, 1995; Bar-on and Zanga, 1996; Berner *et al.*, 2001; Patel *et al.*, 2001; Weisman, 2003). Early recognition that RSV activity is present in the community and institution of appropriate infection control measures have been effective in reducing nosocomial infection in contact infants from rates as high as 40–45% (Hall, 1983; Goldmann, 2001; Greenough, 2001).

RSV nosocomial infections may also involve both staff and adult patients. In immunocompromised patients, especially transplant recipients, RSV infection tends to be serious and difficult to control (Englund *et al.*, 1991; Ljungman, 1997; Whimbey *et al.*, 1997; Champlin and Whimbey, 2001; Goldmann, 2001). Children with mild colds visiting relatives who are patients are often the source. In compromised patients, nosocomially acquired RSV infection frequently is not recognised as being caused by RSV but is thought to be one of the opportunistic infections to which such patients are prone and which often have similar clinical manifestations. The outcome, however, may be as devastating and even fatal.

Hospital personnel may also have a high rate of RSV infection, acquired nosocomially or in the community, which may appear insignificant as, frequently, it is mild enough that absence from work is not required (Hall, 1983). Yet hospital staff may be integral to the continued spread of RSV on wards housing children or adults.

The spread of RSV appears to require close contact with infectious secretions, either by large particle aerosols or by fomites (Hall, 1983). Small particle aerosols, which can traverse greater distances, appear to be an infrequent mode of transmission for RSV. Hospital staff are apt to spread the virus by touching contaminated secretions or objects while caring for an infected patient. Self-inoculation may then occur by the inadvertent rubbing of their eyes or nose, the major portals of entry for RSV. RSV may remain infectious on skin for enough time to allow it to be transmitted by self-inoculation, and to other individuals via contaminated hands. This underscores the observation that good hand washing is the single most effective means of controlling the spread of RSV. This may be accomplished by traditional washing methods with soap and water and by the more recently preferred alcohol-based hand cleansers that provide extended protection (CDC, 2002a).

PATHOGENESIS

The incubation period for RSV is usually 3–6 days, but can be 2–8 days. Inoculation of the virus occurs through the upper respiratory tract, primarily the eyes or nose (Hall, 1983). The virus subsequently spreads along the epithelium of the respiratory tract, mostly by cell-to-cell transfer of the virus along intracytoplasmic bridges. As the virus spreads to the lower respiratory tract it may produce bronchiolitis and/or pneumonia.

Pathology

Early in bronchiolitis a peribronchiolar inflammation with lymphocytes occurs, and the walls, submucosa and adventitial tissue appear oedematous (Figure 7.3) (Hall, 2000b). This progresses to the characteristic necrosis and sloughing of the bronchiolar epithelium, which may also be associated with a proliferative response of the epithelium. Plugging of these small airways results from the sloughed, necrotic material leading to obstruction of the flow of air, the hallmark of bronchiolitis. The tiny lumina of an infant's airways are particularly prone to obstruction from such inflammatory exudate and increased secretion of mucus.

If the bronchiolar lumina are incompletely obstructed, air trapping will occur distal to the sites of partial occlusion. Similar to a ball-and-valve mechanism, airflow is less impeded during the negative pressure of the infant's inspiration, but with the increased pressure of expiration, the airway lumen narrows, causing greater or complete obstruction to the flow of air. The trapped air causes the characteristic hyperinflation of bronchiolitis, which, when adsorbed, results in multiple areas of focal atelectasis.

Resolution of these pathological changes may take weeks. Although the bronchiolar epithelium may show signs of regeneration in 3–4 days, ciliated cells can rarely be found within the first 2 weeks. Other changes in the submucosal glands and types of cells in the airway may persist for even longer periods.

The pathological findings of bronchiolitis may progress or coexist with those of pneumonia during RSV infection. In the latter, infiltration of the interstitial tissue with mononuclear cells is seen. The subsequent oedema and necrosis of the parenchyma result in the filling and collapse of the alveoli.

Immunity

No-one appears to escape infection with RSV. Almost all infections are acquired during the first 3 years of life and essentially all adults possess specific antibody. Hence, passive antibody is present in all newborns and in young infants—the age at which the most severe RSV disease occurs. Lower respiratory tract disease from RSV appears to be limited generally to the first 3 years of life (Henderson *et al.*, 1979; Glezen *et al.*, 1986). Repeated infections may occur throughout life, but generally after 3 years of age they are milder, consisting of upper respiratory tract infections or bronchitis (Hall *et al.*, 1991). Repeated infections may also occur during the first 3 years of life, commonly during the next community outbreak, but even in these young children, second infections are rarely as symptomatic as primary infection. Immunity, although not durable, does afford protection against lower respiratory tract disease with time. The explanation of this is of much recent interest and expanding research.

The normal immune response to primary RSV infection is associated with a specific, but transitory,

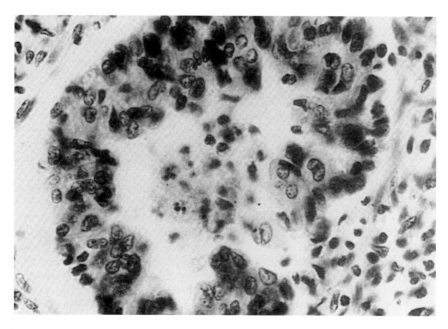

Figure 7.3 Pathological findings of an infant dying with RSV bronchiolitis. The wall of the bronchiole appears inflamed and oedematous and sloughed, necrotic material fills the lumen in the small airway

serum IgM antibody response. IgG antibody is subsequently detected in about the second week after infection, which tends to diminish after 1–2 months. The neutralising antibody response of young infants may be poor and responses to the F and G proteins diminished. These proteins are glycosylated, especially the G protein, and thus are poor immunogens. Maternal antibody also can interfere with the antibody response in infants. An IgA serum antibody response in young infants may not be detectable. After repeated infection an anamnestic response generally occurs in all three immunoglobulin classes.

Specific secretory antibody has also been identified in the secretions of infected infants. IgA, IgG and IgM antibodies bound to epithelial cells and free in nasal secretions have been identified during the course of infection.

Systemic and local cell-mediated immune responses appear to be key to the severity and recovery from RSV infection. This is supported by the observation that children and adults who have deficient cell-mediated responses tend to have prolonged, severe and sometimes fatal infection with RSV (Jarvis et al., 1983; Hall et al., 1986; Champlin and Whimbey, 2001; Ljungman, 1997; Small et al., 2002).

Recognition that the immune response to RSV may be integral in the pathogenesis of disease, indeed more important than the cytopathology engendered by direct viral invasion, came initially from studies aimed at explaining the experience with the first RSV vaccine, the formalin-inactivated vaccine, developed in the 1960s, and second, by the similar characteristics of RSV bronchiolitis and asthma (Welliver, 2000; Openshaw et al., 2003) (see Complications, below).

In the trials of this first vaccine for RSV, those infants who received the formalin-inactivated vaccine, when subsequently exposed to the wild virus, developed more severe disease than did those children who had not received the RSV vaccine (Chin et al., 1969; Fulginiti et al., 1969; Kapikian et al., 1969; Kim et al., 1969). Yet these vaccinees did evoke high levels of circulating antibody to the F and G proteins, measured by enzyme-linked immunosorbent assay, but low levels of neutralising antibody. This suggested a detrimental effect of the formalin on the neutralising epitopes of the surface glycoproteins (Murphy et al., 1986). Furthermore, pathological studies of the vaccinees who unfortunately died with severe RSV infection showed peribronchiolar infiltration and increased levels of eosinophils in the lung (Chin et al., 1969).

Subsequent studies have offered a potential explanation for the abnormal response in the recipients of the inactivated vaccine by delineating the divergent cellular responses elicited by live RSV infection compared to that from inactivated or killed RSV (Graham et al., 1991a, 1993; Bright et al., 1995; Toms, 1995; Mobbs et al., 2002). Live RSV, as with other natural live viral infections, characteristically evokes a Th1 helper cell response, which is associated with IL-2 and IFN-γ production, as well as IgG$_{2a}$ neutralising antibody and CD8$^+$ cytotoxic T cells (CTL). Inactivated RSV and other non-replicating antigens, on the other hand, usually elicit a Th2 cytokine pattern (i.e. IL-4, IL-5, IL-6, IL-10 and IL-13), which promotes the synthesis of IgE and elicits an eosinophilic response in the lungs. The formalin-inactivated vaccine, therefore, may have altered the usual immune response evoked by natural RSV infection to an abnormal one, producing primarily a Th2 type response and affecting multiple components of the immune system. However, analysis of the cytokines present in the respiratory secretions of children with RSV disease have not been closely correlated with the degree of severity of the RSV infection (Welliver et al., 2002).

Animal studies, primarily in BALB/c mice, have further explored and enhanced the role of CD4$^+$ T cells in mediating the immunopathology and exacerbation of RSV disease (Graham et al., 1991b; Alwan et al., 1992; Alwan and Openshaw, 1993). In these animal models the augmented pathology resulting from the formalin-inactivated vaccine was reproduced by priming the mice with either the formalin-inactivated vaccine or with the G glycoprotein expressed by a recombinant vaccinia virus followed by challenge with live RSV (Connors et al., 1992; Openshaw et al., 1992; Tang and Graham, 1994; Waris et al., 1996).

In the same model the F protein or matrix (M2 proteins) could also elicit the pathology characteristic of a memory T cell response in the lung, but the eosinophilia associated with immunisation with the G protein did not occur (Openshaw et al., 1992; Alwan and Openshaw, 1993). These findings suggest that the G protein generates a strong memory response of G protein-specific CD4$^+$ T cells, but not an adequate MHC class 1 restricted CD8$^+$ T cell response. The F protein, on the other hand, does induce a MHC class 1 restricted CTL and Th1 response, but not the Th2 response of CD4$^+$ T cells (Srikiatkhachorn and Braciale, 1997b; Srikiatkhachorn et al., 1999).

The memory response to the G protein in these mice produced a mixture of Th1 and Th2 cytokine-secreting cells, which has also been noted in children hospitalised with RSV infection (Tripp et al., 2002). Thus, a Th2 vs. Th1 response cannot be the full explanation of the immunopathology of RSV disease. Indeed, further studies have suggested that RSV infection may result in a selective priming of a small subset of virus-specific CD4$^+$ T cells, which may be modified by the CD8$^+$ T cell response, and the IFN-γ that is produced via the CD8$^+$ T cell response may be necessary to inhibit the CD4$^+$ T cell eosinophilic response in the lung (Alwan et al., 1994; Hussell et al., 1997; Srikiatkhachorn and Braciale, 1997a). However, in RSV infection this CD8$^+$ T cell response in the lung may be impaired, thus resulting in the more dominant expression of the small set of specific CD4$^+$ T cells elicited.

Many of the recent studies on the immunopathogenesis of RSV infection, as noted above, have focused on the T cell cytokine response, but the immune response to RSV is likely modulated through multiple mechanisms, including neuronal pathways, which then result in selective impairment of both the initial and memory immune responses (van Schaik et al., 2000; Piedimonte, 2002b, 2003). This may partially explain the conundrum of the lack of durable immunity and repeated infections as these potentially variable and selective impairments of the immune response may provide incomplete, but some, protection and allow reinfections of less severity than that of primary infection to occur. Furthermore, the spectrum of impaired functions may be genetically influenced, helping to explain why some children have severe disease and some have recurrent episodes of wheezing.

CLINICAL FEATURES

Infection in Infants and Young Children

The importance of RSV as a cause of lower respiratory tract disease in the young is illustrated by the observation that the periods of peak occurrence of pneumonia and bronchiolitis in young children signal the presence of RSV in the community. RSV has been reported in various studies as causing 10% of croup cases, 5–40% of the pneumonias and bronchitis in young children, and 50–90% of the cases of bronchiolitis. In the USA the estimated hospitalisation rate annually for bronchiolitis attributed to RSV is 51 000–82 000 children within the first year of life and 62 000–100 000 children within the first 5 years of life (Shay et al., 1999). RSV pneumonia contributes another 11 000–44 000 hospitalisations for children under 1 year of age. Worldwide, RSV is estimated to cause 600 000–1 million deaths among children < 5 years of age (Simoes, 1999). In the UK approximately 3% of each year's birth cohort, approximately 20 000 infants, are admitted for bronchiolitis every winter, and 3% of

these children need assisted ventilation (Sharland and Bedford-Russell, 2001). Similar admission rates for bronchiolitis have been estimated for Europe, Australia and North America. However, children with high-risk conditions may have substantially higher rates of admission (Meissner, 2003; Simoes and Carbonell-Estrany, 2003; Weisman, 2003). In the UK and North America, readmission rates for RSV bronchiolitis of premature infants (< 32 weeks gestation) have been reported as about 6–8% and 12–17% for infants with chronic lung disease. The mortality from RSV bronchiolitis, nevertheless, has been significantly reduced in recent years to an estimated 0.13% (Sharland and Bedford-Russell, 2001; PREVENT Study Group, 1997).

Primary RSV Infection

The first RSV infection is almost always symptomatic, but may be as mild as a common cold or as severe as a life-threatening lower respiratory tract infection. The manifestations of RSV infection initially observed in infants are usually those of a febrile upper respiratory tract infection. Lower respiratory tract involvement commonly becomes evident within several days. Although fever is common during the early phase of the illness, the infant may be afebrile by the time the lower respiratory tract disease becomes prominent and hospitalisation is undertaken.

The harbinger of the lower respiratory tract disease is often a worsening cough. As the disease progresses, tachypnoea, and dyspnoea develop, overtly marked by retractions of the chest wall. The hallmarks of bronchiolitis are wheezing and hyperinflation, often associated with a strikingly elevated respiratory rate and sometimes with diffuse crackles. In pneumonia, the crackles may be localised or diffuse and may be accompanied intermittently by wheezes. Indeed, bronchiolitis and pneumonia often appear to represent a continuum and may be difficult to differentiate clinically. The variability in auscultatory findings and in the respiratory rate within short periods of time is common enough in infants with lower respiratory tract infection due to RSV to be considered characteristic. The course of the illness similarly may be variable, lasting from 1 to several weeks, but most infants will show clinical improvement within 3–4 days of the onset of the lower respiratory tract disease.

Evaluation of the severity of the lower respiratory tract disease in these young infants is often problematic. Factors which have been associated with an increased risk of severe disease include first, and most predictive, an oxygen saturation by pulse oximetry of <95%, an appearance of clinical toxicity, and tachypnoea with a respiratory rate of ⩾70 breaths/min. Some studies have also indicated the additional risk factors of atelectasis on chest roentgenogram and a gestational age of <34 weeks or chronologic age of <3 months (Shaw et al., 1991). The observation of these risk factors may be confounded by not realising that the degree of hypoxaemia may not be clinically evident, as cyanosis is present only in a minority of infants. Second, an increased respiratory rate may result from the concurrent presence of fever. Fever and the extent of the wheezing or crackles generally do not correlate with the severity of illness.

The hypoxaemia results from diffuse involvement of the lung parenchyma, causing an abnormally low ratio of ventilation to perfusion, which is characteristic of viral infection in contrast to bacteria infection; however, this may not be evident on chest roentgenogram. Alveolar hypoventilation and progressive hypercarbia may develop but are rare in infants given good oxygenation and supportive care.

The roentgenographic picture in infants with lower respiratory tract disease due to RSV may vary from a virtually normal appearance to one that mimics bacterial pneumonia. However, the severity of the infant's illness generally is not mirrored by the roentgenographic changes. Infants with the typical findings of bronchiolitis, hyperinflation and minimal peribronchial increased markings, may be severely ill and hypoxaemic. The most characteristic findings on the chest radiograph with RSV lower respiratory tract disease are hyperinflation, infiltrates—which are often perihilar, involving more than one lobe—and atelectasis, especially of the right middle or right upper lobes. This latter finding of apparent consolidation is commonly mistaken for bacterial pneumonia.

In the Newcastle upon Tyne (UK) studies of infants hospitalised with lower respiratory tract disease due to RSV, hyperinflation was present in over half the children and increased peribronchial markings in 39% (Simpson et al., 1974). Hyperlucency, which occurred as the sole abnormality in 15% of the cases, was particularly associated with RSV infection. Consolidation was present in approximately one-quarter of the cases and was usually subsegmental in distribution. The roentgenographic abnormalities, and sometimes the hypoxaemia, tend to persist beyond the time of clinical improvement.

RSV infection in newborns had been thought to occur rarely, but is now recognised as being relatively common (Mlinaric-Galinovic and Varda-Brkic, 2000; Heerens et al., 2002). The manifestations of the disease in the newly-born, however, may be atypical and missed clinically (Hall et al., 1979). Neonates, especially in the first 2–3 weeks of life, infrequently have the typical clinical findings of lower respiratory tract disease. More commonly, RSV is initially manifested by such non-specific signs as lethargy and poor feeding. Upper respiratory tract signs may be present in only about half. Premature infants appear to be more susceptible to infection and the mortality may be high in neonatal intensive care units.

Primary infections may also be manifested only as upper respiratory tract disease or tracheobronchitis, especially in older infants. Otitis associated with RSV infection is common, and 20–30% of infants hospitalised with RSV infection manifest otitis media. RSV may be recovered from 0–60% of middle ear aspirates of children with otitis media. It may be the sole pathogen or is sometimes found in conjunction with bacterial agents. Recent studies have indicated that RSV may be a major cause of otitis media in the infant in the first years of life and, furthermore, RSV-associated otitis media may have a more complicated course (Chonmaitree et al., 1992; Anderson, 2001). In general, upper respiratory tract infections associated with RSV, whether primary or recurrent, tend to be more prolonged and severe than the usual cold (Hall, 2001a).

Complications

Apnoea is a frequent complication of RSV infection in young infants, occurring in approximately 20% of hospitalised cases (Church et al., 1984; Openshaw et al., 2003). Apnoea may be the initial sign of RSV infection, preceding overt respiratory signs. The apnoea is most likely to occur in premature infants with a gestation of 32 weeks or less and in those of young postnatal age, less than 44 weeks postconceptional age (Church et al., 1984). A history of apnoea of prematurity has also been identified as a significant risk factor for the development of apnoea with RSV infection. The apnoea associated with RSV infection is non-obstructive and tends to develop at the onset or within the first few days of the illness. Although the prognosis for such infants has not been defined accurately, it does not appear to place the infant at increased risk of subsequent apnoea (Church et al., 1984).

Recently infants with RSV bronchiolitis have been shown to be at high risk for aspiration, which may be clinically manifest as airway hyperreactivity (Hernandez *et al.*, 2002). One recent study conducted over a 12 month follow-up period showed that 83% of infants who have been hospitalised with RSV bronchiolitis developed reactive airway disease if given no ribavirin or therapy for aspiration. However, of infants who were given thickened feedings along with early ribavirin therapy, 45% developed reactive airway, and episodes of reactive airway disease were similarly reduced (Khoshoo *et al.*, 2001). It is of note that the reduction was greater with both ribavirin and thickened feedings than with either therapy alone.

Despite the often prolonged and severe course of lower respiratory tract disease in young children, secondary bacterial infection is an unusual complication (< 1% of cases). Furthermore, antibiotic therapy has been shown not to improve the rate of recovery of infants with RSV lower respiratory tract disease (National Guideline Clearinghouse, 1998). In developing countries, however, concurrent bacterial infection is more common and may be a major factor leading to the high mortality rate in such infants.

Certain groups of children appear to be at risk of developing complicated, severe or even fatal RSV infection (Meissner, 2003; Weisman, 2003). Among these the highest risk groups are those with chronic lung, cardiac and immunosuppressive conditions. In children with nephrotic syndrome and cystic fibrosis, RSV may also cause exacerbations and complications of their underlying disease (MacDonald *et al.*, 1986; Abman *et al.*, 1988).

Infants with underlying pulmonary disease, especially chronic lung disease following prematurity, are at risk of developing prolonged and complicated infection with RSV, even in their second year of life if they have continued to require medical therapy (Groothuis and Nishida, 2002; Meissner, 2003; Weisman, 2003). Another group who are prone to extensive and severe RSV infection are those with immunosuppression, especially from congenital immunodeficiency diseases and bone marrow or solid organ transplantation (Hall *et al.*, 1986; Pohl *et al.*, 1992; Moscona, 2000; Champlin and Whimbey, 2001; Mobbs *et al.*, 2002). These patients may develop lower respiratory tract disease at any age, which may be severe or even fatal and tends to be associated with extended shedding of the virus.

Patients who have other conditions which cause compromise of their immune system, such as those infected with HIV, may also have more severe disease from RSV. Although information on RSV disease in children with varying stages of HIV infection is limited, RSV infection in general does not appear to be as severe as in those with severe immunosuppression associated with transplantation and congenital immune deficiency disease (Chandwani *et al.*, 1990; King, 1997; Madhi *et al.*, 2000, 2001, 2002). In HIV-infected children the degree of immunosuppression tends to correlate with the severity of RSV infection and a longer duration of shedding of RSV, and often involves the lower respiratory tract (Chandwani *et al.*, 1990; King, 1997). However, these findings are confounded by the observation that those children with HIV infection and viral respiratory infections also have a higher rate of bacterial co-infection (Madhi *et al.*, 2000, 2001, 2002). Furthermore, the clinical outcome of viral respiratory infections in general, including influenza, in some studies has not been different between children with or without HIV infection (Madhi *et al.*, 2002).

Infants hospitalised in the first few months of life with uncorrected cyanotic congenital heart disease are potentially at particular peril (Meissner, 2003). Although all the factors or types of cardiac conditions associated with a poor prognosis have not been defined, pulmonary hypertension accompanying congenital heart disease may increase the risk appreciably. Recent surgical and technical advances and early correction currently have substantially reduced the mortality and morbidity in infants with congenital heart disease, although their risk for fatal RSV disease still appears to be more than three- or four-fold greater than that estimated for other infants hospitalised with RSV infection (Navas *et al.*, 1992; Fixler, 1996; Meissner, 2003).

The most frequent sequelae from RSV lower respiratory tract disease in early infancy is recurrent wheezing, sometimes associated with prolonged alterations in pulmonary function. A number of studies have reported rates of subsequent reactive airway disease of approximately 50% (Wennergren and Kristjansson, 2001; Piedimonte, 2002a). In most children these clinical manifestations improve with age; in some, pulmonary function abnormalities may persist but be clinically silent (Martinez, 2003). The link between reactive airway disease and RSV is not clearly defined. Whether RSV lower respiratory tract infection early in life is truly causal of these later sequelae is controversial. Much current research, however, has suggested that potential immune and neuronal pathways, as noted previously, may be the mechanism for a link between RSV and reactive airway disease (Piedimonte, 2002a, 2003; Openshaw *et al.*, 2003).

The similarities in the immune response between asthma and RSV bronchiolitis have suggested this link and possible explanations for the immunopathogenesis of RSV disease (Hacking and Hull, 2002; Holt and Sly,

2002; Openshaw et al., 2002, 2003; Welliver et al., 2002). During RSV infection, transcription factors are activated which result in the release of proinflammatory cytokines and chemokines. Included in these are IL-1β, IL-6, IL-10, IL-11 and the chemokines IL-8, RANTES (regulated on activation, normal T cell expressed and presumably secreted) and MIP-1α (macrophage inflammatory protein 1α). These have been identified both in vitro and, more recently, in the secretions of children with RSV infection (Noah et al., 1995; Saito et al., 1997; Sheeran et al., 1999; Openshaw, 2001; Openshaw et al., 2003; Hacking and Hull, 2002). The interaction and precise role of these cytokines in the immunopathogenesis of RSV is complex and awaits better definition. Clearly they are released at higher concentrations during RSV infection than in controls or during infections with some other viruses. In general, the concentrations of these cytokines correlate with the increase in white blood cells in the secretions of children with RSV infection. A number of studies examining the link between RSV and asthma have focused on those cytokines which are chemotactic for eosinophils, monocytes and T cells, as seen in an allergic response (Welliver et al., 2002; Openshaw et al., 2003). Although these cytokines are also elevated in RSV infection, they have not been clearly correlated with severity of disease. Indeed, studies by Sheeran et al. (1999) have suggested that the concentration of RANTES, IL-8 and IL-10 correlated inversely with severity of disease. In aggregate, these studies indicate that cytokines have a role in the pathogenesis of RSV infection and also in hyperreactivity of the lung.

Determination of the precise role of individual cytokines is further compounded by other factors which may cause a variable response in the host. Among these are a genetic predisposition to hyperreactive lungs, smaller airways or an atopic diathesis (Landau, 1994). Studies in which the initial infection was identified as being caused by RSV and in which the children were prospectively followed have indicated that atopy does not appear to be the major factor in predicting which children will develop such long-term pulmonary abnormalities (Martinez, 2003). In a subgroup of children, however, atopy does appear to be a major factor in increasing their risk of more severe RSV disease and subsequent complications, such as recurrent wheezing (Welliver, 2000; Welliver et al., 1993, 2002).

Genetic heterogeneity in the immune response of children with RSV infection may also explain some of the variation in disease severity. Recent studies investigating the role of gene variants, i.e. polymorph-

isms, in the immune response have supported this. One recent study showed that certain variants of the genes encoding IL-4 and the IL-4 receptor α-chain were associated in a case control study with more severe RSV bronchiolitis (Hoebee et al., 2003).

Infection in Older Children and Adults

Repeated RSV infections occur throughout life, and the interval between infections may be only weeks or months (Hall et al., 1991). In older children and adults these repeated infections are usually manifested as upper respiratory tract infections or sometimes as tracheobronchitis. In a minority of adults, usually less than 15%, the infection may be asymptomatic (Hall, 2001a). Even in young healthy adults, RSV infection may be associated with pulmonary function abnormalities, mostly hyperreactivity of the airway to cholinergic stimulus, which may last for 6 or more weeks.

RSV infection in the elderly may be more severe and have some similarities to infection at the other end of the age spectrum (Nicholson, 1996; Nicholson et al., 1997; Falsey and Walsh, 2000). In older individuals, RSV has been associated with pneumonia, exacerbations of chronic bronchitis, underlying cardiac disease, and can produce a flu-like syndrome indistinguishable from that of influenza. RSV infection in older adults occurs more frequently than is generally recognised and has been shown to have an impact equal to that of non-pandemic influenza. Although the rates of RSV infection in this population is variable from year to year and according to their general health, about 5–10% of those in assisted-living or long-term care facilities will acquire RSV infection each year, and 2–5% will succumb.

On acute medical wards, RSV infections, both nosocomially and community acquired, in adult patients of all ages and staff also are being recognised increasingly (Takimoto et al., 1991; Falsey et al., 1995; Dowell et al., 1996; Champlin and Whimbey, 2001; Goldmann, 2001). Although any patient is at risk for RSV infection, those with the most severe clinical manifestations, similar to children, are generally those with chronic or immunosuppressive underlying conditions.

DIAGNOSIS

RSV infection may be diagnosed by identification of the viral antigen by rapid diagnostic techniques, viral isolation or serology. Rapid diagnosis is important in management for the initiation of proper infection control procedures and for antiviral chemotherapy.

Viral isolation has been the standard upon which other diagnostic methods are usually judged, but viral isolation is dependent on the quality of the laboratory tissue culture techniques, the specimen and the age of the patient. For infants, viral isolation can be sensitive and specific, but for older children and adults tissue culture diagnosis may be less sensitive, as individuals with a recurrent infection shed smaller quantities of virus and for shorter periods.

Nasal washes or tracheal secretions are generally the best specimens for isolation. The specimen should be inoculated onto tissue culture promptly and without subjecting it to major temperature changes. RSV is a relatively labile virus and withstands freezing and thawing poorly. At 37°C approximately 10% of infectivity of the virus in tissue culture medium remains after 24 h. However, at 4°C in certain media, such as veal infusion broth, little loss in virus titre may occur for 2–3 days. Control of the pH of the media is important in preventing loss of infectivity, the optimum pH being 7.5. Specific cytopathic changes usually appear within 3–5 days in sensitive continuous cell lines, such as Hep-2. The use of shell vials allows earlier diagnosis. The sensitivity of such cell lines for growth and recognition of RSV may be variable and the cell lines utilised require constant monitoring. Characteristic cytopathic effect of RSV is most evident in cell lines that are young and lightly seeded at the time of specimen inoculation (Figure 7.4). Heavy growth of the tissue culture may prevent the development of the characteristic RSV CPE.

Commercially available rapid assays for detecting RSV antigen have become plentiful and widely used. Most are based on an enzyme immunosorbent assay (EIA). The sensitivity and specificity of these kits, however, may be variable and results are likely to be considerably less accurate in a busy clinic than those reported in published studies from evaluating laboratories. The sensitivity of the EIA assays against isolation of the virus in cell culture has ranged from about 50% to 95% and the specificity from about 70% to 100%. A major factor in the reported sensitivity of these assays is the quality and sensitivity of the test to which it is being compared, and viral isolation abilities of different laboratories appear to be particularly variable. The type of specimen is also important in the sensitivity of EIA detection. Nasal wash specimens have been reported as positive in 15% compared to 71% of endotracheal secretion specimens and 89% of bronchioalveolar washes in culture-positive patients (Englund *et al.*, 1996).

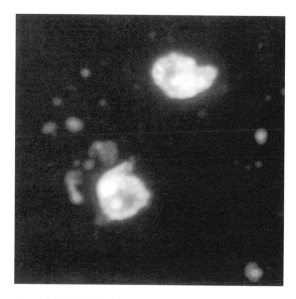

Figure 7.4 Positive indirect immunofluorescent antibody test on nasal secretions from an infant with lower respiratory tract disease due to RSV

Both direct and indirect immunofluorescent reagents, utilising either polyclonal or monoclonal antibodies, are available which possess a high degree of specificity and sensitivity. The direct immunofluorescence assay has the advantage that the patterns of immunofluorescence may be evaluated, providing additional confirmation of specificity. However, this assay also requires specialised equipment and a greater expertise. The fluorescent pattern observed will depend on the antibody used. Monoclonal antibody to the nucleocapsid protein or the phosphoprotein will produce specific large and small cytoplasmic inclusions in RSV-positive cells, while monoclonal antibody to the fusion (F) protein shows diffuse cytoplasmic staining. Polyclonal antiserum produces both specific inclusions and diffuse staining in the cytoplasm (Figure 7.5). The immunofluorescent reagents utilised for RSV may be combined with those specific for other respiratory agents, to allow detection of several agents in one specimen of exfoliated cells from the respiratory secretions.

The recent use of RT-PCR for diagnosis of RSV infections, mostly in research laboratories, has shown much higher rates of specificity and sensitivity than other diagnostic methods, generally 98% (Freymuth *et al.*, 1995). The inclusion of appropriate additional primers allows simultaneous assay for multiple pathogens (Fan *et al.*, 1998; Tang *et al.*, 1999). Currently the

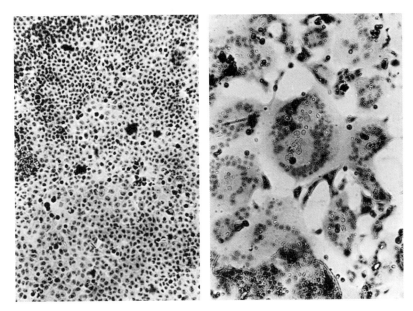

Figure 7.5   Stained preparations of uninfected HeLa cells (left) and cells infected with RSV (right). Syncytial formation is well illustrated by the infected monolayer

commercial availability and feasibility of using these assays in primary care facilities is limited.

Serologic diagnosis by detecting antibody rises in acute and convalescent sera is unlikely to be of help in the management of the patient because of the time required. Furthermore, the serological response in young infants may be poor and not detectable by some antibody assays. Seroconversion usually does not occur for at least 2 weeks and may require 4–6 weeks. Several serological tests are available, mostly in research laboratories. Neutralisation and EIA are most frequently used and offer the possibility of detecting specific antibody classes. Assays for IgM antibodies to RSV are of limited usefulness, as they are commonly not detectable in patients with proven infection and, if present, may appear anywhere from 6 to 40 days from the onset of the illness (Vikerfors *et al.*, 1988; Dowell *et al.*, 1996).

MANAGEMENT

Most infants do well with their RSV infection with no more than the usual care given for fever and to maintain adequate hydration. In the more severely affected infants with lower respiratory tract disease, the quality of the supportive care is most important (Panitch, 2003). Since most hospitalised infants are hypoxaemic, documentation of the blood gases in the more severely ill infant is essential for good management. Most infants respond well to relatively low concentrations of oxygen, since the major parenchymal abnormality is an unequal ratio of ventilation to perfusion. Hypercarbia may develop in the severely ill infant, requiring frequent monitoring of the blood gases and, if progressive, may lead to airway intervention. Hypercarbia and recurrent apnoea are the most frequent reasons for assisted ventilation. Hypoxaemia, unresponsive to oxygen therapy, is less common.

The antiviral agent, ribavirin (1-β-D-ribofuranosyl-1,2,4-triazole-3-carboxamide), has been approved for specific treatment of RSV infection (Jafri, 2003). Ribavirin is a synthetic nucleoside which appears to interfere with the expression of mRNA and is unusual in that its antiviral activity appears to be broad-spectrum, affecting a variety of both RNA and DNA viruses *in vivo* and *in vitro*. No toxicity has been shown with ribavirin therapy (Krilov, 2002) and development of resistance to ribavirin by RSV strains or other viruses has not been observed, even with prolonged treatment. Ribavirin is administered by small-particle aerosol into an oxygen tent, oxygen hood or via a ventilator, usually for 12 or more h/day, but may be in shorter or intermittent periods until clinical improvement, which is usually in 2–5 days. Which infants should receive ribavirin is not entirely clear. Some controlled double-blind studies have shown ribavirin to have a beneficial effect on the clinical course of RSV bronchiolitis and pneumonia in infants who were mostly mildly to moderately ill, as measured by the rate of improvement in illness severity and on the measured levels of the infants' arterial oxygen saturation, as well as the duration of mechanical ventilation and supplemental oxygenation (Smith *et al.*, 1991). However, the days of hospitalisation and short-term outcome in some studies have not been shown to be affected, and the degree of benefit relative to the cost must be considered on an individual basis (American Academy of Pediatrics, COID, 1998). For infants who have underlying conditions which put them most at risk for severe RSV disease, the benefits may outweigh the costs. Recent follow-up studies have indicated that ribavirin treatment may ameliorate the long-term sequelae of diminished pulmonary function and wheezing that frequently follows RSV bronchiolitis (Khoshoo *et al.*, 2002).

Aerosolised bronchodilators have also been employed intermittently for some patients with bronchiolitis (Panitch, 2003). Their use is controversial, as most studies have failed to show that their use, especially in infants under 12–18 months of age, has resulted in improved oxygen saturation, reduced hospital stay or clinical benefit, and side-effects such as tachycardia may occur (Hall, 2002). Hence, routine therapy with bronchodilators for first-time wheezers under 1 year of age is not recommended. Some experts would nevertheless advise that a trial with carefully monitored aerosolised bronchodilator therapy be considered for the more severely affected infants, particularly those above 6 months of age (National Guideline Clearinghouse, 1998; Rodriguez, 1999; Kellner *et al.*, 2000).

Corticosteroids also are not recommended for the routine management of infants who are first-time wheezers. The trials with corticosteroids and RSV infection, mostly bronchiolitis, have had conflicting results for therapy with both inhaled and systemic corticosteroids (Perlstein *et al.*, 1999; van Woensel *et al.*, 2000; Wennergren and Kristjansson, 2001; Hall, 2002; Panitch, 2003). However, one meta-analysis of systemic corticosteroids indicated an improvement in clinical symptoms and length of hospital stay, but few trials could be included and most possessed design defects, suggesting that further trials are required (Kellner *et al.*, 1996; Cade *et al.*, 2000; Patel *et al.*, 2001). The studies evaluating corticosteroids have been mostly with inhaled corticosteroids. In two studies evaluating systemic corticosteroid therapy, no benefit was shown acutely or in follow-up (Springer *et al.*, 1990; van Woensel *et al.*, 2000). Of the aerosolised corticosteroid studies, five showed no benefit initially

or on subsequent wheezing episodes, and two showed benefit, including a diminished incidence of subsequent wheezing (Khoshoo *et al.*, 2002). These conflicting results may be explained by the variable design and efficiencies, the lack of specific aetiology of the bronchiolitis, and the heterogeneity in the children included.

Chest physiotherapy, cool mist therapy, aerosolised therapy with saline, supervised cough and suction, and antibiotics also are not recommended for the routine management of RSV infection (National Guideline Clearinghouse, 1998; Perlstein *et al.*, 1999).

Prevention

For decades now, research has been directed towards the development of a safe and effective vaccine for RSV (Piedra, 2003). A vaccine for this virus, however, poses particular problems. It would have to be administered at a very young age, within the first few weeks of life, and should be able to produce an immunity more durable than that seen after natural infection.

The first vaccine developed—the alum-precipitated, formalin-inactivated vaccine tested in the 1960s—produced high levels of serum antibody but then resulted in augmented disease following infection with the wild virus (Toms, 1995). Subsequently, candidates for subunit and live-attenuated vaccines have been sought. Vaccines developed from both cold-adapted strains and from temperature-sensitive (ts) mutants appeared promising in initial trials, but were later shown to be too reactive, genetically unstable or overly attenuated.

Research recently has focused on the two major surface glycoproteins, the F and G proteins, as the major immunising agents (Oien *et al.*, 1993; Paradiso *et al.*, 1994; Toms, 1995; Piedra, 2002; Simoes *et al.*, 2002). Three generations of the purified fusion protein (PFP1–3) vaccine have been evaluated in clinical trials. These vaccines are made from the F protein of the A2 strain of RSV with aluminium hydroxide. The trials in children have included both normal children and those with underlying disease who have had prior RSV infection (Tristram *et al.*, 1993; Paradiso *et al.*, 1994; Piedra *et al.*, 1996; Groothuis *et al.*, 1998). These vaccines have also been tried in normal healthy adults as well as elderly adults and women in their third trimester of pregnancy or postpartum (Falsey and Walsh, 1996; Englund *et al.*, 1998). In general, these PFP vaccines have been safe and immunogenic in about one-half to two-thirds of the vaccinees, but did not offer protection against RSV infection. However, in two small studies of children with underlying pulmonary disease, some protection against lower respiratory tract disease with RSV was observed (Piedra et al., 1996; Groothuis et al., 1998). Additional potentially more immunogenic and effective candidate subunit F and FG vaccines are being developed from purified viruses with new adjuvants, from recombinant vectors, and from plasmids containing complementary DNA of the F and G genes (Simoes et al., 2001, 2002).

The development of live-attenuated vaccines is of increasing interest and investigation, as they offer the potential advantages of both systemic and mucosal immunity and the ease of intranasal administration (Piedra, 2003). The previous live-attenuated candidate vaccines have been improved by repetitive rounds of chemical mutagenesis, resulting in mutations that provide better attenuation, stability and immunogenicity (Crowe, 2002; Piedra, 2002, 2003).

Generations of new candidate strains with the cold passage and temperature-sensitive attenuating mutations are under development by the use of reverse genetics (Collins and Murphy, 2002; Murphy and Collins, 2002). Clinical evaluation in seropositive subjects thus far indicates that these are promising vaccine candidates for both infants and older individuals. These new recombinant genetic engineering methods can produce full-length RSV complementary DNA which produces infectious RNA transcripts as well as recrafting the genomic soul of RSV to bring precise improvements in immunogenicity and safety (Collins and Murphy, 2002).

Other currently available means of protection are for limited periods and for those most at risk for severe or complicated RSV disease. Prime among these is prevention of severe RSV infection in high-risk infants, by the passive administration of intravenous immunoglobulin containing high levels of RSV neutralising antibody or intramuscular monoclonal antibody (American Academy of Pediatrics, COID, 1998; Sanchez, 2002). In 1996, the Food and Drug Administration in the USA licensed the first such preparation, a polyclonal antibody preparation, which showed clinical benefit for preventing serious RSV disease in high-risk children with prematurity or pulmonary or cardiac disease. The RSV-IVIG was administered once a month (PREVENT Study Group, 1997; Wang and Tang, 2000) and led to an overall reduction of 41% in hospitalisations for RSV disease in these high-risk groups. Because of concerns that this prophylactic treatment may have had adverse effects among children with cyanotic congenital heart disease, the RSV-IVIG was not approved for use in children with

congenital heart disease with a right-to-left shunt. Subsequently a humanised mouse IgG monoclonal antibody (palivizumab), which binds the F protein of RSV, was developed (Impact RSV Study Group and Connor, 1998). Palivizumab has the advantages of easier intramuscular administration and similar effectiveness in the reduction (55%) of hospitalisation in the same high-risk groups of infants as that engendered with prophylaxis by the RSV-IVIG preparation. Furthermore, palivizumab was safe and well tolerated (Impact RSV Study Group and Connor, 1998). Currently in the USA palivizumab is recommended by the American Academy of Pediatrics as prophylaxis that should be considered, for specific groups of children with chronic lung disease who are less than 24 months of age and infants with gestational ages of less than 28 weeks (American Academy of Pediatrics, COID, 1998) (Table 7.2). Recent studies have suggested that palvizumab also may be safe for those children with cyanotic heart disease who meet the other criteria for RSV prophylaxis (Hudak, 2003). Definition of the precise groups that would benefit most, and the relative cost to the benefit, remain controversial (Clark et al., 2000; Sharland and Bedford-Russell, 2001). A number of studies have suggested that further, more limited definition of infants eligible for prophylaxis is necessary to result in a favourable ratio of the benefit to the cost (O'Shea et al., 1998; Joffe et al., 1999; Atkins et al., 2000; Stevens et al., 2000; Thomas et al., 2000; Romero, 2003).

The prevention of RSV infection in normal infants, however, currently is not possible because of the ubiquitous and contagious nature of the virus. Infection control procedures may be effective in limiting nosocomial spread of RSV, but are of limited effectiveness and feasibility in the home.

Table 7.2 American Academy of Pediatrics guidelines for using palivizumab

- Infants younger than 24 months of age with chronic lung disease (CLD) who have required medical therapy within the past 6 months
- Neonates born at 28 weeks gestation or less with CLD and who are < 12 months of age at the start of the RSV season
- Neonates born at > 28 weeks and < 32 weeks gestation without CLD who are < 6 months of age at the start of the RSV season
- Neonates born between 32 and 35 weeks gestation without CLD who are < 6 months of age and who have additional risk factors, including school-aged siblings, crowding in the home, day care attendance, exposure to tobacco smoke in the home and multiple births

Of the infection control procedures employed to limit the nosocomial spread of RSV, annual education of staff and hand washing are the most important (Hall, 2000a). When compliance with consistent and careful hand washing is less than optimal, the use of gloves may be of benefit. The routine use of gowns and masks has not been shown to be of additional benefit. The use of gowns, however, may be advisable during periods of close contact in which an infant's secretions are apt to contaminate the clothing. Since RSV primarily infects via the eyes and nose, masks are of limited value, but eye-nose goggles have been shown to be beneficial (Hall, 2000a).

Other procedures of potential benefit include isolation or cohorting of infected infants and assigning nursing personnel to care for either infected infants or uninfected infants, but not both simultaneously. During epidemic periods the number of patient contacts and visitors should be limited. Cleaning of objects and surfaces contaminated with infant secretions is also advisable. Elective admissions of infants with high-risk conditions should be avoided during the epidemic periods of RSV. For those infants who must be admitted, particular care must be employed to prevent such cross-infections.

REFERENCES

Abman S, Ogle J *et al.* (1988) Role of respiratory syncytial virus in early hospitalizations for respiratory distress of young infants with cystic fibrosis. *J Pediatr*, **113**, 826–830.

Alwan W and Openshaw P (1993) Distinct patterns of T and B cell immunity to respiratory syncytial virus induced by individual viral proteins. *Vaccine*, **11**, 431–437.

Alwan W, Record F *et al.* (1992) CD4$^+$ T cells clear virus but augment disease in mice infected with respiratory syncytial virus. Comparison with the effects of CD8$^+$ T cells. *Clin Exp Immunol*, **88**(3), 527–536.

Alwan WH, Kozlowska WJ *et al.* (1994) Distinct types of lung disease caused by functional subsets of antiviral T cells. *J Exp Med*, **179**, 81–89.

American Academy of Pediatrics, COID (Committee on Infectious Diseases) (1998) Prevention of respiratory syncytial virus infections: indications for use of palivizumab and update on the use of RSV-IVIG. *Pediatrics*, **102**, 1211–1216.

Anderson L (2001) Respiratory syncytial virus vaccines for otitis media. *Vaccine*, **19**, S59–S65.

Anderson L, Hendry R *et al.* (1991) Multicenter study of strains of respiratory syncytial virus. *J Infect Dis*, **163**, 687–692.

Atkins J, Karimi P *et al.* (2000) Prophylaxis for respiratory syncytial virus with respiratory syncytial virus-immunoglobulin intravenous among preterm infants of 32 weeks gestation and less: reduction in incidence, severity of illness and cost. *Pediatr Infect Dis J*, **19**, 138–143.

Bar-on M and Zanga J (1996) Bronchiolitis. *Primary Care*, **23**, 805–819.

Berner R, Schwoerer F *et al.* (2001) Community and nosocomially acquired respiratory syncytial virus infection in a German paediatric hospital from 1988 to 1999. *Eur J Pediatr*, **160**, 541–547.

Bright H, Turnbull T *et al.* (1995) Comparison of the T helper cell response induced by respiratory syncytial virus and its fusion protein in BABL/c mice. *Vaccine*, **13**, 915–922.

Cade A, Brownlee K *et al.* (2000) Randomized placebo controlled trial of nebulized corticosteroids in acute respiratory syncytial viral bronchiolitis. *Arch Dis Child*, **82**, 126–130.

Cane P (2001) Molecular epidemiology of respiratory syncytial virus. *Rev Med Virol*, **11**, 103–116.

Cane P and Pringle C (1995) Evolution of subgroup A respiratory syncytial virus: evidence for progressive accumulation of amino acid changes in the attachment protein. *J Virol*, **69**, 2918–2925.

CDC (Centers for Disease Control and Prevention) (2002a) Guideline for hand hygiene in health-care settings. Recommendations of the Healthcare Infections Control Practices Advisory Committee and the HICPAC/SHEA/APIC/IDSA Hand Hygiene Task Force. *Morbid Mortal Wkly Rep*, **51**(RR-16).

CDC (Centers for Disease Control and Prevention) (2002b) Respiratory syncytial virus activity—United States, 2000–2001 season. *Morbid Mortal Wkly Rep*, **51**, 26–28.

Champlin R and Whimbey E (2001) Community respiratory virus infections in bone marrow transplant recipients: the M.D. Anderson Cancer Center experience. *Biol Blood Marrow Transpl*, **7**, 8S–10S.

Chandwani S, Borkowsky W *et al.* (1990) Respiratory syncytial virus infection in human immunodeficiency virus-infected children. *J Pediatr*, **117**, 251–254.

Chanock R, Roizman B *et al.* (1957) Recovery from infants with respiratory illness of a virus related to chimpanzee coryza agent (CCA): I. Isolation, properties and characterization. *Am J Hyg*, **66**, 281–290.

Chin J, Magoffin R *et al.* (1969) Field evaluation of a respiratory syncytial virus vaccine and a trivalent parainfluenza virus vaccine in a pediatric population. *Am J Epidemiol*, **89**, 449–463.

Chonmaitree T, Owen M *et al.* (1992) Effect of viral respiratory tract infection on outcome of acute otitis media. *J Pediatr*, **120**, 856–862.

Church N, Anas N *et al.* (1984) Respiratory syncytial virus-related apnea in infants: Demographics and outcome. *Am J Dis Child*, **138**, 247–250.

Clark S, Beresford M *et al.* (2000) Respiratory syncytial virus infection in high risk infants and the potential impact of prophylaxis in a United Kingdom cohort. *Arch Dis Child*, **83**, 313–316.

Collins P, McIntosh K *et al.* (1996) Respiratory syncytial virus. *Field's Virology* (eds Fields B, Knipe D and Howley P), pp 1313–1351. Lippincott-Raven, Philadelphia, PA.

Collins P and Murphy B (2002) Respiratory syncytial virus: reverse genetics and vaccine strategies. *Virology*, **296**, 204–211.

Connors M, Kulkarni A *et al.* (1992) Pulmonary histopathology induced by respiratory syncytial virus (RSV) challenge of formalin-inactivated RSV-immunized BALB/c mice is abrogated by depletion of CD4$^+$ T cells. *J Virol*, **66**, 7444–7451.

Crowe J (2002) Respiratory syncytial virus vaccine development. *Vaccine*, **20**, S32–S37.

Dowell S, Anderson L *et al.* (1996) Respiratory syncytial virus is an important cause of community-acquired lower respiratory infection among hospitalized adults. *J Infect Dis*, **174**, 456–462.

Englund J, Anderson L *et al.* (1991) Nosocomial transmission of respiratory syncytial virus in immunocompromised adults. *J Clin Microbiol*, **29**, 115–119.

Englund J, Glezen W *et al.* (1998) Maternal immunization against viral disease. *Vaccine*, **16**, 1456–1463.

Englund J, Piedra P *et al.* (1996) Rapid diagnosis of respiratory syncytial virus infections in immunocompromised adults. *J Clin Microbiol*, 1649–1653.

Falsey A, Cunningham C *et al.* (1995) Respiratory syncytial virus and influenza A infections in the hospitalized elderly. *J Infect Dis*, **172**, 389–394.

Falsey A and Walsh E (1996) Safety and immunogenicity of a respiratory syncytial virus subunit vaccine (PFP-2) in ambulatory adults over age 60. *Vaccine*, **14**, 1214–1218.

Falsey A and Walsh E (2000) Respiratory syncytial virus infections in adults. *Clin Microbiol Rev*, **13**, 371–384.

Fan J, Henrickson K *et al.* (1998) Rapid simultaneous diagnosis of infections with respiratory syncytial virus A and B, influenza viruses A and B, and human parainfluenza virus types 1, 2, and 3 by multiplex quantitative reverse transcription—polymerase chain reaction—enzyme hybridization assay (Hexaplex). *Clin Infect Dis*, **26**, 1397–1402.

Fixler D (1996) Respiratory syncytial virus infection in children with congenital heart disease: a review. *Pediatr Cardiol*, **17**, 163–168.

Freymuth F, Eugene G *et al.* (1995) Detection of respiratory syncytial virus by reverse transcription-PCR and hybridization with a DNA enzyme immunoassay. *J Clin Microbiol*, **33**, 3352–3355.

Fulginiti V, Eller J *et al.* (1969) Respiratory virus immunization I. A field trial of two inactivated respiratory virus vaccines; an aqueous trivalent parainfluenza virus vaccine, and an alum-precipitated respiratory syncytial virus vaccine. *Am J Epidemiol*, **89**, 435–448.

Glezen W, Taber L *et al.* (1986) Risk of primary infection and reinfection with respiratory syncytial virus. *Am J Dis Child*, **140**, 543–546.

Goldmann D (2001) Epidemiology and prevention of pediatric viral respiratory infections in health-care institutions. *Emerg Infect Dis*, **7**, 249–253.

Graham B, Bunton L *et al.* (1991a) Respiratory syncytial virus infection in anti-μ treated mice. *J Virol*, **65**, 4936–4942.

Graham B, Bunton L *et al.* (1991b) Role of T lymphocyte subsets in the pathogenesis of primary infection and rechallenge with respiratory syncytial virus in mice. *J Clin Invest*, **88**, 1026–1033.

Graham B, Henderson G *et al.* (1993) Priming immunization determines T helper cytokine mRNA expression patterns in lungs of mice challenged with respiratory syncytial virus. *J Immunol*, **151**, 2032–2040.

Greenough A (2001) Recent advances in the management and prophylaxis of respiratory syncytial virus infection. *Acta Paediatr*, **436**, 11–14.

Groothuis J, King S *et al.* (1998) Safety and immunogenicity of a purified F protein respiratory syncytial virus (PFP-2) vaccine in seropositive children with bronchopulmonary dysplasia. *J Infect Dis*, **177**, 467–469.

Groothuis J and Nishida H (2002) Prevention of respiratory syncytial virus infections in high-risk infants by monoclonal antibody (palivizumab). *Pediatr Int*, **44**, 235–241.

Hacking D and Hull J (2002) Respiratory syncytial virus— viral biology and the host response. *J Infect*, **45**, 18–24.

Hall C (1983) The nosocomial spread of respiratory syncytial virus infections. *Ann Rev Med*, **34**, 311–319.

Hall C (2000a) Nosocomial respiratory syncytial virus infections: the 'cold war' has not ended. *Clin Infect Dis*, **31**, 590–596.

Hall C (2000b) Respiratory syncytial viral infections: pathology and pathogenicity. *Contemporary Diagnosis and Management of Respiratory Syncytial Virus Infection* (eds Weisman L and Groothuis J), pp 72–93. Handbooks in Health Care (a division of AMA Co), Newtown, PA.

Hall C (2001a) Respiratory syncytial virus infections in previously healthy working adults. *Clin Infect Dis*, **33**, 792–796.

Hall C (2001b) Medical progress: respiratory syncytial virus and parainfluenza virus. *N Engl J Med*, **344**, 1917–1928.

Hall C (2002) *Clinanswers. Bronchiolitis.* Clineguide. Wolters Kluwer, Los Angeles, CA.

Hall C, Kopelman A *et al.* (1979) Neonatal respiratory syncytial viral infections. *N Engl J Med*, **300**, 393–396.

Hall C, Powell K *et al.* (1986) Respiratory syncytial virus infection in children with compromised immune function. *N Engl J Med*, **315**, 77–81.

Hall C, Walsh E *et al.* (1990) Occurrence of groups A and B of respiratory syncytial virus over 15 years: associated epidemiologic and clinical characteristics in hospitalized and ambulatory children. *J Infect Dis*, **162**, 1283–1290.

Hall C, Walsh E *et al.* (1991) Immunity to and frequency of reinfection with respiratory syncytial virus. *J Infect Dis*, **163**, 693–698.

Heerens A, Marshall D *et al.* (2002) Nosocomial respiratory syncytial virus: a threat in the modern neonatal intensive care unit. *J Perinatol*, **22**, 306–307.

Henderson F, Collier A *et al.* (1979) Respiratory syncytial virus infections, reinfections and immunity. *N Engl J Med*, **300**, 530–534.

Hernandez E, Khoshoo V *et al.* (2002) Aspiration: a factor in rapidly deteriorating bronchiolitis in previously healthy infants? *Pediatr Pulmonol*, **33**, 30–31.

Hoebee B, Rietveld E *et al.* (2003) Association of severe respiratory syncytial virus bronchiolitis with interleukin-4 and interleukin-4 receptor α-polymorphisms. *J Infect Dis*, **187**, 2–11.

Holt P and Sly P (2002) Interactions between RSV infection, asthma, and atopy: unraveling the complexities. *J Exp Med*, **196**, 1271–1275.

Hudak M (2003) Palivizumab prophylaxis of RSV disease— results of 5097 children, 2001–2002 Outcome Registry. AAP National Conference and Exhibition, Boston, Abstract 700.

Hussell T, Baldwin C *et al.* (1997) CD8[+] T cells control Th2-driven pathology during pulmonary respiratory syncytial virus infection. *Eur J Immunol*, **27**, 3341–3349.

Impact RSV Study Group and Connor E (1998) Palivizumab, a humanized respiratory syncytial virus monoclonal antibody, reduces hospitalization from respiratory syncytial virus infection in high-risk infants. *Pediatrics*, **102**, 531–537.

Isaacs D (1995) Bronchiolitis. *Br Med J*, **310**, 4–5.

Jafri H (2003) Treatment of respiratory syncytial virus: antiviral therapies. *Pediatr Infect Dis J*, **22**, S89–S93.

Jarvis W, Middleton P et al. (1983) Significance of viral infections in severe combined immunodeficiency disease. *Pediatr Infect Dis J*, **2**, 187–192.

Joffe S, Ray G et al. (1999) Cost-effectiveness of respiratory syncytial virus prophylaxis among preterm infants. *Pediatrics*, **104**, 419–427.

Johnson P, Olmsted R et al. (1987) Antigenic relatedness between glycoproteins of human respiratory syncytial virus subgroups A and B: evaluation of the contributions of F and G glycoproteins to immunity. *J Virol*, **10**, 3163–3166.

Kapikian A, Mitchell R et al. (1969) An epidemiologic study of altered clinical reactivity to respiratory syncytial (RS) virus infection in children previously vaccinated with an inactivated RS virus vaccine. *Am J Epidemiol*, **89**, 405–421.

Kellner J, Ohlsson A et al. (1996) Efficacy of bronchodilator therapy in bronchiolitis: a meta-analysis. *Arch Pediatr Adolesc Med*, **150**, 1166–1172.

Kellner J, Ohlsson A et al. (2000) Bronchodilators for bronchiolitis. *Cochrane Database Syst Rev*, **3**, CD001266.

Khoshoo V, Ross G et al. (2001) Benefits of thickened feeds in previously healthy infants with respiratory syncytial virus bronchiolitis. *Pediatr Pulmonol*, **31**, 301–302.

Khoshoo V, Ross G et al. (2002) Effect of interventions during acute respiratory syncytial virus bronchiolitis on subsequent long term respiratory morbidity. *Pediatr Infect Dis J*, **21**, 468–472.

Kim H, Arrobio J et al. (1973) Epidemiology of respiratory syncytial virus infection in Washington DC I. Importance of the virus in different respiratory tract disease syndromes and temporal distribution of infection. *Am J Epidemiol*, **98**, 216–225.

Kim H, Canchola J et al. (1969) Respiratory syncytial virus disease in infants despite prior administration of antigenic inactivated vaccine. *Am J Epidemiol*, **89**, 422–434.

King J (1997) Community respiratory viruses in individuals with human immunodeficiency virus infection. *Am J Med*, **102**, 19–26.

Krilov L (2002) Safety issues related to the administration of ribavirin. *Pediatr Infect Dis J*, **21**, 479–481.

Landau L (1994) Bronchiolitis and asthma: are they related? *Thorax*, **49**, 293–296.

Ljungman P (1997) Respiratory virus infections in bone marrow transplant recipients: the European perspective. *Am J Med*, **102**, 44–47.

MacDonald N, Wolfish N et al. (1986) Role of respiratory viruses in exacerbations of primary nephrotic syndrome. *J Pediatr*, **108**, 378–382.

Madhi S, Ramasamy N et al. (2002) Lower respiratory tract infections associated with influenza A and B viruses in an area with a high prevalence of pediatric human immunodeficiency type 1 infection. *Pediatr Infect Dis J*, **21**, 291–297.

Madhi S, Schoub B et al. (2000) Increased burden of respiratory viral associated severe lower respiratory tract infections in children infected with human immunodeficiency virus type-1. *J Pediatr*, **137**, 78–84.

Madhi S, Venter M et al. (2001) Differing manifestations of respiratory syncytial virus-associated severe lower respiratory tract infections in human immunodeficiency virus type 1-infected and uninfected children. *Pediatr Infect Dis J*, **20**, 164–170.

Martinez F (2003) Respiratory syncytial virus bronchiolitis and the pathogenesis of childhood asthma. *Pediatr Infect Dis J*, **22**, S76–S82.

McConnochie K, Hall C et al. (1990) Variation in severity of respiratory syncytial virus infections with subtype. *J Pediatr*, **117**, 52–62.

Meissner H (2003) Selected populations at increased risk from respiratory syncytial virus infection. *Pediatr Infect Dis J*, **22**, S40–S45.

Mlinaric-Galinovic G and Varda-Brkic D (2000) Nosocomial respiratory syncytial virus infections in children's wards. *Diagn Microbiol Infect Dis*, **37**, 237–246.

Mobbs K, Smyth R et al. (2002) Cytokines in severe respiratory syncytial virus bronchiolitis. *Pediatr Pulmonol*, **33**, 449–452.

Moscona A (2000) Management of respiratory syncytial virus infections in the immunocompromised child. *Pediatr Infect Dis J*, **19**, 253–254.

Murphy B and Collins P (2002) Live-attenuated virus vaccines for respiratory syncytial and parainfluenza viruses: applications of reverse genetics. *J Clin Invest*, **110**, 21–27.

Murphy B, Prince G et al. (1986) Dissociation between serum neutralizing antibody responses of infants and children who received inactivated respiratory syncytial virus vaccine. *J Clin Microbiol*, **24**, 197–202.

National Guideline Clearinghouse (1998). Evidence based guidelines for the medical management of infants 1 year of age or less with a first time episode of bronchiolitis.

Navas L, Wang E et al. (1992) Improved outcome of respiratory syncytial virus infection in a high-risk hospitalized population of Canadian children. *J Pediatr*, **121**, 348–354.

Nicholson K (1996) Impact of influenza and respiratory syncytial virus on mortality in England and Wales from January 1975 to December 1990. *Epidemiol Infect*, **116**, 51–63.

Nicholson K, Kent J et al. (1997) Acute viral infections of upper respiratory tract in elderly people living in the community: comparative, prospective, population based study of disease burden. *Br Med J*, **315**, 1060–1064.

Noah T, Henderson F et al. (1995) Nasal cytokine production in viral acute upper respiratory infection of childhood. *J Infect Dis*, **171**, 584–592.

Oien N, Brideau R et al. (1993) Vaccination with a heterologous respiratory syncytial virus chimeric FG glycoprotein demonstrates significant subgroup cross-reactivity. *Vaccine*, **11**, 1040–1048.

Openshaw P (2001) Potential mechanisms causing delayed effects of respiratory syncytial virus infection. *Am J Respir Crit Care Med*, **163**, S10–S13.

Openshaw P, Clarke S et al. (1992) Pulmonary eosinophilic response to respiratory syncytial virus infection in mice sensitized to the major surface glycoprotein G. *Int Immunol*, **4**, 493–500.

Openshaw P, Culley F et al. (2002) Immunopathogenesis of vaccine-enhanced RSV disease. *Vaccine*, **20**, S27–S31.

Openshaw P, Dean G et al. (2003) Links between respiratory syncytial virus bronchiolitis and childhood asthma: clinical and research approaches. *Pediatr Infect Dis J*, **22**, S58–S65.

O'Shea M, Sevick M et al. (1998) Costs and benefits of respiratory syncytial virus immunoglobulin to prevent hospitalization for lower respiratory tract illness in very low birth weight infants. *Pediatr Infect Dis J*, **17**, 587–593.

Panitch H (2003) Respiratory syncytial virus bronchiolitis: supportive care and therapies designed to overcome airway obstruction. *Pediatr Infect Dis J*, **22**, S83–S88.

Paradiso P, Hildreth S *et al.* (1994) Safety and immunogenicity of a subunit respiratory syncytial virus vaccine in children 24 to 48 months old. *Pediatr Infect Dis J*, **13**, 792–798.

Patel H, Platt R *et al.* (2001) Glucocorticoids in hospitalized infants and young children with acute viral bronchiolitis (protocol for a Cochrane review). *The Cochrane Library*, Oxford.

Peret T, Hall C *et al.* (1998) Circulation patterns of genetically distinct group A and B strains of human respiratory syncytial virus in a community. *J Gen Virol*, **79**, 2221–2229.

Perlstein P, Kotagal U *et al.* (1999) Evaluation of an evidence-based guideline for bronchiolitits. *Pediatrics*, **104**, 1334–1341.

Piedimonte G (2002a) The association between respiratory syncytial virus infection and reactive airway disease. *Resp Med*, **96**, S25–S29.

Piedimonte G (2002b) Neuroimmune interactions in respiratory syncytial virus-infected airways. *Pediatr Infect Dis J*, **21**, 462–467.

Piedimonte G (2003) Contribution of neuroimmune mechanisms to airway inflammation and remodeling during and after respiratory syncytial virus infection. *Pediatr Infect Dis J*, **22**, S66–S75.

Piedra P (2002) Future directions in vaccine prevention of respiratory syncytial virus. *Pediatr Infect Dis J*, **21**, 482–487.

Piedra P (2003) Clinical experience with respiratory syncytial virus vaccines. *Pediatr Infect Dis J*, **22**, S94–S99.

Piedra P, Grace S *et al.* (1996) Purified fusion protein vaccine protects against lower respiratory tract illness during respiratory syncytial virus season in children with cystic fibrosis. *Pediatr Infect Dis J*, **15**, 23–31.

Pohl C, Green M *et al.* (1992) Respiratory syncytial virus infections in pediatric liver transplant recipients. *J Infect Dis*, **165**, 166–169.

PREVENT Study Group (1997) Reduction of respiratory syncytial virus hospitalization among premature infants and infants with bronchopulmonary dysplasia using respiratory syncytial virus immune globulin prophylaxis. *Pediatrics*, **99**, 93–99.

Rodriguez W (1999) Management strategies for respiratory syncytial virus infections in infants. *J Pediatr*, **135**, S45–S50.

Romero J (2003) Palivizumab prophylaxis of respiratory syncytial virus disease from 1998 to 2002: results from four years of palivizumab usage. *Pediatr Infect Dis J*, **22**, S46–S54.

Saito T, Deskin R *et al.* (1997) Respiratory syncytial virus induces selective production of the chemokine RANTES by upper airway epithelial cells. *J Infect Dis*, **175**, 497–504.

Sanchez P (2002) Immunoprophylaxis for respiratory syncytial virus. *Pediatr Infect Dis J*, **21**, 473–478.

Selwyn B (1990) The epidemiology of acute respiratory tract infection in young children: comparison of findings from several developing countries. Coordinated Data Group of BOSTID Researchers. *Rev Infect Dis*, **12**, S870–S888.

Sharland M and Bedford-Russell A (2001) Preventing respiratory syncytial virus bronchiolitis. *Br Med J*, **322**, 62–63.

Shaw K, Bell L *et al.* (1991) Outpatient assessment of infants with bronchiolitis. *Am J Dis Child*, **145**, 151–155.

Shay D, Holman R *et al.* (1999) Bronchiolitis-associated hospitalizations among US children, 1980–1996. *J Am Med Assoc*, **282**, 1440–1446.

Sheeran P, Jafri H *et al.* (1999) Elevated cytokine concentrations in the nasopharyngeal and tracheal secretions of children with respiratory syncytial virus disease. *Pediatr Infect Dis J*, **18**, 115–122.

Simoes E (1999) Respiratory syncytial virus infection. *Lancet*, **354**, 847–852.

Simoes E and Carbonell-Estrany X (2003) Impact of severe disease caused by respiratory syncytial virus in children living in developed countries. *Pediatr Infect Dis J*, **22**, S13–S20.

Simoes E, Tan D *et al.* (2001) Respiratory syncytial virus vaccine: a systematic overview with emphasis on respiratory syncytial virus subunit vaccines. *Vaccine*, **20**, 954–960.

Simoes E, Tan D *et al.* (2002) Respiratory syncytial virus vaccine: a systematic overview with emphasis on respiratory syncytial virus subunit vaccines. *Vaccine*, **20**, 954–960.

Simpson W, Hacking P *et al.* (1974) The radiological findings in respiratory syncytial virus infection in children. Part II: The correlation of radiological categories with clinical and virological findings. *Pediatr Radiol*, **2**, 155–160.

Small T, Casson A *et al.* (2002) Respiratory syncytial virus infection following hematopoietic stem cell transplantation. *Bone Marrow Transpl*, **29**, 321–327.

Smith D, Frankel L *et al.* (1991) A controlled trial of aerosolized ribavirin in infants receiving mechanical ventilation for severe respiratory syncytial virus infection. *N Engl J Med*, **325**, 24–29.

Springer C, Bar-Yishay E *et al.* (1990) Corticosteroids do not affect the clinical or physiological status of infants with bronchiolitis. *Pediatr Pulmonol*, **9**, 181–185.

Srikiatkhachorn A and Braciale T (1997a) Virus-specific CD8$^+$ T lymphocytes downregulate T helper cell type 2 cytokine secretion and pulmonary eosinophilia during experimental murine respiratory syncytial virus infection. *J Exp Med*, **186**, 421–432.

Srikiatkhachorn A and Braciale T (1997b) Virus-specific memory and effector T lymphocytes exhibit different cytokine responses to antigens during experimental murine respiratory syncytial virus infection. *J Virol*, **71**, 678–685.

Srikiatkhachorn A, Chang W *et al.* (1999) Induction of Th-1 and Th-2 responses by respiratory syncytial virus attachment glycoprotein is epitope and major histocompatibility complex independent. *J Virol*, **73**, 6590–6597.

Stevens T, Sinkin R *et al.* (2000) Respiratory syncytial virus and premature infants born at 32 weeks' gestation or earlier. *Arch Pediatr Adoles Med*, **154**, 55–61.

Takimoto C, Cram D *et al.* (1991) Respiratory syncytial virus infections on an adult medical ward. *Arch Intern Med*, **151**, 706–708.

Tang Y, Heimgartner P *et al.* (1999) A colorimetric microtiter plate PCR system detects respiratory syncytial virus in nasal aspirates and discriminates subtypes A and B. *Diagn Microbiol Infect Dis*, **34**, 333–337.

Tang Y-W and Graham B (1994) Anti-IL-4 treatment at immunization modulates cytokine expression, reduces illness, and increases cytotoxic T lymphocyte activity in mice challenged with respiratory syncytial virus. *J Clin Invest*, **94**, 1953–1958.

Thomas M, Bedford-Russell A *et al.* (2000) Hospitalization for RSV infection in ex-preterm infants—implications for use of RSV immune globulin. *Arch Dis Child*, **83**, 122–127.

Toms G (1990) Respiratory syncytial virus: virology, diagnosis, and vaccination. *Lung*, **168**, 388–395.

Toms G (1995) Respiratory syncytial virus—how soon will we have a vaccine? *Arch Dis Child*, **72**, 1–3.

Tripp R, Moore D *et al.* (2002) Peripheral blood mononuclear cells from infants hospitalized because of respiratory syncytial virus infection express T helper-1 and T helper-2 cytokines and CC chemokine messenger RNA. *J Infect Dis*, **185**, 1388–1394.

Tristram D, Welliver R *et al.* (1993) Immunogenicity and safety of respiratory syncytial virus subunit vaccine in seropositive children 18–36 months old. *J Infect Dis*, **167**, 191–195.

van Schaik S, Welliver R *et al.* (2000) Novel pathways in the pathogenesis of respiratory syncytial virus disease. *Pediatr Pulmonol*, **30**, 131–138.

van Woensel J, Kimpen J *et al.* (2000) Long-term effects of prednisolone in the acute phase of bronchiolitis caused by respiratory syncytial virus. *Pediatr Pulmonol*, **30**, 92–96.

Vikerfors T, Grandien M *et al.* (1988) Detection of an immunoglobulin M response in the elderly for early diagnosis of respiratory syncytial virus infection. *J Clin Microbiol*, **26**, 808–811.

Wang E and Tang N (2000) Immunoglobulin for preventing respiratory syncytial virus infection. *Cochrane Database Syst Rev*, **2**, CD001725.

Waris M, Tsou C *et al.* (1996) Respiratory syncytial virus infection in BALB/c mice previously immunized with formalin-inactivated virus induces enhanced pulmonary inflammatory response with a predominant Th2-like cytokine pattern. *J Virol*, **70**, 2852–2860.

Weisman L (2003) Populations at risk for developing respiratory syncytial virus and risk factors for respiratory syncytial virus severity: infants with predisposing conditions. *Pediatr Infect Dis J*, **22**, S33–S39.

Welliver R (2000) Immunology of respiratory syncytial virus infection: eosinophils, cytokines, chemokines, and asthma. *Pediatr Infect Dis J*, **19**, 780–783.

Welliver R and Duffy L (1993) The relationship of RSV-specific immunoglobulin E antibody responses in infancy, recurrent wheezing, and pulmonary function at age 7–8 years. *Pediatr Pulmonol*, **15**, 19–27.

Welliver R, Garofalo R *et al.* (2002) β-Chemokines, but neither T helper type 1 nor T helper type 2 cytokines, correlate with severity of illness during respiratory syncytial virus infection. *Pediatr Infect Dis J*, **21**, 457–561.

Wennergren G and Kristjansson S (2001) Relationship between respiratory syncytial virus bronchiolitis and future obstructive airway diseases. *Eur Respir J*, **18**, 1044–1058.

West W, Lounsbach G *et al.* (1994) Biological activity, binding site and affinity of monoclonal antibodies to the fusion protein of respiratory syncytial virus. *J Gen Virol*, **75**, 2813–2819.

Whimbey E, Englund J *et al.* (1997) Community respiratory viral infections in the immunocompromised host. *Am J Med*, **102**, 1–80.

8

Adenoviruses

Marcela Echavarría

CEMIC University Hospital, Buenos Aires, Argentina

INTRODUCTION

Adenoviruses, when discovered in 1953, were initially associated with acute respiratory disease. It was soon recognised that in addition to respiratory infections, adenoviruses are responsible for gastrointestinal and ocular infections worldwide. More recently, these viruses have been associated with additional important syndromes, including pharyngitis, pharyngoconjunctival fever, conjunctivitis, pertussis-like syndrome, keratoconjunctivitis, bronchiolitis, pneumonia and acute haemorrhagic cystitis. Less frequently, they also cause hepatitis, meningitis, encephalitis, myocarditis, pericarditis, genital infections, pancreatitis and disseminated fatal disease. Clinical manifestations vary with the host, the site of pathology and the serotype involved.

The virus has been extensively studied. It is an icosohedral, non-enveloped virus that is relatively persistent on environmental surfaces and readily spread in closed populations. To date, 51 adenovirus serotypes have been described. Most of the higher serotypes have been isolated from immunocompromised individuals. Different serotypes have had a predilection for specific clinical manifestations, indicating their different tropisms.

Adenovirus infections are common, especially during childhood. Although frequently asymptomatic or mild and self-limited, disease may be severe, with high mortality rates in some patients. Recently, wider tropisms of adenovirus infections have been increasingly recognised, especially in immunocompromised individuals. These findings may be attributed to a greater awareness of these viruses and their pathogenic role in a range of diseases and to the development of more sensitive diagnostic methods. Therefore, sensitive, rapid and early diagnosis has become important, given the severity of the disease and high mortality rates in some patient populations.

Adenovirus diagnosis can be performed using direct or indirect methods, including virus isolation in cell culture, electron microscopy, antigen detection by immunofluorescence and immunohistochemistry and genome detection, with or without amplification and serology. New and recently developed molecular methods using DNA amplification by polymerase chain reaction (PCR) have increased the sensitivity and rapidity of diagnosis. Although no specific treatment has been evaluated in prospective and controlled clinical trials, there is evidence that some antiviral agents may be useful with early diagnosis

HISTORY

Adenoviruses (AdVs) were initially recognised in the 1950s during active searching for agents that cause respiratory tract infections. In 1953, Rowe *et al.* described an agent that caused spontaneous degeneration of tissue culture cells from adenoidectomies obtained from children. Hilleman and Werner (1954) recovered in cell culture a similar agent from respiratory samples of military recruits with acute respiratory disease or atypical pneumonia. It was shown that the viruses discovered by the two groups were related. They were initially called 'adenoid-degeneration agent' (Rowe *et al.*, 1953) and 'RI-67' 'respiratory infection

Principles and Practice of Clinical Virology, Fifth Edition. Edited by A. J. Zuckerman, J. E. Banatvala, J. R. Pattison, P. D. Griffiths and B. D. Schoub
© 2004 John Wiley & Sons Ltd   ISBN 0 470 84338 1

from recruit No. 67' (Hilleman and Werner, 1954) but in 1956 the term 'adenoviruses' was adopted as they were first recovered from adenoid tissues (Enders *et al.*, 1956).

In 1942, a commission on acute respiratory disease defined the term 'acute respiratory disease' (ARD) as an entity caused by filterable agents with an incubation period of 5–6 days. After the discovery of AdV in military recruits, retrospective serological procedures demonstrated that AdV was present and associated with ARD in soldiers at Fort Bragg during World War II.

TAXONOMY

Adenoviruses (AdVs) are widespread in nature and have been isolated from human and many animal species. The family *Adenoviridae* has been recently subdivided into four genera: *Mastadenovirus*, *Aviadenovirus*, *Atadenovirus* and *Siadenovirus* (Mayo, 2002).

The genus *Aviadenovirus*, from the latin 'avi' meaning 'bird', is limited to viruses of birds.

The genus *Mastadenovirus*, from the Greek 'mastos' meaning 'breast', infects mammals and includes human, simian, bovine, equine, porcine, ovine, canine and opossum viruses.

The genus *Atadenovirus*, named in recognition of the high A + T content in the genome, has been recovered from reptiles, birds, marsupials and ruminants.

The genus *Siadenovirus*, from '*Si*' for '*sialidase*', in recognition of the presence of a putative sialidase homologue gene, infects amphibians and birds.

The regions E1A and E1B, E3 and E4 are present only in the genus *Mastadenovirus*. In the other genera, the location and organisation of these three early regions is very different.

BASIC VIROLOGY

At least 19 species from different animals have been described within the genus *Mastadenovirus*, six of which are human adenoviruses. These six species (formerly called subgenera) are called *Human adenovirus A–F*. The human species A, B (subdivided into subspecies B1 and B2), C, D, E and F were defined based on immunological, biological, and biochemical characteristics, specifically on the basis of oncogenicity in rodents, the differential haemagglutination patterns with erythrocytes from different species, the lengths of their fibres and the percentage of G + C in the genome (Table 8.1). AdV serotype 12 was the first DNA virus shown to cause tumours in animals. Although all AdVs can transform cells in tissue culture, there is no clear evidence that they cause cancer in humans.

Different AdV serotypes are described within one species. A serotype is defined on the basis of its immunological distinctiveness, as determined by quantitative neutralisation with animal antisera. To date, 51 human serotypes have been distinguished by neutralisation (De Jong *et al.*, 1999). Initially, only 24 antigenically distinct adenoviruses have been described. In 1960, serotypes 25–33 were recovered from stool samples and were not associated with known diseases. Types 40 and 41 were associated with gastroenteritis and the last nine serotypes (43–51) were isolated from AIDS patients (De Jong *et al.*, 1999). Within one serotype there may be different genotypes, which suggests changes of the genomic DNA that are not associated with serological changes. Genome typing can be done by restriction endonuclease analysis of full-length viral DNA, by PCR or by sequencing. Forty genotypes for AdV 2, 12 for AdV 7 and 11 for AdV 11 are some of the examples obtained by restriction enzyme analysis (Adrian *et al.*, 1986). The prototype strain is named with the letter 'p' and

Table 8.1 Classification of the 51 human adenovirus serotypes by species characteristics

Species	Serotypes	Oncogenic potential	G + C (%)	Haemagglutination		Fibre length (nm)
				Rhesus	Rat	
A	12, 18, 31	High	48–49	−	+/−	28–31
B1	3, 7, 16, 21, 50	Weak	50–52	+	−	9–11
B2	11, 14, 24, 35	Weak	50–52	+	−	9–11
C	1, 2, 5, 6	None	57–59	−	+/−	23–31
D	8–10, 13, 15, 17, 19, 20, 22–30, 32, 33, 36–39, 42–49, 51	None	58	+/−	+	12–13
E	4	None	57–61	−	+/−	17
F	40, 41	None	57–59	−	+/−	∼29

the subsequent genotypes with letters a, b, c, d, etc. Most of the prototype strains are not currently circulating, probably due to a continuous evolutionary process. Although AdVs are DNA viruses with a DNA polymerase, giving high fidelity due to proof-reading capability, the emergence of new serotypes and genotypes is well known, especially among species D. The appearance of multiple serotypes or genotypes among AdVs and papillomaviruses (another DNA virus) suggests an evolutionary mechanism. Beside homologous recombination as a primary mechanism for evolution, it has been proposed that illegitimate recombination can occur among AdVs (Crawford-Miksza and Schnurr, 1996).

STRUCTURE

There is no common antigenic determinant that characterises the whole family. However, all members of the family *Adenoviridae* have a virus particle of similar size, structure and polypeptide composition. Adenoviruses are non-enveloped viruses, 70–90 nm in diameter, and have 10 structural proteins. The capsid proteins are arranged in an icosahedron with 252 capsomers divided into two principal types: 240 hexons occupying the 20 triangular faces of the virus and 12 pentons at the 12 vertices of the particle. Each penton consists of a base and a fibre, which is a rod-like outward projection of variable length (depending on the serotype) with a terminal knob that is responsible for the interaction with the cellular receptor (Figure 8.1, see plate section). The pentons are especially active in haemagglutination. The polypeptides are numbered with Roman numerals (I–X) and some of their functions are still unknown (Table 8.2). The hexon, penton and fibre (polypeptides II, III and IV,

respectively) are the major components of the capsid and the principal antigenic determinants of the virus (Figure 8.1). Neutralising antibodies are directed against the ε epitope of the hexon. Each hexon has three identical chains of polypeptide II (complex protein of 900 residues) and each fibre has three identical units of polypeptide IV. Polypeptides V and VII are strongly basic proteins and are associated with the viral DNA in the core of the particle. They may be involved in neutralising the charges during the packaging process (Figure 8.1).

AdVs have a linear, non-segmented, double-stranded DNA of about 36 kb. The terminal nucleotide sequences are inverted repetitions and there is a protein of 55 kDa covalently attached to the 5′ end of each strand. Both of these features are related to viral DNA replication, which contains two identical origins.

RESISTANCE TO PHYSICOCHEMICAL AGENTS

As non-enveloped viruses, AdVs are resistant to inactivation at room temperature. They are unusually resistant to physical and chemical agents, resulting in prolonged survival and a great potential for spread. They can spread through water, fomites, instruments and between individuals, including nosocomially. They are stable at low pH and resistant to gastric and biliary secretions, thus allowing the virus to replicate and achieve a high viral load in the gut. They are resistant to ether and isopropyl alcohol. Sodium hypochlorite (500 ppm) for 10 min, or immersion in a water bath at 75°C for 30 s, at 60°C for 2 min or at 56°C for 30 min can be used to inactivate AdV. Serotype 4 is especially heat-resistant. They survive freezing with minimal loss of infectivity.

Table 8.2 Adenovirus proteins

No.	Proteins from the capsid	
	Name	Known functions
II	Hexon monomer	Structural
III	Penton base	Penetration
IIIa	Associated to penton base	Penetration
IV	Fibre	Receptor attachment, haemagglutination
V	Core: associated to DNA and penton base	Histone-like; packaging?
VI	Hexon minor polypeptide	Stability/particle assembly?
VII	Core	Histone-like
VIII	Hexon minor polypeptide	Stability/particle assembly?
IX	Hexon minor polypeptide	Stability/particle assembly?
TP	Genome–terminal protein	Genomic replication

REPLICATION

Adenoviruses initially interact with the host cells via the knobs of the fibre. Most human adenovirus species A, C, D, E and F use the coxsackie-adenovirus receptor (CAR) protein, which is a member of the immunoglobulin superfamily, as the initial receptor (Roelvink *et al.*, 1998).

The species B attachment receptor has not been identified, although recent studies have proposed a species B adenovirus receptor (sBAR) for species B1 and B2 and a specific receptor sB2AR exclusively for species B2 (Segerman *et al.*, 2003). Some adenovirus serotypes use a receptor other than CAR. Adenovirus serotypes 8, 19 and 37 (species D), which cause epidemic keratoconjunctivitis, use sialic acid saccharides as a cellular receptor (Arnberg *et al.*, 2002).

After attachment, the virus migrates to clathrin-coated pits and is internalised in endosomes. Interaction between the penton base protein of the viral capsid and integrins ($\alpha_v\beta_3$ and $\alpha_v\beta_5$) is needed for efficient internalisation. The interaction occurs through an Arg–Gly–Asp (RGD) sequence present in the penton base. Since not all cell types produce α_v integrins, attachment can occur but no efficient replication is achieved. Uncoating of the virus occurs and transport of the genome to the host nucleus is microtubule-mediated. The intracellular trafficking is different for species B and C. AdV 5 (species C) rapidly translocates to the nucleus within 1 h after infection, while AdV 7 (species B) is widely distributed in the cytoplasm. It has been suggested that the fibres not only mediate binding to the cell surface but also modulate intracellular trafficking (Miyazawa *et al.*, 1999).

AdVs conduct a carefully orchestrated programme of gene expression after infecting sensitive cells. Viral proteins are expressed and viral DNA replication, which occurs in the nucleus, starts 12 h post-infection in tissue culture. After maturation, the viruses remain localised in the nucleus (Figure 8.2). During a lytic infection the cells die and the virus particles are liberated.

Virus DNA Replication

The replication cycle is divided into three phases: an immediate early phase, a delayed early phase that precedes viral DNA replication and a late phase that follows DNA replication and is characterised by the expression of the structural proteins of the viral capsid.

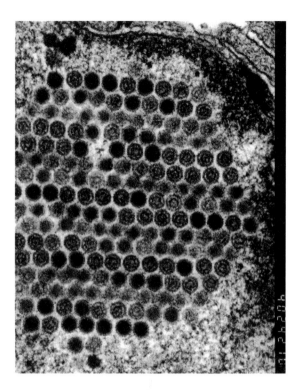

Figure 8.2 Electronic microscopy micrographs of adenovirus in the nucleus. (Provided by Dr L. Asher)

The five early transcription units are E1A, E1B, E2, E3 and E4. E1A and E1B stimulate the infected cell to transcribe and replicate AdV genes (Russell, 2000). E1A blocks interferon-induced gene expression and blocks the ability of the p53 and Rb growth suppressor genes to suppress cell division. E1B proteins inhibit apoptosis in the stimulated cell. The E2 region codes for proteins necessary for viral DNA replication. Several E3 products prevent death due to receptor-mediated apoptosis. E3/14.7K seems to interfere with the cytolytic and pro-inflammatory activities of TNF while E3/10.4K and 14.5K proteins remove Fas and TRAIL receptors from the cell surface by inducing their degradation in lysosomes. These and other functions that may affect granule-mediated cell death might drastically limit lysis by NK cells and cytotoxic T cells. In general, E3 gene products appear to facilitate immune evasion. E4 gene products are diverse and some are required for efficient tripartite splicing used in the transcription of the late genes. The two delayed early units are IX and IVa2 and one late unit that is processed to generate five families of late mRNA (L1, L2, L3, L4 and L5). Not all the late genes are structural. There are also virus-associated (VA) genes transcribed by the RNA polymerase III. The VA RNA is a short, highly structured RNA that interferes with the cell's ability to produce interferon.

Almost all transcription units generate a complex set of alternately spliced mRNAs that encode for multiple proteins. Interestingly, important molecular and cell biological processes such as RNA splicing and cell cycle regulation were discovered while studying adenovirus gene expression.

Assembly of the virion particles occurs in the nucleus, where they form crystalin aggregates like nuclear inclusion bodies (Figure 8.2). The replication cycle takes approximately 30 h and results in the production of 100–10 000 new virus particles/cell.

There are three types of infection: (a) lytic—cell death occurs as a result of virus infection, as in mucoepithelial cells; (b) latent/persistent—the virus remains in the host cell (lymphoid tissue); and (c) oncogenic transformation—the cell grows and the replication continues without cell death. This last mechanism has been observed in hamsters infected with AdV species A.

EPIDEMIOLOGY

AdV infections are transmitted by direct contact, small droplet aerosols, the faecal–oral route, water, ocular instruments and fomites. The mode of transmission in early life is thought to be primarily faecal–oral. A child born in a family with relatives harbouring the virus in the intestine will eventually become an excretor. An infected child may excrete the virus initially from the respiratory tract and later from the gastrointestinal tract. Intermittent excretion in stools can be as prolonged as 906 days (Brandt et al., 1969). AdV infections occur worldwide as epidemic, endemic and sporadic infections.

The most common AdV serotypes causing respiratory infections are serotypes 1, 2 and 5 (species C) and serotypes 3 and 7 (species B). AdV types 1, 2, 5 and 6 are mostly endemic, whereas 4, 7, 14 and 21 cause small epidemics. Respiratory outbreaks have been described in closed communities such as boarding schools, day care centres and military training facilities. For epidemic types (4 and 7) respiratory spread by contact and by aerosols is important.

The epidemiological pattern of AdV respiratory infection in civilian populations is different from the military. Recent publications have described serotypes 4, 7 and 21 as the most prevalent types related to respiratory outbreaks among military recruits in the USA (Kolavic-Gray et al., 2002).

AdV can cause ocular infections, such as pharyngo-conjunctival fever (PCF) and keratoconjunctivitis (KC). PCF has been mostly associated with serotypes 1–7 and less frequently with serotypes 11–17, 19–21 and 29. Serotypes 3, 4 and 7 are commonly associated with swimming pool outbreaks (Turner et al., 1987). AdV 4, causing ocular infections, is common in Asia but uncommon in Western countries. Large epidemics of KC have been associated with serotypes 8, 9 and 37 (Keenlyside et al., 1983). They spread by contact, through contaminated fingers or ophthalmological instruments. These serotypes are often endemic in the poor hygienic conditions of developing countries, but in Western countries occur mostly in epidemics that are sometimes nosocomial.

Infant gastroenteritis has been mostly associated with serotypes 40 and 41, therefore named as 'enteric adenoviruses'. Types 2 and 31, and even less frequently types 1, 3, 5, 7, 12 and 18, can cause acute gastroenteritis (Yolken et al., 1982). Enteric 40 and 41 types spread via the faecal–oral route and gastroenteritis occurs endemically throughout the world.

CLINICAL MANIFESTATIONS

AdV infections are widely distributed and common. Infections occur most frequently during childhood, where they tend to be self-limited and induce type-specific immunity following recovery. Approximately half of the human AdV serotypes are known to cause illness in humans. AdV serotypes have different cell tropisms and cause distinct clinical manifestations (Table 8.3). In addition, some genotypes (e.g. serotype 7h) are more virulent than others, causing unusually severe manifestations and higher mortality rates (Kajon et al., 1996). Although AdV infections were traditionally associated only with respiratory, ocular and gastrointestinal diseases, many other clinical manifestations have been associated with AdV replication, especially in immunocompromised patients. Clinical manifestations depend on the host and the serotype involved and include pharyngitis, pharyngoconjunctival fever, conjunctivitis, pertussis-like syndrome, keratoconjunctivitis, bronchiolitis, pneumonia, acute haemorrhagic cystitis and gastroenteritis. Less frequent clinical syndromes are hepatitis, meningitis, encephalitis, myocarditis, pericarditis, genital infections, pancreatitis and fatal disseminated disease

Table 8.3 Adenovirus infections and serotypes involved

Syndrome	Signs and symptoms		AdV serotypes	
	More frequent	Less frequent	Frequently	Less frequent
Upper respiratory disease	Coryza, pharyngitis, fever, tonsillitis	Otitis media, gastroenteritis	1, 2, 3, 5, 7	4, 6, 11, 18, 21, 29, 31
Lower respiratory disease	Bronchitis, pneumonia, fever, cough	Bronchiolitis	3, 4, 7, 21	1, 2, 5, 35
Pertussis syndrome	Paroxysmal cough, vomiting	Fever, URI	5	1, 2, 3
Acute respiratory disease	Tracheobronchitis, fever, myalgia, coryza	Pneumonia	4, 7	3, 14, 21
Pharyngoconjunctival fever	Pharyngitis, fever, conjunctivitis	Coryza, headache, diarrhoea, rash, nodes	3, 4, 7	1, 11, 14, 16, 19, 37
Epidemic keratoconjunctivitis	Keratitis, headache, preauricular nodes	Coryza, pharyngitis, gastroenteritis	8, 37	3, 4, 7, 10, 11, 19, 21
Haemorrhagic conjunctivitis	Chemosis, follicles, subconjunctival haemorrhages	Preauricular nodes, fever, coryza	11	2–8, 14, 15, 19, 37
Haemorrhagic cystitis	Cystitis	Fever, pharyngitis	11	7, 21, 34, 35
Immunocompromised host disease	Diarrhoea, rash, URI, pneumonia, cystitis	Hepatitis, otitis media, pancreatitis	1, 2, 5, 11, 34, 35	7, 21, 29–31, 37–39, 35, 43
Infant gastroenteritis	Diarrhoea, fever	Nausea, vomiting, mild URI	31, 40, 41	1, 2, 12–17, 21, 25, 26, 29
Neurological disease	Meningitis	Encephalitis, Reye's syndrome	7	3, 32
Venereal disease	Ulcerative genital lesions	Cervicitis, urethritis	2, 37	1, 5, 7, 11, 18, 19, 31

Adapted from Hierholzer (1995).
URI, upper respiratory infection.

(Davis *et al.*, 1988; Swenson *et al.*, 1995; Munoz *et al.*, 1998).

RESPIRATORY INFECTIONS

In Children

Most children become infected with one or more AdV types early in life. These infections are usually self-limited and mild. When symptomatic, the usual signs and symptoms are fever, nasal congestion, coryza, pharyngitis and cough, with or without otitis media. AdV may cause an exudative tonsillitis that is clinically indistinguishable from group A streptococcus. If conjunctivitis accompanies the syndrome, the disease is called pharyngoconjunctival fever. The most frequent serotypes associated with paediatric upper respiratory tract infections are types 1–3 and 5–7. In some cases, there may be a prolonged viral excretion in stools, continuing for months or years, after the onset of symptoms (Brandt *et al.*, 1969). This feature may account for the endemic presence of the virus in paediatric populations. AdV types 1, 2, 5 and 6 may persist in adenoidal and tonsillar tissues (Rowe *et al.*, 1953).

AdV can also cause acute lower respiratory infections (ALRIs) that may require hospitalisation. In children less than 4 years old, 2–7% of acute respiratory infections and 10% of respiratory infections that require hospitalisation are caused by adenoviruses. The syndromes include bronchitis, bronchiolitis, croup, and pneumonia. Severe and even fatal pneumonia, with a fatality rate around 16% or higher that is primarily associated with AdV types 3 and 7, can occur in infants and children (Murtagh *et al.*, 1993). Among survivors, residual lung damage secondary to bronchiolitis obliterans has been reported. Children less than 2 years old are more susceptible to severe primary infections, with occasionally fatal outcomes and long-term sequelae. In general, extrapulmonary manifestations, such as gastroenteritis, renal involvement, hepatosplenomegaly, meningoencephalitis or disseminated disease, have been associated with a higher mortality rate. AdV can be recovered throughout the year although higher frequency is observed in winter and spring.

AdVs are the third most common cause of viral ALRI. In the south cone of America (Argentina, Chile and Uruguay), they are the second most common viral entity (Weissenbacher et al., 1990). In Argentina, the prevalence of AdV in hospitalised children with ALRI is in the range 3–14%, depending on the complexity of the hospital analysed (Videla et al., 1998a; Carballal et al., 2001). The most frequently recovered types were from species B. The genetic variant 7h, initially described in Argentina, was associated with a fatal outcome in 34% of cases during the acute stage of the disease (Murtagh et al., 1993). In this study, none of the patients had been exposed to measles or was immunocompromised, and most were under 1 year of age. In bronchiolitis cases, intense air trapping with parahilar and peribronchiolar infiltrates and with segmental or lobar atelectasis is observed, frequently localised in the right upper lobe. Infiltrates radiate outwards from the hilar regions can be associated with bilateral hilar adenopathies. When multifocal pneumonia develops, fluffy or patchy and dense parenchymal infiltrates, indicating alveolar consolidations scattered throughout both lungs, with ill-defined margins, are observed. With progression of the disease, hazy to totally opaque lungs can be observed. Air leaks can produce pneumothorax or pneumomediastinum (Murtagh et al., 1993). Of those who recover, most have residual chronic pulmonary sequelae. Genotype 7h may have an increased virulent effect compared to other types (Kajon and Wadell, 1994). During 1984–1985, the predominant genotype in Argentina was 7c but in 1986 it switched to 7h (Carballal et al., 2002). In Japan, the first report on 7h occurred in 1996 (Hashido et al., 1999). In the USA, Australia and countries in Europe, the most prevalent genotype has been 7b, although the recent appearance of 7d2 and 7h in North America represents recent introduction of these viruses from previously geographically restricted areas (Erdman et al., 2002).

Severe lung disease after measles infections have also been described. It is suggested that secondary infection with AdV is responsible for causing this lung disease in some patients. Measles virus may have rendered the children more susceptible to serious complications from AdV infection. The many deaths from 'measles pneumonia' in developing countries and the occasional occurrence of post-measles bronchiectasis in some countries may be due to secondary AdV infections (Warner and Marshall, 1976).

Pertussis-like Syndrome

Pertussis syndrome is usually caused by Bordetella pertussis; however, AdVs have been frequently isolated in patients with this syndrome. The rate of AdV infection was statistically significant in patients with pertussis syndrome (23%) vs. control subjects (5%). The frequent association of AdV with pertussis syndrome may play a role in the pathogenesis of this disease. AdV type 5 has been isolated from patients with severe whooping cough that ended fatally. It is not known whether AdV co-infects with B. pertussis or whether that infection may cause conditions favourable to reactivation of latent AdV.

Acute Respiratory Disease in Military Recruits

Adenoviruses were first associated with respiratory outbreaks among military recruits undergoing basic training in 1953 (Hilleman and Werner, 1954). During the 1950s and 1960s, AdV-associated acute respiratory disease (ARD) constituted one of the most important causes of medical morbidity among military recruits in the USA. The serotypes most commonly associated with respiratory disease were types 4 and 7, with types 3, 14 and 21 also detected in these populations. Severe ARD required hospitalisations in 50% of cases at Fort Dix (Top, 1975) and fatal pneumonia with AdV type 7 was reported in three previously healthy military trainees (Dudding et al., 1972).

Since 1980, the routine use of live oral vaccines to serotypes 4 and 7 among military recruits resulted in a significant decrease in ARD morbidity (Figure 8.3). However, in 1996 a discontinuation of production resulted in a resurgence of AdV-associated respiratory disease epidemics at military training centres (Kolavic-Gray et al., 2002). Most recruits presented with fever, sore throat and persistent cough. AdV 4 was the most prevalent type recovered, followed by types 3 and 21.

During the pre-vaccine era, recruits used to develop severe signs and symptoms of lower respiratory tract infection and pneumonia. During recent respiratory outbreaks (1997, 1998, 2000 and 2001), the hospitalisation rates have been 10–21% but were not significantly severe (Kolavic-Gray et al., 2002). The low level of pre-existing immunity for AdV 4 (12–26%) in young adults may reflect the lack of exposure to this serotype during childhood. Type 4 has uncommonly been associated with respiratory disease in civilians. The different epidemiology of AdV among civilian and military groups is not completely understood. It may be due to conditions during military training, where individuals from different geographic areas and backgrounds are subjected to crowding and stress that may potentiate outbreaks. In one study evaluating for AdV carriage at entry, no AdV was recovered by culture in throat swab

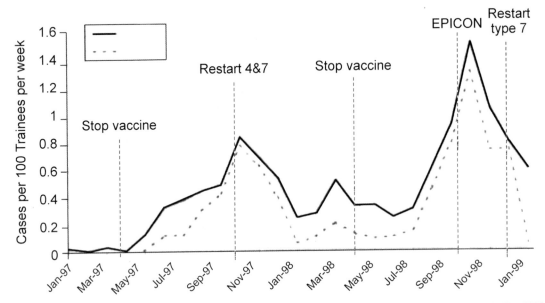

Figure 8.3 Average weekly acute respiratory disease (ARD) and adenovirus (AdV) rates at Fort Jackson, USA (Jan 1997–Jan 1999)

samples, although one individual was weakly positive by PCR (Echavarria *et al.*, 2003).

Interestingly, adenovirus DNA type 4 was detected by PCR from air filters in sleeping barracks during respiratory outbreaks (Echavarria *et al.*, 2000a). Positivity in air filters correlated with the number of hospitalisations due to AdV-ARD during the same period. Environmental control of air-borne spread of AdV may help to reduce the risk of AdV-associated outbreaks during periods of vaccine unavailability.

OCULAR INFECTIONS

Pharyngoconjunctival Fever

Pharyngoconjunctival fever (PCF) is characterised by follicular conjunctivitis and lymphadenopathy as well as fever, pharyngitis and malaise. Headache, diarrhoea and rash can also be present and 5–10% of patients may have involvement of the cornea. Either one or both eyes may be involved. Infected individuals can shed the virus for about 10 days. Complete recovery without sequelae usually occurs. PCF is seen in children and young adults in discrete outbreaks, but sporadic cases occur at all ages. Community outbreaks of PCF have been associated with inappropriate chlorination systems in swimming pools (Turner *et*

al., 1987). Illness was directly related to hours of exposure to the pool and swallowing pool water. AdV serotypes 3 and 7 have been mostly associated with PCF. AdV types 1–7, 11–17, 19 and 21 have also been reported.

Epidemic Keratoconjunctivitis

In contrast to PCF, epidemic keratoconjunctivitis (EKC) is highly contagious and serious. EKC can start with conjunctivitis that may be follicular, followed by oedema of the eyelids, pain, photophobia and lacrimation. Superficial erosions of the cornea may occur, followed by deeper subepithelial corneal infiltrates with a characteristic round shape. A mild respiratory infection may accompany the symptoms. This clinical entity was identified in 1941, before AdV were initially isolated, in the marine shipyards at Pearl Harbor. 'Shipyard eye' was probably transmitted in the medical facilities caring for eye trauma. AdV 8 was the cause of those infections.

The incubation time may be 8–10 days and conjunctivitis may resolve in 2 weeks, although reduced vision, photophobia and foreign body sensation may persist for months to years. Adenoviruses 8, 19 and 37 are the most prevalent serotypes associated with keratoconjunctivitis. In Japan, AdV 4 has also been associated with this condition.

EKC outbreaks have been reported in many countries as an important cause of nosocomial morbidity in ophthalmology clinics. Risk factors for EKC were associated with exposure to contact tonometry (Keenlyside et al., 1983). Ophthalmic solutions, the hands of medical personnel and towels are also vehicles for spread. Direct inoculation into the eye appears to be needed to cause disease. In areas with high levels of air-borne particulates, EKC outbreaks have resulted from eye–fomite–eye inoculation.

In Taiwan and Japan, epidemics of keratoconjunctivitis presumably occur by direct contact between children and family members.

GASTROINTESTINAL INFECTIONS

Adenoviruses are the second most common cause of viral gastroenteritis in children less than 2 years old. The incidence for this disease is 4–12% of cases of diarrhoea and it occurs throughout the year. The route of transmission is the faecal–oral route. During the prodrome, 50% of the patients have respiratory symptoms. Diarrhoea is usually watery, non-bloody and with no faecal leukocytosis. The mean duration is 10 days. It may be associated with mild fever, vomiting and abdominal pain. Gastroenteritis may also be a sign of systemic infection related to serotypes 3 and 7 that cause respiratory symptoms. Subsequent to gastroenteritis due to AdV, some patients become intolerant to lactose-containing products for up to 5–7 months. Other gastrointestinal syndromes associated with AdV have included intussusception, acute mesenteric lymphadenitis and appendicitis. Serotypes 40 and 41, called the enteric adenoviruses, are the most prevalent types that cause acute gastroenteritis (van der Avoort et al., 1989). In patients who develop AdV enteritis, the enteric strains seem to induce disease that persists longer than that caused by strains other than 40 and 41.

HAEMORRHAGIC CYSTITIS

Adenoviruses can cause acute haemorrhagic cystitis (HC) in paediatric populations and in immuncompromised patients. A sudden onset of gross haematuria, dysuria and increased frequency of urination has been described. Serotype 11 is the most prevalent type recovered in these patients (Ambinder et al., 1986). Other serotypes, including 34 and 35, have also been

commonly recovered from immunocompromised patients. AdVs 11, 34 and 35 can cause persistent infection in the kidney and may be reactivated during immunosuppression. HC has been highly associated with AdV in bone marrow transplant recipients and can represent the first clinical manifestation of a disseminated adenoviral disease (Echavarria et al., 1999). HC has also been described in renal transplant recipients.

ADV INFECTIONS IN IMMUNOCOMPROMISED PATIENTS

Adenoviruses are increasingly recognised as viral pathogens that may cause severe disease, including fatal infections in immunocompromised patients. In recent years, populations of immunocompromised patients have expanded due to advances in transplantation technology and treatment, cancer therapy and the AIDS epidemic. The severity of AdV disease differs in immunocompromised patients, in whom the infection tends to be long-term, difficult to treat and may result in fatal outcome. AdV-associated case fatality rates in the immunocompromised have been reported to be as high as 60% for patients with pneumonia, and 50% for those with hepatitis, compared with fatality rates of 15% for pneumonia and 10% for hepatitis in immunocompetent patients (Hierholzer, 1992).

In bone marrow transplant (BMT) recipients, AdV infections are especially frequent. An increasing incidence of 5–14% or higher in adults and 31% in children has recently been described (Table 8.4). Of those with definite or probable AdV disease, the mortality rates varied (12–70%) (Table 8.4). The prevalence of infection and mortality rates vary significantly with the population studied (Table 8.4). Underlying disease, type of transplant, age and serotype involved count for the different prevalence and severity of AdV infection. Some of the risk factors for the development of infection are: lower age, allogeneic transplant, T cell depletion, unmatched donor and total body irradiation. The infection is thought to be due to reactivation of latent virus or transmission of latent virus via donor marrow or transfusion. The clinical manifestations in BMT include haemorrhagic cystitis, pneumonia, hepatitis, colitis, pancreatitis and disseminated disease. AdV detection in plasma has been associated with fatal disseminated disease (Echavarria et al., 2001a). AdV infection can develop between the first and third month post-transplant, although AdV has been

Table 8.4 Prevalence of adenovirus infection among bone marrow and haematopoietic stem cell transplant recipients

Publication	Characteristics	AdV infection (n)	% Fatal
Yolken et al., 1982	BMT	15% (12/78)	42
Shields et al., 1985	A, C, BMT	5% (51/1051)	10
Wasserman et al., 1988	C, Allo, Auto, BMT	18% (17/96)	NA
Ljungman et al., 1989	BMT	6% (5/78)	20
Flomenberg et al., 1994	A, C, Allo, Auto, TCD, TBI, BMT	21% (42/201) [14% A; 31% C]	17
Blanke et al., 1995	Allo, TCD, BMT	14% (10/74)	50
Hale et al., 1999	C, TBI, Allo, Auto BMT	6% (13/206)	50
Howard et al., 1999	A, C, BMT	12% (64/532)	17
Venard et al., 2000	Allo, Auto, TCD, BMT	20% (13/65)	70
Bordigoni et al., 2001	Allo, TCD, BMT	12% (35/303)	41
Runde et al., 2001	A, C, Allo, HSCT	27% (35/130)	0
Hoffman et al., 2001	Allo, HSCT	47% (17/36)	12
La Rosa et al., 2001	A, HSCT	3% (87/2889)	26
Chakrabarti et al., 2002	A, Allo, HSCT	20% (15/76)	13
Schilham et al., 2002	C, HSCT	11% (36/328)	19

A, adults; C, children; Auto, autologous; Allo, allogeneic; BMT, bone marrow transplant; HSCT, haematopoietic stem cell transplant; TBI, total body irradiation; TCD, T cell depletion.

recovered during the first month, even before transplantation, and 1 year post-transplant. The serotypes most frequently recovered from BMT patients in urine are 11, 34 and 35. Other serotypes, such as 1–7, 12, 31 and 41, have been recovered from respiratory samples, blood and stools.

In liver transplant recipients, the most frequent clinical manifestation is hepatitis most commonly associated with AdV species C (serotypes 1, 2 and 5). The mortality rate can be as high as 53%.

In renal transplant recipients, the predominant symptom is haemorrhagic cystitis, mostly related to AdV species B (serotypes 7, 11, 34 and 35) and a 17% fatality rate.

AdV infections are frequent in HIV-infected patients and can range from 7% to 29%. Many of the patients are co-infected with other pathogens. The most frequent sites for AdV recovery are the gastrointestinal and urinary tracts. Prolonged AdV faecal excretion has been associated with low CD4 counts (Khoo et al., 1995).

De Jong et al. (1983) reported a 20% isolation rate of AdV from the urine of AIDS patients, even in the absence of cystitis or haematuria. This frequency is higher when molecular methods are applied (Echavarria et al., 1998). Serotypes 11, 34, 35 and 42–47 have been found in the urine of AIDS patients (Echavarria et al., 2001b). Many of these serotypes, especially those belonging to species D, are rarely isolated from clinical samples from immunocompetent patients or from patients suffering from other kinds of immunodeficiencies.

The introduction of highly active antiretroviral therapy (HAART) has dramatically reduced the incidence and mortality from opportunistic infections, including AdV in AIDS patients. However, the development of viral resistance and difficulties with compliance may lead to the re-emergence of AdV infections.

UNCOMMON CLINICAL MANIFESTATIONS

Adenoviruses have been recovered from cerebrospinal fluid and brain tissue from patients with meningoencephalitis. AdVs 3 and 7 were the most prevalent serotypes associated with this syndrome. Severe encephalitis has also been associated with AdV species B.

AdV can also be the cause of myocarditis. The AdV genome has been detected by PCR in myocardial samples from patients with acute myocarditis.

AdV serotypes 2, 8 and 37 have been isolated in 0.3% of patients with genital lesions attending a sexually transmitted disease clinic (Swenson et al., 1995). These findings have suggested that AdV may be sexually transmissible.

AdV 36 can cause obesity in animals. Studies done in rhesus and marmoset monkeys have demonstrated a significant longitudinal association of positive antibody status to AdV 36 with weight gain (Dhurandhar et al., 2002). Further studies are needed to determine whether such an association exists in humans.

PATHOGENESIS

In vitro, AdVs cause cell rounding, aggregation and accumulation of basophilic nuclear inclusions. The pentons have a toxin-like activity and isolated penton bases produce the detachment of monolayers in cell culture after 2 h incubation. AdVs have the capability to shut down host mRNA and synthesise AdV structural proteins which accumulate in the nucleus, giving the characteristic histopathological intranuclear inclusions.

The reasons for the different organ tropisms and the production of such diverse diseases by AdV serotypes has not been completely elucidated. It has been shown that different fibre specificities demonstrate different receptor attachments.

Studies of the pathophysiology are limited, due to the lack of animal models that faithfully reproduce the diseases seen in humans. Studies on pathogenesis have been done in cotton rats (*Sigmodon hispidus*), as these animals are susceptible to intranasal infection with AdV type 5 and develop pulmonary histopathology similar to that in humans, although the virus is not truly adapted to this animal.

In the cotton rat, the virus replicates in bronchiolar epithelial cells. *In situ* hybridisation also shows early gene expression in macrophage/monocytes in alveoli and hilar lymph nodes (Ginsberg and Prince, 1994). The histopathological response consists of two phases. The early one is a mild to moderate injury of bronchiolar epithelial cells (including cytoplasmic vacuolation and loss of cilia) and diffuse infiltration of the peribronchiolar and alveolar regions with monocytes/macrophages, neutrophils and lymphocytes. The late phase consists of a peribronchiolar and perivascular infiltration composed almost entirely of lymphocytes. The predominant process is the response of the host to infection, rather than direct viral damage to cells.

Only early genes seem to be required to induce pathological changes in cotton rats. It seems that for complete viral replication it is essential only to infect a sufficient number of cells to yield an adequate expression of early gene functions. However, results from the cotton rat should be cautiously extrapolated to humans.

Whether AdV causes a lytic infection still remains controversial. Earlier studies on the mechanism of AdV pathogenesis in cell cultures led to the hypothesis that the basis of cell killing is due to the intranuclear accumulation of viral proteins. Studies in mice and cotton rats showed that neither AdV 2- nor AdV 5-infected epithelial cells are lysed, although they are severely injured and probably die, because early AdV genes shut off DNA and protein synthesis in infected cells.

Studies on pathogenesis in children with fatal AdV infections have shown that TNFα and IL-6 and IL-8 were detected in the serum, while these cytokines were not found in those patients with moderate diseases (Mistchenko *et al.*, 1994). Whether the cell-damaging effects of AdV infection or the host immune responses are responsible for the tissue pathology and clinical manifestations remains unclear.

Latency/Persistence

AdV devotes a significant portion of its genome to gene products whose sole function seems to be the modulation of host immune responses. These mechanisms might play a role in maintaining the virus in a persistent state. AdV mounts an apparently effective defence against the host immune response, as evidenced by the ability of the virus to persist at low levels in the host for long periods of time, with periodic shedding of infectious virus in the faeces and into respiratory secretions. AdVs 1, 2 and 5 persist in the tonsils for years through low-grade replication.

Although the establishment of persistent infections is well documented in several epidemiological studies, the tissue site of replication during asymptomatic periods is enigmatic. In 1973, van der Veen *et al.* isolated AdV types 1, 2, 5 and 6 at low frequency from tonsil- and adenoid-derived lymphocytes. One group reported the presence of AdV nucleic acids sequences in peripheral lymphocytes of healthy adults by *in situ* hybridisation (Horvath *et al.*, 1986). However, amplification studies using PCR have not demonstrated the presence of AdV DNA in peripheral blood from healthy volunteers (Flomenberg *et al.*, 1997; Villamea *et al.*, 2002).

The gp19 kDa and protein 14.7 kDa, play a central role in the ability of subgroup C to produce persistent infections. gp 19 prevents transport of the class I MHC to the surface of infected cells, reducing cytotoxic T cell attack of the infected cells.

IMMUNE RESPONSE

The host has a range of strategies to counteract AdV infection that are efficient and well-orchestrated. Innate defense, including recruitment of macrophages, activation of complement and natural killers, the production of a range of pro-inflammatory cytokines and the orchestration of other signalling pathways play a significant role in clearing AdV infection. The host also produces interferon and the cell can redirect its metabolism to apoptotic circuits. On the other hand, AdVs develop a number of mechanisms to evade the host immune response (see Immune Evasion, below).

In addition, cellular and humoral responses are critical in controlling AdV infection. T cells are effective defences via both CD8 and CD4. CD4 T helpers stimulate proliferation of B cells to synthesised immunoglobulins for the humoral response. It was suggested that CD4 T cells recognise conserved antigens among different serotypes and that the majority of individuals develop long-lived CD4 T cell responses to AdV (Flomenberg et al., 1995). This may play a role in modulating infections with a range of serotypes.

The humoral response is a major component to control AdV infections. After infection, most patients develop group- and type-specific antibodies to the infecting serotype. Group-specific antibodies are not neutralising of viral infectivity but are useful for diagnosis. Type-specific antibodies are measured by neutralisation or inhibition of the haemagglutination. AdV neutralising antibodies are directed against epitopes of the capsid, including the penton, the fibre and the hexon. These antibodies may protect against reinfection with the same serotype. This observation led to the development of effective vaccines for military recruits.

Immune Evasion

AdVs are capable of evading the immune system through different mechanisms (Mahr and Gooding, 1999):

1. Inhibition of interferon (IFN) functions by viral-associated (VA) RNA and E1A. Interferons are often the earliest host response to viral infection. dsRNA produced during viral infection induces antiviral cytokines. The dsRNA-dependent protein kinase (PKR) phosphorylates the translation factor eIF2α. AdVs encode VA RNAs that are transcribed by RNA polymerase III. VA RNA synthesis begins early in infection. They bind and inhibit PKR, preventing the induction of IFN type I. In addition, E1A proteins have also the property to inhibit the function of IFN type I.

2. Inhibition of tumour necrosis factor (TNF) and Fas-mediated apoptosis. TNF is a pro-inflammatory cytokine secreted by activated macrophages and T cells, and can induce cell death. AdV encodes four proteins (E1B19K, E314.7, E310.4K/14 and 5K) that protect AdV-infected cells from TNF and/or Fas-mediated apoptosis.

3. Downregulation of surface class I MHC. Antiviral immune effector mechanisms rely on cytotoxic T lymphocytes (CTLs) to clear virus-infected cells. CD8 CTLs are triggered to lyse virus-infected cells through recognition of viral peptides bound to class I MHC molecules on the cell surface. AdV encodes proteins that inhibit class I presentation. E3 gp 19 and E1A from AdV type 12 bind MHC class I and retains them in the endoplasmic reticulum, thus reducing the transport of class I MHC to the cell surface.

Oncogenicity

Subgroup A are highly oncogenic and subgroup B are weakly oncogenic in newborn hamsters. Despite extensive efforts, no evidence has been found regarding the aetiological role of AdV in human malignancies.

DIAGNOSIS

The syndromes caused by AdV are frequently not clinically distinguishable from other bacterial or viral entities, therefore the laboratory diagnosis of AdV infections becomes important. In addition, virus detection and characterisation are essential for epidemiological studies.

AdVs have been isolated in tissue culture from stool, throat swabs, nasopharyngeal aspirates, conjunctival swabs, urine, cerebrospinal fluid, blood and a variety of biopsy specimens. Sample collection early in the illness is necessary for optimal recovery. The duration of excretion from the onset of symptoms is around 1 week in respiratory infections, 2 weeks from eye specimens in those with pharyngoconjunctival fever, and 2 weeks to 12 months or longer in urine and stool from immunocompromised patients. AdVs are stable and can be transported at room temperature, although prompt shipping to the laboratory is always recommended. Swabs and biopsies should be transported in viral transport media containing serum, albumin or gelatin, and antibiotics/antimycotics. AdV diagnosis can be performed using direct methods (detection of the viral particle, viral antigen or genome) or indirect methods (serology) (Table 8.5).

Current methods for the diagnosis of AdV infections have serious limitations. Culture may be prolonged, inhibited by neutralising antibody or other interfering substances, and electron microscopy and antigen detection methods are relatively insensitive. Serology may be positive due to prior infection, or falsely negative during early disease or with immunosuppression. The development and application of diagnostic methods using molecular techniques have demonstrated to be more sensitive and rapid than conventional methods.

Direct Methods

Virus Isolation

In cell cultures of human origin, virus isolation is used for the recovery of AdV from all clinical specimens. All AdV serotypes, except 40 and 41, grow in human epithelial cell lines and they produce a cytopathic effect (CPE), characterised by clumping and cell rounding with refractile intranuclear inclusion bodies. The rapidity of CPE depends upon the concentration of infectious particles in the sample, the sensitivity of the cell line and the AdV serotype involved. CPE may take from 2–28 days to become evident. CPE needs to be confirmed by indirect immunofluorescence (IF) with monoclonal antibodies, by radioimmunoassay or by ELISA. Primary human embryonic kidney (HEK) cells produce optimal isolation rates for all types except AdVs 40 and 41. However, because HEK cells often are not available, continuous epithelial cell lines, such as Hep-2, HeLa, and A549, are commonly substituted. Serotypes 40 and 41 are fastidious and require the 293 cell line. Cell culture remains the gold standard, although it can be insensitive with many clinical samples (e.g. blood), may have fungal or bacterial contamination, may have inhibitors, or be toxic to the host cells.

Histopathology

Histopathological findings in lung are characterised by diffuse interstitial pneumonitis, necrosis of bronchial epithelial cells, bronchiolitis with mononuclear cell infiltrates, and hyaline membrane formation. Infected cells have enlarged nuclei with basophilic inclusions, surrounded by a thin rim of cytoplasm, and are called 'smudge' cells, which are typical of AdV infection.

Direct Antigen Detection

Immunofluorescence. This uses monoclonal antibodies usually directed against the hexon protein. It is especially useful for respiratory specimens, swabs or biopsies. The advantage of this method is rapidity, as a result can be obtained within 2–4 h. However, it lacks sensitivity, depending on sample quality, timing and type of monoclonal antibody used. Sensitivities of 30–60% in comparison to cell culture have been described.

EIA. EIA is particularly useful for diagnosing enteric AdV in faecal samples, where the antigen is not intracellular. It lacks sensitivity for other types of samples.

Immunohistochemistry. This method is used on tissue sections using AdV monoclonal antibody directed against the hexon antigen. This method is specific but also lacks sensitivity.

Direct Particle Detection

Electron microscopy. The EM morphology of adenoviruses is unique, allowing for rapid identification of the virus. EM is mainly used for diagnosis of AdV acute gastroenteritis due to the high number of viral particles excreted (10^6–10^8 particles/ml). It requires an electron microscope and highly-trained personnel and lacks sensitivity.

Direct Detection of Viral Genome

DNA detection can be performed using molecular methods with or without amplification.

Hybridisation. Hybridisation is a molecular method without amplification that has proved to be an appropriate tool for diagnosis especially in tissue sections, although its lack of sensitivity has been recognised. In situ hybridisation has proved useful, not only for diagnosis but also for studies of pathogenesis.

Polymerase chain reaction (PCR). Amplification of the viral genome, using methods such as the polymerase chain reaction (PCR), has been shown to increase sensitivity and rapidity compared to conventional classical methods. The usefulness and application of this method in the clinical setting has significantly increased in recent years. Until 1997, only a few PCR methods for stools and swabs were available for clinical diagnosis (Allard *et al.*, 1990; Morris *et al.*, 1996). Later, different generic and type-specific assays were developed and tested on a range of different clinical samples (Echavarria *et al.*, 1998; Xu *et al.*, 2000; Allard *et al.*, 2001). For clinical diagnosis, assays should be capable of detecting all AdV serotypes. PCR primers from the hexon region or VA I and II regions are usually chosen because of their extensive homology among serotypes. The hexon gene is located between 0.51 and 0.6 of the genome and has three different segments: a central variable region (nucleotides 403–1356) and two highly conserved regions flanking the central one. There are seven hypervariable regions inside the variable region, which differ in sequence and length. Hypervariable region 1 has the higher variability and is related to viral tropism (Crawford-Miksza and Schnurr, 1996).

When developing new PCR assays, they should be tested for their analytical and microbiological sensitivity, including cross-reactivity to other viruses that can be detected in the same clinical site. Clinical specificity should also be evaluated and the positive and negative predictive values should be determined for the populations for which the test is to be applied. Some PCR assays proved to have high clinical specificity as determined by studying urine, respiratory samples and blood from healthy asymptomatic immunocompetent individuals (Echavarria *et al.*, 2003; Villamea *et al.*, 2002).

In patients with disseminated disease, PCR has proved to detect the virus in the bloodstream while other methods could not (Echavarria *et al.*, 1999). Recent studies have evaluated AdV detection by PCR in serum or plasma. The presence of adenoviral DNA in serum was found to be associated with severe or fatal adenovirus infection in bone marrow transplant recipients (Echavarria *et al.*, 2001a).

Since proper management of these patients is dependent on early diagnosis and differentiation from other conditions, PCR assays can offer a valuable tool as an early marker for disease. These sensitive methods can contribute to the management of life-threatening infections, especially in complex immunocompromised patients who may be thought to have an alternative diagnosis.

Since higher AdV levels in blood have been correlated with a fatal outcome, current studies are using 'real-time' amplification methods for the rapid determination and quantification of the virus in different clinical samples (Schilham *et al.*, 2002; Lankester *et al.*, 2002). Further studies are necessary to determine the usefulness and clinical significance of applying quantitative methods for AdV detection.

Indirect Methods

Serology

AdV infections can be diagnosed by the presence of specific IgM or IgG seroconversion (at least a four-fold rise in IgG titre between acute and convalescent sera). Some of the methods utilised include complement fixation (CF), ELISA, haemagglutination inhibition and neutralisation. CF uses common antigens from the hexon and detects responses to many serotypes. ELISA and IF are the methods more frequently used in the diagnostic laboratory. Serum neutralisation assays or haemagglutination–inhibition assays are used for detecting specific antibodies against each AdV serotype.

Some of the limitations of serology are: (a) specific IgM is detected in only 20–50% of infections; (b) false negative results may occur due to a poor serological response; (c) false positive results may occur due to heterotypic anamnestic responses; (d) when testing seroconversion, the diagnosis is retrospective. Nevertheless, serology is useful and important for epidemiological studies.

PREVENTION

Prevention of AdV infections is not yet possible in community or institutional settings, although feasible in hospitals and eye clinics. AdV spreading in hospitals can be reduced by isolating infected patients, using good hand-washing practices, and cleaning and appropriately disinfecting instruments and equipment. Adequate chlorination of swimming pools has also prevented keratoconjunctivitis epidemics.

Vaccines

To prevent acute respiratory disease among military recruits, live oral AdV types 4 and 7 vaccines were developed in the 1960s. The vaccine serotypes are packaged together in enteric capsules, which bypass the stomach and only replicate once they reach the intestine. These vaccines were licensed in 1980 only to US recruits who were routinely immunised (Top,

Table 8.5 Diagnostic methods for adenovirus infections

Direct methods	
Cell culture isolation in	HeLa, HEp-2, KB, HEK, HNK, A549, Graham-293, HLF
CPE and identification by	Immunofluorescence, neutralisation, complement fixation
Detection:	
Viral antigens	IF, EIA, RIA, immunohistochemistry
Viral particle	Electron microscopy
Viral genome	Hybridisation, PCR
Indirect methods	Seroconversion
	Specific IgM

1975). Until recently, these vaccines were highly successful in preventing AdV-associated acute respiratory disease; however, with interruptions of the vaccine supply due to the manufacturer's decision to terminate production, AdV-associated acute respiratory disease has re-emerged at military basic training facilities (Kolavic-Gray et al., 2002).

The use of AdV vaccines has not been extended to young children, although this age group is at particular risk. The lack of attenuation and concern about potential oncogenicity have prevented their use as routine vaccines in civilians.

AdV as Vectors for Vaccination and Gene Therapy

For gene therapy, several E1, E3 deleted vectors containing foreign genes have been constructed. The advantages of using AdV as vectors are that they can be produced in large amounts which transduce in both replicating and non-replicating cells.

AdV vectors for the treatment of genetic diseases carrying the cystic fibrosis transmembrane regulator (CFTR) gene and others with the dystrophin gene have been constructed. Human trials with the CFTR gene have not been particularly promising, due to inefficient gene delivery to target cells and short-lived expression. Since AdVs do not integrate into the host chromosome, the expression is usually transient (Russell, 2000). Other studies for the treatment of cancer used the p53 inserted in AdV vectors to restore the antioncogenic effect. Although preliminary evidence of efficacy has been reported, definite results are not yet available (Russell, 2000).

A variety of recombinant AdV-expressing exogenous genes for vaccination use have been constructed for HIV and rabies. Human trials are still under investigation.

This is an active field of research and significant progress is expected in the future for both gene therapy and recombinant vaccines.

TREATMENT

At present, there are no proven effective therapies for the treatment of AdV disease or publications on prospective randomised controlled trials. Antiviral agents such as ganciclovir, vidarabine and ribavirin have shown conflicting results. More experience has been obtained with ribavirin and cidofovir. Ribavirin is a wide-spectrum antiviral agent related to guanosine, with in vitro activity against RNA and DNA viruses. The most common adverse effect is reversible mild anaemia. Successful use was described in the treatment of AdV haemorrhagic cystitis, pneumonia, enteritis after BMT and hepatitis in a liver transplant recipient (Arav-Boger et al., 2000; Howard et al., 1999). Other authors, however, have described its therapeutic failure (Hale et al., 1999; Chakrabarti et al., 1999). Success seems to be related to early treatment. No real benefit will be seen if therapy is begun late in the course of the infection. Therefore, early identification, e.g. by PCR, of those patients at risk of disseminated disease, may permit earlier antiviral treatment.

Cidofovir, a nucleoside and phosphonate analogue is a broad-spectrum anti-DNA viral agent. It is nephrotoxic. Some publications based on case reports and a prospective trial have described the successful outcome of AdV disease in paediatric haematopoietic stem cell transplant recipients with haemorrhagic cystitis, pneumonia, hepatitis or enteritis (Hoffman et al., 2001). The small number of patients treated and the lack of a control group limits the significance of these findings. Prospective controlled clinical trials and systematic studies of the efficacy of these antivirals are needed.

Another therapeutic alternative is the use of immunotherapy. Donor lymphocyte infusion has been successfully applied to a few bone marrow transplant patients with severe AdV infection (Chakrabarti et al., 2000). In vitro production of specific CTL to control AdV infections constitutes an active area of research.

FUTURE PROSPECTS

Given the severity and prevalence of AdV diseases among immunocompromised patients, there is a need for effective and non-toxic anti-AdV therapy. Large multicentre prospective controlled clinical trials in different patient populations are required to determine the benefits and adverse effects of different antiviral drugs and immunotherapy.

No AdV vaccines are available for civilian populations. The live oral vaccine approved only for US military recruits has been discontinued. Current studies to re-establish the production and usage in the military population are under development. New studies are needed in order to develop new and safe vaccines, especially for young children and immunocompromised patients.

AdV vectors offer good promise for gene therapy and vaccination. Although no significant clinical success has yet been shown with earlier first- and second-generation vectors, third-generation ones are now being studied.

The new highly sensitive molecular methods for AdV detection have proven usefulness in the early diagnosis and monitoring of AdV disease, especially among transplant recipients. They will also be useful to achieve a better understanding of pathogenic mechanisms, such as latency, persistence and cyclical reactivation of the virus. Quantitative molecular methods using real-time PCR may prove to be valuable in assessing the clinical significance of determining the viral load in different clinical samples and in predicting disease.

The knowledge of this virus is rapidly expanding at present. It is clear that its clinical importance is only beginning to be fully defined.

REFERENCES

Adrian T, Wadell G, Hierholzer JC and Wigand R (1986) DNA restriction analysis of adenovirus prototypes 1 to 41. *Arch Virol*, **91**, 277–290.

Allard A, Albinsson B and Wadell G (2001) Rapid typing of human adenoviruses by a general PCR combined with restriction endonuclease analysis. *J Clin Microbiol*, **39**(2), 498–505.

Allard A, Girones R, Per J and Wadell G (1990) Polymerase chain reaction for detection of adenoviruses in stool samples. *J Clin Microbiol*, **28**, 2659–2667.

Ambinder RF, Burns W, Forman M *et al.* (1986) Hemorrhagic cystitis associated with adenovirus infection in bone marrow transplantation. *Arch Intern Med*, **146**, 1400–1401.

Arav-Boger R, Echavarria M, Forman M *et al.* (2000) Clearance of adenoviral hepatitis with ribavirin therapy in a pediatric liver transplant recipient. *Pediatr Infect Dis J*, **19**, 1097–1100.

Arnberg N, Edlund K, Pring-Akerblom P *et al.* (2002) Sialic acid is a cellular receptor for the ocular adenoviruses types

8, 19 and 37. Abstract V-100. XII International Congress of Virology, Paris.

Blanke C, Clark C, Broun ER *et al.* (1995) Evolving pathogens in allogeneic bone marrow transplantation: increased fatal adenoviral infections. *Am J Med*, **99**, 326–328.

Bordigoni P, Carret AS, Venard V *et al.* (2001) Treatment of adenovirus infections in patients undergoing allogeneic hematopoietic stem cell transplantation. *Clin Infect Dis*, **32**(9), 1290–1297.

Brandt CD, Kim HW, Vargosko A (1969) Infections in 18 000 infants and children in a controlled study of respiratory tract disease. I. Adenovirus pathogenicity in relation to serologic type and illness syndrome. *Am J Epidemiol*, **90**(6), 485–500.

Carballal G, Videla C, Espinosa MA *et al.* (2001) Multi-centered study of viral acute lower respiratory infections in children from four cities of Argentina, 1993–1994. *J Med Virol*, **64**, 167–174.

Carballal G, Videla C, Misirlian A *et al.* (2002) Adenovirus type 7 associated with severe and fatal acute lower respiratory infections in Argentine children. *BioMed Central Pediatrics*, **2**(6), 1–7.

Chakrabarti S, Collingham KE, Fegan CD *et al.* (2000) Adenovirus infections following haematopoietic cell transplantation: is there a role for adoptive immunotherapy? *Bone Marrow Transpl*, **26**, 305–307.

Chakrabarti S, Collingham KE, Fegan CD and Milligan DW (1999) Fulminant adenovirus hepatitis following unrelated bone marrow transplantation: failure of intravenous ribavirin therapy. *Bone Marrow Transplant*, **23**, 1209–1211.

Chakrabarti S, Mautner V, Osman H *et al.* (2002) Adenovirus infections following allogeneic stem cell transplantation: incidence and outcome in relation to graft manipulation, immunosuppression, and immune recovery. *Blood*, **100**(5), 1619–1627.

Crawford-Miksza L and Schnurr D (1996) Adenovirus serotype evolution is driven by illegitimated recombination in the hypervariable regions of the hexon protein. *Virology*, **224**, 357–367.

Davis D, Henslee PJ and Markesbery WR (1988) Fatal adenovirus meningoencephalitis in a bone marrow transplant patient. *Ann Neurol*, **23**, 385–389.

De Jong JC, Wermenbol AG, Verweij-Uijterwaal MW *et al.* (1999) Adenoviruses from human immunodeficiency virus-infected individuals, including two strains that represent new candidate serotypes Ad50 and Ad51 of species B1 and D, respectively. *J Clin Microbiol*, **37**, 3940–3945.

De Jong PJ, Valderrama G, Spigland L and Horwitz MS (1983) Adenovirus isolates from urine of patients with acquired immunodeficiency syndrome. *Lancet*, **I**, 1293–1296.

Dhurandhar NV, Whigham LD, Abbott DH *et al.* (2002) Human adenovirus Ad-36 promotes weight gain in male rhesus and marmoset monkeys. *J Nutr*, **132**(10), 3155–3160.

Dudding BA, Wagner SC, Zeller JA *et al.* (1972) Fatal pneumonia associated with adenovirus type 7 in three military trainees. *N Engl J Med*, **286**, 1289–1292.

Echavarria M, Forman M, Schnurr D *et al.* (2001b) Association of adenovirus types 11, 34 and 35 with parenteral exposure and earlier death in AIDS patients. The 1st IAS Conference on HIV Pathogenesis and Treatment, Buenos Aires, Argentina.

Echavarria M, Forman M, Ticehurst J *et al.* (1998) PCR method for detection of adenovirus in urine of healthy and human immunodeficiency virus-infected individuals. *J Clin Microbiol*, **36**, 3323–3326.

Echavarria M, Forman M, van Tol MJ *et al*. (2001a) Prediction of severe disseminated adenovirus infection by serum PCR. *Lancet*, **358**, 384–385.

Echavarria M, Kolavic SA, Cersovsky S *et al*. (2000a) Detection of adenoviruses (AdV) in culture-negative environmental samples by PCR during an AdV-associated respiratory disease outbreak. *J Clin Microbiol*, **38**, 2982–2984.

Echavarria MS, Ray SC, Ambinder R *et al*. (1999) PCR detection of adenovirus in a bone marrow transplant recipient: hemorrhagic cystitis as a presenting manifestation of disseminated disease. *J Clin Microbiol*, **37**, 686–689.

Echavarria M, Sanchez JL, Kolavic SA *et al*. (2003) Adenovirus detection in throat swab specimens by a generic PCR during a respiratory disease outbreak among military recruits. *J Clin Microbiol*, **41**(2), 810–812.

Echavarria M, Villamea L, Videla C *et al*. (2000b) Performance characteristics of an adenovirus PCR method during a fatal respiratory outbreak in Argentina. Virology Lab, Centro de Educación Medica e Investigaciones Clínicas (CEMIC), XVI Clinical Virology Symposium, Clearwater.

Enders JF, Bell JA, Dingle JH *et al*. (1956) Adenoviruses. Group name proposed for new respiratory-tract viruses. *Science*, **124**, 119–120.

Erdman DD, Xu W, Gerber SI *et al*. (2002) Molecular epidemiology of adenovirus type 7 in the United States, 1966–2000. *Emerg Infect Dis*, **8**(3), 269–277.

Flomenberg P, Babbitt J, Drobyski WR *et al*. (1994) Increasing incidence of adenovirus disease in bone marrow transplant recipients. *J Infect Dis*, **169**, 775–781.

Flomenberg P, Gutierrez E, Piaskowski V and Casper JT (1997) Detection of adenovirus DNA in peripheral blood mononuclear cells by polymerase chain reaction assay. *J Med Virol*, **51**, 182–188.

Flomenberg P, Piaskowski V, Truitt R and Casper J (1995) Characterization of human proliferative T cells responses to adenovirus. *J Infect Dis*, **171**, 1090–1096.

Ginsberg HS and Prince GA (1994) The molecular basis of adenovirus pathogenesis. *Infect Ag Dis*, **3**, 1–8.

Hale GA, Heslop HE, Krance RA *et al*. (1999) Adenovirus infection after pediatric bone marrow transplantation. *Bone Marrow Transpl*, **23**, 277–282.

Hashido M, Mukouyama A, Sakae K *et al*. (1999) Molecular and serological characterization of adenovirus genome type 7h isolated in Japan. *Epidemiol Infect*, **122**(2), 281–286.

Hierholzer JC (1992) Adenoviruses in the immunocompromised host. *Clin Microbiol Rev*, **5**, 262–274.

Hierholzer JC (1995) Adenoviruses. In *Diagnostic Procedure for Viral, Rickettsial and Chlamydial Infections*, 7th edn (eds Lennette EH, Lennette DA and Lennette ET), pp 169–188. American Public Health Association, Washington DC.

Hilleman MR and Werner J (1954) Recovery of new agent from patients with acute respiratory illness. *Proc Soc Exp Biol Med*, **85**, 183–188.

Hoffman JA, Shah AJ, Ross LA and Kapoor N (2001) Adenoviral infections and a prospective trial of cidofovir in pediatric hematopoietic stem cell transplantation. *Biol Blood Marrow Transplant*, **7**, 388–394.

Horvath J, Palkonyay L and Weber J (1986) Group C adenovirus DNA sequences in human lymphoid cells. *J Virol*, **59**, 189–192.

Howard DS, Phillips GL II, Reece DE *et al*. (1999) Adenovirus infections in hematopoietic stem cell transplant recipients. *Clin Infect Dis*, **29**, 1494–1501.

Kajon A and Wadell G (1994) Genome analysis of South American adenovirus strains of serotype 7 collected over a 7-year period. *J Clin Microbiol*, **32**, 2321–2323.

Kajon AE, Mistchenko AS, Videla C *et al*. (1996) Molecular epidemiology of adenovirus acute lower respiratory infections of children in the south cone of South America (1991–1994). *J Med Virol*, **48**, 151–156.

Keenlyside RA, Hierholzer JC and D'Angelo LJ (1983) Keratoconjunctivitis associated with adenovirus type 37: an extended outbreak in an ophthalmologist's office. *J Infect Dis*, **147**(2), 191–198.

Khoo SH, Bailey AS, de Jong JC and Mandal BK (1995) Adenovirus infections in human immunodeficiency virus-positive patients: clinical features and molecular epidemiology. *J Infect Dis*, **172**, 629–637.

Kolavic-Gray SA, Binn LN, Sanchez JL *et al*. (2002) Large epidemic of adenovirus type 4 infection among military trainees: epidemiological, clinical, and laboratory studies. *Clin Infect Dis*, **35**(7), 808–818.

Lankester AC, van Tol M, Claas E *et al*. (2002) Quantification of adenovirus DNA in plasma for management of infection in stem cell graft recipients. *Clin Infect Dis*, **34**, 864–867.

La Rosa A, Champlin R, Mirza N *et al*. (2001) Adenovirus infections in adult recipients of blood and marrow transplants. *Clin Inf Dis*, **32**, 871–876.

Ljungman P, Gleaves CA and Meyers JD (1989) Respiratory virus infection in immunocompromised patients. *Bone Marrow Transpl*, **4**, 35–40.

Mahr JA and Gooding LR (1999) Immune evasion by adenoviruses. *Immunol Rev*, **168**, 121–130.

Mayo MA (2002) ICTV at the Paris ICV: results of the plenary session and the binomial ballot. *Arch Virol*, **147**, 2254–2260.

Mistchenko A, Diez RA, Mariani AL *et al*. (1994) Cytokines in adenoviral disease in children. Association of interleukin 6, interleukin 8 and tumor necrosis factor alpha levels with clinical outcome. *J Pediatr*, **124**, 714.

Miyazawa N, Leopold PL, Hackett NR *et al*. (1999) Fiber swap between adenovirus subgroups B and C alters intracellular trafficking of adenovirus gene transfer vectors. *J Virol*, **73**(7), 6056–6065.

Morris DJ, Cooper RJ, Barr T and Bailey AS (1996) Polymerase chain reaction for rapid diagnosis of respiratory adenovirus infection. *J Infect*, **32**, 113–117.

Munoz FM, Piedra PA and Demmler GJ (1998) Disseminated adenovirus disease in immunocompromised and immunocompetent children. *Clin Infect Dis*, **27**, 1194–1200.

Murtagh P, Cerqueiro C, Halac A *et al*. (1993) Adenovirus type 7h respiratory infections: a report of 29 cases of acute lower respiratory disease. *Acta Paediatr*, **82**(6–7), 557–561.

Roelvink PW, Lizonova A, Lee JG *et al*. (1998) The coxsackievirus-adenovirus receptor protein can function as a cellular attachment protein for adenovirus serotypes from subgroups A, C, D, E, and F. *J Virol*, **72**(10), 7909–7915.

Rowe WP *et al*. (1953) Reported recovery of an agent from human adenoid tissue. *Proc Soc Exp Biol Med*, **84**, 570.

Runde V, Ross S, Trenschel R *et al*. (2001) Adenoviral infection after allogeneic stem cell transplantation (SCT): report on 130 patients from a single SCT unit involved in a prospective multi center surveillance study. *Bone Marrow Transpl*, **28**, 51–57.

Russell WC (2000) Update on adenovirus and its vectors. *J Gen Virol*, **81**, 2573–2604.

Schilham MW, Claas EC, van Zaane W *et al.* (2002) High levels of adenovirus DNA in serum correlate with fatal outcome of adenovirus infection in children after allogeneic stem-cell transplantation. *Clin Infect Dis*, **35**(5), 526–532.

Segerman A, Arnberg N, Erikson A *et al.* (2003) There are two different species B adenovirus receptors: sBAR, common to species B1 and B2 adenoviruses, and sB2AR, exclusively used by species B2 adenoviruses. *J Virol*, **77**(2), 1157–1162.

Shields AF, Hackman RC, Fife KH *et al.* (1985) Adenovirus infections in patients undergoing bone-marrow transplantation. *N Engl J Med*, **312**, 529–533.

Swenson P, Lowens M, Connie C and Hierholzer J (1995) Adenovirus types 2, 8 and 37 associated with genital infections in patients attending a sexually transmitted disease clinic. *J Clin Microbiol*, **Oct**, 2728–2731

Top FH Jr (1975) Control of adenovirus acute respiratory disease in US Army trainees. *Yale J Biol Med*, **48**, 185–195.

Turner M, Istre GR, Beauchamp H *et al.* (1987) Community outbreak of adenovirus type 7a infections associated with a swimming pool. *South Med J*, **80**(6), 712–715.

van der Avoort HG, Wermenbol AG, Zomerdijk TP *et al.* (1989) Characterization of fastidious adenovirus types 40 and 41 by DNA restriction enzyme analysis and by neutralizing monoclonal antibodies. *Virus Res*, **12**(2), 139–157.

van der Veen J and Lambriex M (1973) Relationship of adenoviruses to lymphocytes in naturally infected human tonsils and adenoids. *Infect Immun Apri*, **7**(4), 604–609.

Venard V, Carret A, Corsaro D *et al.* (2000) Genotyping of adenoviruses isolated in an outbreak in a bone marrow transplant unit shows that diverse strains are involved. *J Hosp Infect*, **44**, 71–74.

Videla C, Carballal G, Misirlian A and Aguilar M (1998a) Acute lower respiratory infections due to respiratory syncytial virus and adenovirus among hospitalized children from Argentina. *Clin Diagn Virol*, **10**, 17–23.

Videla C, Corazza R, Clary A *et al.* (1998b) Viral study of an acute lower respiratory outbreak in hospitalized children from Eva Perón Hospital. VIIIth Congreso Argentino de Microbiología, Buenos Aires, Argentina.

Villamea L, Echavarria M, Ricarte C *et al.* (2002) Absence of adenovirus detection by culture and PCR in peripheral blood leukocytes from healthy donors. 18th Annual Clinical Virology Symposium, April 2002. Clearwater Beach, FL.

Warner JO and Marshall WC (1976) Crippling lung disease after measles and adenovirus infection. *Br J Dis Chest*, **70**(2), 89–94.

Wasserman R, August CS and Plotkin SA (1988) Viral infections in pediatric bone marrow transplant patients. *Pediatr Infect Dis J*, **7**, 109–115.

Weissenbacher MG, Carballal M, Avila H *et al.* (1990) Etiologic and clinical evaluation of acute lower respiratory tract infections in young Argentinian children: an overview. *Rev Infect Dis* (Suppl 8), S889–S898.

Xu W, McDonough MC and Erdman DD (2000) Species-specific identification of human adenoviruses by a multiplex PCR assay. *J Clin Microbiol*, **38**(11), 4114–4120.

Yolken RH, Bishop CA, Townsend TR *et al.* (1982) Infectious gastroenteritis in bone-marrow-transplant recipients. *N Engl J Med*, **306**, 1010–1012.

9

Rhinoviruses

Nikolaos G. Papadopoulos[1] and Sebastian L. Johnston[2]

[1]*University of Athens, Greece, and* [2]*Imperial College of Science, Technology and Medicine, London, UK*

INTRODUCTION

Rhinoviruses (Figure 9.1) are the major cause of the common cold. Although the majority of infections produce only mild disease, their impact on overall morbidity and their economic cost worldwide is considerable. More recently, their role in acute exacerbations of asthma and other airway disease has been demonstrated, revealing a less benevolent nature than previously thought. Therefore, in addition to physician visits, use of medication (including so-called 'alternative preparations'), loss of school and work, etc., the cost of complications should be added, making the overall economic and disease burden enormous.

While the recorded history of the common cold is over 2000 years old, already known and commented on by Hippocrates around 400 BC, rhinoviruses were first propagated in 1953 in tissue cultures whose supernatants were able to produce common cold symptoms in volunteers. The first rhinovirus was initially isolated from patients with colds and named in 1957, while 3 years later cytopathogenic viruses were recovered using human embryo kidney cell cultures (Tyrrell and Parsons, 1960). Other susceptible cell lines were subsequently discovered and used to identify additional serotypes to study rhinovirus biology and their role in disease. Recently, the genomes of several serotypes have been sequenced and their three-dimensional structure has been revealed in atomic resolution. Molecular technologies are rapidly progressing in the development of novel diagnostic tools and will hopefully aid the so far unsuccessful search for an effective treatment.

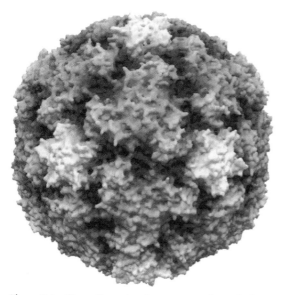

Figure 9.1 Three-dimensional computer-enhanced electron micrography of *Human rhinovirus-14*. Courtesy of Dr J.Y. Sgro

TAXONOMY

Rhinoviruses are small RNA viruses belonging to the family *Picornaviridae* (pico = small + RNA), which also includes the enteroviruses, e.g. polio, coxsackie and echo viruses; cardioviruses, e.g. the rodent encephalomyocarditis virus; and aphthoviruses, or foot and

Principles and Practice of Clinical Virology, Fifth Edition. Edited by A. J. Zuckerman, J. E. Banatvala, J. R. Pattison, P. D. Griffiths and B. D. Schoub
© 2004 John Wiley & Sons Ltd ISBN 0 470 84338 1

mouth disease viruses. Rhinoviruses are more closely related to enteroviruses than the other genera. They are the most numerous of the *Picornaviridae*, with over

Table 9.1   Rhinovirus serotypes

Serotype	Prototype strain	Serotype	Prototype strain
1A	Echo-28	51	F01-4081
1B	B632	52	F01-3772
2	HGP	53	F01-3928
3	FEB	54	F01-3774
4	16/60	55	WIS 315E
5	Norman	56	CH82
6	Thompson	57	CH47
7	68-CV 11	58	21-CV 20
8	MRH-CV 12	59	611-CV 35
9	211-CV 13	60	2268-CV 37
10	204-CV 14	61	6669-CV 39
11	1-CV 15	62	1963-CV 40
12	181-CV 6	63	6360-CV 40
13	353	64	6258-CV 44
14	1059	65	425-CV 47
15	1734	66	1983-CV 48
16	11757	67	1857-CV 51
17	33342	68	F02-2317-Wood
18	5986-CV 17	69	F02-2513-Mitchinson
19	6072-CV 18	70	F02-2547-Treganza
20	15-CV 19	71	SF365
21	47-CV 21	72	K2207
22	127-CV 22	73	107E
23	5124-CV 24	74	328A
24	5146-CV 25	75	328F
25	5426-CV 12	76	H00062
26	5660-CV 27	77	130-63
27	5870-CV 28	78	2030-65
28	6101-CV 29	79	101-1
29	5582-CV 30	80	277G
30	106F	81	483F2
31	140F	82	03647
32	363	83	Baylor 7
33	1200	84	432D
34	137-3	85	50-525-CV-54
35	164A	86	121564-Johnson
36	342H	87	F02-3607-Corn
37	151-1	88	CVD-01-0165-Dambrauskas
38	CH79	89	41467-Gallo
39	209	90	K2305
40	1794	91	JM1
41	56110	92	SF-1662
42	56822	93	SF-1492
43	58750	94	SF-1803
44	71560	95	SF-998
45	Baylor 1	96	SF-1426
46	Baylor 2	97	SF-1372
47	Baylor 3	98	SF-4006
48	1505	99	604
49	8213	100	K6579
50	A2 No. 58		

100 serotypes identified and numbered by specific antisera in a collaborative programme supported by the World Health Organisation (Hamparian *et al.*, 1987) (Table 9.1). New virus types are continually emerging by a process of random mutation and immune selection (Patterson and Hamparian, 1997; Savolainen *et al.*, 2002b). Rhinoviruses are divided into major (90%) and minor (10%) groups, according to their cellular receptor usage (Uncapher *et al.*, 1991). An alternative classification, dividing the viruses into groups A and B, based on sensitivity to antiviral compounds and correlating with sequence similarities and pathogenicity, has also been proposed (Andries *et al.*, 1990).

STRUCTURE

The Capsid

Rhinoviruses are among the simplest infectious agents. Their virion consists of a non-enveloped capsid surrounding a single-stranded positive-sense genomic RNA. In 1985 X-ray crystallography revealed the structure of rhinovirus-14 and poliovirus-1 at atomic resolution (Rossmann *et al.*, 1985). These and subsequent studies showed considerable structural similarities amongst picornaviruses, such as prominent β-sheets forming a β-barrel, even though the sequence of each virus differs considerably from others in the group. The rhinovirus capsid is composed of 60 identical subunits, arranged as 12 pentamers in an icosahedron. Each subunit consists of all four structural proteins of the virus, named VP1–VP4, with molecular masses of 32, 29, 26 and 7 kDa, respectively. VP1, 2 and 3 are surface proteins interacting with antibody and corresponding to the part of the genome with the highest variability. VP4 is confined to the interior of the capsid and is closely associated with the viral RNA. The arrangement of these structural proteins can be seen in Figure 9.2. Around the five-fold axis of symmetry of the capsid there is a 2.5 nm-deep depression shaped by the five VP1 units, forming a 'canyon' (Figure 9.1). In most rhinoviruses, VP1 also contains a hydrophobic 'pocket' under the canyon, containing an incompletely characterised fatty-acid 'pocket factor'. This pocket is thought to be involved in virus uncoating and is the major target of antiviral compounds (Hadfield *et al.*, 1997).

The conformation of the canyon, being physically unreachable by the immunoglobulin Fabs, led to the hypothesis that this was the receptor binding site. Evidence in favour of this hypothesis has been

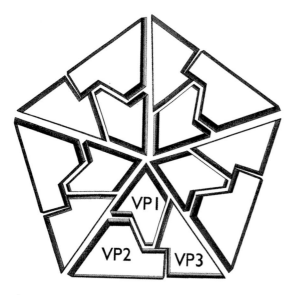

Figure 9.2 Arrangement of the three main structural rhinovirus proteins. The fourth structural protein, VP4, is confined in the interior and hence is not visualised

produced (Colonno *et al.*, 1988), demonstrating that the amino acid sequences at the base of the canyon are very well conserved, while the edges of the canyon and the most external portions of the virus capsid are hypervariable and correspond to neutralising immunogenic sites (Rossmann and Palmenberg, 1988).

Antigenicity

Four such sites, localised in different areas of the capsid of HRV14 along the edge of the canyon, were characterised by RNA sequencing of mutants that escaped neutralisation by specific antisera (Sherry *et al.*, 1986). Nim-1a, Nim-1b on VP1 are positioned above the canyon, while Nim-2 on VP2 and Nim-3 on VP3, are positioned below. HRV2 has a slightly different pattern: nevertheless, the antigenic sites are still located on the most protrusive regions of the virion. A peptide from VP2 (156–170) of HRV2, structured like a random coil in solution, was shown to contain enough information to direct the production of neutralising antibodies against the serotype (Molins *et al.*, 1998). High variability of these regions is implied by the large number of distinguishable serotypes and has been, to a certain extent, molecularly characterised (Horsnell *et al.*, 1995).

Expression of foreign peptides, such as peptides from respiratory syncytial virus or HIV, has been successful, and resulted in an immune response against the specific peptide (Zhang *et al.*, 1999). Such chimaeric viruses may become potent tools for mucosal immunisation.

Receptors

An important function of the viral capsid is to deliver the genomic material intact into a cell following attachment to a cell-surface receptor. Initially, it has been shown that almost 90% of rhinoviruses (major group) bind to one receptor on HeLa cells, while the remaining (HRV 1a, 1b, 2, 29, 30, 31, 44, 47, 49 and 62) use another (Colonno *et al.*, 1986). The major group receptor was independently identified by three different groups (Greve *et al.*, 1989; Staunton *et al.*, 1989; Tomassini *et al.*, 1989) as intercellular adhesion molecule 1 (ICAM-1). ICAM-1 is a 95 kDa glycoprotein, a member of the immunoglobulin superfamily, physiologically acting as a receptor for the lymphocyte-function associated antigen-1 (LFA-1, CD11a/CD18) and Mac-1, found on leukocytes. It facilitates the interaction of lymphocytes with antigen presenting cells as well as their migration to inflammatory sites. The binding sites of LFA-1 and major rhinoviruses on the ICAM molecule are distinct but significantly overlapping (Staunton *et al.*, 1990). Furthermore, cryo-electron microscopy proved that the rhinovirus binding site is positioned in the canyon, verifying the 'canyon hypothesis' (Rossmann, 1994). Recently, the three-dimensional atomic structure of the two amino-terminal domains (D1 and D2) of ICAM-1 has been determined. Rhinovirus attachment is confined to the BC, CD, DE and FG loops of the amino-terminal immunoglobulin-like domain (D1) at the end distal to the cellular membrane (Bella *et al.*, 1999). Binding of rhinoviruses to ICAM-1 blocks LFA-1–ICAM-1 interaction, possibly downregulating the local immune response and upregulating the viral receptor itself (Papi and Johnston, 1999), while there is evidence that at the same time rhinovirus–ICAM-1 binding induces conformational changes promoting viral uncoating and cell entry (Casasnovas and Springer, 1994).

The minor group viruses bind to members of the low-density lipoprotein receptor family (LDLR), including the VLDLR and α2-macroglobulin receptor/LDLR related protein (α2MR/LRP) (Hofer *et al.*, 1994). The minor receptor binds to the small star-shaped dome on the icosahedral five-fold axis, in contrast to the major group, where the receptor site for ICAM-1 is located at the base of a depression around each five-fold axis (Hewat *et al.*, 2000). Minor-group viruses, exemplified by rhinovirus-2, transfer their genomic RNA to the cytoplasm through a pore in the endosomal membrane (Schober *et al.*, 1998). Interestingly, rhinovirus 89, a major group virus, was adapted in culture to replicate in ICAM-1-devoid cells, and LDLR-soluble fragments could not inhibit such replication, suggesting the possibility of additional receptors (Reischl *et al.*, 2001).

Replication

Rhinovirus RNA has a molecular weight of approximately 2 MDa, consisting of some 7200 nucleotides (Duechler *et al.*, 1987). A 5′ non-coding region of around 620 bases in length and a 3′ non-coding region of 50 bases before a polyadenylated tail are characteristic of all currently sequenced serotypes (Figure 9.3). The long 5′ untranslated region is highly conserved and contains several AUG codons upstream of that used to initiate translation. These sequences are within a complex structure, termed the internal ribosome entry site or IRES, which can bind ribosomal subunits directly, without the requirement for a free 5′ end or a cap-binding protein (Stoneley *et al.*, 2000). The organisation of the genome is shown in Figure 9.3. The structural proteins VP1–4 derive from the P1 region, while P2 and P3 code for the enzymes required for virus replication. The non-structural proteins, seven in total, include two proteases with specific viral cleavage sites (2A, 3C), an RNA-dependent RNA-polymerase (3D) and a small protein Vpg (3B), which is covalently bound to the 5′ end of the RNA and possibly acts as a primer for RNA synthesis (Rowlands, 1995). The remaining non-structural proteins (2B, 2C, 3A) are associated with RNA replication. Interestingly, an internal *cis*-acting replication element (*cre*), located within the genome segment encoding the capsid proteins, is required for RNA replication (McKnight and Lemon, 1998).

The single-stranded, positive-sense RNA can act as messenger RNA and is also infectious. Similarly to the other picornaviruses, the genome is translated into a polyprotein from a single long open reading frame. This polyprotein is processed into the mature proteins by several cleavage steps performed by virus-specific proteases. With the polymerase, a negative-sense copy of the genome is produced, from which further positive strands are made by viral RNA polymerase, and these can act either as messenger RNA, being subsequently translated, or can be incorporated as genomic RNA in the progeny virus.

Translation requires cellular *trans*-acting factors that are absent from, or limiting in, rabbit reticulocytes, but are more abundant in HeLa cell extracts. At least two such factors have been identified, polypyrimidine tract-binding protein (PTB) and a complex of unr, an RNA-binding protein with five cold-shock domains and a 38 kDa protein, named UNRIP (unr-interacting protein) (Hunt *et al.*, 1999).

Infection results in shut-off of host protein synthesis, a procedure mediated by the cleavage of host proteins, such as the eukaryotic initiation factor 4G (eIF4G) and poly(A)-binding protein (PABP), by viral proteases (Kerekatte *et al.*, 1999).

Rhinoviruses are capable of completing numerous replicative cycles within 6–8 h with a yield of up to 100 000 viruses/cell (Belsham and Sonenberg, 1996).

PHYSICAL PROPERTIES

Rhinoviruses are small, with a diameter of 28–34 nm. Their total molecular weight is approximately 8–8.5 MDa and their buoyant density in caesium chloride is 1.38–1.42 g/ml as fully infectious particle or 1.29 g/ml as empty capsids.

They are resistant to inactivation by organic solvents, including ether and chloroform, due to the absence of a lipid envelope around the virion. They are also unaffected by 70–95% ethanol, 5% phenol and trichlorofluorethane (Macnaughton, 1982). However, weak hypochlorite solution (common bleach) rapidly inactivates infectivity, provided that there is not a high

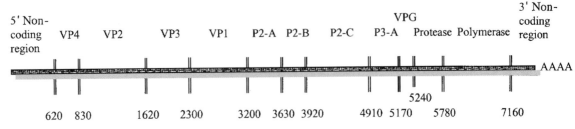

Figure 9.3 Diagrammatic representation of the rhinovirus genome

concentration of organic matter present. Rhinoviruses are characteristically susceptible to extreme pH due to irreversible conformational changes, being inactivated at pH < 5 as well as at pH 9–10. Acid sensitivity, together with lipid solvent stability tests, have been used for the identification of rhinoviruses. In addition, ultraviolet radiation is inactivating for rhinoviruses, while cationic substances such as $MgCl_2$ are favourable for the replication of most serotypes, appearing to stabilise the virions, especially at high temperatures (Blough et al., 1969).

Viability steadily decreases at room temperature, while it remains stable for days at 4°C, months at −20°C and indefinitely at −70°C or lower. Rhinoviruses show considerable variation in their ability to resist heat inactivation at 50–56°C, with some serotypes completely inactivated at lower temperatures and others quite resistant. Optimal culture temperature is in the range 33–35°C (Killington et al., 1977) but most serotypes are able to productively infect and replicate in HeLa cells at 37°C (Papadopoulos et al., 1999b).

INCUBATION AND TRANSMISSION

Infection with a rhinovirus can be initiated by small doses if the inoculum is effectively delivered to the nasopharynx. In experimental human transmission studies the frequency of virus shedding after inoculation varied by inoculum size and the titre of the subject's serum specific antiserotype antibodies. All subjects with no neutralising antibody could be infected with an inoculum of 10^4 $TCID_{50}$ (Johnston and Tyrrell, 1995). The mode of person-to-person transmission has been debated but it is likely that both direct hand–surface–hand contact (Gwaltney and Hendley, 1978) and aerosol inhalation (Meschievitz et al., 1984) are involved. Rhinoviruses are capable of surviving on surfaces for several hours under ambient conditions (Sattar et al., 1993) and transfer of rhinovirus through hand touch can occur in only a few seconds, so that direct inoculation by rubbing the nares or eyes with infected hands can readily occur. Furthermore, the viral load in oral and pharyngeal secretions is considerably lower in comparison to nasal mucus. On the other hand, there is good experimental (Dick et al., 1987) and epidemiological evidence favouring the predominance of the inhaled route (Johnston et al., 1996).

The incubation period is 1–4 days, commonly 2–3 days. Generally, viral shedding peaks 2–4 days post-infection, lasting usually for 7–10 days although it can

persist for as long as 3 weeks. Viral clearance may be suboptimal in atopic subjects, with around half of them still bearing the virus 2 weeks after an experimental infection (Gern et al., 2000). Natural transmission increases in relation to high virus titres in nasal secretions, increased symptoms, time spent in contact and social factors such as crowding and poor hygiene. In families, the interval between the initial and secondary infections relates to the quantity and duration of shedding, ranging up to 10 days with an average of 3 days (Foy et al., 1988).

HOST RANGE

Rhinoviruses are in general extremely host-specific. Human viruses have not been recovered from animals. Under experimental conditions, chimpanzees have been infected, developing a common cold-like disease, as well as gibbons, which do not exhibit symptoms. Other primates are less susceptible. Mice, although they develop an immune response to parenterally administered rhinoviruses (Hastings et al., 1991), do not become infected. An attempt to adapt a serotype for the purpose of a mouse model had very limited success (Yin and Lomax, 1986). Bovine and equine strains are not pathogenic to humans.

PATHOGENESIS

The nose is the main portal for rhinovirus entry. Alternatively, the eye and possibly the mouth may serve as entry routes. Whether or not an infection can begin in the lower airways is not as yet clearly determined. The nasal epithelium is the primary site of infection. A series of upper airway biopsies suggested that rhinovirus infection may be initiated in the nasopharynx, in the area of the adenoids (Winther et al., 1986). Rhinovirus replication occurs primarily in the nose, as inferred from comparative titrations of nasal, pharyngeal and oral secretions as well as of droplets from coughs and sneezes. Nevertheless, the fact that rhinovirus replication occurs in the lower airways has been confirmed in several studies (Gern et al., 1997b; Papadopoulos et al., 2000; Mosser et al., 2002) and evidence suggests that this is the norm rather than an exception following infection of the upper airways. Viraemia is not detected in normal adults.

Rhinovirus infection does not produce extensive (or even detectable in some cases) cytopathology of the nasal mucus membrane; however, the extent correlates with the titre of recoverable virus. *In vitro*, exposure of human primary bronchial epithelial cells to rhinovirus may result in extensive CPE, depending on serotype and culture conditions (Schroth *et al.*, 1999; Papado-poulos *et al.*, 2000). Mucosal oedema with sparse infiltration of inflammatory cells, mainly neutrophils, are the predominant histological changes. Nasal mucociliary clearance is reduced, as a result of a reduced ciliary beat frequency and loss of ciliated epithelium (Wilson *et al.*, 1987).

Nasal secretions of infected individuals have increased plasma proteins such as albumin and IgG, as well as glandular proteins (lactoferrin, lysozyme and secretory IgA, 7F10 immunoreactive mucin) (Igarashi *et al.*, 1993; Yuta *et al.*, 1998). These findings reflect both increased vascular permeability, usually mediated by vasoactive amines, and glandular secretion, com-monly induced by cholinergic reflexes and neuropeptides. However, the detailed involvement of any such mediators remains to a great extent spec-ulative (Figure 9.4). Kinins are generated in nasal

secretions during natural and experimental colds, while their intranasal instillation causes sore throat (Naclerio *et al.*, 1988). The list of both proinflammatory (IL-1β, IL-2, IL-4, IL-6, IL-8, IL-11, IL-12, IL-13, IL-16, G-CSF, GM-CSF, TNFα and IFN-γ) and antiinflamma-tory (IL-1Ra, IL-10) cytokines, induced either *in vitro* or *in vivo* by rhinovirus infections, is already long and is growing (Einarsson *et al.*, 1996; Zhu *et al.*, 1996; Teran *et al.*, 1997; Johnston *et al.*, 1998; Zhu *et al.*, 1999). Several chemokines, able to attract neutrophils and eosinophils, are also induced after RV infection of bronchial epithelium, including RANTES, Groα, ENA-78, eotaxin and eotaxin-2 (Papadopoulos *et al.*, 2001). Rhinoviruses are also able to directly activate airway smooth muscle cells *in vitro*; however, it is not clear whether the virus could reach these cells *in vivo* (Grunstein *et al.*, 2001). The presence of these proinflammatory mediators is supportive of an immune rather than a cytopathic basis of rhinoviral common cold symptomatology. Oxidative stress and the activation of inflammation-related transcription factors, such as nuclear factor kappa-B (NF-κB),

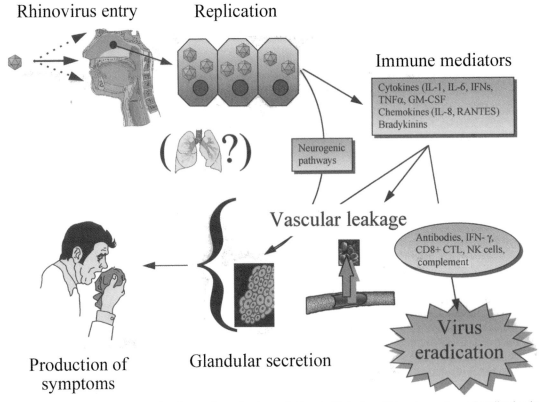

Figure 9.4 Schematic representation of pathogenetic mechanisms of rhinoviral infection. Rhinovirus entry and replication in the nasopharynx induces immune mediators and neurogenic pathways. Viruses are eradicated, but the concurrent vascular leakage and glandular secretion result in the well-known symptomatology

mediate the elaboration of several RV-induced cytokines and chemokines (Zhu *et al.*, 1997; Biagioli *et al.*, 1999). This is also the case for ICAM-1, which is also significantly upregulated by RV infection via an NF-κB-mediated mechanism (Papi and Johnston, 1999). A possible pathway may be through the stress-activated protein kinase p38 (Griego *et al.*, 2000).

The involvement of histamine is uncertain and conflicting results have been obtained from clinical trials of antihistamines. First-generation antihistamines could relieve sneezing and nasal discharge, but these compounds have H1 blocking, anticholinergic and other CNS activities, in contrast to second-generation agents which are less effective in colds. Elevated histamine levels were detected after experimental and wild-type infection in allergic patients but not in normal subjects (Igarashi *et al.*, 1993). Nevertheless, the second-generation antihistamines loratadine and desloratadine were able to inhibit rhinovirus-induced ICAM-1 upregulation in airway epithelial cells *in vitro* (Papi *et al.*, 2001).

The arachidonic acid pathways are also involved, suggested by induction of 5-lipoxygenase and cyclooxygenase-2-positive cells in bronchial biopsies of experimentally infected volunteers (Seymour *et al.*, 2002).

As far as the nervous system is concerned, parasympathetic blockade is able to reduce some symptoms of rhinoviral colds (Jacoby and Fryer, 1999). Furthermore, unilateral inoculation and infection results in bilateral symptomatology, favouring a neural pathway activation (Winther *et al.*, 1986).

Vascular leakage and mucus secretion result in nasal blockage and stimulation of the sneeze and cough reflexes, resulting in the well-known common cold symptomatology.

Mucosal oedema resulting from vascular leakage, venous sinusoidal engorgement and mucosal inflammatory cell infiltration is a prominent feature, and may lead to complications such as otitis and sinusitis. Indeed, CT scans obtained during and after acute rhinoviral infection have clearly demonstrated that paranasal sinus occlusion is a common event in rhinovirus colds (Gwaltney *et al.*, 1994).

The mechanisms of asthma exacerbations induced by viral infections in susceptible individuals is another currently investigated issue in rhinovirus pathophysiology. Rhinovirus infection seems to potentiate allergic responses (Calhoun *et al.*, 1994) but the precise mechanisms have yet to be determined. Inflammatory mediators such as kinins, and proinflammatory cytokines induced by rhinovirus infection (see list above), altered cell-mediated immunity, virus-specific IgE and

other mechanisms have been proposed, but the relative importance of each of these currently remains unclear (Papadopoulos and Johnston, 2001b).

IMMUNITY

Both cellular and humoral immunity are activated in response to rhinovirus infection. Virus-specific IgG and IgA serum antibodies remain low for the first week after inoculation and subsequently begin to increase to reach their peak approximately a month later. IgG antibodies stay at high levels for at least a year, while IgA declines slowly but remains detectable during the same period. Nasal IgA is also produced, becoming detectable 2 weeks post-inoculation, reaching its peak 1 week later and slowly declining to its original levels by 1 year (Barclay *et al.*, 1989). The late rise in antibody titres indicates that humoral immunity is not essential for recovery from viral illness. On the other hand, existing antibodies, especially in high titres, are associated with protection against reinfection with the same serotype and/or lessened signs and symptoms (Alper *et al.*, 1998). Possible ways for antibody-mediated virus inactivation include virus aggregation, activation of the complement cascade, prevention of binding to receptor as well as inhibition of uncoating (Rowlands, 1995).

An important role in virus eradication has been attributed to cellular immunity; however, the mechanisms involved are not yet understood in detail. In contrast to the high specificity of humoral immunity, rhinovirus-specific T cells can recognise both serotype-restricted and shared viral epitopes (Gern *et al.*, 1997a). Peripheral blood lymphocyte counts are decreased during infection, followed by recovery or even leukocytosis (Skoner *et al.*, 1993). An increased production of IL-2 and IFN-γ after mitogen stimulation, as well as increased natural killer cytotoxicity, have been found in peripheral blood mononuclear cells after experimental rhinovirus infection (Hsia *et al.*, 1990). Lymphocytes can be activated both specifically and non-specifically through a monocyte-dependent mechanism (Gern *et al.*, 1996a). Rhinoviruses enter, but do not replicate inside, monocytes and airway macrophages, indicating a potentially direct effect of these cells in antiviral immunity (Gern *et al.*, 1996b). The production of type 1 (IFN-γ, IL-12) as well as type 2 (IL-4 and IL-10) cytokines has been documented, and atopic asthmatic individuals appear to respond with relatively deficient type 1 cytokine production (Parry *et al.*, 2000; Papadopoulos *et al.*, 2002b).

Locally produced soluble factors by activated immune cells, such as IFNs or TNFs, have potent antiviral activities.

EPIDEMIOLOGY

The common cold is probably the most frequent illness afflicting mankind and certainly the most common cause for primary care consultations and absenteeism from work or school. The average number of yearly infections in adults is estimated to be between two and five, while this number increases up to 12 in children. A simple estimation would suggest that a normal individual spends 1–2 years of his life suffering from colds! At least one-quarter of 6 month-old infants have antibodies against rhinoviruses, while over 90% have such antibodies at the age of 2 years (Blomqvist et al., 2002).

Rhinoviruses cause about 35–60% of common colds. Interestingly, in contrast to the popular belief, early studies were unable to demonstrate any increase in susceptibility to rhinoviral infections after exposure to cold temperatures (Douglas et al., 1967). However, several other epidemiological factors are involved. Age is certainly important. Infections increase significantly from the second year of life and throughout school age, decreasing subsequently, probably due to neutralising antibodies induced by previous exposures (Monto, 1995). Increased morbidity and complications reappear in the elderly (Nicholson et al., 1997). Apart from the age-related susceptibility to the virus, socio-economic factors such as nutrition and population density, but most importantly family structure, strongly influence the incidence of rhinovirus infections. An infection is usually introduced by a child to other siblings and parents at home. Mothers are more susceptible than fathers, possibly because of increased exposure. School and day-care transmission is also very high, due to overcrowding, low immunity and children's unhygienic habits (Goldmann, 1992).

A seasonal pattern has been documented in temperate climates, with two peaks occurring, one in autumn, coinciding with the opening of schools, and another in late spring. During winter the occurrence of rhinovirus infections is reduced. School attendance is the major factor in determining seasonal patterns; infections occur throughout the winter months, peaking in the first 2–3 weeks after children return to school (Johnston et al., 1996). Depending on season and population and on the sensitivity of the PCR assay, 3–30% of asymptomatic subjects may be found positive by PCR (Marin et al., 2000; Nokso-Koivisto et al., 2002).

All populations are affected. The prevalent serotypes vary from year to year. It is possible that a small number of serotypes may cause most of the illnesses (Monto et al., 1987) but virus isolation and serotyping techniques are still cumbersome and insufficient for detailed evaluation. However, there is evidence of a striking genetic diversity of HRV strains circulating in a given community during a short time (Savolainen et al., 2002a).

There is a well-documented epidemiological relationship between various aspects of psychological stress and the susceptibility to rhinovirus infection (Cohen et al., 1997; Takkouche et al., 2001), the mechanisms of which are still speculative.

The question of whether atopic individuals are more susceptible to colds, develop more severe colds or clear rhinoviruses less effectively than normal subjects is still incompletely understood. There is evidence for incomplete virus clearance (Gern et al., 2000; Papadopoulos et al., 2002b) and augmented colds in atopic asthmatic subjects (Bardin et al., 1994). A recent, well-designed longitudinal study could not find differences between atopic asthmatic and normal subjects with respect to frequency, duration, or severity of rhinovirus colds in terms of upper respiratory symptoms, although there were significantly increased lower respiratory symptoms and falls in lung function in the asthmatic subjects (Corne et al., 2002). An epidemiological study has confirmed a synergistic interaction between respiratory virus infections and allergen exposure in risk of asthma exacerbations (Green, 2002). Surprisingly, in one report, experimental allergen challenge was able to protect from subsequent rhinovirus infection, suggesting a more complicated interaction (Avila et al., 2000). The explanations for these apparently contradictory findings will require further study.

CLINICAL FEATURES

The symptoms easiest to describe are those that everybody has experienced. Rhinoviruses produce the symptoms of the common cold, including rhinorrhoea, sneezing, nasal obstruction, sore throat and cough. General malaise and headache may occur, while fever is less common. Mood and mental functioning are also affected, with reduced alertness and slowed reaction times (Smith et al., 1998). Sleep is also significantly impaired (Drake et al., 2000). The course of the disease correlates with virus titres. Symptoms appear after a 24–48 h incubation period, reach their peak 2–3 days later and last for 5–7 days in total, persisting occasionally for as long as 2–4 weeks. Symptom severity is highly variable; on many occasions the disease may be hardly noticed, while around 20% of non-influenza flu-like illness can be attributed to rhinoviruses (Boivin et al., 2002). In patients hospitalised with respiratory problems, rhinovirus-related clinical presentations include bronchiolitis and pneumonia at ages < 5 years, asthma exacerbations in older children and young adults and pneumonia, COPD exacerbations and congestive heart failure in older adults (El-Sahly et al., 2000). The presence of rhinovirus, either alone or in combination with RSV, may be related to a more severe clinical presentation of acute bronchiolitis in infants (Papadopoulos et al., 2002a).

On the other hand, rhinovirus infections may cause significant morbidity in specific patient groups. Infants with bronchopulmonary dysplasia may develop serious respiratory illness, necessitating intensive care unit admission and occasionally mechanical ventilation (Chidekel et al., 1997). This is also the case for children with primary immunodeficiencies (Crooks et al., 2000). Myelosuppressed individuals frequently develop fatal pneumonia (Ghosh et al., 1999). Pulmonary function abnormalities, disease progression and secondary bacterial infections can result in children with cystic fibrosis (Collinson et al., 1996). Senior persons, especially residents of nursing homes, are also prone to severe disease that can exceptionally prove fatal (Wald et al., 1995).

COMPLICATIONS

Acute otitis media (AOM) is the most common complication of viral upper respiratory infection in children. Negative middle ear pressure develops in the majority of common colds in healthy individuals (Winther et al., 2002). Using PCR, rhinoviruses are detected in the middle ear fluid of 25–40% of episodes of AOM. Rhinoviruses were also present in 20% of middle ear fluids of patients with otitis media with effusion, at the time of tympanostomy tube placement (Pitkaranta et al., 1998). As previously mentioned, sinus involvement is detected by CT scan in a considerable percentage of rhinovirus infections, while there is evidence suggesting a causal role of the virus in as many as 50% of episodes of community-acquired sinusitis (Pitkaranta et al., 1997). In both

instances, the viruses may also facilitate or contribute to concurrent bacterial infections.

The role of rhinovirus infection in the exacerbations of asthma has been well documented in recent studies. Upper respiratory tract infections are associated with up to 80% of asthma episodes in schoolchildren, with rhinovirus being the most commonly isolated causal agent (Johnston et al., 1995) (Figure 9.5). In adults the figures are less, possibly due to diminished viral shedding; however, recent studies using sensitive molecular methodology indicate an involvement in at least half of the exacerbations (Nicholson et al., 1993; Teichtahl et al., 1997). Time trend analysis suggests that viral infections are indeed important in exacerbations in adults as well as children (Johnston et al., 1996). The mechanisms by which rhinoviruses exacerbate asthma are under investigation; they include bronchial epithelium-mediated inflammation, induction of an abnormal immune response, neural mechanisms and more, which are reviewed elsewhere (Papadopoulos and Johnston, 2001b).

Rhinoviruses are also implicated in acute and chronic bronchitis (Seemungal et al., 2000), bronchiolitis and pneumonia, although these areas have yet to be adequately studied (Papadopoulos and Johnston, 2001a; Papadopoulos et al., 2002a).

DIAGNOSIS

Virus cultures, serological tests and, more recently, nucleic acid detection have been used in the diagnosis of rhinoviruses. The former is cumbersome, time consuming and relatively insensitive, so that its diagnostic value is very limited in a clinical setting. Serology is totally impractical as a result of the large number of serotypes. Nucleic acid techniques, mainly the polymerase chain reaction (PCR), can potentially overcome these difficulties and have become the methods of choice for viral detection; a considerable number of protocols are currently under evaluation.

Virus Isolation

The optimal specimen for virus isolation is a nasal washing or a nasal aspirate. Throat or nasal swabs are used as an alternative in the field, or from children where nasal washings are difficult to obtain. Samples should be transported to the laboratory in virus transport medium as soon as possible and put immediately into culture or stored frozen at −70°C.

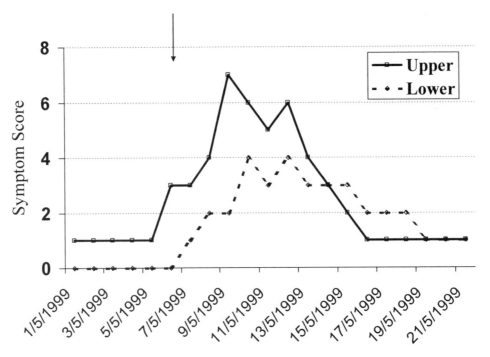

Figure 9.5 Upper and lower airway symptom score charts during rhinovirus infection. The arrow indicates the time a nasal wash was obtained and rhinovirus aetiology was confirmed with PCR. In this patient, lower airway symptoms follow shortly after the upper respiratory symptoms

Rhinoviruses replicate in several human embryonic and monkey tissues. However, they replicate best in human fetal lung fibroblasts (WI38, MRC5) and strains of HeLa cells. Samples are inoculated in cell cultures in tubes and are incubated in a roller drum at 33°C. They are then monitored under low-field magnification daily for the development of a cytopathic effect (CPE). Rhinoviral CPE is characterised by shrinkage and rounding of cells, cellular destruction and detachment of the cell layer (Figure 9.6). This can be noticed as early as 24 h post-inoculation, while the majority of positive samples develop CPE within 8 days. A second passage after this time is usually performed to identify less potent strains (Johnston and Tyrrell, 1995). Confirmation of rhinovirus identity can be performed by acid stability testing and of individual serotypes by neutralisation tests, using serotype-specific antisera.

Serology

Serological methods can be used for the detection of antiviral antibodies. Neutralisation tests can be done in combination with any culture system and have been the only standardised method for a number of years. They are used for antibody detection and quantification once the serotype is known, as in the case of experimental studies with volunteers inoculated with a known serotype, or with a virus isolated from the same patient. Pre-infection and post-infection serum titres are compared. Unfortunately, due to the large number of serotypes (> 100), these tests are only of limited practical value and are not used in routine clinical diagnosis.

Haemagglutination-inhibition tests are possible with a subset of rhinoviruses that agglutinate red blood cells. Their results are comparable to those of the neutralisation assays, but they are not widely used as they require a large amount of virus and can be applied only to a subset of serotypes.

ELISA is faster and much easier to perform, offers better sensitivity and can be readily adapted to measure different antibody isotypes in both serum and nasal secretions (Barclay and Al-Nakib, 1987). However, as with the other serological assays, ELISA is diagnostically useful only when the rhinovirus serotype is already known.

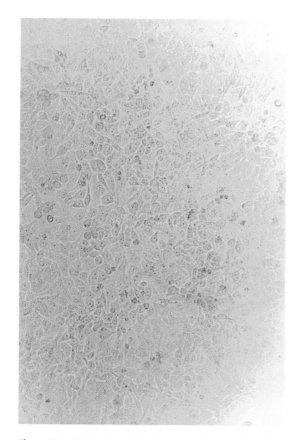 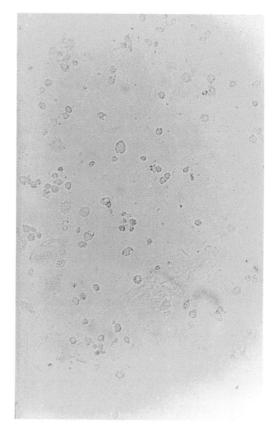

Figure 9.6 Rhinovirus-infected primary human bronchial epithelial cells developing a characteristic cytopathic effect (right) in comparison to control cells (left)

Recently, optically coated silicon surfaces have been used in a multiserotype detection system using polyclonal antibodies against the rhinovirus 3C protease (Ostroff *et al.*, 2001). This assay was successful in detecting 87% of laboratory-grown rhinovirus serotypes tested, but has not yet been tested in field studies.

Nucleic Acid Detection

Molecular methods for infectious agent identification are steadily becoming more widely applied in regard to a vast array of microorganisms, including rhinoviruses. Different approaches based on PCR have been investigated in order to optimise the method for research as well as clinical purposes (Andeweg *et al.*, 1999; Blomqvist *et al.*, 1999; Steininger *et al.*, 2001). Most sets of primers derive from the 5′ non-coding region that is the most conserved between different serotypes. Sensitivity is markedly improved in comparison to virus culture (Johnston *et al.*, 1993; Hyypia *et al.*, 1998). A problem has arisen from the fact that in several instances these procedures could not distinguish rhinoviruses from the closely related enteroviruses. Several approaches, including nested designs, differential hybridisation or restriction fragment length polymorphism have addressed this problem successfully (Mori and Clewley, 1994; Papadopoulos *et al.*, 1999a) (Figure 9.7). Nucleic acid sequence-based amplification (NASBA) (Samuelson *et al.*, 1998) and real-time PCR are also in development. Thin-film technology has been used to increase sensitivity and versatility of amplicon detection (Jenison *et al.*, 2001). Finally, multiplex-PCR approaches for the simultaneous detection of different respiratory viral pathogens, including rhinoviruses, which would greatly facilitate epidemiological studies as well as clinical diagnosis, are also in development. A database containing information on virus-specific oligonucleotides and primers has been developed and published on the Internet (Onodera and Melcher, 2002).

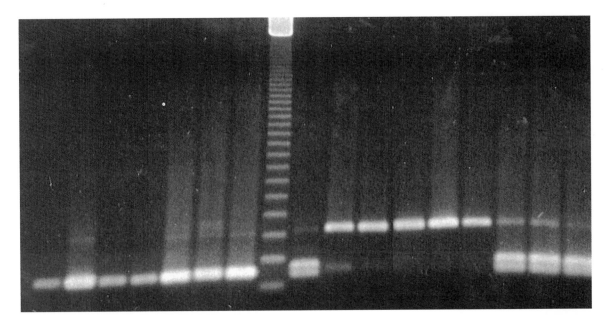

Figure 9.7　Agarose gel electrophoresis of PCR products reveal a band at 190 bp in the case of rhinovirus (lanes 1–7) and a 380 bp band or a double 180–200 bp band in the case of enteroviruses (lanes 9–17), after RFLP digestion of picornavirus PCR amplicons. Lane 8 is a ladder

PREVENTION AND TREATMENT

Intensive efforts during the last 40–50 years for the development of treatment or prevention strategies against rhinovirus common colds have so far been without encouraging results. The approaches that have been investigated include non-specific and empiric therapies, antiviral and antimediator drug treatments and vaccines. Very frequently, inappropriate and costly remedies have been used (Bertino, 2002).

The major obstacle for vaccine development is the large number of serotypes which do not produce heterotypic humoral immunity. Initial attempts with inactivated viruses have achieved serotype-specific protection in volunteers. A decavalent vaccine was also tested in humans resulting in variable responses to the included serotypes and insufficient heterotypic immunity (Hamory *et al.*, 1975). The protective duration of any responses was also undefined. The design of peptide vaccines, especially against T cell epitopes, which seem to be more conserved, is promising but still at an early stage (Francis *et al.*, 1987).

Among the pharmacological antiviral agents, IFN-α has been the first and most widely investigated. IFN is effective if given intranasally before or shortly after exposure to the virus, both in experimental infections in volunteers and in family outbreaks (Douglas and Betts, 1974). However, its high cost and local bleeding and discharge after long-term prophylactic use have been the major drawbacks to its clinical use.

A large number of compounds able to inhibit rhinovirus infection by preventing virus uncoating and/or cell entry have been investigated (Table 9.2). Unfortunately, to date no effective drug has emerged from this research, due to problems in potency, delivery and toxicity of the compounds and the emergence of resistant viral strains (Arruda and Hayden, 1996).

Since much of the symptomatology of the common cold is produced through inflammatory mediators, drugs antagonising these mediators have been investigated. Little benefit was demonstrated by antihistamine treatment, a bradykinin antagonist showed negative results, while anticholinergic sprays are able to reduce rhinorrhoea and sneezing (Johnston, 1997). Corticosteroids were found to have a marginal effect on symptoms but a rebound appeared when treatment was stopped; moreover, they have been associated with increases in viral titres. Speculations on the potential use of macrolide antibiotics, due to their *in vitro*

Table 9.2 Efforts towards an antirhinoviral therapy

General	
Ascorbic acid, zinc gluconate, inhalation of hot air, echinacea, NSAIDs	Questionable benefit
Antiinflammatory	
Corticosteroids (oral or inhaled)	Effective in reducing symptoms only in high doses, for a short period and with a rebound effect
Cromolyns	Reduce symptoms and duration of disease. Unkown mechanisms
Antihistamines	Little benefit. Some improvement in sneezing and rhinorrhoea
Anticholinergic nasal sprays	Reduce sneezing and rhinorrhoea
Antiviral	
IFN-α	Able to prevent symptoms, but expensive and with significant side-effects
Combination therapies	Combination of IFN-α, ipratropium and naproxen was effective in one clinical trial
Experimental therapies	
Antirhinoviral compounds	Enviroxime, WIN compounds, chalcones, pyridazinamines and other. Prevent viral uncoating. Some are currently under clinical trials
Soluble ICAM-1	Inhibits viral attachment of major type viruses to their receptors. Promising in initial clinical trials
Antisense oligonucleotides, 3C antiproteinases, DNA vaccines	Potential routes of future intervention

antiinflammatory effects (Suzuki *et al.*, 2002), were not confirmed in a clinical trial (Abisheganaden *et al.*, 2000).

The inadequacy of specific therapies, in addition to the frequency of the problem, have supported the emergence of non-specific treatments. These include the use of ascorbic acid, zinc gluconate, echinacea and the inhalation of humidified hot air. For all these remedies the mechanisms are speculative and the evidence frequently contradictory. Despite several blinded studies and meta-analyses, the usefulness of zinc preparations is, at best, marginal (Turner and Cetnarowski, 2000). However, *in vitro* addition of zinc salts is able to potentiate the antirhinoviral activity of IFN-α by 10-fold (Berg *et al.*, 2001). Substances with antioxidant properties are also able to inhibit *in vitro* the rhinovirus-induced ICAM-1 upregulation, suggesting a possible mechanism of action for ascorbic acid. Ascorbic acid in relatively high doses seems to have a modest benefit in reducing duration of cold symptoms, but potential prophylactic effects have not been confirmed (Douglas *et al.*, 2002). Although promising results were obtained with the use of cromolyns, which were able to reduce cold symptoms and shorten the duration of the illness (Aberg *et al.*, 1996), these have not been reconfirmed or further exploited.

A combination approach was also proposed involving the administration of antiviral (IFN-α), anticholinergic (ipratropium) and antiinflammatory (naproxen) drugs (Gwaltney, 1992). A significant therapeutic result was achieved, together with a decrease in viral shedding.

The advances in molecular biological techniques have renewed interest in novel therapeutic approaches. New antiviral compounds are synthesised by computer-aided design (Joseph-McCarthy *et al.*, 2001), such as drugs that can fit in the hydrophobic pocket of VP1, stabilising the capsid proteins and preventing uncoating, or rhinovirus protease inhibitors (Tsang *et al.*, 2001; Johnson *et al.*, 2002). Another possibility includes the use of antisense oligonucleotides, which anneal *in vitro* to viral RNA and are subsequently degraded by RNases (Johnston, 1997). A considerable number of such compounds are currently being evaluated *in vitro*, while some, such as pleconaril and AG7088 (Witherell, 2000), are undergoing clinical trials. These compounds are reviewed elsewhere (McKinlay, 2001).

Most interestingly, a soluble form of the major rhinovirus receptor ICAM-1 can inhibit viral entry and inactivate the virus in most experimental settings. Soluble ICAM-1 was able to prevent rhinovirus infection in chimpanzees (Huguenel *et al.*, 1997) and initial human trials have shown promising results (Turner *et al.*, 1999). Recombinant low-density lipoprotein receptor fragments are also able to inhibit minor group rhinovirus infection *in vitro* (Marlovits *et al.*, 1998), suggesting that receptor blockage could be an important antirhinovirus strategy.

REFERENCES

Aberg N, Aberg B and Alestig K (1996) The effect of inhaled and intranasal sodium cromoglycate on symptoms of upper respiratory tract infections. *Clin Exp Allerg*, **26**, 1045–1050.

Abisheganaden JA, Avila PC, Kishiyama JL *et al.* (2000) Effect of clarithromycin on experimental rhinovirus-16 colds: a randomized, double-blind, controlled trial. *Am J Med*, **108**, 453–459.

Alper CM, Doyle WJ, Skoner DP *et al.* (1998) Prechallenge antibodies moderate disease expression in adults experimentally exposed to rhinovirus strain hanks. *Clin Infect Dis*, **27**, 119–128.

Andeweg AC, Bestebroer TM, Huybreghs M *et al.* (1999) Improved detection of rhinoviruses in clinical samples by using a newly developed nested reverse transcription-PCR assay. *J Clin Microbiol*, **37**, 524–530.

Andries K, Dewindt B, Snoeks J *et al.* (1990) Two groups of rhinoviruses revealed by a panel of antiviral compounds present sequence divergence and differential pathogenicity. *J Virol*, **64**, 1117–1123.

Arruda E and Hayden F (1996) Update on therapy of influenza and rhinovirus infections. *Adv Exp Med Biol*, **394**, 175–187.

Avila PC, Abisheganaden JA, Wong H *et al.* (2000) Effects of allergic inflammation of the nasal mucosa on the severity of rhinovirus 16 cold. *J Allerg Clin Immunol*, **105**, 923–932.

Barclay W and Al-Nakib W (1987) An ELISA for the detection of rhinovirus-specific antibody in serum and nasal secretion. *J Virol Methods*, **15**, 53–64.

Barclay W, Al-Nakib W, Higgins P and Tyrrell D (1989) The time course of the humoral immune response to rhinovirus infection. *Epidemiol Infect*, **103**, 659–669.

Bardin P, Fraenkel D, Sanderson G *et al.* (1994) Amplified rhinovirus colds in atopic subjects. *Clin Exp Allerg*, **24**, 457–464.

Bella J, Kolatkar PR, Marlor CW *et al.* (1999) The structure of the two amino-terminal domains of human intercellular adhesion molecule-1 suggests how it functions as a rhinovirus receptor. *Virus Res*, **62**, 107–117.

Belsham G and Sonenberg N (1996) RNA–protein interactions in regulation of picornavirus RNA translation. *Microbiol Rev*, **60**, 499–511.

Berg K, Bolt G, Andersen H and Owen TC (2001) Zinc potentiates the antiviral action of human IFN-α ten-fold. *J Interferon Cytokine Res*, **21**, 471–474.

Bertino JS (2002) Cost burden of viral respiratory infections: issues for formulary decision makers. *Am J Med*, **112**(6A), 42S–49S.

Biagioli MC, Kaul P, Singh I and Turner RB (1999) The role of oxidative stress in rhinovirus-induced elaboration of IL-8 by respiratory epithelial cells. *Free Radic Biol Med*, **26**, 454–462.

Blomqvist S, Roivainen M, Puhakka T *et al.* (2002) Virological and serological analysis of rhinovirus infections during the first two years of life in a cohort of children. *J Med Virol*, **66**, 263–268.

Blomqvist S, Skytta A, Roivainen M and Hovi T (1999) Rapid detection of human rhinoviruses in nasopharyngeal aspirates by a microwell reverse transcription-PCR-hybridization assay. *J Clin Microbiol*, **37**, 2813–2816.

Blough H, Tiffany J, Gordon G and Fiala M (1969) The effect of magnesium on the intracellular crystallization of rhinovirus. *Virology*, **38**, 694–698.

Boivin G, Osterhaus AD, Gaudreau A *et al.* (2002) Role of picornaviruses in flu-like illnesses of adults enrolled in an oseltamivir treatment study who had no evidence of influenza virus infection. *J Clin Microbiol*, **40**, 330–334.

Calhoun W, Dick E, Schwartz L and Busse W (1994) A common cold virus, rhinovirus 16, potentiates airway inflammation after segmental antigen bronchoprovocation in allergic subjects. *J Clin Invest*, **94**, 2200–2208.

Casasnovas J and Springer T (1994) Pathway of rhinovirus disruption by soluble intercellular adhesion molecule 1 (ICAM-1): an intermediate in which ICAM-1 is bound and RNA is released. *J Virol*, **68**, 5882–5889.

Chidekel A, Rosen C and Bazzy A (1997) Rhinovirus infection associated with serious lower respiratory illness in patients with bronchopulmonary dysplasia. *Pediatr Infect Dis J*, **161**, 43–47.

Cohen S, Doyle W, Skoner D *et al.* (1997) Social ties and susceptibility to the common cold. *J Am Med Assoc*, **277**, 1940–1944.

Collinson J, Nicholson KG, Cancio E *et al.* (1996) Effects of upper respiratory tract infections in patients with cystic fibrosis. *Thorax*, **51**, 1115–1122.

Colonno R, Callahan P and Long W (1986) Isolation of a monoclonal antibody that blocks attachment of the major group of human rhinoviruses. *J Virol*, **57**, 7–12.

Colonno R, Condra J, Mizutani S *et al.* (1988) Evidence for the direct involvement of the rhinovirus canyon in receptor binding. *Proc Natl Acad Sci USA*, **85**, 5449–5453.

Corne JM, Marshall C, Smith S *et al.* (2002) Frequency, severity and duration of rhinovirus infections in asthmatic and non-asthmatic individuals: a longitudinal cohort study. *Lancet*, **359**, 831–834.

Crooks BN, Taylor CE, Turner AJ *et al.* (2000) Respiratory viral infections in primary immune deficiencies: significance and relevance to clinical outcome in a single BMT unit. *Bone Marrow Transpl*, **26**, 1097–1102.

Dick E, Jennings L, Mink K (1987) Aerosol transmission of rhinovirus colds. *J Infect Dis*, **156**, 442–448.

Douglas R, Chalker E and Treacy B (2002) Vitamin C for preventing and treating the common cold (*Cochrane Review*). The Cochrane Library, Issue 4, 2003.

Douglas RCJ, Couch R and Lindgren K (1967) Cold doesn't affect the 'common cold' in study of rhinovirus infections. *J Am Med Assoc*, **199**, 29–30.

Douglas RGJ and Betts R (1974) Effect of induced interferon in experimental rhinovirus infections in volunteers. *Infect Immun*, **9**, 506–510.

Drake CL, Roehrs TA, Royer H *et al.* (2000) Effects of an experimentally induced rhinovirus cold on sleep, performance, and daytime alertness. *Physiol Behav*, **71**, 75–81.

Duechler M, Skern T, Sommergruber W *et al.* (1987) Evolutionary relationships within the human rhinovirus genus: comparison of serotypes 89, 2, and 14. *Proc Natl Acad Sci USA*, **84**, 2605–2609.

Einarsson O, Geba G, Zhu Z *et al.* (1996) Interleukin-11: stimulation *in vivo* and *in vitro* by respiratory viruses and induction of airways hyperresponsiveness. *J Clin Invest*, **97**, 915–924.

El-Sahly HM, Atmar RL, Glezen WP and Greenberg SB (2000) Spectrum of clinical illness in hospitalized patients with 'common cold' virus infections. *Clin Infect Dis*, **31**, 96–100.

Foy H, Cooney M, Hall C *et al.* (1988) Case-to-case intervals of rhinovirus and influenza virus infections in households. *J Infect Dis*, **157**, 180–182.

Francis M, Hastings G, Sangar D *et al.* (1987) A synthetic peptide which elicits neutralizing antibody against human rhinovirus type 2. *J Gen Virol*, **68**(10), 2687–2691.

Gern J, Dick E, Kelly E *et al.* (1997a) Rhinovirus-specific T cells recognize both shared and serotype-restricted viral epitopes. *J Infect Dis*, **175**, 1108–1114.

Gern J, Vrtis R, Kelly E *et al.* (1996a) Rhinovirus produces nonspecific activation of lymphocytes through a monocyte-dependent mechanism. *J Immunol*, **157**, 1605–1612.

Gern JE, Dick EC, Lee WM *et al.* (1996b) Rhinovirus enters but does not replicate inside monocytes and airway macrophages. *J Immunol*, **156**, 621–627.

Gern JE, Galagan DM, Jarjour NN *et al.* (1997b) Detection of rhinovirus RNA in lower airway cells during experimentally induced infection. *Am J Respir Crit Care Med*, **155**, 1159–1161.

Gern JE, Vrtis R, Grindle KA *et al.* (2000) Relationship of upper and lower airway cytokines to outcome of experimental rhinovirus infection. *Am J Resp Crit Care Med*, **162**, 2226–2231.

Ghosh S, Champlin R, Couch R *et al.* (1999) Rhinovirus infections in myelosuppressed adult blood and marrow transplant recipients. *Clin Infect Dis*, **29**, 528–532.

Goldmann D (1992) Transmission of infectious diseases in children. *Pediatr Rev*, **13**, 283–293.

Green RM, Custovic A, Sanderson G *et al.* (2002) Synergism between allergens and viruses and risk of hospital admission with asthma: case–control study. *Br Med J*, **324**, 763.

Greve JM, Davis G, Meyer AM *et al.* (1989) The major human rhinovirus receptor is ICAM-1. *Cell*, **56**, 839–847.

Griego SD, Weston CB and Adams JL (2000) Role of p38 mitogen-activated protein kinase in rhinovirus-induced cytokine production by bronchial epithelial cells. *J Immunol*, **165**, 5211–5220.

Grunstein MM, Hakonarson H, Whelan R *et al.* (2001) Rhinovirus elicits proasthmatic changes in airway responsiveness independently of viral infection. *J Allerg Clin Immunol*, **108** 997–1004.

Gwaltney JMJ (1992) Combined antiviral and antimediator treatment of rhinovirus colds. *J Infect Dis*, **166**, 776–782.

Gwaltney JMJ and Hendley J (1978) Rhinovirus transmission: one if by air, two if by hand. *Am J Epidemiol*, **107**, 357–361.

Gwaltney JMJ, Phillips C, Miller R and Riker D (1994) Computed tomographic study of the common cold [see comments]. *N Engl J Med*, **330**, 25–30.

Hadfield A, Lee W, Zhao R *et al.* (1997) The refined structure of human rhinovirus 16 at 2.15 A resolution: implications for the viral life cycle. *Structure*, **5**, 427–441.

Hamory B, Hamparian V, Conant R and Gwaltney JMJ (1975) Human responses to two decavalent rhinovirus vaccines. *J Infect Dis*, **132**, 623–629.

Hamparian V, Colonno R, Cooney M *et al.* (1987) A collaborative report: rhinoviruses—extension of the numbering system from 89 to 100. *Virology*, **159**, 191–192.

Hastings GZ, Rowlands DJ and Francis MJ (1991) Proliferative responses of T cells primed against human rhinoviruses to other rhinovirus serotypes. *J Gen Virol*, **72**, 2947–2952.

Hewat EA, Neumann E, Conway JF *et al.* (2000) The cellular receptor to human rhinovirus 2 binds around the 5-fold axis and not in the canyon: a structural view. *EMBO J*, **19**, 6317–6325.

Hofer F, Gruenberger M, Kowalski H *et al.* (1994) Members of the low density lipoprotein receptor family mediate cell entry of a minor-group common cold virus. *Proc Natl Acad Sci USA*, **91**, 1839–1842.

Horsnell C, Gama R, Hughes P and Stanway G (1995) Molecular relationships between 21 human rhinovirus serotypes. *J Gen Virol*, **76**(10), 2549–2555.

Hsia J, Goldstein A, Simon G *et al.* (1990) Peripheral blood mononuclear cell interleukin-2 and interferon-γ production, cytotoxicity, and antigen-stimulated blastogenesis during experimental rhinovirus infection. *J Infect Dis*, **162**, 591–597.

Huguenel E, Cohn D, Dockum D *et al.* (1997) Prevention of rhinovirus infection in chimpanzees by soluble intercellular adhesion molecule-1. *Am J Resp Crit Care Med*, **155**, 1206–1210.

Hunt SL, Hsuan JJ, Totty N and Jackson RJ (1999) unr, a cellular cytoplasmic RNA-binding protein with five cold-shock domains, is required for internal initiation of translation of human rhinovirus RNA. *Genes Dev*, **13**, 437–448.

Hyypia T, Puhakka T and Ruuskanen O (1998) Molecular diagnosis of human rhinovirus infections: comparison with virus isolation. *J Clin Microbiol*, **36**, 2081–2083.

Igarashi Y, Skoner D, Doyle W *et al.* (1993) Analysis of nasal secretions during experimental rhinovirus upper respiratory infections. *J Allerg Clin Immunol*, **92**, 722–731.

Jacoby DB and Fryer AD (1999) Interaction of viral infections with muscarinic receptors. *Clin Exp Allerg*, **29**(2), 59–64.

Jenison R, Rihanek M and Polisky B (2001) Use of a thin film biosensor for rapid visual detection of PCR products in a multiplex format. *Biosens Bioelectron*, **16**, 757–763.

Johnson TO, Hua Y, Luu HT *et al.* (2002) Structure-based design of a parallel synthetic array directed toward the discovery of irreversible inhibitors of human rhinovirus 3C protease. *J Med Chem*, **45**, 2016–2023.

Johnston SL (1997) Problems and prospects of developing effective therapy for common cold viruses. *Trends Microbiol*, **5**, 58–63.

Johnston SL, Papi A, Bates PJ *et al.* (1998) Low grade rhinovirus infection induces a prolonged release of IL-8 in pulmonary epithelium. *J Immunol*, **160**, 6172–6181.

Johnston SL, Pattemore PK, Sanderson G *et al.* (1995) Community study of role of viral infections in exacerbations of asthma in 9–11 year-old children. *Br Med J*, **310**, 1225–1228.

Johnston SL, Pattemore PK, Sanderson G *et al.* (1996) The relationship between upper respiratory infections and hospital admissions for asthma: a time-trend analysis. *Am J Resp Crit Care Med*, **154**, 654–660.

Johnston SL, Sanderson G, Pattemore PK *et al.* (1993) Use of polymerase chain reaction for diagnosis of picornavirus infection in subjects with and without respiratory symptoms. *J Clin Microbiol*, **31**, 111–117.

Johnston SL and Tyrrell DAJ (1995) Rhinoviruses. In *Diagnostic Procedures for Viral, Rickettsial and Chlamydial Infections* (ed Lennette ET), pp 553–563. American Public Health Association, Washington.

Joseph-McCarthy D, Tsang SK, Filman DJ *et al.* (2001) Use of MCSS to design small targeted libraries: application to picornavirus ligands. *J Am Chem Soc*, **123**, 12758–12769.

Kerekatte V, Keiper BD, Badorff C *et al.* (1999) Cleavage of poly(A)-binding protein by coxsackievirus 2A protease *in vitro* and *in vivo*: another mechanism for host protein synthesis shut-off? *J Virol*, **73**, 709–717.

Killington RA, Stott EJ and Lee D (1977) The effect of temperature on the synthesis of rhinovirus type 2 RNA. *J Gen Virol*, **36**, 403–411.

Macnaughton M (1982) The structure and replication of rhinoviruses. *Curr Top Microbiol Immunol*, **97**, 1–26.

Marin J, Jeler-Kacar D, Levstek V and Macek V (2000) Persistence of viruses in upper respiratory tract of children with asthma. *J Infect*, **41**, 69–72.

Marlovits TC, Zechmeister T, Schwihla H *et al.* (1998) Recombinant soluble low-density lipoprotein receptor fragment inhibits common cold infection. *J Mol Recogn*, **11**, 49–51.

McKinlay MA (2001) Recent advances in the treatment of rhinovirus infections. *Curr Opin Pharmacol*, **1**, 477–481.

McKnight KL and Lemon SM (1998) The rhinovirus type 14 genome contains an internally located RNA structure that is required for viral replication. *RNA*, **4**, 1569–1584.

Meschievitz C, Schultz S and Dick E (1984) A model for obtaining predictable natural transmission of rhinoviruses in human volunteers. *J Infect Dis*, **150**, 195–201.

Molins MA, Contreras MA, Fita I and Pons M (1998) Solution conformation of an immunogenic peptide from HRV2: comparison with the conformation found in a complex with a Fab fragment of an anti-HRV2 neutralizing antibody. *J Pept Sci*, **4**, 101–110.

Monto A (1995) Viral respiratory infections in the community: epidemiology, agents, and interventions. *Am J Med*, **99**, 24S–27S.

Monto A, Bryan E and Ohmit S (1987) Rhinovirus infections in Tecumseh, Michigan: frequency of illness and number of serotypes. *J Infect Dis*, **156**, 43–49.

Mori J and Clewley JP (1994) Polymerase chain reaction and sequencing for typing rhinovirus RNA. *J Med Virol*, **44**, 323–329.

Mosser AG, Brockman-Schneider R, Amineva S *et al.* (2002) Similar frequency of rhinovirus-infectible cells in upper and lower airway epithelium. *J Infect Dis*, **185**, 734–743.

Naclerio R, Proud D, Lichtenstein L *et al.* (1988) Kinins are generated during experimental rhinovirus colds. *J Infect Dis*, **157**, 133–142.

Nicholson KG, Kent J, Hammersley V and Cancio E (1997) Acute viral infections of upper respiratory tract in elderly people living in the community: comparative, prospective, population based study of disease burden. *Br Med J*, **315**, 1060–1064.

Nicholson KG, Kent J and Ireland DC (1993) Respiratory viruses and exacerbations of asthma in adults. *Br Med J*, **307**, 982–986.

Nokso-Koivisto J, Kinnari TJ, Lindahl P *et al.* (2002) Human picornavirus and coronavirus RNA in nasopharynx of children without concurrent respiratory symptoms. *J Med Virol*, **66**, 417–420.

Onodera K and Melcher U (2002) VirOligo: a database of virus-specific oligonucleotides. *Nucleic Acids Res*, **30**, 203–204.

Ostroff R, Ettinger A, La H *et al.* (2001) Rapid multiserotype detection of human rhinoviruses on optically coated silicon surfaces. *J Clin Virol*, **21**, 105–117.

Papadopoulos N and Johnston S (2001a) The rhinovirus—not such an innocent? *Qu J Med*, **94**, 1–3.

Papadopoulos N and Johnston S (2001b) The role of viruses in the induction and progression of asthma. *Curr Allerg Asthma Rep*, **1**, 144–152.

Papadopoulos NG, Bates PJ, Bardin PG *et al.* (2000) Rhinoviruses infect the lower airways. *J Infect Dis*, **181**, 1875–1884.

Papadopoulos NG, Hunter J, Sanderson G *et al.* (1999a) Rhinovirus identification by BglI digestion of picornavirus RT-PCR amplicons. *J Virol Methods*, **80**, 179–185.

Papadopoulos NG, Moustaki M, Tsolia M *et al.* (2002a) Association of rhinovirus infection with increased disease severity in acute bronchiolitis. *Am J Resp Crit Care Med*, **165**, 1285–1289.

Papadopoulos NG, Papi A, Meyer J *et al.* (2001) Rhinovirus infection upregulates eotaxin and eotaxin-2 expression in bronchial epithelial cells. *Clin Exp Allergy*, **31**, 1060–1066.

Papadopoulos NG, Sanderson G, Hunter J and Johnston SL (1999b) Rhinoviruses replicate effectively at lower airway temperatures. *J Med Virol*, **58**, 100–104.

Papadopoulos NG, Stanciu LA, Papi A *et al.* (2002b) A defective type 1 response to rhinovirus in atopic asthma. *Thorax*, **57**, 328–332.

Papi A and Johnston SL (1999) Rhinovirus infection induces expression of its own receptor intercellular adhesion molecule 1 (ICAM-1) via increased NF-kappaB-mediated transcription. *J Biol Chem*, **274**, 9707–9720.

Papi A, Papadopoulos NG, Stanciu LA *et al.* (2001) Effect of desloratadine and loratadine on rhinovirus-induced inter-cellular adhesion molecule 1 upregulation and promoter activation in respiratory epithelial cells. *J Allerg Clin Immunol*, **108**, 221–228.

Parry DE, Busse WW, Sukow KA *et al.* (2000) Rhinovirus-induced PBMC responses and outcome of experimental infection in allergic subjects. *J Allerg Clin Immunol*, **105**, 692–698.

Patterson L and Hamparian V (1997) Hyper-antigenic variation occurs with human rhinovirus type 17. *J Virol*, **71**, 1370–1374.

Pitkaranta A, Arruda E, Malmberg H and Hayden F (1997) Detection of rhinovirus in sinus brushings of patients with acute community-acquired sinusitis by reverse transcription-PCR. *J Clin Microbiol*, **35**, 1791–1793.

Pitkaranta A, Jero J, Arruda E *et al.* (1998) Polymerase chain reaction-based detection of rhinovirus, respiratory syncytial virus, and coronavirus in otitis media with effusion. *J Pediatr*, **133**, 390–394.

Reischl A, Reithmayer M, Winsauer G *et al.* (2001) Viral evolution toward change in receptor usage: adaptation of a major group human rhinovirus to grow in ICAM-1-negative cells. *J Virol*, **75**, 9312–9319.

Rossmann M (1994) Viral cell recognition and entry. *Protein Sci*, **3**, 1712–1725.

Rossmann M, Arnold E, Erickson J *et al.* (1985) Structure of a human common cold virus and functional relationship to other picornaviruses. *Nature*, **317**, 145–153.

Rossmann M and Palmenberg A (1988) Conservation of the putative receptor attachment site in picornaviruses. *Virology*, **164**, 373–382.

Rowlands DJ (1995) Rhinoviruses and cells: molecular aspects. *Am J Resp Crit Care Med*, **152**, S31–S35.

Samuelson A, Westmoreland D, Eccles R and Fox JD (1998) Development and application of a new method for amplification and detection of human rhinovirus RNA. *J Virol Methods*, **71**, 197–209.

Sattar S, Jacobsen H, Springthorpe V et al. (1993) Chemical disinfection to interrupt transfer of rhinovirus type 14 from environmental surfaces to hands. Appl Environ Microbiol, 59, 1579–1585.

Savolainen C, Blomqvist S, Mulders MN and Hovi T (2002a) Genetic clustering of all 102 human rhinovirus prototype strains: serotype 87 is close to human enterovirus 70. J Gen Virol, 83, 333–340.

Savolainen C, Mulders MN and Hovi T (2002b) Phylogenetic analysis of rhinovirus isolates collected during successive epidemic seasons. Virus Res, 85, 41–46.

Schober D, Kronenberger P, Prchla E et al. (1998) Major and minor receptor group human rhinoviruses penetrate from endosomes by different mechanisms. J Virol, 72, 1354–1364.

Schroth MK, Grimm E, Frindt P et al. (1999) Rhinovirus replication causes RANTES production in primary bronchial epithelial cells. Am J Resp Cell Mol Biol, 20, 1220–1228.

Seemungal TA, Harper-Owen R, Bhowmik A et al. (2000) Detection of rhinovirus in induced sputum at exacerbation of chronic obstructive pulmonary disease. Eur Resp J, 16, 677–683.

Seymour ML, Gilby N, Bardin PG et al. (2002) Rhinovirus infection increases 5-lipoxygenase and cyclooxygenase-2 in bronchial biopsy specimens from nonatopic subjects. J Infect Dis, 185, 540–544.

Sherry B, Mosser A, Colonno R and Rueckert R (1986) Use of monoclonal antibodies to identify four neutralization immunogens on a common cold picornavirus, human rhinovirus 14. J Virol, 57, 246–257.

Skoner D, Whiteside T, Wilson J et al. (1993) Effect of rhinovirus 39 infection on cellular immune parameters in allergic and nonallergic subjects. J Allerg Clin Immunol, 92, 732–743.

Smith A, Thomas M, Kent J and Nicholson K (1998) Effects of the common cold on mood and performance. Psychoneuroendocrinology, 23, 733–739.

Staunton D, Dustin M, Erickson H and Springer T (1990) The arrangement of the immunoglobulin-like domains of ICAM-1 and the binding sites for LFA-1 and rhinovirus [published errata appear in Cell 1990, 61(2), t1157 and Cell, 66(6), 1311ff]. Cell, 61, 243–254.

Staunton D, Merluzzi V, Rothlein R et al. (1989) A cell adhesion molecule, ICAM-1, is the major surface receptor for rhinoviruses. Cell, 56, 849–853.

Steininger C, Aberle SW and Popow-Kraupp T (2001) Early detection of acute rhinovirus infections by a rapid reverse transcription–PCR assay. J Clin Microbiol, 39, 129–133.

Stoneley M, Subkhankulova T, Le Quesne JP et al. (2000) Analysis of the c-myc IRES; a potential role for cell-type specific trans-acting factors and the nuclear compartment. Nucleic Acids Res, 28, 687–694.

Suzuki T, Yamaya M, Sekizawa K et al. (2002) Erythromycin inhibits rhinovirus infection in cultured human tracheal epithelial cells. Am J Resp Crit Care Med, 165, 1113–1118.

Takkouche B, Regueira C and Gestal-Otero JJ (2001) A cohort study of stress and the common cold. Epidemiology, 12, 345–349.

Teichtahl H, Buckmaster N and Pertnikovs E (1997) The incidence of respiratory tract infection in adults requiring hospitalization for asthma. Chest, 112, 591–596.

Teran LM, Johnston SL, Schröder JM et al. (1997) Role of nasal interleukin-8 in neutrophil recruitment and activation in children with virus-induced asthma. Am J Resp Crit Care Med, 155, 1362–1366.

Tomassini J, Graham D, DeWitt C et al. (1989) cDNA cloning reveals that the major group rhinovirus receptor on HeLa cells is intercellular adhesion molecule 1. Proc Natl Acad Sci USA, 86, 4907–4911.

Tsang SK, Cheh J, Isaacs L et al. (2001) A structurally biased combinatorial approach for discovering new anti-picornaviral compounds. Chem Biol, 8, 33–45.

Turner RB and Cetnarowski WE (2000) Effect of treatment with zinc gluconate or zinc acetate on experimental and natural colds. Clin Infect Dis, 31, 1202–1208.

Turner RB, Wecker MT, Pohl G et al. (1999) Efficacy of tremacamra, a soluble intercellular adhesion molecule 1, for experimental rhinovirus infection: a randomized clinical trial. J Am Med Assoc, 281, 1797–1804.

Tyrrell DAJ and Parsons R (1960) Some virus isolations from common colds. III. Cytopathic effects in tissue cultures. Lancet 1, 239–242.

Uncapher C, DeWitt C and Colonno R (1991) The major and minor group receptor families contain all but one human rhinovirus serotype. Virology, 180, 814–817.

Wald T, Shult P, Krause P et al. (1995) A rhinovirus outbreak among residents of a long-term care facility. Ann Intern Med, 123, 588–593.

Wilson R, Alton E, Rutman A et al. (1987) Upper respiratory tract viral infection and mucociliary clearance. Eur J Respir Dis, 70, 272–279.

Winther B, Gwaltney JMJ, Mygind N et al. (1986) Sites of rhinovirus recovery after point inoculation of the upper airway. J Am Med Assoc, 256, 1763–1767.

Winther B, Hayden FG, Arruda E et al. (2002) Viral respiratory infection in schoolchildren: effects on middle ear pressure. Pediatrics, 109, 826–832.

Witherell G (2000) AG-7088 Pfizer. Curr Opin Invest Drugs, 1, 297–302.

Yin F and Lomax N (1986) Establishment of a mouse model for human rhinovirus infection. J Gen Virol, 67(11), 2335–2340.

Yuta A, Doyle WJ, Gaumond E et al. (1998) Rhinovirus infection induces mucus hypersecretion. Am J Physiol, 274, L1017–1023.

Zhang A, Geisler SC, Smith AD et al. (1999) A disulfide-bound HIV-1 V3 loop sequence on the surface of human rhinovirus 14 induces neutralizing responses against HIV-1. Biol Chem, 380, 365–374.

Zhu Z, Homer RJ, Wang Z et al. (1999) Pulmonary expression of interleukin-13 causes inflammation, mucus hypersecretion, subepithelial fibrosis, physiologic abnormalities, and eotaxin production. J Clin Invest, 103, 779–788.

Zhu Z, Tang W and Gwaltney JMJ (1997) Rhinovirus stimulation of interleukin-8 in vivo and in vitro: role of NF-κB. Am J Physiol, 273, L814–824.

Zhu Z, Tang W, Ray A et al. (1996) Rhinovirus stimulation of interleukin-6 in vivo and in vitro. Evidence for nuclear factor κ B-dependent transcriptional activation. J Clin Invest, 97, 421–430.

10

Coronaviruses and Toroviruses

David Cavanagh

Institute for Animal Health, Newbury, UK

INTRODUCTION

Until early in 2003, human coronaviruses were usually thought of in the context of the common cold and, indeed, these viruses are responsible for approximately 25% of colds. Then, in late February 2003, Dr Carlo Urbani of the World Health Organisation (WHO) notified the WHO of cases of atypical pneumonia in Hanoi, Vietnam. The disease, subsequently named severe acute respiratory syndrome (SARS), was rapidly identified as being caused by a previously unknown coronavirus, *SARS coronavirus*. The first known cases of SARS were in Guangdong Province, People's Republic of China, in November 2002, although this did not become widely known until February of the following year. The disease spread to neighbouring Hong Kong and thence to several other countries. By the end of June 2003 there had been 8460 cases of SARS, 808 of them fatal. In addition to pneumonia, *SARS coronavirus* was often associated with diarrhoea, which has also been associated with infection by strains of the previously known human coronaviruses.

The long-known coronaviruses can grow in some neural cells *in vitro* and have been associated with cases of multiple sclerosis (MS), although the role of the coronavirus in such cases is not clear. The alimentary tract is certainly a site of replication of toroviruses, including those of humans; these viruses morphologically resemble coronaviruses, with which they may be confused.

Coronaviruses were first isolated in humans in the mid-1960s (Tyrrell and Bynoe, 1965; Hamre and Procknow, 1966). The original coronavirus strains were passaged in organ cultures of human embryonic trachea or nasal epithelium and in primary human kidney cell cultures. Subsequently, several other human coronaviruses (HCoVs) have been isolated in organ or cell cultures. The majority of HCoVs studied to date are serologically related to one of two reference strains, 229E and OC43. Molecular analysis has shown that these two viruses differ extensively from each other; they are distinct species of coronavirus (*Human coronavirus 229E* and *Human coronavirus OC43*), not simply variants of each other. Similarly, *SARS coronavirus* has a genome organisation distinct from these and other coronaviruses, and structural proteins that have only low amino acid identity with the HCoVs.

Toroviruses were first isolated from cases of diarrhoea in horses in 1972 (Berne virus, the type strain of *Equine torovirus*, EqTV) and neonatal calves 1982 (Breda virus, type strain of *Bovine torovirus*, BTV; Weiss and Horzinek, 1987). Subsequently particles resembling these two viruses were observed by electron microscopy in the stools of children and adults with diarrhoea (*Human torovirus*, HTV; Beards *et al.*, 1984). More recent studies have confirmed the presence of HTV, especially associated with gastroenteritis.

A feature of coronaviruses and toroviruses is recombination, both of the homologous (with viruses of the same species and other coronaviruses) and heterologous type (with viruses of other genera, although this is rare) (Lai and Cavanagh, 1997).

THE VIRUSES

Coronavirus and *Torovirus* are the two genera within the family *Coronaviridae*, order *Nidovirales* (Enjuanes

Principles and Practice of Clinical Virology, Fifth Edition. Edited by A. J. Zuckerman, J. E. Banatvala, J. R. Pattison, P. D. Griffiths and B. D. Schoub
© 2004 John Wiley & Sons Ltd   ISBN 0 470 84338 1

et al., 2000). Both genera have genomes which are non-segmented, single-stranded RNA of approximately 30 000 nucleotides and positive polarity (Enjuanes *et al.*, 2000) and have similar gross appearance. The coronaviruses are largely associated with respiratory and enteric infections in mammals and birds (Lai and Cavanagh, 1997; Siddell, 1995) whilst to date the fewer known toroviruses have been associated with diarrhoea (Koopmans *et al.*, 1997; Jamieson *et al.*, 1998).

The large surface projections of the coronaviruses gave them an appearance reminiscent of a crown, hence the name 'coronaviruses' (Latin *corona*, crown; Figures 10.1 and 10.2). The doughnut shape sometimes seen within torovirus particles resulted in the use of the root 'toro', from the Latin *torus*, the lowest convex moulding in the base of a column (Figures 10.1 and 10.2). The dozen or so known coronaviruses, of mammalian and avian species (Table 10.1), cause respiratory or enteric illnesses (Enjuanes *et al.*, 2000). *SARS coronavirus* was associated not only with pneumonia but also with diarrhoea, e.g. in 38% of cases referred to the Prince of Wales Hospital, Hong Kong. If it is demonstrated that the virus was directly responsible for the pathology in both respiratory tract and gut, it will be the first strain of a coronavirus that has caused pathology in both regions. Some avian coronaviruses can cause nephritis (Cavanagh *et al.*, 2002) whilst *Feline coronavirus* (FCoV) can infect macrophages, sometimes leading to infectious peritonitis. *Murine hepatitis virus* (MHV) strains can infect the liver, and replicate in cells of the central nervous system, causing encephalitis and demyelination (Stohlman and Hinton, 2001; Matthews *et al.*, 2002). *Haemagglutinating encephalomyelitis virus* (HEV) of pigs also selectively infects neuronal tissue. Coronaviruses have been assigned to one of groups 1, 2 and 3 (Table 10.1) on the basis of group-specific (usually non-structural) proteins, genome organisation and amino acid sequence identity, supported to some extent by antigenic analyses (Enjuanes *et al.*, 2000; González *et al.*, 2003). The low degree of amino acid identity between the proteins of *SARS coronavirus* and those of groups 1, 2 and 3 have suggested that it be placed in a new group, 4. There is a school of thought that suggests that *SARS coronavirus* be included in group 2, on the basis of features of the proteins encoded by gene 1.

Electron Microscopic Appearance

Coronaviruses and toroviruses are pleiomorphic, ether-labile, enveloped viruses with diameters of approximately 120 nm and a buoyant density in

Table 10.1 Coronavirus groups

Group 1
  Human coronavirus 229E
  Canine enteric coronavirus
  Feline coronavirus
  Porcine transmissible gastroenteritis coronavirus
  Porcine epidemic diarrhoea coronavirus

Group 2
  Human coronavirus OC43
  Bovine coronavirus
  Canine respiratory coronavirus
  Porcine haemagglutinating encephalomyelitis coronavirus
  Murine hepatitis coronavirus

Group 3
  Infectious bronchitis coronavirus
  Turkey coronavirus
  Pheasant coronavirus

Group 4
  SARS coronavirus[a]

[a]SARS coronavirus has been placed in a new group on the basis of the extremely low amino acid identity between its proteins and nature and organisation of its non-structural protein genes and those of the other three groups, consistent with the criteria used to assign coronaviruses to groups 1, 2 and 3. It has also been suggested that *SARS coronavirus* might be placed into group 2, on the basis that its gene 1b-encoded proteins are phylogenetically closer to those of group 2 members than to groups 1 and 3.

sucrose of 1.15–1.18 g/ml. Toroviruses are variously described as being doughnut-, disc-, kidney- or rod-shaped, depending on the angle of view (Figure 10.1). Particles of both genera have club-shaped surface projections or spikes (S) of up to 20 nm in length, although the shape varies among the species. Particles may be seen with few or no spikes visible (Weiss *et al.*, 1983). Electron microscopy of BTV revealed few of the 20 nm spikes but rather an intact fringe of smaller spikes, some 7–9 nm in length (Woode *et al.*, 1982; Cornelissen *et al.*, 1997). Toroviruses isolated from human faeces had an intact fringe of 10 nm spikes (Duckmanton *et al.*, 1997) that resembled those seen on human toroviruses by Beards *et al.* (1984). The latter reported observing the 20 nm spikes only rarely. It is possible that the 10 nm spikes are the haemagglutinin esterase (HE) protein. BTV has an HE protein which forms a fringe of spikes approximately 6 nm in length (Cornelissen *et al.*, 1997).

Composition of Virions

The S protein is a type I glycoprotein, most probably trimeric (see Lewicki and Gallagher, 2002). The

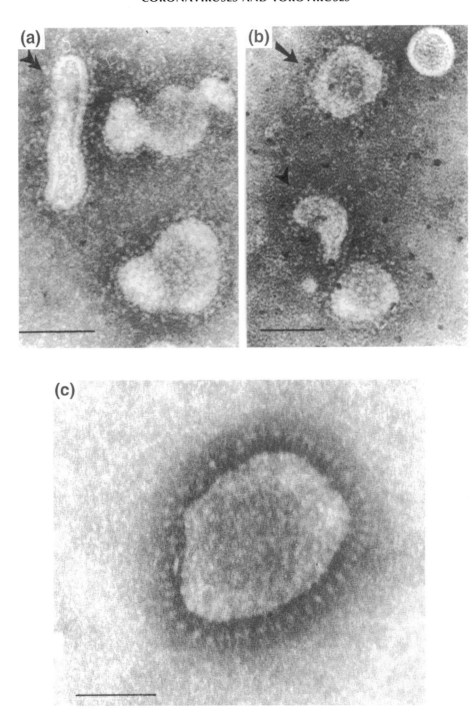

Figure 10.1 Electronmicrographs of (a, b) human enteric torovirus showing torus (arrow), crescent (arrow-head) and rod (double arrow-head) and (c) a human enteric coronavirus. The latter has spikes which are more prominent and readily discernible than those of the torovirus. The shorter, 10 nm, projections on the torovirus particles may be the haemagglutinin-esterase protein (HE). Bar = 100 nm. Reprinted by permission from Duckmanton *et al.* (1997), © 1997 Elsevier

(a)

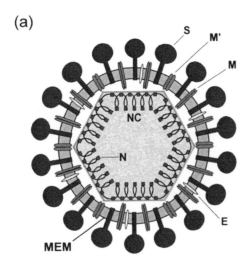

(b)

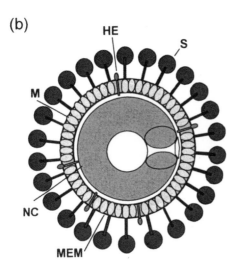

Figure 10.2 Diagrammatic representation of the virions of (a) a coronavirus and (b) a torovirus. Both types of virus have a lipid membrane (MEM), prominent spike proteins (S) and an integral membrane protein (M). HCoV-OC43, but not HCoV-229E, and some toroviruses have an HE protein. Coronaviruses, but not toroviruses, contain a small number of molecules of an E protein. (a) Cryoelectron microscopy has indicated the presence of a core structure in coronaviruses, comprising a nucleocapsid (NC, N protein plus genomic RNA) and the endodomain of the M protein (in the nexo-cendo orientation; Risco et al., 1996). Some of the M molecules (M′) are in the nexo-cexo orientation. (b) The nucleocapsid of toroviruses has the appearance of a torus. Reprinted by permission of Springer-Verlag from González et al. (2003)

membrane-spanning region is near the carboxy(C)-terminus, the actual C-terminus being within the lumen of the virion. Viruses of both genera contain, in addition to S, a smaller integral membrane glycoprotein (M) largely embedded in the virus envelope, tiny amounts of a third, even smaller membrane-associated non-glycosylated protein, E (for envelope) and a nucleocapsid (N) protein that surrounds the genome (Figure 10.2).

The M protein, a type III glycoprotein, has a short (20 amino acids or so) glycosylated amino(N)-terminus at the surface of the virion, followed by three hydrophobic membrane-spanning regions, an amphipathic region and finally a C-terminal tail in the lumen of the virion. The amphipathic and tail regions may be referred to as the endodomain. Studies with transmissible gastroenteritis virus (TGEV) have indicated that two-thirds of the M protein has a nexo-cendo orientation, i.e. N-terminus on the outside of the virion, the C-terminus in the lumen, whilst one-third has a nexo-cexo orientation i.e. both termini on the outside (Escors et al., 2001a). Cryoelectron microsope visualisation of unstained TGEV in vitreous ice has revealed the presence of a core structure in TGEV (Risco et al., 1996). It has been proposed that the TGEV virion comprises (a) a core, made of the nucleocapsid (N protein plus genome) and the endodomain of M, and (b) the envelope, containing S, E and M. The M molecules in the nexo-cendo orientation are those that remain with the core when it is purified (Escors et al., 2001b).

The E protein, comprising only 76–110 amino acids, is present in only trace amounts in virions.

Human coronaviruses of the OC43, but not 229E, species, as with other members of coronavirus group 2, contain an additional HE glycoprotein, which forms a 5 nm layer of surface projections. As described above, BoTV has an HE protein which is absent from equine torovirus (EqTV), as this virus has an incomplete HE gene (Cornelissen et al., 1997). The BoTV HE protein has approximately 30% amino acid sequence identity with that of coronaviruses and influenza C virus. In addition to the HE protein, which is not essential for replication in vitro, the toroviruses have three structural proteins; N, M, S (Figure 10.2). The S protein is highly glycosylated (N-linked glycans), as for the coronavirus S protein, and is proteolytically processed, like the coronavirus S protein, into S1 (amino-terminal) and S2 subunits.

The reader is referred to several chapters in Siddell (1995) and to Lai and Cavanagh (1997) and Cornelissen et al. (1997) for comprehensive reviews of coronavirus and torovirus proteins.

Assembly of Virions

The coronavirus glycoproteins are synthesised at the rough endoplasmic reticulum and are then translocated to the endoplasmic reticulum–Golgi intermediate compartment. This is the budding compartment, where immature virus particles containing the viral ribonucleoprotein (genome plus nucleocapsid protein) form (Salanueva *et al.*, 1999). The particles progress to the *cis*-, medial, *trans*-Golgi compartments and then to the *trans*-Golgi network. Secretory vesicles then transport the virus particles to the cell surface, the vesicles presumably fusing with the plasma membrane to release the virus particles.

The coronavirus M protein is not translocated beyond the Golgi compartments, hence this is where virus particles form, not at the plasma membrane. The C-terminal domain is crucial for virus particle formation whilst glycosylation appears to be non-essential (de Haan *et al.*, 1998). The M protein of toroviruses is also thought to determine the site of virus particle formation. In the case of the coronaviruses, E protein is also essential for the formation of virus particles. It is integrated into membranes without involvement of a cleaved signal peptide, the C-terminus being within the lumen of virus particles, the molecule spanning the membrane once, possibly twice (Raamsman *et al.*, 2000). As the E protein occurs in only trace amounts in virions, it is considered that interaction of M protein molecules with each other is the main inducer of particle formation (de Haan *et al.*, 2000).

The S protein can be transported to the cell surface but some of it remains in the Golgi as a consequence of interaction with the M protein (Opstelten *et al.*, 1995) via the transmembrane region and C-terminal tail of the S protein (Kuo *et al.*, 2000). The amphipathic domain, but not the C-terminal tail, of M is particularly involved in the M–S interaction (de Haan *et al.*, 1998).

RNA Replication and Transcription

Investigation of HCV-229E took a great leap forward by the development of a reverse-genetic system: a DNA copy of the full-length genome was assembled *in vitro* and cloned in the vaccinia virus genome (Thiel *et al.*, 2001). This permits the precise modification of any part of the genome, followed by recovery of recombinant HCV-229E. Reverse-genetic systems have been developed for coronaviruses in each of the three groups (Casais *et al.*, 2001).

The genome organisation of HCV-229E, HCV-OC43 and *SARS coronavirus* are shown in Figure 10.3. They all differ with respect to the number and location of genes that encode proteins believed to be non-structural, i.e. not present in virus particles. In HCoV-OC43 all the genes are monocistronic, whilst in HCoV-229E and *SARS coronavirus* there are one and four dicistronic genes (Thiel *et al.*, 2003), although it has not been demonstrated that all the second cistrons of *SARS coronavirus* are expressed. Interestingly, the genome of the *SARS coronavirus* isolated from Himalayan palm civet cats and racoon dogs, and one early human isolate in Guangdong Province, has 29 extra nucleotides compared to the other human isolates (Yi Guan, WHO meeting, Kuala Lumpur, June 2003). This results in there being only one open reading frame (ORF) in gene 8, compared to two in most of the human isolates.

Some of the other coronaviruses contain non-structural protein genes that do not have homologues in any of the three HCoVs, including SARS. Members of a given coronavirus group tend to have similar non-structural protein genes located in the same positions of the genome. Hence they are also referred to as being group-specific genes, whose roles are not known. De Haan *et al.* (2002a) made recombinant MHVs that lacked one or more of the group 2-specific genes. Infectivity *in vitro* was the same or near that of the wild-type virus; these genes are not essential for infectivity *per se*. Consequently, they have also been referred to as accessory genes. It is believed that they play a role *in vivo*; deletion of these genes from MHV attenuated the pathogenicity of the virus (de Haan *et al.*, 2002a). Rearrangement of the gene order had little effect on infectivity of MHV (de Haan *et al.*, 2002b). Toroviruses do not have any non-structural protein genes, other than gene 1 (Figure 10.3).

Gene 1 of the coronaviruses ($\sim$20 000 nucleotides) and toroviruses encodes various proteins required for RNA replication and transcription. In both genera it comprises two overlapping ORFs, the second one, 1b, being translated by a frameshifting mechanism. This, and the subsequent processing of the gene polyproteins, have been reviewed (Lai and Cavanagh, 1997; de Vries *et al.*, 1997).

Transcription in both genera involves the production of a 3′ co-terminal nested set of mRNAs (Figure 10.3b). At the 5′ end of each coronavirus gene is a transcription-associated sequence (TAS; also known as a transcription regulatory sequence), whilst at the 5′ terminus of the genome is a leader sequence of up to approximately 98 nucleotides (at the 3′ end of which is also a TAS). The subgenomic mRNAs have a copy of the leader sequence fused at the TAS region. The sequence of the TAS varies amongst the coronaviruses. There is a central conserved core TAS of six, seven or

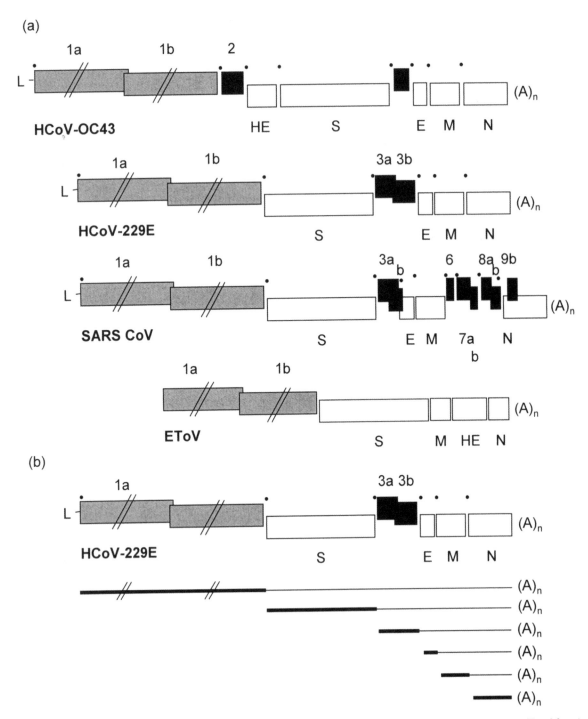

Figure 10.3 (a) Genome organisation of the HCoV-OC43 (group 2), HcoV-229E (group 1), *SARS coronavirus* (Frankfurt 1 strain; Thiel *et al.*, 2003) and equine torovirus. The replicase/polymerase-encoding gene 1, structural protein genes and the group-differentiating non-structural protein genes are shown by grey, white and black rectangles, respectively. (b) The 3′ co-terminal nested set arrangement of coronavirus mRNAs, illustrated for HCoV-229E. The thick black lines indicate the part of each mRNA that is translated. Filled black circles show the position of the core of the TAS sequences

eight nucleotides; ACGAAC, UCUCAAC and UCUAAAC in *SARS coronavirus*, HCoV-229E and HCoV-OC43, respectively (Herold *et al.*, 1993; Thiel *et al.*, 2003). An undetermined number of different nucleotides on both sides of each core TAS affect transcription. It is generally believed that the TASs function as terminators of the progression of the RNA polymerase during synthesis of negative-sense RNA from the positive-sense genome RNA (Sawicki and Sawicki, 1990, 1998). The nascent subgenomic negative-sense RNAs are then 'finished' by acquisition of an anti-sense leader transcribed from the 5′ end of the genomic RNA, by a discontinuous transcription process. The resultant negative-sense mRNAs are believed to be copied to produce the positive-sense RNAs (Sawicki and Sawicki, 1998). According to this model, the replicase pauses at a TAS; it might terminate transcription immediately, to generate an mRNA, or continue to the next TAS, and so on.

Toroviruses have TAS-like sequences (UCUUUAGA in EqTV) at the 5′ end of the M, HE and N genes but, unlike coronaviruses, the mRNAs corresponding to these genes do not have a leader sequence fused at their 5′ end (van Vliet *et al.*, 2002). However, the S gene, which does not have an obvious TAS sequence, does have an mRNA with a leader sequence, albeit a short one (18 nucleotides) from the 5′ end of the genome (van Vliet *et al.*, 2002).

Sequence of HCoV and Torovirus Proteins

Several HCoV genes have been cloned and sequenced. The heavily glycosylated S glycoproteins of HCoV-229E, *SARS coronavirus* and HCoV-OC43 comprise 1173, 1255 and 1353 amino acids, respectively (Raabe *et al.*, 1990; Mounir and Talbot, 1993; Marra *et al.*, 2003; Rota *et al.*, 2003). Whereas the S proteins of some coronaviruses, e.g. infectious bronchitis virus (IBV), are efficiently cleaved into two subunits, S1 and S2 (S2 being a little longer than S1), the S of HCoV-229E grown in human embryonic lung cells is not cleaved. In accordance with this, sequencing shows that the HCoV-229E S protein (and that of *SARS coronavirus*) lacks a highly basic sequence such as occurs in IBV at the S1–S2 cleavage site. Most of the S of HCoV-OC43 grown in a human rectal tumour cell line is not cleaved but addition of trypsin cleaves S into S1 and S2. This indicates that the extent to which the S of HCoV-OC43 is cleaved in various cell types depends in part on the presence in the cells of proteases which cleave adjacent to a basic S1–S2 connecting peptide, a situation which also applies to MHV. S1 and S2 are not linked by disulphide bonds.

The S protein of EqTV comprises 1581 amino acids and, like S of HCoV strains, has a M_r of about 200 000

when glycosylated. It has a highly basic S1–S2 connecting peptide and occurs as two subunits in virions.

The M proteins of *SARS coronavirus*, HCoV-229E, OC-43 and EqTV torovirus comprise 221, 225, 230 and 233 amino acids, respectively, of which probably only 10%, associated with one N-linked oligosaccharide in the case of HCoV-229E (*SARS coronavirus* has one potential N-linked glycosylation site) and potentially several O-linked oligosaccharides for HCoV-OC43, protrudes at the virion surface.

The N proteins also vary in size; 229E (389 amino acids), *SARS coronavirus* (422) and OC43 (448 residues). The N protein of 229E is very similar in size to that of TGEV (both are group 1 coronaviruses), with 46% amino acid identity within the first third of the protein, while that of OC43 is identical in size to that of BCV (both are group 2 viruses) and shares 97.5% identity overall. The N protein of EqTV is much smaller than that of any coronavirus, comprising only 160 amino acids.

The degree of amino acid identity between the S, E, M and N proteins of *SARS coronavirus* and those of the other coronaviruses are in the ranges 21–24%, 18–23%, 27–40% and 23–33%, respectively (Rota *et al.*, 2003).

Strain OC43, in common with other coronaviruses in group 2 (Table 10.1), has an HE glycoprotein that has 95% amino acid identity with the HE of BCV strain G95. Remarkably, the coronavirus and torovirus HE proteins have 30% sequence identity with the haemagglutinin–esterase fusion (HEF) protein of influenza C virus. Two functions have been assigned to coronavirus HE protein, receptor-binding and receptor-destroying (see below). Nevertheless, the HE proteins of coronaviruses and toroviruses are not essential for replication *in vitro*. The human toroviruses of Duckmanton *et al.* (1997) agglutinated rabbit and human erythrocytes. Coronavirus 229E lacks HE, in common with other group 1 members, group 3 viruses and *SARS coronavirus* (Table 10.1). The structural proteins are reviewed in detail in several chapters in Siddell (1995).

Antigenic Structure

Virus-neutralising (VN) antibodies and haemagglutination-inhibiting antibodies are induced by both the S and HE proteins of coronaviruses and toroviruses and some antibodies against the coronavirus M protein neutralise virus in the presence of complement.

Epitope mapping of coronaviruses has been done mostly for S and has shown that VN epitopes are formed largely by the amino-terminal S1 half of the protein, which correlates with the much greater amino acid sequence variation in S1 than in S2 (Siddell, 1995). Removal of glycans from S of IBV greatly diminished the binding of VN monoclonal antibodies. The structural proteins of HCoV-229E, -OC43 and *SARS coronavirus* are not related antigenically (indeed, HCoV-229E is not antigenically related to other members of group 1). An early report that *SARS coronavirus* was antigenically related to members of group 1 should be viewed with caution (Ksiazek *et al.*, 2003).

The S protein has been shown to be a major inducer of protective immunity although the other structural proteins, particularly the nucleocapsid protein, contribute. In the case of feline infectious peritonitis virus (FIPV) it is the immune response to S that exacerbates the disease. It is thought that FIPV attached to anti-S antibody remains infectious and is more readily taken up by macrophages (antibody-dependent enhancement), in which FIPV replicates, than is virus without antibody (de Groot and Horzinek, 1995).

Immune electron microscopy has revealed relationships between the toroviruses of humans, equines and bovines (Beards *et al.*, 1984; Duckmanton *et al.*, 1997). Much remains to be done to establish the extent of variation among human toroviruses.

Growth *In Vitro*

Previously, OC43 and serologically related strains of HCoV were considerably more difficult to propagate in cell culture than 229E-related strains and so organ cultures were used for OC43, hence the letters 'OC'. Now, however, cell lines are available for the propagation of both of the *laboratory-adapted* HCoV types, although primary isolation remains difficult. Cultures of fetal and adult astrocytes were infected by both types of HCoV but infectious virus was only released from the fetal cells (Bonavia *et al.*, 1997). *SARS coronavirus* has been isolated using fetal rhesus kidney cells and Vero E6 cells, although the latter rapidly became the cell of choice for virus isolation and subsequent characterisation (Ksiazek *et al.*, 2003; Peiris *et al.*, 2003). Human *torovirus* has not been grown *in vitro*.

INITIATION OF INFECTION

Cell Attachment Proteins

The S protein serves to attach the virus to cells. The extent to which the HE protein, when present, is also responsible for cell attachment is not clear. The HE proteins, in contrast to the S proteins, of both

coronaviruses and toroviruses are not required for replication *in vitro* (Popova and Zhang, 2002). Experiments using soluble truncated histidine-tagged S proteins, produced using baculovirus expression vectors, showed that the region of the HCoV-229E S protein from amino acids 417–547 was required for binding to its cell receptor (Bonavia *et al.*, 2003). That the S protein is a determinant of host cell range has been elegantly demonstrated using recombinant coronaviruses expressing heterologous S proteins. For example, MHV expressing the FCoV S protein was able to successfully infect and replicate in feline cells, previously refractory to MHV infection (Kuo *et al.*, 2000). It is the S1 part of S that determines receptor specificity (Tsai *et al.*, 2003). Experiments with recombinant MHVs showed that the extent of replication of the virus and the degree of hepatitis in the liver was determined largely by the S protein (Navas *et al.*, 2001). Gallagher and Buchmeier (2001) have reviewed virus entry and pathogenesis for MHV.

Cell Receptors for Coronaviruses

The attachment of a virus to host cells is a crucial early step in infection and specificity of attachment can be a major factor in determining host cell range and hence pathogenesis. This has been elegantly demonstrated by the transfer of coronavirus receptors from susceptible cells to other cells, rendering the latter susceptible to infection. This topic has been reviewed in Siddell (1995) and Lai and Cavanagh (1997).

Human aminopeptidase N (APN) has been identified as a receptor for HCoV-229E (Tresnan *et al.*, 1996). This protein is a metalloprotease located on the surface of epithelial cells, including those of the intestine, lung and kidney. Human cells that were not susceptible to canine coronavirus (CCoV) or FCoV became susceptible when transfected with a human/canine chimaera of APN (Benbacer *et al.*, 1997). The critical carboxy-terminal domain was formed by amino acids 643–841 of the canine APN. When amino acids 255–348 of porcine APN were replaced by amino acids 260–353 of human APN, the resulting chimaeric protein was able to function as a receptor for HCoV-229E (Kolb *et al.*, 1996). Thus, different parts of APN molecules may function as receptors for different coronaviruses within viruses of group 1. Expression of feline APN in rodent cells rendered the cells susceptible not only to FCV but also to HCoV-229E, CCV and TGEV (Tresnan *et al.*, 1996). Previous work had shown, however, that human APN would bind HCoV-229E but not TGEV, whilst porcine APN would bind TGEV but not HCoV.

The metalloprotease angiotensin-converting enzyme 2, on Vero cells, has been shown to act as a receptor for SARS CoV (Li *et al.*, 2003). It remains to be demonstrated, not only for SARS CoV but also for the other coronaviruses, which molecules act as receptors for coronaviruses in host animals.

The cellular receptor for MHV (a group 2 coronavirus, like HCV-OC43) is a member of the carcinoembryonic antigen (CEA) family of glycoproteins in the immunoglobulin superfamily (reviewed by Lai and Cavanagh, 1997). This CEA protein, previously of several names but now named CEACAM 1, is a 424 amino acid glycoprotein with four immunoglobulin-like domains (see Lewicki and Gallagher, 2002). A soluble form of this protein has been crystallised and an atomic structure deduced (Tan *et al.*, 2002).

Chen *et al.* (1997) transfected COS-7 cells, which lack a functional receptor for MHV, with genes of human CEACAM and human biliary glycoprotein; the cells were then susceptible to MHV. Experiments with chimaeras of human and murine CEACAM proteins revealed that the immunoglobulin loop of human CEACAM conferred virus-binding specificity. Different isoforms of murine CEACAMs exist. These have extensive differences in the amino-terminal immunoglobulin-like domain to which MHV binds and bind MHV to different extents. Analysis of chimaeras indicated that amino acids 38–43 were key elements for binding MHV and virus-induced membrane fusion (Rao *et al.*, 1997). Interestingly, when MHV had established a persistent infection in murine 17 Cl 1 cells, which express very low levels of the CEACAM 1 receptor, there was selection of mutant MHVs that were better able to use other molecules as receptors (Schickli *et al.*, 1997).

Much less work has been done on receptors for HCoV-OC43.

Involvement of Glycans on Receptors

Both the S and HE proteins of BCoV bind to cell surface components, a vital component of which is the glycan component N-acetyl-9-*O*-acetylneuraminic acid (Neu5,9Ac$_2$). This residue acts as a receptor not only on erythrocytes but also on susceptible cell cultures (Schultze and Herrler, 1992). The S protein binds more efficiently than HE to Neu5,9Ac$_2$ and it has been proposed that the BCV S protein is responsible for the primary attachment to cells.

Attachment of coronaviruses might be a two-step process. Primary attachment might be mediated by a first receptor, e.g. Neu5,9Ac$_2$, for some coronaviruses, a second receptor, e.g. APN or CEACAM proteins, bringing the virus and cell membranes closer together for subsequent membrane fusion. Some receptors might fulfil both functions for some coronaviruses.

The role played by the HE protein, where present, e.g. in HCoV-OC43, is not clear. Although it can mediate binding to erythrocytes, the main function of HE might be to remove neuraminic acid from the virus and cell surface. The esterase activity of the HE, and HEF protein of influenza C, specifically cleaves Neu5,9Ac$_2$.

The Cell Attachment and Fusion Processes

Lewicki and Gallagher (2002) have indicated that soluble S1 fragments of MHV were dimers and that CEACAM binding was entirely dependent on this quaternary structure. Unexpectedly, only a single CEACAM bound to an S1 dimer. This binding induced separation of S1 from S2, and altered the conformation of S1, generating alternative disulphide linkages within S1. The fusion-inducing domain of S is formed by S2 (see Luo *et al.*, 1999). Lewicki and Gallagher (2002) have proposed two models for the attachment and subsequent fusion process.

CLINICAL FEATURES

Although generally associated with the common cold, HCoVs have also been investigated in recent years in the context of asthma exacerbations and hospitalised patients with severe respiratory illness. Unlike these viruses, which are rarely associated with lower respiratory tract disease, *SARS coronavirus* is associated with pneumonia and diarrhoea. A higher incidence of HCoV RNA in the brains of MS patients compared with controls has been reported in some, although not all, studies. Human toroviruses are associated with gastroenteritis.

Upper Respiratory Tract Disease and Otitis Media

Most information on the clinical features of HCoV infections in man has been obtained from volunteers experimentally infected with HCoVs. HCoVs generally cause mild upper respiratory tract infections in man and are believed to be second only to rhinoviruses with respect to the percentage (approximately 25%; Makela *et al.*, 1998) of colds that they cause.

The incubation period of HCoV infections is relatively short, with a range of 2–5 days. Illness—nasal discharge, mild sore throat, sneezing, general malaise, perhaps with headache—then lasts for an average of 6–7 days, sometimes lasting for 18 days. Fever and coughing may be exhibited in 10% and 20% of cases, respectively. No difference is observed between 229E and OC43 strains in the pathology of infection. Generally, symptoms are indistinguishable from those of colds caused by rhinoviruses. Virus excretion reaches a detectable level at the time symptoms begin and lasts for 1–4 days. Subclinical or very mild infections are common and can occur throughout the year.

In a study of children with otitis media with effusion, HCoVs were associated with 10% of them, respiratory syncytial virus being associated in approximately 30% of cases (Pitkranta et al., 1998).

Lower Respiratory Tract Disease and Asthma

There have been some reports indicating a more serious lower tract involvement of HCoVs in young children and old people. It is not clear that HCoVs infect the lower respiratory tract but the occurrence of HCoV upper respiratory tract infections coupled with other factors may cause more serious disease. Up to 30% of acute wheezing episodes in asthmatic children may be due to coronavirus infection. Mckean et al. (2001) have established an experimental model for viral wheeze, involving volunteers (some atopic, others not) with and without a history of viral wheeze. Over half developed colds after inoculation with HCoV-229E. The viral wheezers reported more upper respiratory tract symptoms than controls. Over half of the wheezers, but none of the controls, reported lower respiratory tract symptoms (wheeze, chest tightness and shortness of breath).

A study in a neonatal intensive care unit revealed that all premature infants infected with coronaviruses had symptoms of bradycardia, apnoea, hypoxaemia, fever or abdominal distention. Chest X-ray revealed diffuse infiltrates in two cases. In a study of nosocomial viral respiratory infections (NVRI) in neonates (up to 1 month of age) who had been hospitalised, it was concluded that the incidence of NVRI with common respiratory viruses was low, HCoV being the most important pathogen in NVRI in the study (Gagneur et al., 2002). Elderly patients who had been hospitalised because of cardiopulmonary illnesses, and who tested negative for influenza and respiratory syncytial viruses, were examined further. Approximately 8% were

identified as having either HCoV-229E or -OC43 (Falsey et al., 2002).

Infections with respiratory viruses, of which HCoVs are but one, are commonly associated with asthma exacerbation. Coronavirus was detected in approximately 5% of children (Freymuth et al., 1999) and 22% of adults hospitalised because of asthma (Atmar et al., 1998). Allergic patients with a common cold, associated with a number of viruses including HCoVs (25%), had prolonged nasal eosinophil influx (van Benten et al., 2001). Whether that would increase the risk of subsequent allergen-induced hypersensitivity reactions is not known.

The clinical signs and other changes associated with SARS coronavirus infection were described in several of the early reports on this disease (Poutanen et al., 2003; Tsang et al., 2003; Chan-Yeung and Yu, 2003; Peiris et al., 2003; Lee et al., 2003). The incubation period was 3–5 days but could be up to 10 days. Case definitions published by the WHO very soon after the first reports of SARS to that body were subsequently revised and may be revised again (http://www.who.int/csr/sars/casedefinitions). The definition, current in June 2003, of a suspect case included high fever ($>38°C$) and cough or breathing difficulty and potential epidemiological links, e.g. contact with a SARS case or travel to a SARS area (however, it is believed that not all SARS cases had a temperature of $>38°C$). A probable case was defined as a suspect case with radiographic evidence of infiltrates consistent with pneumonia or respiratory distress syndrome on chest X-ray. Alternatively, a suspect case that was positive for SARS coronavirus by one or more assays would also be considered as a probable case. This allows for cases in which, although there is infection by SARS, there may be less serious clinical signs.

Other manifestations of SARS include dyspnoea, malaise, headache and hypoxaemia. Virus was observed in the villi of gut cells by electron microscopy. In Hong Kong 38% of SARS patients referred to the Prince of Wales hospital had diarrhoea, often severe, whilst 73% of patients from the Amoy Gardens apartment blocks, Hong Kong, had diarrhoea (Sung, 2003). A higher proportion of those with diarrhoea required respiratory support, including intensive care.

Early radiographic changes were indistinguishable from those associated with other causes of broncho-pneumonia. Conventional and high-resolution CT images of the thorax were useful for diagnosing SARS. Frequently observed were ill-defined, ground-glass opacification in the periphery of the affected lung parenchyma, usually in a subpleural location. In patients with clinical deterioration there was progression of pulmonary infiltrates 7–10 days after admission. There was diffuse alveolar damage, hyaline membrane formation and minimal mononuclear cell infiltration. These changes, combined with no evidence for a substantial presence of the virus in the lung, led to the suggestion that part of the lung damage was due to cytokines induced by the virus (Chan-Yeung, 2003). This remains a hypothesis; nevertheless, it was the basis for therapeutic action (described below).

Epidemiology

Generally HCoV epidemics occur during the winter and early spring but the peak period may vary by several months. However, other periods of high infection rates have been observed and it appears that major peaks may occur at any time of the year. All age groups are infected with HCoVs and infection rates have been shown to be relatively uniform. This is different from the situation with some other respiratory viruses, such as respiratory syncytial virus, where there is a distinct decrease in infection rates with increase in age. Reinfection of individuals with the same HCoV serotype often occurs within 4 months of the first infection, suggesting that homologous HCoV antibodies are protective for about 4 months. In addition, there are indications that antibodies to one HCoV group may not be protective against infection with viruses from the other HCoV group; cross-protection would not be expected, as the 229E and OC43 virus proteins have very different amino acid sequences.

SARS coronavirus is most likely to have been transmitted to humans from an animal reservoir in Guangdong Province, People's Republic of China, where the first known human cases occurred in November 2002. Several species of wild animals, for sale in live animal markets, were tested for the presence of the virus. Six of six Himalayan civet palm cats (*Paguma larvata*; not related to the domestic cat) and one of one racoon dog (*Nyctereutes procyonoides*; distantly related to the domestic dog) were found to be positive for *SARS coronavirus*, either by RT–PCR, virus isolation in Vero E6 cells, or both, and had antibodies detectable by a virus neutralisation test (Guan *et al.*, 2003). The incidence of SARS virus antibodies in the animal handlers was much greater than in the surrounding community in Guanzhi, Guangdong Province. However, the gene sequences of the animal and human viruses were not identical. They had 99.7% nucleotide identity over the whole genome, and 99% nucleotide identity in the spike protein gene (Guan *et al.*, 2003). Whilst this is a very

high degree of identity, 99% has been observed between group 2 coronaviruses isolated from cattle and humans. Thus, it cannot be concluded that the epidemic in Guangdong Province was started by transmission from either the civet cats or racoon dogs in which the virus was detected, although that is possible. It is also possible that there is one or more other species that are a reservoir for the virus. It has not been excluded that the virus might have been present in an isolated human community prior to November 2002.

Much of the following account was obtained at WHO meetings in Kuala Lumpur and Singapore in June 2003. Detailed epidemiological investigations suggested that close contact (distances of <1 metre) were required for transmission amongst people, with aerosols being an unlikely component. Most cases could be traced back to close contact with earlier cases. Health care workers (HCWs), especially those associated with hospitals, were the hardest-hit group of people. Thus, 53% and 58% of the SARS cases in Vietnam and Hong Kong, respectively, were HCWs. Indeed, hospitals were the major place for transmission in some countries, being described as 'major disease amplifiers'.

Fomites were not excluded as agents of transmission but there was not much evidence of a prolonged risk. Faecal contamination has not been eliminated as a possible route of transmission; indeed, in the outbreak at the Amoy Gardens residences, Hong Kong, there was a breakdown of the sewage system. An environmental study indicated that there was a single index case within the apartments. Faeces released into a common sewage vent went into the apartments via the toilets, and spread thereafter, aided by extractor fans. Over 300 cases were traced back to the Amoy Gardens index case.

Survival of the virus in the environment depends, as would be expected, on various parameters. Virus in cell culture fluid remained infectious for 0.5–3 days, depending on the surface, whilst virus experimentally added to faeces was infectious for 1–4 days. Faeces released from patients were still positive for the virus in almost all cases 2 weeks after infection, about twice the rate of detection in respiratory material, e.g. sputum.

The mortality rate during the March–June epidemic, worldwide, was not evenly distributed amongst age groups: <1% of <24 year-olds; 6% of 25–44 year-olds; 15% of 45–64 year-olds; and >50% of >64 year-olds. The reasons are not clear, although a high number of unrelated illnesses in the oldest age group were likely contributing factors.

The term 'super-spreader' was coined to describe those patients who were recognised as having transmitted the disease to large numbers of people, e.g. five patients accounted for spread to 103 of 205 probable SARS cases in Singapore. However, there was no evidence that these five people were more infectious than the majority. Rather it might have been that various circumstances (super-spreader events, SSEs) contributed to the high rate of successful transmission.

Lipsitch *et al.* (2003) and Riley *et al.* (2003) analysed the transmission of SARS during the first 2 months after its spread beyond China. Both teams estimated that during the early weeks of the epidemic, excluding SSEs, a single infectious case of SARS infected approximately three secondary cases, transmissions in hospitals contributing greatly to this figure. Control of nosocomial transmission was crucial. The transmission rate declined as control measures were instigated. In addition to good practice in hospitals and basic public hygiene, these included isolation of SARS cases and quarantine of their asymptomatic contacts. SARS virus was considered to be moderately transmissible, capable of causing a very large epidemic. However, this was not inevitable if isolation, tracing and quarantine of contacts and travel restrictions were put in place (Dye and Gay, 2003).

There was concern that there might have been asymptomatic virus shedders during the epidemic; some people were antibody- and RT–PCR-positive but had no clinical signs. Also, it was conceivable that some recovered patients might have been persistently infected, with the possibility of renewed shedding of virus months later. Persistent infections have been reported for IBV in experimentally infected chickens (Jones and Ambali, 1987) and in cats naturally infected with feline coronavirus, 13% of 151, of which became asymptomatic chronic shedders of the initial virus (Addie and Jarrett, 2001; Addie *et al.*, 2003).

As of mid-June 2003 there had been 8460 cases of SARS worldwide, 808 of them fatal. Asia accounted for 95% of cases (84% in People's Republic of China), with 3.8% in North America (mostly associated with Canada). All cases beyond China were spread by travellers from that region, and their subsequent contacts. The 2003 epidemic was declared over by early July of the same year. The global population was susceptible at the start of the epidemic and essentially remained so.

Host Range of Coronaviruses

It should not have come as a surprise that viruses with >99% nucleotide identity with *SARS coronavirus* from humans were identified in animals (Himalayan palm civet cats and racoon dogs) during the SARS epidemic in China. Although coronaviruses have been

described as being fastidious with regard to their hosts, this is true *in vitro* but not *in vivo*. Thus, it has been very difficult to obtain cell cultures to grow some coronaviruses, e.g. HCoV-OC43 strains, and turkey coronavirus. However, the host range of coronaviruses is greater *in vivo*. Some HCoV isolates, of the OC43 genotype, have >99% amino acid identity in their S and HE proteins with the corresponding proteins of BCoV (Zhang *et al.*, 1994). A recently discovered respiratory canine coronavirus is a group 2 coronavirus (Erles *et al.*, 2003), the S protein of which had 96% and 95% amino acid identity with that of BCoV and HCoV-OC43, respectively. Cross-infection by these viruses has not been studied but a broad host range for them is a possibility. Turkeys are naturally infected with a coronavirus that is genetically very similar to IBV, a group 3 coronavirus (Cavanagh *et al.*, 2002). Notwithstanding, turkeys have been successfully infected with BCoV, leading to diarrhoea (Ismail *et al.*, 2001).

Group 1 coronaviruses include TGEV, FCoV and enteric CCoV. CCoV experimentally applied orally to pigs replicated in them, inducing antibodies although not causing disease (Woods and Wesley, 1992). When hysterotomy-derived pigs were infected orally by these three viruses, virulent FCoV type I caused villous atrophy in the jejunum and ileum, resulting in clinical signs typical of a virulent TGEV infection and death of 3/12 pigs (Woods *et al.*, 1981). Cell culture-adapted FCoV and virulent CCoV produced less severe lesions and no mortality. Replication of these coronaviruses was confirmed by immunofluorescence. FCoV type II is a recombinant of FCoV type I and enteric canine coronavirus (Herrewegh *et al.*, 1998).

Within 2 months of the emergence of SARS in Hong Kong, Fouchier and colleagues (2003) had demonstrated that *SARS coronavirus* replicated and caused SARS-like disease in cynomolgus macaques (*Macaca fascicularis*). This fulfilled Koch's postulates, as modified by Rivers for viral diseases, for *SARS coronavirus*. Subsequently these same researchers demonstrated that ferrets (*Mustela furo*) and domestic cats (*Felis domesticus*) were susceptible to, and transmitted, SARS CoV (Martina *et al.*, 2003). Virus was detected in the respiratory, gastrointestinal and urinary tracts of both species.

Coronaviruses Associated with the Human Enteric Tract

Before the appearance of SARS there were reports describing coronavirus-like viruses isolated from faecal specimens from humans (Duckmanton *et al.*, 1997).

Some of these viruses were isolated from infants with necrotising enterocolitis, patients with non-bacterial gastroenteritis and from homosexual men with diarrhoea who were symptomatic and seropositive for human immunodeficiency virus. Some isolates were shown to be serologically related to OC43. The discovery that a protein found in enterocytes functions as a receptor for HCoV-229E strengthens the likelihood that coronaviruses might replicate in the human alimentary tract.

Toroviruses Associated with the Human Enteric Tract

Evidence has increased that toroviruses are associated with gastroenteritis in humans. In a case–control study of children, an antigen capture ELISA revealed torovirus in stools from 27% (9/33) of children with acute diarrhoea, 27% (11/41) with persistent diarrhoea and none in controls (Koopmans et al., 1997). Enteraggregative Escherichia coli was commonly found in assocation with the torovirus. In another childhood study, electron microscopy revealed a torovirus incidence of 35% (72/206) and 15% in gastroenteritis cases and controls, respectively (Jamieson et al., 1998). Those infected with torovirus were more frequently immunocompromised (43% vs. 16%) and nosocomially infected (58% vs. 31%), experienced less vomiting (47% vs. 68%) and had more bloody diarrhoea (11% vs. 2%).

Coronaviruses in the Central Nervous System

Multiple sclerosis is a chronic disease of the central nervous system (CNS) involving multifocal regions of inflammation and myelin destruction. A number of environmental factors have been proposed for triggering MS, foremost among them being infectious agents. A number of enveloped and non-enveloped, RNA and DNA viruses have been associated with demyelination in humans and rodents, including coronaviruses (Stohlman and Hinton, 2001) Not only has coronavirus RNA been detected in the brains of humans but also many human neural cell lines have been shown to support the replication of both OC43 and 229E types of HCoV. Murine hepatitis virus infection in mice and rats has long been a model for coronavirus-induced demyelination, although the exact mechanism(s) by which MHV induces demyelination and the role of the immune system in the pathology is not known (Matthews et al., 2002). Several inflammatory mol-

ecules, e.g. interleukin-1β, tumour necrosis factor and IL-6, have been detected during MHV-induced chronic demyelination. Another possibility is that MHV infection induces an immune response that cross-reacts with myelin proteins. Peripheral cross-reactive T cell clones recognising both HCoV and a myelin antigen have been detected in MS patients. Arbour et al. (2000) hypothesised that HCoV RNA might sometimes lead to a low level of viral protein synthesis that could be involved in the stimulation of immune responses within the CNS, exacerbating the effect of coronaviral infection in MS patients.

Stewart et al. (1992) analysed RNA from brain tissue of MS patients using PCRs specific for the nucleocapsid (N) protein gene of HCoVs OC43 and 229E. RNA of the latter type was detected in 4/11 MS patients and in none of six neurological and five normal controls. No OC43 RNA was detected. In a more recent study combining RT-PCR and Southern hybridisation, brains of 90 people with various neurological diseases were analysed (Arbour et al., 2000). The 229E type of HCoV was detected in 51% of MS donors but this was not significantly different from the incidence in normal donors (44%). In contrast, OC43 was detected in 36% of MS donors, which was significantly different from normal donors (20%). RNA of OC43 was demonstrated in an MS brain by in situ hybridisation, and the N protein mRNA of OC43 was detected by Northern blotting in two cases. In contrast, Dessau et al. (2001), using RT-PCR, did not detect either OC43 or 229E RNA in the brains of 25 MS patients or 36 controls. However, a number of studies have now revealed the persistence of coronavirus RNA in human brains.

Experiments have shown that both OC43 and 229E can establish acute infections in many human neural cell lines; astrocytoma, neuroblastoma, neuroglioma, oligodendrocyte and microglial cell lines (Arbour et al., 1999). Persistent infections were established in some of the lines.

DIAGNOSIS

Diagnosis of HCoV and HTV infections is not routinely done in most diagnostic virus laboratories. In part this is because HCoV and HTV infections are largely of minor clinical significance. In addition they are difficult to grow in the laboratory. However, the increased application of polymerase chain reaction (PCR) technology in medical diagnostic laboratories has made it easier to detect HCoVs, and may prove to do so for HTVs. Nucleic acid technology played a major role in the identification of the aetiological agent of SARS and subsequent diagnosis. Electron microscopy revealed the presence of a coronavirus-like virus in early cases. Further support for a coronavirus being the aetiological agent was obtained by DeRisi and colleagues, using a recently developed microarray for viruses (Wang *et al.*, 2002). Subsequently RT-PCRs were performed on material from patients, using oligonucleotides designed after comparison of the ORF1b part of gene one, the most conserved part of the genome amongst coronaviruses of groups 1, 2 and 3 (Stephensen *et al.*, 1999). Oligonucleotides for the RT-PCR could be designed, synthesised and put into operation for diagnosis within a couple of days of a coronaviral aetiology being suspected. Maximum excretion of SARS coronavirus was not reached until approximately 10 days after infection, and virus-specific IgG was not detected until this time (Drosten *et al.*, 2003). In SARS cases confirmed by clinical and epidemiological criteria in Hong Kong, 92% and 63% were positive by immunofluorescence and RT-PCR, respectively (Peiris, 2003). An imperative identified by the WHO in mid-2003 was the development of diagnostic tests with greater sensitivity, to enable detection within the first few days. Rapid diagnosis was crucial to implementation of the measures described above (see Epidemiology) for the interruption of the transmission of SARS in early to mid-2003.

Virus Isolation

Isolation of respiratory HCoVs can be done from nasal and throat swabs, and nasopharyngeal aspirates taken from infected individuals.

229E and related strains can be isolated in roller culture monolayers of human embryonic lung fibroblasts, such as W138 and MRC5 cells. In virus-positive cultures, a gradual cytopathic effect consisting of small, granular, round cells appears throughout the monolayers, although especially around the periphery of the monolayers. However, cell sheets are rarely destroyed completely on initial isolation. Other cell types that have been used are described by Myint in Siddell (1995).

Vero E6 cells rapidly became the cells of choice for the isolation of *SARS coronavirus* (Drosten *et al.*, 2003; Ksiazek *et al.*, 2003), although fetal rhesus kidney cells were also used successfully (Peiris *et al.*, 2003). A few syncytia were observed. Interestingly, Thiel *et al.* (2003) discovered that within three passages in Vero cells of the Frankfurt strain, a variant emerged with a 45 nucleotide deletion in gene 7. An early

comparison of the complete genomes of 14 *SARS coronavirus* isolates revealed 129 sequence variations. Most of these might have occurred during replication in Vero cells (Ruan *et al.*, 2003). Sixteen changes were considered to have happened during the spread of the virus in humans. Two-thirds of these differences were within gene 1; the latter accounts for two-thirds of the size of the genome.

OC43-related strains usually cannot be grown in cell cultures, at least on initial isolation, and for these strains isolation has been performed in organ cultures of human embryonic tissues. Small pieces of tracheal or nasal epithelium, with the ciliated surface uppermost, are inoculated with the respiratory specimens and the culture examined for ciliary activity daily for up to 2 weeks.

HTVs have not been grown in culture.

Electron Microscopy

Electron microscopy has been used to detect HCoVs, e.g. in epithelial cells shed from the nasopharynx of patients, and after attempted isolation in cell culture (229E strains) and organ culture (OC43 type), including immune electron microscopy using convalescent sera from patients. Electron microscopy contributed to the early identification of the aetiological agent of SARS as being a coronavirus, including demonstration with bronchoalveolar lavage fluid (Ksiazek *et al.*, 2003) and lung biopsy samples (Peiris *et al.*, 2003).

Enteric HCoVs and HTVs have also been sought in faeces using electron and immune electron microscopy (Duckmanton *et al.*, 1997; Jamieson *et al.*, 1998). The two types of virus are of similar size. HTVs are pleiomorphic, sometimes exhibiting a torus (doughnut) appearance and an irregular rod shape. The spikes of coronaviruses, and possibly of toroviruses, are not always clearly revealed by negative staining and can resemble toroviruses morphologically. Thus the two viruses can be confused if only electron microscopy is used; corroborative evidence is required (Cornelissen *et al.*, 1998).

Serological Analysis

Antigen-capture ELISAs have been used to detect HCoV antigens in nasal and throat swabs and nasopharyngeal aspirates and to detect HTVs in stools (Koopmans *et al.*, 1997). Immunofluorescence tests, using patients' sera with *SARS coronavirus*-infected Vero E6 cells, confirmed the presence in 92% of cases in Hong Kong, whereas only 63% of them were confirmed by RT-PCR.

Jamieson *et al.* (1998) purified HTV from the stool of a patient (Duckmanton *et al.*, 1997) and used this in an haemagglutination-inhibition assay to detect antibodies to HTV in nosocomial cases of gastroenteritis; acute and convalescent sera were examined, revealing rises in antibody titres. Duckmanton *et al.* (1999, 2001) dotted HTV proteins from patients onto nitrocellulose and probed them with antisera against BTV. The bovine serum cross-reacted with the human TVs, showing that BTV antisera could be used for human diagnostic purposes. Human convalescent HTV serum reacted with the HE protein of BTV in Western blots.

RT-PCR

Fundamental studies of the RNA genomes of HCoVs 229E and OC43 have provided the gene sequence data necessary for the application of reverse transcriptase (RT) PCR technology to the detection of these viruses. Many studies have used this technology in recent years to assess the incidence of these viruses in respiratory infections, often in conjunction with PCRs for other respiratory viruses (Freymuth *et al.*, 1999; Macek *et al.*, 1999; Vabret *et al.*, 2001). It is possible that these studies might have underestimated the incidence of HCoVs, as the oligonucleotide primers used in the RT–PCRs are based on gene sequence data derived largely from one isolate, obtained many years ago, of each of the two HCoV species. Little is known of the sequence heterogeneity exhibited by HCoVs. It is possible that the oligonucleotide primers used to date will not function with some HCoVs. The respiratory coronavirus of chickens, IBV, exhibits extensive sequence and antigenic variation, with consequences for reinfection, prophylaxis and virus detection (Cavanagh and Naqi, 2003).

Stephensen *et al.* (1999) designed a 'consensus PCR assay for the genus *Coronavirus*' using pairs of degenerate oligonucleotides corresponding to regions of the 1b part of gene 1 (replicase gene). An RT-PCR with these oligonucleotides amplified HCoV 229E and OC43 and eight other coronaviruses from all three coronavirus groups. A similar approach was taken by Ksiazek *et al.* (2003) for the detection of *SARS coronavirus*, followed by the synthesis of *SARS coronavirus*-specific oligonucleotides corresponding to ORF1b sequences. Prior to the identification of the aetiological virus, Peiris *et al.* (2003) performed PCRs with RNA from uninfected and virus-infected fetal rhesus kidney cells with oligonucleotides in which the six 3′-most nucleotides were random. PCR products unique to the infected cells were cloned and sequenced. Drosten *et al.* (2003) actually used degenerate oligonucleotides designed to detect yellow fever virus and the polymerase gene of members of the family *Paramyxoviridae*, followed by reamplification, using the same primers without degeneracy, and sequencing. Three fragments encoded amino acid sequences with homology to coronavirus ORF 1b sequences.

The complete genomes of over a dozen SARS isolates have been sequenced and are accessible in the nucleotide sequence databanks (Ruan *et al.*, 2003).

The application of PCR technology for the detection of HTVs awaits gene sequence data.

MICROARRAY ANALYSIS

In October 2002 Wang *et al.* described a microarray for the detection of many genera and species of virus. Although this was principally for the detection and study of human viruses, the coronavirus element of the array included sequences (70-mer oligonucleotides) of several species of coronavirus. Probes were made by RT-PCR from clinical material of early SARS cases. Probing of the microarray provided some of the earliest evidence for the involvement of a coronavirus in SARS. There is no doubt that microarrays will increasingly feature prominently in the early stages of investigations of future epidemics where the aetiology is not certain and where more than one pathogen might be involved.

PROPHYLAXIS

There are no vaccines for the group 1 and 2 HCoVs, although vaccine development against *SARS coronavirus* was recommended by the WHO in 2003. Vaccines against coronaviruses of veterinary interest have had limited success. They have been developed against three group 1 coronaviruses, TGEV, FCoV and CCoV. Views differ as to their efficacy; they are not used universally. The primary purpose of the live TGEV vaccine is to induce high levels of antibody in sows, which is passed to neonates in colostrum, providing some protection during the greatest at-risk period. There are both live and killed vaccines against enteric CCoV, although the disease caused is of less concern than that caused by FCoV in cats. Although 80% of cats develop diarrhoea, from which they recover, up to 10% can develop infectious peritonitis (actually a vasculitis), which is invariably fatal (de Groot and Horzinek, 1995; Addie and Jarrett, 2001; Addie *et al.*, 2003). Although there is a temperature-sensitive vaccine, other vaccines against FCoV, whether live or killed, have actually exacerbated the disease; they have induced antibodies, especially when there has been a weak cell-mediated immune response, and have potentiated the uptake of the virus by macrophages, resulting in replication therein in addition to dissemination.

The most widely and successfully used coronavirus vaccines are those against IBV of chickens (Cavanagh and Naqi, 2003). Unfortunately, inactivated IB induces protection in only approximately 30% of birds (Cavanagh et al., 1986), so they are used after first priming chicks with live attenuated vaccine, after which the inactivated vaccine induces longer lasting protection.

Attenuation, currently by serial passage (50–120) in embryonated chicken eggs, is a trade-off between apathogenicity and efficacy. If chickens are to be vaccinated more than once, the first vaccination may be with a highly attenuated strain, to minimise vaccine reactions, whilst revaccination might be with a less attenuated strain. Live attenuated IB vaccines are applied by spray on the day of hatching. Experiments over many decades have demonstrated that they induce protection against the homologous virulent strain in virtually 100% of chicks, as measured by failure to recover the challenge virus or observation of an intact ciliated tracheal epithelium. Immunity is short-lived, the percentage of birds susceptible to challenge increasing from 2 months after vaccination. Chicks may be revaccinated, by spray or in drinking water, at 2–3 weeks of age in areas of high challenge. IBV exists as scores of serotypes, cross-immunity being generally poor. A second vaccination may, therefore, be with a vaccine of a serotype distinct from that of the initial vaccine, which sometimes induces better cross-protection against other serotypes than either vaccine alone.

Breeding stock and eating–egg layers not only get two or three live vaccinations but also inactivated, oil emulsion vaccine. This is not only to protect them against IBV infection, which would lead to loss of egg production, but also to raise a sustained serum antibody level, antibody being transmitted in the yolk sac to give some protection to the neonate chick.

Recently the IBV S1 spike protein subunit has been expressed from a fowl adenovirus vector. A single oral application induced 90–100% protection (Johnston et al., 2003).

THERAPY

Notwithstanding research in this area, drugs are not used for control of the 'common cold' caused by

HCoVs in coronavirus groups 1 and 2. The great seriousness of many cases of SARS led to the application of drugs. The nature of the lung damage in extreme cases, combined with the detection of only a little virus in the lung, led to the suggestion that some of the damage was caused by cytokines induced by the virus. Consequently, some patients were treated with corticosteroids (e.g. hydrocortisone, prednisolone). In addition, the antiviral agent ribavirin was applied orally or intravenously (Chan-Yeung and Yu, 2003; Lee et al., 2003; Poutanen et al., 2003; Tsang et al., 2003). These were not case-controlled studies, so it was not possible to determine to what extent, if any, the recovery of those who did not die was a consequence of the intervention with drugs. Experiments with an animal model might clarify this important issue. Ferrets (Mustela furo) and domestic cats (Felis domesticus) are susceptible to SARS CoV (Martina et al., 2003). Pulmonary lesions were induced, although these were milder than in macaques (Macaca fascicularis; Fouchier et al., 2003). Notwithstanding, the ferret and domestic cat have promise as models for SARS CoV infection and testing of therapeutics and prophylactics. During the 2003 epidemic over 300 000 compounds were tested for anti-SARS coronavirus activity and, notably, ribavirin had no activity in vitro.

ACKNOWLEDGEMENTS

The author acknowledges financial support from the Department of Food, Rural Affairs and the Environment, and the Biotechnology and Biological Sciences Research Council, UK.

REFERENCES

Addie DD and Jarrett O (2001) Use of a reverse-transcriptase polymerase chain reaction for monitoring the shedding of feline coronavirus by healthy cats. Vet Rec, 148, 649–653.

Addie DD, Schaap IAT, Nicolson O and Jarrett O (2003) Persistence and transmission of natural type 1 feline coronavirus infection. J Gen Virol, 84, 2735–2744.

Arbour N, Coté G, Lachance C et al. (1999) Acute and persistent infection of human neural cell lines by human coronavirus OC43. J Virol, 73, 3338–3350.

Arbour N, Day R, Newcombe J and Talbot PJ (2000) Neuroinvasion by human respiratory coronaviruses. J Virol, 74, 8913–8921.

Atmar RL, Guy E, Guntupalli KK et al. (1998) Respiratory tract viral infections in inner-city asthmatic adults. Arch Intern Med, 158, 2453–2459.

Beards GM, Hall C, Green J et al. (1984) An enveloped virus in stools of children and adults with gastroenteritis that resembles the Breda virus of calves. Lancet, 12, 1050–1052.

Benbacer L, Kut E, Besnardeau L *et al.* (1997) Interspecies aminopeptidase-N chimeras reveal species-specific receptor recognition by canine coronavirus, feline infectious peritonitis virus, and transmissible gastroenteritis virus. *J Virol*, **71**, 734–737.

Bonavia A, Arbour N, Yong VW and Talbot PJ (1997) Infection of primary cultures of human neural cells by human coronaviruses 229E and OC43. *J Virol*, **71**, 800–806.

Bonavia A, Zelus BD, Wentworth DE *et al.* (2003) Identification of a receptor-binding domain of the spike glycoprotein of human coronavirus HCoV-229E. *J Virol*, **77**, 2530–2538.

Breslin JJ, Mork I, Smith MK *et al.* (2003) Human coronavirus 229E: receptor binding domain and neutralization by soluble receptor at 37 degrees C. *J Virol*, **77**, 4435–4438.

Casais R, Thiel V, Siddell S *et al.* (2001) A reverse genetics system for the avian coronavirus infectious bronchitis virus. *J Virol*, **75**, 12359–12369.

Cavanagh D, Davis PJ, Darbyshire JH and Peters RW (1986) Coronavirus IBV: virus retaining spike glycopolypeptide S2 but not S1 is unable to induce virus-neutralising or haemagglutination-inhibiting antibody, or induce chicken tracheal protection. *J Gen Virol*, **67**, 1435–1442.

Cavanagh D, Mawditt K, Welchman D *et al.* (2002) Coronaviruses from pheasants (*Phasianus colchicus*) are genetically closely related to coronaviruses of domestic fowl (infectious bronchitis virus) and turkeys. *Avian Pathol*, **31**, 81–93.

Cavanagh D and Naqi S (2003) Infectious bronchitis. In *Diseases of Poultry*, 11th edn (eds Saif YM, Barnes HJ, Glisson JR, *et al.*), pp 101–119. Iowa State Press: Ames, IO.

Chan-Yeung M and Yu WC (2003) Outbreak of severe acute respiratory syndrome in Hong Kong Special Administrative Region: a case report. *Br Med J*, **326**, 850–852.

Chen DS, Asanaka M, Chen FS *et al.* (1997) Human carcinoembryonic antigen and biliary glycoprotein can serve as mouse hepatitis virus receptors. *J Virol*, **71**, 1688–1691.

Cornelissen LAHM, Wierda CMH, van der Meer FJ *et al.* (1997) Hemagglutinin-esterase, a novel structural protein of torovirus. *J Virol*, **71**, 5277–5286.

Cornelissen LAHM, van Woensel PAM, de Groot RJ *et al.* (1998) Cell culture-grown putative bovine respiratory torovirus identified as a coronavirus. *Vet Rec*, **142**, 683–686.

de Groot RJ and Horzinek MC (1995) Feline infectious peritonitis. In *The Coronaviridae* (ed. Siddell SG), pp 293–315. Plenum, New York.

de Haan CAM, Kuo L, Masters PS *et al.* (1998) Coronavirus particle assembly: primary structure requirements of the membrane protein. *J Virol*, **72**, 6838–6850.

de Haan CAM, Masters PS, Shen X-L *et al.* (2002a) The group-specific murine coronavirus genes are not essential, but their deletion, by reverse genetics, is attenuating in the natural host. *Virology*, **296**, 177–189.

de Haan CAM, Vennema H and Rottier PJ (2000) Assembly of the coronavirus envelope: homotypic interactions between the M proteins. *J Virol*, **74**, 4967–4978.

de Haan CAM, Volders H, Koetzner CA *et al.* (2002b) Coronaviruses maintain viability despite dramatic rearrangments of the strictly conserved genome organization. *J Virol*, **76**, 12491–12502.

de Vries AAF, Horzinek MC, Rottier PJM and de Groot RJ (1997) The genome organization of the *Nidovirales*: similarities and differences between arteri-, toro- and coronaviruses. *Semin Virol*, **8**, 33–47.

Dessau RB, Lisby G and Frederiksen JL (2001) Coronaviruses in brain tissue from patients with multiple sclerosis. *Acta Neuropathol*, **101**, 601–604.

Drosten C, Gunther S, Preiser W *et al.* (2003) Identification of a novel coronavirus in patients with severe acute respiratory syndrome. *N Engl J Med*, **348**, 1967–1976.

Duckmanton L, Luan B, Devenish J *et al.* (1997) Characterization of torovirus from human faecal specimens. *Virology*, **239**, 158–168.

Duckmanton L, Tellier R, Richardson C and Petric M (1999) The novel hemagglutinin-esterase genes of human torovirus and Breda virus. *Virus Res*, **64**, 137–149.

Duckmanton L, Tellier R, Richardson C and Petric M (2001) Notice of retraction to 'The novel hemagglutinin-esterase genes of human torovirus and Breda virus' [*Virus Res*, **64**, 1999, 137–149]. *Virus Res*, **81**, 167.

Dye C and Gay N (2003) Modelling the SARS epidemic. *Science*, **300**, 1884–1885.

Enjuanes L, Brian D, Cavanagh D *et al.* (2000) Coronaviridae. In *Virus Taxonomy* (eds Regenmortel MHV, Fauquet CM, Bishop DHL *et al.*), pp 835–849. Academic Press, New York.

Erles K, Toomey C, Brooks HW and Brownlie J (2003) Detection of a group 2 coronavirus in dogs with canine infectious respiratory disease. *J. Virol*, **310**, 216–223.

Escors D, Camafeita E, Ortego J *et al.* (2001a) Organization of two transmissible gastroenteritis coronavirus membrane protein topologies within the virion and core. *J Virol*, **75**, 12228–12240.

Escors D, Ortego J, Laude H and Enjuanes L (2001b) The membrane M protein carboxy-terminus binds to transmissible gastroenteritis coronavirus core and contributes to core stability. *J Virol*, **75**, 1312–1324.

Falsey AR, Walsh EE and Hayden FG (2002) Rhinovirus and coronavirus infection-associated hospitalisations among older adults. *J Infect Dis*, **185**, 1338–1341.

Fouchier RA, Kuiken T, Schutten M *et al.* (2003) Koch's postulates fulfilled for SARS virus. *Nature*, **423**, 240.

Freymuth F, Vabret A, Brouard J *et al.* (1999) Detection of viral, *Chlamydia pneumoniae* and *Mycoplasma pneumoniae* infections in exacerbations of asthma in children. *J Clin Virol*, **13**, 131–139.

Gagneur A, Sizun J, Vallet S *et al.* (2002) Coronavirus-related nosocomial viral respiratory infections in a neonatal and paediatric intensive care unit: a prospective study. *J Hosp Infect*, **51**, 59–64.

Gallagher TM and Buchmeier MJ (2001) Coronavirus spike proteins in viral entry and pathogenesis. *Virology*, **279**, 371–374.

González JM, Gomez-Puertas P, Cavanagh D *et al.* (2003) Taxonomical relations within the family *Coronaviridae* based on sequence identity analyses. *Arch Virol*, **148**, 2207–2235.

Guan Y (2003) World Health Organization meeting, Kuala Lumpur, June.

Hamre D and Procknow JJ (1966) A new virus isolated from the human respiratory tract. *Proc Soc Exp Biol Med*, **121**, 190–193.

Hays JP and Myint SH (1998) PCR sequencing of the spike genes of geographically and chronologically distinct human coronaviruses 229E. *J Virol Methods*, **75**, 179–193.

Herold J, Raabe T, Schelle-Prinz B and Siddell SG (1993) Nucleotide sequence of the human coronavirus 229E RNA polymerase locus. *Virology*, **195**, 680–691.

Herrewegh AAPM, Smeenk I, Horzinek MC *et al.* (1998) Feline coronavirus type II strains 79-1683 and 79-1146 originate from a double recombination between feline coronavirus type I and canine coronavirus. *J Virol*, **72**, 4508–4514.

Ismail MM, Cho KO, Ward LA *et al.* (2001) *Avian Dis*, **45**, 157–163.

Jamieson FB, Wang EEL, Bain C *et al.* (1998) Human torovirus: a new nosocomial gastrointestinal pathogen. *J Inf Dis*, **178**, 1263–1269.

Johnston MA, Pooley C, Ignjatovic J and Tyack SG (2003) A recombinant fowlpox virus adenovirus expressing the S1 gene of infectious bronchitis virus protects against challenge with infectious bronchitis virus. *Vaccine*, **21**, 2730–2736.

Jones RC and Ambali AG (1987) Re-excretion of an enterotropic infectious bronchitis virus by hens at point of lay after experimental infection at day old. *Vet Rec*, **120**, 617–618.

Kolb AF, Maile J, Heister A and Siddell SG (1996) Characterization of functional domains in the human coronavirus HCoV 229E receptor. *J Gen Virol*, **77**, 2515–2521.

Koopmans MP, Goosen ES, Lima AA *et al.* (1997) Association of torovirus with acute and persistent diarrhea in children. *Pediatr Infect Dis J*, **16**, 504–507.

Ksiazek TG, Erdman D, Goldsmith C *et al.* (2003) A novel coronavirus associated with severe acute respiratory syndrome. *N Engl J Med*, **348**, 1953–1966.

Kuo L, Godeke GJ, Raamsman MJ *et al.* (2000) Retargeting of coronavirus by substitution of the spike glycoprotein ectodomain: crossing the host cell species barrier. *J Virol*, **74**, 1393–1406.

Lai MMC and Cavanagh D (1997) The molecular biology of coronaviruses. *Adv Virus Res*, **48**, 1–100.

Lee N, Hui D, Wu A *et al.* (2003) A major outbreak of severe acute respiratory syndrome in Hong Kong. *N Engl J Med*, **348**, 1986–1994.

Lewicki DN and Gallagher TM (2002) Quaternary structure of coronavirus spikes in complex with carcinoembryonic antigen-related cell adhesion molecule cellular receptors. *J Biol Chem*, **277**, 19727–19734.

Li W-H, Moore MJ, Vasilieva N *et al.* (2003) Angiotensin-converting enzyme 2 is a functional receptor for the SARS coronavirus. *Nature*, **426**, 450–454.

Lipsitch M, Cohen T, Cooper B *et al.* (2003) Transmission dynamics and control of severe acute respiratory syndrome. *Science*, **300**, 1966–1970.

Luo Z, Matthews AM and Weiss SR (1999) Amino acid substitutions within the leucine zipper domain of the murine coronavirus spike protein cause defects in the oligomerization and the ability to induce cell-to-cell fusion. *J Virol*, **73**, 8152–8159.

Macek V, Dakhama A, Hogg JC *et al.* (1999) PCR detection of viral nucleic acid in fatal asthma: is the lower respiratory tract a reservoir for common viruses? *Can Respir J*, **6**, 37–43.

Makela MJ, Puhakka T, Ruuskanen O *et al.* (1998) Viruses and bacteria in the etiology of the common cold. *J Clin Microbiol*, **36**, 539–542.

Marra MA, Jones SJM, Astell CR *et al.* (2003) The genome sequence of the SARS-associated coronavirus. *Science*, **300**, 1399–1404.

Martina BEE, Haagmans BL, Kuiken T *et al.* (2003) SARS virus infection of cats and ferrets. *Nature*, **425**, 915.

Matthews AE, Weiss SR and Paterson Y (2002) Murine hepatitis virus—a model for virus-induced CNS demyelination. *J Neurovirol*, **8**, 76–85.

Mckean MC, Leech M, Lambert PC *et al.* (2001) A model of viral wheeze in non-asthmatic adults: symptoms and physiology. *Eur Respir J*, **18**, 23–32.

Mounir S and Talbot PJ (1993) Molecular characterization of the S protein gene of human coronavirus OC43. *J Gen Virol*, **74**, 1981–1987.

Navas S, Seo S-H, Chua M-M *et al.* (2001) Murine coronavirus spike protein determines the ability of the virus to replicate in the liver and cause hepatitis. *J Virol*, **75**, 2452–2457.

Opstelten DJ, Raamsman MJ, Wolfs K *et al.* (1995) Envelope glycoprotein interactions in coronavirus assembly. *J Cell Biol*, **131**, 339–349.

Peiris M (2003) World Health Organization meeting, Kuala Lumpur, June.

Peiris M, Lai ST, Poon LLM *et al.* (2003) Coronavirus as a possible cause of severe acute respiratory syndrome. *Lancet*, **361**, 1319–1325.

Popova R and Zhang X (2002) The spike but not the hemagglutinin/esterase protein of bovine coronavirus is necessary and sufficient for viral infection. *Virology*, **294**, 222–236.

Poutanen SM, Low DE, Henry B *et al.* (2003) Identification of severe acute respiratory syndrome in Canada. *N Engl J Med*, **348**, 1995–2005.

Pitkranta A, Jero J, Arruda E *et al.* (1998) Polymerase chain reaction-based detection of rhinovirus, respiratory syncytial virus, and coronavirus in otitis media with effusion. *J Pediatr*, **133**, 390–394.

Raabe T, Schelle-Prinz B and Siddell SG (1990) Nucleotide sequence of the gene encoding the spike glycoprotein of human coronavirus HCV 229E. *J Gen Virol*, **71**, 1065–1073.

Raamsman MJ, Locker JK, de Hooge A *et al.* (2000) Characterization of the coronavirus mouse hepatitis virus strain A59 small membrane protein E. *J Virol*, **74**, 2333–2342.

Rao PV, Kumari S and Gallagher TM (1997) Identification of a contiguous 6-residue determinant in the MHV receptor that controls the level of virion binding to cells. *Virology*, **229**, 336–348.

Riley S, Fraser C, Donnelly CA *et al.* (2003) Transmission dynamics of the etiological agent of SARS in Hong Kong: impact of public health interventions. *Science*, **300**, 1961–1966.

Risco C, Anton IM, Enjuanes L and Carrascosa JL (1996) The transmissible gastroenteritis coronavirus contains a spherical core shell consisting of M and N proteins. *J Virol*, **70**, 4773–4777.

Rota PA, Oberste MS, Monroe SS *et al.* (2003) Characterization of a novel coronavirus associated with severe acute respiratory syndrome. *Science*, **300**, 1394–1399.

Ruan Y-J, Chia LW, Ling AE *et al.* (2003) Comparative full-length genome sequence of 14 SARS coronavirus isolates and common mutations associated with putative origins of infection. *Lancet*, **361**, 1779–1785.

Salanueva IJ, Carrascosa JL and Risco C (1999) Structural maturation of the transmissible gastroenteritis coronavirus. *J Virol*, **73**, 7952–7964.

Sawicki SG and Sawicki DL (1990) Coronavirus transcription: subgenomic mouse hepatitis virus replicative intermediates function in RNA synthesis. *J Virol*, **64**, 1050–1056.

Sawicki SG and Sawicki DL (1998) A new model for coronavirus transcription. *Adv Exp Med Biol*, **440**, 215–219.

Schickli JH, Zelus BD, Wentworth DE *et al.* (1997) The murine coronavirus mouse hepatitis virus strain A59 from persistently infected murine cells exhibits an extended host range. *J Virol*, **71**, 9499–9507.

Schultze B and Herrler G (1992) Bovine coronavirus uses N-acetyl-9-*O*-acetylneuraminic acid as a receptor determinant to initiate the infection of cultured cells. *J Gen Virol*, **73**, 901–906.

Siddell SG (1995) The Coronaviridae: an introduction. In *The Coronaviridae* (ed. Siddell SG), pp 1–10. Plenum, New York.

Stephensen CB, Casebolt DB and Gangopadhyay NN (1999) Phylogenetic analysis of a highly conserved region of the polymerase gene from 11 coronaviruses and development of a consensus polymerase chain reaction assay. *Virus Res*, **60**, 181–189.

Stewart JN, Mounir S and Talbot PJ (1992) Human coronavirus gene expression in the brains of multiple sclerosis patients. *Virology*, **191**, 502–505.

Stohlman SA and Hinton DR (2001) Viral induced demyelination. *Brain Pathol*, **11**, 92–106.

Sung JJY (2003) World Health Organization meeting, Kuala Lumpur, June.

Tan K, Zelus BD, Meijers R *et al.* (2002) Crystal structure of murine sCEACAM1a[1,4]: a coronavirus receptor in the CEA family. *EMBO J*, **21**, 2076–2086.

Thiel V, Herold J, Schelle B and Siddell SG (2001) Infectious RNA transcribed *in vitro* from a cDNA copy of the human coronavirus genome in vaccinia virus. *J Virol*, **82**, 1273–1281.

Thiel V, Ivanov KA, Putics A *et al.* (2003) Mechanisms and enzymes involved in SARS coronavirus genome expression. *J Gen Virol*; http:dx.doi.org/10.1099/vir.0.19424-0.

Tresnan DB, Levis R and Holmes KV (1996) Feline aminopeptidase N serves as a receptor for feline, canine, porcine, and human coronaviruses in serogroup I. *J Virol*, **70**, 8669–8674.

Tsai JC, Zelus BD, Holmes KV and Weiss SR (2003) The N-terminal domain of the murine coronavirus spike glycoprotein determines the CEACAM1 receptor specificity of the virus strain. *J Virol*, **77**, 841–850.

Tsang KW, Ho PK, Ooi GC *et al.* (2003) A cluster of cases of severe acute respiratory syndrome in Hong Kong. *N Engl J Med*, **348**, 1977–1985.

Tyrrell DAJ and Bynoe ML (1965) Cultivation of a novel type of common cold virus in organ cultures. *Br Med J*, **1**, 1467–1470.

Vabret A, Mouthon F, Mourez T *et al.* (2001) Direct diagnosis of human respiratory coronaviruses 229E and OC43 by the polymerase chain reaction. *J Virol Methods*, **97**, 59–66.

Van Benten IJ, KleinJan A, Neijens HJ *et al.* (2001) Prolonged nasal eosinophilia in allergic patients after common cold. *Allergy*, **56**, 949–956.

Van Vliet ALW, Smits SL, Rottier PJM and de Groot RJ (2002) Discontinuous and non-discontinuous subgenomic RNA transcription in a nidovirus. *EMBO J*, **21**, 6571–6580.

Wang D, Coscoy L, Zylberberg M *et al.* (2002) Microarray-based detection and genotyping of viral pathogens. *Proc Natl Acad Sci USA*, **99**, 15687–15692.

Weiss M and Horzinek MC (1987) The proposed family *Toroviridae*: agents of enteric infections. *Arch Virol*, **92**, 1–15.

Weiss M, Steck F and Horzinek MC (1983) Purification and partial characterization of a new enveloped RNA virus (Berne virus). *J Gen Virol*, **64**, 1849–1858.

Woode GN, Reed DE, Runnels PL *et al.* (1982) Studies with an unclassified virus isolated from diarrhoeic calves. *Vet Microbiol*, **7**, 221–240.

Woods RD, Cheville NF and Gallagher JE (1981) Lesions in the small intestine of newborn pigs inoculated with porcine, feline, and canine coronaviruses. *Am J Vet Res*, **42**, 1162–1169.

Woods RD and Wesley RD (1992) Seroconversion of pigs in contact with dogs exposed to canine coronavirus. *Can J Vet Res*, **56**, 78–80.

Zhang XM, Herbst W, Kousoulas KG and Storz J (1994) Biological and genetic characterization of a hemagglutinating coronavirus isolated from a diarrhoeic child. *J Med Virol*, **44**, 152–161.

11

Measles

Sibylle Schneider-Schaulies and Volker ter Meulen

University of Würzburg, Würzburg, Germany

INTRODUCTION

Acute measles is normally a mild disease contracted by children and young adults as a result of infection by the highly contagious measles virus (MV; ter Meulen and Billeter, 1995). MV is an efficient pathogen, persisting in nature in populations large enough to support it, even though it is able to cause an acute infection in any individual only once in a lifetime. Despite this, the virus is distributed worldwide and virological procedures have been unable to demonstrate significant differences between isolates from different locations. With the advent of molecular epidemiology, however, the existence of about 22 MV genotypes, which cluster into eight clades, has been confirmed. Thus, measles is a highly successful virus, which has efficiently exploited its potential for spread. Unlike other viruses (e.g. influenza viruses), MV has no animal reservoir and, although monkeys are susceptible to infection, transmission from animals is not an important means of introducing the disease into a community. Furthermore, although MV may persist for years in a single individual, these persistent infections are rare and are not associated with periodic shedding of infectious virus, as in herpesvirus infections. A single attack of measles is sufficient to confer lifelong immunity to clinical disease upon reinfection, even in the absence of re-exposure to the virus. Consequently, in order to remain endemic in a given community, the virus must rely on the infection of the young who are still susceptible. So efficient is the process that the first known report of measles (in Egyptian hieroglyphics) failed to recognise the infectious nature of the illness and described it as a normal part of child growth and development.

In the prevaccine era in developed countries the maximum incidence of measles was seen in children aged 5–9 years. Infections and epidemics centred around elementary schools, and younger children acquired measles as secondary cases from their school-age siblings. By the age of 20, approximately 99% of subjects tested had been exposed to the virus. With the introduction of the measles vaccine, the age incidence and percentage of measles cases in different age groups has changed markedly. In countries with optimal vaccine utilisation, measles infection has shifted to the teenage group, whereas in areas with an ineffective vaccine programme children up to 4 years of age show a high primary measles attack rate (Centers for Disease Control, 1991, 1996). In contrast, in Third World countries measles has its greatest incidence in children under 2 years of age. Here the disease is a serious problem with a high mortality (up to 10%) and it has been found that the severity of acute measles and mortality correlate in general with the severity of malnutrition. Therefore, the pattern of epidemiology observed differs markedly in different parts of the world, and a thorough understanding of this is essential to the development of successful vaccination programmes.

THE VIRUS

Although measles has been known for centuries, it was only with the isolation of the virus by Enders and Peebles in 1954 that experimentation became possible. The development of tissue culture systems, the availability of monoclonal antibodies and molecular

Principles and Practice of Clinical Virology, Fifth Edition. Edited by A. J. Zuckerman, J. E. Banatvala, J. R. Pattison, P. D. Griffiths and B. D. Schoub
© 2004 John Wiley & Sons Ltd   ISBN 0 470 84338 1

biological approaches have since then permitted a greater dissection of the virus structure and replication strategy. Experimental approaches to define MV protein functions in detail have long been limited, due to the lack of a system that allows a reverse genetic approach. With the development of a plasmid-based system to rescue infectious MV in tissue culture, the introduction of stable alterations into the viral genome became possible and thus the contribution of any single viral gene product in the MV life cycle can now be unravelled and to determine precisely how its functions are exerted (Radecke *et al.*, 1995). Moreover, recombinant MVs are now available which additionally express fluorescent (such as GFP) or enzymatically active proteins (such as the CAT gene) and these tools have proved instrumental in following MV spread in tissue culture and in experimentally infected animals.

Measles virus (MV) is a member of the newly introduced group, *Mononegavirales*, which includes the *Rhabdo-*, *Filo-*, *Henipa-*, *Borna-* and *Paramyxoviridae*. As a paramyxovirus, MV reveals structural and biochemical features associated with this group; however, it lacks a detectable virion-associated neuraminidase activity. Therefore it has been grouped into a separate genus, the morbilliviruses, of which it is the type species. Other members of this group include: 'peste de petit ruminants' (PPRV), which infects sheep and goats; rinderpest virus (RPV), which infects cattle; canine distemper virus (CDV), which infects dogs; phocine distemper virus (PDV), which infects seals and sea-lions; dolphin morbillivirus (DMV); and porpoise morbillivirus (PMV). All these viruses exhibit antigenic similarities, and all produce similar diseases in their host species. Both MV and CDV can persist in the CNS in their natural hosts and produce chronic neurological diseases.

Virus Morphology

MV particles consist of a lipid envelope surrounding the viral RNP complex, which is composed of genomic RNA associated with proteins (Figure 11.1a). Both viral transmembrane proteins [fusion (F) and haemagglutinin (H) proteins] are present on the envelope surface and appear as projections from the particle. Portions of both the F and H proteins extend through the virion envelope (transmembrane) and appear on its inside surface (Fraser and Martin, 1978). It is the amino-terminus of the H protein that protrudes through the cytoplasmic and viral membranes (type II glycoprotein), while the F protein is anchored near

the carboxy-terminus (type I glycoprotein). One or both of the cytoplasmic domains are believed to interact physically and functionally with the matrix (M) protein which, in turn, links the envelope to the RNP core structure. The viral genomic RNA is fully encapsidated by N (nucleocapsid) protein to form the RNP core structure, which resists RNAse degradation. There is recent evidence from *in vitro* experimentation that the virion is able to package more than one genome as long as the 'rule of six' (see below) is maintained (Rager *et al.*, 2002). As the viral genome cannot serve as mRNA, the viral polymerase complex consisting of the P (phospho-) and the L (large) proteins is part of the RNP core complex. Their location within this complex has not yet been resolved. The same holds true for cellular actin, which is also known to be packaged into the virion structure.

The virions are highly pleomorphic, with an average size of 120–250 nm, and both filamentous and irregular forms are known. The virion shown in an electron micrograph (Figure 11.2a) is bounded by a lipid envelope which bears a fringe of spike-like projections (peplomers) 5–8 nm long. The membrane below the spikes is 10–20 nm in thickness and encloses the helical viral RNP core, which has a diameter of 17 nm and a regular pitch of 5 nm. Immediately below the membrane, M proteins appear as a shell of electron-dense material.

Genome Structure

The viral genome is a non-segmented RNA molecule of negative polarity that is about 16 kb in length. The genome, completely sequenced for the MV Edmonston (ED) strain and a Japanese wild-type isolate, encodes six structural genes, for which the reading frames are arranged linearly and without overlap in the following order: 3' nucleoprotein (N, 60 kDa), phosphoprotein (P, 70 kDa), matrix protein (M, 37 kDa), fusion protein (F, disulphide linked 41 kDa F_1 and 22 kDa F_2 proteins, cleavage products of a 60 kDa precursor F_0 protein), haemagglutinin protein (H, 80 kDa, existing as disulphide-linked homodimer) and the large protein (L, 220 kDa) encoded on its 5' end (Figure 11.1b) (Rima *et al.*, 1986).

The genome is flanked by non-coding 3' leader and 5' trailer sequences that are thought to contain specific encapsidation signals and the viral promoters used for viral transcription and/or replication (Parks *et al.*, 2001). The genomic RNA molecule is entirely complexed with N protein, with one N molecule covering

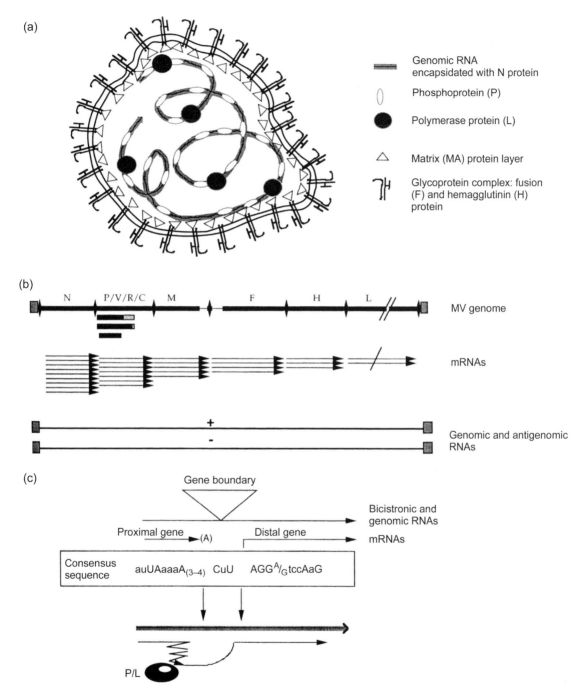

Figure 11.1 (a) A diagrammatic representation of the measles virus particle. (b) MV mRNAs are sequentially transcribed from the genome with decreasing efficiency and encode the structural proteins. In addition, the second gene (the P gene) encodes three non-structural viral proteins, C, R and V. (c) At the gene boundaries, MV genes are separated by conserved intergenic regions, where the polymerase complex polyadenylates the proximal mRNA and subsequently reinitiates transcription of the downstream gene. Alternatively, these signals are neglected by the polymerase when bi- or polycistronic mRNAs are transcribed, as well as during genome replication

(a)

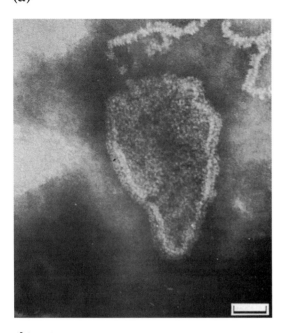

(b)

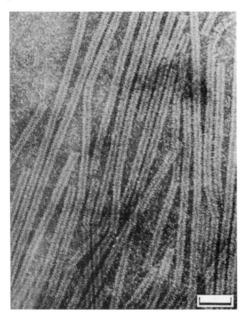

Figure 11.2 (a) Electron micrograph of the measles virion (bar = 50 nm). (b) Electron micrograph of purified MV nucleocapsids (bar = 50 nm); both are negatively stained with phosphotungstic acid. Reproduced from Meadeley (1973) published by Churchill Livingstone

six nucleotides (referred to as the 'rule of six'). This is thought to be the reason why only viral genomes (also including recombinant measles viruses carrying extra transcription units) whose number of nucleotides is a multimer of six are efficiently replicated by the viral polymerase. Within the 3′ leader sequence, transcription of the viral monocistronic mRNAs from the encapsidated genome is initiated. The coding regions of the viral genome are separated by conserved intergenic regions which consist of a polyadenylation signal at the 3′ of each gene, a conserved trinucleotide (CUU, except for CGU at the H/L gene boundary) and a reinitiation signal for the distal gene (Figure 11.1c) (Parks *et al.*, 2001). From the P gene, three non-structural proteins, C (20 kDa), V (46 kDa) and R (46 kDa) are expressed. Whereas the genetic information for the C protein is encoded by a separate reading frame (Bellini *et al.*, 1985), V protein can only be translated from edited P mRNAs in which a G residue not encoded by the viral genome has been co-transcriptionally inserted at a particular site. It thus shares a common amino-terminal domain with P, while a zinc finger-like domain is present on the carboxy-terminus of V. About 50% (to yield V) and 1.5% (to yield R) of the P mRNAs are edited, and it has been established that editing is an intrinsic activity of the MV polymerase. This is because P mRNAs, once synthesised, are not edited, and editing of P-gene transcripts is not performed by heterologous polymerases such as that of vaccinia virus. At the M–F gene boundary a GC-rich region of about 1 kb in length spans the 3′ end of the M gene and the 5′ end of the F gene. Several open reading frames have been predicted for this region which could only be accessed by translation from a rare bicistronic transcript by ribosomal reinitiation. None of the putatively encoded proteins has yet been detected in infected cells.

MV Protein Functions

The Viral RNP and Non-structural Proteins

The fully encapsidated MV genomic RNA serves as a unique target for the viral polymerase to initiate transcription and replication. The N protein, which is phosphorylated at serine and threonine residues, is the most abundant of the MV proteins and acts to condense the viral genomic and antigenomic RNAs into a smaller, more stable and more readily packaged form. This gives the nucleocapsid its helical form and its 'herringbone' appearance in the electron micrograph (Figure 11.2b). In addition, there is evidence for the formation of N–V complexes (Tober, 1998).

When expressed in the absence of viral RNA, N proteins self-aggregate into nuclear and cytoplasmic nucleocapsid-like structures, which are thought to contain encapsidated cellular RNAs. The amino-terminal 398 amino acids are important for self-aggregation and RNA interaction, while the carboxy-terminal 125 amino acids protrude from the nucleocapsid. This particular domain has recently been found to have an intrinsically disordered structure (Longhi *et al.*, 2003) and to interact with cellular proteins such as Hsp72 and IRF-3. It is the formation of high-affinity protein complexes with the phosphorylated P protein, however, by which self-aggregation and nuclear localisation of N proteins, as well as encapsidation of cellular RNAs, are prevented during replication of the viral genome. It is upon the interaction with the P protein that folding of the carboxy-terminal domain of the N protein occurs (Johannson *et al.*, 2003). Both carboxy-terminal and amino-terminal domains of P protein are involved in N–P complex formation, while another carboxy-terminal domain within the P protein was found essential for its dimerisation. The P protein is phosphorylated on serine residues and this was found important for its ability to function as polymerase co-factor in transcription and replication. Equally important for these processes, stable complexes between P and L have to be formed, and apparently L protein is stabilised by this interaction. Moreover, P acts as a transactivator, regulating L protein functions. The L protein is a multifunctional RNP-specific RNA polymerase producing mRNAs, replicative intermediates and progeny viral genomic RNAs. Capping, methylation, editing and polyadenylation are thought to be mediated by the polymerase protein in addition to initiating, elongating and terminating ribonucleotide polymerisation. Active sites within the protein have not yet been determined; however, conserved motifs that suggest a linear arrangement of the functional domains have been identified. The non-structural proteins C, V and R are expressed in the cytoplasm of infected cells, with no association with the virion structure. Their role in MV replication has not been defined. With the availability of the recombinant MV cDNA, viruses have been constructed that are defective in both V and C protein functions. Deletion of either of these gene products apparently did not affect the capacity of the recombinant viruses to replicate in tissue culture (Radecke and Billeter, 1996; Schneider *et al.*, 1997). However, there is evidence that they affect the efficiency of MV replication in peripheral blood cells or modulate the cellular interferon response (Palosaari *et al.*, 2003; Takeuchi *et al.*, 2003; Escoffier *et al.*, 1999). Not surprisingly, absence of these proteins affects MV virulence in animal models (Tober *et al.*, 1998; Valsamakis *et al.*, 1998).

The Envelope Proteins

The RNP core structure is enclosed by a lipid envelope which contains two proteins on its external surface, the haemagglutinin (H) and the fusion (F) proteins, that are organised as functional complexes and constitute the spikes observed in the EM. The H protein mediates binding of the virus to receptors on the surface of the target cells, while the F protein causes the virus envelope to fuse with the cell, thus delivering the RNP core into the cytoplasm. Both H and F are glycoproteins and after infection it is to these polypeptides that neutralising antibodies are raised. These proteins are protease-sensitive, as virions appear smooth under the EM following protease treatment. Both types of spikes can be isolated following gentle detergent lysis of the virion, although F tends to remain strongly associated with cellular actin. Both spikes have the tendency to aggregate; this is presumably mediated by the hydrophobic tail of each molecule, which normally serves to anchor the spike in the lipid bilayer.

The H protein can be isolated as a tetrameric complex from the cell membrane and its ability to agglutinate red blood cells from sheep and monkeys, but not humans, has long been recognised. Glycosylation sites are bunched within a region of 70 amino acids, and glycosylation has been shown to be essential for haemadsorption, probably by stabilising the highly complex tertiary structure of the protein. In analogy to the structure of the related NDV HN protein, the ectodomain of the MV H protein is thought to be organised into a membrane-proximal stalk and a membrane-distal globular head region, composed of a six-winged propeller structure (Crennell, 2000). Seven residues located within the globular head domain were found to be essential for oligomerisation and folding of the H protein, while a cysteine residue in the stalk regions is important for the formation of disulphide-linked dimers. In addition, amino acids involved in binding of the H protein to the MV receptors, CD46 and CD150 (see below), were identified. These are located in the ectodomain and include residues 451, 481, 546 and 473–477.

As revealed by transfection experiments, the H protein also exerts a helper function in F-mediated membrane fusion, probably by directing the fusion domain into the optimal distance to the target cell membrane and stabilising the interaction.

Synthesised as a precursor protein (F_0), F protein is cleaved in the Golgi compartment by subtilisin-like proteases to yield two disulphide-linked subunits, F_1 and F_2, a structure common to many virus proteins with membrane fusion activity. Glycosylation of the F_0 precursor is an essential prerequisite for cleavage, and it is only the F_2 subunit that contains all the potential N-glycosylation sites. Mutations of any of these sites affect cell surface transport, proteolytic cleavage, stability and fusogenic activity of the F protein. The F_1 subunit reveals an amino-terminal stretch of hydrophobic residues (the fusion domain) and two amphipatic α-helical domains, one of which is adjacent to the fusion domain (HRA), the other (containing a leucine-zipper motif) amino-terminal to the transmembrane region (HRB). There are still only theoretical explanations as to why the fusogenic amino-terminus of the F_1 subunit fails to induce membrane fusion during intracellular transport. Most likely, the fusogenic domain is masked during this process by intramolecular folding to a distal domain within the F_1 protein. A central region is thought to mediate interaction with the H protein. Homo- and hetero-oligomerisation of both glycoproteins occurs in the ER and the strength of F–H interaction and the fusogenic activity of the complex are also influenced by their cytoplasmic tails, both independently of and dependent on their interaction with the M protein (Plemper et al., 2002). The fully processed F_1 or F_2 protein is incorporated into the cell membrane as an oligomer. In the intact virion the active site of each protein is presumably carried at the tip of the spike and orientated outwards, away from the hydrophobic tail and towards any possible target cell.

The M protein is thought to interact with the viral RNP and with the plasma membrane in which the glycoproteins are inserted to stabilise the virion structure. Recombinant MVs carrying deletions of major parts of the M gene were found to bud highly inefficiently, thus supporting the initial suggestions that this protein might be essential in this process. A physical interaction between MV M and other viral structural proteins has not yet been demonstrated; however, the M protein modulates the fusogenic activity of the F–H complex and interactions of M with the glycoprotein cytoplasmic tails allow M-glycoprotein co-segregation to the apical surface in polarised cells. The generation of a recombinant MV defective for the expression of the MV glycoproteins (and expressing instead the glycoprotein of *Vesicular stomatitis virus*) revealed that the presence of the MV glycoproteins was required for packaging the M protein into mature budding virions, thus indicating that either F or H, or both, would at least transiently have to interact with M protein.

The Replication Cycle

MV Receptor Usage and Tropism

One of the most important parameters determining viral tropism is the availability of specific receptors on the surface of susceptible target cells that allow viral attachment and penetration. MV is highly species-specific, in that it does not naturally replicate in non-primate hosts. *In vivo* it reveals a pronounced tropism for cells of the haematopoetic lineage but at later stages can replicate productively in a variety of cell types, as it does in tissue culture. Thus, the receptor would be expected to be expressed by most human cells both *in vivo* and *in vitro*. This is in fact the case for one of the MV receptors identified (Griffin and Bellini, 1996), CD46 (MCP; membrane co-factor protein), a member of the 'regulators of complement' (RCA) gene family. Moesin (membrane-organising external spike protein), which is tightly associated with CD46, may have a co-receptor function. CD46 reveals a wide tissue distribution *in vivo*, and it is of note that CD46 is only expressed on monkey but not on human erythrocytes. Several isoforms of CD46 (due to alternative splicing of a precursor mRNA) are expressed in a tissue-specific manner and all of them can support MV uptake. CD46 contains four repetitive conserved domains, of which the two most distal from the cell membrane were found to be essential for binding MV or MV-H protein. The molecule's physiological ligand(s), complement components C3b/C4b, bind to other domains located proximal to the membrane (Figure 11.3, see plate section). As a member of the RCA gene family, CD46 is essentially involved in protecting uninfected cells from lysis by activated complement by recruiting the C3b/C4b components, rendering them accessible to degradation by serum proteases and thus interfering with the formation of membrane attack complexes. It is considered of pathogenic importance that CD46 is downregulated from the surface of infected cells or following interaction with MV-H protein, as these cells are significantly less protected against complement-mediated lysis *in vitro* (Schneider-Schaulies *et al.*,

1995). The inability of certain MV strains, predominantly those that have been exclusively isolated and passaged on lymphocytes, to use CD46 as entry receptor and to downregulate this protein from the cell surface soon indicated that an additional MV receptor should exist. That was identified as CD150 (also referred to as SLAM; signalling lymphocyte activation molecule), a CD2-like molecule of the Ig superfamily (Tatsuo and Yanagi, 2002). CD150 is expressed by activated and memory T and B cells and immature thymocytes, but not by freshly isolated monocytes and immature dendritic cells; it can, however, be induced on these cells upon stimulation. For monocytes, this induction can be mediated by interaction of the H protein of wild-type MV strains with Toll-like receptor 2 (TLR2), which itself does not serve as an entry receptor (Bieback et al., 2002). As with CD46, the most membrane distal portion of CD150, the V domain, is important for MV binding and the molecule is also downregulated by MV infection or H protein interaction. In addition, the cytoplasmic domain of both CD46 and CD150 have signalling properties, which might be modulated by MV H interaction. The ability of CD150, in contrast to CD46, to confer susceptibility to infection with any MV strain tested and its expression pattern, restricted to cells of the haematopoietic lineage, suggests that alternative MV entry receptors should exist. This hypothesis is supported by the property of wild-type MV to enter into CD150-negative cell types such as endothelial, epithelial (during acute measles) and brain cells (as a prerequisite for CNS persistence). Evidence for MV entry independent of CD46 and CD150 has also been recently provided by tissue culture experiments.

The contribution of the MV receptors to MV tissue tropism and pathogenicity is not yet understood. Rodents genetically modified to express CD46 cell are not susceptible to MV infection unless the virus is intrathecally applied, and it is likely that this will also be observed with CD150 transgenic animals. The failure to support MV replication in these animals is most likely due to unknown intracellular factors which restrict MV in rodent cells (a phenomenon which has long been observed in tissue culture). Infection of brain cells in vivo, on the other hand, can occur independently of CD46 expression as documented in mice or rats after intracerebral infection with an attenuated, rodent brain-adapted MV strain. In cotton rats (Sigmodon hispidus), which are susceptible to intranasal infection with both attenuated and wild-type MV strains (as documented by virus isolation from peripheral blood mononuclear cells, development of interstitial pneumo-

nia and immunosuppression), tissue distribution of potential CD150 and CD46 orthologues has not yet been possible to evaluate, due to the lack of appropriate reagents. However, it has been shown in these animals that infection with the wild-type MV strain or recombinant viruses expressing the wild-type MV H glycoprotein leads to preferential infection of secondary lymphoid tissues and pronounced immunosuppression. These findings lend strong support to the essential role of the interaction of the MV H protein with its receptors in MV pathogenesis in vivo.

Intracellular Replication

The time taken for MV replication in a suitable host cell is highly variable and becomes shorter as the virus adapts to growth in vitro. For instance, the Edmonston strain replicates well in Vero cells, a permanent cell line derived from the kidney of a green monkey. Growth is complete within 6–8 h and is accompanied by effective inhibition of host cell macromolecular synthesis. However, other strains, particularly freshly derived isolates, grow more slowly and replication times of 7–15 days are not uncommon. Such viruses often have very little inhibitory effect on the biosynthesis of the host cell. The origin and activation stage of the host cells also influence the efficiency of MV replication, e.g. it has been shown that productive MV infection in primary lymphocytes only occurs if the cells are activated and does not generally occur in most rodent cells, even after host cell penetration.

MV replication is confined to the cytoplasmic compartment. Following delivery of the viral RNP complex into the cytoplasm of a susceptible host cell, viral transcription is initiated after specific attachment of the polymerase complex to the promoter located within the $3'$ end of the genome and progresses to the $5'$ end by transcribing mono- and bicistronic mRNAs (Figure 11.4). At each gene boundary, the polymerase complex resumes transcription of the distal gene or, controlled by unknown factors, leaves the template to reinitiate at the promoter region. As a consequence, a polar gradient is established for the frequency of viral mRNAs, with the N-specific mRNA being the most abundant and the L-specific mRNA the least represented (Figure 11.1b). At the $3'$ end of each gene, poly(A) tracts are added to the mRNA transcripts, most probably by a polymerase stuttering mechanism at the termination signals (Figure 11.1c). This stuttering again reflects the RNA editing activity of the viral polymerase and the introduction of non-templated

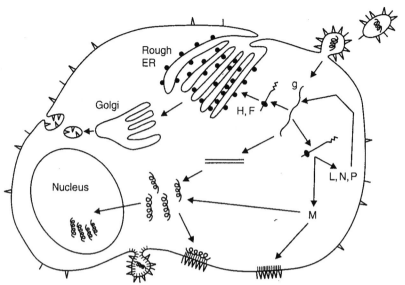

Figure 11.4 A schematic representation of the events occurring in measles virus replication

nucleotides in primary transcripts. In addition, bi- and polycistronic polyadenylated transcripts spanning two or more adjacent genes are produced. In the replication mode, the polymerase complex has to read through the intergenic boundaries to yield a positive copy of the entire viral genome, the replicative intermediate, which is about 100-fold less abundant than that of negative polarity. It is not known how the polymerase complex decides whether to interrupt transcription at the gene boundaries and polyadenylate the nascent transcripts, or to read through and continue transcription to full genomic length. Transcripts of positive polarity containing the encapsidation signal at their $5'$ ends joined to the N gene sequence are thought to be indicative of replication of the antigenome. Replication of, but not primary transcription from, viral genomic RNA is dependent on protein synthesis, and it is thought that the switch to the replication mode is determined by the accumulation levels of N protein that has to encapsidate the nascent genome and may act as an antiterminating protein.

The viral mRNAs direct the synthesis of viral proteins by host ribosomes. Those encoding the glycoproteins F and H become membrane-bound in the rough endoplasmic reticulum. Protein products are translocated and modified through the Golgi apparatus (acquisition of N-linked glycosylation and proteolytic cleavage of the F_0 protein) and finally inserted into the plasma membrane. As established, the F protein associates preferentially with membrane

microdomains (also referred to as lipid rafts) and drags the H protein into these structures, from where the virus subsequently buds. Progeny RNA interacts with N protein to form the nucleocapsid, and P and L proteins bind to these structures in the perinuclear area. Late in infection, nucleocapsids may also enter the cellular nucleus. M protein combines with some of the cytoplasmic nucleocapsids but also complexes with the plasma membrane and draws together the dispersed virus glycoproteins. It is quite possible that M protein also interacts with cytoskeletal components during this process, as well as during intracellular transport of viral RNPs. Progeny nucleocapsid structures line up beneath these modified areas of membrane and are pinched off in the budding process.

The mechanism of budding is unclear, but the ability of M to aggregate in a crystalline array could confer upon it the capacity to distort the membrane into an outward-facing bulge, and ultimately to bud off the nucleocapsid inside a small vesicular structure—the new virion (Figure 11.4). M is thought to act as a trigger in this process, and lack of this protein, and possibly of glycoproteins, is considered to be crucial in the pathogenesis of subacute sclerosing panencephalitis (SSPE).

During the replication process the large amount of glycoprotein inserted into the cell membrane causes it to develop the capacity to haemadsorb, whilst the F protein promotes fusion with adjacent cells. Multinucleate giant cells are thus formed which are pathognomonic for measles infection. This fusion kills the cells more rapidly than the virus, and if it is prevented the cells survive longer and yields of virus are increased.

BIOLOGICAL PROPERTIES OF MV

Stability

The structure of the virion explains much of the early data concerning the stability of the virus. The particle is dependent upon the integrity of the envelope for infectivity and is inactivated by any procedure which disrupts this structure. Hence, the virus is sensitive to detergents or other lipid solvents, such as acetone or ether. Particles are acid-labile and inactivated below pH 4.5, although they remain infective in the range pH 5–9. The virus is also thermolabile. It may remain infective for 2 weeks at 4°C but it is completely inactivated after 30 min at 56°C. At 37°C it has a half-life of 2 h. Thermolability is probably due to an effect on the internal structure of the particle, since haemagglutinin is relatively temperature-resistant. Virus can be stored for prolonged periods at −70°C and also freeze-dries well. These properties have important consequences for the transport and storage of vaccine.

Haemagglutinin

Unlike other members of the morbilliviruses, MV displays haemagglutination activity. This is easily demonstrated using monkey erythrocytes from the rhesus, patas and African green monkey and baboon. Human erythrocytes are not agglutinated. The virus H protein acts as a means of attachment to susceptible cells. Consequently, the ability to cross-link erythrocytes, which do not support virus replication, represents an unnatural process in virus multiplication. Thus the inability to agglutinate erythrocytes from the primary host, which is based on the lack of the major MV receptor component CD46 on these cells, is not surprising. Morbilliviruses are not thought to reveal neuraminidase activity and there is no evidence that they attach to receptors containing sialic acid. Consequently, once attached to a red blood cell, MV does not re-elute rapidly.

H protein inserted into any membranous structure is active in the haemagglutination test (HA). Virus particles separated by isopyknic centrifugation have a buoyant density of $1.23 \, \mathrm{g/cm^3}$, and HA activity is detected in this area of the gradient. A large amount of haemagglutinating material is also found in the upper regions of the gradient (termed 'light haemagglutinin'), which probably represents H protein inserted into empty membranous fragments of the infected cell, or defective virus particles. Haemagglutinating activity in this fraction can exceed that associated with the intact particles. It is of note, however, that recent MV wild-type strains (isolated on B lymphoid cells and not adapted to grow on Vero cells) have very low haemagglutination activity, which may be caused by the presence of an additional N-linked glycosylation site within their H proteins, but is best explained by their inability to interact with CD46 on monkey erythrocytes.

H is the major immunogen of the virus, and antibodies directed against this polypeptide have both haemagglutination-inhibiting (HI) and virus-neutralising (NT) activities. This is presumably accomplished by blocking the attachment of virus to target cells. However, these antibodies cannot prevent the progressive cell-to-cell spread of the virus mediated by the F protein. The function of H as the major viral attachment protein to host cell receptor(s) has already been outlined (see above) as has the property of H proteins from certain MV strains to modulate the expression of CD46, and all MV strains that of CD150. This latter modulation has been shown to occur after mere surface interaction between MV H protein and its receptors, and is thus also observed independent of infection. Although not defined so far, this process is thought to involve membrane signalling, as it has also been found that cross-linking of CD46 by various compounds including MV particles, leads to an inhibition of IL-12 synthesis in monocytes/macrophages in tissue culture (see below).

Haemolysis (HL)

The ability to lyse red blood cells once the virus has bound is mediated by the viral F protein. This ability is also artificial in the same sense as haemagglutination, since the F protein is not normally called upon to lyse a target cell before productive infection is accomplished. Nevertheless, HL provides a convenient measure of F protein activity which is more sensitive to both pH and temperature than haemagglutination. The optimum temperature for HL is 37°C and the optimum pH is 7.4. The ability of the paramyxoviruses to fuse at neutral pH accounts for the characteristic cytopathic effect (CPE) induced by these viruses, the formation of giant cells.

Proteolytic activation of the F protein is vital for its fusion activity; although uncleaved molecules can be inserted into mature virus particles, these have lost the ability to fuse with target cells and are therefore not infectious. The mechanism of F protein activity is not understood. Most likely, interaction of H protein with its receptor triggers a structural rearrangement of the F protein that allows insertion of its fusion domain into the cell membrane. This is also thought to have a destabilising effect on the local structure of the envelope. The importance of the fusion domain in this process is underlined by the fact that synthetic peptides with similarity to this region, but also those corresponding to the heptad repeat regions (which inhibit back-folding of the F_1 subunit into its fusion active conformation after MV receptor interaction), efficiently impair cell fusion. The requirement for F protein cleavage could be interpreted as necessary to permit the free movement of the two chains during the conformational change. Antibodies directed against the F protein are required for effective containment of virus infection, because local infection can be maintained by cell–cell fusion.

EPIDEMIOLOGY AND RELATEDNESS OF DIFFERENT VIRUS ISOLATES

The efficient spread of the virus is mediated by aerosol droplets and respiratory secretions, which can remain infectious for several hours. The disease incidence in the northern hemisphere tends to rise in winter and spring, when lowered relative humidity would favour this form of transmission. In equatorial regions, epidemics of measles are less marked but can occur in the hot dry seasons. Acquisition of the infection is via the upper respiratory tract, the nose and, possibly, the conjunctivae. Virus is also shed in the urine but this is unlikely to be an important means of transmission.

The spread of measles has been used as a convenient example to illustrate the principles of epidemiology, and it has been calculated that any community of less than 500 000 is unlikely to have a high enough birth rate to supply the number of susceptible children required for the continuous maintenance of the virus in the population. In fact, the complete elimination of measles from isolated groups has been documented. Such communities remain free of the disease until MV is reintroduced from outside, and susceptible individuals are once more at risk. Measles often leads to a more serious disease in such communities experiencing the illness for the first time, because all age groups are susceptible to the infection. In general, measles mortality is highest in children under 2 years of age and in adults. Death from uncomplicated measles is rare in the developed world, but the introduction of the virus to the Fiji Islands in 1875 resulted in an epidemic with a fatality rate of 20–25%, and introduction into Greenland in 1951 produced an epidemic which infected 100% of the susceptible population and resulted in a death rate of 18 per 1000.

MV isolates have been obtained from many different locations and from patients with different clinical conditions. Much effort has been invested in attempts to distinguish between these viruses and, in particular, to identify any strains which might be predisposed toward the production of encephalitis or SSPE. Conventional serological techniques applying polyclonal antibodies have, so far, failed to demonstrate any significant differences. Thus, infection by any one MV confers immunity to them all.

Measles virus is monotypic in nature, i.e. only a single serotype of the virus has been described. Antigenic differences, as observed with monoclonal antibodies between vaccine and wild-type viruses, need further study as it is not clear how much this affects the ability of wild-type strains to replicate and be transmitted from persons with waning titres of immunity generated by vaccination with a different genotype. The monotypic nature of MV in serological terms has masked the existence of a set of genotypes which accumulate mutations continuously. During the recent past, the molecular epidemiology of MV has been intensely studied. This has been undertaken to reveal whether there are MV strains with different pathogenic potential (lymphotropism and neurovirulence, the latter more likely to cause SSPE) or to monitor potential antigenic drift in wild-type MV strains that may impair the protective effect of the current vaccine. Moreover, in populations where mass vaccination campaigns have been undertaken, it is important to define whether any single measles case would be due to an imported virus or represent a still inadequate vaccine coverage or vaccine failure. Thus, in 1995, 60% of the 309 cases of measles reported in the USA were either directly imported or were found to be directly linked to an imported case by routine investigation or molecular epidemiology methods (Rota et al., 1992).

Sequence analysis of vaccine and wild-type MV strains, as well as SSPE isolates, have enabled researchers to establish the relationship of these various MVs into lineage groups, which are referred to as 'clades' (numbered A–H), and within those different genotypes can be distinguished. The assignment to a given clade and genotype (in general terms, the genotyping) of any given measles strain is based on the sequence of the COOH-terminal 151 amino acids of the N protein. Within this region, up to 7.2% divergence in the coding sequence and 10.6% divergence in the amino acid sequence between the most unrelated strains can occur. For most of the recent isolates, the sequence of the full-length H gene is also available, which provides information on their receptor usage. MV strains fall into different genotypes, some of which are extinct (i.e. have not been isolated for at least 15 years) or others which are still co-circulating in the human population. The activity within a given clade is directly mirrored by the heterogeneity of genetically related recent isolates which are drifting on a genetic level. It is indicative of MV reimportation into regions where transmission of indigenous MV is interrupted that MVs of different, genetically unrelated genotypes are isolated during an outbreak. In this respect, MV does not differ from other paramyxoviruses, such as human respiratory syncytial virus, human parainfluenza virus type 3 and mumps virus. Genetic characterisation of MV has proved to be a powerful adjunct to the standard epidemiological techniques that are used to study the transmission of measles. Molecular data help to confirm the sources of virus or suggest a source for unknown source cases. These data can also help to establish links, or lack thereof, between cases and outbreaks. Molecular surveillance is most beneficial when it is possible to observe the change in virus genotypes over time in a particular region, because this information, when analysed in conjunction with standard epidemiological data, has helped to document the interruption of transmission of endemic measles. Thus, molecular characterisation of measles viruses has provided a valuable tool for measuring the effectiveness of measles control programmes. The MV vaccine strains (which all fall within clade A) widely differ from the wild-type isolates, and SSPE-derived sequences were much more similar to those seen in wild-type viruses. Based on these sequence similarities, it was even possible to identify wild-type MVs having circulated in a given population as likely infectious agents found later in SSPE brain material. In the late 1980s and early 1990s of the last century, reimportation of wild-type measles of a known genotype into the USA caused about 50 000 cases. As shown by a recent study, after a typical interval of about 10 years, seven cases of SSPE were noted, which, upon sequence analyses, could clearly be assigned to the wild-type MV having caused the acute infection. These findings resulted in three important conclusions: first, SSPE develops more frequently than previously thought, second, SSPE develops after infection with a wild-type MV and not following vaccination; and third, circulating wild-type viruses, and not particular neurotropic strains, initially infect the CNS. So far, evidence indicates that measles is an antigenically stable virus and that the development of complications is not determined solely by the virus. Susceptibility of the host, age and immune status at the time of infection, and possibly other factors, are almost certainly more significant than the invading virus. The biological importance of the fact that all vaccine strains have a genotype substantially different from the currently co-circulating wild-type viruses is unclear. There is, however, no evidence to suggest that the currently used vaccines are not able to control MV infection with viruses of differing genotypes.

CLINICAL MANIFESTATIONS

Acute Measles

Measles was an inevitable disease of childhood prior to the vaccine era. It has been studied in detail and the clinical features are well documented. The course of acute measles is illustrated diagrammatically in Figure 11.5. MV first gains entry into the body through the upper respiratory tract or conjunctiva. Replication is assumed to occur at the site of entry. It is unknown as yet whether epithelial cells in the respiratory epithelium support MV replication, or if the first target cells are professional antigen-presenting cells (such as monocytes or tissue resident macrophages or dendritic cells). The first sign of infection is normally virus replication in the draining lymph nodes and destruction of lymphoid tissue. The virus then spreads to the rest of the reticuloendothelial system and respiratory tract through the blood (primary viraemia). Giant cells containing inclusion bodies (Warthin–Finkeldey cells) are formed in lymphoid tissue and also on the epithelial surfaces of the trachea and bronchi. About 5 days after the initial infection, the virus overflows from the compartments in which it has previously been replicating, to infect the skin and viscera, kidney and bladder (secondary viraemia). Giant cells are formed in all infected tissues. Unlike other viruses, measles infection is characterised by lymphoid hyperplasia and inflammatory mononuclear cell infiltrates in all infected organs.

After 10–11 days of incubation the patient enters the prodromal phase, which lasts 2–4 days. The initial symptoms consist of fever, malaise, sneezing, rhinitis, congestion, conjunctivitis and cough. These symptoms increase over the next days and are quite troublesome. At the beginning of the prodromal stage, a transitory rash can sometimes develop which has an urticarial or macular appearance, but disappears prior to the onset of the typical exanthem. At this time giant cells are present in the sputum, nasopharygeal secretions and urinary sediment cells. Virus is present in blood and secretions, and the patient is highly infectious. During this period Koplik's spots, the pathognomonic enanthem of measles, appear on the buccal and lower labial mucosa opposite the lower molars. These raised spots with white centres are characteristic of measles and begin to fade some 2–4 days after the onset of the prodromal phase as the rash develops.

The distinctive maculopapular rash appears about 14 days after exposure and starts behind the ears and on the forehead. From there the exanthem spreads within 3 days and involves the face, neck, trunk and upper and lower extremities. Once the entire body is covered, the rash fades on day 3 or 4 and a brownish discolouration occurs, sometimes accompanied by a fine desquamation. Histologically, the rash is characterised by vascular congestion, oedema, epithelial necrosis and round cell infiltrates. Once the exanthem has reached its height, the fever usually falls and the conjunctivitis as well as the respiratory symptomatology begins to subside. Antibody titres rise and virus shedding decreases from this point. Normally, the patient shows a rapid improvement. Continuation of clinical symptoms of the respiratory tract of fever suggests complications.

Modified Measles

This disease occurs in partially immunised children. These may be infants with residual maternal antibodies or individuals who have received immune serum globulin for protection. Occasionally, this infection has also been seen in the course of live vaccine failure. In general, the illness is mild and follows the regular sequence of events seen in acute measles, but with a very reduced symptomatology.

Atypical Measles

This form of a measles is established after incomplete measles vaccination prior to the exposure to natural MV. The majority of reported cases received either several doses of inactivated vaccine or a combination of inactivated vaccine followed by attenuated live vaccine. After an incubation period of about 7–14

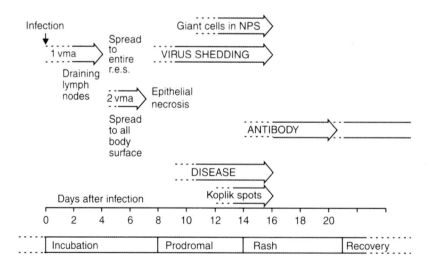

Figure 11.5 The course of clinical measles. The events occurring in the spread of the virus within the body are shown in lower case lettering. As the virus spreads by primary and secondary viraemia (vma) from the lymph node to the entire reticuloendothelial system (r.e.s.) and finally to all body surfaces, epithelial cell necrosis occurs and disease. The characteristics of the disease are given in upper case lettering

days, high fever with headache, abdominal pain and myalgia characterise the sudden onset of the disease. In addition, a dry cough and a pleuritic chest pain are common prior to the rash. In contrast to typical measles, the exanthem develops on the distal extremities and spreads. The rash itself is initially erythematous and maculopapular, but can later be purpuric, vesicular or urticarial. Frequently, oedema of the extremities develop. It is noteworthy that the exanthem involves the palms and soles with a prominent appearance on the wrists and ankles. The majority of cases develop a pneumonia with a lobular or segmental appearance, accompanied by pleural effusion, resulting in respiratory distress with dyspnoea. Recovery from the pulmonary symptomatology is rather slow, and pulmonary lesions can sometimes still be seen by X-ray months after onset of the disease. Marked hepatosplenomegaly, hyperaesthesia, numbness or paraesthesia are occasionally found. The pathogenesis of this disease is still unknown. At the onset, patients may or may not have low anti-measles antibody titres, which rise dramatically during the clinical disease to amounts not seen in acute measles. So far, MV has not been isolated from patients with atypical measles, probably due to pre-existing antibodies which, however, cannot prevent infection by natural measles. Immunological studies have suggested that these patients lack antibodies to measles virus F protein and therefore cannot block virus spread occurring by cell fusion. It was therefore believed that the F protein of killed measles vaccine was no longer immunogenic, as a result of the inactivation procedure. More recently, experimentation in monkeys has provided evidence that this might not be the case. F-specific antibodies, with all biological properties tested for, could be documented in animals that had been vaccinated with the killed vaccine. It was rather shown that the animals had a strong anamnestic humoral antibody response after challenge with wild-type virus, albeit the antibodies were preferentially of low avidity, complement-fixing and non-protective. In these animals, deposition of immune complexes in the lung and a pronounced eosinophilia was noted (Polack et al., 2003).

Complications of Measles Infection

Complications of acute measles are relatively rare, and result mainly from opportunistic secondary infection of necrotic surfaces, such as those in the respiratory tract. Bacteria and other viruses can invade to cause pneumonia or other complications, such as otitis media and bronchitis. The most severe complications caused directly by measles virus are giant cell pneumonia and subacute measles encephalitis, both of which occur in the immunocompromised patient as well as acute measles postinfectious encephalitis (AMPE) and SSPE, in which no underlying susceptibility factor has been identified. Other unusual manifestations which may complicate acute measles are myocarditis, pericarditis, hepatitis, appendicitis, mesenteric lymphadenitis and ileocolitis. If measles infection occurs during pregnancy, spontaneous abortions or stillbirth may occur, as well as an increased rate of low-birth-weight infants. Congenital malformations have also been reported.

Giant Cell (Hecht) Pneumonia

In immunocompromised patients, with immunodeficiencies as a result of an immunosuppressive regimen or underlying diseases, MV itself may lead directly to a life-threatening pneumonia, characterised by the formation of giant cells, squamous metaplasia of the bronchiolar epithelia and alveolar lung cell proliferation. Measles infection in such patients is thus a serious threat, usually severe with a protracted course, and is frequently fatal.

Measles Inclusion Body Encephalitis

This condition has been recognised only in immunosuppressed patients. It is most common in children with leukaemia undergoing axial radiation therapy. The incubation period ranges from a few weeks to 6 months and the patients often present without a rash, since generation of the rash requires an antiviral immune response. The condition commences with convulsions, mainly myoclonic jerks, and is frequently confused with SSPE (see below). The seizures are often focal and localised to one site. Other findings include hemiplegia, coma or stupor, depending on the localisation of the infectious disease process within the CNS. The disease course is much more rapid than in SSPE and proceeds to death within weeks or a few months. Furthermore, no or only low titres of measles antibodies are detectable in the CSF. This kind of infection is probably best regarded as an opportunistic MV infection.

Acute Measles Postinfectious Encephalitis (AMPE)

Acute encephalitis during the course of measles is a severe complication. It is observed at a frequency of about 1 in 1000–5000 cases of acute measles, although the incidence, the frequency of sequelae and the mortality rate of this CNS disease vary among the available reports. In general, about 15% of cases are fatal, and 20–40% of those who recover are left with lasting neurological sequelae. Encephalitis usually develops when exanthem is still present within a period of 8 days after the onset of measles. Occasionally this CNS complication may occur during the prodromal stage. The encephalitis is characterised by resurgence of fever, headache, seizures, cerebellar ataxia and coma. In common with postinfectious encephalitis induced by other viruses, this condition reveals demyelination, perivascular cuffing, gliosis, and the appearance of fat-laden macrophages near the blood vessel walls. Petechial haemorrhages may be present and in some cases inclusion bodies have been observed in brain cells. CSF findings in measles encephalitis consist usually of mild pleocytosis and absence of measles antibodies. Long-term sequelae include selective brain damage with retardation, recurrent convulsive seizures, hemi- and paraplagia.

Subacute Sclerosing Panencephalitis (SSPE)

SSPE is a rare, fatal, slowly progressing degenerative disease of the brain. It is generally seen in children and young adults and follows measles after an interval of 6–8 years, although SSPE cases have also occurred up to 20–30 years after primary infection. Boys are more likely to develop SSPE than girls but the overall incidence is low: based on recent findings (see above) it should be indicated with 1 case in 10^4 cases of acute measles rather than 1 in 10^6. Half the SSPE patients have contracted measles before the age of 2 years, which is a remarkably high figure considering the proportion of actual measles cases in these young children. No unusual features of the acute measles have ever been demonstrated and other factors are presumed important.

The course of SSPE is remarkably variable but seems to start with a generalised intellectual deterioration or psychological disturbance. This may last for weeks or months and may not be recognised as illness until more definite signs appear. These are neurological or motor dysfunctions and may take the form of dyspraxia, generalised convulsions, aphasia, visual disturbances or mild, repetitive simultaneous myoclonic jerks. The invasion of the retina by the virus leads, in 75% of cases, to a chorioretinitis, often affecting the macular area, followed by blindness. Finally, the disease proceeds to progressive cerebral degeneration, leading to coma and death. The progression of the disease is highly variable, remissions are common and some stages may overlap so that the progression of symptoms may not be as described. The illness lasts 1–3 years and inevitably leads to death. Much more rapid forms which lead to death in a matter of months are also known.

Neuropathological investigations reveal a diffuse encephalitis affecting both the white and the grey matter, characterised by perivascular cuffing and diffuse lymphocytic infiltration. Glial cells may proliferate, and fibrous astrocytes, neurons and oligodendroglial cells contain intranuclear inclusion bodies, which may occupy practically the entire nucleus. These have been shown to contain MV nucleocapsid structures. Giant cell formation or membrane changes consistent with virus maturation have not been observed. The neuropathological lesions lead to characteristic EEG changes, consisting of periodic high-amplitude slow-wave complexes which are synchronous with myoclonic jerks recurring at 3.5–20 s intervals. These periodic complexes are remarkably stereotyped, in that their form is similar in any case. They are bilateral, usually synchronous and symmetrical. Moreover, they usually consist of two or more delta waves and are biphasic or polyphasic in appearance. The pathophysiology of this abnormal EEG pattern is as yet poorly understood, but most investigators regard these complexes in SSPE as characteristic and even pathognomic. It is noteworthy that this EEG pattern is variable within the course of the disease and from one patient to another. Moreover, these typical complexes may disappear as the disease progresses.

Another important and pathognomic finding is the state of hyperimmunity against measles virus as well as the prominent γ-globulin increase in CSF. High measles antibody titres, except against the M protein (see 'Pathogenesis', below), are present in both serum and CSF. The isotypes of MV-specific antibodies found in CSF include IgG, IgA and IgD, and in this compartment the immune response is of restricted heterogeneity. Isoelectric focusing experiments have indicated that it is oligoclonally restricted. This is thought to be due to a restricted number of antibody-secreting cells which have migrated into the CNS and synthesise their antibodies there.

Osteitis Deformans and Otosclerosis

Viral-like nuclear and cytoplasmic inclusions that react with antibodies against paramyxoviruses, including MV, have been detected in multinucleated osteoclasts, osteoblasts, osteocytes, fibroblasts and lymphomonocytes of patients with Paget's disease (Baslé *et al.*, 1986). The mechanisms responsible for viral persistence are still unclear, particularly as the disease persists for many years and remains highly localised, with new lesions rarely if ever developing in previously unaffected bones. As revealed by recent studies, MV N-specific transcripts were successfully amplified from mononuclear cells and osteoclast-like multinucleated cells formed in long-term bone marrow cultures as well as osteoclast precursors and PBMCs of patients, but not of controls (Reddy *et al.*, 1996). Similarly, by ultrastructural and immunohistochemical studies, MV-like structures and MV antigens and, by RT-PCR, MV N-specific transcripts were detected in bone material from patients with otosclerosis, a disease that shares clinical and histopathological findings with Paget's disease (Arnold *et al.*, 1996; McKenna *et al.*, 1996). Since the aetiology of both Paget's disease and otosclerosis is largely unknown, it is unclear whether the observation of measles virus in bone tissue is of pathogenetic significance or merely an epiphenomenon.

PATHOGENESIS OF MEASLES AND ITS COMPLICATIONS

Measles is a remarkable pathogen: it is able to replicate in a variety of tissues, including cells of the immune system. Indeed, its interaction with the immune system is itself responsible for some of the key features of the disease. A delayed hypersensitivity reaction is implicated in the production of the rash, and could also be involved in the tissue damage observed in AMPE. Furthermore, there is evidence to suggest that interaction with the immune system may be responsible for the modification of the disease process observed in SSPE.

MV pathogenesis is not easily assessed in animal models. As yet, only primates have been found permissive for MV following intranasal infection and clinically develop measles, whereas attempts to induce measles-like disease processes in small animals by this route have largely failed. Apparently, MV replication in rodents is impaired due to intracellular restriction, as both rats and mice genetically engineered to express CD46 fail to replicate the virus after peripheral infection. For unknown reasons, only cotton rats (*Sigmodon hispidus*) reveal a certain permissivity, as infectious virus can be reisolated from lung tissue following intranasal infection. Moreover, as with acute measles, experimental infection of these animals is accompanied by a marked immunosuppression (see below). In addition, experimentally induced CNS infections have been described after intracerebral infection with certain MV strains in both mice and rats, which has led to a better understanding of both virological and immunological parameters of MV-induced CNS diseases.

Acute Measles

One of the earliest signs of infection is a pronounced lymphopenia and a defect in cell-mediated immunity is observed, as demonstrated in tuberculin-positive individuals who become tuberculin-negative. These effects are the result of virus interactions with cells of the lymphoid system (see below). After gaining entry to the body, the virus exhibits pronounced lymphotropism, and replication is normally detected in the draining lymph nodes rather than at the site of entry. *In vitro*, replication of MV is only observed in mitogen-activated lymphocytes, whereas monocytes apparently do not support productive replication at all. *In vivo*, the virus remains highly cell-associated and can be isolated from lymphocytes in the early stages of infection. Again, this is greatly assisted if the cells are mitogenically stimulated. Only a small proportion of the patient's lymphocytes are infected, and these include B and T cells as well as monocytes. Particularly in late stages of the infection, MV is almost exclusively found in monocytes.

Following extensive replication in the lymphoid tissue, virus is spread through a secondary viraemia, and replication continues in the epithelia of the lung and buccal cavity. The epithelia of the respiratory tract and conjunctiva are relatively thin, with about one or two cell layers. These soon begin to break down, and inflammatory reaction leads to the symptoms observed at the beginning of the prodromal phase—runny nose, conjunctivitis, malaise and fever. The thicker mucosal surfaces of the buccal cavity are then affected and Koplik spots appear about 11 days after infection. The appearance of these spots marks the commencement of a delayed-type hypersensitivity reaction, similar to that which gives rise to the rash. The spots fade some 3 days after their appearance as the rash itself develops. The mechanism underlying the production of both the spots and the rash is thought to be the same. Unlike other sites of replication, virus antigen is absent from the lesions themselves. Virus antigen can be detected in the skin, but it is concentrated near blood vessels and in the endothelial cells of the dermal capillaries themselves. The rash is characterised by vascular congestion, oedema, epithelial necrosis and round cell infiltration, but giant cells are absent. Virus replication does not break through the skin and virus is not shed from this surface. The containment of infection in the skin is thought to be due to the development of cytotoxic T cells, which destroy infected tissue, and to interferon production, which acts to promote cellular resistance to infection. More recently, the importance of CD8$^+$ T cells in controlling the acute infection has been directly demonstrated in experimentally infected rhesus monkeys (Permar et al., 2003). The rash itself results from accumulated damage to the vascular walls caused by this delayed-type hypersensitivity reaction, and is thus mostly not observed in the immunosuppressed.

Although antibody titres are normally rising at this stage of the illness, they are not thought to be the major factor in promoting recovery. MV-infected cells are lysed inefficiently by the classic pathway of the complement activation, although more so by the alternative pathway. Furthermore, patients with agammaglobulinaemia handle measles virus infection normally and recover. However, those with T cell deficiencies do not usually develop the rash and can be severely ill.

MV-induced Immunosuppression

Evidently, measles infection in the immunocompetent host triggers an efficient virus-specific immune response that leads to the clearance of the virus from peripheral blood and the establishment of a lifelong immunity against reinfection. Paradoxically, at the same time a general suppression of responsiveness to other pathogens is established that has been recognised long before the virus was isolated, and which is the major reason for the constantly high morbidity and mortality rate associated worldwide with acute measles. Typically, the patients are highly susceptible to opportunistic infections and reveal a marked lymphopenia affecting both B and T cells. As seen in a recent study, this is not due to reduced thymic output of lymphocytes (Permar et al., 2003), although another study done in SCID mice engrafted with human thymic material suggests massive thymocyte apoptosis.

It has also been documented by in vitro experimentation that MV can target CD34$^+$ stem cells directly (Manchester et al., 2002), which, if also happening in vivo, could also contribute to lymphopenia. It is, however, also likely that lymphocytes are lost due to viral infection, which may initially proceed quite extensively. In addition, it has been proposed that activated T cells expressing high levels of LFA-1 are preferentially lost from the peripheral blood and that this results from an aberrant homing to tissues. Immunosuppression, however, is still observed weeks after the onset of the rash, when the lymphocyte counts have returned to normal and MV-infected cells are present with only low frequency or are no longer detectable. Key features of MV-induced immunosuppression are inhibition of delayed-type hypersensitivity responses and a restricted ability of lymphocytes to proliferate in response to recall-antigens, as well as allogenic and mitogenic stimulation (Figure 11.6a). As only a few infected cells are usually detected, several hypotheses have been put forward to explain this finding, which include the production of inhibitory factors by infected cells that have not yet been identified (Oldstone and Fujinami, 1982). It was shown that the interaction of the viral glycoproteins with the surface of uninfected cells may interfere with the production of stimulatory cytokines, such as IL-12 by monocyte/macrophages (Karp et al., 1996). Whether this also accounts for the observed suppression of stimulated IL-12 release from dendritic cells in culture (Fugier-Vivier et al., 1997) or in vivo (Atabani et al., 2001) is unknown as yet. The MV glycoprotein complex has also been found to induce, in a dose-dependent manner, a cell cycle arrest in uninfected lymphocytes, both in vitro and after transfer in cotton rats (Sanchez-Lanier et al., 1988; Schlender et al., 1996; Niewiesk et al., 1997) (Figure 11.6b). Interestingly, professional antigen-presenting cells, such as dendritic cells (DCs), have also been found to impair rather than stimulate activation of T cells in vitro once they express viral glycoproteins on their surface (Schnorr et al., 1997; Klagge et al., 2000; Dubois et al., 2001). As for the fusogenic activity of this complex, the proteolytic activation of the F protein is also a prerequisite for its immunosuppressive activity. It was found by both in vitro and in vivo experimentation that negative signalling by the MV glycoprotein complex profoundly interferes with the activation of intracellular signalling cascades in uninfected T cells, but does not induce T cell apoptosis (Schneider-Schaulies et al., 2003). Dendritic cells with functional characteristics of epidermal Langerhans cells form a continuous network within the epithelial lining of the conductive airways, and are the most potent type of antigen presenting cells (APCs) for activation of naive and memory T cells once they have homed to the local lymph nodes. Thus, these MV-infected cells confer a negative rather than a positive signal to lymphocytes in the T cell areas of the lymph node and could play a central role in the induction of a widespread immune suppression. It appears particularly important in this setting that wild-type MV strains and recombinant MVs expressing the wild-type MV H protein reveal a pronounced tropism for secondary lymphatic tissues and are of higher immunosuppressive activity (Ohgimoto *et al.*, 2001). *In vivo* infection of dendritic cells in the course of measles or after vaccination has, however, not been confirmed as yet. In contrast, MV-infected follicular dendritic cells (FDCs) have been found in the B cell areas of lymph nodes of experimentally infected rhesus macaques, and generation of secondary follicles was largely impaired in areas where infected FDCs were observed.

The role of the MV receptors in immunosuppression is not yet understood. The ability of certain MV strains (either by surface contact or infection) to downregulate CD46 from the cell surface was found to enhance susceptibility to complement-mediated lysis of the affected cells, and this might limit viral spread by cellular depletion. As this property is mainly confined to attenuated MV strains, this may represent an attenuation marker rather than contributing to immunosuppression. Consequences of MV-mediated downregulation of CD150 have not yet been established. As this molecule is predominantly expressed on activated lymphocytes, it has been suggested that these might be efficiently eliminated by MV infection. It has already been mentioned above that both CD46 and CD150 have also signalling properties and thus MV interaction with either of them could probably alter cellular signalling independent of infection. In T cells, however, antibody ligation of either of these molecules was found to provide co-stimulatory rather than inhibitory signals. It is, however, essentially clear that induction of T cell unresponsiveness by surface interaction with the MV glycoprotein complex does not require one or both of the MV receptors.

Acute Measles Postinfectious Encephalitis (AMPE)

It is likely that CNS involvement, even in uncomplicated measles, is common. Transient abnormality of the EEG is detected in about 50% of patients, headache is common and CSF pleocytosis is also observed. The question of whether and how MV may reach the CNS in the course of the acute infection is still a matter of controversy. MV is highly lymphotropic and could be carried into the CNS, even in cases where encephalitis has not been recognised. However, only exceptionally can MV be isolated from the brain tissue of AMPE patients. In the majority of cases studied, neither MV antigen nor RNA have been found in the CNS. Therefore, current theories favour an autoimmune reaction as the possible cause of CNS damage, since AMPE patients may exhibit a proliferative T lymphocyte response to basic myelin protein (MBP). In addition in CSF specimens of such patients, MBP was detected as a consequence of myelin breakdown. Such MBP-specific lymphoproliferative responses have not only been seen after measles but also in patients with postinfectious encephalomyelitis following rubella, varicella or after rabies immunisation (Johnson and Griffin, 1986). The latter disorder is probably the human equivalent of experimental allergic encephalitis (EAE), since such patients received rabies vaccine prepared in brain tissue. Since AMPE is characterised by demyelinating lesions in association with blood vessels, as in EAE, it is therefore not surprising that the finding of an MBP-specific lymphoproliferative response in measles infection is considered to be of pathogenetic importance. How measles virus leads to a T cell-mediated autoimmune response is still unknown. At present, the possibilities of molecular mimicry or a deregulation of autoreactive cells occurring secondary to viral infections of lymphocytes are being considered.

Measles Inclusion Body Encephalitis (MIBE)

As this condition arises in patients with underlying immunodeficiencies, it is not usually accompanied by intrathecal antibody synthesis, and the unprotected cells develop massive inclusion bodies, consisting of virus nucleocapsids in both nucleus and cytoplasm. The condition can develop following exposure to measles or develop later. Infectious virus has not been isolated by conventional methods from brain tissue, suggesting defects in replication. This assumption has been supported by immunohistological and molecular biological studies on brain tissue of a case of MIBE. Of the five major structural proteins of MV, only N and P proteins were consistently detected in infected brain cells, whereas the envelope proteins were missing. In contrast, the mRNAs specific for the five viral proteins were detectable in

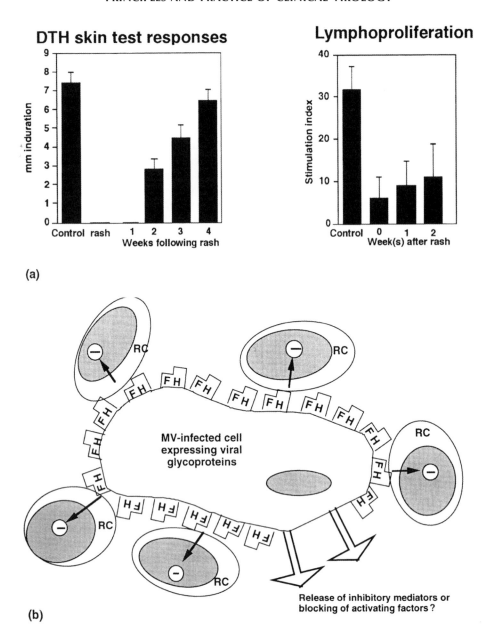

Figure 11.6 (a) In the course of and following measles, both delayed type hypersensitivity reactions (DTH) as measured by tuberculin test and *in vitro* proliferative responses of lymphocytes to mitogen stimulation are suppressed. Data from Tamashiro *et al.* (1987) and Hirsch *et al.* (1984). (b) A schematic representation of current models to explain MV-induced immunosuppression. RC means responder cells, which are uninfected lymphocytes

brain-derived total RNA samples by Northern blot analyses, although the mRNAs for the envelope proteins were underrepresented in comparison with lytically infected cells. *In vitro*, N and P proteins were efficiently synthesised from their corresponding mRNAs, indicating a restriction of the expression of the MV envelope proteins in MIBE (Baczko *et al.*, 1988). Partially, this restriction has been explained by sequence analyses, which revealed a high rate of mutations distributed over the entire MV genome.

For the MV M gene, mutations have eliminated the initiation codon, which explains the failure of MV M protein synthesis in infected MIBE brain tissue (Cattaneo *et al.*, 1988). Defects in MV mRNA transcription and envelope protein synthesis apparently do not largely affect the activity of the RNP complex, which spreads to different areas of the patient's brain. As infectious virus particles may never be formed, due to the restriction of the envelope proteins required for assembly and budding, and giant cell formation has never been observed, the spread is thought to occur by microfusion events.

Subacute Sclerosing Panencephalitis (SSPE)

MV was first implicated in the aetiology of this disease by immune fluorescence in 1967 and this has since been confirmed by electron microscopy, immunoelectron microscopic (IEM) methods, and finally by the successful rescue of virus by co-cultivation techniques (ter Meulen and Hall, 1978; ter Meulen and Carter, 1984). Despite this, the manner in which the persistent infection is first established in the brain, and exactly how this leads to the production of disease, are still largely unknown. The virus is thought to gain entry to the CNS during viraemia in acute measles or by infected lymphocytes, but once there, replication proceeds only slowly and a widespread encephalitis is not established. It is also not known to what extent virus replication *per se* is responsible for the development of lesions, or what part is played by the immune system.

Virological Aspects

Important clues have come from the study of MV replication. The virus normally replicates with the production of giant cells and release of infectious progeny. In SSPE, free infectious virus has never been isolated from either brain or CSF, and histopathological examinations have consistently failed to reveal the morphological changes associated with virus maturation (ter Meulen *et al.*, 1983, Schneider-Schaulies and ter Meulen, 1992). As with MIBE, giant cells and thickening of the plasma membrane at points of budding have never been observed, suggesting the absence of viral glycoproteins. Viral nucleocapsids present in the cytoplasm are randomly scattered and show no sign of regular alignment beneath the plasma membrane. As budding viral particles and infectious virus are not detected, the infection may spread slowly, strictly in a cell-associated manner. MV-specific antibodies produced in the CNS are oligoclonal, as opposed to the polyclonal response observed in the serum (Dörries *et al.*, 1988). This suggests that antibody in the CSF is made locally by a much smaller population of lymphocytes which have invaded this compartment in response to antigens present in the CNS. This is further supported by the finding that only MV-specific antibody titres are tremendously elevated, titres against other viruses being normal. In serum specimens, antibodies with specificity to all MV proteins are present, although recognition of the M protein is low or sometimes absent, whereas antibodies in CSF samples generally fail completely to detect M protein.

In SSPE brain sections, only the expression of the MV N and P proteins, and not of the envelope proteins, was consistently detected in infected cells by immunohistochemistry. Molecular biological studies on SSPE brain tissue revealed extensive transcriptional and translational alterations, affecting mainly MV M, F and H genes (Carter *et al.*, 1983; Sheppard *et al.*, 1986; Liebert *et al.*, 1986; Baczko *et al.*, 1986; Cattaneo *et al.*, 1986). As in MIBE, the envelope protein-specific mRNAs were only detected at low copy numbers (Cattaneo *et al.*, 1987) and were highly impaired in directing the synthesis of the corresponding gene products *in vitro* (Figure 11.7). Sequence analyses revealed a high rate of mutations located all over the MV genome, although different genes were affected at different levels. The highest number of alterations were found in the M gene, followed by F, H, P and N genes, which were mutated to about the same extent, whereas the L gene was most conserved. Mutations introduced were either point mutations, most probably accumulating due to the infidelity of the viral polymerase, or appeared as clustered transitions, which are thought to result from the activity of a cellular enzyme complex that actively modifies viral genetic information. As a result of either of these events, translation of viral mRNAs was completely abolished or led to the synthesis of truncated or unstable MV proteins. These molecular biological data explain the absence of infectious MV particles and the lack of a budding and a cell-fusion process in infected SSPE brain tissue, since for these events biologically active MV envelope proteins are required. Although infectious virus is not present in the CNS, virus can occasionally be rescued from brain tissue obtained post mortem by co-cultivation (Wechsler and Meissner, 1982). So-called SSPE isolates can be of two different types: cytolytic budding or cell-associated viruses, the latter spreading through the culture with a gradually enlarging area of cytopathic effect (CPE). In the second type of isolate, mRNAs for the MV envelope proteins are detectable in infected cells, although their function is impaired, since these proteins are not synthesised in infected cells or in *in vitro* translation experiments. As revealed by recent sequence analyses, some of the SSPE isolates are probably contaminations and are in fact ordinary laboratory MV strains. It is still unclear whether those that are true SSPE isolates may represent a small subpopulation of replication/maturation-competent viruses or revertants that have been selected by the isolation procedure and may not be representative for the dominant virus population in the infected brain.

These virological and molecular biological findings in SSPE help in understanding the absence of MV particles in brain tissue and explain the failure of the humoral immune response to eliminate infected brain cells. Factors involved in the establishment of persistence by a non-defective MV in brain tissue are largely unknown, since these studies have been carried out on autopsy material. In tissue culture experiments with cells of neural origin and in brain material of experimentally infected animals, evidence has been provided that intracellular factors intimately control the efficiency of MV replication (Schneider-Schaulies *et al.*, 1990). This applied particularly to attenuation of viral transcription as well as to translational control exerted predominantly on MV-specific and not on cellular mRNAs in brain cells *in vitro*. In addition, the cellular enzyme activity actively modifying the primary sequence of viral RNAs has been demonstrated in these cells. Thus, it is a likely assumption that intracellular factors present in brain cells act to slow down viral replication after primary infection, thus preventing a rapid host cell destruction. Whether these control mechanisms efficiently control the maintenance of the persistent infection, or other factors, such as the introduction of mutations into the viral genome, are required, has not been resolved.

Immunological Aspects

One of the immunological hallmarks in SSPE is the hyperimmune response to MV antigens, which includes neutralising antibodies in serum and CSF, yet this immune response fails to control virus infection. This phenomenon has led to the proposal that measles antibodies may support persistence, rather than interfere with it. In tissue culture, MV-specific antibodies act to cross-link viral proteins expressed on the surface of infected cells, which subsequently aggregate at the pole of the cell to form so-called 'cap-structures'. These caps are internalised and thus removed from the cell surface. During this process, M protein co-caps with the viral glycoproteins. Since complement-mediated lysis is of low efficiency in the brain as a result of low complement concentration in this compartment, it is likely that the major effect of antibody in brain tissue would be to promote clearance of antigen from the brain cell surfaces, rather than lysis of the infected cells. This process might explain the lack of membrane glycoproteins on the surface of brain cells but cannot explain the lack of intracellular envelope proteins. Yet some evidence has been obtained in tissue culture experiments, which suggest that the capping process could interfere with viral protein synthesis. It has been shown that antibody directed against the haemagglutinin of influenza viruses can exert an inhibitory effect on the activity of the viral polymerase. Similar observations have been made in cell lines persistently infected with MV or in MV-infected rats. In the latter experiment, passive transfer of neutralising monoclonal antibodies directed against the MV H protein led to the development of a subacute MV encephalitis by preventing an acute CNS infection (Liebert *et al.*, 1990). Molecular biological analysis revealed a transcriptional restriction of viral mRNAs. Thus, in SSPE the host immune response could contribute to the production of this serious fatal disease.

It is well known that cell-mediated immunity (CMI) is far more significant in the control of MV infection than the humoral immune response. This has led to considerable interest in the CMI response mounted by SSPE patients. In general, no evidence for a general impairment of CMI in these patients was obtained. T cells are present in normal amounts, and lymphoproliferation and interleukin synthesis in response to a variety of antigens are normal. Similarly, skin grafts are rejected in a normal fashion. It is possible that the response to MV antigens is impaired, since anamnestic skin tests with measles antigens are often negative. A disparity of results was obtained by using MV antigens in assays for CMI. Depending on the test system employed and on the potency and purity of the virus antigens used, a minor inhibition of CMI or normal reactions in comparison to controls can be observed in SSPE patients.

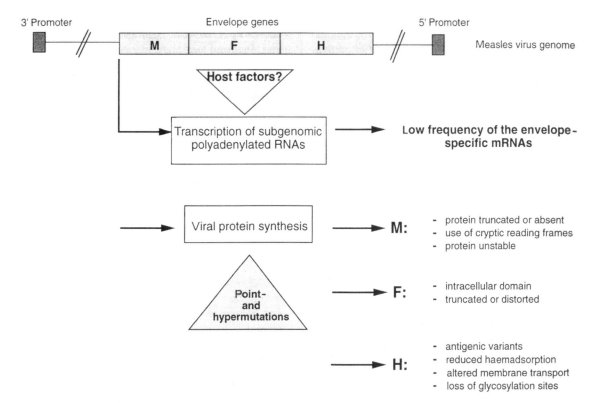

Figure 11.7 Schematic representation of restrictions of MV gene expression found in SSPE brain tissue. MV mRNAs encoding the viral envelope proteins are expressed at low frequency (most probably due to host cell control mechanisms) and, in addition, harbour mutations that prevent the synthesis of functional translation products

DIAGNOSIS

The symptoms of acute measles are so distinctive that a virus laboratory is seldom called upon to make a diagnosis. As the vaccination programme takes effect, physicians may become less familiar with the disease, and vaccination itself has led to the emergence of atypical forms of measles. Diagnosis of these manifestations may require laboratory work. Furthermore, as more patients are placed on immunosuppressive regimens, the need for diagnosis of MV may well increase. Several procedures are available, which are described below.

Microscopy

Direct Examination

Production of multinucleate giant cells with inclusion bodies is pathognomic for measles during the prodromal phase. Such cells are detectable in the nasopharyngeal secretions (NPS). Clear identification of giant cells is facilitated if the smear is first fixed in formalin and then stained with haematoxylin and eosin. The Cowdry inclusion bodies are then easily discerned.

Fluorescence Microscopy

Both direct and indirect immunofluorescence (IF) have been widely used to stain cells shed in nasal secretions, although it may be necessary to remove antibodies which already coat virus antigens with a low pH buffer. Stained cells include macrophages and ciliated cells as well as giant cells. Urinary sediment cells have also been examined with a high degree of success. IF-positive cells may be shed in the urine from 2 days before to up to 5 days after the appearance of the rash. This method may therefore be more applicable in later stages than examination of NPS specimens. Such cells may also be present in the urine 4–16 days after vaccination with the live vaccine. IF is useful for the diagnosis of measles in the pre-eruptive phase or in children vaccinated with killed vaccine, where rash development is atypical. Immunoperoxidase histochemical stains have also been used, and the use of monoclonal antibodies has improved sensitivity and reliability of virus detection.

Serological Methods

In common with other infections, diagnosis of measles may be made if antibody titres rise by more than fourfold between the acute and the convalescent phases or if measles-specific IgM is found. Several methods are available for this determination and are also useful for the assessment of immune status. The tests most commonly used are haemagglutination-inhibition (HI), neutralisation (NT), haemolysin-inhibition (HLI), complement fixation (CF) and enzyme-linked immunosorbent assay (ELISA). NT is the most sensitive and specific of these tests, but it is not very practical and therefore is rarely used. HI, HLI, ELISA and CF are more useful in practice, although the decreased sensitivity of the CF test renders it not useful for testing immune status. ELISA tests are usually applied for measles-specific IgG and IgM. Other tests, such as gel precipitation are rarely used. In general, titres of 8 or higher are indicative of immunity. In the case of SSPE, it is important that CSF is also tested.

Virus Isolation and Detection of Viral RNA

Both virus isolation and RT-PCR-based detection of viral RNA should be applied only in specific instances, such as suspected infection of the immunosuppressed in the absence of rash (when only limited antiviral immunoglobulins might be expected), developing pneumonia without a rash, or unexplained encephalitis. Finally, both techniques can be attempted as a means of retrospective diagnosis using tissue obtained post mortem.

RT-PCR analyses using MV N and/or F gene-specific primers are mostly performed on serum, nasopharygeal aspirates and urine sediment cells, can, however, also be applied to tissue samples such as brain material. This technique requires an RNA extraction step prior to reverse transcription and subsequent PCR amplification.

In acute measles, virus isolation is difficult and the success rate may be low. Isolation is most likely to be achieved from material (such as throat or conjunctival washings, sputum, urinary sediment cells and lymphocytes) taken during the prodromal phase and is unlikely to succeed once antibody titres have started to rise. Isolation is therefore only usually attempted in unusual cases. For virus isolation, washings and swabs are collected and mixed with buffered salt solution (pH 7.2) containing antibiotics. Urinary sediment cells are collected by low-speed sedimentation and treated similarly. Measles can be isolated directly from blood but efficiency is increased if lymphocytes are first separated on a Ficoll gradient and stimulated with mitogen before use. Samples are then inoculated in triplicate on susceptible tissue cultures, such as primary human embryo kidney (HEK) cells and primary monkey kidney cells. In the latter case, the monkeys should have been serologically tested, since some animals harbour monkey intranuclear inclusion agent (MINIA), which is similar to measles. Continuous cells lines derived from green monkey kidney cells (Vero or CV-1) are also suitable. These are less likely to be successful than primary cell culture. Given the low ability of wild-type MV strains to interact with CD46, Epstein–Barr virus-transformed B lymphoblastoid cell lines (B95a, BJAB) are widely used for MV isolation (Kobune et al., 1990). It was shown that these cells revealed a significantly higher susceptibility to MV present in clinical specimens than Vero cells. Moreover, MV isolated in B95a cells differed in some biological properties from those adapted to Vero cells, suggesting that the MV is subject to host cell-mediated selection. It is therefore recommended by WHO to use these cell lines for isolation of wild-type strains. Cytopathic effects (CPE) develop usually between 48 h and 15 days, and consist either of a broad syncytium or of a stellate form. Both types reveal inclusion bodies, which may be present in both nucleus and cytoplasm. It is not known what governs the different forms of CPE, but the availability of cellular nutrients as well as the type of virus has an effect. Uninoculated identical cultures should also be maintained as controls. If CPE is slow or not clear, it is possible to test whether the cells have acquired the ability to haemadsorb monkey erythrocytes or contain MV antigens or RNA.

Diagnosis of SSPE

The diagnosis of SSPE presents certain problems. Formerly, brain biopsy was performed routinely and tissue thus obtained was examined for inclusion bodies and virus antigen by immunofluorescence. After recognition of the characteristic intrathecal antibody synthesis, determination of measles antibody titres in the CSF may be sufficient with, if necessary, demonstration of MV-specific heterogeneity by isolectric focusing in combination with an immunoblot technique (Dörries and ter Meulen, 1984). Virus isolation from SSPE brain tissue is complicated. Expression of virus must be restored by growing cells derived from brain tissue with cells susceptible to MV infection, or fusing them together directly. It is therefore necessary that samples from SSPE brain contain viable cells. As MV replication only occurs within brain cells and viral particles are not released, MV-specific sequences can generally not be amplified by RT-PCR in CSF samples.

MANAGEMENT

Measles

Measles is an acute self-limiting disease which, in the absence of complications, will run its course without the need for specific intervention. Infection of the undernourished, the immunocompromised, or children suffering from chronic debilitating diseases is more serious. Such patients, as well as children of less than 1 year of age and pregnant women after household contacts, can be protected by the administration of human anti-measles γ-globulin (0.25–0.5 ml/kg). If this is given within the first 3 days after exposure, it is usually effective. The effectiveness is diminished if the globulin is given 4–6 days after exposure, and abolished if more than 6 days have elapsed.

Measles Pneumonia

Respiratory tract infections cause considerable damage to the ciliated epithelium and this may lead to superimposed bacterial infections. In the case of a pneumonia it is sometimes difficult to distinguish between primary viral infections and the superimposed bacterial infection. In any case, treatment with antibiotics is required.

Encephalitis

Treatment of acute measles postinfectious encephalitis is only symptomatic and supportive, and does not differ from any other postinfectious encephalitis. Careful attention to fluid and electrolyte balance is essential. Seizure control requires anticonvulsive drugs. Application of steroids has not been shown to be beneficial. No specific therapy is known for subacute measles encephalitis.

A variety of approaches to the treatment of SSPE have been attempted. As yet, no convincing effects have been demonstrated and almost all cases have proved fatal. Evaluation of the effectiveness of treatment is extremely difficult. First, the course of SSPE is highly variable and spontaneous remissions are common. Second, SSPE is a rare disease; clinical trials are therefore inevitably based on a very small number of patients and interpretation is difficult.

The aim of any therapy must be to prevent the spread of virus within the CNS and to aid the body's immune system to bring about the ultimate elimination of the virus from the body. The disease is extremely difficult to treat because no antiviral drugs which are effective against MV yet exist. Furthermore, access is limited because of the anatomical and physiological pecularities of the brain. Therefore, most attempts at treatment have aimed towards the activation of potentiation of the immune defence in the brain. A possible deficiency in the CMI to measles virus has already been discussed, and the following regimens have been used with no or doubtful effects: removal of blocking factors by complete CSF exchange, potentiation of helper T cell activity, isoprinosine (inosiplex), levamisole (L-tetramisole) and interferon treatment. In the case of inosiprinosine, it seems likely that treatment may lengthen survival time if given early in the disease. This effect becomes less pronounced if the drug is administered later.

PREVENTION

Since MV has no animal reservoir, it is an obvious target for a controlled campaign aimed at the eradication of the virus (Mitchell and Balfour, 1985). In the USA and Canada, where vaccination of all children is required at or before commencing school, quite startling results have been achieved. Case reports have fallen by over 99% but eradication has not yet been achieved. In Germany and the UK, where vaccination is not mandatory, distrust of vaccination has led to a lower acceptance rate and less dramatic results have been achieved. In developing countries, where the consequences of MV infection are most severe, considerable effort has been expended with comparatively little return. Any vaccine used must be safe, as measles is not normally a severe illness, and cheap enough for mass administration. Its effectiveness should also be long-lasting. Natural immunity is known to last for at least 65 years in the total absence of restimulation from virus in the environment. In 1781, measles disappeared from the Faroe Islands following an epidemic. It was not reintroduced until 1846. Individuals old enough to have experienced the disease 65 years previously were still protected. This unusual persistence of immunity, even in the absence of re-exposure from the environment, has suggested that MV may normally persist inside the body, possibly in lymphocytes, and thus restimulate immunity from within.

Inactivated Vaccine

This vaccine was intended for use in young children less than 1 year of age, who are most prone to serious complications. It was therefore considered desirable to avoid the use of a live vaccine. With the formalin-killed virus preparation, it was found that at least three vaccinations were necessary to elicit a suitable antibody response. Titres were lower than those induced by natural measles and soon waned. This left vaccinees open to virus attack, but the nature of their partial immunity led to serious hypersensitivity reactions to infection and the disease course was modified (see 'Atypical Measles'). The problems could perhaps be overcome, but, in view of the rapid decline in induced antibody, live vaccination is now recommended, and individuals previously immunised with the killed vaccine should be reimmunised with the live attenuated strain of virus. Even this procedure is not without risk and adverse reactions to the live vaccine may be seen in as many as 50% of the revaccinees. A similar phenomenon occurs in the case of live and killed vaccinia virus vaccines, where the killed virus lacks an important antigen found only on mature released virus.

Live Vaccine

The first attenuated vaccine strain was the Edmonston B strain, produced by serial passage of the virus in human kidney cells, human amnion cells, chick chorioallantoic membrane and, finally, duck embryo cells. This vaccine was administered intramuscularly or subcutaneously 12–18 months after the disappearance of maternal antibodies. It was effective and achieved seroconversion in 95% of recipients, but side-effects of mild measles were common (5–10%). In order to oppose this, γ-globulin was administered. The amount of γ-globulin was crucial: too little and side-effects could occur; too much could promote vaccine failure. In 1966 a Medical Research Council (MRC) trial conducted in the UK followed 36 000 children. Measles incidence fell 84% in the first 9 months and decreased by 14% in the next 2 years. A follow-up study showed that the vaccine remained effective for at least 12 years.

The side-effects and necessity to provide γ-globulin led to the development of the further attenuated and less reactogenic Schwartz and Moraten (Enders) strains. These were derived from the Edmonston B vaccine by further passage in the chick embryo at lowered temperature. Further MRC trials demonstrated that these were indeed less reactogenic and the incidence of postvaccination febrile convulsions was reduced from 7.7 to 1.9/1000 recipients. Both vaccines produced a 95% seroconversion rate, although antibody titres induced by the Schwartz strain declined more rapidly than those produced in response to the Moraten strain, but remained at protective levels. In recent years, the Edmonston strain was further attenuated by passing it in human diploid cells. This vaccine, referred to as Edmonston Zagreb strain, has been shown to produce higher seroconversion rates than the Schwartz vaccine when administered at the same age. Similar observations have been made with the AIK-C vaccine, produced in Japan. Titres of protective antibodies were seen to decline in isolated communities but were still detectable 14 years later. Children living in an open environment showed serological evidence of subclinical re-exposure which acted to boost their immunity. The attenuated strains now in use are so reduced in virulence that encephalitis has only been noted in about 1 in 1 million vaccine recipients, as compared to 1 in 1000–5000 children with natural measles. The measles vaccine is administered subcutaneously, usually at age 9–20 months for primary vaccination. Humoral immune responses, as defined by HI, NT and ELISA, are good and protective as long as the vaccine is given after waning of the maternal antibodies. As with acute measles, the major isotype of MV-specific antibodies is IgG1. Levels of antibodies induced are generally lower than after measles and may decay more rapidly, but are still measurable in most individuals 15 years after immunisation in the absence of boosting infections. Activation of cell-mediated immunity is generally thought to be similar to that of acute measles, in that both MV-specific CD4 and CD8 T cells are stimulated, although CTL responses after restimulation in vitro are considerably lower than after natural infection. Also similar to acute measles, administration of live measles vaccine is associated with transient lymphopenia, loss of DTH skin test responses to recall antigen and decreased *in vitro* proliferative responses to mitogens. Both mild leukopenia and atypical lymphocytosis have also been found after revaccination. In general, however, the immunosuppression observed after vaccination is less pronounced than that of acute measles, and is usually not associated with complications. Recent reports that both measles (contracted early in childhood) and measles vaccine would predispose to the later development of intestinal bowel diseases, such as Morbus Crohn or ulcerative colitis, have not been substantiated (Feeney *et al.*, 1997).

Effectiveness of Vaccination in the Control of Measles

In the prevaccine era, an estimated 4–5 million cases occurred annually in the USA and by the age of 15 years 95% of the population was seroconverted. Following the rigorous implementation of the MV vaccination programme, the case reports have fallen dramatically from 500 000 annually to 26 000 in 1978 and 1500 in 1983; during 1984–1988 only 3700 cases were registered. As a result of measles vaccination, the mortality and AMPE have also declined and the available experience indicates that SSPE can also be prevented by measles vaccination. However, in 1989 and 1990 a dramatic increase in acute measles cases was observed in the USA, which rose in 1989 to 18 193 and in 1990 to 27 786 cases (Atkinson and Orenstein, 1992). Measles cases typically occur in two distinct cohorts, preschool children aged less than 5 years and school children aged 5–19. In the former group, failure to obtain recommended vaccination is prominent, while in the latter, the majority of patients are infected despite previous vaccination. This indicated that lifelong immunity may not be induced by the application of live measles vaccine. The reasons for vaccine failure may be administration of the vaccine in the presence of maternal antibodies or an inadequate response to vaccination (primary vaccine failure) or loss of immunity in time (secondary vaccine failure). Molecular biological studies of contemporary MV strains revealed sequence changes to past strains which may be associated with different biological properties, although vaccine-induced MV antibodies still neutralise MV isolates from current epidemics. As a result of these measles epidemics, the American Academy of Pediatrics (AAP) and the Immunisation Practices

Advisory Committee of the USA (ACIP) recommended a change from a one-dose to a two-dose schedule for measles vaccination, which is expected to be optimal for measles control and eventual elimination. The first dose of measles vaccination, should be administered at 15 months of age, as delayed primary measles vaccination (at age 15 months or later) significantly reduces measles risk at later ages. Initial vaccination at age 12 months is recommended for children living in high-risk areas (areas with a large inner-city urban population, where more than five cases among preschool-aged children occurred during each of the last 5 years, or with recent outbreaks among unvaccinated preschool-aged children). Of course, initial vaccination of infants aged 12–14 months is also recommended before travelling to areas in which measles is endemic or epidemic. ACIP recommend a second dose with an interval of at least 2 months after primary immunisation up to 4–6 years of age, which is expected to provide protection to most persons who do not respond to their initial vaccination. Persons who received inactivated vaccine and are therefore at risk of developing severe atypical measles after exposure to natural measles should receive two doses of live vaccine, separated by not less than 1 month. It is of note that up to 55% of these vaccinees may reveal reactions to the live vaccine, such as local swelling and low-grade fever.

Side-effects of Live Vaccination, Adverse Reactions, Precautions and Contraindications

The vaccine has an excellent record of safety (National Vaccine Advisory Committee, 1991). Although on rare instances a transient rash or low-grade fever are observed after 5–12 days in some vaccinees, these remain otherwise asymptomatic, as for the vast majority of recipients. As with the administration of any agent that can induce fever, some children may have a febrile seizure. Although children with a history of seizures are at increased risk for developing idiopathic epilepsy, febrile seizures following vaccinations do not increase the probability of subsequent epilepsy or neurological disorders. Most convulsions following measles vaccination are simple febrile seizures, and they affect children without known risk factors. Nevertheless, parents of children who have a personal or family history of seizures should be advised of the small increased risk of seizures following measles vaccination which is, however, by far outweighed by the benefits of the protective effects. CNS conditions such as encephalitis and encephalopathy have been reported with a frequency of less than 1 per million doses administered, an incidence which is lower than that of encephalitis of unknown aetiology. This finding suggests that the reported severe neurological disorders temporally associated with measles vaccination were not caused by the vaccine.

Live measles vaccine should not be administered to women who are pregnant or who are considering becoming pregnant within the next 3 months, because of the theoretical risk of fetal infection. The decision to administer or delay vaccination because of a current febrile illness depends on the cause of the illness and the severity of symptoms. Hypersensitivity reactions following the administration of live measles vaccine are rare and usually occur at the injection site. Persons with a history of anaphylactic reactions following egg ingestion should, however, be vaccinated with extreme caution, and individuals who have experienced anaphylactic reactions to neomycin should not be given the vaccine. Unlike with natural measles, exacerbation of tuberculosis has not been observed after measles vaccination.

Vaccination of Immunocompromised and HIV-infected Individuals

Replication of vaccine viruses can be enhanced in persons with immune deficiency diseases and in those with immunosuppression, as occurs with leukaemia, lymphoma, generalised malignancy, or therapy with alkylating agents, antimetabolites, radiation or large doses of corticosteroids. Thus, patients with such conditions or therapies (except for HIV infection) should not be given live measles vaccine. Short-term corticosteroid therapy does not contraindicate live measles vaccination. The increasing number of infants and preschoolers with HIV infection in certain countries has directed special attention to the appropriate immunisation of these children. Asymptomatic children in need of measles live vaccination should receive it without prior evaluation of HIV infection state. Moreover, vaccination should be considered for all symptomatic HIV-infected children, including those with AIDS, since measles in these children can be severe. Limited data on measles vaccination among both asymptomatic and symptomatic HIV-infected children indicate that the vaccine has not been associated with severe or unusual adverse events (Moss et al., 2002). Exposed symptomatic HIV-infected (as well as other immunocompromised) persons should receive high doses of measles Ig, regardless of their previous vaccination status.

Vaccination in Developing Countries

In developing countries 1–1.5 million measles-related deaths are reported per year. Measles seems more severe in Africa than on other continents, with a number of countries reporting case fatality ratios higher than in most areas. Infants are at special risk for measles and case fatality ratios are high both during the acute phase and a 9-month following period. Malnutrition aggravates measles infection, and major complications are pneumonia and diarrhoea, which lead to an overall two- or four-fold increase in mortality. Administration of vitamin A has been shown to reduce measles morbidity and mortality.

Vaccination in these areas has so far failed to yield dramatic results. This is largely due to the epidemiology of measles in these areas. Interrupting transmission through vaccination would require high vaccination coverage rates ($>80\%$), and even with extremely high vaccination coverage rates outbreaks can be expected to occur. Measles is particularly severe in infants. The peak incidence of measles occurs in the very young, less than age 2 years, and 97% of cases occur below the age of 5. Vaccination should therefore be performed on younger children than in industrialised countries and frequent revisits to the same area are essential in order to prevent a large population of susceptible infants appearing through births in a single year. The time of waning of maternal antibodies, the incidence of measles infection in early life and the efficiency of measles vaccination are determinants of the earliest possible age for vaccination against measles. Vaccination is generally performed in industrialised countries at age 12 months. This is to some extent a compromise between vaccinating at 15 months (when seroconversion would be efficient (95%) but a large number of children would already have contracted measles), and vaccination earlier, before infection (when the success rate of vaccination is lower, 50–75% in 6 month-old children), and the risk of side-effects is greater). There is still an ongoing debate over the optimum age at which vaccination should be performed, particularly since recent trials with a high-titre vaccine at the age of 5–6 months suggested an increase in child mortality over control groups (Garenne et al., 1991). The basis for this has not yet been resolved.

Future studies will undoubtedly lead to further elucidation of the regulatory mechanisms involved in the normal replication of MV. This should in turn lead to a greater understanding of the events preceding measles invasion of the CNS and possible new avenues of therapy. Moreover, progress made in the molecular biology of MV could lead to the development of genetically engineered measles vaccines or subunit vaccines, which should be free of side-effects and possibly suitable for the immunisation of individuals currently at greatest risk, such as young infants or those suffering from chronic debilitating diseases.

REFERENCES

Arnold W, Niedermayer HP, Lehn N *et al.* (1996) Measles Virus in Otosclerosis and the specific immune response of the inner ear. *Acta Otolaryngol*, **116**, 705–709.

Atabani SF, Byrnes AA, Jaye A *et al.* (2001) Natural measles causes prolonged suppression of interleukin-12 production. *J Infect Dis*, **184**, 1–9.

Atkinson WL and Orenstein WA (1992) The resurgence of measles in the United States, 1989–1990. *Ann Rev Med*, **43**, 451–463.

Baczko K, Liebert UG, Billeter M *et al.* (1986) Expression of defective measles virus genes in brain tissues of patients with subacute sclerosing panencephalitis. *J Virol*, **59**, 472–478.

Baczko K, Liebert UG, Cattaneo R *et al.* (1988) Restriction of measles virus gene expression in measles virus inclusion body encephalitis. *J Infect Dis*, **158**, 144–150.

Baslé MF, Fournier JG, Rozenblatt S *et al.* (1986) Measles virus RNA detected in Padget's disease bone tissue by *in situ* hybridization. *J Gen Virol*, **67**, 907–913.

Bellini WJ, Englund G, Rozenblatt S *et al.* (1985) Measles virus P gene codes for two proteins. *J Virol*, **53**, 908–919.

Bieback K, Lien E, Klagge IM *et al.* (2002) Hemagglutinin protein of wild-type measles virus activates toll-like receptor 2 signaling. *J Virol*, **76**, 8729–8736.

Carter MJ, Willcocks MM and ter Meulen V (1983) Defective translation of measles virus matrix protein in a subacute sclerosing panencephalitis cell line. *Nature*, **305**, 153–155.

Cattaneo R, Rebmann G, Baczko K *et al.* (1987) Altered ratios of measles virus transcripts in diseased human brains. *Virology*, **160**, 523–526.

Cattaneo R, Schmid A, Eschle D *et al.* (1988) Biased hypermutation and other genetic changes in defective measles viruses in human brain tissues. *Cell*, **55**, 255–265.

Cattaneo R, Schmid A, Rebmann G *et al.* (1986) Accumulated measles virus mutations in a case of subacute sclerosing panencephalitis: interrupted matrix protein reading frame and transcription alteration. *Virology*, **154**, 97–107.

Centers for Disease Control (1991) Measles—United States 1990. *Morbid Mortal Wkly Rep*, **40**, 369–372.

Centers for Disease Control (1996) Measles—United States 1995. *Morbid Mortal Wkly Rep*, **45**, 415–418.

Crennell S, Takimoto T, Portner A and Taylor G (2000) Crystal structure of the multifunctional paramyxovirus hemagglutinin-neuraminidase. *Nature Struct Biol*, **7**, 1068–1074.

Dörries R, Liebert UG and ter Meulen V (1988) Comparative analysis of virus-specific antibodies and immunoglobulins in serum and cerebrospinal fluid of subacute measles virus-induced encephalomyelitis (SAME) in rats and subacute sclerosing panencephalitis (SSPE). *J Neuroimmunol*, **19**, 339–352.

Dörries R and ter Meulen V (1984) Detection and identification of virus-specific, oligoclonal IgG in uncon-centrated cerebrospinal fluid by immunoblot technique. *J Neuroimmunol*, **7**, 77–89.

Dubois B, Lamy PJ, Chemin K *et al.* (2001) Measles virus exploits dendritic cells to suppress CD4$^+$ T cell proliferation via expression of surface viral glycoproteins independently of T cell trans-infection. *Cell Immunol*, **214**, 173–183.

Escoffier C, Manie S, Vincent S *et al.* (1999) Non-structural C protein is required for efficient measles virus replication in human peripheral blood cells. *J Virol*, **73**, 1695–1698.

Feeney M, Clegg A, Winwood P and Snook J (1997) A case-control study of measles vaccination and inflammatory bowel disease. *Lancet*, **350**, 764–766.

Fraser KB and Martin SJ (1978) *Measles Virus and Its Biology*. Academic Press, London.

Fugier-Vivier I, Servet-Delprat C, Rivailler P *et al.* (1997) Measles virus suppresses cell-mediated immunity by interfering with the survival and functions of dendritic and T cells. *J Exp Med*, **186**, 813–823.

Garenne M, Leroy O, Beau J-P and Sene I (1991) Child mortality after high-titre measles vaccines: prospective study in Senegal. *Lancet*, **338**, 903–907.

Griffin DE and Bellini WJ (1996) Measles Virus. In *Field's Virology*, 3rd edn (eds Fields BN, Knipe DM and Howley PM), p 1267. Lippincott-Raven, Philadelphia.

Hirsch HL, Griffin DE, Johnson RT *et al.* (1984) Cellular immune responses during complicated and non-uncompli-cated measles virus infections of man. *Clin Immunol Immunopathol*, **31**, 1–12.

Johansson K, Bourhis JM, Campanacci V *et al.* (2003) Crystal structure of the measles virus phosphoprotein domain responsible for the induced folding of the C-terminal domain of the nucleoprotein. *J Biol Chem*, **278**, 44567–44573.

Johnson RT and Griffin DE (1986) Virus induced auto-immune demyelinating disease of the CNS. In *Concepts in Viral Pathogenesis* (eds Notkins AL and Oldstone MBA), pp 203–209. Springer Verlag, New York.

Karp CL, Wysocka M, Wahl LM *et al.* (1996) Mechanism of suppression of cell-mediated immunity by measles virus. *Science*, **273**, 228–231.

Klagge IM, ter Meulen V and Schneider-Schaulies S (2000) Measles virus-induced promotion of dendritic cell matura-tion by soluble mediators does not overcome the im-munosuppressive activity of viral glycoproteins on the cell surface. *Eur J Immunol*, **30**, 2741–2750.

Kobune F, Sakata H and Sugiura A (1990) Marmoset lymphoblastoid cells as a sensitive host for isolation of measles virus. *J Virol*, **64**, 700–705.

Liebert UG, Baczko K, Budka H and ter Meulen V (1986) Restricted expression of measles virus proteins in brains from cases of subacute sclerosing panencephalitis. *J Gen Virol*, **67**, 2435–2444.

Liebert UG, Schneider-Schaulies S, Baczko K and ter Meulen V (1990) Antibody-induced restriction of viral gene expres-sion in measles encephalitis in rats. *J Virol*, **64**, 706–713.

Longhi S, Receveur-Brechot V, Karlin D *et al.* (2003) The C-terminal domain of the measles virus nucleoprotein is intrinsically disordered and folds upon binding to the C-terminal moiety of the phosphoprotein. *J Biol Chem*, **278**, 18638–18648.

Manchester M, Smith KA, Eto DS *et al.* (2002) Targeting and hematopoietic suppression of human CD34$^+$ cells by measles virus. *J Virol*, **76**, 6636–6642.

McKenna MJ, Kristiansen AG and Haines J (1996) Polymerase chain reaction amplification of a measles virus sequence from human temporal bone sections with active otosclerosis. *Am J Otol*, **17**, 827–830.

Meadeley CR (1973) *Virus Morphology*. Churchill Livingstone, Edinburgh.

Mitchell CD and Balfour HH (1985) Measles control: so near and yet so far. *Progr Med Virol*, **31**, 1–42.

Moss WJ, Monze M, Ryon JJ *et al.* (2002) Prospective study of measles in hospitalized, human immunodeficiency virus (HIV)-infected and HIV-uninfected children in Zambia. *Clin Infect Dis*, **35**, 189–196.

National Vaccine Advisory Committee (1991) The measles epidemic: the problems, barriers, and recommendations. *J Am Med Assoc*, **266**, 1547–1552.

Niewiesk S, Eisenhuth I, Fooks A *et al.* (1997) Measles virus induced immune suppression in the cotton rat (*Sigmodon hispidus*) model depends on viral glycoproteins. *J Virol*, **71**, 7214–7219.

Ohgimoto S, Ohgimoto K, Niewiesk S *et al.* (2001) The haemagglutinin protein is an important determinant of measles virus tropism for dendritic cells *in vitro*. *J Gen Virol*, **82**, 1835–1844.

Oldstone MBA and Fujinami RS (1982) Virus persistence and avoidance of immune surveillance: how measles viruses can be induced to persist in cells, escape immune assault and injure tissues. In *Virus Persistence* (eds Mahy BWT, Minson AC and Darby GK), pp 185–202. Cambridge University Press, Cambridge.

Palosaari H, Parisien JP, Rodriguez JJ *et al.* (2003) STAT protein interference and suppression of cytokine signal transduction by measles virus V protein. *J Virol*, **77**, 7635–7644.

Parks CL, Lerch RA, Walpita P *et al.* (2001) Analysis of the non-coding regions of measles virus strains in the Edmonston vaccine lineage. *J Virol*, **75**, 921–933.

Permar SR, Klumpp SA, Mansfield KG *et al.* (2003a) Role of CD8(+) lymphocytes in control and clearance of measles virus infection of rhesus monkeys. *J Virol*, **77**, 4396–4400.

Permar SR, Moss WJ, Ryon JJ *et al.* (2003b) Increased thymic output during acute measles virus infection. *J Virol*, **77**, 7872–7879.

Plemper RK, Hammond AL, Gerlier D *et al.* (2002) Strength of envelope protein interaction modulates cytopathicity of measles virus. *J Virol*, **76**, 5051–5061.

Polack FP, Hoffman SJ, Crujeiras G and Griffin DE (2003) A role for non-protective complement-fixing antibodies with low avidity for measles virus in atypical measles. *Nature Med*, **9**, 1209–1213.

Radecke F and Billeter MA (1996) The non-structural C protein is not essential for multiplication of Edmonston B strain measles virus in tissue culture cells. *Virology*, **217**, 418–421.

Radecke F, Spielhofer P, Schneider H *et al.* (1995) Rescue of measles viruses from cloned cDNA. *EMBO J*, **14**, 5773–5784.

Rager M, Vongpunsawad S, Duprex WP and Cattaneo R (2002) Polyploid measles virus with hexameric genome length. *EMBO J*, **21**, 2364–2372.

Reddy S, Singer F, Mallette L and Roodman GD (1996) Detection of measles virus nucleocapsid transcripts in circulating blood cells from patients with Paget's disease. *J Bone Min Res*, **11**, 1602–1607.

Rima BK, Baczko K, Clarke DK *et al.* (1986) A complete transcriptional map for morbilliviruses. *J Gen Virol*, **67**, 1971–1978.

Rota JS, Hummel KB, Rota PA and Bellini WJ (1992) Genetic variability of the glycoprotein genes of current wild-type measles isolates. *Virology*, **188**, 135–142.

Sanchez-Lanier M, Guerin P, McLaren LC and Bankhurst AD (1988) Measles virus-induced suppression of lymphocyte proliferation. *Cell Immunol*, **116**, 367–381.

Schlender J, Schnorr JJ, Spielhofer P *et al.* (1996) Interaction of measles virus glycoproteins with the surface of uninfected peripheral blood lymphocytes induces immunosuppression *in vitro*. *Proc Natl Acad Sci USA*, **93**, 13194–13199.

Schneider H, Kaelin K and Billeter MA (1997) Recombinant measles viruses defective for RNA editing and V protein synthesis are viable in cultured cells. *Virology*, **227**, 314–322.

Schneider-Schaulies S, Klagge IM and ter Meulen V (2003) Dendritic cells and measles virus infection. *Curr Top Microbiol Immunol*, **276**, 77–101.

Schneider-Schaulies S, Liebert UG, Baczko K and ter Meulen V (1990) Restricted expression of measles virus in primary rat astroglial cells. *Virology*, **177**, 802–806.

Schneider-Schaulies J, Schnorr JJ, Brinckmann U *et al.* (1995) Receptor usage and differential downregulation of CD46 by measles virus wildtype and vaccine strains. *Proc Natl Acad Sci USA*, **92**, 3943–3947.

Schneider-Schaulies S and ter Meulen V (1992) *Molecular Aspects of Measles Virus-induced Central Nervous System Diseases* (ed. Ross RP), pp 449–472. Humana Press, Totowa, NJ.

Schnorr JJ, Xanthakos S, Keikavoussi P *et al.* (1997) Induction of maturation of human blood dendritic cell precursors by measles is associated with immunosuppression. *Proc Natl Acad Sci USA*, **94**, 5326–5331.

Sheppard RD, Raine CS, Bornstein MB and Udem SA (1986) Rapid degradation restricts measles virus matrix protein expression in a subacute sclerosing panencephalitis cell line. *Proc Natl Acad Sci USA*, **83**, 7913–7917.

Takeuchi K, Kadota SI, Takeda M *et al.* (2003) Measles virus V protein blocks interferon (IFN)-α/β but not IFN-γ signaling by inhibiting STAT1 and STAT2 phosphorylation. *FEBS Lett*, **545**, 177–182.

Tamashiro VG, Perez HH and Griffin DE (1987) Prospective study of the magnitude and duration of changes in tuberculin reactivity during complicated and uncomplicated measles. *Pediatr Infect Dis J*, **6**, 451–454.

Tatsuo H and Yanagi Y (2002) The morbillivirus receptor SLAM (CD150). *Microbiol Immunol*, **46**, 135–142.

ter Meulen V and Billeter MA (eds) (1995) *Current topics in Microbiology and Immunology: Measles Virus*, vol 191. Springer Verlag, Berlin.

ter Meulen V and Carter MJ (1984) Measles virus persistency and disease. *Progr Med Virol*, **30**, 44–61.

ter Meulen V and Hall WW (1978) Slow virus infections of the nervous system: virological, immunological and pathogenetic considerations. *J Gen Virol*, **41**, 1–25.

ter Meulen V, Stephenson JR and Kreth HW (1983) Subacute sclerosing panencephalitis. *Compr Virol*, **18**, 105–159.

Tober C, Seufert M, Schneider H *et al.* (1998) Expression of measles virus V protein is associated with pathogenicity and control of viral RNA synthesis. *J Virol*, **72**, 8124–8132.

Valsamakis A, Schneider H, Auwaerter PG *et al.* (1998) Recombinant measles viruses with mutations in the C, V, or F gene have altered growth phenotypes *in vivo*. *J Virol*, **72**, 7754–7761.

Wechsler SL and Meissner HC (1982) Measles and SSPE viruses: similarities and differences. *Progr Med Virol*, **28**, 65–95.

12

Rubella

Jennifer M. Best and Jangu E. Banatvala

Guy's, King's and St Thomas' School of Medicine, London, UK

HISTORICAL INTRODUCTION

Rubella was known initially as 'German measles' because it was first described by two German physicians in the mid-eighteenth century and was initially known by a German name, 'Roteln'. For many years German measles was confused with other diseases causing a rash, such as measles and scarlet fever. It was eventually recognised as a distinct disease by an International Congress of Medicine in London in 1881. The name 'rubella' was accepted at about that time. The main historical events associated with rubella are summarised in Table 12.1. Being a generally mild disease, it received comparatively little attention after 1881, until its association with congenital defects was recognised in 1941 by N. McAlister Gregg, an Australian ophthalmologist. He observed that 78 babies with a similar type of congenital cataract, some also with heart disease, were born after an extensive rubella epidemic in 1940 (Gregg, 1941). All but 10 of the mothers had a history of rubella, usually in the first or second month of pregnancy. These findings were confirmed by other Australian workers, who also observed deafness and microcephaly. Deafness occurred in infants whose mothers were infected slightly later in pregnancy (mean 2.1 months' gestation), whereas congenital cataracts occurred in infants whose mothers had had rubella on average at 1.5 months' gestation. Other retrospective studies in Australia and other countries confirmed these findings (reviewed by Hanshaw *et al.*, 1985).

These retrospective studies, in which the starting point for investigations was an infant with congenital deformities, suggested that a very high proportion of mothers who had had rubella during pregnancy were delivered of infants with congenital malformations. For example, Gregg, in a more extensive survey, reported that 122 of 128 (95%) children whose mothers had had rubella before the 16th week of gestation had congenital defects. He also reported the birth of six normal infants following rubella in early pregnancy.

Prospective studies, which were designed to give a more accurate assessment of the risk of maternal rubella, were carried out in the 1950s and early 1960s. These studies showed that the incidence of congenital malformation following maternal rubella was 10.2–54.2%, much less than that shown by retrospective studies. However, these studies were based on a clinical diagnosis of maternal rubella, which is now known to be unreliable, particularly during non-epidemic periods. Consequently, the incidence of congenital malformation was underestimated, since many women who did not have rubella and who were delivered of normal babies were probably included. More recent studies involving pregnant women with serologically proven rubella are discussed on pp 438–440.

Virological Studies

Early work on the characteristics and transmission of rubella was carried out in monkeys and human volunteers. It was first demonstrated that rubella could be transmitted by bacteria-free filtrates in 1938. Between 1949 and 1953, further experimental studies using human volunteers showed that the incubation

Principles and Practice of Clinical Virology, Fifth Edition. Edited by A. J. Zuckerman, J. E. Banatvala, J. R. Pattison, P. D. Griffiths and B. D. Schoub

Table 12.1　Main historical events

1881	Rubella accepted as a distinct disease by International Congress of Medicine
1938	First evidence to show that rubella was caused by a virus
1941	Teratogenic effects of rubella first recognised by Gregg in Australia
1962	Rubella virus isolated in cell cultures. Neutralisation test developed
1963–1964	Extensive epidemics of rubella in USA and Europe
1965–1967	Development of attenuated vaccine strains and first vaccine trials
1967	Rubella virus shown to haemagglutinate. Haemagglutination-inhibition (HAI) test developed
1967	Rubella virus first visualised by electron microscopy
1969	USA: HPV77.DE5 and Cendehill vaccine strains licensed. Vaccination offered to all pre-school children
1970	UK: Cendehill vaccine strain licensed. Vaccination offered to all 11–14 year-old schoolgirls
1971	USA: MMRI* licensed
1972	UK: Rubella vaccination extended to all susceptible adult women of child-bearing age including women attending antenatal clinics. Susceptible pregnant women offered vaccination in the immediate postpartum period
1977	USA: National Childhood Immunization initiative—intensification of rubella vaccination of teenagers and susceptible adult women
1978–1979	UK: Rubella epidemics; 124 cases of congenitally acquired rubella and 1405 terminations of pregnancy due to rubella or rubella contact
1979	USA: RA27/3 replaced other vaccine strains
1983	UK: Rubella epidemic. Further intensification of vaccination campaign
1988	UK: Vaccination policy augmented by offering MMR to pre-school children of both sexes. MMR II licensed
1996	UK: Schoolgirl vaccination discontinued; children offered second dose of MMR before school entry
1997	USA: Change in policy: children offered first dose of MMR at 12–15 months and second dose at 4–6 years of age
1986	Rubella virus genome sequenced
2000	WHO recommends immunisation policies for elimination of CRS
2002	123/212 (57%) of countries/territories include rubella vaccination in national immunisation programmes

MMR, measles, mumps and rubella vaccine.

period of rubella was 13–20 days. Subclinical infection was demonstrated, since secondary cases of rubella occurred in contacts of volunteers inoculated with serum who had not themselves developed a rash.

Rubella virus (RV) was not isolated in cell cultures until 1962, when two groups of workers simultaneously published methods for the isolation of RV. Parkman and his colleagues (1962) inoculated primary vervet monkey kidney (VMK) cultures with throat washings obtained from military recruits when rash was present. Although no cytopathic effect (CPE) was observed, when cultures were challenged 7–14 days after inoculation with 10^4 TCID$_{50}$ *Echovirus 11* (EV11), the distinct CPE produced by this virus was not observed, suggesting the presence of an interfering agent. The interfering agent was neutralised by rabbit antiserum raised against one of the isolates. Weller and Neva (1962) also isolated the virus from blood and urine taken from typical cases of rubella in primary human amnion cultures. After specimens were passed once or twice in these cell cultures, a characteristic CPE with cytoplasmic inclusions was observed. These effects were neutralised by serum obtained from patients convalescent from rubella. The agents isolated in the different cell cultures by these two groups of workers were exchanged and found to be identical.

It was subsequently shown that RV induced interference in continuous lines of monkey kidney cells and that viruses other than EV11 (e.g. *Coxsackievirus A9*, *Bovine enterovirus M-6* and *Vesicular stomatitis virus*) could be used to challenge rubella-infected cell cultures. Many other primary and continuous cultures were subsequently shown to support the growth of RV.

Rubella-neutralising antibodies were detected by Parkman and his colleagues (1962), who demonstrated that convalescent sera neutralised the interference effect produced by a standard inoculum of RV. The presence of neutralising antibodies was shown to be associated with protection against reinfection. This technique was used extensively for diagnostic purposes and serological surveys. Studies conducted in different countries showed that the acquisition of rubella antibodies was related to age, social class and geographical location, and that approximately 80% of women of childbearing age living in urban areas in Western countries were immune. Initial attempts to develop a haemagglutination-inhibition (HAI) test were unsuccessful, since it was not appreciated that inhibitors of haemagglutination, shown to be serum lipoproteins, were present both in the serum incorporated in culture medium and in the test sera. Details of a successful HAI test were published in 1967 (Stewart *et al.*, 1967).

Clinical and virological investigations carried out during the extensive rubella epidemic in the USA during the winter and spring of 1963–1964 led to a greater understanding of the pathogenesis of congenital rubella syndrome (CRS) as well as a further appreciation of its clinical features and sequelae. During this epidemic many pregnant women were inevitably infected and this resulted in the delivery of about 30 000 rubella-damaged babies (Cooper, 1975). Studies at the time revealed that multisystem involvement was common and the range of abnormalities much wider than previously reported. When maternal rubella occurred in early pregnancy, a generalised infection developed in the fetus, which persisted during the remainder of gestation and into infancy, despite the presence of rubella antibodies. Many infected infants excreted virus and transmitted virus to susceptible contacts. This epidemic highlighted the importance of developing a vaccine.

THE VIRUS

Classification

RV is classified as a non-arthropod-borne togavirus and is the only member of the genus *Rubivirus*. The overall structure and strategy of replication of RV is similar to that of the alphaviruses of the *Togaviridae*, such as Semliki-Forest and Sindbis (Frey, 1994). By HAI, however, no antigenic relationship has been shown between rubella and more than 200 alphaviruses and flaviviruses.

Structure

The virus particle is 58 ± 7 nm in diameter, while the nucleocapsid is 33 ± 1 nm in diameter and surrounds the RNA genome (Figure 12.1). The virion consists of two membrane-bound glycoproteins, E1 (58 kDa) and E2 (42–47 kDa), and C, a non-glycosylated capsid protein. The symmetry of the nucleocapsid was difficult to establish due to its instability, but an icosahedron with 32 capsomers has been described. The lipoprotein envelope bears surface spikes of 5–8 nm composed of the two glycoproteins. The non-rigid delicate character of the envelope results in the virus particle being pleomorphic; elliptical and oblong virus particles and particles bearing finger-like protrusions have been described.

Genome Structure and Function

The RV genome is comprised of a positive sense 40S strand of RNA, 9762 nucleotides (nt) in length, which is capped at the 5′ end and polyadenylated at the 3′ end (Frey, 1994; Pugachev *et al.*, 1997). The cap serves as a ribosome recognition site and is required for efficient translation. The RNA is infectious when extracted under appropriate conditions. The base composition of the genome is G 30.8%, C 38.7%, A 14.9% and U 15.4%. The genome consists of two non-overlapping open reading frames (ORFs) separated by an untranslated region of 123 nucleotides, and has some features in common with the alphaviruses. The 5′ proximal ORF extends between nt 41–6388 (total 6348 nt) and codes for a polyprotein precursor of the non-structural proteins (NSP). The 3′ proximal ORF extends between nt 6512–9700 (total 3189 nt) and codes for the polyprotein precursor of the structural proteins. The gene order for the 40S RNA is 5′-p150-p90-C-E2-E1-3′ (Figure 12.2).

Genetic Variation

The complete genomes of several strains of RV have been sequenced. Sequencing has been difficult due to the high GC content of the genome (69%) and several errors appeared in early sequence data (Frey, 1994; Pugachev *et al.*, 1997). RA27/3 differs from M33 and Therien at 36 nucleotides, 18 of which are silent with respect to amino acid coding. As sequence differences are maintained in virus recovered from vaccinees who received the RA27/3 vaccine, they can be used to identify this attenuated strain in clinical specimens (Pugachev *et al.*, 1997). Other sequencing studies, which have concentrated on the E1 ORF, have shown that most available isolates belong to one genotype, but that some isolates from China and India differ from isolates from Europe, North America and Japan by 8–10% of nucleotides, although by only 1–3% at the amino acid level. These have been classified as genotype 2 (Bosma *et al.*, 1996; Frey *et al.*, 1998). There is no evidence that reinfection is due to an antigenic variant, but two viruses isolated from joints exhibit changes in antigenic epitopes in E1 (Bosma *et al.*, 1996; Frey *et al.*, 1998). Thus, the level of diversity is low when compared with some alphaviruses and other RNA viruses, such as HIV and poliovirus, and there is no evidence of antigenic drift, even in highly vaccinated populations (Best *et al.*, 1993; Frey *et al.*,

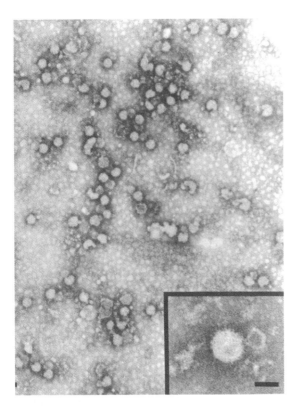

Figure 12.1 Negatively stained preparation of rubella virus. Inset: an enlarged particle, showing spikes (bar = 50 nm). Kindly provided by Dr I. Chrystie. Reproduced from Banatvala and Best (1998) published by Edward Arnold, London,

1998). A comparison of NSP coding sequences shows that the 1970–2360 nt region of p150 is also variable.

Replication

RV probably enters the cell by receptor-mediated endocytosis. Although the cellular receptor for the virus has not been identified, membrane phospholipids and glycolipids are probably involved, which may explain the wide tissue tropism of the virus. The reproductive cycle takes place in the cytoplasm and probably resembles that of the alphaviruses. The virion is transported to the endosomal compartment, where the low pH brings about the uncoating of the viral genome and fusion of the E1 and E2 glycoproteins with the endosomal membranes, allowing the viral genome to be released into the cytoplasm. Vesicles are formed within the endosome, which provide a protected environment for the synthesis of viral RNA. The endosome probably fuses with a lysosome to form a replication complex, similar to those found in alphavirus-infected cells.

Four RNA species can be found in RV-infected cells; a single-stranded 40S genomic RNA, a 24S subgenomic RNA, a 21S replicative intermediate with partially double-stranded (ds) RNA and viral replicative forms of 19–20S full ds RNA. The 40S genomic RNA is translated to produce the 2116 amino acid polyprotein (p200) encoded by the 5′ proximal ORF. This polyprotein is cleaved by a viral protease to give two products of 150 and 90 kDa. The p150 contains the proposed methyltransferase and protease motifs, while the p90 contains amino acid motifs indicative of replicase and helicase activity (Figure 12.2). An X motif of unknown function is also present, which is a short region of homology between RV and the alphavirus NSP3. P200 is required for synthesis of the negative-sense genome. This is used as a template for the production of both full-length 40S progeny genomes and 24S subgenomic RNA, for which p150 and p90 are required. The 24S subgenomic RNA, which is capped, methylated and polyadenylated, is translated to produce a 110 kDa polyprotein, which is cleaved by a host cell signal peptidase to produce the three structural proteins C, E2 and E1 (Figure 12.2). All three structural proteins are transported to the Golgi complex. E1 and E2 form heterodimeric complexes, while the C protein forms dimers, which are stabilised by disulphide bond formation shortly before virus release.

In cell cultures RV is released by budding from intracellular membranes (e.g. Golgi, endoplasmic reticulum) and from the plasma membrane. The RNA-containing nucleocapsid cores become visible for the first time before they bud from the cellular membranes, where they form mature virus particles by acquiring an envelope consisting of the E1 and E2 glycoproteins and host-cell lipids. The ability to bud from intracellular vacuoles allows the virus to evade the host's immune response, which may enable the virus to establish persistent infections (Chantler et al., 2001).

In vertebrate cell cultures the replication of RV is slow and less efficient than the alphaviruses. In Vero cells viral genomic and subgenomic RNA are first detected 12 h after infection and virus production reaches a peak at 48 h after infection at high multiplicities of infection (Hemphill et al., 1988). No effect on total cell RNA or protein synthesis has been noted within 72 h after infection. Defective interfering RNAs have been detected. Membrane alterations and cytoplasmic vacuoles are observed in infected cells by electron microscopy.

The structure and replication of RV have been reviewed in more detail by Frey (1994), Lee and Bowden (2000) and Chantler *et al.* (2001).

Physical and Chemical Properties

Physical properties of RV have been reviewed in detail by Horzinek (1981) and Banatvala and Best (1998). The virus is stable at $4°C$ for $\geqslant 7$ days, but is inactivated at $0.1–0.4 \log_{10} TCID_{50/0}$ 1 ml/h at $37°C$ and at $1.5–3.5 \log_{10} TCID_{50/0}$ 1 ml/h at $56°C$. It is stable at $-70°C$ and when stored freeze-dried at $4°C$. Stability is enhanced by the addition of proteins to the suspending medium. $MgSO_4$ appears to improve the thermostability of the virus.

RV is inactivated by detergents and organic solvents, since the viral envelope contains lipid. The effects of these and other chemicals have been extensively reviewed elsewhere (Norrby, 1969; Herrmann, 1979; Frey, 1994).

Antigenic Characteristics

Only one serotype of rubella virus has been identified. Early work on RV identified haemagglutinating (HA), complement-fixing, platelet aggregating and haemolytic activity (Banatvala and Best, 1998). The HA is composed of almost equal proportions of the E1 and E2 glycoproteins. Methods for producing HA and complement-fixing antigens have been reviewed elsewhere (Banatvala and Best, 1998; Best and O'Shea, 1995).

Humoral and cell-mediated responses are produced against all three structural proteins, although E1 appears to immunodominant (Cusi *et al.*, 1989; Chaye *et al.*, 1992). Information on immunoreactive regions within the structural proteins has been obtained using monoclonal antibodies to map epitopes and by measuring antibody reactivity and T cell proliferative responses to synthetic peptides and recombinant proteins. E1 has been shown to have at least six independent linear epitopes including two or three neutralising epitopes within the amino acid region 214–285. However, conformation-dependent epitopes, which may also play an important role in the induction of immune responses, have not been identified. The E2 glycoprotein in the mature virion appears to be relatively inaccessible to the immune response, but a number of B cell epitopes have been identified (Wolinsky *et al.*, 1991; Mitchell *et al.*, 1993). Strain-specific antigens have been identified on E1 and E2 using Western blotting (Dorsett *et al.*, 1985; Cusi *et al.*, 1989). Human sera react with synthetic peptides comprising residues 214–285 of the E1 protein and a recombinant protein containing these epitopes was recognised by most rubella antibody-positive sera (Starkey *et al.*, 1995). At least 17 T cell epitopes have been described on the structural proteins.

Antigenic characteristics of RV have been reviewed in more detail by Chantler *et al.* (2001).

Growth in Cell Cultures

Although humans are the only natural host, RV grows in a wide range of primary and continuous cell cultures (Herrmann, 1979). It induces a CPE only in such continuous cell cultures as RK13 (rabbit kidney), SIRC (rabbit cornea), and Vero (VMK), provided that conditions are controlled carefully. These cell cultures, together with primary VMK cell cultures, have been used most frequently for virus isolation. Virus is identified in primary VMK by interference. Vero cells are useful for virus isolation because they do not produce interferon, and virus can therefore replicate more rapidly to high titre. Since RV does not produce CPE in all sublines of Vero cells, passage into another cell line has been used for virus identification. Although RV produced a characteristic CPE in RK13 and SIRC cells, the virus may be identified more reliably in both these and Vero cell cultures by immunofluorescence (IF) or polymerase chain reaction (PCR) (p 446). The CPE has been shown to be due to rubella-induced caspase-dependent apoptosis in a number of continuous cell lines (Hofmann *et al.*, 1999; Duncan *et al.*, 2000). The exact mechanism of apoptosis has not been elucidated, but it is dependent on virus replication and is initiated within 12 h of infection (Pugachev and Frey, 1998; Hoffman *et al.*, 1999; Cooray *et al.*, 2003). Recent work suggests that the p53 pathway is not involved (Domegan and Atkins 2002; Cooray S, Jin L and Best JM, unpublished results).

BHK-21 and Vero cell cultures are used extensively for producing high titres of RV, which are required for use as antigens in serological tests (Best and O'Shea, 1995).

Rubella-induced interference is probably associated with the interferon pathway, although interferon is not always detected in infected cell cultures. RV also induces intrinsic interference, i.e. resistance to superinfection by high multiplicities of Newcastle disease virus in human fibroblasts, induced by the viral genome.

The growth of RV in cell cultures and organ cultures has been reviewed by Herrmann (1979) and Banatvala and Best (1990).

Pathogenicity for Animals

RV infects rhesus (*Cercopithicus aethiops*), vervet (*Macaca mulatta*) and *Erythrocebus patas* monkeys, marmosets (*Sanguinus* species), chimpanzees, baboons, suckling mice, hamsters, ferrets and rabbits (reviewed by Herrmann, 1979; Banatvala and Best, 1990). Monkeys usually develop a subclinical infection with viraemia, virus excretion and an immune response, similar to that in humans (p 436). Viraemia and humoral and cell-mediated immune responses have been detected in 6–8 week-old BALB/c mice, which remain asymptomatic (Chantler *et al.*, 2001). Persistent infection has been established in suckling mice, adult hamsters, ferrets and rabbits. Vaccinia-expressed E1 and E2 proteins have induced autoantibodies to pituitary cells and autoimmune lymphocytic hypophysitis in Syrian hamsters (Yoon *et al.*, 1992).

Attempts to reproduce the teratogenic effects of RV in an animal model have produced inconsistent results. The monkey is the only animal whose reproductive process is similar to that of humans, but even in these animals results have not been reproducible. Thus, some workers isolated rubella from conceptuses but no malformations were observed. An increased rate of spontaneous abortion and lenticular changes were observed in some studies, whilst others failed to isolate virus or to find evidence of malformation, although they showed that an immune response developed *in utero*. Congenital infection has been reported in rabbits, ferrets and rats, but these reports could not be confirmed, the occurrence of malformations being inconsistent. Insufficient attention was given in these studies to the use of adequate controls and such factors as virus passage history, species adaptation, route of inoculation, nutrition and the effects of increased handling of the animals.

POSTNATALLY ACQUIRED INFECTION

Epidemiology

Humans are the only known hosts for RV, which had a worldwide distribution before the introduction of rubella vaccination programmes (pp 450–454). In temperate climates outbreaks usually occurred in the spring and early summer. Infection is uncommon in pre-school children, but outbreaks involving school-children and young adults living in institutional population groups are common. Women of child-bearing age are often infected as a result of exposure to children within their household or as a result of

occupational exposure. Unlike measles, rubella does not exhibit characteristic periodicity. Occasionally, extensive worldwide pandemics have occurred, e.g. in the early 1940s and again in 1963–1965, when a high incidence was reported in the USA, the UK and Australia. More commonly, rubella exhibits an increased incidence every 3–4 years, although within a particular country epidemics may be localised to certain areas only. Thus, in the UK, extensive outbreaks of rubella occurred in 1978–1979, 1982–1983, 1993 and more recently in 1996 (Figure 12.3). The augmentation of the rubella vaccination programme in 1988, in which measles, mumps and rubella (MMR) vaccine was offered to pre-school children of both sexes (pp 452–453), resulted in a marked reduction in the incidence of rubella, with the lowest-ever number of cases reported in 1992 (Miller *et al.*, 1993). The 1996 outbreak was largely confined to 17–24 year-old males who had never been offered rubella vaccine; about 16% of males in this age group were susceptible. Fortunately, transmission of rubella to pregnant women was limited, since 98–99% were immune, either as a result of naturally acquired infection or vaccination as schoolgirls or postpartum (Miller *et al.*, 1997).

Since rubella is not a notifiable disease in many countries, and the clinical diagnosis is unreliable, seroepidemiological studies provide a more accurate assessment of the incidence of rubella in different age groups and in different geographical areas. Despite serological tests being carried out by different techniques in different laboratories, surveys have produced remarkably consistent results. Thus, in temperate climates before the introduction of rubella vaccination, the proportion of seropositive persons increased progressively with age. In general, about 50% of 9–11 year-old children and about 80–85% of women of childbearing age had rubella antibodies.

Rubella in Developing Countries

Although CRS is now a rare disease in those developed countries which have adopted rubella vaccination programmes, the burden induced by CRS imposes a considerable strain on scarce health and educational resources in many developing countries. Unfortunately, this is insufficiently appreciated. The proportion of susceptible women in many developing countries, although exhibiting considerable variation even within different parts of a country, shows that the proportion of rubella-susceptible women (15–20%) is little different from those in industrialised countries in the pre-vaccine era (Cutts *et al.*, 1997; Robertson *et al.*,

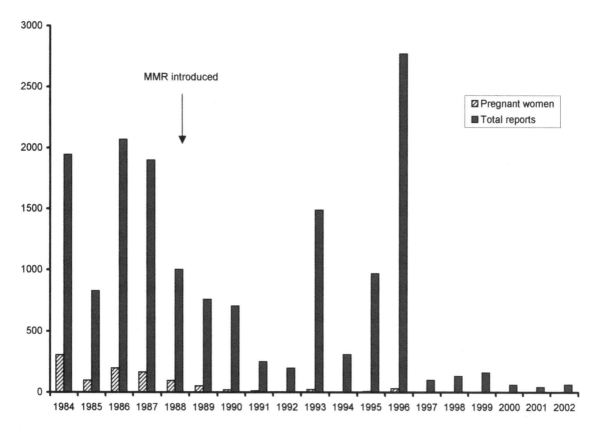

Figure 12.3   Laboratory reports of rubella in England and Wales, 1984–2002. Data kindly provided by the Dr E. Miller, Health Protection Agency, UK

1997). Susceptibility rates of more than 25% were reported from 12 of the 45 developing countries surveyed (Figure 12.4). Particularly high susceptibility rates occurred in island populations, e.g. Trinidad and Tobago and Jamaica, which have now adopted rubella vaccination programmes (p 454).

Although outbreaks of rubella may not always be recognised in developing countries, or rubella-induced rashes misdiagnosed, the incidence of CRS has recently been reported to have been considerably higher (range 0.6–2.2/1000 live births) than during the early years of the rubella vaccination programme in the UK (0.14/1000 during epidemics; at other times, 0.08/1000). Mathematical modelling from five WHO regions, excluding Europe, estimated that there were approximately 236 000 cases of CRS in developing countries during non-epidemic years; following epidemics the number might show as much as a 10-fold increase (Salisbury and Savinykh, 1991).

Clinical and Virological Features of Primary Infection

Clinical Features

Rubella is spread mostly by droplets via the respiratory route. High concentrations of virus ($> 10^5$ TCID$_{50}$/0.1 ml) may be excreted, but close and prolonged contact is usually required for virus to be transmitted to susceptible persons. The epithelium of the buccal mucosa and the lymphoid tissue of the nasopharynx and upper respiratory tract probably represent the site of initial virus replication, following which rubella spreads to the lymphatic system and establishes a systemic infection. It is likely that mononuclear cells are involved in dissemination of virus to different parts of the body, although extracellular virus may be detected in serum.

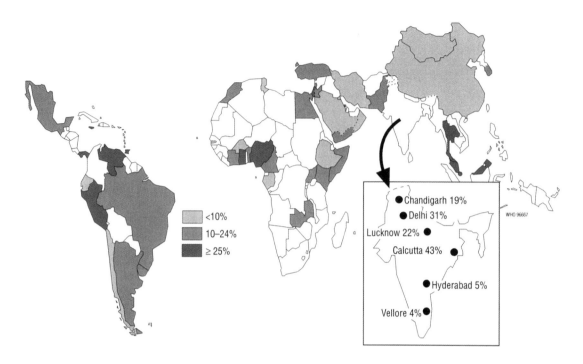

Figure 12.4   Rubella susceptibility in women of childbearing age: selected studies in developing countries prior to use of vaccine. The designations employed and the presentation of material on this map do not imply the expression of any opinion whatsoever on the part of the World Health Organization concerning the legal status of any country, territory, city or area or of its authorities, or concerning the delimitation of its frontiers or boundaries. Dotted lines represent approximate border lines for which there may not yet be full agreement. Reproduced by permission of the World Health Organization from Cutts *et al.* (1997)

Rubella has an incubation period of 13–20 days, following which the characteristic rash may appear. Lymphadenopathy may appear up to a week before the rash and persist for 10–14 days after the rash has disappeared. Lymphadenopathy may be generalised, but the suboccipital, postauricular and cervical lymph nodes are affected most frequently. Among children, onset is usually abrupt with the appearance of rash and constitutional symptoms usually mild or absent. The rash is at first discrete, and is in the form of pinpoint macular lesions. It appears first on the face and spreads rapidly to the trunk and then to the limbs. Lesions may coalesce, but the rash seldom lasts for more than 3 days; in many cases it is fleeting. Adults may experience a prodromal phase with such constitutional features as malaise or fever for a day or two before rash develops. At this time an erythematous pinpoint enanthem may be visible on the soft palate. Although the mechanism by which RV induces rash has not been established, an immunopathological mechanism is suggested by the finding that virus can be isolated from skin biopsies

taken from areas with and without rash as well as from the skin of patients with subclinical infections.

Complications

Joint involvement is the most common complication of naturally acquired rubella as well as rubella vaccination, usually developing as the rash subsides. Although relatively uncommon among prepubertal females and males, it may occur in up to 70% of postpubertal females. Symptoms may vary in severity from a transient stiffness of the joints to an arthritis with pain, swelling and limitation of movement. This usually lasts for 3–4 days, but may occasionally persist for up to 1 month. The finger joints, wrists, knees and ankles are most frequently affected. Arthralgia may be the result of direct viral invasion of the synovium, since virus has been isolated from joint aspirates of patients with naturally acquired rubella and vaccinees with vaccine-induced

Table 12.2 Differential diagnosis of postnatal rubella in different geographical regions

Virus infection	Geographical distribution								Key features
	Africa	Asia	Australia	Europe	North America	Central America	South America	Pacific	
Rubella	+	+	+	+	+	+	+	+	
Parvovirus B19	+	+	+	+	+	+	+	+	Erythema infectiosum
Human herpes viruses 6 and 7	+	+	+	+	+	+	+	+	Exanthem subitum. Predominantly <2 years
Measles	+	+	+	+	+	+	+	+	Prodrome with cough, conjunctivitis, coryza
Enteroviruses	+	+	+	+	+	+	+	+	Echovirus 9, coxsackie A9 most frequent
Dengue	+	+	+	−	−	+	+	+	Joint and back pain, haemorrhagic complications in children
West Nile	+	+	−	+	+	−	−	−	⎫
Chickungunya	+	+	−	−	−	−	−	−	⎬ Joint pain
Ross River	−	−	+	−	−	−	−	+	⎪
Sindbis	+	+	+	+	−	−	−	−	⎭

Reproduced with permission from Elsevier. Banatvala and Brown (2003), *The Lancet*

arthritis. *In vitro* studies have shown that wild-type and attenuated strains of rubella will replicate in human synovial membrane cell cultures. Immune mechanisms may be involved, however, for in addition to virus, high levels of rubella-specific IgG have been detected in joint aspirates. This suggests that joint symptoms may be mediated by immune complexes; indeed, the presence of immune complexes in the sera of vaccinees has been associated with a high incidence of joint symptoms. Hormonal factors may also be involved, since in addition to being commonest in postpubertal females, joint symptoms are most likely to develop within 7 days of the onset of the menstrual cycle in vaccinees. It has been suggested that rubella or rubella vaccination might be a cause of chronic joint disease, as RV or its antigens have been detected in the synovial fluid or synovium of patients with rheumatoid arthritis and sero-negative arthritis (rheumatoid factor-negative), but more recent studies have failed to confirm these findings. RV may persist in the synovium, as virus has very occasionally been detected in both the synovial fluid and cells of patients with chronic joint disease, including some who were immunosuppressed (Bosma *et al.*, 1998).

Very rarely rubella is associated with other complications. A post-infectious encephalopathy may develop in 1 in 5000–10000 cases within a week of onset of rash. In contrast with measles, the prognosis is usually good, with recovery within 7–30 days, and death is rare (Chantler *et al.*, 2001). The CSF usually contains cells, mostly lymphocytes, but CSF protein levels are normal. The encephalopathy may be immune-mediated, since infectious virus or its nucleic acid has been detected only rarely (Frey, 1997) and is not associated with demyelination or inflammatory damage, which is present in other post-infectious encephalitides. Guillain–Barré syndrome is an even rarer complication of rubella.

Thrombocytopenia is also a rare complication of rubella, in which a purpuric rash, epistaxis, haematuria and gastrointestinal bleeding have been reported.

Differential Diagnosis

In up to 25% of cases, rubella infection is subclinical. Conversely, typical rubelliform rashes may result from infection by other viruses (e.g. enteroviruses, measles, HHV-6 and 7). Infections by such viruses as the human parvovirus (B19) and some arboviruses (e.g. Dengue, Chikungunya and Ross River viruses) may cause both rubelliform rashes and arthralgia (Table 12.2). Because clinical diagnosis is unreliable, it is essential that all women who have been exposed to, or develop, rubella-like illnesses in pregnancy be assessed virologically (pp 444–445); a past history of rubella without laboratory confirmation of the diagnosis must never be accepted as indicative of previous infection and consequent immunity.

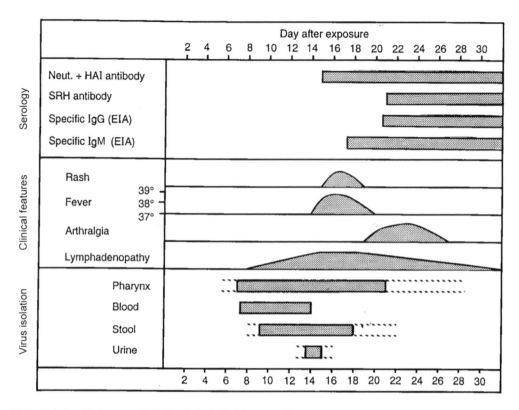

Figure 12.5 Relationship between clinical and virological features of postnatally acquired rubella. Reproduced from Banatvala and Best (1998) published by Edward Arnold, London

Virological and Immunological Features

The relationship between the clinical and virological features of infection is shown in Figure 12.5. Patients are potentially infectious over a prolonged period; pharyngeal excretion may be present for up to 1 week before the onset of rash, and for 7–10 days thereafter. Although virus may be recovered from the stools and urine, excretion from these sites is more transient. Such specimens are therefore less suitable for virus isolation and do not play an important role in the transmission of virus. Viraemia is present for about a week before the onset of rash but, as rubella antibodies develop, viraemia ceases. IgG antibodies detected by enzyme immunoassay (EIA) and single radial haemolysis (SRH) usually develop 6–7 days after onset of rash, while antibodies detected by HAI and neutralisation appear a few days earlier. Differing results have been obtained by the various workers who have examined IgG subclasses. Thomas and Morgan-Capner (1988) compared the use of different sources of rubella antigens in EIAs and reported IgG_1 in all sera

containing rubella antibodies detectable by SRH or latex agglutination (LA) and IgG_3 in most sera from cases of recent naturally acquired rubella. IgG_4 has been detected in sera collected many years after infection.

Reinfection

Natural infection is followed by a very high order of protection from reinfection. However, reinfection does occur and is defined by a significant rise in rubella IgG concentration and/or detection of specific IgM in a patient with pre-existing antibodies (p 446). It is more likely to occur in those with vaccine-induced immunity than in those who have been naturally infected. It may be difficult to distinguish between primary infection and reinfection, particularly if blood was not obtained shortly after contact or if sera taken prior to contact (e.g. for screening purposes) are not available.

Reinfection would provide a hazard to the fetus if associated with viraemia, but this has only rarely been documented. Several well-documented cases of rubella reinfection have been reported in which RV was isolated from the products of conception or children with congenital rubella were born (Best *et al.*, 1989), although previous reports suggested that asymptomatic reinfection in early pregnancy was unlikely to be associated with fetal infection. Morgan-Capner *et al.* (1991) have calculated that the risk of fetal infection is approximately 8% following reinfection in the first 16 weeks of pregnancy, but fetal malformations are rare. Rubella reinfection is not associated with a lack of neutralising antibodies or a specific defect in rubella-specific lymphoproliferative responses (O'Shea *et al.*, 1994), but a failure to produce epitope-specific antibodies is possible. RV strains isolated from cases of reinfection do not appear to have sequence changes in the E1 ORF (Bosma *et al.*, 1996; Frey *et al.*, 1998). The diagnosis of rubella reinfection is discussed on p 446 and reinfection following rubella vaccination on p 449.

CONGENITALLY ACQUIRED INFECTION

Pathogenesis

If acquired at an early gestational age, rubella is likely to induce a generalised and persistent fetal infection, resulting in multisystem disease. This is a reflection of the inefficiency of the placenta to act as a barrier as well as the fact that the fetus is unable to mount an immune response to eliminate virus. Töndury and Smith (1966) conducted classic histopathological studies, which demonstrated the probable mechanism by which RV induces fetal damage. The earliest lesions are found in the placenta, which is almost certainly infected during the maternal viraemic phase. However, since rubella is also excreted via the cervix for at least 6 days after the onset of rash, and since it is possible that virus may multiply elsewhere in the genital tract following an acute infection, placental infection by direct contact from an ascending genital infection cannot be excluded. Töndury and Smith (1966) suggested that rubella enters the fetus via the chorion, since necrotic changes to the epithelial cells and in the endothelial lining of the blood vessels were present as early as the 10th day after maternal rash. Damaged endothelial cells may then be desquamated into the lumen of the vessel and transported into the fetal circulation in the form of virus-infected 'emboli', to infect the various fetal organs. Damage to fetal endothelial cells may be extensive and is the result of

viral replication rather than any immunopathological mechanism, since extensive lesions are present at an early gestational age, before fetal immune mechanisms are sufficiently mature to be activated. The marked absence of any inflammatory cellular response following rubella during the early gestational period was characteristic. Anomalies were present in 68% of 57 fetuses when maternal rubella was contracted during the first trimester. Eighty per cent were abnormal when rubella was contracted during the first month of pregnancy, with sporadic foci of cellular damage in the heart, lens, inner ear, teeth and skeletal muscle. In addition to virus-induced tissue necrosis, RV induces a retardation in cell division. It has been suggested that this is due to a rubella-specific protein, which reduces the rate of mitosis in infected cells. If this occurs during the critical phase of organogenesis, the organs will contain fewer cells than those of uninfected infants and multiple developmental defects are likely to occur. Although the rubella-specific protein has not been identified, human embryonic cells persistently infected with rubella *in vitro* have an altered responsiveness to the growth-promoting properties of epidermal growth factor and a decreased capacity for the synthesis of collagen (Yoneda *et al.*, 1986). It has also been demonstrated that rubella induces caspase-dependent apoptosis (p 431) and this may contribute to the pathogenesis of congenital rubella. Additional damage to such malformed organs as the liver, myocardium and organ of Corti results from the damage caused to endothelial cells, which may result in haemorrhages in small blood vessels, causing tissue necrosis over a prolonged time.

Viral antigens and RNA can almost always be detected in the products of conception of virologically-confirmed cases of maternal rubella during the first trimester (Cradock-Watson *et al.*, 1989; Bosma *et al.*, 1995a). This demonstrates that the fetus is almost invariably infected regardless of when maternal infection occurred during this period. Should such pregnancies proceed to term, the rubella-infected infants would almost certainly be excreting RV at birth and for some months thereafter. However, virus is isolated infrequently from neonates whose mothers acquired rubella after the first trimester, probably because fetal immune mechanisms can then be activated and effectively terminate infection. That fetal infection occurs following post-first trimester rubella, however, is apparent from the finding that serological evidence of fetal infection has been obtained in 25–33% of infants whose mothers acquired maternal rubella between weeks 16 and 28 of gestation (Cradock-Watson *et al.*, 1980; Miller *et al.*, 1982).

Virus Persistence

Following intrauterine infection in early pregnancy, RV persists throughout gestation and can be isolated from most organs obtained at autopsy from infants who die in early infancy with severe and generalised infections. In infancy virus may also be recovered from the nasopharyngeal secretions, urine, stools, CSF and tears. RV can be isolated from nasopharyngeal secretions of most neonates with severe congenitally acquired disease, but by the age of 3 months the proportion excreting virus declines to 50–60% and by 9–12 months to 10% (Cooper and Krugman, 1967). During the first few weeks after birth, those with severe disease may excrete high concentrations of virus and readily transmit infection to rubella-susceptible contacts. RV may persist in infants with congenitally acquired disease in some sites for even longer. Thus, RV has been recovered from a cataract removed from a 3 year-old child and detected by PCR in lens aspirates from children with CRS up to the age of 12 months (Bosma *et al.*, 1995a). RV has also been detected in the CSF of children with CNS involvement up to the age of 18 months. Rubella antigen was detected by IF in the thyroid from a 5 year-old child with Hashimoto's disease, and by co-cultivation techniques RV was recovered from the brain of a child who developed rubella panencephalitis at the age of 12 years. Experimental studies have shown that, within the CNS, the astrocyte is the main cell type in which virus replicates, high levels of virus being expressed. Intrauterine infection involving these cells may perhaps induce focal areas of necrosis resulting in the pattern of neurological deficit observed in CRS (Chantler *et al.*, 1995).

The mechanism by which RV persists throughout gestation and for a limited period during the first year of life has not been clearly established. Suggested mechanisms include defects in cell-mediated immunity (CMI), poor interferon synthesis and the possibility that a limited number of infected fetal cells give rise to infected clones which persist for a limited period. It has also been suggested that selective immune tolerance to the RV E1 protein may play a role (Mauracher *et al.*, 1993). Studies *in vitro* show that RV replicates in T lymphocytes and macrophages and can also persist in B lymphocytes, causing inhibition of host-cell protein synthesis. Infection of macrophages may interfere with their interactions with T cells.

Postnatally acquired rubella causes a transient reduction in lymphocyte responses to phytohaemagglutinin as well as a decrease in the numbers of T cells. CRS might be expected to cause an even greater reduction in responsiveness. Indeed, significantly diminished lymphoproliferative responses to phytohaemagglutinin and rubella antigen, as well as diminished interferon synthesis, have been demonstrated in 40 congenitally infected children aged 1–12 years (Buimovici-Klein *et al.*, 1979). Impairment of CMI responses was related to the gestational age at which maternal infection occurred, and was greatest in infants whose mothers acquired rubella in the first 8 weeks of pregnancy. Hosking and colleagues (1983) suggested that children with nerve deafness due to CRS could be distinguished from those with immunity due to postnatally acquired rubella by their failure to produce lymphoproliferative responses to rubella antigen. O'Shea *et al.* (1992) reported that 10 of 13 (80%) children with CRS under the age of 3 years failed to mount a lymphoproliferative response. Congenitally infected infants have also been shown to have impaired natural killer cell activity and persistent T cell abnormalities. It is of interest that the defective CMI responses may persist into the second decade of life, well beyond the time when RV can be recovered from accessible sites.

Risks to the Fetus

Maternal Rubella in the First Trimester

Maternal rubella may result in fetal death and spontaneous abortion, the delivery of a severely malformed infant, an infant with minimal damage or a healthy infant. The outcome depends on a combination of factors. These include the level of maternal viraemia, perhaps the genetic susceptibility of fetal cells to rubella infection, but most importantly the gestational age at which maternal infection occurs.

Studies which have included virological confirmation of the diagnoses of maternal rubella and congenital rubella suggest that the incidence of defects following maternal infection in the first trimester is more than 75%, much higher than had hitherto been realised. If maternal rubella is acquired during the first 8 weeks of pregnancy, spontaneous abortion may occur in up to 20% of cases. Figure 12.6 relates the type of rubella-induced congenital anomaly with the gestational age at which infection occurred among 376 infants infected *in utero* during the 1964 USA epidemic. Cardiac and eye defects are likely to result when maternal infection is acquired during the critical phase of organogenesis, in the first 8 weeks of pregnancy, whereas retinopathy and hearing defects

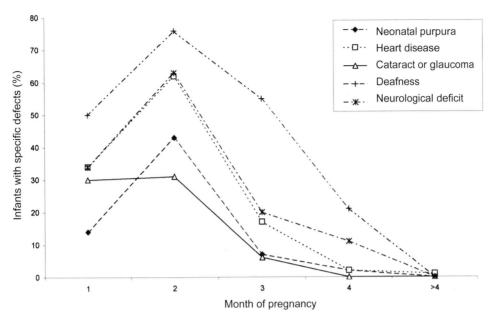

Figure 12.6 Relationship between the gestational age at time of maternal infection and clinical manifestations of congenital rubella. Extrapolated from Cooper *et al.* (1969)

are more evenly distributed throughout the first 16 weeks of gestation.

Risk of Maternal Rubella after the First Trimester

RV is seldom isolated from infants whose mothers acquired rubella after the first trimester, although *in vitro* studies have shown that fetal tissues, regardless of gestational age, are susceptible to infection. Indeed, serological studies confirm that a high proportion of infants are infected following maternal post-first trimester rubella, rubella-specific IgM being detected in 25–33% of infants whose mothers had rubella between the 16th and 20th weeks of pregnancy (Cradock-Watson *et al.*, 1980; Miller *et al.*, 1982). However, because organogenesis is complete by 12 weeks and in more mature fetuses immune responses may limit or terminate infection, such infants rarely have severe or multiple anomalies. The results of four studies conducted in different countries are shown in Table 12.3. Most surveys have shown that deafness and retinopathy, which *per se* does not affect vision,

Table 12.3 Incidence of rubella-induced effects in infants infected *in utero* after the first trimester

	Gestational age (weeks)		
	13–16	17–20	>20
Peckham (1972)[a]	7/73 (10%)	4/40 (10%)	1/11 (9.1%)
Vejtorp and Mansa (1980)[b]	0/4	1/14 (7%)	1/16 (6.2%)
Miller *et al.* (1982)	9/26 (35%)	0/10	0/53
Grillner *et al.* (1983)	4/17 (23%)	2[c]/54 (3.7%)	0/35
Total	20/120 (16.7%)	7/118 (5.9%)	2/115 (1.7%)

[a]These children were normal at birth.
[b]Children followed up for 6 months only.
[c]One additional case of deafness reported since 1983.
Reproduced from Collier and Timbury (1990).

are likely to be the only anomalies commonly associated with post-first trimester rubella (reviewed by Banatvala and Best, 1998). Figure 12.6 shows that deafness is usually the sole clinical manifestation of fetal infection occurring between 13 and 16 weeks, and is relatively common, but deafness or any other defect is only rarely encountered after this time. These findings emphasise the importance of conducting careful follow-up studies on infants with serological evidence of intrauterine infection as a result of maternal infection occurring between 13 and 16 weeks, particular importance being directed towards the recognition of hearing defects.

Risks of Preconceptual Rubella

If conception occurs shortly after the appearance of rash, there should be little risk of the conceptus being infected, because the development of the rash coincides with the immune response and the termination of viraemia. However, because RV may persist elsewhere after the onset of rash, e.g. in the genital tract, infection of the conceptus via this route is a possibility. Although occasional case reports prior to 1984 suggested that maternal infection occurring as long as 21 days prior to conception resulted in intrauterine infection, it is encouraging that the definitive study conducted in Germany and the UK showed that preconceptual rubella did not result in transmission of RV to the fetus. Thus, there was no serological or clinical evidence of intrauterine infection in 38 infants whose mothers' rash appeared before or within 11 days after their last menstrual period (LMP). However, fetal infection occurred when there was an interval of 12 days between LMP and rash and all 10 mothers who developed rash 3–6 weeks after their LMP transmitted infection to their fetuses (Enders et al., 1988).

Clinical Features

The frequency and importance of congenital defects involving the heart, eyes and ears were emphasised in the early retrospective as well as in most prospective studies. However, following the extensive 1963–1964 epidemic in the USA, as well as in subsequent epidemics in other parts of the world, a much broader range of rubella-induced congenital anomalies was observed. This phenomenon is more likely to be due to more careful and prolonged observation than to any change in the biological behaviour or teratogenic potential of the virus. Thus, careful examination of the case notes of infants with congenitally acquired disease who were born before this outbreak showed that such anomalies as thrombocytopenic purpura and osteitis occurred fairly frequently, even though not recorded in the literature. In addition, careful and prolonged follow-up studies showed that CRS was not a static disease, since some features of intrauterine infection might not be apparent for months or indeed years (e.g. perceptive deafness, IDDM).

Clinical features of the congenital rubella syndrome (CRS) have been categorised into those which are transient or permanent, some of which may be delayed to appear months or even years later (Table 12.4). The National Congenital Surveillance Programme in the UK classify suspected cases of congenital rubella according to the criteria shown in Table 12.5. Criteria used in the USA were updated in 2001 (Centers for Disease Control, 2001a).

Transient Anomalies

Transient anomalies, usually present during the first few weeks of life, do not recur and are not associated with permanent sequelae. Their pathogenesis has not been established, but such features as intrauterine growth retardation (small-for-dates babies), cloudy cornea, thrombocytopenic purpura (Figure 12.7), hepatosplenomegaly and haemolytic anaemia are common. About 60% of infected infants fall below the 10th growth percentile and 90% below the 50th. The above features, which often result from infection acquired at an early gestational age, seldom occur without such other manifestations of congenital disease as heart and eye defects, and reflect extensive infection, which may result in high perinatal mortality rates. Infants with thrombocytopenic purpura have platelet counts of $3–100 \times 10^9/1$ (normal $= 310 \pm 68 \times 10^9/1$). This is associated with a decrease in the number of megakaryocytes in the bone marrow, although they are morphologically normal. If severely affected infants survive, their platelet count rises spontaneously during the first few weeks of life; rarely, infants may die from such complications of thrombocytopenia as intracranial haemorrhage.

Bony lesions may be present in about 20% of congenitally infected infants. The metaphyseal portion of the long bones are usually involved and radiologically appear as areas of translucency. These lesions, which are due to a disturbance in bone growth rather than an inflammatory response, usually resolve without residual sequelae within the first 1–2 months of age.

Table 12.4 Clinical features of congenital rubella syndrome

	Early transient features	Permanent features, some recognised late	Use in surveillance*
Ocular defects			
Cataracts (uni-/bilateral)		+	A
Glaucoma		+	A
Pigmentary retinopathy		+	A
Microphthalmia		+	
Iris hypoplasia		+	
Cloudy cornea	+		
Auditory defects			
Sensorineural deafness (uni-/bilateral)		+	A
Cardiovascular defects			
Persistent ductus arteriosus		+	A
Pulmonary artery stenosis		+	A
Ventricular septal defect		+	A
Myocarditis	+		
Central nervous system			
Microcephaly		+	B
Pyschomotor retardation		+	
Meningoencephalitis	+		B
Behavioural disorders			
Speech disorders			
Intrauterine growth retardation	+		
Thrombocytopenia, with purpura	+		B
Hepatitis/hepatosplenomegaly	+		B
Bone 'lesions'	+		B
Pneumonitis	+		
Lymphadenopathy	+		
Diabetes mellitus		+	
Thyroid disorders		+	
Progressive rubella panencephalitis		+	

*For surveillance, a clinically confirmed case is defined as one in which two complications from group A or group B or one from group A or one from group B are present (World Health Organization, 1999).
Adapted from Banatvala and Brown (2003), *The Lancet*. Reproduced with permission from Elsevier.

About 25% of infants who present at birth with clinical manifestations of CRS also have CNS involvement, this usually being in the form of meningoencephalitis. At birth, these infants may be either irritable or lethargic with a full fontanelle and CSF changes consistent with a meningoencephalitis. Although about 25% of infants presenting at birth with a severe neonatal encephalitis may, by the age of 18 months, be severely retarded and have communication problems, ataxia or spastic diplegia, some infants progress well neurologically despite poor development during their first few months of life.

Late-onset disease. Between the ages of about 3 and 12 months, some congenitally infected infants may develop a chronic rubella-like rash, persistent diarrhoea and pneumonitis, which is referred to as 'late-onset disease'. Mortality is high, but some infants improve dramatically if treated with corticosteroids. Circulating immune complexes are probably responsible for inducing this syndrome (reviewed by Hanshaw *et al.*, 1985).

Permanent Defects

The major permanent defects which may be present at birth are cardiac and ocular defects and damage to the organ of Corti. These and other defects are listed in Table 12.4. Cardiovascular and ocular anomalies provide the greatest problems.

Cardiac defects. Cardiac defects are responsible for much of the high perinatal mortality associated with

Table 12.5 Congenital rubella: case classification criteria (Miller *et al.*, 1994)

Congenital rubella infection	
No rubella defects but congenital infection confirmed by isolation of virus, or detection of specific IgM or persistent IgG in infant	
Congenital rubella syndrome	
Confirmed	Typical rubella defect(s) plus virus-specific IgM or persistent IgG in infant; or two or more rubella defects plus confirmed maternal infection in pregnancy
Compatible	Two or more rubella defects with inconclusive laboratory data; or single rubella defect plus confirmed maternal infection in pregnancy
Possible	Compatible clinical findings with inconclusive laboratory data, e.g. single defect plus probable maternal infection in pregnancy
Unclassified	Insufficient information to confirm or exclude

Reproduced by permission of the PHLS Communicable Disease Surveillance Centre ©1994 PHLS; and from Banatvala and Best (1998), ©1998 Edward Arnold.

CRS, the commonest lesions being the persistence of patent ductus arteriosus, proximal (valvular) or peripheral pulmonary artery stenosis or a ventricular septal defect. In association with such anomalies, a neonatal myocarditis may occasionally occur. RV may also cause proliferation and damage to the intimal lining of the arteries and this may cause obstructive lesions of the pulmonary and renal arteries.

Ocular defects. Most of the classical ocular defects seen in CRS were described by Gregg (1941), who drew particular attention to the pigmented retinopathy and cataract. Although usually present at birth, cataracts may not be visible until several weeks later. They are unilateral in about 50% of patients, and may be subtotal, consisting of a dense pearly white central opacity (Figure 12.8), or total, with a more uniform density throughout the lens. Microphthalmia may be present in eyes with cataract. Glaucoma occurs much less frequently than cataract, but glaucoma and cataract do not seem to be present in the same eye. Retinopathy is present in about 50% of congenitally infected infants and its presence may provide a useful clinical diagnostic marker. Retinopathy is not the result of an inflammatory response but is due to a defect in pigmentation and usually involves the macular areas. Hyperpigmented and hypopigmented areas give the retina a 'salt and pepper' appearance. Chronic uveitis, choroidal neovascularisation, corneal hydrops and keratoconus have also been described.

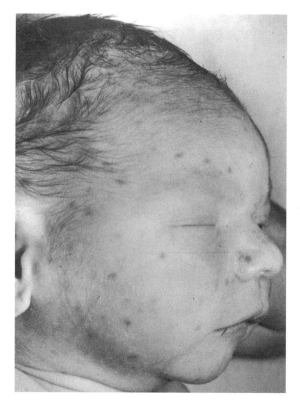

Figure 12.7 Purpuric rash in newborn infant with congenitally acquired rubella, who was subsequently found to have congenital heart disease and cataract. Reproduced from Banatvala and Best (1998) published by Edward Arnold, London

The mechanisms involved may include damage induced by viral persistence causing reduced cell growth rate and lifespan, virally induced vascular damage or autoimmune phenomena (reviewed by Arnold *et al.*, 1994).

Hearing defects. Rubella-induced deafness may be unilateral, with no characteristic audiometric pattern. Prior to the introduction of vaccination programmes, CRS probably represented the commonest cause of congenital deafness in most developed countries, its impact being insufficiently appreciated since there may have been no history of maternal rubella. Deafness may be the only anomaly present, particularly if maternal infection occurred after the first trimester. Thus, in a study on a large number of children aged 6 months to 4 years who attended the Nuffield Hearing and Speech Centre in London, it was estimated that

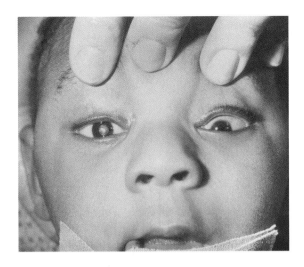

Figure 12.8 Congenital rubella cataract in a 9 month-old infant. Cataract was also present in the left eye but was removed surgically. Reproduced from Banatvala and Best (1984) published by Hodder Arnold, London

about 15% of all cases of sensorineural deafness were the result of CRS.

Late-onset Manifestations

Some defects may take months or years before becoming apparent, but persist indefinitely. Failure to recognise them may not merely be the result of difficulty in their detection, for there is evidence to show that such defects as perceptive deafness, some CNS anomalies and some ocular defects may actually develop later or become progressively more severe.

Hearing defects. Audiological examination has shown that some infants, although having apparently normal hearing at 9–12 months of age, are found to have severe sensorineural deafness a few months later. Improvements in technology, such as otoacoustic emissions and auditory brainstem responses, may be of value in assessing hearing defects in early infancy (van Straaten *et al.*, 1996).

Insulin-dependent diabetes mellitus (IDDM). IDDM (juvenile-onset; type 1) is the most frequent endocrine disorder among children with congenital rubella. It was thought originally to be a rare complication of congenital rubella, but it is now recognised that clinical manifestations may be delayed until adolescence or adult life. A follow-up study of patients in New South Wales who were born with CRS in the 1940s showed that 20% eventually developed IDDM. Follow-up studies in New York on children, most of whom were infected *in utero* during the 1963–1964 epidemic, have shown that 30 of 242 (12.4%) had developed IDDM, although a higher proportion (20%) had pancreatic islet cell antibodies, suggesting that more of these patients were likely to develop IDDM (reviewed in Burke *et al.*, 1985). The mean age of children developing IDDM in this US study was 9 years, while all of the Australian patients were in their 20s (reviewed by Banatvala and Best, 1990). Lymphocytic infiltration of the pancreas of an infant with CRS but without IDDM may suggest that RV can initiate the train of events, which subsequently results in IDDM in later life. RV has been shown to induce a depression of immunoreactive secreted insulin in human fetal islet cells without being cytolytic (Numazaki *et al.*, 1990). Several experimental studies support the role for autoimmune mechanisms. Thus, Karounos *et al.* (1993) showed that immunoreactive epitopes in the RV capsid shared antigenicity (molecular mimicry) with islet β cell protein. Ou *et al.* (1999), using clones of T cells from patients with CRS, have described HLA-restricted cytotoxic responses to a β cell autoantigen, GAD65. The HLA types in patients with IDDM are typical of those with autoimmune disease, there being a significant increase in prevalence of HLA-DR3 (reviewed in Burke *et al.*, 1985). Islet cell antibodies have been detected in 20% of these patients; these antibodies have a cytotoxic effect on cultured islet cells and predict the diabetic state. The mechanism by which RV may trigger autoimmune responses remains to be established, since studies on pathogenesis are limited by the lack of a suitable animal model.

Other endocrine disorders. Thyroid autoantibodies have been detected in 20–40% cases of CRS, but it is not clear if CRS is associated with thyroid dysfunction. Growth hormone deficiency has also been reported in CRS, suggesting pituitary dysfunction.

Central nervous system. The progressive nature of congenital acquired rubella is emphasised by reports that occasionally children with previously clinically stable congenitally acquired disease may develop a widespread subacute panencephalitis, which is invariably fatal (Frey, 1997; Chantler *et al.*, 2001). About 50 cases have been described in association with CRS and very rare cases following postnatally acquired rubella. Clinical and laboratory features are analogous to measles-induced subacute sclerosing panencephalitis, since, in addition to intellectual deterioration, spasticity and ataxis occur. Histological studies revealed a panencephalitis with a perivascular inflammatory response as well as a vasculitis. RV has been isolated from the brains of such patients and has also been recovered from their lymphocytes. Rubella antigens have not been detected by immunofluorescence in sections of brain. High levels of rubella-specific IgG and, occasionally, IgM may be present in the serum, whilst in the CSF there are elevated levels of protein and immunoglobulin, and oligoclonal bands are found. There is also a high CSF:serum rubella antibody titre ratio. It has been postulated that post-rubella panencephalitis may be a disease mediated by immune complexes or by RV-mediated autoreactivity to brain antigens.

Outlook for children with congenital rubella. As a result of the extent and severity of rubella-induced congenital malformations, any surviving children require continuous and specialised medical care, rehabilitation and education. However, assessment of 25 year-old patients whose mothers acquired rubella during the extensive epidemic in Australia in the early 1940s showed that many had developed far better than had been anticipated in early childhood, despite the presence of hearing and eye defects. Most were of average intelligence, employed, and some had married and had normal children (Menser *et al.*, 1967). In contrast, studies on children with CRS resulting from the 1963–1964 US epidemic showed that they had fared less favourably (Cooper, 1975). This difference is probably due to the survival of children with some of the more severe manifestations of congenital infection, which reflects more modern, vigorous and sophisticated methods of treatment that were not available previously. Other studies have reported a prevalence of diabetes, thyroid disorders, early menopause and osteoporosis that is higher than that in general population (Munroe, 1999; Forrest *et al.*, 2002).

LABORATORY TECHNIQUES AND DIAGNOSIS

Serological Assessment of Women Exposed to or Developing Rubella-like Illnesses in Pregnancy

It is essential that, before attempting to interpret serological results on sera from women who have been exposed to or who have developed rubella-like illness in pregnancy, accurate information is obtained relating to date and duration of exposure, and date of onset of illness, including the presence and distribution of rash, lymphadenopathy and arthralgia. A history of rubella vaccination as well as results of previous rubella antibody screening tests, together with the techniques by which they were carried out, are also relevant.

Blood should be collected from pregnant women with features of a rubella-like illness as soon as possible after the onset of symptoms. A significant rise in antibody titre can often be detected within 7 days, although occasionally the response may be delayed, in which case it may be necessary to test additional blood samples at 3–4 day intervals. Although HAI antibodies may be present during the acute phase of the illness, antibodies detected by SRH and the IgG response detectable by EIA may not be present until 6–7 days after the onset of rash (see Figure 12.5). Tests for rubella-specific IgM should also be carried out; these tests are of particular value when patients present in the post-acute phase of their illness, at which time IgG antibody levels may already have reached their maximum. It is important to stress that, regardless of technique employed, no particular titre of antibody can be regarded as indicative of recent or current infection. Although the presence of rubella-specific IgM used to be considered indicative of a recent primary infection, it is now recognised that, if sensitive techniques are employed, low and transient concentrations of rubella-specific IgM may persist for several years and may also be detected in reinfection. Such findings, and the occurrence of occasional false positive rubella IgM results, emphasise the importance of assessing clinical and serological data carefully before making a diagnosis of primary rubella infection, the consequences of which may result in termination of a precious pregnancy (Best *et al.*, 2002).

Women who give a history of exposure to a rubella-like illness are much more likely to acquire infection if exposure is close and prolonged, e.g. within their own household or, in the case of a school teacher, to children in class. Although rubella contacts may give a history of rubella vaccination or have been found to have rubella antibodies when screened during a previous pregnancy, it is still advisable to investigate such persons serologically if they have been exposed recently to rubella-like illness. Thus, some vaccinees may fail to develop an immune response following rubella vaccination (p 449) and very occasionally the result of a screening test may be recorded incorrectly. In addition, rubella screening, if carried out by HAI, may be unreliable, giving rise to false positive results (p 445). Blood should be obtained from pregnant women for rubella antibody screening when they first book at antenatal clinics. It is advisable to store these specimens for at least a year, so that this pre-exposure specimen can be tested in parallel with later serum samples should a patient subsequently give a history of exposure to a rubella-like illness. In addition, should an infant be delivered with clinical features compatible with an intrauterine infection, serum obtained in early pregnancy can be tested in parallel with that obtained after delivery and the infant's cord or neonatal blood (Department of Health, 2003; http://www.phls.org.uk/topics_az/rashes/rash.pdf). Tests may be carried out for evidence of congenital infection, not only by rubella but also by such organisms as cytomegalovirus, parvovirus B19 and *Toxoplasma gondii*.

If a history of exposure to a rubella-like illness is given prior to attending the first antenatal clinic, or if no earlier blood sample is available, it is important that blood be obtained as soon as possible after contact. The presence of antibodies in such a sample suggests that any antibody present is long-standing, resulting from infection in the past, provided that the sample was obtained well within the incubation period of rubella (e.g. within 10–14 days of last exposure). Nevertheless, it is advisable to collect more blood in 7–10 days, to ensure that there is no change in rubella antibody concentration. Patients who present for virological investigations some time after exposure to possible rubella are more difficult to assess, since it cannot be determined whether antibody is long-standing or the result of recently acquired infection. This can be established, however, by testing sera for rubella-specific IgM. Women who are seronegative should be followed up for 1 month after the date of the last contact to ensure that seroconversion does not occur. Many of these women experience considerable anxiety during this period, which may be allayed by testing the index case for rubella IgM in serum or oral fluid (see p 446) to determine whether or not the infection was indeed rubella. Patients who have been followed up but who remain seronegative should be offered rubella vaccination postpartum.

Serological Techniques Used for Rubella Antibody Screening

Extensive rubella antibody screening of adult women is carried out in order to identify susceptibles who require vaccination. EIA, SRH and latex agglutination (LA) are the techniques used most frequently for screening purposes. HAI is not recommended, since it is time consuming, labour intensive and false positive results may occur, this being due to failure to remove all serum lipoprotein inhibitors from test sera (PHLS, 1988).

Many tests for rubella antibody screening are available commercially. EIAs are used widely because they are readily automated and can be used in automated antenatal screening. LA has the advantage of providing a result within a few minutes and may be used to confirm negative results. SRH is still used in some UK laboratories, commercially available reagents being used to prepare plates in the laboratory. These techniques have been described in detail by Best and O'Shea (1995). Vaccination should be offered to women with antibody concentrations <10–12 IU/ml (Skendzel, 1996) and this is the cut-off in most commercial assays. Negative results should be confirmed using a different assay in order to identify sampling errors and monitor the first assay (Department of Health, 2003; http://www.phls.org.uk/topics_az/rashes/rash.pdf;). Some women fail to produce antibody levels >10 IU/ml even after several vaccinations. Many laboratories therefore consider women with a well-documented history of more than one vaccination to be immune, if low levels of antibodies are detectable by two reliable assays.

Rubella-specific IgG antibodies have been detected in oral fluid by IgG capture radioimmunoassay (GACRIA) (Perry *et al.*, 1993). Thus, oral fluid may be used instead of serum for seroepidemiological studies, especially those involving children and in developing countries (Eckstein *et al.*, 1996).

Serological Techniques Used for Diagnosis

Detection of Rubella-specific IgM

Serological methods are used for the diagnosis of rubella acquired postnatally, since RV is slow to grow and difficult to identify in cell cultures. A diagnosis is usually made by detection of rubella-specific IgM, but in the case of a pregnant woman it is advisable to confirm that diagnosis by demonstrating a rise in specific IgG concentration or by detecting specific IgM in a second serum. Rubella-specific IgM may be detected by commercial EIAs. The M-antibody capture format is generally preferred to indirect assays, for which serum pretreatment is required due to the possibility of false positive results due to IgM antiglobulins, such as rheumatoid factor. Care should be taken to ensure that the test employed has a high level of sensitivity and specificity (Hudson and Morgan-Capner, 1996). The performance of commercial assays may differ, but it is possible usually to detect specific IgM antibodies within 4 days of onset of rash and for 4–12 weeks thereafter.

Detection of a Significant Rise in Antibody Titres

A significant rise in antibody titre can be detected by a quantitative EIA, HAI or LA titration. Seroconversion can be detected by SRH. Although HAI antibodies may develop 1–2 days after onset of symptoms, IgG antibodies detected by EIA, LA or SRH may be delayed until 7–8 days (see Figure 12.5).

Use of Oral Fluid

Rubella-specific IgG and IgM antibodies may be detected in oral fluid using antibody capture immunoassays, and the results correlate well with serum antibodies (Ramsay et al., 1998). The optimum time for detecting specific IgM is 1–5 weeks after onset of illness. Using saliva, it has been possible to demonstrate that rubella-like illnesses in children under 1 year of age are due to other viruses, such as parvovirus B19 (Ramsay et al., 2002). Optimum methods for collection, extraction and preservation of samples have been established (Mortimer and Parry, 1988).

Diagnosis of Reinfection

Rubella reinfection may be diagnosed by a significant rise in rubella IgG concentrations, sometimes to very high levels, or detection of specific IgM in a patient with pre-existing antibodies. If serum samples obtained before reinfection are not available for retesting, evidence of pre-existing antibody may be accepted if there are at least two laboratory reports of antibodies >10 IU/ml obtained by a reliable technique (not HAI). A documented history of rubella vaccination, followed by at least one test for rubella antibodies >10 IU/ml is also acceptable (Best et al., 1989). The rubella-specific IgM response is usually lower and more transient than following primary infection.

It is often possible to distinguish reinfection from primary infection by examining the antigen-binding avidity of specific IgG. Sera taken from cases of recent primary rubella reinfection have low IgG avidity, while sera taken from persons with distant infection, including cases of rubella reinfection, have higher avidity (Thomas and Morgan-Capner, 1990). Low-avidity IgG can also be detected in oral fluid (Akingbade et al., 2003). Immunoblotting may also be useful as antibodies to E2 do not appear until about 3 months after primary infection (Pustowoit and Liebert, 1998).

Detection of RV

RV may be detected in clinical samples by isolation in cell culture or by reverse transcription nested PCR (RT-nPCR), but these techniques are only available in specialised laboratories. RT-nPCR is of value for postnatal and prenatal diagnosis of congenital rubella (see below) and has been described in detail by Bosma et al. (1995a, 1995b) and Revello et al. (1997).

RV can be identified by cytopathic effect in RK13 or certain sublines of Vero cells (reviewed by Best and O'Shea, 1995; Banatvala and Best, 1998). In our experience, the technique of choice is two passages in Vero cells and a third passage in RK13 cells, in which RV can be detected by indirect immunofluorescence. Alternatively, RT-nPCR can be used to identify virus after two passages in Vero cells.

Virological Diagnosis of Congenitally Acquired Infection

Postnatal Diagnosis

Results of laboratory tests are required for case classification of congenital rubella (see Table 12.5). The most common methods for diagnosing congenital rubella are as follows.

Detection of rubella-specific IgM in cord blood or serum samples taken in infancy. Rubella-specific IgM antibodies synthesised by the fetus *in utero* are present at birth. The detection of rubella-specific IgM in cord, neonatal or infant sera by an M-antibody capture assay is the method of choice for the diagnosis of CRS. If other IgM assays are used, rubella-specific IgM may not always be detected at birth and further serum samples should be tested if indicated. Specific IgM has been detected by M-antibody capture RIA in all confirmed cases to the age of 3 months, 86% of infants aged 3–6 months, 62% infants aged 6 months–1 year, 42% children aged 1 year–18 months, but

rarely in children over 18 months of age (Chantler *et al.*, 1982). The sensitivity of commercially available M-antibody capture EIAs have not usually been established for the diagnosis of congenital rubella. However, the absence of specific IgM by M-antibody capture assays in the neonatal period virtually excludes symptomatic congenital rubella. If a low or equivocal result is obtained by any assay, a further specimen of serum should be examined and other techniques employed.

Detection of a persistent rubella IgG response in the infant. Maternally derived rubella-specific IgG antibodies, as well as specific IgG, will be present at birth. The presence of rubella antibody at a time beyond which maternal antibody would normally have disappeared (approximately 6 months of age) is suggestive of congenital infection. The detection of specific IgG may be of value when tests for specific IgM have not been conducted in early infancy. Since rubella is uncommon under the age of 2 years, specific IgG detected between the ages of 8 months and 2 years may be suggestive of congenital rubella. However, each case must be assessed individually, taking into account such factors as age, maternal history, presence of clinical findings suggestive of or compatible with congenital rubella, and rubelliform illnesses since birth. Detection of low-avidity IgG_1 may also assist the diagnosis in children up to the age of 3 years, as the avidity matures more slowly in children with congenital rubella than following postnatal infection (Thomas *et al.*, 1993).

Detection of RV in samples (such as nasopharyngeal swabs) from infected infants during the first few months of life. Virus may be detected by isolation in cell culture, or more rapidly by RT-nPCR. Specimens can be sent on dry ice or in formol saline for RT-nPCR in a distant laboratory. This has been used in our laboratory to test lens aspirates and to confirm the diagnosis of congenital rubella in children in India (Bosma *et al.*, 1995a, 1995b). Certain types of filter paper may also be used to collect fluids for RT-PCR.

As discussed on p 438, RV may be isolated from nasopharyngeal secretions from most neonates with severe CRS which results from maternal infection in the first trimester, but by the age of about 3 months the proportion excreting virus has declined to 50–60%; and at 13–20 months to 3% (Cooper and Krugman, 1967). However, it is possible that virus excretion may be detectable for a longer time if RT-nPCR is used and

studies are in progress to assess this method of diagnosis.

Other tests. Although rubella-specific IgG detected by SRH and EIA may persist indefinitely, studies on 223 children with congenital rubella following the 1963–1964 US epidemic showed that the HAI antibodies declined more rapidly among congenitally-infected children than among their mothers; by the age of 5, 20% of infants with congenital rubella no longer had HAI antibodies. Nevertheless, seronegative children failed to develop an HAI response or excrete virus when challenged with an attenuated vaccine. More recent studies suggest a decreased production of antibodies to the epitopes on the E1 glycoprotein which induce HAI antibodies in some children with congenital rubella, and Forrest *et al.* (2002) reported that at age 60 years 41% patients with congenital rubella had no detectable rubella antibodies. Thus, in order to determine the immune status of such children in later life, it may be necessary to test sera by EIA, LA or immunoblotting (Meitsch *et al.*, 1997). Rubella-specific lymphoproliferative assays may also help to provide a retrospective diagnosis of CRS in children aged 1–3 (O'Shea *et al.*, 1992).

Risk of Cross-infection

Infants with severe disease, particularly during the first few weeks after birth, often excrete high titres of virus and may readily transmit infection to rubella-susceptible persons. Women of childbearing age, some of whom may be in early stages of pregnancy, must be dissuaded from visiting such infants unless they have had rubella vaccine or serological tests confirm that they are immune. It is important that midwives and nursing staff who may have to care for such infants are also shown to be immune to rubella; it must be appreciated that midwives and nurses who originate from countries without rubella vaccination programmes may be more likely to be susceptible to rubella, as they may not have been offered rubella vaccination (p 453).

Prenatal Diagnosis

Prenatal diagnosis of suspected congenital infection is of value when the mother is reluctant to have therapeutic abortion following rubella in the first trimester, when maternal infection has occurred after the first trimester, in cases of possible maternal reinfection and where equivocal serological results were obtained, such as when the mother presents some time after a rubella-like illness.

A prenatal diagnosis may be made by detecting rubella RNA by RT-nPCR in amniotic fluid or fetal blood obtained by cordocentesis. When RT-nPCR is used, a result can be available within 48 h. Rubella-specific IgM may also be detected in fetal blood. It is usually advisable to use all available assays to exclude a diagnosis of CRS (Enders, 1998).

The detection of rubella RNA in amniotic fluid by RT-nPCR has a sensitivity of 87–100% (Revello et al., 1997; Enders, 1998). Amniotic fluid should be taken after 15 weeks' gestation and $\geqslant 8$ weeks after onset of maternal rubella infection. However, as false negative results may be obtained occasionally if the sample is taken too early, it may be necessary to test a second sample at 22–23 weeks' gestation. Detection of virus in chorionic villus biopsies should be interpreted with caution, as the detection of RV in the placenta may not always reflect fetal infection (Bosma et al., 1995a).

Rubella-specific IgM may be detected in fetal blood following infection in early pregnancy, but the fetus may not produce sufficient IgM before the 22nd week of gestation, and even at 23 weeks' gestation false negative results may be obtained, as concentrations of fetal rubella-specific IgM may be too low to be detected. Thus, it is advised to test fetal blood for rubella-specific IgM by more than one assay.

PREVENTION—RUBELLA VACCINATION

Development and Use of Attenuated Vaccines

The first attenuated strain of RV was developed at the National Institutes of Health in the USA by passage of a virus isolated from a military recruit with rubella in VMK cells. Seventy-seven passages resulted in the strain being attenuated (HPV77) and preliminary trials in primates showed that the attenuated strain was well tolerated, induced an immune response and, following challenge, was protective. Five further passages in duck embryo cultures were carried out to give HPV77-DE5 and this vaccine was also shown to be well tolerated, immunogenic and protective.

Further vaccine strains were prepared, being attenuated in primary rabbit kidney (Cendehill) and in human diploid cell cultures (RA27/3). The latter vaccine strain was originally isolated from the fetal kidney of a rubella-infected conceptus and is now the most widely used vaccine world-wide. The Japanese

and Chinese use attenuated strains developed in their own countries. The development and use of rubella vaccines has been reviewed (Best, 1991; Best and O'Shea, 2003). Rubella vaccine is often given to children in the combined MMR vaccine.

Immune Responses

About 95% of vaccinees develop an immune response some 20–28 days post-vaccination, although occasionally it may be delayed for up to 2 months.

Failure to respond may result from not complying with the manufacturer's instructions during storage or following reconstitution (with consequent inactivation of virus or loss of potency), or pre-existing low levels of antibody. Passively acquired antibody via blood transfusion or administration of human immunoglobulin may suppress the replication of attenuated rubella vaccines. It is therefore advisable to avoid the administration of such live vaccines as rubella for a period of 3 months following transfusion or administration of immunoglobulins.

Rubella-specific IgG and IgA responses can be detected, while virus-specific IgM is detected in about 70% of vaccines 3–8 weeks after immunisation and may occasionally persist for 6 months and rarely for up to 4 years (O'Shea et al., 1985). Rubella-specific 7S IgA responses persist for up to 10–12 years but the oligomeric 10S response is transient. The RA27/3 vaccine induces a secretory IgA response which can be detected in nasopharyngeal secretions for up to 5 years post-vaccination. Antibodies against E1 and C recombinant proteins can readily be detected, but antibodies to recombinant E2 are weak or absent (Nedeljkovic et al., 1999).

Serum antibodies are long-lasting and it is expected that they will provide lifelong protection in most vaccinees. Thus, antibodies detected by HAI and SRH have been shown to persist for at least 21 years, although in about 10% of vaccinees they decline to low ($< 15 \, \text{mIU/ml}$) or even undetectable levels within 5 years. Up to 23% of young women in the USA and Nova Scotia, where there has been little circulation of rubella, have been shown to lack antibodies to rubella. Nevertheless, when 19 volunteers with low or undetectable antibody levels were challenged intranasally with high-titre RA27/3, only one was viraemic, this being transient and at a low level (O'Shea et al., 1983). Lymphoproliferative responses are difficult to detect after vaccination (Buimovici-Klein and Cooper, 1985).

Virus Excretion

Provided that sensitive assays are used, RV may be detected in the nasopharyngeal secretions of virtually all vaccinees 6–29 days post-vaccination. Vaccine strains may also be detected in the breast milk of lactating women. However, vaccine strains are not transmitted. This may reflect the low concentrations of virus excreted, or attenuation may result in alteration of the biological properties of the virus to make it less transmissable.

Vaccine Reactions

Rubella vaccines are generally well tolerated. Lymphadenopathy, rash and joint symptoms may occur some 10–30 days post-vaccination, although they are usually much less severe than following naturally acquired infection. Lymphadenopathy is often not noticed by vaccinees and, should rash be present, it is usually faint, macular and evanescent. Joint symptoms are rare in children of both sexes but up to 40% of postpubertal females may develop an arthralgia. The small joints of the hands are most commonly affected but such other joints as the wrists, knees and ankles may also be involved. Some vaccinees may experience a vaccine-induced arthritis with swelling and limitation of joint movement. Symptoms rarely persist for longer than about a week and, although recurrences may occur, this is a rare event. Rubella vaccine strains have been isolated from the joint fluids of vaccinees with arthritis. Mitchell *et al.* (1998) have shown that there was a significantly higher frequency of HLA-DR2 and -DR5 and lower frequencies of -DR4 and -DR6 in RA27/3 vaccinees with arthropathy than in placebo recipients. Hormonal changes may also affect the development of joint symptoms (p 435).

It has been claimed that the combined MMR vaccine is associated with chronic inflammatory bowel disease and autism. This has generated considerable public concern about the safety of MMR. However, it should be emphasised that there is no good scientific evidence to support the association and a number of expert groups who have examined the evidence did not support it (http://www.doh.gov.uk/mmr/index.html; Institute of Medicine 2001: WHO, 2003a).

Vaccine Failures

Rubella is a labile virus and is therefore inactivated by exposure to heat and light. Manufacturers recommend that vaccine be stored at 2–8°C and that after reconstitution it should be kept at that temperature, protected from light and used within 1 hour. Failure to adhere to these instructions is the most frequent reason for vaccinees failing to seroconvert. Approximately 5% of vaccinees fail to respond for unexplained reasons, but usually respond satisfactorily if revaccinated. A few may fail to do so, or respond poorly, because they have a pre-existing low level of antibody, which is undetectable by some techniques. Seroconversion after vaccination should be assessed normally at about 8 weeks after vaccination, but occasional vaccinees may experience a delayed response, antibodies appearing even later. Passively acquired antibody, whether from blood transfusion, immunoglobulin or maternally acquired, may interfere with vaccine uptake. Vaccination should be delayed for 3 months following blood transfusion or administration of immunoglobulin (but see below).

Reinfection

Evidence of reinfection is usually obtained serologically by demonstrating a significant rise in antibody titre (p 446). Experimental studies suggest that reinfection is more likely to occur in those whose immunity is vaccine-induced rather than naturally acquired (reviewed in Best, 1991). A transient rubella-specific IgM response may be detected, sometimes at only a low level, if serum is tested by a sensitive technique within 6 weeks of exposure. Viraemia has very occasionally been detected in vaccinees who have been reinfected naturally or experimentally. The risk of such reinfection resulting in fetal damage is small (p 437).

Contraindications

As with other live vaccines, patients who are immunocompromised as a result of disease or its treatment (including cytotoxic drugs, corticosteroids or radiotherapy) should not be vaccinated. Contraindications should also be extended to those with thrombocytopenia.

HIV-positive patients who are mildly asymptomatic or without symptoms may be vaccinated, since they do not appear to suffer complications following the administration of attenuated vaccines for polio or measles and, if unprotected, may experience severe infections (particularly with measles) (http://www.cdc.gov/nip/publications/pink/rubella.pdf). Since rubella vaccine is usually administered as MMR, HIV-positive persons (particularly children) should benefit from being afforded protection (Department of Health, 1996).

If another live vaccine is to be administered at the same time, both should be given simultaneously but at different sites (except in the case of MMR). Alternatively, both vaccinations should be separated by an interval of at least 3 weeks. A 3 week interval should also be allowed between the administration of rubella and BCG. If the patient is suffering from a febrile illness, it is better to delay rubella vaccination. The manufacturer's leaflet should be studied carefully when patients with known hypersensitivity are to be vaccinated, since rubella vaccines contain traces of antibiotics (neomycin and/or kanamycin or polymyxin). There is increasing evidence that MMR vaccine can be given safely to children with an allergy to egg. Pregnancy should be avoided for 1 month after administration of rubella and MMR vaccines (Department of Health, 1996; Centers for Disease Control, 2001b). Although passively acquired antibodies may interfere with antibody responses following rubella vaccination, if anti-D is required, it may be given at the same time, but at different sites and from different syringes. Anti-D does not interfere with vaccine induced antibody responses (Department of Health, 1996).

Vaccination during Pregnancy

Pregnancy should be avoided for 1 month after rubella vaccination, but if a pregnant woman is inadvertently vaccinated there is no indication for therapeutic abortion (Department of Health, 1996; Centers for Disease Control, 2001b). Thus, although RV has been recovered from the products of conception following vaccination of susceptible pregnant women, it is encouraging that of 657 infants followed up only one had a transient abnormality (heart murmur) compatible with CRS (Table 12.6). Examination of the products of conception of rubella-susceptible women inadvertently vaccinated during pregnancy has shown that RV may be recovered from the placenta, kidney and bone marrow for up to 94 days after vaccination, indicating that vaccine virus can cross the placenta and establish persistent fetal infection. Follow-up studies on women who elected to go to term following inadvertent vaccination during pregnancy, or within 3 months before conception, revealed no abnormalities compatible with congenital rubella among 684 babies delivered by these women. However,

a specific-IgM response provided virological evidence of congenital infection in 16 of the 405 (3.95%) babies tested (Table 12.6). In the US study 212/324 babies were born to women who had received the RA27/3 vaccine strain. It should be noted, however, that only 293/661 (44.3%) women in the combined series were vaccinated in the high-risk period between 2 weeks before and 6 weeks after conception (Table 12.6). If rubella vaccines were to induce congenital defects, it may be necessary for infection to occur during a much shorter period than following naturally acquired infection. Many of the cases included in these follow-up studies were vaccinated within the 3 months before conception, which is probably of minimal risk. The theoretical maximum risk of rubella-induced major malformations among infants delivered of susceptible mothers who were vaccinated in the high-risk period has been calculated to be 1.3% (Centers for Disease Control, 2001b). This is less than the risk of major malformation occurring in 'normal' pregnancies (approximately 3%). The lack of teratogenicity may well be due to a lower viral load rather than a difference in teratogenicity of the attenuated viruses. One case of vertical transmission with prolonged virus shedding from the infant has been described, but the infant had no signs of CRS (Hofmann et al., 2000).

Antibody screening prior to vaccination should considerably reduce the number of women who might be inadvertently vaccinated during pregnancy. On the other hand, the two-stage procedure involving screening and vaccination may be counterproductive, deterring patients and their doctors from achieving higher immunisation rates. This could be overcome by ensuring that a woman was using effective contraception; there would then be relatively little risk of vaccination during pregnancy. Even if the vaccinee was subsequently found to be pregnant, it would be possible to determine prior immune status retrospectively by testing serum samples obtained after vaccination for rubella-specific IgM.

Vaccination Programmes

Rubella vaccination programmes have had a major impact in preventing CRS in countries which have implemented rubella vaccination programmes. The aim of these programmes is to prevent women acquiring rubella while they are pregnant. Initially, the USA adopted universal childhood immunisation. This programme resulted in a more than 99% decrease in the number of cases of rubella reported between 1969 and

Table 12.6   Combined data for risk of CRS in infants born to susceptible women whose pregnancies were complicated by rubella vaccination

Country	Live births to women receiving rubella immunisation			
	Within 3 months of conception or during pregnancy	In the high-risk period[a]	Evidence of infection[b]	Abnormalities compatible with CRS
USA	324	113	6/222 (2.7%)	0/324
Germany	257[c]	155	6/126 (4.8%)	0/257
Sweden	5	NK	0/5	0/5
UK	75[d]	25	4[e]/52 (7.7%)	1[f]/75
Totals	661	293 (44.3%)	16/405 (3.95%)	1[f]/661

NK, not known.

[a]USA used between 1 week before and 4 weeks after conception, UK used 1–6 weeks after LMP; 69 cases from Germany were between 1 week before and 4 weeks after conception and 86 cases were between 2 weeks before to 6 weeks after conception.

[b]Number with evidence of infection/number tested. Data from Germany: IgM positive in 6/126 cord bloods tested with information on health at birth and telephonic information on health at birth in 131 cases.

[c]Gisela Enders, personal communication, 2003.

[d]Pat Tookey, personal communication, 2000. Includes one set of twins.

[e]Three of the rubella IgM-positive infants were born to mothers who were inadvertently immunised within the 6 weeks after LMP.

[f]One rubella IgM-positive infant had a heart murmur which had resolved by 2 months of age.

1988 (Figure 12.9). However, as a number of rubella outbreaks occurred among adolescents and young adults in the late 1970s, further emphasis was placed on vaccinating susceptibles in these older age groups, which resulted in a further decline in rubella notifications.

Vaccination in the USA

Since 1978 the decline in the incidence of CRS in the USA paralleled the decline in postnatally acquired rubella. Although there was substantial underreporting

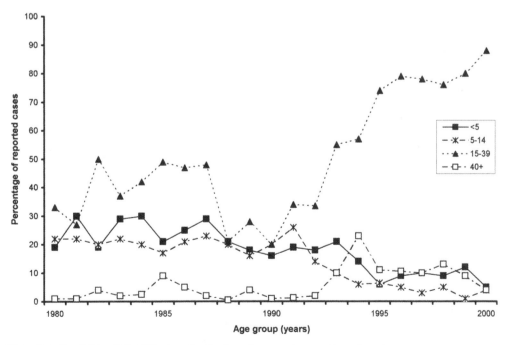

Figure 12.9   Rubella—USA, 1980–2000. Age distribution of reported cases. Data from http://www.cdc.gov/nip/publications/pink/rubella.pdf

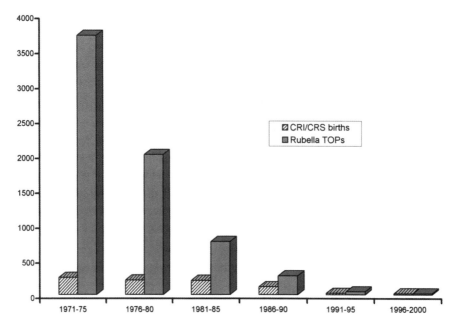

Figure 12.10   Congenital rubella births and rubella-associated terminations of pregnancy (TOPs) in England and Wales. From National Congenital Rubella Surveillance Programme (2003)

of CRS, it was anticipated that CRS was on the verge of elimination in the USA in the 1980s. However, in 1989–1990 there was a resurgence of CRS in southern California and among the Amish population in Pennsylvania. This was the result of missed opportunities for rubella screening or vaccination; many of the cases of maternal rubella could have been prevented if postpartum immunisation had been carried out following previous pregnancies. The USA policy results in a financial saving: cost–benefit analysis shows that the cost of rubella in an unvaccinated population is approximately 11 times more than the cost of the vaccination policy.

Vaccination in the UK

The UK initially adopted a selective vaccination programme, in order to protect women during their childbearing years. In the UK during 1970–1988, vaccination was directed towards prepubertal school-girls and rubella-susceptible women of childbearing age. The selective vaccination programme was replaced by universal immunisation of children in 1988, since some of the remaining susceptible pregnant women (2–3%) were infected during outbreaks as rubella

continued to circulate among children. In the UK and USA, rubella vaccine is now offered as MMR to children at 12–15 months and at 4–5 years of age; however, it is possible to give the two doses 3 months apart in order to improve uptake. Vaccination of susceptible women continues.

In order to eliminate rubella, it is necessary to monitor the efficacy of rubella vaccination programmes. In the UK this is done by seroprevalence studies in different age-groups, including pregnant women, reporting of congenital rubella cases and therapeutic abortions due to rubella in pregnancy, and monitoring uptake of MMR in children. In the UK in 1994–1995 only 2% of nulliparous and 1.2% of parous women were rubella-susceptible and this, together with the decline in circulation of rubella among young children, has resulted in termination of pregnancy because of maternal rubella and CRS is now rare in Britain (Figure 12.10) (Miller *et al.*, 1997; Tookey and Peckham, 1999). However, women who come to the UK from countries that do not have an effective rubella vaccination programme are more likely to be susceptible. In North London during 1996–1999 it was shown that susceptibility was about 5% in women born outside the UK, with the highest rates of susceptibility among women from Asia and Africa; 23.3% of Sri Lankan women in their first

Table 12.7 Summary of recommendations from WHO for elimination of rubella and congenital rubella

1. Countries undertaking measles elimination should take the opportunity to eliminate rubella through the use of measles–rubella or MMR vaccine in their childhood immunisation programmes, as well as through campaigns. All countries undertaking rubella elimination should ensure that women of childbearing age are immune and that routine coverage in children is sustained at 80% or above
2. Countries that currently include rubella in their childhood immunisation programmes should ensure that women of childbearing age are immune and should move towards rubella elimination
3. If a global measles eradication goal is established, rubella should be included
4. Rubella vaccine should be considered as a priority for initiatives to introduce new or under-utilised vaccines in developing countries

Reproduced by permission of the World Health Organization from Hinman *et al.* (2002).

pregnancy were susceptible to rubella (Tookey *et al.*, 2002). Many of the recent reported cases have acquired rubella abroad. Seven cases of CRS were born between January 2000 and December 2001; six of the seven mothers had been born abroad and five had acquired rubella abroad in their countries of origin (Rahi *et al.*, 2001; Tookey P, personal communication, 2002). This emphasises the importance of questioning women who come from developing countries when pregnant, about any illness experienced in early pregnancy, so that appropriate tests can be carried out (Department of Health, 2003).

Although the uptake of MMR among children was 92% in 1995, it has dropped to 84% in England and Wales in 2002, due to unnecessary public concern about the safety of MMR (p 449). This has resulted in measles outbreaks in 2002 and 2003 and may put unvaccinated girls at risk of rubella in the future.

Other European Countries

Initially selective vaccination programmes were adopted in other countries in Western Europe.

Subsequently MMR has been introduced into childhood vaccination programmes and many countries now offer a second dose. Sweden and Finland have already eliminated rubella by the use of two-dose MMR vaccination programmes (Böttiger and Forsgren, 1997; Peltola *et al.*, 1994).

Recently uptake rates of rubella vaccine have been poor in parts of Eastern Europe and Italy and this has resulted in an increase in the number of cases of CRS (Tookey P, personal communication, 2003).

Developing Countries

Rubella vaccination strategies are unsatisfactory in many developing countries (Robertson *et al.*, 1997) and there is a considerable burden of CRS in many countries (p 432). In 2000 WHO proposed strategies for rubella elimination (World Health Organization, 2000) which have been summarised by Hinman *et al.* (2002), as shown in Table 12.7. The major thrust of the proposal was to 'piggy back' rubella with measles (MR) or measles and mumps (MMR) vaccines. It was emphasised that, in order to be effective, programmes

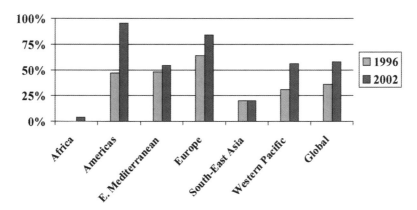

Figure 12.11 Percentage of countries/territories, by WHO region and globally, with rubella vaccine in the national immunisation system, 1996 and 2002. Reproduced by permission of the World Health Organization from Robertson *et al.* (1997)

should be directed towards women of childbearing age as well as children. By 2002 rubella vaccination was included in national immunisation programmes of 123 (57%) countries/territories, an increase of 14% since 1996 (Figure 12.11), with the most impressive coverage seen in the PAHO region (about 90%). By 2002, 41/44 countries in the PAHO region had incorporated MR or MMR into their childhood immunisation programmes. This has been combined with immunisation of adult females or males and females in some countries, in order to avoid shifting the age of infection to susceptible adults (World Health Organization, 2003b).

Caution must be expressed about the introduction of rubella vaccination in countries with relatively low measles uptake rates, e.g. parts of Africa with uptake rates of about 60%. Intermediate rubella vaccination rates will only increase the average age of infection and, consequently, lead to more cases in young adults, including pregnant women, which would lead to an increase in the incidence of CRS. It is now recognised that children of both sexes and susceptible adult women should be vaccinated in order to eliminate rubella and avoid an increase in incidence of congenital rubella. The danger of low rubella or MMR vaccination coverage of children was illustrated by an epidemic of rubella in Greece in 1993, with a resulting incidence of CRS of 24.6/100 000 live births (Panagiotopoulos et al., 1999).

Passive Immunisation

Women who come into contact with rubella and for whom a termination would be unacceptable may be offered normal human immmunoglobulin or high-titred rubella immunoglobulin. Although normal human immunoglobulin may reduce the incidence of clinically overt infection, subclinical infection may still occur. Since subclinical infection is accompanied by viraemia, there is still a risk of fetal infection. It has been shown that the infants of women who experienced subclinical rubella in early pregnancy following administration of normal immunoglobulin were less likely to be infected in utero, or, if infected, less severely affected, than infants of mothers not given this preparation. It is proposed that the immunoglobulin decreased viraemia and there was consequently less damage (reviewed by Hanshaw et al., 1985). Although high-titred rubella immunoglobulins have been developed and gave encouraging results in experimental studies, they have not been properly evaluated in the field (reviewed by Best and Banatvala, 2000).

REFERENCES

Akingbade D, Cohen BJ and Brown DWG (2003) Detection of low-avidity immunoglobulin G in oral fluid samples: new approach for rubella diagnosis and surveillance. Clin Diagn Lab Immunol, 10, 189–190.

Arnold JJ, McIntosh ED, Martin FJ et al. (1994) A fifty-year follow-up of ocular defects in congenital rubella: late ocular manifestations. Austr NZ J Ophthalmol, 22, 1–6.

Banatvala JE and Best JM (1984) Topley and Wilson's Principles of Bacteriology, Virology and Immunity, 7th edn, vol 4. Hodder Arnold, London.

Banatvala JE and Best JM (1990) Rubella. In Topley and Wilson's Principles of Bacteriology, Virology and Immunity, 8th edn, vol 1 (eds Collier L and Timbury M), pp 501–531. Edward Arnold, London.

Banatvala JE and Best JM (1998) Rubella. In Topley and Wilson's Microbiology and Microbial Infections, 9th edn, vol 1 (eds Mahy BJ and Collier L), pp 551–577. Edward Arnold, London.

Banatvala JE and Brown DWG (2003) Rubella. Lancet (in press).

Best JM (1991) Rubella vaccines—past, present and future. Epidemiol Infect, 107, 17–30.

Best JM and Banatvala JE (2000) Rubella. In Principles and Practice of Clinical Virology, 4th edn (eds Zuckerman AJ, Banatvala JE and Pattison JR), pp 387–418. Wiley, Chichester.

Best JM, Banatvala JE, Morgan-Capner P and Miller E (1989) Foetal infection after maternal reinfection with rubella: criteria for defining re-infection. Br Med J, 299, 773–775.

Best JM, Cooray S and Banatvala JE (2004) Rubella. In Topley and Wilson's Microbiology and Microbial Infections, 10th edn, Virology Volume (eds Mahy B and ter Meulen V). Arnold, London (in press).

Best JM and O'Shea S (1995) Rubella virus. In Diagnostic Procedure for Viral, Rickettsial and Chlamydial Infections, 7th edn (eds Lennette EH, Lennette DA and Lennette ET), pp 583–600. American Public Health Association, Washington, DC.

Best JM and O'Shea S (2003) Disease states and vaccines: rubella. In The Vaccine Book (eds Bloom B and Lambert P-H), pp 197–209. Academic Press, San Diego.

Best JM, O'Shea S, Tipples G et al. (2002) Interpretation of rubella serology in pregnancy—pitfalls and problems. Br Med J, 325, 147–148.

Best JM, Thomson A, Rey Nores J et al. (1993) Rubella virus strains show no major antigenic differences. Intervirology, 34, 164–168.

Bosma TJ, Best JM, Corbett KM et al. (1996) Nucleotide sequence analysis of a major antigenic domain of the E1 glycoprotein of 22 rubella virus isolates. J Gen Virol, 77, 2523–2530.

Bosma TJ, Corbett KM, Eckstein MB et al. (1995a) Use of PCR for prenatal and postnatal diagnosis of congenital rubella. J Clin Microbiol, 33, 2881–2887.

Bosma TJ, Corbett KM, O'Shea S *et al.* (1995b) Use of the polymerase chain reaction for the detection of rubella virus RNA in clinical samples. *J Clin Microbiol*, **33**, 1075–1079.

Bosma TJ, Etherington J, O'Shea S *et al.* (1998) Rubella virus and chronic joint disease: is there an association? *J Clin Microbiol*, **36**, 3524–3526.

Böttiger M and Forsgren M (1997) Twenty years' experience of rubella vaccination in Sweden: 10 years of selective vaccination (of 12 year-old girls and of women postpartum) and 13 years of a general two-dose vaccination. *Vaccine*, **15**, 1538–1544.

Buimovici-Klein E and Cooper LZ (1985) Cell-mediated immune response in rubella infections. *Rev Infect Dis*, **7** (1), S123–S128.

Buimovici-Klein E, Lang PB, Ziring PR and Cooper LZ (1979) Impaired cell mediated immune response in patients with congenital rubella: correlation with gestational age at time of infection. *Pediatrics*, **64**, 620–626.

Burke JP, Hinman AR and Krugman S (eds) (1985) International symposium on prevention of congenital rubella infection. *Rev Infect Dis*, **7** (1).

Centers for Disease Control (2001a) Control and prevention of rubella: evaluation and management of suspected outbreaks, rubella in pregnant women, and surveillance for congenital rubella syndrome. *Morbid Mortal Wkly Rep*, **50** (RR-12), 1–23.

Centers for Disease Control (2001b) Revised ACIP recommendation for avoiding pregnancy after receiving a rubella-containing vaccine. *Morbid Mortal Wkly Rep*, **50** (49), 1117.

Chantler JK, Smymis L and Tai G (1995) Selective infection of astrocytes in human glial cell cultures by rubella virus. *J Lab Invest*, **72**, 334–340.

Chantler J, Wolinsky JS and Tingle A (2001) Rubella Virus. In *Field's Virology*, 4th edn (eds Knipe DM, Howley PM *et al.*), pp 963–990. Lippincott, Williams & Wilkins, Philadelphia, PA.

Chantler S, Evans CJ, Mortimer PP *et al.* (1982) A comparison of antibody capture radio- and enzyme immunoassays with immunofluorescence for detecting IgM antibody in infants with congenital rubella. *J Virol Methods*, **4**, 305–313.

Chaye H, Chong P, Tripet B *et al.* (1992) Localization of the virus neutralising and hemagglutinin epitopes of E1 glycoprotein of rubella virus. *Virology*, **189**, 483–492.

Collier L and Timbury M (eds) (1990) Topley and Wilson's Principles of Bacteriology, Virology and Immunity, 8th edition, vol. 1. Edward Arnold, London.

Cooper LZ (1975) Congenital rubella in the United States. In *Infections of the Fetus and the Newborn Infant, Progress in Clinical and Biological Research*, vol 3 (eds Krugman S and Gershon AA), pp 1–21. Alan R. Liss, New York.

Cooper LZ and Krugman S (1967) Clinical manifestations of postnatal and congenital rubella. *Arch Ophthalmol*, **77**, 434–439.

Cooper LZ, Zirling PR *et al.* (1969) Rubella: clinical manifestations and management. *Am J Dis Child*, **118**, 18–29.

Cooray S, Best JM and Jin L (2003) Time-course induction of apoptosis by wild-type and attenuated strains of rubella virus. *J Gen Virol*, **84**, 1275–1279.

Cradock-Watson JE, Miller E, Ridehalgh MKS *et al.* (1989) Detection of rubella virus in fetal and placental tissues and in the throats of neonates after serologically confirmed rubella in pregnancy. *Prenatal Diagn*, **9**, 91–96.

Cradock-Watson JE, Ridehalgh MKS, Anderson MJ *et al.* (1980) Fetal infection resulting from maternal rubella after the first trimester of pregnancy. *J Hygiene*, **85**, 381–391.

Cusi MG, Metelli R, Valensin PE *et al.* (1989) Immune responses to wild and vaccine rubella viruses after rubella vaccination. *Arch Virol*, **106**, 63–72.

Cutts FT, Robertson SE, Diaz-Ortega J-L and Samuel R (1997) Control of rubella and congenital rubella syndrome (CRS) in developing countries, Part 1: burden of disease from CRS. *Bull World Health Org*, **75**, 55–68.

Department of Health (2003) *Screening for Infectious Diseases in Pregnancy*. Stationery Office, London.

Department of Health, Welsh Office, Scottish Office Department of Health, D.H.S.S. (Northern Ireland) (1996) *Immunisation Against Infectious Disease*. HMSO, London.

Domegan LM and Atkins GJ (2002) Apoptosis induction by the Therien and vaccine RA27/3 strains of rubella virus causes depletion of oligodendrocytes from rat neural cell cultures. *J Gen Virol*, **83**, 2135–2143.

Dorsett PH, Miller DC, Green KU and Byrd FI (1985) Structure and function of the rubella virus proteins. *Rev Infect Dis*, **7**, S150–S156.

Duncan R, Esmaili A, Law LMJ *et al.* (2000) Rubella virus capsid protein induces apoptosis in transfected RK13 cells. *Virology*, **275**, 20–29.

Eckstein MB, Brown DWG, Foster A *et al.* (1996) Congenital rubella in south India: diagnosis using saliva from infants with cataract. *Br Med J*, **312**, 161.

Enders G (1998) Fetale Infektionen. In (eds Hansmann M, Feige A and Saling E) *Pränatal-und Geberutsmedizin*, Berichte vom 5th Kongress der Gesellschaft für Pränatal-und Geburtsmedizin, 21–23 February 1997. Meckenheim: DCM Druck Center, pp 76–82.

Enders G, Nickerl-Pacher U, Miller E and Cradock-Watson JE (1988) Outcome of confirmed periconceptional maternal rubella. *Lancet*, **I**, 1445–1446.

Forrest JM, Turnbul FM, Sholler GF *et al.* (2002) Gregg's congenital rubella patients 60 years later. *Med J Austr*, **177**, 664–667.

Frey TK (1994) Molecular biology of rubella virus. *Adv Virus Res*, **44**, 69–160.

Frey TK (1997) Neurological aspects of rubella virus infection. *Intervirology*, **40**, 167–175.

Frey TK, Abernathy ES, Bosma TJ *et al.* (1998) Molecular analysis of rubella virus epidemiology across three continents, North America, Europe and Asia, 1961–1997. *J Infect Dis*, **178**, 642–650.

Gregg NMcA (1941) Congenital cataract following German measles in mother. *Trans Ophthalmol Soc Austr*, **3**, 35–46.

Grillner L, Forsgren M, Barr B *et al.* (1983) Outcome of rubella during pregnancy with special reference to the 17–24th weeks of gestation. *Scand J Infect Dis*, **15**, 321–325.

Hanshaw JB, Dudgeon JA and Marshall WC (1985) *Viral Diseases of the Fetus and Newborn*, 2nd edn. W.B. Saunders, Philadelphia, PA.

Hemphill ML, Forng R-Y, Abernathy ES *et al.* (1988) Time course of virus-specific macromolecular synthesis during rubella virus infection in Vero cells. *Virology*, **162**, 65–75.

Herrmann KL (1979) Rubella virus. In *Diagnostic Procedures for Viral, Rickettsial and Chlamydial Infections*, 5th edn (eds Lennette EH and Schmidt NJ), pp 725–766. American Public Health Association, Washington, DC.

Hinman AR, Irons B, Lewis M and Kandola K (2002) Economic analyses of rubella and rubella vaccines: a global review. *Bull World Health Org*, **80**, 264–270.

Hofmann J, Kortung M, Pustowoit B *et al.* (2000) Persistent fetal rubella vaccine virus infection following inadvertent vaccination during early pregnancy. *J Med Virol*, **61**, 155–158.

Hofmann J, Pletz MW and Leibert UG (1999) Rubella virus-induced cytopathic effect *in vitro* is caused by apoptosis. *J Gen Virol*, **80**, 1657–1664.

Horzinek MC (1981) *Non-arthropod-borne Togaviruses*. Academic Press, London.

Hosking CS, Pyman C and Wilkins B (1983) The nerve deaf child—intrauterine rubella or not? *Arch Dis Child*, **58**, 327–329.

Hudson P and Morgan-Capner P (1996) Evaluation of 15 commercial enzyme immunoassays for the detection of rubella-specific IgM. *Clin Diagn Virol*, **5**, 21–26.

Institute of Medicine (2001) Immunization Safety Review: Measles–Mumps–Rubella Vaccine and Autism. http://search.nap.edu/books/0309074479/html/

Karounos DG, Wolinsky JS and Thomas JW (1993) Monoclonal antibody to rubella virus capsid protein recognises a β-cell antigen. *J Immunol*, **150**, 3080–3085.

Lee J-Y and Bowden DS (2000) Rubella virus replication and links to teratogenicity. *Clin Microbiol Rev*, **13**, 571–587.

Mauracher CA, Mitchell LA and Tingle AJ (1993) Selective tolerance to the E1 protein of rubella virus in congenital rubella syndrome. *J Immunol*, **151**, 2041–2049.

Meitsch K, Enders G, Wolinsky JS *et al.* (1997) The role of rubella-immunoblot and rubella-peptide EIA for the diagnosis of the congenital rubella syndrome during the prenatal and newborn periods. *J Med Virol*, **51**, 280–283.

Menser MA, Dods L and Harley JD (1967) A twenty-five year follow-up of congenital rubella. *Lancet*, **ii**, 1347–1350.

Miller E, Cradock-Watson JE and Pollock TM (1982) Consequences of confirmed maternal rubella at successive stages of pregnancy. *Lancet*, **ii**, 781–784.

Miller E, Tookey P, Morgan-Capner P *et al.* (1994) Rubella surveillance to June 1994: third joint report from the PHLS and the National Congenital Rubella Surveillance Programme. *Commun Dis Rep*, **4**, R146–152.

Miller E, Waight PA, Gay N *et al.* (1997) The epidemiology of rubella in England and Wales before and after the 1994 measles and rubella vaccination campaign: fourth joint report from the PHLS and the National Congenital Rubella Surveillance Programme. *Commun Dis Rep*, **7** (review 2), R26–R32.

Miller E, Waight PA, Vurdien JE *et al.* (1993) Rubella surveillance to December 1992: second joint report from the PHLS and the National Congenital Rubella Surveillance Programme. *Commun Dis Rep*, **3**, R35–R40.

Mitchell LA, Decarie D, Tingle AJ *et al.* (1993) Identification of immunoreactive regions of rubella virus E1 and E2 envelope proteins by using synthetic peptides. *Virus Res*, **29**, 33–57.

Mitchell LA, Tingle AJ, MacWilliam L *et al.* (1998) HLA-DR Class II associations with rubella vaccine-induced joint manifestations. *J Infect Dis*, **177**, 5–12.

Morgan-Capner P, Miller E, Vurdien JE and Ramsay MEB (1991) Outcome of pregnancy after maternal reinfection with rubella. *Commun Dis Rep*, **1**, R57–R59.

Mortimer PP and Parry JV (1988) The use of saliva for viral diagnosis and screening. *Epidemiol Infect*, **101**, 197–201.

Munroe S (1999) *A Survey of Late-emerging Manifestations of Congenital Rubella in Canada*. Canadian Deaf-blind and Rubella Association, Brantford, Canada.

National Congenital Rubella Surveillance Programme (2003) Available from: http://www.ich.ucl.ac.uk/ich/html/academicunits/paed_epid/ncrsp.htm

Nedeljkovic J, Jovanovic T, Mladjenovic S *et al.* (1999) Immunoblot analysis of natural and vaccine-induced IgG responses to rubella virus proteins expressed in insect cells. *J Clin Virol*, **14**, 119–131.

Norrby E (1969) *Rubella Virus*. Virology Monographs, vol 7, pp 115–174. Springer-Verlag, Vienna.

Numazaki K, Goldman H, Seemayer T *et al.* (1990) Infection by human cytomegalovirus and rubella of cultured human fetal islets of Langerhans. *In Vivo*, **4**, 49–54.

O'Shea S, Best JM and Banatvala JE (1983) Viremia, virus excretion, and antibody responses after challenge in volunteers with low levels of antibody to rubella virus. *J Infect Dis*, **148**, 639–647.

O'Shea S, Best JM and Banatvala JE (1992) A lymphocyte transformation assay for the diagnosis of congenital rubella. *J Virol Methods*, **37**, 139–148.

O'Shea S, Best JM, Banatvala JE and Shepherd WM (1985) Development and persistence of class specific serum and nasopharyngeal antibodies in rubella vaccinees. *J Infect Dis*, **151** (1), 89–98.

O'Shea S, Corbett KM, Barrow SM *et al.* (1994) Rubella re-infection; role of neutralising antibodies and cell-mediated immunity. *Clin Diagn Virol*, **2**, 349–358.

Ou D, Jonsen LA, Metzger DL and Tingle AJ (1999) CD4 and CD8 T cell clones from congenital rubella syndrome patients with IDDM recognise overlapping GAD65 protein epitopes. *Human Immunology*, **60**, 652–664.

Panagiotopoulos T, Antoniadou I and Valassi-Adam E (1999) Increase in congenital rubella occurrence after immunisation in Greece: retrospective survey and systematic review. *Br Med J*, **319**, 1462–1466.

Parkman PD, Buescher EL and Artenstein MS (1962) Recovery of rubella virus from army recruits. *Proc Soc Exp Biol Med*, **111**, 225–230.

Peckham CS (1972) Clinical and laboratory study of children exposed *in utero* to maternal rubella. *Arch Dis Child*, **47**, 571–577.

Peltola H, Heinonen OP, Valle M *et al.* (1994) The elimination of indigenous measles, mumps, and rubella from Finland by a 12-year, two-dose vaccination program. *N Engl J Med*, **331**, 1446–1447.

Perry KR, Brown WG, Parry JV *et al.* (1993) Detection of measles, mumps and rubella antibodies in saliva using antibody capture radioimmunoassay. *J Med Virol*, **40**, 235–240.

PHLS Working Party on the Laboratory Diagnosis of Rubella (1988) Summary of the Recommendations. *Microbiol Dig*, **5**, 49–51.

Pugachev KV, Abernathy ES and Frey TK (1997) Genomic sequence of the RA27/3 vaccine strain of rubella virus. *Arch Virol*, **141**, 1165–1180.

Pugachev KV and Frey TK (1998) Rubella virus induces apoptosis in culture cells. *Virology*, **250**, 359–370.

Pustowoit B and Liebert UG (1998) Predictive value of serological tests in rubella virus infection during pregnancy. *Intervirology*, **41**, 170–177.

Rahi J, Adams G, Russell-Eggitt I and Tookey P (2001) Epidemiological surveillance of rubella must continue. *Br Med J*, **323**, 112.

Ramsay ME, Brugha R, Brown DWG *et al.* (1998) Salivary diagnosis of rubella: a study of notified cases in the United Kingdom, 1991–1994. *Epidemiol Infect*, **120**, 315–319.

Ramsay M, Reacher M, O'Flynn C *et al.* (2002) Causes of morbilliform rash in a highly immunised English population. *Arch Dis Child*, **87** (3), 202–206.

Revello MG, Baldanti FS, Sarasini A *et al.* (1997) Prenatal diagnosis of rubella virus infection by direct detection and semiquantitation of viral RNA in clinical samples by reverse transcription–PCR. *J Clin Microbiol*, **35**, 708–713.

Robertson SE, Cutts FT, Samuel R and Diaz-Ortega J-L (1997) Control of rubella and congenital rubella syndrome (CRS) in developing countries, part 2: vaccination against rubella. *Bull World Health Org*, **75**, 69–80.

Salisbury DM and Savinykh AI (1991) Rubella and congenital rubella syndrome in developing countries. Document EPI/GAG/91/WP.15. Presented at the EPI Global Advisory Group Meeting, Antalya, Turkey, 14–18 October 1991.

Skendzel LP (1996) Rubella immunity—defining the level of protective antibody. *Am J Clin Pathol*, **106**, 170–174.

Starkey WG, Newcombe J, Corbett KM *et al.* (1995) Use of rubella E1 fusion proteins for the detection of rubella antibodies. *J Clin Microbiol*, **33**, 270–274.

Stewart GL, Parkman PD, Hopps HE *et al.* (1967) Rubella virus hemagglutination-inhibition test. *N Engl J Med*, **276**, 554–557.

Thomas HIJ and Morgan-Capner P (1988) Rubella-specific IgG subclass concentrations in sera using an enzyme-linked immunosorbent assay (ELISA): the effect of different sources of rubella antigen. *Epidemiol Infect*, **101**, 599–604.

Thomas HIJ and Morgan-Capner P. (1990) The avidity of specific IgM detected in primary rubella and re-infection. *Epidemiol Infect*, **104**, 489–497.

Thomas HIJ, Morgan-Capner P, Cradock-Watson J *et al.* (1993) Slow maturation of IgG₁ avidity in congenital rubella: implications for diagnosis and immunopathology. *J Med Virol*, **41**, 196–200.

Töndury G and Smith DW (1966) Fetal rubella pathology. *J Pediatr*, **68**, 867–879.

Tookey PA, Cortina-Borja M and Peckham CS (2002) Rubella susceptibility among pregnant women in North London, 1996–1999. *J Publ Health Med*, **24**, 211–216.

Tookey PA and Peckham CS (1999) Surveillance of congenital rubella in Great Britain, 1976–1996. *Br Med J*, **318**, 769–770.

Van Straaten HL, Groote ME and Oudesluys-Murphy AM (1996) Evaluation of an automated auditory brainstem response infant hearing screening method in at risk neonates. *Eur J Pediatr*, **155** (8), 702–705.

Vejtorp M and Mansa B (1980) Rubella IgM antibodies in sera from infants born after maternal rubella later than the 12th week of pregnancy. *Scand J Infect Dis*, **12**, 1–5.

Weller TH and Neva FA (1962) Propagation in tissue culture of cytopathic agents from patients with rubella-like illness. *Proc Soc Exp Biol Med*, **111**, 215–225.

World Health Organization (1999) *Guidelines for Surveillance of Congenital Rubella Syndrome and Rubella.* Field Test Version, WHO/V&B/99.22. WHO, Geneva.

World Health Organization (2000) Report of a meeting on preventing congenital rubella syndrome: immunisation strategies, surveillance needs. Unpublished document WHO/V&B/00; available from http://www.who.int/vaccines-documents

World Health Organization (2003a) Global Advisory Committee on Vaccine Safety, 16–17 December 2002. *Wkly Epidemiol Rec*, **78**, 17–18.

World Health Organization (2003b) Accelerated control of rubella and prevention of congenital rubella syndrome, WHO region of the Americas. *Wkly Epidemiol Rec*, **78**, 50–54.

Wolinsky JS, McCarthy M, Allen-Cannady O *et al.* (1991) Monoclonal antibody-defined epitope map of expressed rubella virus protein domains. *J Virol*, **65**, 3986–3994.

Yoneda T, Urade M, Sakuda M and Miyazaki TC (1986) Altered growth, differentiation, and responsiveness of epidermal growth factor human embryonic mesenchymal cells of palate by persistent rubella virus infection. *J Clin Invest*, **77**, 1613–1621.

Yoon J-W, Choi D-S, Liang H-C *et al.* (1992) Induction of an organ-specific autoimmune disease, lymphocytic hypophysitis, in hamsters by recombinant rubella virus glycoprotein and prevention of disease by neonatal thymectomy. *J Virol*, **66**, 1210–1214.

13

Mumps

Pauli Leinikki

National Public Health Institute, Helsinki, Finland

INTRODUCTION

Mumps is an acute infectious disease of children and young adults, caused by a paramyxovirus. The description by Hippocrates in the fifth century BC of an epidemic disease with swelling near the ear and painful enlargement of the testis is usually cited as the first description of mumps. Over the last two centuries the disease has been reported from most countries of the world. Outbreaks in military personnel have received special attention, and mumps has been a considerable health problem for the armed forces until recently. In 1918, during the First World War, the mortality rate among the US and French armies was as high as 75/1000 men, causing as serious a problem as the opposing army.

Johnson and Goodpasture (1934) were able to show that the disease could be transmitted to rhesus monkeys by means of a filterable agent. Habel (1945) cultured the virus in chick embyro, and as early as in the mid-1940s both live attenuated and inactivated vaccines were tried in experimental animals and human volunteers (Enders *et al.*, 1946; Henle *et al.*, 1951).

THE VIRUS

Mumps virus is taxonomically located in the family *Paramyxoviridae* where, along with *Newcastle disease virus* and *Simian virus 5* it forms a separate genus called *Rubulavirus* (Bellini *et al.*, 1998).

Paramyxovirus virions are enveloped spherical particles with surface spikes projecting from the envelope (Figure 13.1). Inside, there is a large, helically arranged nucleocapsid. The virus is sensitive to lipid solvents and is labile, 90–99% of infectivity being lost in 2 h at 4°C in protein-free medium.

Comprehensive details of the structure of *Mumps virus* have been given by Kelen and McLeod (1977) and Strauss and Strauss (1983). The size of the virion shows considerable variation. Usually the diameter is 150–200 nm but bigger virions are occasionally seen (up to 340 nm). A 220 nm filter which is commonly used in virological laboratories to remove bacteria from biological fluids may, in certain conditions, retain a large proportion of viral activity. A few virions contain multiple copies of nucleocapsid. The biological function of these 'supervirions' is not known.

Chemical analysis of the virion reveals that less than 1% of the total weight of the virion is RNA, 73% protein, 20% lipids and 6% carbohydrate.

The RNA is a single molecule, located in a helical nucleocapsid composed of the RNA and predominantly one protein species, the nucleoprotein (NP). The RNA is not infectious if inserted into a cell in naked form—the virus is a negative-stranded RNA virus. If, however, a nucleocapsid is used instead of naked RNA, infection of the target cell follows, indicating that nucleocapsid proteins play an essential role in the replicative cycle of the virus.

The genome has about 16 000 nucleotides. The virion contains RNA polymerase, haemagglutinin and neuraminidase activities and the following peptides have been identified in it: L (large polymerase, molecular weight > 160 kDa), HN (haemagglutinin-neuraminidase, 65–74 kDa), three fusion proteins (F_0, 60–68 kDa; F_1, 48–59 kDa; F_2, 10–15 kDa), NP (nucleocapsid protein, 56–61 kDa), M (matrix protein,

Principles and Practice of Clinical Virology, Fifth Edition. Edited by A. J. Zuckerman, J. E. Banatvala, J. R. Pattison, P. D. Griffiths and B. D. Schoub
© 2004 John Wiley & Sons Ltd   ISBN 0 470 84338 1

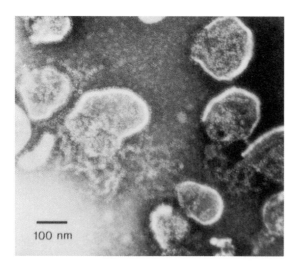

Figure 13.1 Electron micrograph of disrupted mumps virions, revealing the enveloped structure and unfolded nucleocapsid

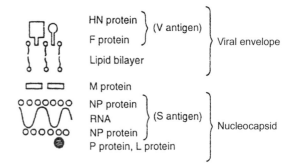

Figure 13.2 Structure components of the mumps virion

34–41 kDa), P (phosphoprotein, 44–84 kDa and SH (function unknown, 5 kDa) (Figure 13.2). In addition, at least four non-structural proteins, designated C, V, W and I are coded by the viral genome (Bellini *et al.*, 1998). The gene order (from the 3′ end) is NP–P/V–M–F–SH–HN–L (Elango *et al.*, 1998).

NP plays a central role in the encapsidation, transcription and replication of viral RNA. It is the most abundant protein of the virion and of the infected cells. P proteins serve an important role in RNA synthesis. They are components of viral polymerase complexes and probably bind both to NP and L proteins. The M protein forms the structure which underlies the viral envelope. It is important for the assembly of the virions during the replicative cycle. The HN glycoproteins agglutinate red cells of many species. Haemagglutination of avian cells is widely used in the diagnostic methods for mumps. A separate part of the molecule carries neuraminidase activity, which mediates the attachment of the virion to target cells via receptor molecules of the cell which contain sialic acid. The protein also plays a role in the fusion of plasma membranes and viral envelope working together with the F protein.

F protein is actually made of two subunits, F_1 and F_2, which are formed as a result of proteolytic cleavage of a larger precursor molecule called F_0. The F proteins play an essential role in the fusion of membranes. Antibodies reacting with F proteins inhibit haemolysis caused by *Mumps virus* and neutralise it. The F proteins are probably crucial in determining the spread of the virus in a cell population and also in the body. The proteolytic cleavage of F_0 to subunits is a host cell function. Failure of this cleavage due either to host cell malfunction or to change in the amino acid composition of F_0 results in the production of non-infectious viruses.

In purified virions actin is frequently found. M protein has a strong affinity for actin but the biological role of this virus-associated actin is unknown.

The function of SH protein is still unknown. The SH genome has been used for genetic distinction of mumps virus strains. Geographically restricted lineages have been identified which seem to be stable over time but which do not show similar progressive strain evolution as in influenza (Afzal *et al.*, 1997).

Antigenic Structure of the Virus

Only a single serotype of mumps virus is known (Hopps and Parkman, 1979). It cross-reacts considerably with other members of the genus *Paramyxovirus*. In serum samples derived from mumps patients, significant rises in antibody titres are often seen against heterologous viruses, most often against parainfluenza type 1. The viral glycoproteins HN and F are responsible for the crossreactivity, while NP and M proteins elicit a more type-specific response. Two different antigenic preparations are used in the diagnostic laboratory. Mumps V antigen consists predominantly of HN glycoprotein, while mumps S antigen is largely NP. In mumps infections antibodies develop first against S antigen and only later against V antigen. By measuring antibodies to the two antigens it is possible to make a specific laboratory diagnosis quite early in the course of infection (p 464).

Antibodies against HN and F proteins neutralise infectious virus but immunoblot analysis reveals that all components of the virion are immunogenic.

Replicative Cycle of Mumps

The virion attaches to its specific cellular receptor followed by a fusion of the viral envelope with the plasma membrane. Replication occurs exclusively in the cytoplasm. The genome is arranged in a single linear sequence from where the transcription proceeds, so that the polymerase stops and reinitiates mRNA synthesis at each gene junction. Accumulation of viral proteins leads to a switch from transcription to virion maturation. Regulation of the various steps of transcription is a complex process involving different viral proteins. For viral assembly complete nucleocapsids must be formed that are engulfed into the viral envelope by a budding process whose details are poorly understood (Bellini *et al.*, 1998).

Several details of the molecular biology of mumps still await experimental confirmation. Understanding the events in viral infections at a molecular level will help us to understand the mechanisms whereby *Mumps virus* can produce acute or chronic infection and which components are crucial for establishing protective immunity.

PATHOGENESIS

Mumps is transmitted by droplet spread or by direct contact, and the primary site of replication for the virus is the epithelium of the upper respiratory tract or eye (Feldman, 1982). The first infected cells form the primary focus, from which the virus spreads to local lymphoid tissues. Further multiplication within this restricted area results eventually in the primary viraemia, during which the virus is seeded to distant sites. The parotid gland is usually involved but so may be the central nervous system (CNS), testis or epididymis, pancreas or ovary. A few days after the onset of clinical parotitis, virus can again be isolated from blood, indicating that virus multiplication in target organs leads to a secondary viraemia (Figure 13.3). As a result, virus may again spread to various target organs. The clinical course of mumps virus infection is quite variable: meningitis may precede parotitis by a week, the disease may manifest with orchitis only, with a combination of pancreatitis and orchitis, and so on. Nevertheless, parotitis is the most

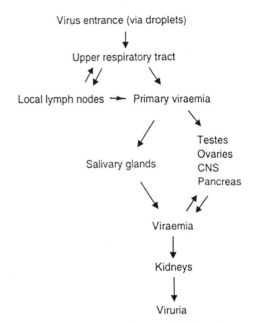

Figure 13.3 Pathogenesis of mumps infection. Primary and secondary viraemia can both lead to infection of target organs other than salivary glands

frequent presentation, occurring in 95% of those with clinical symptoms.

Virus is excreted in the urine in infectious form starting at any time during the 2 weeks following the onset of clinical disease. It is not known whether virus actually multiplies in renal tissues or whether the virus is of haematogenous origin, but in most cases slight abnormalities can be detected in renal function, such as microscopic haematuria and proteinuria. Virus is also excreted in breast milk, and it has been suggested that the virus multiplies in the lactating breast.

Interferon probably plays an important role in the pathogenesis. Highest concentrations can be detected within the first few days. Interferon can also be found in saliva and cerebrospinal fluid (CSF). Mumps infection results in a marked increase of specific antibodies of IgG, IgM and IgA antibody classes. It also stimulates a cell-mediated immune reaction which can be demonstrated *in vitro* for a few months after the infection. Which of these responses is most important for protective immunity is not known. Mumps is not a clinical problem in immunocompromised children.

Pathological changes induced by the virus in various organs are non-specific. In the parotid glands they include serofibrinous exudate and polymorphonuclear cells in the connective tissue and within the ducts. The ductal cells show degeneration but inclusion bodies have not been described. In infected testes the changes may be more pronounced, with marked congestion and punctate haemorrhages. Similar changes have been described in the pancreatic tissue.

Within the CNS the lesions are not well known. In meningitis, electroencephalograms usually show little alteration, suggesting the lesions are located predominantly in the meninges. In the rare cases where encephalitis occurs as a complication of mumps, lesions are found in the spinal cord and brain tissue. It seems evident that the lesions are produced from the combined effect of direct viral cytopathic effect and immunopathological destruction of CNS cells. Involvement of the CNS may be associated with symptoms compatible with paralytic disease and deafness. The exact pathogenesis is not known.

On several occasions prolonged involvement of the CNS after clinically manifested mumps meningo-encephalitis has been described (Julkunen *et al.*, 1985). Whether this reflects a true replication of virus within the brain tissue over an unusually long period or whether the clinical condition is a result of prolonged immunological damage is not known.

Mumps virus can multiply *in vitro* in human pancreatic islet cells (Parkkonen *et al.*, 1992). The virus can also grow in cell cultures from human joint tissues, causing chronic infection associated with an incomplete replicative cycle (Huppertz and Chantler, 1991).

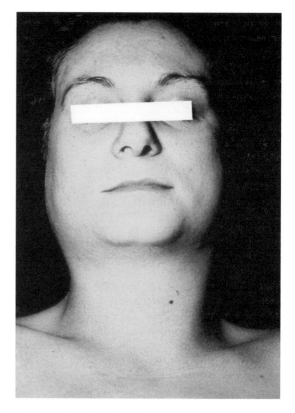

Figure 13.4   A patient with mumps parotitis

CLINICAL PICTURE

Classic Parotitis

The incubation period is 16–18 days but may vary from 14 to 25 days. Parotid swelling appears in 95% of those who develop clinical disease (Figure 13.4). The rate of subclinical infections varies somewhat with age but is, on average, 30%. In a small proportion the symptoms may resemble only mild respiratory tract illness. Patients with classic mumps develop enlargement of one parotid gland which, in 75% of cases, is followed 1–5 days later by enlargement of the contralateral gland. For 1–2 days prodromal symptoms may dominate; these include malaise, myalgia, headache and low-grade fever.

Vaccination status of the affected population may influence the clinical presentation of the disease by shifting the prevalent age distribution or affecting the course of the disease by pre-existing immunity. In an outbreak affecting both vaccinated and unvaccinated individuals at all age groups, 57% of the clinically

affected people were males and 43% were females, 58% had fever, 57% general malaise, 39% headache, 1% rash. Meningitis was seen in 1%, and orchitis in 7% of the male cases. Complications seem to be less common in vaccinated children (6% vs. 1%; Visser *et al.*, 1998).

The parotid involvement initially causes local tenderness and sometimes earache, and a few days later clinically apparent swelling. This involves the entire gland, including the area in front of the ear lobe. The orifice of the glandular duct becomes red and oedematous, and direct pressure on the glands yields only clear fluid, if anything. Submandibular and sublingual glands are occasionally also involved but practically never without parotid infection.

The parotid swelling starts to subside after 4–7 days. Virus shedding into saliva begins a couple of days before clinical parotitis and ends 7–8 days later. Glandular swelling is followed by constitutional symptoms such as fever, which seldom exceeds 40°C, and pain. These diminish when the swelling has reached its maximum and the general feeling of the patient starts improving. Recovery is rapid unless followed by a complication. Sometimes presternal oedema and sublingual and laryngeal swelling may alter the classic picture. This is thought to result from lymphatic obstruction in the cervical and mandibular areas. Severe anorexia and photophobia have been described.

Complications

The course of mumps infection may be extremely variable, as described in the section on pathogenesis. Diseases such as orchitis or pancreatitis could therefore be regarded as systemic manifestations of mumps rather than true complications. However, since classic parotitis is so characteristic and clinically dominating, all other clinical features are often regarded as complications. For a further description of the clinical aspects of mumps virus infection see Marcy and Kibrick (1983) and Christie (1974).

Meningitis

Aseptic meningitis is a common complication of mumps patients. As many as 50% may show pleocytosis of the CSF and clinical signs are seen in 1–10%. Mumps meningitis can be associated with parotid swelling but can also occur in its absence, thus causing problems in differential diagnosis. *Mumps virus* used to be the most common virologically confirmed causative agent of aseptic meningitis before general vaccinations were started. It is two to three times more frequent in males than in females and the age distribution is the same as for mumps parotitis.

Symptoms are indistinguishable from other types of aseptic meningitis and they can start from 1 week before parotid swelling to 3 weeks after it. Sometimes the clinical picture is more severe, 6–18% of hospitalised patients having symptoms resembling encephalitis (see below).

Laboratory examination of CSF reveals pleocytosis (usually <500 lymphocytes/ml, sometimes up to 1000), normal or slightly decreased sugar. Virus can be isolated from the CSF during the first 2–3 days after the onset. Later, intrathecal synthesis of mumps antibodies can be demonstrated. Symptoms of meningitis subside 3–10 days after onset, and recovery is complete.

Encephalitis

Clinical features suggesting encephalitis are convulsions, focal neurological signs, movement disorders and changes in sensory perception. Sometimes polio-like paralysis ensues and even fatalities have been reported. Probably both direct viral invasion and allergic inflammatory reactions lie behind the nervous tissue damage. The incidence of encephalitis is about 1/6000 cases of mumps.

Other Neurological Manifestations

Before vaccinations, mumps used to be one of the leading causes of hearing loss in children and young adults. According to a study from military forces in Finland, 4% of mumps cases among military recruits were associated with deafness or significant hearing loss (Vuori *et al.*, 1962). In most cases the condition was transient but in a few permanent dysfunction ensued. Hearing problems did not correlate with meningitis. The incidence of permanent hearing loss has been estimated to be 1/15 000 cases of mumps. Sometimes Ménière's disease is a late complication.

Orchitis and Oophoritis

After puberty the incidence of orchitis is 20–30%, and in 20–40% of cases there is bilateral involvement. Symptoms are acute, with pain and tenderness accompanied by fever, nausea and vomiting. The testis may enlarge three- to four-fold within 4–5 days. There is associated epididymitis in 85% of cases. Late sequelae include atrophy of testicular tissue, which may lead, in cases with bilateral disease, to infertility. Late sequelae of prepubertal orchitis are not known.

In females oophoritis is evident in approximately 5% of postpubertal cases. No correlation with infertility has been recorded. The condition may present with pelvic tenderness and cause problems of differential diagnosis from acute appendicitis.

Pancreatitis

The exact frequency of pancreatitis is difficult to determine but figures as high as 5% have been proposed. Clinical signs, such as epigastric pain and tenderness accompanied by vomiting, may lead to the diagnosis, which can be confirmed by serum amylase determination. Although the clinical picture may be quite dramatic, the outcome is almost invariably good.

Other Manifestations

Sometimes such glands as the lacrimal, thyroid or prostate become affected by *Mumps virus*, producing unusual clinical presentations.

Arthralgia or monoarthritis, involving a large joint, are complications of mumps which may develop about 2 weeks after parotitis. They are most frequent in young male adults.

Myocarditis can usually be found only upon electrocardiographic examination. In 10–15% of all mumps patients typical changes are seen. No late sequelae are known.

Transient renal dysfunction is a frequent feature of clinical mumps. In very rare instances severe nephritis and thrombocytopenia may ensue, with a fatal outcome on occasion.

If a pregnant woman contracts mumps she has an increased risk of abortion. This is thought to be due to hormonal imbalance caused by viral infection. No evidence of an increased risk of congenital malformations has been documented in humans, although paramyxoviruses cause CNS abnormalities of the developing fetus in monkeys and *Mumps virus* can cause abnormalities in the developing chick lens.

Endocardial fibroelastosis, a rare condition affecting the inner lining of the heart, is associated with a positive skin test for mumps antigen. However, a link between *Mumps virus* and the condition is doubtful.

LABORATORY DIAGNOSIS

Virus Antibody Assays

Different serological tests have been used to demonstrate a rise in the specific antibody titres or the presence of IgM class antibodies. Complement fixation test employing S and V antigens prepared from the virions was earlier frequently used as the most common test. However, due to problems in reagent stability, this technique has been replaced in many laboratories by enzyme immunosorbent assay (EIA) tests. EIA antibody levels correlate with levels of neutralising antibodies, suggesting that EIA could also reflect the immune status of the individual (Leinikki *et al.*, 1979). However, the extent of cross-reactivity from exposure to closely related paramyxoviruses may cause problems in interpretation of the results in individual

cases. The specificity of IgM antibody assays is greatly enhanced by using IgM capture techniques, where IgM class antibodies are separated in an additional incubation step from other serum constituents (Morgan-Capner, 1983).

Haemagglutination-inhibition and neutralisation antibody assays can be used as supplemental tests for both diagnostic cases and in immunity studies. Other tests, such as haemolysis in gel, can also be applied in virological laboratories.

Virus Detection

Mumps virus can be isolated from clinical samples using cell cultures or embryonated eggs. Both saliva and urine can be used as samples for diagnostic or epidemiological investigations. Mumps antigen has also been demonstrated from saliva samples by immunofluorescence or EIA techniques, allowing easy processing of large numbers of samples. Polymerase chain reaction (PCR) applications may provide even more rapid and accurate diagnostic tools in the near future.

EPIDEMIOLOGY AND CONTROL

Mumps is a disease of childhood. In unvaccinated populations the highest incidence is in children between 5 and 9 years of age. The disease is somewhat less contagious than other childhood diseases, such as measles and varicella, and quite a number of children seem to escape the infection before puberty and even beyond. The proportion of seronegatives among medical students was less than 10% in a study of an unvaccinated population. According to a survey in the USA, one-tenth of the population had mumps during each of the first 5 years of life, 74% had had it by the age of 10 and 95% by 20 years of age (Feldman, 1982).

General vaccinations have changed the epidemiological pattern profoundly. Prior to vaccination mumps used to be common in most urban areas, while in some less densely populated areas it caused widespread epidemics at 2–4 year intervals. A few descriptions of outbreaks in isolated areas have been published where the affected population had no preexisting immunity. As can be expected, age as such did not protect; however, the proportion of subclinical infections increased with age, with the exception of the youngest children (2–3 years of age), in whom subclinical infections were also very frequent. Up to 90% of infections at the age of 10–14 years were associated with clinical symptoms, while practically all infections were subclinical beyond 60 years of age. Although the clinical symptoms are usually more severe in adolescents and young adults than in children, the frequency of complications follows closely the frequency of mumps in general. Two well-known exceptions are orchitis and oophoritis, which have a much higher frequency after puberty than before, and meningoencephalitis, which is two to three times more common in males than in females.

In temperate zones of the northern hemisphere a clear-cut seasonal variation is evident. From June to September the number of reported cases is on the average less than one-third of the figures from January to May, according to a survey of 12 years and more than 150 000 cases. The peak months were February and March. No such seasonal variation is reported from tropical countries.

Only one serotype of mumps virus exists and one would expect a lifelong immunity after natural infection. However, reinfections have been reported in up to 1–2% of cases. This could indicate that mumps infection is not able to induce a lifelong protective immunity. Another explanation is that other microbes cause similar clinical pictures: in a recent study of clinically suspected mumps cases in a low-prevalence population in about half of the cases a virus other than mumps was the causative agent. Viruses such as EBV, adenovirus, parainfluenza and even enteroviruses were found (Davidkin *et al.*, 2002, personal communication). A third explanation may come from divergent genomic lineages of mumps virus that have been identified by comparing RNA sequences of strains from different outbreaks (Stöhle *et al.*, 1996).

Vaccinations Against Mumps

Control of mumps by immunisation can be very successful. In USA, the number of cases notified to the Centers for Disease Control and Prevention has dropped from over 150 000 annual cases to around 1500 cases in 20 years (Centers for Disease Control and Prevention, 1995). In Finland, with a very high childhood vaccination coverage, the endemic disease has been eradicated (National Public Health Institute, Finland, 2001). Large outbreaks of mumps in the neighbouring Russian territories have not led to local outbreaks in Finland in spite of frequent travel across the border.

However, vaccinated populations have also encountered outbreaks of mumps in recent years (Briss *et al.*,

Table 13.1 Likely problems eliminated by mumps vaccine (Finland 1971 vs. 1997)

	Cases/year 1997	Cases/year 1971*
Number of notified cases	0	22 980
Absent from school or work (person years)	0	650
Meningitis	0	6400
Encephalitis	0	160
Orchitis	0	1600
Bilateral	0	500
Male sterility	0	125
Mastitis	0	1800
Temporary hearing problems	0	920
Permanent hearing problems	0	25
Thryoiditis	0	250
Pancreatitis	0	80
Myocarditis	0	30

*The year 1971 was an epidemic year. Finland has a population of about 5 million. Reproduced from Peltola *et al.* (1999).

1994; Dias *et al.*, 1996; Visser *et al.*, 1998). Analysis of the genomic sequence has shown that multiple lineages of virus have co-circulated, suggesting lack of immunity due to either vaccine failures or low vaccination coverage.

A strain called Jeryl Lynn has been used in most vaccinations worldwide since the 1970s. Vaccines containing this strain have proved to be effective in protecting against clinical disease and even led to eradication in some countries (Peltola *et al.*, 1994). Serious complications are extremely rare: less than 1 child/1 million vaccines is affected by aseptic meningitis (Patja *et al.*, 2000).

Another strain called Urabe was introduced as a vaccine in the 1980s. Unfortunately, it proved to be associated with increased frequency of CNS complications and has been withdrawn in most countries. Another vaccine strain, called Leningrad-Zagreb attenuated mumps virus strain, was recently found to be associated with an increase of aseptic meningitis and clinical mumps after mass vaccination campaigns in Brazil (da Cunha *et al.*, 2001). The risk for aseptic meningitis was approximately 1 case/10 000 doses of vaccine; for mumps it was 1 case/300 doses. Leningrad strain has also been detected in cases of aseptic meningitis in St. Petersburg recently (Davidkin *et al.*, unpublished).

A strain used widely in vaccines, the Rubini strain, has been found to give insufficient protection against wild mumps virus and outbreaks of mumps in previously vaccinated populations have been described (Tabin *et al.*, 1993; Germann *et al.*, 1996).

Even though general vaccination of children against mumps virus has led to significant public health achievements (Table 13.1), mumps remains a challenge to clinical virology. With lowering vaccine coverage among children and variations in the efficacy of the vaccine strains, individual cases and even outbreaks are probable. In particular, individual cases without an obvious epidemiological link may pose significant diagnostic problems and emphasise the importance of virological laboratory diagnosis.

REFERENCES

Afzal MA, Buchanan J, Heath AB *et al.* (1997) Clustering of mumps virus isolates by SH gene sequence only partially reflects geographical origin. *Arch Virol*, **142**, 227–238.

Bellini WJ, Rota PA and Anderson LJ (1998) Paramyxoviruses. In *Topley and Wilson's Microbiology and Microbial Infections* (eds Collier L, Balows A and Sussman M), pp 435–461. Edward Arnold, London.

Briss PA, Fehrs LJ, Parker RA *et al.* (1994) Sustained transmission of mumps in a highly vaccinated population: assessment of primary vaccine failure and waning vaccine-induced immunity. *J Infect Dis*, **169**, 77–82.

Centers for Disease Control and Prevention (1995) Mumps surveillance—United States, 1988–1993. *Morbid Mortal Wkly Rep*, **44** (SS-3), 1–14.

Christie AB (1974) Mumps. In *Infectious diseases: Epidemiology and Clinical Practice*, pp 454–483. Livingstone, Edinburgh.

da Cunha SS, Rodrigues LC, Barreto ML and Dourado I (2001) Outbreak of aseptic meningitis and mumps after mass vaccination with MMR vaccine using Leningrad-Zagreb mumps strain. *Vaccine*, **2972**, 1–7.

Dias JA, Cordeiro M, Afzal MA *et al.* (1996) Mumps epidemic in Portugal despite high vaccine coverage—preliminary report. *Eurosurveillance*, **1**(4), 25–28.

Elango N, Varsanyi TM, Kövamees J *et al.* (1988) Molecular cloning and characterization of six genes, determination of gene order and intergenic sequences and leader sequence of mumps virus. *J Gen Virol*, **69**, 2893–2900.

Enders JF, Levens JH, Stokes J Jr *et al.* (1946) Attenuation of virulence with retention of antigenicity of mumps virus after passage in the embryonated egg. *J Immunol*, **54**, 283–291.

Feldman HA (1982) Mumps. In *Viral Infections of Humans: Epidemiology and Control* (ed. Evans AS), pp 419–435. Plenum Medical, New York.

Germann D, Ströhle A, Eggenberger K *et al.* (1996) An outbreak of mumps in a population partially vaccinated with the Rubini strain. *Scand J Infect Dis*, **28**, 235–238.

Habel K (1945) Cultivation of mumps virus in the developing chick embryo and its application to studies of immunity to mumps in man. *Publ Health Rep*, **60**, 201–212.

Henle G, Henle W, Burgoon JS *et al.* (1951) Studies on the prevention of mumps. I. The determination of susceptibility. *J Immunol*, **66**, 535–549.

Hopps HE and Parkman PD (1979) Mumps. In *Diagnostic Procedures for Viral, Rickettsial and Chlamydial Infections* (eds Lennette EH and Schmidt NJ), pp 633–663. American Public Health Assocation, Washington, DC.

Huppertz HI and Chantler JK (1991) Restricted mumps virus infections of cells derived from normal human joint tissue. *J Gen Virol*, **72**, 339–347.

Johnson CD and Goodpasture EW (1934) An investigation of the aetiology of mumps. *J Exp Med*, **59**, 1–19.

Julkunen I, Koskiniemi M-L, Lehtokoski-Lehtiniemi E *et al.* (1985) Chronic mumps virus encephalitis. *J Neuroimmunol*, **8**, 167–175.

Kelen EE and McLeod DA (1977) Paramyxoviruses: comparative diagnosis of parainfluenza mumps, measles and respiratory syncytial virus infections. In *Comparative Diagnosis of Viral Diseases* (eds Kurstak E and Kurstak C), pp 503–607. Academic Press, New York.

Leinikki P, Shekarchi I, Tzan N *et al.* (1979) Evaluation of enzyme-linked immunosorbent assay (ELISA) for mumps virus antibodies. *Proc Soc Exp Biol Med*, **160**, 363–367.

Marcy SM and Kibrick S (1983) Mumps. In *Infectious Diseases* (ed. Hoeprich P), pp 737–744. Harper & Row, New York.

Morgan-Capner P (1983) The detection of rubella-specific antibody. *Publ Health Lab Serv Microbiol Dig*, **1**, 6–11.

National Public Health Institute, Helsinki, Finland (2001) Infectious diseases. In *Infectious Diseases in Finland 1995–2000*, pp. 1–32.

Parkkonen P, Hyöty H, Koskinen L *et al.* (1992) Mumps virus infects β cells in human fetal islet cell cultures upregulating the expression of HLA class I molecules. *Diabetologia*, **35**, 63–69.

Patja A, Davidkin I, Kurki T *et al.* (2000) Serious adverse events after measles–mumps–rubella vaccination during a 14 year prospective follow-up. *Pediatr Inf Dis J*, **19**, 1127–1134.

Peltola H, Davidkin I, Paunio M *et al.* (2000) Mumps and rubella eliminated from Finland. *J Am Med Assoc*, **284**, 2643–2647.

Peltola H, Heinonen OP, Valle M *et al.* (1994) The elimination of indigenous measles, mumps, and rubella from Finland by a two-year, two-dose vaccination program. *N Engl J Med*, **331**, 1397–1402.

Peltola H, Davidkin I, Paunio M *et al.* (1999) Indigenous mumps eliminated from Finland. 39th Interscience conference on Antimicrobial Agents and Chemotherapy (ICAAC), 26–29 September, San Francisco, CA (abstr 158 G/HS).

Stöhle A, Bernasconi C and Germann D (1996) A new mumps virus lineage found in the 1995 mumps outbreak in Western Switzerland by nucleotide sequence analysis of the SH gene. *Arch Virol*, **141**, 733–741.

Strauss EG and Strauss JH (1983) Replication strategies of the single stranded RNA viruses of eukaryotes. *Curr Top Microbiol Immunol*, **105**, 45–79.

Tabin R, Berclaz J-P, Dupuis G and Peter O (1993) Rèponse immune à divers vaccins anti-ourliens. *Rev Mèd Suisse Rom*, **113**, 981–984.

Visser LE, Gonzales Peres LC, Tejera R *et al.* (1998) An outbreak of mumps in the province of León, Spain, 1995–1996. *Eurosurveillance*, **3**, 14–18.

Vuori M, Lahikainen EA and Peltonen T (1962) Perceptive deafness in connection with mumps. *Acta Oto-Laryngol*, **55**, 231–236.

14

Enteroviruses

Philip D. Minor[1] and Peter Muir[2]

[1]*NIBSC, Potters Bar and* [2]*Health Protection Agency South West, Bristol, UK*

INTRODUCTION

The enteroviruses belong to a genus of the family *Picornaviridae*. At least 66 enterovirus serotypes have been isolated from humans. Their normal site of replication is the intestinal tract, where infection may often be clinically inapparent, or result in a mild non-specific illness. However, in a proportion of cases the virus spreads to other organs, causing severe illnesses, the characteristics of which are often typical of individual enterovirus types. Poliomyelitis is one of the most severe diseases caused by an enterovirus but members of the genus are also implicated in aseptic meningitis, encephalitis, myocarditis, rashes and conjunctivitis. They may cause particularly severe disease in neonates. This chapter describes the virological properties of enteroviruses, and the pathogenesis and clinical aspects of the diseases which they cause. Prevention is, so far, limited to poliomyelitis. Although numerous agents with anti-picornaviral activity have been described, to date only one, pleconaril, shows promise as a chemotherapeutic agent.

THE VIRUSES

Viruses of the *Picornaviridae* show similar morphological, structural and molecular properties and replication strategies. They are divided into nine genera: the rhinoviruses, which are one of the causative agents of the common cold (Chapter 9); the enteroviruses, which are surprisingly closely related to the rhinoviruses; the parechoviruses, a recently recognised group which currently consists of two serotypes formerly classified as enteroviruses but now known to be genetically and biologically distinct; the cardioviruses, which cause diseases of mice and other animals; the aphthoviruses, which are causative agents of foot-and-mouth disease of cattle; the hepatoviruses, a genus encompassing hepatitis A viruses (Chapter 3); the teschoviruses (formerly porcine enteroviruses) and two genera which currently contain a single species representative: the kobuviruses and erboviruses (Minor *et al.*, 1995). The human enteroviruses include the polio, Coxsackie, enterocytopathic human orphan (echo) viruses and more recently isolated enteroviruses, designated enteroviruses 68–71. This total of 66 human enteroviruses is currently classified into five species which will be detailed later. The various members of the group differ in their cultural characteristics, antigenic properties and certain features of their replication cycle, such as the receptor sites by which they gain access to the host cell. In all cases the normal habitat and primary site of replication of the virus are thought to be the intestinal tract.

Physical Characteristics of the Virus Particle

The virion is a largely featureless, symmetrical particle, approximately 27 nm in diameter when examined electron microscopically (Figure 14.1a). Non-infectious empty capsids, unlike virions, are penetrated by stain, revealing the virion shell to be approximately 2.5 nm in thickness (Figure 14.1b). The essentially spherical appearance of the particle is consistent with icosahedral symmetry, and this has been broadly confirmed by particle shadowing, which produces

Principles and Practice of Clinical Virology, Fifth Edition. Edited by A. J. Zuckerman, J. E. Banatvala, J. R. Pattison, P. D. Griffiths and B. D. Schoub
© 2004 John Wiley & Sons Ltd   ISBN 0 470 84338 1

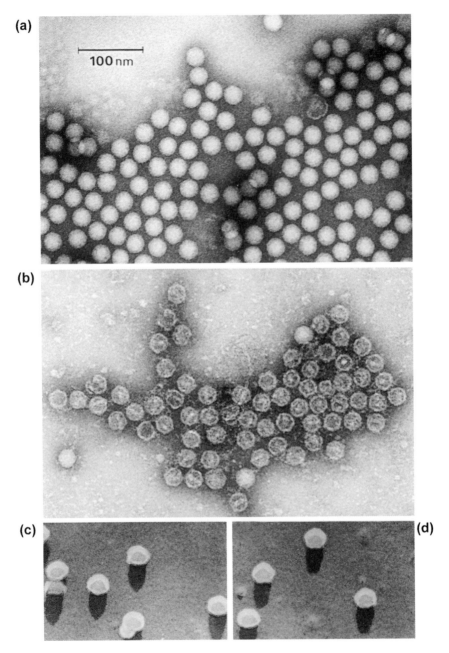

Figure 14.1 Electron micrograph of poliovirus, negatively stained with 4% sodium silicotungstate: (a) whole virus particles (D antigen) approximately 30 nm in diameter; (b) empty capsids, showing penetration of stain; (c) shadowed virus (print reversed to give black shadows) producing pointed shadows; (d) shadowed virus (print reversed to give black shadows) producing blunt-ended shadows

pointed and blunt shadows (Figure 14.1c,d). The sedimentation coefficient of the intact virus on centrifugation is 155–160S, while that of the empty capsid is 70–80S. The buoyant density of the virion in caesium chloride gradients is 1.34 g/ml. A particle with the chemical composition of an enterovirus virion would be expected to have a density of 1.47 g/ml if freely permeable to caesium ions; the low density of the enteroviruses implies that the virion is essentially impermeable, consistent with the failure of electron microscopic stains to penetrate infectious particles (Figure 14.1a). In the past, the behaviour of the viruses on isopyknic centrifugation has been used as a criterion for differentiating enteroviruses from rhinoviruses and aphthoviruses, both of which have a higher buoyant density in caesium chloride. The enteroviruses are stable to acid pH, also unlike the rhinovirus and aphthoviruses, which are inactivated by brief exposure to pH 2. This has also been used as a criterion for the identification of a picornavirus as an enterovirus.

Biochemical Structure of the Virus Particle

The infectious particle consists of a capsid constructed of 60 copies of each of four proteins, VP1, VP2, VP3 and VP4, arranged with icosahedral symmetry around a single-stranded positive (messenger)-sense RNA genome of approximately 7300 bases. Like many eukaryotic messenger RNA molecules, the genomic RNA terminates in a sequence of 40–100 adenylic acid residues at the 3′ end [the poly(A) tract]. At the 5′ end, however, it bears a small virally-encoded protein (VPg), approximately 22 amino acids long, covalently linked to the RNA by the hydroxyl group of a tyrosine residue. The complete genomic sequences of several enteroviruses are now known. The virion is believed to be entirely devoid of carbohydrate and lacks a lipid membrane, although, as described below, lipid molecules form an integral part of the structure. The particle has a relative molecular mass (M_r) of 8×10^{-6}, of which the RNA provides 32% and the protein 68% by weight. The four principal structural proteins of the virion are of M_r approximately 30 000 (VPI), 27 000 (VP2), 24 000 (VP3) and 7000 (VP4). VP2 and VP4 are formed by the cleavage of a precursor protein, VP0, as the last stage in the maturation of a virus particle, probably in an autocatalytic process resulting from the encapsidation of the nucleic acid genome.

The absence of a lipid layer has made it possible to obtain crystals suitable for X-ray diffraction studies, and the molecular structures of poliovirus (Hogle *et al.*, 1985) and other picornaviruses have been resolved, such that the interactions involved in maintaining the structural features of the infectious virion are now clear. The three largest virion proteins, VP1, VP2 and VP3, have a very similar core structure in which the peptide backbone of the protein loops back on itself to form a barrel of eight strands held together by hydrogen bonds (the β barrel). This core forms a

wedge shape, and the amino acid sequences between the sequences forming the β barrel and the sequences at the N- and C-terminal portions of the protein contain elaborations which include the main antigenic sites involved in the neutralisation of viral infectivity.

The proteins are arranged with icosahedral symmetry, with VP1 molecules at the pentameric apices of the icosahedron, orientated such that the pointed end of the wedge-shaped protein points towards the apex. The other two proteins, VP2 and VP3, alternate about the centre of the triangular face of the icosahedron (the three-fold axis of symmetry). There are extensive interactions between the three large proteins, and also with the fourth protein, VP4, which is internal. In particular, the N terminus of VP1 lies under VP3, and the N terminus of VP3 under VP1. The apical structure formed by VP1 is separated from the plateau formed by VP2 and VP3 by a cleft or canyon; the peak of the VP1 structure is 16.5 nm from the virion centre, whilst the plateau made up of VP2 and VP3 is approximately 15 nm from the centre. The base of the cleft is of the order of 11 nm from the centre, and it has been postulated that this cleft may contain the regions of the virus to which the cellular receptor attaches. The interactions between the component proteins that form the most stable unit of the structure is a pentamer made up of five copies each of VP1, VP2, VP3 and VP4; it seems likely that this is the basic unit from which the virus is assembled. A diagrammatic representation of the three-dimensional structure of the capsid proteins of poliovirus type 1 is shown in Figure 14.2.

In addition to the protein components of the virus, lipid molecules are also found in the structure. Myristic acid is found covalently attached to the N terminus of the smallest capsid protein, VP4. The aliphatic chain penetrates the apex of the icosahedron and it is possible that this forms a structural support for the virion. Myristic acid has been found attached to virion proteins in other viruses, including retroviruses and rotaviruses. A second lipid moiety, not yet identified, is present in the structures of poliovirus type 1 and type 3. It has a 16-carbon aliphatic chain which lies in the pocket formed by the β barrel of VP1. The other end of the molecule has not been observed. Rhinovirus 14 has no such insert, and it is not yet clear how general a feature of enteroviruses this lipid molecule is. However, certain antiviral compounds insert into the corresponding region of rhinovirus 14 and, in so doing, prevent uncoating. It is therefore possible that the lipid plays a part in uncoating or assembly of enteroviruses.

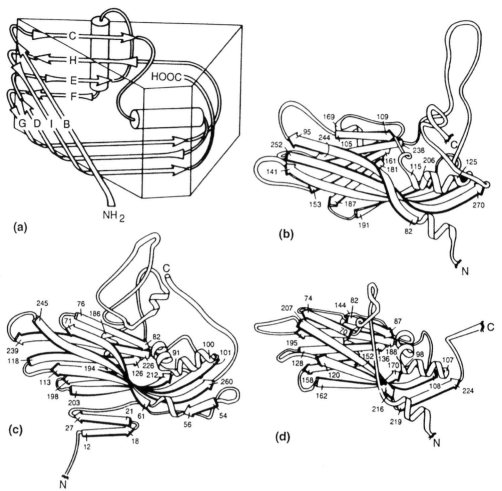

Figure 14.2 Three-dimensional structure of the capsid proteins of poliovirus. The numbers indicate positions of amino acid residues: (a) core structure common to capsid proteins; (b) VP1; (c) VP2; (d) VP3. Reprinted with permission from Hogle *et al.* (1985) The three dimensional structure of poliovirus at 2.9Å resolution. *Science*, **229**, 1358. American Association for the Advancement of Science.

Antigenic Structure of the Virus

The antigenic properties of the enteroviruses provide one of the main methods of differentiating them. In most cases serotype-specific antisera neutralise only virus isolates or strains of the homologous serotype, but this is not always so. For every picornavirus studied in detail, it has been shown that empty capsids prepared under appropriate conditions present major antigenic determinants differently from those of the infectious virus. Moreover, the infectious virus can be readily denatured by relatively mild conditions, such as treatment with ultraviolet light, heating to 56°C for 10 min or attachment to a plastic surface in solid phase enzyme immunoassays. The infectious particle is said

to express D or N antigenic character, and the empty capsid or denatured virus C or H antigenic character. C antigen is less specific to a particular virus than is D antigen. Thus, there is evidence for cross-reaction of C antigen-specific monoclonal antibodies with poliovirus of types 1, 2 and 3, whereas cross-reaction by neutralising monoclonal antibodies or those reacting with D antigen is rare. Monoclonal antibodies able to neutralise both type 1 and type 2 poliovirus have been reported (Uhlig *et al.*, 1990) and priming for a secondary response to type 1 or type 3 by previous injection with type 2 is documented. Similarly, there is evidence for cross-reaction of echoviruses 11, 16 and parechovirus 1 with poliovirus with appropriate C-specific antibodies. In addition, some epitopes present on VP1 appear to be conserved among most or all human enteroviruses, and monoclonal antibodies to such epitopes have been used as pan-enterovirus detection reagents (Trabelsi *et al.*, 1995). The difference between particles expressing D and C antigen is due to the conformation of the proteins, rather than to the loss of a protein; cross-reactive epitopes are internalised in the infective virion, but become surface-exposed and thus able to bind antibody following denaturation. Thus, methods based on virus neutralisation by antibody are required to determine serotype-specific humoral immunity, while solid phase EIA or immunoblot methods detect both type-specific and cross-reactive antibody (Muir and Banatvala, 1990).

The antigenic structures involved in the neutralisation of picornavirus infectivity have been the subject of much study and have been clarified by the resolution of the molecular structures of poliovirus and rhinovirus and representatives of the other genera outlined above. Neutralising epitopes have been identified by the isolation of antigenic variants resistant to monoclonal antibodies, able to neutralise a parental strain, and then characterised by sequencing the genomic RNA. This has revealed four major sites to which neutralising antibodies bind, formed from a number of exposed surface loops. For type 3 poliovirus they include: (a) a sequence of VP1 about one-third of the way in from the N terminus, involving residues 89–100, together with sequences from three other loops from VP1, including amino acids 142, 166 and 253; (b) a complex site involving residues 220–222 of VP1 and 160–170 of VP2 and the C terminus of VP2; (c) a complex site involving residues 286–290 of VP1 and 58–60 of VP3 (Minor, 1990). The fourth site involves residues in different pentamers and is therefore only found in the intact virion, while the other sites are also found in some viral subunits. For poliovirus type 1, the site located at residues 89–100 of VP1 has been implicated in virus neutralisation, although to a far lesser extent than for type 3, where the homologous region is the principal target for neutralising antibodies in sera from immunised animals. The site involving VP3 is the next most common target of antibodies, including most of the antibodies showing extreme strain specificity for poliovirus, whilst the site involving VP2 is the least common.

The antigenic structure of poliovirus type 2 virus has been less well characterised. The site to which cross-reactive antibodies bind appears to involve sequences around 200–210 of VP3 and 239–245 of VP2, and may be linked to the strain-specific site involving VP1 and VP3 (Uhlig *et al.*, 1990).

Cellular Receptor Sites

Enteroviruses attach to and enter cells by specific cell-surface receptors. This was first shown for poliovirus by the observation that purified genomic RNA was infectious for rabbit cells, whereas the virus itself was not. Competition experiments between different viruses have shown, for example, that all three poliovirus serotypes utilise the same cellular receptor, which is distinct from that for the Coxsackie B viruses. This phenomenon has been confirmed in a number of cases by the isolation of monoclonal antibodies, which will specifically block the attachment of certain types of virus by reacting with the host cell rather than with the virus (Minor *et al.*, 1984).

The enteroviruses and picornaviruses in general are responsible for a range of diseases with different target organs. These include the heart (Coxsackie viruses), nerve tissue (polioviruses), liver (HAV) and others, as well as the intestinal tract. It is possible that the expression of the receptor sites in specific tissues plays a part in the tropism of the virus, although it is unlikely to be the only factor. This may suggest a novel chemotherapeutic approach for enterovirus infections using synthetic receptor analogues.

The cellular gene encoding the receptor for poliovirus has been identified (Mendelsohn *et al.*, 1989) as a previously unknown three-domain protein of the immunoglobulin superfamily termed CD155. The terminal domain is required for activity. Transgenic mice carrying the gene for the human receptor for poliovirus (Ren *et al.*, 1990; Koike *et al.*, 1991) are susceptible to poliovirus infection, with pathology similar to that observed in primates. Mouse cells are not normally susceptible to infection with poliovirus or most other human enteric viruses. When stably transfected with the human gene for the poliovirus receptor, however, they are rendered sensitive, and can thus be used to identity polioviruses in the presence of other viruses. This is of value in clinical studies related to the programme to eradicate poliomyelitis, as described later.

The receptor for echovirus 1 has been isolated and identified as the integrin VLA-2, a known surface molecule (Bergelson *et al.*, 1992). DAF (decay accelerating factor; CD55), a cell surface protein involved in the complement pathway, is a receptor site for many echoviruses (Bergelson *et al.*, 1994) some Coxsackie B viruses (Shafren *et al.*, 1995), and enterovirus 70 (Karnauchow *et al.*, 1996). Coxsackie virus B1–6 serotypes also use a common receptor, also used by some adenoviruses (the Coxsackie–adenovirus receptor), identified as a probable cellular adhesion

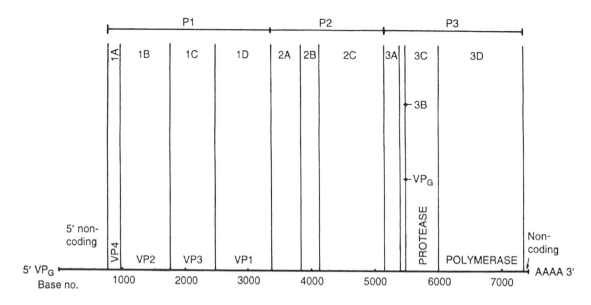

Figure 14.3 Organisation of the genome of poliovirus, a typical enterovirus showing the two non-coding regions and the location of the regions coding for the various virus proteins. In the formal nomenclature (Rueckert and Wimmer, 1984), the P1 region encodes the structural capsid proteins, and the P2 and P3 regions encode non-structural proteins found only in infected cells

molecule which contains two immunoglobulin-like domains, and is expressed preferentially in brain, heart and pancreas (Bergelson *et al.*, 1997). Coxsackie viruses A10, 15, 18 and 21 employ ICAM-1, as does the major rhinovirus group. Coxsackie virus B3 also uses nucleolin, and Coxsackie virus A9 αvβ3 integrin.

Strategy of Replication

The genome of the virus is a single positive-strand RNA molecule, and thus acts as a messenger RNA for the synthesis of the proteins found in infected cells. The genome can be divided into three regions, a 5′ non-translated region (NTR) of about 750 bases, followed by a large open reading frame encoding a polyprotein which comprises most of the genome, then a second short 3′ NTR terminated by a poly(A) tail. The open reading frame can be divided into three regions, termed P1–3, which correspond to the primary cleavage products of the polyprotein (see below). The P1 region encodes virion structural proteins, while the P2 and P3 regions encode non-structural proteins necessary for virus replication, such as the RNA polymerase. This arrangement is summarised in Figure 14.3. The NTRs are highly conserved, reflecting their importance in virus replication.

The 5′ NTR of eukaryotic messenger RNA usually terminates in a methylated guanosine cap, which is important in binding ribosomes and thus translation of the RNA into protein. Thus, most eukaryotic messenger RNA molecules require a free 5′ terminus, and initiation of translation internally is not possible. However, it has been shown that the 5′ NTRs of poliovirus and other picornaviruses contain an internal ribosomal entry site (IRES), which enables ribosomal binding in the absence of a free 5′ capped terminal structure (Pelletier and Sonnenberg, 1988). In fact, poliovirus infection results in the cessation of cap-dependent translation. The mechanism of internal initiation involves binding of cellular proteins, including the eukaryotic translation initiation factors, a pyrimidine tract binding protein and poly(rC) binding proteins to the IRES (Hellen *et al.*, 1993). There is evidence that additional cell type-specific proteins also interact with the IRES, and the ability of a given IRES to interact with such non-canonical translation initiation factors may in part determine the susceptibility of a given cell type to infection with a particular enterovirus (Malnou *et al.*, 2002), since it is known that the availability of cellular receptor proteins is not the sole determinant of tissue tropism.

The viral proteins are translated as a single polyprotein. This precursor protein includes two known sequences which act as proteolytic enzymes and digest the protein at specific positions during the course of translation. The first (P2A) acts to cleave the structural (P1) from the non-structural (P2–3) proteins (Figure 14.3), whilst the second completes all the other processing of the protein, except the final maturational cleavage of VP0 to VP2 and VP4. The non-structural proteins include proteases (2A, 3C and the intermediate cleavage product 3CD), a polymerase (3D), nucleotide triphosphatase (2C) and the small protein VPg (3B), which is covalently attached to the 5' terminus of both positive- and negative-sense viral RNA. Proteins 2B and 2BC induce extensive rearrangement of intracellular membranes into vesicles, which are a required component of viral replication complexes. The 2C protein coding sequence also contains a highly conserved stem–loop RNA structure which is a *cis*-acting replication element (CRE) required for viral RNA synthesis.

In the early stages of the infection process the genome is used predominantly for translation of viral proteins. However as the pool of viral proteins increases, protease 3CD binds to the 5' NTR, repressing translation and favouring RNA synthesis. The positive-sense genomic RNA acts as a template for the synthesis of a negative-sense copy. Negative strand synthesis requires circularisation of the genome, in which a ribonucleoprotein complex formed at the 5' NTR interacts with poly(A) binding protein bound to the 3' poly(A) tail. The viral polymerase (3D) then catalyses the uridylation of the VPg, using the poly(A) tail of the viral genome as template. The resulting VPg-poly(U) primes the synthesis of negative-sense RNA. This gives rise to a double-stranded replicative intermediate, which associates with membranous vesicles to form replication complexes. The replicative intermediate acts as a template for further positive-sense strand synthesis. Positive-strand synthesis also requires a uridylated VPg primer, but in this instance adenosine residues within the loop of the CRE RNA structure serve as the template for uridylation, in a complex between the 5' and 3' NTRs, the CRE and the 3C and 3CD proteins. The resulting uridylated protein [VPgpUpU(OH)] presumably associates with the 3' terminus of the negative-sense RNA and primes positive-strand synthesis. It is likely that the increasing excess of VPgpUpU(OH) over VPg during the course of infection favours synthesis of the positive over the negative strand. Thus, the different mechanisms involved in uridylation of VPg and the initiation of transcription for positive- and negative-strand synthesis leads to asymmetrical replication of viral RNA. Positive-sense RNA is the major species made after the early stages of infection and is used both for translation and for packaging into virus.

The assembly of the virus particle involves the synthesis of VP0, VP1 and VP3 as a single unit, which is then assembled into pentamers, followed by the association of 12 pentamers into the virion, a process which involves host factors. The X-ray crystallographic structure of the virus implies that the final maturation cleavage of VP0 to VP2 and VP4 is autocatalytic. Thus, a serine residue is found close to the N-terminus of VP2. A number of serine proteases are known, and it may be concluded that as soon as the proton donor, such as the genomic RNA, is brought into the vicinity of the serine residue the final cleavage will take place. The virus is released from the cell by lysis.

Sequence Comparisons of Enteroviruses

Complete genomic sequences for a number of enteroviruses and other picornaviruses have been determined (Stanway, 1990). Comparison of such sequences reveals a surprisingly close relationship between the enteroviruses and rhinoviruses, the genomes of which show a high degree of homology. In contrast hepatitis A has no significant homology with enteroviruses at the nucleic acid level. Similarly, parechovirus 1 (formerly echovirus 22) is also unique in the sequence, showing no homology with other enteroviruses.

The human enteroviruses can be divided into two genetic clusters on the basis of sequence comparisons of the 5' NTR (Pöyry *et al.*, 1996; Hyypiä *et al.*, 1997). One includes polioviruses, Coxsackie viruses A21 and A24 and enterovirus 70, while Coxsackie B, Coxsackie viruses A9 and A16, enterovirus 71, echovirus 11, echovirus 12 and all partially sequenced echoviruses form the second cluster. Similar sequence comparisons of the coding region and 3' NTR reveal four major genetic clusters of the human enteroviruses, and this genetic analysis now forms the basis of a new human enterovirus (HEV) species classification (Table 14.1). Although the polioviruses fall within the same genetic cluster as HEV-C, they have been assigned to a distinct species in recognition of their biological uniqueness as agents of poliomyelitis (Minor *et al.*, 1995), although this may not be justified in other ways. Viruses within a particular human enterovirus group are apparently able to recombine readily. Thus, the non-structural parts of the genome are not informative in attempting to identify a group C enterovirus as a poliovirus, for example. There is good evidence for recombination between vaccine strains of poliovirus and unidentified

Table 14.1 Phylogenetic classification of human enteroviruses

Human enterovirus species	Historical grouping	Serotypes
Human enterovirus A (HEV-A)	Coxsackie virus A	2, 3, 5, 7, 8, 10, 12, 14, 16
	Enterovirus	71
Human enterovirus B (HEV-B)	Coxsackie virus A	9
	Coxsackie virus B	1, 2, 3, 4, 5, 6
	Echovirus	1, 2, 3, 4, 5, 6, 7, 8, 9, 11, 12, 13, 14, 15, 16, 17, 18, 19, 20, 21, 24, 25, 26, 27, 29, 30, 31, 32, 33
	Enterovirus	69
Human enterovirus C (HEV-C)	Coxsackie virus A	1, 11, 13, 15, 17, 18, 19, 20, 21, 22, 24
Human enterovirus D (HEV-D)	Enterovirus	68, 70
Poliovirus (PV)	Poliovirus	1, 2, 3

enteroviruses of group C, probably Coxsackie A viruses, in a number of small outbreaks, to be described later.

Sequenced animal enteroviruses, such as bovine enteroviruses, form groups distinct from the human enteroviruses when either the 5′ NTR or the remainder of the genome is considered. Different regions of the genome vary in their homology between enteroviruses and other picornaviruses. Certain sections in the 5′ NTR of the genome are identical in all enteroviruses examined, implying some definite functional constraint; this identity may carry over into the rhinoviruses, but it is possible to identify sequences which are apparently enterovirus-specific. It is further possible to identify regions such as the 3′ NTR which are strongly conserved for a particular species, such as a poliovirus. Finally, certain regions, including those areas encoding the capsid protein VP1, are extremely strain-specific. In principle, as described later, it is possible to exploit these various types of region to devise genomic probes or polymerase chain reaction (PCR) primers which are specific either for enteroviruses in general, for a particular species of enterovirus, for a particular enterovirus serotype or even for a particular strain. Such probes are valuable in clinical and epidemiological studies.

PATHOBIOLOGICAL AND CLINICAL ASPECTS OF HUMAN ENTEROVIRUSES

Enterovirus serotypes are defined on the basis of homotypic seroneutralisation, and exhibit a wide range of biological and pathogenic properties which are often characteristic of individual enterovirus groups. An extensive literature of up-to-date and authoritative reviews on the clinical, pathological and epidemiological properties of individual groups of human

enteroviruses is available (Tracy *et al.*, 1991; Rotbart, 1995; Melnick, 1996), to which the reader is referred for further detailed information.

Historically, the enteroviruses were divided into five groups: polioviruses, Coxsackie virus group A, Coxsackie virus group B, echoviruses and recently characterised human enteroviruses. The virus types comprising each group are summarised in Table 14.2, together with the major diseases with which they are associated and their cultural characteristics.

The historical classification of the enteroviruses closely followed the history of the development of knowledge on the aetiology of the diseases they cause. Poliovirus was first identified in 1909 by inoculation of monkeys with specimens from cases of paralytic poliomyelitis. Following the discovery by Enders *et al.* (1949) that poliovirus could be grown in cell cultures, the importance of the enteroviruses as a cause of human disease came to be appreciated. In 1948 Dalldorf and Sickles (1948) recovered a new group of agents by inoculation into newborn mice of faecal extracts from two children with paralytic disease. These agents were named Coxsackie viruses after the town in New York State where the isolations were made. Coxsackie virus types A and B were identified on the basis of the histopathological changes they produced in newborn mice and their capacity to grow in cell cultures. Later a third group, the echoviruses, was identified, which was also associated from time to time with human diseases. Echoviruses were found to be non-pathogenic for subhuman primates and newborn mice, but produced cytopathic changes in cell cultures. Within a few years it was found that all three groups of virus were antigenically distinct and consisted of several and, in some cases, numerous serological subtypes.

Since 1970, new enterovirus types have been allocated sequential numbers (68–71) following those allocated previously to enteroviruses. In the future it is likely that newly identified enterovirus serotypes will

Table 14.2 Types and characteristics of human enteroviruses

Group	Virus types	Cytopathic effects in cell cultures		Pathology in newborn mice	Major disease associations
		Monkey kidney	Human cell culture		
Poliovirus	3 types (poliovirus 1–3)	+	+	−	Paralytic poliomyelitis; aseptic meningitis; febrile illness
Coxsackie virus group A	23 types (A1–A22, A24)	− or ±	− or ±	+	Aseptic meningitis; herpangina; febrile illness; conjunctivitis (A24); hand, foot and mouth disease
Coxsackie virus group B	6 types (B1–B6)	+	+	+	Aseptic meningitis; severe generalised neonatal disease; myopericarditis; encephalitis; pleurodynia (Bornholm disease); febrile illness
Echovirus	31 types (types 1–9, 11–27, 29–33)	+	±	−	Aseptic meningitis, rash, febrile illness; conjunctivitis; severe generalised neonatal disease
Enteroviruses	4 types (types 68–71)	+	+	−	Polio-like illness (E71); aseptic meningitis (E71); hand, foot and mouth disease (E71); epidemic conjunctivitis (E70)

be assigned to one of the new genetically defined HEV species as described above.

The enteroviruses have a worldwide distribution and collectively cause a considerable impact in morbidity and mortality. The extraordinarily wide range of diseases included in their clinical 'repertoire' contributes to their attraction as subjects for study by the molecular virologist, pathologist, clinician and epidemiologist alike.

Although there is little documented evidence of progressive antigenic variation, antigenically unusual strains can be isolated (Magrath et al., 1986), e.g. type 3 polioviruses isolated from patients with paralytic poliomyelitis in Finland in 1984 were antigenically clearly distinguishable from classic poliovirus type 3 strains isolated in the 1950s. It may be significant that the cases of poliomyelitis from which the viruses were isolated occurred in persons who were 'immunised' with inactivated vaccine. Other evidence of antigenic heterogeneity among viruses of a single serotype is the finding that Coxsackie virus B5 strains isolated in 1973 in the USA are clearly distinguishable from the prototype 1952 strains (Melnick, 1996). There is also evidence that recombination between heterologous enterovirus serotypes occurs, and this may result in strains with biological properties distinct from those of the progenitor strains.

The host range of the enteroviruses varies between groups and types. Table 14.2 summarises the ability of the viruses to replicate and produce cytopathogenic effects in cell cultures of monkey kidney and human origin and their pathogenesis for suckling mice. Poliovirus, unlike other enteroviruses, causes flaccid paralysis in monkeys and chimpanzees when administered into the brain or spinal cord. A feature of Coxsackie viruses not shared by other enteroviruses is their pathogenicity for suckling mice. Coxsackie A viruses produce widespread myositis in the skeletal muscles of newborn mice, resulting in flaccid paralysis without other obvious lesions. Coxsackie B viruses also produce myositis but generally of more focal distribution than that caused by group A viruses. In addition they cause necrotising lesions of the brown fat pads (intrascapular cervical and cephalic pads) and, in the case of certain strains, encephalitis with spastic paralysis, pancreatitis, myocarditis, endocarditis and hepatitis in both infant and adult mice. Coxsackie A viruses, unlike Coxsackie B strains, replicate poorly if at all in monkey kidney cell cultures. As already mentioned, most echoviruses are non-pathogenic in primates and mice.

The common portal of entry for enteroviruses is generally thought to be the alimentary tract via the mouth. Replication of virus in the cells lining the alimentary tract may be preceded by, or accompany, oropharyngeal replication.

A viraemic phase is followed by infection of target organs, e.g. spinal cord and brain, meninges, myocardium or skin. Incubation periods before onset of disease vary widely from 2 days to 30–40 days depending on the clinical manifestation. The pathogenesis of poliomyelitis has been studied extensively (Minor, 1996) but is still not fully understood. According to Bodian, the virus, having entered via the alimentary tract, multiplies locally at the initial sites of virus colonisation (tonsils, Peyer's patches) and associated lymph nodes. At this stage virus may be isolated from both throat and faeces. Secondary spread of virus apparently occurs via the blood to other susceptible tissues (e.g. other lymph nodes, brown fat pads and nervous tissue). On the other hand, Sabin held the view that the virus replicates chiefly in the mucosal layers of the intestine or oropharynx, seeding the associated lymphoid tissues, where it does not necessarily replicate. After a low-level, possibly undetectable viraemia, replication at distant unidentified sites leads to a secondary viraemia, which may result in infection of either the peripheral or central nervous system (for further details, see Minor, 1996).

Within the central nervous system the virus appears to spread along nerve fibres. If local multiplication is extensive, motor neurons are destroyed and paralysis results. The anterior horn cells of the spinal cord are most prominently involved but in severe poliomyelitis the posterior horn and dorsal root ganglia are affected. Shedding of virus occurs from the throat and in faeces and thus transmission of infection occurs independently of invasion of the nervous system.

The pathogenesis of Coxsackie B virus-induced myocarditis is also well studied in murine models, and is discussed below. The major clinical aspects of enterovirus infection are now summarised.

CNS Infections

Paralytic Poliomyelitis

The clinical features and epidemiology of this disease have been reviewed in detail by Minor (1996). Progress towards its eradication is described later.

Poliovirus infection may be asymptomatic or mild and only about 1% of infections result in illness with neurological involvement. Cases of abortive polio-myelitis, often accompanied by fever, malaise, headache, nausea or vomiting, are followed by uneventful recovery. Some patients develop aseptic meningitis with clinical features similar to those caused by other enteroviruses (non-paralytic poliomyelitis). In a small number of cases, paralytic poliomyelitis occurs.

Most cases occur without evidence of an earlier phase of illness. The most predominant sign is acute flaccid paralysis, resulting from lower motor neuron damage. Painful spasms and incoordination of non-paralysed muscles may also occur. Death may be due to respiratory paralysis. In those who survive, some recovery of muscular function is common but may take 6 months or longer. In epidemics in developed countries in the early 1950s, typically 5% of cases were fatal, 10% showed full recovery with no sequelae, while the remainder showed permanent paralysis to some degree. Isolation of a poliovirus from a patient with acute flaccid paralysis confirms the diagnosis of paralytic poliomyelitis in the absence of any other cause. Poliomyelitis, when epidemic, occurs primarily in the summer months in temperate zones. Non-polio enteroviruses, particularly Coxsackie virus A7 and enterovirus 71, occasionally cause polio-like illness, and in some regions where wild polioviruses have been eradicated, enterovirus 71 is emerging as an important cause of acute flaccid paralysis (Alexander et al., 1994; da Silva et al., 1996).

Many years after maximal recovery from the original attack of poliomyelitis, some patients develop further muscle weakness, the post-poliomyelitis syndrome. There have been suggestions that in some cases this may be due to persistent poliovirus infection of neural cells, based on the detection of intrathecal poliovirus antibody and the presence of poliovirus RNA in cerebrospinal fluid (Leparc-Goffart et al., 1996), although there are alternative hypotheses, such as ageing (Munsat, 1991). Persistence of poliovirus or other enterovirus infection of the central nervous system has also been implicated in the aetiology of motor neuron disease, and the presence of enterovirus RNA in cerebrospinal fluid or neural tissue has been reported in small numbers of patients (Woodall et al., 1994; Leparc-Goffart et al., 1996). However, two other studies found that, while enterovirus RNA can be detected in post-mortem brain and spinal cord tissue of patients with post-poliomyelitis syndrome or motor neuron disease, viral RNA was also detectable in patients with other neurological or non-neurological diseases (Muir et al., 1996; Giraud et al., 2001), and was therefore unlikely to be related to chronic neurological disease.

Aseptic Meningitis

Aseptic meningitis occurs most frequently in young children. Enteroviruses are the commonest cause of aseptic meningitis in countries where mumps has been controlled by vaccination. A febrile illness may be followed by meningeal signs, with stiffness of the neck or back, and muscle weakness, clinically reminiscent of mild poliomyelitis, may occur (Rotbart, 1995). However, in infections caused by non-polio enteroviruses there is almost always complete recovery from paresis. Coxsackie viruses of both group A and group B (especially types B1–B6, A7 and A9), many echoviruses (notably types 4, 6, 11, 14, 16, 25, 30 and 31) as well as enterovirus 71 have been associated with aseptic meningitis.

Patients with aseptic meningitis have a clear CSF which is usually under normal, or slightly increased, pressure. A pleocytosis, usually of the order of 10–500/ mm^{-3}, mainly of lymphocytes is often, although not invariably present. During the first day or so after the onset of symptoms, polymorphonuclear leukocytes may predominate. The protein concentration is normal or slightly increased and the CSF glucose concentration is generally within normal limits. Thus, a normal CSF does not exclude enterovirus infection. Enteroviruses can be cultured from CSF, although viral RNA detection by PCR is more sensitive, as described below. In neonates and infants, PCR detection of viral RNA in serum or urine also provides useful evidence of systemic infection.

Encephalitis

Although herpes simplex virus is the most commonly identified pathogen in patients with encephalitis (see Chapter 2A), enteroviruses are increasingly recognised as encephalitic agents (Modlin et al., 1991). Enteroviral encephalitis may be associated with aseptic meningitis, or may present with absent or minimal meningeal involvement. Children and young adults are most frequently affected. Although most patients recover uneventfully, a few have neurological sequelae or damage to the hypothalamic–pituitary axis, which causes endocrine disturbance. CSF findings are similar to those occurring in aseptic meningitis. Again, a normal CSF does not exclude enterovirus infection. Viral detection in CSF by PCR is considered proof of aetiology, although the sensitivity of PCR in this setting has not been established. Viral detection at

peripheral sites, or viral serology may be required to provide evidence of recent enterovirus infection.

Patients with hypogammaglobulinaemia may develop persistent infections following enterovirus infection, associated with chronic meningeal irritation, encephalitis, insidious intellectual impairment or, sometimes, a dermatomyositis-like syndrome (Wilfert et al., 1977). Although some patients recover, there is a high mortality rate. Many echoviruses and Coxsackie viruses B have been shown to cause such persistent infections; occasionally, multiple serotypes may be involved. Patients with hypogammaglobulinaemia may also develop paralytic disease following administration of attenuated live polio vaccine. Virus may be recovered from the CSF, sometimes intermittently, although high concentrations are often present. Treatment with high-titre specific immunoglobulin has not been shown to be particularly effective in eradicating virus from the CNS, although combination treatment with immunoglobulin and the antipicornaviral drug pleconaril (described later) is anecdotally reported to be more successful.

Heart Disease

Myocarditis

A wide range of viruses may cause myocarditis, including ortho- and paramyxoviruses, togaviruses, herpesviruses and adenoviruses. However, Coxsackie B viruses are the most commonly identified cause. In addition, current understanding of pathogenesis in viral myocarditis derives mainly from studies of Coxsackie B virus infection, including both clinical studies in humans and experimental studies of Coxsackie B3 virus-induced murine myocarditis. Other enteroviruses, including polioviruses, Coxsackie A viruses and echoviruses, may also cause myocarditis, and the relative importance of other non-polio enteroviruses may have been underestimated in recent years because of the wider availability of serological tests for Coxsackie virus B infection.

Acute myocarditis is an inflammatory disease of the heart muscle. Diagnosis therefore requires histological examination of endomyocardial biopsy or autopsy tissue. As this is often not available, it is likely that myocarditis is underdiagnosed. Clinical features are non-specific and variable.

Neonatal myocarditis can be rapidly fatal, and may be confused with congenital heart disease. Other systemic symptoms may be present. The pathological changes vary with the duration of illness. In infants who die early after infection (2–5 days), left ventricular dilatation is present. The endocardium and valves are normal, even though the myocardium is pale. Late in infection (9–11 days of illness) the size of the heart is increased, largely due to dilatation of the left, and occasionally the right, ventricle. Microscopically, myofibre necrosis and inflammation are evident. Initially the inflammatory infiltrate is composed of polymorphonuclear leukocytes, but by day 5 or 6 mononuclear inflammatory cells are found.

In contrast to the abrupt, severe and often fatal disease seen in the neonatal period, viral myocarditis in adolescents and adults usually has a delayed onset, often following an upper respiratory (typically influenza-like) or gastrointestinal illness. Acute heart disease may become evident a week to 10 days later and has a presentation that can mimic myocardial infarction, coronary artery occlusion or progressive heart failure. Some patients do not present with heart disease but manifest non-specific symptoms and signs, such as fever, myalgia and headache; often, cardiac involvement is suspected only because of typical ECG changes. In a proportion the main presenting feature is pericarditis, characterised by acute, often severe, retrosternal chest pain. Other clinical findings include shortness of breath, tachycardia, arrhythmias, murmurs, rubs and cardiomegaly (due to ventricular dilatation or pericardial effusion). Death can supervene due to arrhythmias or congestive heart failure, but this is relatively uncommon. As in the neonatal infection, manifestations of systemic disease in adults may be noted. In Coxsackie virus B infections these may include pleurodynia, meningitis, hepatitis, orchitis, lymphadenopathy and splenomegaly. There may be recrudescences following the acute episode; up to 20% of patients in whom the major presenting feature is pericarditis will experience one or more relapsing episodes in the following months or years (Muir *et al.*, 1989). Acute myocarditis may also lead to chronic myocarditis or dilated cardiomyopathy (DCM), as described below.

Viral infection of the myocardium is believed to be a prerequisite to myocarditis, although antiviral cellular immune responses and autoreactive T cells activated following local tissue damage and release of sequestered autoantigen are likely to be important effectors of myocardial pathology (Horwitz *et al.*, 2000). At present there is a lack of consensus on the most appropriate treatment for DCM. Thus, while steroid therapy has been used in patients with myocarditis, evidence of efficacy is lacking (Mason *et al.*, 1995) and concerns remain that immunosuppressive therapy may

result in increased viral replication and persistence (Heim *et al.*, 1994).

Virological investigations including virus isolation, PCR and serological studies, as described later, can assist in establishing a viral aetiology but often give negative or inconclusive findings. Even if cardiac biopsy samples are taken early or the patient dies during the acute phase, it is exceptionally rare to isolate virus or detect virus antigen in heart tissue, although enterovirus RNA may be detected. Because myocarditis may present some time after the initiating viral infection, specific antibody titres may have already peaked. Thus, serological investigation using paired acute and convalescent samples may fail to demonstrate a diagnostic rise in titre. Enterovirus IgM testing may be used in the absence of suitably paired sera or isolation samples, but IgM seroprevalence in the community can be significant, especially during high-activity seasons, reflecting asymptomatic infection. Thus, a positive result provides only circumstantial evidence of aetiology.

Dilated Cardiomyopathy

Dilated cardiomyopathy is a postinflammatory disease which is a significant cause of heart failure and sudden cardiac death, and one of the commonest reasons for requiring cardiac transplantation. Enteroviruses are the most commonly identified agents of acute myocarditis, and there is now strong evidence that they also cause persistent infection associated with chronic myocarditis and chronic DCM (reviewed by Muir and Archard, 1994). There is evidence that viral persistence after the initial infection is directly involved in the evolution of DCM (Bowles *et al.*, 1986), although immunopathological mechanisms, including the development of cardiac autoimmunity, may also contribute to chronic disease (Liu and Mason, 2001).

Infectious virus or viral antigens cannot be detected in cardiomyopathic hearts, although a proportion of patients have elevated neutralising antibody titres (Cambridge *et al.*, 1979) and persistent enterovirus-specific IgM responses (Muir *et al.*, 1989). Viral RNA can be detected in cardiac muscle of a proportion of cases by nucleic acid hybridisation (Bowles *et al.*, 1986; Kandolf *et al.*, 1990) or reverse transcriptase-PCR (Schwaiger *et al.*, 1993; Kämmerer *et al.*, 1994; Archard *et al.*, 1998). Small numbers of patients with myocarditis or DCM have been treated with IFN-α, either alone or in combination with IFN-β, with evidence of viral clearance and clinical improvement in some.

Characteristics of Murine Coxsackie B Viral Disease

Experimentally, Coxsackie viruses B replicate and produce inflammatory lesions in the heart, pancreas, liver, spleen and brain in several strains of mice. Studies in weanling and adult animals with Coxsackie viruses B have shown that parenteral infection results in viraemia and then replication in target organs. Viraemia is detected within 24 h and usually persists until day 3. The virus grows in various target organs, with maximum levels achieved by day 3 or 4. After maximum virus growth is established, virus titres decline and are usually undetectable by 7–10 days, presumably due to the induction of neutralising antibody. Nevertheless, viral RNA may persist in heart and other organs for several weeks or months after clearance of viral infectivity (Reetoo et al., 2000). Murine models may therefore be useful for understanding the molecular basis and pathogenetic consequence of viral persistence following acute myocarditis. The details of viral pathogenesis in murine models vary according to both viral strain and host physiology and immunogenetics. Different host–pathogen combinations are characterised by differences in disease severity, and in susceptibility to persistent infection and chronic disease. The relative contribution of direct virus-mediated pathology, immune-mediated pathology and autoimmunity also varies, as do the cellular and humoral immune effectors. It is likely that this pathogenetic diversity reflects that which occurs in human disease.

Neonatal Infection

Coxsackie viruses B and echoviruses, particularly types 6, 7 and 11, may cause severe and often fatal infection in newborn infants (Modlin, 1988; Abzug et al., 1995). Although there have been occasional reports of intrauterine death resulting from maternal enterovirus infection, there is no confirmed association with congenital abnormalities. Infection may be transmitted transplacentally in late pregnancy, the infant developing heart failure from a severe myocarditis or a meningoencephalitis soon after delivery. More frequently, infection is transmitted perinatally from the mother, or postnatally from other virus-infected infants in nurseries for the newborn or special care baby units. Some infected neonates may be asymptomatic, but others will develop manifestations at 3–7 days of age, ranging from a mild febrile illness to fulminating multisystem involvement and death. Myocarditis, pneumonia and meningoencephalitis may be present. A severe hepatitis with jaundice, which results in an increased prothrombin time, and profuse haemorrhage may also occur. These features are indicative of a generalised infection, and neonatal enterovirus infection may be confused with other causes of neonatal sepsis. Enterovirus may be detected in stool, urine, serum, brain, spinal cord and myocardium. It is essential to establish a diagnosis as rapidly as possible in order to guide patient management and institute appropriate infection control measures. In outbreaks of neonatal infection there is some evidence that administration of human convalescent serum containing a high neutralising antibody titre to the virus may be of value in preventing or attenuating infection in susceptible neonates (Modlin, 1988; Abzug et al., 1995).

Bornholm Disease (Epidemic Pleurodynia)

Coxsackie viruses B are the commonest cause of this syndrome, but echovirus serotypes including 1, 6, 9, 16 and 19, and Coxsackie A viruses such as A4, 6, 9 and 10, have also been implicated. Outbreaks involving families are common; more extensive community-wide epidemics have also been reported. The disease usually presents abruptly with fever and chest pain due to involvement of the intercostal muscles, or abdominal pain which results from involvement of the muscles of the upper part of the abdomen. This may be sufficiently severe to mimic an acute surgical condition requiring laparotomy, or myocardial infarction. Some patients have pain localised to the limbs. There is usually muscle tenderness and in some patients swelling may be seen or palpated in affected muscles. Most patients recover within a week, although about 25% of patients may experience relapses, usually within a few days of being symptom-free. Enterovirus isolation from stool and strongly positive virus-specific IgM responses provide evidence of concurrent enterovirus infection.

Enteroviruses have also been implicated in various types of chronic inflammatory myopathies (Bowles et al., 1987), but more recent studies using PCR have failed to demonstrate enterovirus RNA in muscle (Leff et al., 1992).

Herpangina

Coxsackie virus types A1–6, 8, 10 and 22 are associated with herpangina. The illness affects primarily children aged 2–10 years and is characterised by fever, sore throat and pain on swallowing, often associated with vomiting and abdominal symptoms. Small vesicular lesions occur on the fauces, pharynx, palate, uvula and tonsils. Recovery is generally uneventful. Detection of enterovirus in vesicle fluid or other samples may help differentiate this condition from primary HSV infection.

Exanthemata

Hand, Foot and Mouth Disease

An ulcerative exanthem of the buccal mucosa accompanied by mild fever is followed by painful vesicular lesions on the hands or feet. Less commonly, lesions may be present on the buttocks and genitalia. Family outbreaks are common. This disease has been associated with several enteroviruses, but most commonly with Coxsackie virus A16 and, less frequently, with A4, 5 and 9, and B2 and 5. Enterovirus 71 also causes outbreaks of hand, foot and mouth disease. In recent years large enterovirus 71 epidemics have occurred in the Asian and Pacific regions, with complications including aseptic meningitis, acute flaccid paralysis, brainstem encephalitis associated with pulmonary oedema or haemorrhage, myocarditis and herpangina (Chang et al., 1999; Ho et al., 1999). Case fatality rates of up to 0.1% in infants have been reported and significant numbers of survivors have residual neurological sequelae. Enterovirus can be detected in vesicle fluid or stool, although suckling mouse inoculation or PCR may be required to detect noncultivatable group A coxsackieviruses.

Rubelliform Rashes

A fine rubella-like maculopapular rash is often a feature of some Coxsackie A and echovirus infections. Enterovirus infection should thus be considered in the investigation of women exposed to or presenting with rubelliform rash during pregnancy, after exclusion of other causes (see Chapter 12). Most frequently, echovirus 9 is implicated but often other echovirus serotypes and Coxsackie virus A9 may also be involved. Summer outbreaks, most frequently affecting children, are common. Fever, malaise and cervical lymphadenopathy may also occur in patients with rash. Patients generally make an uneventful recovery. Enterovirus detection in stool or throat swab, or the presence of virus-specific IgM, provides evidence of aetiology in the absence of another cause.

Respiratory Infections

Several enteroviruses have been associated with mild illness of the upper respiratory tract, including rhinitis, particularly during the summer and autumn. These include Coxsackie virus A2, 10, 21 (Coe virus), 24 and B2 and 5. Coe virus has caused epidemics of pharyngitis in military recruits. Among the echoviruses which have been isolated from cases of respiratory illness are included types 1, 11, 19, 20 and 22. These viruses most commonly cause outbreaks in young children, in whom pneumonia and bronchiolitis may sometimes occur. Enteroviruses can be detected in nasopharyngeal aspirates, although the interpretation of a positive result must take account of the possibility of a coincidental infection, since enteroviruses can also be detected in respiratory samples from healthy infants.

Conjunctivitis

Several enterovirus serotypes are associated with conjunctivitis. Echovirus 7 and 11 and Coxsackie virus B2 have been isolated from conjunctiva in sporadic cases. Since the early 1970s, major epidemics of acute haemorrhagic conjunctivitis have been described in Africa, the Americas and the Far East. Some epidemics are due to a variant of Coxsackie virus A24 or adenovirus 11, but many are due to enterovirus 70, a virus first identified in 1969.

Unlike most other enterovirus infections, conjunctivitis may result from direct inoculation of virus as a result of hand-to-eye contact, without passage through the intestinal tract. Subconjunctival haemorrhage is more common with enterovirus 70 than with Coxsackie virus A24. There is a high attack rate amongst family members and a short incubation period of 1–2 days. Recovery is usually complete within 1–2 weeks and, for Coxsackie virus A24, sequelae are rare. Coxsackie virus A24 and enterovirus 70 can be isolated from conjunctival scrapings, and neutralising antibody tests may be helpful.

Neurological complications may, in a few cases, accompany conjunctivitis due to enterovirus 70, and occasionally a polio-like paralytic illness ensues. One in 10 000 patients, mainly adult males, may suffer a residual paralysis. The neurological involvement may develop 2 or more weeks after the onset of conjunctivitis. The potential for neurovirulence is a worrying feature of enterovirus 70 and this calls for vigilance in the investigtion of epidemics of conjunctivitis.

Diabetes and Pancreatitis

Type 1 diabetes is an autoimmune disorder in which the insulin-secreting pancreatic islet cells are progressively destroyed. The disease has an extended preclinical incubation period in which islet cell autoantibodies (ICAs) can be detected. Type 1 diabetes occurs more commonly in genetically susceptible individuals, but environmental 'triggers' are also believed to play a role. Although definitive proof is lacking, seroepidemiological evidence, animal model studies and anecdotal case reports all support the hypothesis that enterovirus infections may act as such a trigger. Prospective studies of siblings of cases, who themselves have an increased risk of developing type 1 diabetes, have found that individuals who subsequently develop disease have a higher incidence of enterovirus infections in the prediabetic phase than those who remain asymptomatic (Hyöty et al., 1995). These studies also documented a temporal association between ICA seroconversion and preceding enterovirus infection, and enterovirus infections were particularly frequent during the 6-month period preceding the first detection of autoantibodies (Hiltunen et al., 1997; Salminen et al., 2003). This suggests that enterovirus infection may be involved in the initiation and progression of islet cell damage. Retrospective serological studies of maternal blood samples collected at delivery have reported a higher prevalence of enterovirus-specific IgM in mothers whose infants subsequently developed type 1 diabetes (Hyöty et al., 1995), suggesting that disease initiation may occur in utero. However, enterovirus infection may also precipitate disease onset, as suggested by the presence of enterovirus-specific IgM or enterovirus RNA in serum in a proportion of patients at the time of clinical onset of type 1 diabetes (King et al., 1983; Banatvala et al., 1985; Clements et al., 1995a).

Autoimmunity may arise due to molecular mimicry between viral and host antigens, and molecular mimicry between an epitope of the 2C non-structural enterovirus protein and the islet cell antigen glutamic acid decarboxylase has been demonstrated. However, recent studies in susceptible mouse strains suggest that this may be insufficient in itself to induce type 1 diabetes and that destruction of exocrine pancreas by a pancreatotropic enterovirus infection may release sequestered islet cell antigens, which restimulate autoreactive memory T cells (Horwitz et al., 1998). Thus, successive enterovirus infections may result in frequent restimulation of islet cell-autoreactive T cells, resulting in cumulative loss of islet cells, which eventually culminates in clinical type 1 diabetes.

Although an acute pancreatitis is a predominant feature of Coxsackie B virus infections in mice, there is comparatively little evidence linking this disease with infection with Coxsackie viruses B in humans. However, the pancreas is often involved in generalised neonatal infection, and Coxsackie virus B4 has occasionally been implicated as a cause of pancreatitis in adults; subclinical involvement of the pancreas has been reported in 31% and 23% of Coxsackie B5 virus and Coxsackie virus A infections.

Chronic Fatigue Syndrome

Chronic fatigue syndrome (CFS) has a number of alternative names: myalgic encephalomyelitis (ME), Royal Free disease, Iceland disease, post-viral fatigue syndrome and neuromyasthenia. It occurs as both sporadic and epidemic cases. Although it is a poorly characterised illness, the cardinal feature is excess fatiguability of skeletal muscle, which may be accompanied by muscle pain. Many other symptoms may be present, including headaches, inability to concentrate, paraesthesiae, impairment of short-term memory and poor visual accommodation. Focal neurological signs are rare. Evidence of myopericarditis may be present occasionally.

The clinical spectrum of CFS is broad and diagnosis may be difficult. Physical examination is usually not helpful, although there may be some lymphadenopathy. A history of an initiating non-specific 'virus' illness may be elicited, and such a corroborated history defines postviral fatigue syndrome. Routine laboratory investigations are usually non-contributory. Some groups, however, have described abnormalities of T cell function and muscle structure (necrosis and increase in size and number of type II fibres) and function (abnormal jitter potentials and early intracellular acidosis on exercise), although these findings are not consistent. Recovery within a few weeks or months is usual, but in some patients the syndrome persists and may be relapsing.

There is a continuing debate on the aetiologies. Much attention has focused on a viral aetiology, although it is likely that those ascribed to be suffering from the syndrome are a heterogenous group with organic and functional components contributing in varying degree (Straus, 1996). In Europe, most attention has focused on a possible enteroviral aetiology, while in the USA, various herpesviruses have been implicated. CFS occasionally follows confirmed virus infections, such as varicella zoster, influenza A and infectious mononucleosis, and rarely bacterial and protozoal infections such as *Toxoplasma gondii*, *Leptospira hardjo* and Q fever. Chronic fatigue may also be a prominent feature of chronic hepatitis C, and CFS may be diagnosed if hepatitis C is not suspected. In the majority of cases, however, the initiating viral illness cannot be diagnosed.

Viruses have been implicated not only as a trigger but also as a persistent active infection, although no evidence to support this hypothesis has been forthcoming in recent years. Although some cases may follow infectious mononucleosis, a significant role for chronic EBV infection is no longer considered likely (Straus, 1996). There is some evidence supporting a persistent enterovirus infection. In some studies, but not all, patients with CFS have a higher prevalence of elevated Coxsackie virus B neutralising antibody titres and specific IgM compared with controls (Behan *et al.*, 1985; Mawle *et al.*, 1995). In one study, approximately 50% of patients had circulating immune complexes containing an enterovirus VP1 antigen detectable with a group-reactive monoclonal antibody. Enteroviruses were isolated only occasionally from faeces by routine methods, but were isolated from approximately 20% of patients when the faeces were acidified to disrupt virus–antibody complexes prior to cell culture (Yousef *et al.*, 1988). However others have been unable to reproduce these findings. Skeletal muscle biopsies from 96 patients have been examined with an enterovirus-specific DNA probe and 20 were positive (Archard *et al.*, 1988), suggesting enterovirus persistence.

Enterovirus RNA has also been detected in serum of patients with CFS (Clements *et al.*, 1995b), and the detection of near-identical viral sequences in sequential samples collected several months apart provides further evidence for persistence (Galbraith *et al.*, 1995). However, others have been unable to detect enterovirus sequences in patients with chronic fatigue syndrome (Lindh *et al.*, 1996; McArdle *et al.*, 1996).

Thus, there is some evidence that in those cases of CFS with an organic origin enteroviruses may be implicated not only as a trigger but as a persisting infection. Although many treatments have been tried, such as normal human immunoglobulin, plasmapheresis and inosine pranobex, no evidence of efficacy has been presented.

LABORATORY DIAGNOSIS OF ENTEROVIRUS INFECTIONS

Diagnosis of enterovirus infections is useful where exclusion of serious or treatable conditions with overlapping clinical presentation is required. Thus, demonstration of an enteroviral aetiology in patients with meningitis or encephalitis may be helpful in excluding bacterial meningitis or herpes simplex encephalitis, while diagnosis of neonatal enterovirus infection may exclude other causes of sepsis-like illness, such as neonatal herpes simplex or group B streptococcal infection. Diagnosis may also play a role in infection control and epidemiological surveillance. As enterovirus-active antiviral agents become available, viral diagnosis will be necessary to guide appropriate therapy and for assessing therapeutic response. A combination of virus isolation and serological tests has traditionally been used to diagnose enterovirus infections, although molecular diagnosis now provides more rapid and sensitive viral detection in most settings. Timely submission of appropriate isolation samples and paired serum samples maximises diagnostic yield. In general, demonstration of virus in samples taken from the site of infection provides the most conclusive proof of aetiology. Such samples are not always available, e.g. in patients with myocarditis, and in such circumstances demonstration of concurrent viral excretion at peripheral sites, or serological diagnosis, can be used as circumstantial evidence of aetiology. However, it should be remembered that apparently healthy infants and children frequently excrete enteroviruses: indeed, in tropical countries up to 40% of children up to the age of 2 years may be excreting enteroviruses at any one time. Also, those who have been recently immunised with live attenuated poliovirus vaccine are likely to excrete virus from the upper respiratory tract and faeces for some time. Thus, the possible significance of isolating poliovirus can only be assessed by knowing the vaccine history and clinical features.

Virus Isolation

Enteroviruses can be cultured from solid tissue, blood, CSF, urine, stool and respiratory samples, although the diagnostic significance of enterovirus detection at a normally virologically sterile site is considerably greater than merely detecting virus in faeces or nasopharyngeal secretions, as discussed above. The most sensitive isolation specimens are faecal samples or rectal swabs. Virus excretion is often intermittent and more than one specimen should be collected, with an interval of 24–48 h. Faecal excretion of virus commences within a few days of infection and may continue for weeks, especially with polio and Coxsackie viruses, although it rarely exceeds 1 month with the echoviruses. Concentrations of virus of 10^5–10^6 tissue culture infectious doses per g faeces are not uncommon.

Isolation from the pharynx is possible during the acute phase of the illness, especially in cases with respiratory symptoms (e.g. Echovirus 9, Coxsackie virus A21 and enterovirus 71). The period with the highest rate of isolation is some 5 days before to 5 days after the onset of symptoms.

Viral culture of CSF generally gives a low diagnostic yield, and has largely been replaced by PCR testing, as described below, although during certain echovirus epidemics up to 80% of CSF specimens have yielded virus.

In fatal cases, autopsy specimens of brain, spinal cord, heart and spleen, or other lymphoid tissue, are useful, especially where there is a recent history of oral polio vaccination, where investigations of the origin of the strain may be required.

Polioviruses, Coxsackie B viruses, echoviruses and some Coxsackie A viruses (e.g. A9 and A16) are readily isolated in cell cultures prepared from the kidneys of rhesus, *Cynomolgus* or *Cercopithecus* monkeys. Other useful cultures include human embryo kidney and amnion, primary liver carcinoma, rhabdomyosarcoma (RD) cells, or strains of diploid cells from human fetal lung. Possibly the most generally useful regimen is the inoculation of cell cultures of primary monkey kidney and human embryo lung fibroblasts. Enteroviruses cannot be readily differentiated by their growth in cell cultures, as all produce a similar cytopathic effect (CPE). Infected cells become rounded, refractile and ultimately shrink before detaching from the cell surface. Once a cytopathic agent has been isolated in cell culture, serological tests must be performed to identify the type. Because of the number of potential strains, neutralisation tests using individual type-specific sera are not satisfactory, and it

is usual to employ either a single-stage procedure using antiserum pools containing selected antisera or a two-step method, first identifying the isolate as belonging to one of four groups followed by a second test to identify the type. Because of the labour-intensive nature of serotyping procedures, many laboratories now confirm enterovirus isolates by direct immunofluorescence using enterovirus group-reactive monoclonal antibodies (Trabelsi *et al.*, 1995). Further identification is often not performed, but may also be achieved by immunofluorescent staining with serotype-specific monoclonal antibodies.

Some enteroviruses, notably most Coxsackie A viruses, are not readily detected in cell cultures: if a Coxsackie virus A infection is suspected, specimens can be injected into two or more litters of mice by intracerebral, intraperitoneal and subcutaneous routes. However suckling mouse inoculation is no longer widely available. Neither polio nor echoviruses can be isolated in mice.

Twelve of the echoviruses possess the ability to agglutinate human group O erythrocytes. This activity is integral to the viral particle; spontaneous elution may occur at 37°C but this does not destroy the cell receptors, a property which differentiates the echoviruses from the ortho- and paramyxoviruses. The presence of haemagglutination activity helps reduce the number of possibilities when attempting to identify an enterovirus strain, although this is rarely employed nowadays.

Serological Diagnosis

Neutralisation tests are generally employed for such seroepidemiological purposes as determining the exposure and immunity of a population group to different enteroviruses, including responses to polio vaccination. These tests are labour-intensive and the results are seldom available in less than 3–4 days. They are no longer widely available, although poliovirus-specific testing may be employed in investigating possible poliomyelitis cases. Antibody titres are compared in paired sera, the first being collected within 5 days of onset of symptoms, and the second some days later. Significant rises in antibody titre are detected only occasionally and this has led to significance being attached to elevated neutralising antibody titres. However, elevated titres frequently occur in normal individuals, and so do not confirm recent infection. Significant antibody rises are particularly rare in cardiac disease, probably because cardiac events are a relatively late consequence of enterovirus infection.

Serological diagnosis of recent enterovirus infection has also been achieved by detecting virus-specific IgM using M-antibody capture techniques (Bell *et al.*, 1986). IgM responses are frequently directed against group-reactive determinants, thus allowing an assay employing antigens from a limited range of serotypes to be used to detect responses elicited by a wide range of serotypes. The older the patient, the more likely that such heterotypic responses will occur. Enterovirus-specific IgM responses generally last for 8–12 weeks, but in some patients may persist for much longer, occasionally for some years. It has been suggested that such a prolonged response in, for instance, cases of recurrent pericarditis, may indicate persistence of the infecting enterovirus. Approximately 30–40% of patients with myocarditis, 60–70% of patients with aseptic meningitis and 30% of patients with postviral fatigue syndrome give positive results for Coxsackie virus B-specific IgM. However, approximately 10% of normal adults also give a positive result, presumably reflecting recent asymptomatic infection.

Complement fixation tests and enzyme immunoassays have also been employed to detect enterovirus-specific IgG, but the high prevalence of antibody in the general population, as measured using these group-reactive tests, and the difficulty in obtaining paired sera to demonstrate rising titres, limits diagnostic utility and these tests are no longer widely available. A rising titre of IgG antibody to polioviruses must be treated with caution, as type 1 or type 3 infections may produce a significant boost to type 2 antibody in individuals previously primed to this type.

Molecular Diagnosis

Complementary DNA probes made by reverse transcription of purified Coxsackie B virus genomic RNA have been used to detect enterovirus RNA in infected cell cultures, infected mice and human tissue biopsies. Although prepared against a single Coxsackie virus B serotype, the probes included RNA sequences which are highly conserved amongst enteroviruses and are thus group-specific. They have been used to detect enterovirus RNA, both in RNA extracts from tissue and by *in situ* hybridisation, although infectious virus or viral antigen is rarely detected in these tissues. PCR is technically more straightforward and quicker than nucleic acid hybridisation methods, and is therefore more suitable for viral diagnosis. Identification of extremely conserved sequences within the 5′ NTR of

the enterovirus genome has allowed the design of PCR primers which allow detection of most enteroviruses (Rotbart, 1990) and numerous studies have shown that enterovirus PCR is more sensitive than viral culture for detection of enteroviruses in diverse clinical specimens. In many diagnostic laboratories examination of CSF by enterovirus PCR has replaced virus isolation for diagnosis of enteroviral meningitis, raising the possibility of more rapid diagnosis, which in turn may have greater impact on patient treatment (Schlesinger *et al.*, 1994). Enterovirus PCR is also useful for diagnosis of neonatal infections, and enterovirus myocarditis (Martin *et al.*, 1994; Nicholson *et al.*, 1995) if biopsy or autopsy tissue is available.

These enterovirus PCR protocols do not allow serotypic identification. Although serotypic identification is usually of less clinical urgency, the ability to differentiate polio and non-polio enteroviruses is important for investigation of suspected poliomyelitis cases, for diagnosis of non-polio enterovirus infection in patients recently vaccinated with live polio vaccine, and for monitoring wild poliovirus circulation in endemic regions. The ability to differentiate between wild-type and vaccine strains of poliovirus, and between attenuated and neurorevertant vaccine virus is also crucial to the investigation of suspected vaccine-associated paralytic poliomyelitis. A number of PCR methods have been described for group or serotypic identification of polioviruses (Kilpatrick *et al.*, 1996), or intratypic differentiation of wild and vaccine-strain polioviruses (Yang *et al.*, 1991). These assays are available at WHO poliovirus reference laboratories. Similar serotype-specific assays have also been described for other enteroviruses, and these may be of particular use in outbreak investigation once a particular outbreak strain has been identified. In recent years several groups have described 'molecular serotyping' systems in which capsid coding regions of enterovirus isolates are amplified and sequenced. Comparison of the sequence with published sequences of known serotype allows the serotype of the unknown isolate to be inferred (Caro *et al.*, 2001; Oberste *et al.*, 1999; Palacios *et al.*, 2002).

PREVENTION AND TREATMENT OF ENTEROVIRUS INFECTIONS

Vaccination

Vaccination against echoviruses and Coxsackie viruses is not available. The multiplicity of antigenic types and the usually mild nature of the diseases make the production of vaccines impractical. The only effective measures for their control are high standards of personal and community hygiene. Quarantine is not effective because of the high frequency of inapparent infections.

The observation that there are only three poliovirus types and the discovery that they will grow in cell cultures of non-nervous tissue from monkeys made possible the development of vaccines against poliomyelitis. By 1954, some 12 000 volunteers had been vaccinated with a formalin-inactivated suspension of polioviruses, developed by Dr Jonas Salk in the USA. Dr Albert Sabin and others adopted a different approach and developed attenuated strains of the three poliovirus types capable of inducing immunity by the oral route.

Natural infection with polioviruses is by the oral route and results in viral replication in the mucosa of the pharynx and alimentary tract, causing viraemia and stimulating virus-specific IgA and IgG. The route by which the virus gains access to the CNS is not clear; although there is some experimental evidence that it does so by travelling along autonomic nerve pathways from the site of replication, the greater body of evidence suggests that invasion of the CNS occurs via the bloodstream and may be prevented by circulating antibody. The aim of vaccination is to induce local or systemic immunity to prevent systemic spread and neuroinvasion.

antibody titre at the time of infection. The presence of detectable IgG reduced pharyngeal shedding from 75% to 33% of children, but faecal shedding was reduced only when the titre of antibody was high, in excess of 1:128. The high standards of hygiene in The Netherlands and Scandinavia, where pharyngeal shedding of poliovirus is probably the major source of infection, may explain the success of IPV in these countries.

A small outbreak of poliomyelitis with wide circulation of the type 3 strains occurred in Finland, a country which had relied exclusively on IPV and in which poliomyelitis had been unknown for 20 years. The level of type 3 antibody in the community was known to be low and the absence of poliomyelitis was attributed to persisting immunological memory, since revaccination of seronegative individuals induced rapid booster-like responses. The poliovirus strains isolated in the outbreak were antigenically unusual and, in comparison with other type 3 poliovirus strains, less well neutralised by antisera to reference strains of type 3 virus (Magrath et al., 1986).

The spread of the type 3 strain in Finland may have resulted from the unusual antigenic structure of the virus, resulting in poor immune recognition in vaccines and consequent delayed development of a booster response in many infected subjects, with low initial serum titres. The age of modern high potency vaccines is likely to prevent this in future.

Inactivated Poliovirus Vaccine

The inactivated vaccine for parenteral injection (IPV) has been used extensively in Sweden, Finland, Iceland and The Netherlands and, with acceptance rates of 90% or better, has virtually eliminated poliomyelitis. Surveys also show that the circulation of poliovirus in the community has been dramatically reduced, despite the fact that the vaccine does not induce detectable levels of secretory IgA and, in theory, would not be expected to prevent alimentary tract infections. Sabin has argued that the absence of polioviruses in countries using IPV is due to the use of OPV in neighbouring countries (Sabin, 1982) but studies in The Netherlands and Sweden have shown that during outbreaks of infection within religious sects refusing vaccination there was little virus circulation in the surrounding community with which they were in contact.

It has been observed that the pattern of virus shedding following virus infection of children previously vaccinated with IPV was related to the

Oral Poliovirus Vaccine

The availability in the early 1960s of the live attenuated vaccine, which was cheaper to produce and administer, easier to manufacture in quantity and which had some theoretical advantages over inactivated vaccine, led to its rapid adoption worldwide. The vaccine administered by the oral route parallels the natural infection and stimulates both local secretory IgA in the pharynx and alimentary tract and circulating IgG. Virus is excreted in the faeces for several weeks and possibly for several days in pharyngeal secretions. During this period the vaccine may spread to close contacts, inducing or boosting immunity in them but also, rarely, causing vaccine-associated paralytic poliomyelitis in non-immune contacts (see below).

Oral polio vaccine (OPV) is administered as part of ongoing vaccination programmes in many countries, such that individuals receive vaccine as they reach specific ages, in the UK typically at 2, 4 and 6 months.

This strategy has been extremely effective in reducing the incidence of paralytic poliomyelitis to essentially zero in developed countries, but in other countries it had very little impact.

Reports show that children in warm climates who have been given OPV often respond poorly; indeed, cases of paralytic poliomyelitis have been reported in infants who had received a full course of OPV. Interference by other enteroviruses in the gut, the presence of inhibitors in gastrointestinal secretions and suppression of OPV replication by maternal antibody are among mechanisms which have been proposed. However, it is more likely that failure to control poliomyelitis in developing countries is due partly to failure to reach a sufficiently high proportion of the target population and partly to the use of vaccine which has lost potency due to suboptimal storage.

These difficulties have been countered by the use of national immunisation days (NIDs), in which the aim is to immunise all children under the age of 5 in a country or region within a short period, usually a few days, and then to repeat the process a few weeks later. This results in a higher coverage with fresh vaccine, and the colonisation of susceptible individuals with vaccine virus, so breaking transmission. The strategy, which is usually run in parallel with the programmed strategy used elsewhere, has resulted in the eradication of poliomyelitis in the Americas, declared free of indigenous poliovirus in 1994, and where the last case due to wild-type poliovirus was seen in 1992, in Peru. The western Pacific region was declared poliovirus-free in 2000 and the European region in 2002 (Anonymous, 2003). At the time of writing, poliomyelitis was endemic in only seven countries in the world, including India, Pakistan and Nigeria. The WHO initially declared its intention of eliminating poliomyelitis due to wild-type poliovirus from the world by the year 2000, now revised to 2005, and, although a large poliovirus type 1 epidemic in India in 2002 resulted in an increase in reported cases for that year (John et al., 2003), it is likely that the goal will be achieved close to this date (see the polio eradication website of WHO: www.polioeradication.org). One index of success in controlling transmission comes from molecular analysis of isolates, which can be classified into different genotypes, which disappear one by one as transmission is broken and they die out. Type 2 poliovirus is completely eliminated first, followed by type 1 and then type 3.

The success of the eradication programme has focused attention on the few cases of poliomyelitis apparently caused by the vaccine. Nkowane et al. (1987) estimated the risk in the USA as 1/530 000 primary vaccinees and $1/2 \times 10^6$ overall. Cases associated with the type 1 strain are 10-fold less than with the type 2 and type 3 strain taken together. This incidence should be taken in the context of more than 10 000 cases/year in the USA before the use of vaccines. The rate is the same in India, at the time of writing, to within a factor of two.

Thus a time will come when poliomyelitis will only be caused by the vaccine, raising the question of how vaccination can be safely stopped in view of the excretion of virus, which may be prolonged, especially in the case of hypogammaglobulinaemic individuals, who may shed virus for several years. Approximately 20 cases of long-term excretion are known at present and the incidence of long-term excretion in patients inadvertently or deliberately given the vaccine is probably of the order of 1%. In countries where the routine vaccine coverage is poor, so that immunised and unimmunised children mix freely, transmissible strains can be selected and have been implicated in four small outbreaks, in Hispaniola, Egypt, Madagascar and the Philippines. In all cases the viruses were recombinant strains whose genome included a large sequence unrelated to the vaccine, probably derived from a non-polio enterovirus of group C. It may be possible to deal with circulating vaccine-derived strains of poliovirus by stopping routine vaccination campaigns of poor coverage with a final national immunisation day. Successful treatments for long-term excreters of vaccine strains have not been identified, although many stop excreting virus spontaneously.

In view of these considerations, developed countries are increasingly replacing OPV with IPV in order to limit excretion of vaccine-strain virus.

When poliovirus as well as poliomyelitis is eradicated there is the possibility that it will re-emerge, either from laboratory or other unrecognised reservoirs, or by deliberate release by bioterrorists, or conceivably by the evolution of a Coxsackie A virus to fill the vacated niche. It is thus necessary to maintain a stock of polio vaccine to deal with future emergencies. How this is to be done and how the stock is to be used have not been fully worked out as yet.

Antiviral Therapy

It has long been recognised that picornavirus infection in cell culture could be inhibited by agents which bind stably to the virion, preventing cellular attachment, uncoating and intracellular delivery of the viral genome. Although a series of such compounds has been developed, to date only one agent, pleconaril, has sufficiently low toxicity to be a promising therapeutic agent (Romero, 2001). Pleconaril (3-[3,5-dimethyl-4[[3-(3-methyl-5-isoxazolyl)propyl]oly]phenyl]-5-(trifluoro-methyl)-1,2,4-oxadiazole; Picovir) reduces viral replication and morbidity in animal models of enter-ovirus disease and, in a Phase II clinical trial, reduced the duration and severity of picornavirus-related respiratory infections. Pleconaril is also effective in children and adults with enteroviral meningitis, although no benefit was observable in a study of infants under 1 year with meningitis. At present pleconaril is available on a compassionate use basis for life-threatening infections, and reports of such treatments suggest a measure of efficacy in immuno-compromised patients with persistent infection, and in neonates with fulminant infection. Although drug-resistant viruses have been isolated in cell culture, they appear to be attenuated with respect to virulence in animal models.

Future Prospects

Poliomyelitis is the most significant disease caused by a human enterovirus, and enormous progress has been made towards its eradication. It is anticipated that complete eradication of disease caused by the wild-type virus will be achieved in the near future. Other enteroviruses remain and contribute significantly to human disease. New research methods, including the use of genetically cloned and modified viruses and transgenic and genetic knockout animal models, will increase our understanding of viral pathogenesis and may suggest novel therapeutic strategies. The advent of molecular diagnosis will enable the diagnostic labora-tory to issue results within a time frame that influences patient management in a way not previously possible using slower methods. The case for developing new vaccines against non-polio enteroviruses continues to be made, particularly where a particular serotype is associated with severe disease or public health risk, although the costs involved are a major obstacle. In the meantime, it is likely that additional antiviral agents will be developed, targeting viral enzymes involved in the replication process as well the structural compo-nents of virus particles. Here too, though, the costs of development, licensing and marketing may prove a significant barrier to affordable, widely available treatment for enterovirus infections.

REFERENCES

Abzug JM, Keyserling HL, Lee ML *et al.* (1995) Neonatal enterovirus infection: virology, serology and effects of intravenous immune globulin. *Clin Infect Dis*, **20**, 1201–1206.

Alexander JP, Baden L, Pallansch MA *et al.* (1994) Enterovirus 71 infections and neurological disease. United States 1987–1991. *J Infect Dis*, **169**, 905–908.

Anonymous (2003) Progress toward global eradication of poliomyelitis, 2002. *Morbid Mortal Wkly Rep*, **52**, 366.

Archard LC, Bowles NE, Behan PO *et al.* (1988) Postviral fatigue syndrome: persistence of enterovirus RNA in muscle and elevated creatinine kinase. *J R Soc Med*, **81**, 326.

Archard LC, Khan MA, Soteriou BA *et al.* (1998) Characterisation of coxsackie B virus RNA in myocardium from patients with dilated cardiomyopathy by nucleotide sequencing of reverse-transcription-nested polymerase chain reaction products. *Hum Pathol*, **29**, 578.

Banatvala JE, Schernthaner G, Schober E *et al.* (1985) Coxsackie B, mumps, rubella and cytomegalovirus specific IgM responses in patients with juvenile-onset insulin-dependent diabetes mellitus in Britain, Austria and Australia. *Lancet*, **i**, 1049.

Behan PO, Behan WMH and Bell EJ (1985) The postviral fatigue syndrome: an analysis of the findings in 50 cases. *J Infect*, **10**, 211.

Bell EJ, McCartney RA and Banatvala JE (1986) The routine use of μ-antibody capture ELISA for the serological diagnosis of Coxsackie B virus infections. *J Med Virol*, **19**, 205.

Bergelson JM, Chan M, Solomon K *et al.* (1994) Decay-accelerating factor (CD55), a glycosylphosphotidylinositol-anchored complement regulation protein, is a receptor for many echoviruses. *Proc Natl Acad Sci USA*, **91**, 6245.

Bergelson JM, Cunningham JA, Droguett G *et al.* (1997) Isolation of a common receptor for coxsackie B viruses and adenoviruses 2 and 5. *Science*, **275**, 1320.

Bergelson JM, Shepley MP, Chan BMC *et al.* (1992) Identification of the integrin VLA-2 as a receptor for echovirus 1. *Science*, **255**, 1718.

Bowles NE, Dubowitz V, Sewry CA *et al.* (1987) Dermato-myositis, polymyositis and coxsackie-B-virus infection. *Lancet*, **i**, 1004.

Bowles NE, Richardson PJ, Olsen EG *et al.* (1986) Detection of coxsackie-B-virus-specific RNA sequences in myocardial biopsy samples from patients with myocarditis and dilated cardiomyopathy. *Lancet*, **i**, 1120.

Cambridge G, MacArthur CGC, Waterson AP *et al.* (1979) Antibodies to coxsackie B viruses in primary congestive cardiomyopathy. *Br Heart J*, **41**, 692.

Caro V, Guillot S, Delpeyroux F and Crainic R (2001) Molecular strategy for 'serotyping' of human enteroviruses. *J Gen Virol*, **82**, 79.

Chang LY, Lin TY, Hsu KH *et al.* (1999) Clinical features and risk factors of pulmonary oedema after enterovirus-71-related hand, foot, and mouth disease. *Lancet*, **354**, 1682.

Clements GB, Galbraith DN and Taylor KW (1995a) Coxsackie B virus infection and onset of childhood diabetes. *Lancet*, **346**, 221–223.

Clements GB, McGarry F, Nairn C *et al.* (1995b) The detection of enterovirus specific RNA in serum: the relationship to chronic fatigue. *J Med Virol*, **45**, 151.

Dalldorf G and Sickles GM (1948) An unidentified filtrable agent isolated from the faeces of children with paralysis. *Science*, **108**, 61.

da Silva EE, Winkler MT and Pallansch MA (1996) Role of enterovirus 71 in acute flaccid paralysis after the eradication of poliovirus in Brazil. *Emerg Infect Dis*, **2**, 231.

Enders JF, Weller TH and Robbins FC (1949) Cultivation of the Lansing strain of poliomyelitis virus in cultures of various human embryonic tissues. *Science*, **109**, 85.

Figulla HR, Stille-Siegener M, Mall G et al. (1995) Myocardial enterovirus infection with left ventricular dysfunction: a benign disease compared with idiopathic dilated cardiomyopathy. *J Am Coll Cardiol*, **25**, 1170.

Galbraith DN, Nairn C and Clements GB (1995) Phylogenetic analysis of short enteroviral sequences from patients with chronic fatigue syndrome. *J Gen Virol*, **76**, 1701.

Giraud P, Beaulieux F, Ono S et al. (2001) Detection of enteroviral sequences from frozen spinal cord samples of Japanese ALS patients. *Neurology*, **56**, 1777

Heim A, Stille-Siegener M, Kandolf R et al. (1994) Enterovirus-induced myocarditis: hemodynamic deterioration with immunosuppressive therapy and successful application of interferon-α. *Clin Cardiol*, **17**, 563–565.

Hellen CU, Witherell GW, Schmid M et al. (1993) A cytoplasmic 57 kDa protein that is required for translation of picornavirus RNA by internal ribosomal entry is identical to the nuclear pyrimidine tract-binding protein. *Proc Natl Acad Sci USA*, **90**, 7642.

Hiltunen M, Hyöty H, Knip M et al. (1997) Islet cell antibody seroconversion in children is temporally associated with enterovirus infections. Childhood Diabetes in Finland (DiMe) Study Group. *J Infect Dis*, **175**, 554.

Ho M, Chen ER, Hsu KH et al. (1999) An epidemic of enterovirus 71 infection in Taiwan. Taiwan Enterovirus Epidemic Working Group. *N Engl J Med*, **341**, 929.

Hogle JM, Chow M and Filman DJ (1985) The three dimensional structure of poliovirus at 2.9 Å resolution. *Science*, **229**, 1358.

Horwitz MS, Bradley LM and Harbertson J (1998) Diabetes induced by coxsackie virus: initiation by bystander damage and not molecular mimicry. *Nature Med*, **4**, 781.

Horwitz MS, La Cava A, Fine C et al. (2000) Pancreatic expression of interferon-gamma protects mice from lethal coxsackievirus B3 infection and subsequent myocarditis. *Nature Med*, **6**, 693.

Hyöty J, Hiltunen M, Knip M et al. (1995) A prospective study of the role of coxsackie B and other enterovirus infections in the pathogenesis of IDDM. Childhood Diabetes in Finland (DiMe) Study Group. *Diabetes*, **44**, 652.

Hyypiä T, Hovi T, Knowles NJ et al. (1997) Classification of enteroviruses based on molecular and biological properties. *J Gen Virol*, **78**, 1.

John TJ, Thacker N and Deshpande JM (2003) Setback in polio eradication in India in 2002: Reasons and remedies. *Ind Pediatr*, **40**, 195.

Kämmerer U, Kunkel B and Korn K (1994) Nested polymerase chain reaction for specific detection and rapid identification of human picornaviruses. *J Clin Microbiol*, **32**, 285.

Kandolf R, Canu A, Klingel K et al. (1990) Molecular studies on enteroviral heart disease. In *New Aspects of Positive Strand RNA Viruses* (eds Brinton MA and Heinz FX),

pp 340–348. American Society for Microbiology, Washington, DC.

Karnauchow TM, Tolson DL, Harrison BA et al. (1996) The HeLa cell receptor for enterovirus 70 is decay-accelerating factor (CD55). *J Virol*, **70**, 5143.

Kilpatrick DR, Nottay B, Yang C-F et al. (1996) Group-specific identification of polioviruses by PCR using primers containing mixed-base or deoxyinosine residues at positions of codon degeneracy. *J Clin Microbiol*, **34**, 2990.

King ML, Shaikh A, Bidwell D et al. (1983) Coxsackie-B-virus-specific IgM response in childen with insulin dependent (juvenile-onset, type I) diabetes mellitus. *Lancet*, **i**, 1397.

Koike S, Taya C, Kurata T et al. (1991) Transgenic mice susceptible to poliovirus. *Proc Natl Acad Sci USA*, **88**, 951.

Leff RL, Love LA, Miller FW et al. (1992) Viruses in idiopathic inflammatory myopathies: absence of candidate viral genomes in muscle. *Lancet*, **339**, 1192.

Leparc-Goffart I, Julien J, Fuchs F et al. (1996) Evidence of presence of poliovirus genomic sequences in cerebrospinal fluid from patients with postpolio syndrome. *J Clin Microbiol*, **34**, 2023.

Lindh G, Samuelson A, Hedlund KO et al. (1996) No findings of enteroviruses in Swedish patients with chronic fatigue syndrome. *Scand J Infect Dis*, **28**, 305.

Liu PP and Mason JW (2001) Advances in the understanding of myocarditis. *Circulation*, **104**, 1076.

Magrath DI, Evans DMA, Ferguson M et al. (1986) Antigenic properties of type 3 poliovirus responsible for an outbreak of poliomyelitis in a vaccinated population. *J Gen Virol*, **67**, 899.

Malnou CE, Pöyry TAA, Jackson RJ and Kean KM (2002) Poliovirus internal ribosome entry segment structure alterations that specifically affect function in neuronal cells: molecular genetic analysis. *J Virol*, **76**, 10617.

Martin AB, Webber S, Fricker FJ et al. (1994) Acute myocarditis. Rapid diagnosis by PCR in children. *Circulation*, **90**, 330.

Mason JW, O'Connell JB, Herskowitz S et al. (1995) A clinical trial of immunosuppressive therapy for myocarditis. *N Engl J Med*, **333**, 269–275.

Mawle AC, Nisenboum R, Dobbins J-G et al. (1995) Seroepidemiology of chronic fatigue syndrome: a case control study. *Clin Infect Dis*, **21**, 1386–1389.

McArdle A, McArdle F, Jackson MJ et al. (1996) Investigation by polymerase chain reaction of enteroviral infection in patients with chronic fatigue syndrome. *Clin Sci*, **90**, 295.

Melnick JL (1996) Enteroviruses: polioviruses, coxsackieviruses, echoviruses, and newer enteroviruses. In *Field's Virology*, 3rd edn (eds Fields BN, Knipe DM, Howley PM et al.), pp 655–712. Lippincott-Raven, Philadelphia, PA.

Mendelsohn C, Wimmer E and Racaniello VR (1989) Cellular receptor for poliovirus: molecular cloning, nucleotide sequence and expression of a new member of the immunoglobulin superfamily. *Cell*, **56**, 855.

Minor PD (1990) Antigenic structure of picornaviruses. *Curr Top Microbiol Immun*, **161**, 122.

Minor PD (1996) Poliovirus. In *Viral Pathogenesis* (eds Nathanson N, Ahmed R, Gonzalez-Scarano F et al.), pp 555–574. Lippincott-Raven, Philadelphia, PA.

Minor P, Brown F, Domingo E et al. (1995) Picornaviridae. In *Virus Taxonomy. Classification and Nomenclature of Viruses. Sixth Report of the International Committee on Taxonomy of Viruses Virology Division, International Union of Microbiological Societies* (eds Murphy FA, Fauquet CM, Bishop DHL *et al.*).

Minor PD, Pipkin PA, Hockley D *et al.* (1984) Monoclonal antibodies which block cellular receptors of poliovirus. *Virus Res*, **1**, 203.

Modlin JF (1988) Echovirus infections of newborn infants. *J Paediatr Infect Dis*, **7**, 311.

Modlin JF, Dagan R, Berlin LE *et al.* (1991) Focal encephalitis with enterovirus infections. *Pediatrics*, **88**, 841.

Muir P and Banatvala JE (1990) Reactivity of enterovirus-specific IgM with infective and defective coxsackie B virions in patients with monotypic and multitypic IgM responses. *J Virol Meth*, **29**, 209.

Muir P and Archard LC (1994) There is evidence for persistent enterovirus infections in chronic medical conditions in humans. *Rev Med Virol*, **4**, 245.

Muir P, Nicholson F, Tilzey AJ *et al.* (1989) Chronic relapsing pericarditis and dilated cardiomyopathy: serological evidence of persistent enterovirus infection. *Lancet*, **i**, 804.

Muir P, Nicholson F, Spencer GT *et al.* (1996) Enterovirus infection of the central nervous system of humans; lack of association with chronic neurological disease. *J Gen Virol*, **77**, 1469.

Munsat TL (1991) Poliomyelitis: new problems with an old disease. *N Engl J Med*, **324**, 1206.

Nicholson F, Ajetunmobi JF, Li M *et al.* (1995) Molecular detection and serotypic analysis of enterovirus RNA in archival specimens from patients with acute myocarditis. *Br Heart J*, **74**, 522.

Nkowane BM, Wassilak SG, Oversteen WA *et al.* (1987) Vaccine associated paralytic poliomyelitis in the United States: 1973–1984. *J Am Med Assoc*, **257**, 1335.

Oberste MS, Kaija Maher K, Kilpatrick DR *et al.* (1999) Typing of human enteroviruses by partial sequencing of VP1. *J Clin Microbiol*, **37**, 1288.

Palacios G, Casas I, Tenorio A and Freire C (2002) Molecular identification of enterovirus by analyzing a partial VP1 genomic region with different methods. *J Clin Microbiol*, **40**, 182.

Pelletier J and Sonnenberg N (1988) Internal initiation of translation of eukaryotic mRNA directed by a sequence derived from poliovirus RNA. *Nature*, **334**, 320.

Pöyry T, Kinnunen L, Hyypiä T *et al.* (1996) Genetic and phylogenetic clustering of enteroviruses. *J Gen Virol*, **77**, 1699.

Reetoo KN, Osman SA, Illavia SJ *et al.* (2000) Quantitative analysis of viral RNA kinetics in coxsackievirus B3-induced murine myocarditis: biphasic pattern of clearance following acute infection, with persistence of residual viral RNA throughout and beyond the inflammatory phase of disease. *J Gen Virol*, **81**, 2755.

Ren R, Costantini FC, Gorgaez EJ *et al.* (1990) Transgenic mice expressing a human poliovirus receptor: a new model for poliomyelitis. *Cell*, **63**, 353.

Romero JR (2001) Pleconaril: a novel antipicornaviral drug. *Expert Opin Invest Drugs*, **10**, 369.

Rotbart HA (1990) Enzymatic RNA amplification of the enteroviruses. *J Clin Microbiol*, **28**, 438.

Rotbart HA (1995) Enteroviral infections of the central nervous system. *Clin Infect Dis*, **20**, 971–981.

Rueckert RR and Wimmer E (1984) Systematic nomenclature of picornavirus proteins. *J Virol*, **50**, 957.

Sabin AB (1982) Vaccine control of poliomyelitis in the 1980s. *J Biol Med*, **55**, 383.

Salminen K, Sadeharju K, Lonnröt M *et al.* (2003) Enterovirus infections are associated with the induction of β-cell autoimmunity in a prospective birth cohort study. *J Med Virol*, **69**, 91.

Schlesinger Y, Sawyer MH and Storch GA (1994) Enteroviral meningitis in infancy: potential for polymerase chain reaction in patient management. *Pediatrics*, **94**, 157.

Schwaiger A, Umlauft F, Weyrer K *et al.* (1993) Detection of enterovirus ribonucleic acid in myocardial biopsies from patients with idiopathic dilated cardiomyopathy by polymerase chain reaction. *Am Heart J*, **126**, 406.

Shafren DR, Bates RC, Agrez MV *et al.* (1995) Coxsackievirus B1, B3, and B5 use decay-accelerating factor as a receptor for cell attachment. *J Virol*, **69**, 3873.

Stanway G (1990) Structure, function and evolution of picornaviruses. *J Gen Virol*, **71**, 2483–2501.

Straus SE (1996) Chronic fatigue syndrome. *Br Med J*, **313**, 831–832.

Trabelsi A, Grattard F, Nejmeddine M *et al.* (1995) Evaluation of an enterovirus group-specific anti-VP1 monoclonal antibody, 5-D8/1, in comparison with neutralization and PCR for rapid identification of enteroviruses in cell culture. *J Clin Microbiol*, **33**, 2454.

Tracy S, Chapman NM and Beck MA (1991) Molecular biology and pathogenesis of coxsackie B viruses. *Rev Med Virol*, **1**, 145.

Uhlig J, Wiegers K and Dernick R (1990) A new antigenic site of poliovirus recognised by an intertypic cross-neutralizing monoclonal antibody. *Virol*, **178**, 606.

Why HJF, Meany BT, Richardson PJ *et al.* (1994) Clinical and prognostic significance of detection of enteroviral RNA in the myocardium of patients with myocarditis or dilated cardiomyopathy. *Circulation*, **89**, 2582.

Wilfert CM, Buckley RH, Mohanakumar T *et al.* (1977) Persistent and fatal central nervous system echovirus infections in agammaglobulinaemia. *N Engl J Med*, **296**, 1485.

Woodall CJ, Riding MH, Graham DI *et al.* (1994) Sequences specific for enteroviruses detected in spinal cord from patients with motor neurone disease. *Br Med J*, **308**, 1541.

Yang CF, De L, Holloway BP *et al.* (1991) Detection and identification of vaccine-related polioviruses by the polymerase chain reaction. *Virus Res*, **20**, 159.

Yousef GE, Bell EJ, Mann GF *et al.* (1988) Chronic enterovirus infection in patients with post-viral fatigue syndrome. *Lancet*, **i**, 146.

15

Poxviruses*

Inger Damon[1], Peter Jahrling[2] and James LeDuc[1]

[1]*Centers for Disease Control and Prevention, Atlanta, GA, USA;* [2]*USAMRIID, Maryland, USA*

INTRODUCTION

This chapter deals only with those poxviruses that cause human infection. The last naturally occurring case of smallpox occurred in 1977; the last cases as a result of a laboratory exposure occurred in 1978. Concern for the potential malevolent use of variola has led to increased efforts in clinical education for the recognition of smallpox and other poxvirus infections in general. The remaining human poxvirus infections are largely less clinically significant, although occasional severe infection and even death may occur. With the exception of molluscum contagiosum, existing human poxvirus infections are acquired from animals. This, and the fact that some are restricted geographically, is of value when possible cases are being investigated (Table 15.1). However, increased global travel and commerce will require enhanced clinical vigilance and knowledge of the appearance of poxvirus infections in previously unanticipated geographical locations, e.g. the recent occurrence of monkeypox in the USA (MMWR, 2003).

Because of the concern for emerging and re-emerging infectious diseases, there is still considerable interest in poxviruses, despite the eradication of smallpox. Fundamental and applied work with these viruses generates additional knowledge of them and opens up opportunities for their utilisation, including: studies on gene expression, including the expression of foreign genes and particularly gene products that may

help the virus to evade the host's defence mechanisms; the use of poxviruses as vaccine vectors; the natural evolution of diseases such as myxomatosis; the maintenance of diseases such as monkeypox, cowpox and possibly buffalopox in wildlife populations; the possible effects of such viruses on their wildlife reservoirs; evaluation of the importance of human monkeypox; and the development of improved vaccines for animal poxvirus infections (Moss, 2001; Baxby, 1998). Although perhaps less important than foot and mouth disease and rinderpest, poxviruses of domestic animals, such as sheeppox, camelpox and avianpox, can cause considerable problems for communities dependent on these animals (Baxby, 1988, 1998).

THE VIRUSES

The poxviruses of vertebrates are separated into eight genera, and species within each genus are very closely related. Some poxviruses have yet to be assigned to genera, and the relationships of some viruses within genera need further clarification (Moyer *et al.*, 2000; Baxby, 1998).

Genetic hybridisation can occur within a genus, and the serological relationship between species is very close. Traditionally, virus isolates have been identified on the results of biological tests. These methods are still used for presumptive identification, but increasing use is being made of nucleic acid signature detection and genome analysis. Fortunately, the validity of species established on biological criteria has in general been endorsed by genome analysis. The human

---

*Contains significant material from the 4th edition chapter on Poxviruses by Derrick Baxby, University of Liverpool, UK.

Principles and Practice of Clinical Virology, Fifth Edition. Edited by A. J. Zuckerman, J. E. Banatvala, J. R. Pattison, P. D. Griffiths and B. D. Schoub
© 2004 John Wiley & Sons Ltd   ISBN 0 470 84338 1

Table 15.1 Poxviruses pathogenic for humans

Genus	Virus	Reservoir host	Animals naturally infected	Geographical distribution	Comment
Orthopoxvirus	Smallpox	Humans	—	Formerly worldwide	Last endemic case 1977. Eradication confirmed 1979
	Monkeypox	Squirrels?	Squirrels African rodent species Monkeys	West and Central Africa	Rare zoonosis. Overall mortality 10%. Limited case-to-case spread. Recent importation to non-endemic area (USA)
	Cowpox	Rodents	Cats Cattle	Europe, West CIS (USSR)	Rare zoonosis. Contact with cattle unusual
	Vaccinia (buffalopox)	Buffalo? Rodents?	Buffalo	India	Variant of vaccinia. Established in nature
Parapoxvirus	Orf Pseudocowpox	Sheep Goats Cattle	Sheep Goats Cattle	Worldwide	Common trivial zoonoses Occupational hazards
Molluscipoxvirus	Molluscum	Humans	—	Worldwide	Trivial infections. Often sexually transmitted
Yatapoxvirus	Tanapox	Monkeys	Monkeys	Kenya, Zaire, (Democratic Republic of Congo)	Rare trivial zoonosis. Obtain travel history

pathogens are reasonably well-characterised species and are distributed among four genera (Table 15.1) (Moyer *et al.*, 2000).

Structure and Replication

Morphology

In general, a poxvirus may be recognised as such by its large size and brick-shaped morphology. Most work has been done on vaccinia, which can be taken as representative of orthopoxviruses, molluscum and tanapox viruses. Virions are 200–250 × 250–300 nm, basically brick-shaped but somewhat pleomorphic; parapoxviruses are slightly smaller and somewhat narrower (c. 160 nm) (Figure 15.1a, b). Virions released naturally from cells ('extracellular enveloped virus'; EEV) have an outer envelope which is soon lost on manipulation and not found on virions released artificially ('intracellular mature virus'; IMV) (Figures 15.1a,b and 15.2b). A small portion of IMVs may be further processed to acquire a bilayer envelope of Golgi intermediate compartment membrane that contains specific viral proteins. The intracellular enveloped IMV (IEV) then moves along cellular microtubules to the cell surface, where actin polymerises behind IEV. IEVs exit the cell via distinctive microvilli by fusing the outermost lipoprotein layer with the plasma membrane, thereby releasing the IMV within the inner

lipoprotein layer. The released particle is the extracellular enveloped virion (EEV); EEVs that stay attached to the outer surface of the cell are termed cell-associated EEVs (CEVs). IMVs, EEVs and CEVs are mature infectious particles, each with distinct surface antigenic properties. The extra envelope has antigens not present in IMV, and EEV plays an important role in pathogenesis (Smith *et al.*, 1997, 2003; Payne, 1980). The appearance of both EEV and IMV in the electron microscope is affected by stain penetration. The majority of virions have short surface tubules c. 10 nm in diameter and are referred to as M ('mulberry') forms (Figure 15.1b); a minority, slightly larger and electron-dense, appear to have a thick (c. 20–25 nm) membrane or capsule (hence 'C' forms) (Figure 15.1c). The M form of parapoxvirus is covered by one long tubule which winds round the virion (Figure 15.1a). This gives the characteristic criss-cross effect due to superimposition of the images of the top and bottom surfaces of the virion when seen in the electron microscope. All the forms described (EEV-M, EEV-C, IMV-M, IMV-C) are infectious.

Thin sections show a central dumbbell-shaped core or nucleoid, flanked by two 'lateral bodies'. Inside the cell, virions are often bounded by double or multiple membranes (Figure 15.2a). When released naturally, the outer membranes fuse with the cell or Golgi membranes and the virion is extruded from the cell, invested by the envelope described above (Figure 15.2b).

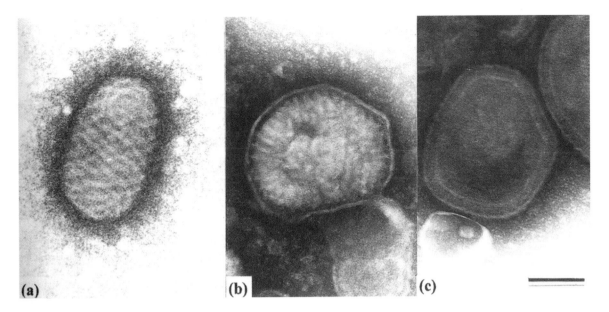

Figure 15.1 (a) Mulberry (M) form of non-enveloped parapox virion; (b) naturally-released (extracellular) M form of *Vaccinia virus*; (c) capsule (C) form of *Vaccinia virus* (negative stain; bar = 150 nm)

Chemical Structure

The genome of poxviruses is one long piece of double-stranded DNA which varies in size from 130 kb (parapoxvirus) to 260 kb (fowlpox virus). The molecule has cross-linked inverted terminal segments and, on denaturation, forms a closed circle of single-stranded DNA (Moss, 2001). The central portion is highly conserved but differences in the terminal regions of different species provide a means for separating them (Esposito and Knight, 1985). The complete sequences of some strains of vaccinia and smallpox virus and considerable sequences of other poxviruses have been determined, and the location and function of the genes is usually related to the *Hin*dIII restriction map of the Copenhagen strain of vaccinia virus (Figure 15.3) (Johnson *et al.*, 1993). The DNA is not infectious *per se*. The virion contains a number of virus-coded enzymes, in particular a DNA-dependent RNA polymerase, which transcribe the viral genome (Moss, 2001).

The virions contain many polypeptides; over 100 have been detected by two-dimensional polyacrylamide electrophoresis, and there is coding potential for c. 200. Some are glycolysated and some of these are found in the envelope of EEV (Moss, 2001).

Antigenic Structure

Poxviruses are antigenically complex. Extracts of infected tissue contain a number of precipitating antigens, the precise number of which is unknown. Such extracts will fix complement and react in ELISA and RIA tests, but it is not known how many antigens take part in these reactions. Virus neutralisation is a complicated process: analysis with monoclonal antibodies has detected nine neutralising epitopes distributed among the IMV of the different species of orthopoxviruses (Czerny *et al.*, 1994). Extra antigens are present on the outer envelope of EEV, although for technical reasons progress here has been less rapid (Vanderplasschen *et al.*, 1997; Baxby, 1998). Orthopoxviruses produce a haemagglutinin antigen which reacts with erythrocytes from certain fowls. This antigen is present on the envelope of EEV and can also be detected in virus-free supernatants.

Replication and Cultivation

Only the briefest summary can be given here but an authoritative and extensively referenced account has been published recently (Moss, 2001).

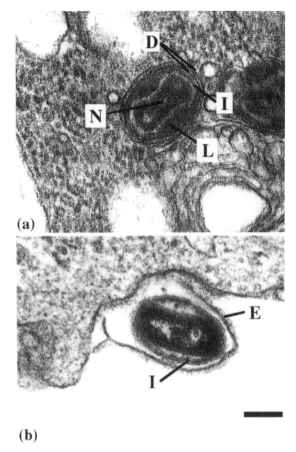

(a)

(b)

Figure 15.2 Thin sections of *Vaccinia virus*. (a) Virion within cell, invested with double membrane; (b) extracellular virion showing outer envelope, partly detached. D, double membrane; E, outer envelope; I, inner membrane; L, lateral body; N, nucleoid or core (bar = 100 nm)

Virions are taken into the cell by pinocytosis and/or phagocytosis, and there is increasing evidence that IMV and EEV attach to different receptors (Vanderplasschen and Smith, 1997). Constitutive cellular enzymes initiate virus uncoating, but virion-coded enzymes are essential for the final stages.

Transcription and translation are under close control; poxvirus genes cannot be controlled by mammalian promoters and there are differences between early, intermediate and late poxvirus-specific promoters. Many gene products are subject to post-transcriptional modification, e.g. by glycosylation and proteolytic cleavage.

Replication takes place in cytoplasmic factories referred to as B-type inclusions, in which virions at various stages of assembly are seen. Cells infected with some poxviruses (e.g. cowpox, avian poxviruses) also contain electron-dense A-type inclusions, usually containing mature virions; A-type inclusions are easily seen by light microscopy (Figure 15.4).

Molluscum contagiosum virus (MCV) has never been cultivated *in vitro*, although some early antigens and a non-transmissible cytopathic effect may be detected in cell culture (Birthistle and Carrington, 1997). DNA and antigens may persist in a primary human fibroblast system for long periods of time (Bugert *et al.*, 2001). The remaining human pathogens can usually be cultivated in easily obtained cell cultures (including Vero, other monkey kidney cell lines, A549 and others), and orthopoxviruses will produce pocks on the chorioallantoic membrane (CAM) of 12 day-old chick embryos. Methods for isolation and identification of individual virus species have been reviewed recently (Damon and Esposito, 2002; Ropp *et al.*, 1995; Meyer *et al.*, 1997, 1998).

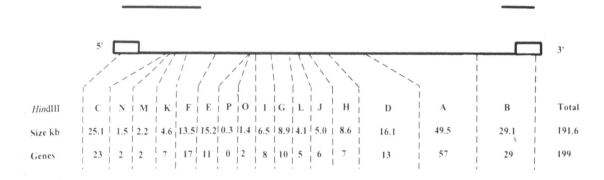

*Hin*dIII	C	N	M	K	F	E	P	O	I	G	L	J	H	D	A	B	Total
Size kb	25.1	1.5	2.2	4.6	13.5	15.2	0.3	1.4	6.5	8.9	4.1	5.0	8.6	16.1	49.5	29.1	191.6
Genes	23	2	2	7	17	11	0	2	8	10	5	6	7	13	57	29	199

Figure 15.3 Representation of the genome of Copenhagen vaccinia showing *Hin*dIII restriction fragments labelled A–P according to decreasing size, inverted terminal repeats (boxes) and two large non-essential regions (horizontal bars) are indicated. Redrawn from Baxby (1998). Published by Edward Arnold (Publishers) Ltd

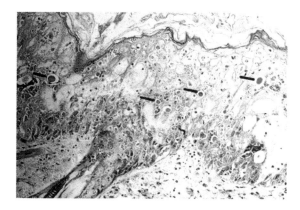

Figure 15.4 Section of cowpox-infected cat skin showing hypertrophy, hyperplasia, leukocyte infiltration and conspicuous intracytoplasmic A-type inclusions (some indicated). Reproduced from Baxby *et al.* (1994) published by Blackwell Science Ltd

Table 15.2 Examples of non-essential poxvirus gene products that contribute to 'virulence'

Gene[a]	Product[b]	Comment
C3L	C4b receptor	Binds C4b. Negative mutants attenuated
C11L	EGF	Promotes cell proliferation. Inactivation attenuates
(C22L)	TNF receptor	Binds TNF, contributes to virulence (disrupted in CopVac)
B5R	EEV antigen	Essential for EEV production
B8R	INF-γ receptor	Bind IFN-γ. Blocks host defences
(B13/14R)	Serpin	Inhibits inflammation (non-functional in CopVac)
B16R	IL-1β	Binds IL-1β. Inhibits febrile response
(CHO)	Host range	Host range gene in cowpox. Non-expression causes apoptosis in CHO cells

[a]With reference to the genome of Copenhagen vaccinia [CopVac]. Initial letter denotes *Hind*III fragment, number and final letter indicate gene number within fragment and direction of transcription. CHO, Chinese hamster ovary. Bracketed entries, gene non-functional or not present in CopVac (see column 3).
[b]C4b, complement component; EGF, epidermal growth factor; TNF, tumour necrosis factor; EEV, extracellular enveloped virus; INF, interferon; Serpin, serine protease inhibitor; IL, interleukin.

Poxvirus Gene Products and Pathogenesis

There has always been interest in the 'virulence' (i.e. safety) of vaccinia virus, particularly given its close relationship to variola. Although some empirical studies showed that, for example, TK minus mutants were attenuated for some hosts, it was apparent that virulence was a complex multifactorial system. Analysis of the genome has identified genes whose expression is not necessary for replication, and strains which do or do not express some of these genes have been compared *in vivo* and *in vitro*. The nucleotide and amino acid sequences and the observed or predicted properties of these gene products provide evidence for their demonstrated or predicted role in pathogenesis. Some examples are given in Table 15.2, and further details are provided elsewhere (Smith *et al.*, 1997; Johnston and McFadden, 2003; Seet *et al.*, 2003). Gene products identified include some which help the virus to evade the immune system by binding components of, for example, complement (gene C3L), interferon (B8R) or interleukins (B16R), or which inhibit inflammation (B13/14R). Other products determine host range and control apoptosis (gene CHO) or promote cell proliferation (C11L). The febrile response to infection is mediated by interleukin 1β and is inhibited by a virus-coded gene product (B16R), which binds this cytokine. The dissemination of naturally-released virions (EEV) is an important aspect of pathogenesis and genes have been identified (e.g. B5R) which code for proteins necessary for the proper development of EEV and expression of virulence. In addition, host cell factors are involved in EEV dissemination (Smith *et al.*, 2003).

SMALLPOX

In 1980, the WHO General Assembly accepted the conclusion of an independent commission that smallpox had been eradicated; destruction of the remaining virus stocks, scheduled for 1999 and then for 2002, has been delayed in an effort to permit research for improved preparedness in the event that smallpox recurs as the result of the malevolent use of variola virus. The importance of smallpox should not be forgotten. It had a measurable impact on the development of civilisation, was the first virus disease for which vaccination became available, and was the first and only disease to be eradicated. Authoritative information on all aspects of smallpox is available in the comprehensive account by Fenner *et al.* (1988).

Naturally acquired variola virus infection causes a systemic febrile rash illness. For ordinary smallpox, the most common clinical presentation, after an asymptomatic incubation period of 10–14 days (range 7–17 days), was fever, quickly rising to about 103°F, sometimes with dermal petechiae. Associated constitutional symptoms included backache, headache, vomiting and prostration. Within 1–2 days after incubation, a systemic rash appeared that was characteristically centrifugally distributed (i.e. lesions were present in greater numbers on the oral mucosa, face, and extremities than on the trunk). Initially, each rash lesion appeared macular, then papular, enlarging and progressing to a vesicle by day 4–5 and to a pustule by day 7; the lesions were encrusted and scabby by day 14 and sloughed off. Skin lesions were deep-seated and in the same stage of development in any one area of the body. Milder and more severe forms of the rash were also documented. Less severe manifestations (modified smallpox or variola sine eruptione) occurred in some vaccinated individuals, whereas haemorrhagic or flat-pox types of smallpox are thought to have developed as a result of impaired immune response of patients.

Variola major smallpox was differentiated into four main clinical types: (a) ordinary smallpox (∼90% of cases) produced viraemia, fever, prostration, and rash; mortality rates were generally proportionate with the extent of rash and, using the WHO classification, ranged from <10% for ordinary discrete to 50–75% for the rarer ordinary confluent presentation; (b) (vaccine)-modified smallpox (5% of cases) produced a mild prodrome with few skin lesions in previously vaccinated people and a mortality rate well under 10%; (c) flat smallpox (5% of cases) produced slowly developing focal lesions with generalised infection and a ∼50% fatality rate; and (d) haemorrhagic smallpox (<1% of cases) induced bleeding into the skin and the mucous membranes and was invariably fatal within a week of onset. A discrete type of the ordinary form, with typical febrile prodrome and rash, resulted from alastrim variola minor infection (Fenner et al., 1988). The WHO established a classification system for smallpox case types based on disease presentation and rash burden. Haemorrhagic and flat smallpox are briefly described below. Ordinary smallpox was subgrouped into three categories, based on the extent of rash on the face and the body. In ordinary confluent smallpox, no area of skin was visible between the vesiculo-pustular rash lesions on the trunk or the face. Patches of normal skin were visible between rash lesions on the trunk in ordinary-semi-confluent disease, as well as on the face in ordinary discrete disease. (Vaccine)-modified disease presented with sparse numbers of lesions.

Prior to its eradication, smallpox as a clinical entity was relatively easy to recognise, but other exanthematous illnesses were mistaken for this disease (Fenner et al., 1988) e.g. the rash of severe chickenpox, caused by varicella-zoster virus, was often misdiagnosed as that of smallpox. However, chickenpox produces a centripetally distributed rash and rarely appears on the palms and soles. In addition, in the case of chickenpox, prodromal fever and systemic manifestations are mild, if manifest at all; the lesions are superficial in nature; and lesions in different developmental stages may present in the same area of the body. Other diseases confused with vesicular-stage smallpox included monkeypox, generalised vaccinia, disseminated herpes zoster, disseminated herpes simplex virus infection, drug reactions (eruptions), erythema multiforme, enteroviral infections, scabies, insect bites, impetigo and molluscum contagiosum. Diseases confused with haemorrhagic smallpox included acute leukaemia, meningococcaemia and idiopathic thrombocytopenic purpura. The Centers for Disease Control and Prevention (CDC), in collaboration with numerous professional organisations, has developed an algorithm for evaluating patients for smallpox. The algorithm and additional information are available at http://www.bt.cdc.gov/agent/smallpox/diagnosis/evalposter.asp and at www.bt.cdc.gov/EmContact/index.asp.

MONKEYPOX

Monkeypox virus was so-named because it was first detected in captive Asiatic monkeys; however, the virus has only been found naturally in Africa and evidence points to squirrels (Funisciurus spp., Heliosciurus spp.) as important reservoir hosts. Recently, a Gambian rat (Cricetomys gambiensis), rope squirrel (Funisciuris spp.) and dormouse (Graphiuris spp.) from the African shipment originating in Ghana and implicated in the US monkeypox outbreak were found to be infected with monkeypox by viral isolation and nucleic acid detection (PCR) (MMWR, 2003). Initial surveys in Zaire (now Democratic Republic of Congo) detected monkeypox-specific antibodies in 85/347 (25%) squirrels sampled but from none of 233 terrestrial rodents. Monkeypox-specific antibody has been detected in very few monkeys, which, like humans are probably only occasional hosts (Khodakevich et al., 1988). Subsequent work (Hutin et al., 2001) in the Democratic Republic of Congo found evidence of orthopoxvirus seroreactivity in some terrestrial rodents tested, including Gambian rats (Cricetomys emini) and elephant shrews (Petrodromus tetradactylus).

Particular attention was focused on monkeypox from 1970, when smallpox surveillance activities in Africa revealed cases of human monkeypox, clinically indistinguishable from smallpox, particularly in Zaire.

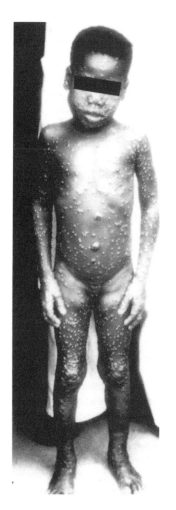

Figure 15.5 Human monkeypox on the 8th day of rash. Note the submaxillary and inguinal lymphadenopathy. Reproduced from Fenner *et al.* (1988) by permission of WHO

Sporadic outbreaks continue to occur and cause concern (Heymann *et al.*, 1998; Bremen, 2000), but most information is available about cases that occurred prior to 1988. More recently, monkeypox infection of humans was identified in the USA, as a result of exposure to ill prairie dogs, probably infected after exposure to infected West African small mammals imported as exotic pets (MMWR, 2003).

Pathogenesis

The pathogenesis of human monkeypox is essentially the same as that of smallpox, i.e. an acute febrile exanthem with an incubation period of about 12 days. During the incubation period virus is distributed initially to internal organs and then to the skin (Fenner *et al.*, 1988; Jezek and Fenner, 1988). The main differences are a greater degree of lymphadenopathy and a lower capacity for case-to-case spread. The major problems concern the source of infection and the mode of transmission.

Clinical Features

In general the clinical features of disease as seen in Central Africa are those of a classical or modified case of smallpox. The most obvious difference is the pronounced lymphadenopathy, which involves the submandibular, cervical and sublingual regions (Figure 15.5).

Most cases occur in unvaccinated children. In Zaire during 1981–1986, 291 cases (86%) occurred in children < 10 years old and only 12 (4%) of these had vaccination scars. The illness lasts 2–4 weeks. Of 292 unvaccinated patients, 22 (7.5%) had a mild illness with < 25 skin lesions and were not incapacitated; 55 (19%) had 25–99 lesions, were incapable of most physical activity and required nursing; and 218 (75%) had > 100 lesions, were totally incapacitated and required intensive nursing. Complications occurred in about 40% of patients: the most common were bacterial skin infections (16%) and respiratory (12%) and gastrointestinal (5%) disorders. The overall mortality was approximately 10%; however, all the deaths occurred in unvaccinated children, in which group mortality is around 15% (Jezek and Fenner, 1988; Jezek *et al.*, 1988). Disease in the 2003 outbreak in the USA appears to have been milder, and only two of the 37 laboratory cases had complications, one with keratitis and one with encephalopathy (MMWR, 2003).

Diagnosis

Until 2003, human monkeypox had not been detected outside Africa. Clinical diagnosis may present a problem because fewer physicians now have experience with smallpox, which human monkeypox closely resembles. Access to a virus diagnostic laboratory should permit detection of virus by electron microscopy and molecular methods, and this provides a sensitive presumptive diagnosis. In some circumstances it may be important to distinguish between monkeypox and tanapox (see below). In the past it was essential to differentiate between monkeypox and variola, which could be done by examination of pock appearance (haemorrhagic or not) and presence of pocks produced on the CAM at 39°C, a temperature which inhibits smallpox. Currently, an array of molecular diagnostic techniques permits the speciation of these viruses (Ibrahim, 2003; Meyer *et al.*, 1997, 1998; Ropp *et al.*, 1995; Loparev *et al.*, 2001).

At the same time, detailed analysis of monkeypox DNA has detected minor differences among different strains which may be of value in epidemiological investigations (Douglas *et al.*, 1994). The close serological relationships among orthopoxviruses makes detection of monkeypox-specific antigens difficult but methods are available and being refined which may be of value, particularly for epidemiological studies of monkeypox virus in its natural reservoirs (Khodacevich *et al.*, 1988).

Of human cases in the 1981–1986 Zaire survey, 74% were confirmed by detection of virus by electron microscopy and virus isolation, and in another 22% retrospectively by serology.

Epidemiology and Control

Management of individual cases is supportive, with case-to-case spread reduced by isolation and, if available, the use of smallpox vaccine for contacts. Potential use of newer therapeutics will be discussed at the end of this chapter.

Human cases in Africa occur in villages in the rainforests where a variety of animals are captured for food. Infection of children might be explained by their playing with carcasses. The results of the comprehensive surveys carried out in the 1980s indicated that those infected were principally unvaccinated children and that case-to-case spread was unusual. Control measures are based in interposing a buffer zone of cleared land between the arboreal reservoir and cultivated land, the development of animal husbandry as a source of meat, and on education in the handling of wildlife, with emphasis on any trapping done by those previously vaccinated; continued vaccination was not thought necessary (Khodakevich *et al.*, 1988).

Only occasional human cases were reported from Central Africa following cessation of routine surveillance activities post-smallpox eradication, but there was a resurgence in 1996–1997 which has not yet been fully explained. Increased political unrest would lead to population displacement and breakdown of routine control measures, and the levels of vaccine-induced immunity will decline with time. A potentially serious finding which requires clarification is the observation that case-to-case transmission appears to have occurred more frequently during 1996–1997 than earlier (Heymann *et al.*, 1998). Monkeypox continues to be sporadically reported (Meyer *et al.*, 2002). Comparison of the genomes of smallpox virus and monkeypox virus strains isolated up to 1986 suggested that they have evolved separately (Douglas and Dumbell, 1992) and the results of complete genome analysis (Shchelkunov *et al.*, 2002) confirm this observation.

Laboratory workers studying monkeypox virus should be vaccinated with vaccinia and handle the virus in safety cabinets. BSL-2 containment, per the BMBL definition, should at a minimum be used. BSL-3 laboratory practices provide additional biosafety.

VACCINIA

Vaccination

Smallpox vaccination, although an efficient prophylactic against smallpox, was not without well-documented risks. These ranged from rare but severe complications, such as generalised vaccinia, which occurred in about 200/million primary vaccinees, to relatively mild but still troublesome satellite lesions or nondescript rashes, which occurred in about 8% of vaccinees (Baxby, 1993; Fulginetti *et al.*, 2003). Routine use of smallpox vaccine is now discontinued; however, to enhance response preparedness to the potential malevolent reintroduction of smallpox, a number of public health personnel have recently been vaccinated. Policies for vaccine use in laboratory personnel working with orthopoxviruses varies internationally. It is necessary for those working with monkeypox virus, but policies about its use for those working with cowpox virus and vaccinia virus vary (Baxby, 1993). Vaccinia immune globulin (Cono *et al.*, 2003) is recommended for use in certain instances of adverse events associated with vaccination.

Buffalopox

Attention has been drawn to 'buffalopox' in water buffaloes and their handlers, particularly in India. Some outbreaks have certainly been caused by typical strains of vaccinia virus. However, studies on isolates obtained after the cessation of routine vaccination suggest that cases continue to be caused by a virus different from vaccinia (Dumbell and Richardson, 1993). These isolates, unlike vaccinia, do not produce pocks on the CAM above 39°C. Their DNA is sufficiently similar to that of vaccinia virus to regard them as variants or subspecies of it (Dumbell and Richardson, 1993; Moyer *et al.*, 2000). However, at present it is not known whether buffaloes are the reservoir host or whether wildlife reservoirs are involved, as in the case of cowpox (see below).

Recombinant Poxvirus Vaccines

'Foreign' genes have been inserted into poxviruses, particularly vaccinia. The resultant recombinant strains retain their infectivity and, in general, the inserted genes are expressed properly. Thus, the use of such recombinants as vaccines has been advocated. Most work has been done on vaccinia as a vector, and vaccinia recombinant vaccines have been used to control wildlife rabies in Europe (Pastoret and Brochier, 1996), and in the USA (Rupprecht, 2001). Human infection with such vectored vaccines has been rarely reported (Rupprecht, 2001). Such concerns have led to the development of severely attenuated vaccinia vectors (Staib and Sutter, 2003; Smith *et al.*, 1997). Other poxviruses are being considered as vaccine vectors, in particular, the use of avian poxviruses as vectors for mammalian vaccines. These are of interest because avian poxviruses induce a good immune response to the foreign gene product without initiating productive infection in mammals (Limbach and Paoletti, 1996).

COWPOX

Cowpox is a relatively unimportant zoonosis, of interest principally because of recent re-evaluation of its epidemiology. Despite its name, cowpox virus is not enzootic in cattle. The virus is maintained in a variety of European rodents, and the most commonly reported victim is the domestic cat, from which source human infections are acquired (Baxby and Bennett, 1997b).

Pathogenesis

Most information is available about cowpox in the domestic cat, an accidental host in which a relatively mild generalised disease occurs following primary infection via a bite or scratch (Bennett *et al.*, 1990).

Human infection, similarly acquired, usually remains localised and is characterised by a marked inflammatory and erythematous response (Baxby *et al.*, 1994). The bulk of the lesion is caused by hypertrophy and proliferation of the basal cell layer of the epidermis, together with massive inflammatory infiltration. Infection usually spreads into follicles and typical A-type inclusions are usually seen (Figure 15.4). By analogy with smallpox vaccination, a transient viraemia might be expected.

Clinical Features

Most information is available from a detailed analysis of 54 human cases investigated during 1969–1993 (Baxby *et al.*, 1994). Lesions are generally restricted to the hands and face and most patients (72%) have only one lesion. Multiple lesions may be caused by multiple primary inoculations, autoinoculation, and very occasionally by lymphatic or viraemic spread.

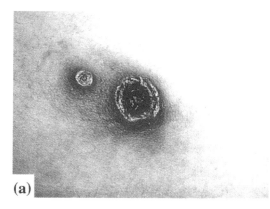 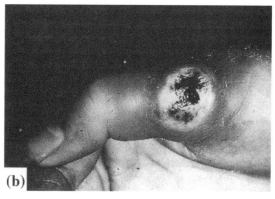

(a) **(b)**

Figure 15.6 Human cowpox. (a) Primary and secondary lesions; the former at the early eschar stage, the latter at the early vesicular stage; (b) at the late vesicular–early pustular stage showing a haemorrhage lesion with marked oedema and erythema. (a) Reproduced from Baxby *et al.* (1994) published by Blackwell Science Ltd. (b) From Baxby D (1982) The natural history of cowpox. *Bristol Medico-Chirurgical Journal*, **97**, 12; reproduced by permission of the Editor

Occasionally, a very severe infection and death may occur, usually in immunosuppressed individuals.

The lesion passes through macular, papular, vesicular and pustular stages before forming a hard black crust (Figure 15.6a). The lesion is usually very painful and erythema and oedema are common at the late vesicular and pustular stages (Figure 15.6b). There is usually lymphadenitis, fever and general malaise, often referred to as 'flu-like'. These features are usually severe in children, and absence from school or work is common; 16/54 patients (30%) were hospitalised. Most cases take 6–8 weeks to recover; in some cases it may take > 12 weeks. Scarring is usually permanent.

Diagnosis

Clinical

The main drawback to clinical diagnosis of cowpox is its rarity and the failure to appreciate important epidemiological information (see below). Cowpox, which is restricted geographically (Table 15.1), should be considered in anyone, including young children, presenting with a painful haemorrhagic lesion or black eschar, with or without erythema and oedema, accompanied by lymphadenopathy and a systemic 'flu-like' illness. This applies particularly to patients seen in July–October and/or who have had contact with cats (see below). Attempts to establish contact with cattle are usually counterproductive. Differential diagnoses include parapoxvirus (see below), herpes and anthrax. Colour illustrations of all these lesions are available (Baxby et al., 1994), which, together with a properly taken history, should help clinical diagnosis. Unfortunately, the rarity of human cowpox means that general practitioners or even consultants seldom have an opportunity to investigate a second case.

Laboratory

Electron microscopy of vesicle fluid or extracts of crusts is particularly valuable because it will differentiate between parapox, herpes and presumptive cowpox infections. Of 24 cases of cowpox where adequate material was available, electron microscopy was successful in 23. Molecular diagnostics (Meyer et al., 1997, 1998; Ropp et al., 1995; Loparev et al., 2001) may also be used to identify cowpox.

If necessary, virus may be isolated on the CAM, where the production of intensely haemorrhagic pocks is diagnostic. Cytopathic effect occurs in many cell lines (Vero, MRC-5, RK13) and detection of A-type inclusions is diagnostic, as it would be if found in biopsy material. Not all strains of cowpox are identical and genome analysis may show differences of epidemiological value.

Epidemiology

As indicated above, cowpox is maintained in rodents; in the UK these are bank voles and woodmice (Crouch et al., 1995; Baxby and Bennett, 1997b). The domestic cat is the most common source of human infection and this probably explains the occurrence of cases in children; 26% of 54 cases were in children < 12 years. Most feline and human cases occur between July and October, with only occasional cases between January and June. Human cases occur in which no source is traced, but despite detailed enquiries only three human cases in the UK since 1968 have been traced to a bovine source, and no case of bovine cowpox has been detected since 1976.

Cowpox virus has a wide host range, and an interesting finding has been the occurrence of cowpox in a variety of captive exotic species in European zoos. Victims have included cheetahs, lions, anteaters, rhinoceros, elephants and okapi, and infection has occasionally been transmitted to animal handlers (Pilaski and Rösen-Wolff, 1988; Baxby and Bennett, 1997b).

Control

Much evidence, albeit circumstantial, suggests that cowpox virus is of low infectivity for humans (Baxby and Bennett, 1997b). Careful handling of infected cats prevents cat-to-human transmission and no case has occurred in a handler after diagnosis of the feline case. Person-to-person transmission has not been reported. Management is supportive, with antibiotics to control any bacterial superinfection. Serious infections could be treated with vaccinia immune-globulin, if available. Aciclovir has no activity against poxviruses. Corticosteroids are contraindicated: when used they have exacerbated infection and delayed recovery. Therapeutics are discussed in more depth at the end of this chapter.

PARAPOXVIRUS

Parapoxvirus infections are widespread in sheep, goats and cattle. Human infections from these sources are a common occupational hazard for those in contact with infected animals.

Parapoxvirus infection in sheep and goats is usually referred to as 'contagious pustular dermatitis' or 'orf', and the corresponding human infection as 'orf'. Parapoxvirus infection of cattle is usually referred to as 'paravaccinia', 'pseudocowpox' or 'ring sores', and the human equivalent as 'paravaccinia', 'pseudocowpox' or 'milker's nodes'.

Pathogenesis

Infection occurs via cuts and scratches and usually remains localised. Lesions are produced by hypertrophy and proliferation of epidermal cells, often marked, and leukocyte infiltration. Histological examination shows many small multilocular vesicles within the dermis; true macrovesicles rarely occur (Johanneson *et al.*, 1975; Yirrell and Vestey, 1994). Lymphadenopathy, malaise and generalised lesions are relatively uncommon and the immune response is poor (Leavell *et al.*, 1968; Yirrell *et al.*, 1994).

Clinical Features

The progressive stages of human infection have been described in detail (Leavell *et al.*, 1968; Johanneson *et al.*, 1975; Yirrell and Vestey, 1994) and illustrations provided (Baxby *et al.*, 1994; Diven, 2001). Lesions start as erythematous papules and progress to a 'target' stage (Figure 15.7a). This, seen 1–2 weeks after infection, has a red centre surrounded by a white halo and an outer inflamed halo. This progresses to a nodular, then papillomatous stage, which often has a 'weeping' surface. In some patients this may enlarge and persist for some weeks before resolving (Figure 15.7b), and may cause some concern (see Diagnosis, below). The lesion resolves via a crusting stage (Figure 15.7c), which may last some weeks (Johanneson *et al.*, 1975; Yirrell and Vestey, 1994). Occasionally very large granulomatous lesions occur which may need surgical removal (Pether *et al.*, 1986).

Most patients have only one lesion, but multiple primary lesions may occur. Systemic reaction is relatively uncommon and the lesion is often not particularly painful. Attention has been drawn to erythema multiforme as a common complication of orf but, because most ordinary cases go unreported, the actual incidence of erythema is probably low. The immune response in natural human infection has been investigated (Yirrel *et al.*, 1994). There is a vigorous

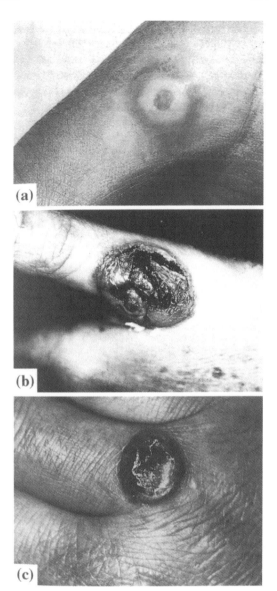

Figure 15.7 Parapoxvirus infection showing lesions in different patients. (a) At the 'larger' stage; (b) an ulcerated granulomatous lesion which could be misdiagnosed as a malignancy; (c) crusting lesion. (a) From Baxby D (1982) The natural history of cowpox. *Bristol Medico-Chirurgical Journal*, **97**, 12; reproduced by permission of the Editor. (b) Kindly supplied by Dr M S Lewis-Jones. (c) Reproduced from Baxby D *et al.* (1994) published by Blackwell Science Ltd

but short-lived cell-mediated response and a relatively poor and short-lived humoral response. This is consistent with the occurrence of second attacks in 8–12% of individuals (Robinson and Peterson, 1983; Yirrell and Vestey, 1994).

Diagnosis

Clinical

The viruses which cause orf and paravaccinia are closely related (Moyer et al., 2000; Mercer et al., 1997) and in the UK human cases are reported as 'orf/paravaccinia', whatever the animal source (Baxby and Bennett, 1997a). Clinical diagnosis of uncomplicated cases in patients with a known animal contact should not cause difficulties. However, farm workers, etc. recognise the infection and tend not to seek medical attention for routine cases. Consequently, a disproportionately large number of reported cases have no known contact with infected animals. Of approximately 500 cases surveyed during 1978–1995, some 45% had no such contact. Clinical diagnosis of such cases, particularly if severe or prolonged, may cause difficulties. In particular, large weeping granulomatous or papillomatous lesions may be misdiagnosed as malignancies, resulting in one case in unnecessary amputation (Johanneson et al., 1975).

Laboratory

Virions with the characteristic morphology of parapoxviruses are usually easily seen by EM in lesion extracts, and this provides a rapid, certain diagnosis. The virus can be grown in cell culture but this is not attempted routinely. Some nucleic acid detection techniques are published (Torfason and Gunadottir, 2002).

Epidemiology

Human infection is an occupational hazard of farmworkers, abattoir workers, veterinary surgeons and students and others with frequent exposure to sheep, cattle or goats. It is most common in the lambing and calving seasons, and more commonly reported in sheep workers than cattle workers; this probably reflects differences in animal husbandry. Of 191 cases with a known source surveyed during 1978–1995, 84% had an ovine source and 16% were from cattle. During the same period 32 cases occurred in abattoir workers (Baxby and Bennett, 1997a).

Control

Most workers at risk get infected at some stage and reinfection is not uncommon. The impact of human infection in the farming and meat industries occasionally causes concern, and has led to industrial disputes (Johanneson et al., 1975; Robinson and Petersen, 1983). Individuals should take care not to spread infection by autoinoculation or to contacts, including animals. The vaccine used to control orf in sheep is fully virulent and has caused human infection.

MOLLUSCUM CONTAGIOSUM

Although lesions resembling molluscum and containing poxvirions have been detected in, for example, horses, human molluscum contagiosum is regarded as a specifically human infection and there is no evidence of transmission between humans and other animals. Molluscum contagiosum is a benign skin tumour which occurs worldwide. It has been the subject of a comprehensive recent review (Birthistle and Carrington, 1997).

Pathogenesis

After a variable, sometimes lengthy, incubation period, papules develop, formed by epidermal hypertrophy. This produces a nodule and also extends the dermis downwards, but the basement membrane usually remains intact. Characteristic inclusions (Henderson–Paterson bodies) are formed in the prickle cell layer and gradually enlarge as the cells age and migrate to the surface. These cells are replaced by hyperplasia of the basal cell layer. The inclusion is a well-defined sac packed with virions (Shelly and Burmeister, 1986). The lesion is circumscribed by a connective tissue capsule and the dermis, apart from distortion, remains essentially normal. Occasionally an inflammatory infiltration of the dermis may occur (Brown et al., 1981).

Clinical Features

Infection is via trauma to the skin. The characteristic lesion begins as a small papule and, when mature, is a discrete, waxy, smooth, dome-shaped pearly or flesh-coloured nodule, often umbilicated (Figure 15.8). There are usually 1–20 lesions but occasionally there may be hundreds. They may become confluent along the line of a scratch and satellite lesions are occasionally seen.

In children, lesions occur mainly on the trunk and proximal extremities. In adults they tend to occur on

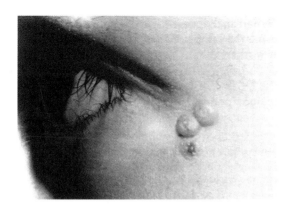

Figure 15.8 Molluscum contagiosum lesions showing umbilication. From a transparency kindly supplied by Dr J Verbov

the trunk, pubic area and thighs, but in all cases infection may be transmitted to other parts by autoinoculation (Brown *et al.*, 1981). Individual lesions last for about 2 months but the disease usually lasts 6–9 months (Steffen and Markman, 1989). More severe and prolonged infection tends to occur in individuals with impaired cell-mediated immunity, including human immunodeficiency virus (HIV) infection (Birthistle and Carrington, 1997).

Diagnosis

The appearance of lesions in normal cases is generally sufficiently characteristic to permit clinical diagnosis. Virions can usually be seen in large numbers if material expressed from the lesion is examined by electron microscopy. The lack of a marked inflammatory response and failure to isolate an agent in cell culture or CAM should eliminate other poxvirus infections.

Epidemiology

Restriction endonuclease analysis of molluscum virus DNA has detected three main subtypes. Their incidence varies from 80–90% for MCV-I to ca. 1% for MCV-III but all subtypes cause similar lesions and infect the same anatomical sites (Scholtz *et al.*, 1989; Porter *et al.*, 1992).

The virus occurs worldwide and tends to be more common in socially deprived areas. Traditional modes

of transmission are associated with mild skin trauma, such as contact sports and shared towels; however, there is increasing evidence that the disease is sexually transmitted and that genital lesions are more common (Birthistle and Carrington, 1997).

Control

Infection is benign and recovery usually spontaneous, but treatment may be sought for cosmetic reasons, particularly for facial or multiple lesions. Various treatments have been tried (Birthistle and Carrington, 1997). Chemical treatments include phenolics, silver nitrate, trichloroacetic and glacial acetic acid. Physical methods include curettage and cryotherapy. Mild trauma may induce a cure, which may be due to release of virus-infected cells accessible to the immune system.

Prevention in developed countries is based on attention to personal hygiene, and in developing countries to this and to general improvements in living conditions. Although relatively unimportant *per se*, the possibility that molluscum may act as a marker for more serious conditions has been raised (Oriel, 1987).

TANAPOX

Human infection with tanapox virus was first recognised in the Lake Tana area of Kenya in 1957, and particular attention was paid to it during post-eradication smallpox surveillance. An account of 264 laboratory-confirmed cases from Zaire (Democratic Republic of Congo), with colour illustrations, is available (Jezek *et al.*, 1985), as is information on the virus itself (Knight *et al.*, 1989). Recent anecdotal reports of human disease outside Africa have been published and illustrate the need to consider poxvirus aetiologies of illness in travellers returning from and emigrants from endemic areas (Croitoru *et al.*, 2002; Stich *et al.*, 2002).

Pathogenesis and Clinical Features

Infection is via the skin. The lesion is characterised by pronounced epidermal hyperplasia with little involvement of the dermis. There is a short prodromal illness with fever and malaise. The lesion starts as a macule and progresses to a raised nodule, which becomes umbilicated (Figure 15.9). The lesions are relatively large (~ 10 mm) and usually break down to form ulcers (Figure 15.9b). There is usually erythema and oedema and lymphadenopathy is common. The lesions generally disappear within 6 weeks. Most (78%) patients have only one lesion, and very few have more than two. They may occur on any exposed area but the head tends to be spared.

Diagnosis

For diagnosis of tanapox the limited geographical distribution should be considered, as well as travel history. The solid nodular/ulcerated lesions are larger and develop more slowly than those of monkeypox, but are smaller and develop more rapidly than those of tropical ulcers.

Virus can be detected by electron microscopy but this would not exclude morphologically similar viruses; nucleic acid tests (Stich *et al.*, 2002) or diagnostic serological tests on lesion extract would do this. Tanapox virus grows in a number of cell lines (e.g. owl monkey kidney, Vero, MRC-5, BSC-1) but not on CAM.

Epidemiology and Control

The virus probably has a simian reservoir and is restricted to Africa, principally Kenya and Zaire (Democratic Republic of Congo). Human-to-human transmission does not occur naturally, and it is thought that transmission from monkeys occurs mainly due to overcrowding during flooding, unrest, etc. With the exception of vaccination, measures for the prevention of monkeypox would be applicable to tanapox; however, the mild and sporadic nature of the infection probably means that specific measures are unnecessary.

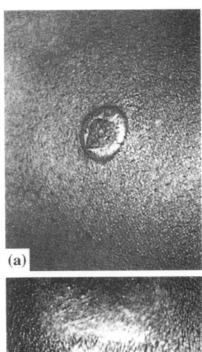
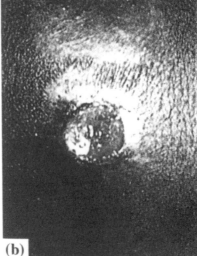

Figure 15.9 Human tanapox lesions. (a) After 10 days, showing oedema and umbilication; (b) after 26 days, showing ulcer formation. Reproduced from Jezek *et al.* (1985) by permission of WHO

DIAGNOSIS

When considering a diagnosis of poxvirus infection, the restricted geographical distribution and potential animal source are important features to consider. In many cases the differential diagnosis is between a particular poxvirus infection and other infections, e.g. herpes, tropical ulcers, anthrax, bacterial abscess, rather than between two different poxviruses.

Summary of Diagnostic Approaches

Electron microscopy is important in rapid diagnosis and will confirm parapox infection or exclude pox infection altogether if herpes virus is seen. Further information, if required, can be obtained by virus isolation in cell culture and/or CAM, often making use of efficiency of growth at elevated temperatures. Virus-specific antigens may be detected by a variety of techniques, and nucleic acid detection tests for virus-specific gene products by polymerase chain reaction (PCR) are now widely used (Ibrahim *et al.*, 2003; Meyer *et al.*, 1997, 1998; Ropp *et al.*, 1995).

Poxviruses will remain infective at ambient temperatures, particularly if kept dry. If specimens cannot be tested 'on the spot', infectivity is retained during transport by first class mail without the need for special transport medium. Vesicle fluid should be smeared on a slide and air-dried. On receipt the material can be reconstituted in buffer. Scrapings from molluscum and parapox lesions can be treated similarly. The infectivity of virus in dried crusts is retained for long periods. Virus may be extracted from such material by freeze–thawing and ultrasonic treatment. However, if the differential diagnosis includes pathogens less resistant than poxviruses, greater care should be taken and appropriate transport medium, etc. used.

Therapeutics

An active area of research involves the development of and evaluation of therapeutics for orthopoxvirus infections. A comprehensive review of the history and recent developments in the development of poxvirus antivirals has been recently published (Neyts and Clercq, 2003). In addition, work testing such compounds on experimental models of variola-infected non-human primates is ongoing (LeDuc *et al.*, 2002), in addition to other animal models of orthopoxvirus infections (Bray *et al.*, 2000). Cidofovir (and potentially its derivatives), an antiviral in use for treatment of cytomegalovirus infections in immunosuppressed patients, appears to show promise as an antiviral for treatment of some poxvirus infections (Kern *et al.*, 2002). The use of vaccinia-immune globulin (VIG) is best described for treatment of certain complications of vaccinia (smallpox) vaccine administration (Cono *et al.*, 2003), but may have utility in the treatment of certain other orthopoxvirus infections. No clear benefit has been shown for this product alone in the treatment of smallpox (Fenner *et al.*, 1988).

REFERENCES

Baxby D (1982) The natural history of cowpox. *Bristol Med Chirurg J*, **97**, 12.

Baxby D (1988) Poxvirus infections in domestic animals. In *Diseases in Laboratory and Captive Animals* (ed. Darai G), pp 17–35. Nijhoff, Boston.

Baxby D (1993) Indications for smallpox vaccination: policies still differ. *Vaccine*, **11**, 395–399.

Baxby D (1998) Poxviruses. In *Topley and Wilson's Microbiology and Microbial Infections*, vol 1 (eds Collier LH, Balows A and Sussman M), pp 367–383. Edward Arnold, London.

Baxby D and Bennett M (1997a) Poxvirus zoonoses. *J Med Microbiol*, **46**, 17–20.

Baxby D and Bennett M (1997b) Cowpox: a re-evaluation of the risks of human infection based on new epidemiological information. *Arch Virol*, **13**(suppl), 1–12.

Baxby D, Bennett M and Getty B (1994) Human cowpox 1969–93; a review based on 54 cases. *Br J Dermatol*, **131**, 598–607.

Bennett M, Gaskell CJ, Baxby D *et al.* (1990) Feline cowpox infection. *J Small Animal Pract*, **31**, 167–173.

Birthistle K and Carrington D (1997) Molluscum contagiosum virus. *J Infect*, **34**, 21–28.

Bray M, Martinez M, Smee DF *et al.* (2000) Cidofovir protects mice against lethal aerosol or intranasal cowpox virus challenge. *J Infect Dis*, **181**, 10–19.

Bremen JG (2000) Monkeypox: an emerging infection for humans? In *Emerging Infections*, vol 4 (eds Scheld WM, Craig WA and Hughes JM), pp 45–67. ASM Press, Washington, DC.

Brown ST, Nalley JF and Kraus SJ (1981) Molluscum contagiosum. *Sex Transm Dis*, **8**, 227–234.

Bugert JJ, Melquiot N and Kehm R (2001) Molluscum contagiosum virus expresses late genes in primary human fibroblasts but does not produce infectious progeny. *Virus Genes*, **22**, 27–33.

Cono J, Casey C and Ball D (2003) Smallpox vaccination and adverse reactions. *Morbid Mortal Wkly Rep*, **52**, RR04.

Croitoru AG, Birge MB, Rudikoff D *et al.* (2002) Tanapox virus infection. *Skinmed*, **1**, 156.

Crouch AC, Baxby D, McCracken CM *et al.* (1995) Serological evidence for the reservoir hosts of cowpox virus in British wildlife. *Epidemiol Infect*, **115**, 185–191.

Czerny C-P, Johann S, Hölzle L *et al.* (1994) Epitope detection in the envelope of intracellular mature orthopox viruses and identification of encoding genes. *Virology*, **200**, 764–777.

Damon IK and Esposito JJ (2002) Poxvirus infections in humans. In *Manual of Clinical Microbiology*, 8th edn (eds Murray PR, Tenover F, Baron EJ *et al.*), pp 1583–1591. American Society for Microbiology, Washington, DC.

Diven DG (2001) An overview of poxviruses. *J Am Acad Dermatol*, **44**, 1–16.

Douglas NJ and Dumbell KR (1992) Independent evolution of monkeypox and variola viruses. *J Virol*, **66**, 7565–7567.

Douglas NJ, Richardson M and Dumbell KR (1994) Evidence for recent genetic variation in monkeypox viruses. *J Gen Virol*, **75**, 1303–1309.

Dumbell KR and Richardson M (1993) Virological investigations of specimens from buffaloes affected by buffalopox in Maharashtra State, India, between 1985 and 1987. *Arch Virol*, **128**, 257–267.

Esposito JJ and Knight JC (1985) Orthopoxvirus DNA: a comparison of restriction profiles and maps. *Virology*, **135**, 230–251.

Fenner F, Henderson DA, Arita I *et al.* (1988) *Smallpox and Its Eradication*. World Health Organisation, Geneva.

Fulginetti V, Papier A, Lane JM *et al.* (2003) Smallpox vaccination: a review, Part II. Adverse events. *Clin Infect Dis*, **37**, 251–271.

Heymann DL, Szczeniowski M and Esteves K (1998) Re-emergence of monkeypox in Africa: a review of the past six years. *Br Med Bull*, **54**, 693–702.

Hutin YJF, Williams RJ, Malfait P *et al.* (2001) Outbreak of human monkeypox, Democratic Republic of Congo, 1996–1997. *Emerg Infect Dis*, **7**(3), 434–438.

Ibrahim MS, Kulesh DA, Saleh SS *et al.* (2003) Real-time PCR assay to detect smallpox virus. *J Clin Microbiol*, **41**(8), 3385–3839.

Jezek Z, Arita I, Szczeniowski M *et al.* (1985) Human tanapox in Zaire: clinical and epidemiological observations on cases confirmed by laboratory studies. *Bull WHO*, **63**, 1027–1035.

Jezek Z and Fenner F (1988) Human monkeypox. In *Monographs in Virology*, vol 17. Karger, Basel.

Jezek Z, Grab B, Szczeniowski M *et al.* (1988) Human monkeypox: secondary attack rates. *Bull WHO*, **66**, 465–470.

Johanneson JV, Krogh HK, Solberg I *et al.* (1975) Human orf. *J Cutan Pathol*, **2**, 265–283.

Johnson GP, Goebel SJ and Paoletti E (1993) An update on the vaccinia virus genome. *Virology*, **196**, 381–401.

Johnston JB and MacFadden G (2003) Poxvirus immuno-modulatory strategies: current perspectives. *J Virol*, **77**(11), 6093–6100.

Keith KA, Hitchcock MJ, Lee WA *et al.* (2003) Evaluation of nucleoside phosphonates and their analogs and prodrugs for inhibition of orthopoxvirus replication. *Antimicrob Ag Chemother*, **47**(7), 2193–2198.

Kern ER, Hartline C, Harden E *et al.* (2002) Enhanced inhibition of orthopoxvirus replication by alkoxyalkyl esters of cidofovir and cyclic cidofovir. *Antimicrob Ag Chemother*, **46**, 991–995.

Khodacevich L, Jezek Z and Messinger D (1988) Monkeypox virus: ecology and public health significance. *Bull WHO*, **66**, 747–752.

Knight JC, Novembre FJ, Brown DR *et al.* (1989) Studies on tanapox virus. *Virology*, **172**, 116–124.

Leavell UW, McNamara MJ, Muelling R *et al.* (1968) Orf: report of 19 human cases with clinical and pathological observations. *J Am Med Assoc* **204**, 657–664.

LeDuc J, Damon I, Meegan J *et al.* (2002) Smallpox research activities: US Interagency Collaboration. *Emerg Infect Dis*, **8**(7), 742–745.

Limbach P and Paoletti E (1996) Non-replicating expression vectors: application in vaccine development and gene therapy. *Epidemiol Infect*, **116**, 241–246.

Loparev VN, Massung RF, Esposito JJ and Meyer H (2001) Detection and differentiation of Old World orthopox-viruses: restriction length polymorphism of the crmB gene region. *J Clin Microbiol*, **39**, 94–100.

Mercer A, Fleming S, Robinson A *et al.* (1997) Molecular genetics analyses of parapoxviruses pathogenic for humans. *Arch Virol*, **13**(suppl), 25–34.

Meyer H, Perrichot M, Stemmler P *et al.* (2002) Outbreaks of disease suspected of being due to human monkeypox virus infection in the Democratic Republic of Congo in 2001. *J Clin Microbiol*, **40**, 2919–2921.

Meyer H, Ropp SL and Esposito JJ (1997) Gene for A-type inclusion body protein is useful for a polymerase chain reaction assay to differentiate orthopoxviruses. *J Virol Meth*, **64**, 217–22.

Meyer H, Ropp SL and Esposito JJ (1998) Poxviruses. In *Methods in Molecular Biology: Diagnostic Virology Protocols* (eds Warnes A and Stephenson J), pp 199–211. Humana Press, Totowa, NJ.

MMWR (2003) Update: multistate outbreak of monkeypox—Illinois, Indiana, Kansas, Missouri, Ohio, and Wisconsin, 2003. *Morbid Mortal Wkly Rep*, **52**(27), 642.

Moss B (2001) Poxviridae and their replication. In *Field's Virology*, 4th edn (eds Fields BN, Knipe DM and Howley PM), pp 2849–2883. Raven, New York.

Moyer RW, Arif BM, Black DN *et al.* (2000) Poxviridae. In *Virus Taxonomy: Classification and Nomenclature of Viruses. Seventh Report of the International Committee on Taxonomy of Viruses* (eds van Regenmortel MHV, Faquet CM, Bishop DHL *et al.*), pp 137–157. Academic Press, San Diego, CA.

Neyts J and Clercq ED (2003) Therapy and short term prophylaxis of poxvirus infections: historical background and perspectives. *Antiviral Res*, **57**, 25–33.

Oriel JD (1987) The increase in molluscum contagiosum. *Br Med J*, **294**, 74.

Pastoret PP and Brochier B (1996) The development and use of a vaccinia recombinant oral vaccine for the control of wildlife rabies. *Epidemiol Infect*, **116**, 235–240.

Payne LG (1980) Significance of extracellular enveloped virus in the *in vitro* and *in vivo* dissemination of vaccinia. *J Gen Virol*, **50**, 89–100.

Pether JVS, Guerrier CJW, Jones SM *et al.* (1986) Giant orf in a normal individual. *Br J Dermatol*, **115**, 497–499.

Pilaski J and Rösen-Wolff A (1988) Poxvirus infection in zoo-kept mammals. In *Virus Diseases in Laboratory and Captive Animals* (ed. Darai G), pp 84–100. Martenjus Nijhoff, Boston, MA.

Porter CD, Blake NW, Cream JJ *et al.* (1992) Molluscum contagiosum virus. In *Molecular and Cell Biology of Sexually Transmitted Diseases* (eds Wright D and Archard L), pp 233–257. Chapman and Hall, London.

Robinson AJ and Petersen GV (1983) Orf virus infection of workers in the meat industry. *N Z Med J*, **96**, 81–85.

Ropp SL, Jin Q, Knight JC *et al.* (1995) PCR strategy for identification and differentiation of smallpox and other orthopoxviruses. *J Clin Microbiol*, **33**, 2069–2076.

Rupprecht CE, Blass L, Smith K *et al.* (2001) Human infection due to recombinant vaccinia-rabies glycoprotein virus. *N Engl J Med*, **345**, 582–586.

Scholtz J, Rosen-Wolff A, Bugert J *et al.* (1989) Epidemiology of molluscum contagiosum using genetic analysis of the viral DNA. *J Med Virol*, **27**, 87–90.

Seet BT, Johnston JB, Brunetti CR *et al.* (2003) Poxviruses and immune evasion. *Ann Rev Immunol*, **21**, 377–423.

Shchelkunov SN, Totmenin AV, Safronov PF *et al.* (2002) Analysis of the monkeypox genome. *Virology*, **297**, 172–194.

Shelly WB and Burmeister V (1986) Demonstration of a unique viral structure: the molluscum viral colony sac. *Br J Dermatol*, **115**, 557–562.

Smith GL, Symons JA, Khanna A *et al.* (1997) Vaccinia virus immune evasion. *Immunol Rev*, **159**, 137–154.

Smith GL, Vanderplasschen A and Law M (2003) The formation and function of extracellular enveloped vaccinia virus. *J Gen Virol*, **83**, 2915–2931.

Staib C and Sutter G (2003) Live viral vectors: vaccinia virus. *Meth Mol Med*, **87**, 51–68.

Steffen C and Markman J (1989) Spontaneous disappearance of molluscum contagiosum. *Arch Dermatol*, **116**, 923–924.

Stich A, Meyer H, Kohler B and Fleischer K (2002) Tanapox: first report in a European traveller and identification by PCR. *Trans R Soc Trop Med Hyg*, **96**, 178–179.

Torfason EG and Gunadottir S (2002) Polymerase chain reaction for laboratory diagnosis of orf virus infections. *J Clin Virol*, **24**, 79–84.

Vanderplasschen A, Hollinshead M and Smith GL (1997) Antibodies against vaccinia virus do not neutralize extracellular enveloped virus but prevent release from infected cells and comet formation. *J Gen Virol*, **78**, 2041–2048.

Vanderplasschen A and Smith GL (1997) A novel binding assay using confocal microscopy: demonstration that the intracellular vaccinia virions bind to different cellular receptors. *J Virol*, **71**, 4032–4041.

Yirrell DL and Vestey JP (1994) Human orf infections. *J Eur Acad Dermatol Venereol*, **3**, 451–459.

Yirrell DL, Vestey JP and Norval M (1994) Immune responses of patients to orf virus infection. *Br J Dermatol*, **130**, 438–443.

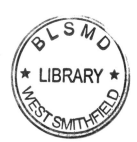

16

Alphaviruses

Graham Lloyd

Health Protection Agency, Porton Down, Salisbury, UK

INTRODUCTION

In 1967 the World Health Organization (WHO, 1967) defined arboviruses as:

> ... viruses which are maintained in nature principally, or to an important extent, through biological transmission between susceptible vertebrate hosts by haematophagous arthropods: they multiply and produce viraemia in the vertebrates, multiply in the tissues of arthropods, and are passed on to new vertebrates by the bites of arthropods after a period of extrinsic incubation.

The definition was therefore based on biological criteria. The arboviruses were initially divided into group A (later known as alphaviruses) and group B (later known as flaviviruses), but this was followed by the recognition of further antigenically related groups of arboviruses. Alphaviruses and flaviviruses were later included as two separate genera in the family *Togaviridae* (Weaver *et al.*, 2000). More recently, however, flaviviruses have been classified as a separate family, the *Flaviviridae*.

All medically important vector-borne togaviruses are members of the genus *Alphavirus*. Alphaviruses are transmitted to their vertebrate hosts by arthropods (Figure 16.1) and have defined geographic distributions. The Eastern equine encephalitis (EEE) and Venezuelan equine encephalitis (VEE) lineages are closely related and restricted to the New World, while the Sindbis-like (with the exception of Aura), Semliki

Forest (with the exception of Mayaro and Una), Barmah Forest, Middelburg and Ndumu lineages occur in the Old World. Natural vertebrate hosts include birds and rodents. Infection in the vertebrate is usually inapparent but can, under certain circumstances, cause disease and death. Transmission may also occur to domestic animals and humans. Here again the spectrum of disease varies from a clinically inapparent infection to a severe disease and even death.

MORPHOLOGY

The alphaviruses are essentially spherical, 60–70 nm in diameter (Figure 16.2) and sensitive to ether and detergent. The viron consists of three components: an outer glycoprotein shell, a lipid bilayer and an RNA-containing core or nucleocapsid (Peters and Dalrymple, 1990). The lipid bilayer is derived from the host-cell plasma membrane. The viral-encoded glycoproteins, designated E1 and E2, form the outer surface of the virus and interact with cellular receptors and host-derived antibodies. The glycoproteins are arranged in an icosahedral surface lattice (Harrison, 1986). Complete sequence information available suggests that the viral genome is 11–12 kb in size and encodes four non-structural proteins (NSP1, NSP2, NSP3 and NSP4) at the 5' end and the five structural proteins (C, E3, E2, 6K and E1) at the 3' end. The nsPs are translated from genomic RNA, and the structural proteins from subgenomic RNA. Electron cryomicroscopy and image reconstruction of Sindbis, Semliki Forest, Ross River and Aura viruses show that the envelope

Principles and Practice of Clinical Virology, Fifth Edition. Edited by A. J. Zuckerman, J. E. Banatvala, J. R. Pattison, P. D. Griffiths and B. D. Schoub
© 2004 John Wiley & Sons Ltd   ISBN 0 470 84338 1

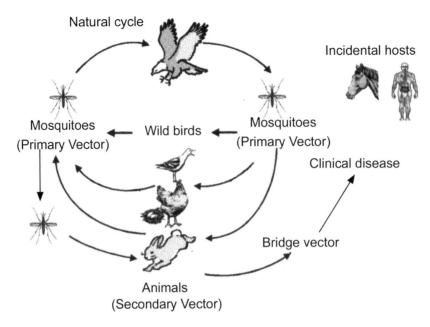

Figure 16.1 Schematic transmission and maintenance cycles

glycoproteins form a T = 4 icosahedral lattice (Cheng *et al.*, 1995; Mancini *et al.*, 2000). The capsid proteins form a T = 4 icosahedral nucleocapsid arranged in distinct pentameric and hexameric capsomeres on the exterior of the nucleocapsid.

BIOCHEMICAL AND BIOPHYSICAL PROPERTIES

The nucleic acid of the alphaviruses consists of a single-stranded (ss) positive-sense RNA, almost 12 000 nucleotides in length, which is capped at the 5′ end and polyadenylated at the 3′ end (Figure 16.3). The naked genome is infectious (Strauss and Strauss, 1986). The sedimentation coefficient has been reported to be 42–49. The genome is divided into two regions; the 5′ two-thirds of the viral genome codes for the non-structural proteins and the 3′ third encodes the structural proteins (Strauss *et al.*, 1984). Both the structural and non-structural proteins are translated as polyprotein precursors. The non-structural polyprotein precursor is cleaved into four non-structural proteins, NSP1, NSP2, NSP3 and NSP4, which function as the replicase–transcriptase of the virus (Strauss and Strauss, 1986). The structural polyprotein precursor is cleaved to form three major polypeptides. The capsid protein C (30–40 kDa) and the envelope glycoproteins E1 and E2 (45–59 kDa) are found in

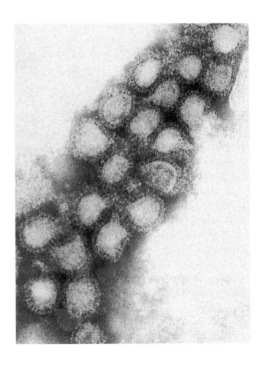

Figure 16.2 Electron micrograph of a preparation of Sindbis virus (3% potassium phosphotungstate, pH 7.0; final magnification × 200 000). Micrograph courtesy of Professor C. R. Madeley, The Royal Victoria Infirmary, Newcastle upon Tyne, UK

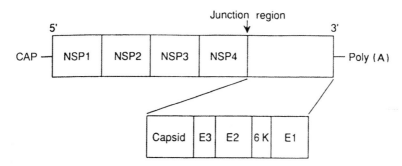

Figure 16.3 Organisation of the alpha virus genome. The 5' two-thirds of the viral genome encode the non-structural proteins, NSP1, NSP2, NSP3 and NSP4. The 3' third encodes the structural proteins. The capsid and envelope glycoproteins (E1 and E2) are present in mature alphavirus particles. A third glycoprotein, E3, has been demonstrated in purified SFV. The 6 K polypeptide is not known to be a structural protein

mature alphavirus particles. In addition, a small glycoprotein, termed E3, has been demonstrated in Semliki Forest virus (Garoff *et al.*, 1974). A further small 6 K polypeptide is also encoded, but has not been demonstrated in any alphavirus particles.

REPLICATION

Viral attachment to a host cell occurs via the glycoprotein spikes on the viral surface. The envelope glycoproteins have receptors that are essential to initiate infection. Alphaviruses are able to infect both vertebrate and arthropod hosts and enter the host cell by endocytosis or direct fusion with the plasma membrane. After endocytosis the capsid is thought to be released by low-pH catalysed membrane fusion, initiated by the E1 glycoprotein (Wang *et al.*, 1992). Once released, the positive-sense ssRNA probably serves as an mRNA. A virus-encoded transcriptase transcribes the positive-sense RNA into minus-stranded RNA, which then forms a template for the synthesis of the positive-stranded progeny RNA. Nucleocapsids are assembled in the cytoplasm and maturation occurs by budding through host cell membranes.

ANTIGENIC AND GENOTYPIC PROPERTIES

The alphaviruses have a group-reactive nucleoprotein. Complex and type-specific reactivity is determined by the envelope glycoproteins. This antigenic comparison of alphaviruses has been conducted using haemagglutination-inhibition (HI) and complement fixation tests (CF), as well as cross-protection tests in mice and neutralisation tests in cell culture (Calisher *et al.*, 1980). The E1 glycoprotein of Sindbis virus contains the antigen responsible for haemagglutination (Chanas *et al.*, 1982). It is assumed that this is also the case for other members of the genus *Alphavirus*. The E2 glycoprotein induces virus-specific neutralising antibody. On the basis of this, alphaviruses have been divided into six antigenic complexes: Western equine encephalitis (WEE), Venezuelan equine encephalitis (VEE), Eastern equine encephalitis (EEE), Semliki Forest (SF), Middelburg and Ndumu viruses (Peters and Dalrymple, 1990). A further virus, Barmah Forest virus, has been shown to be biochemically typical of the genus, but is not related serologically to members of the six antigenic complexes (Table 16.1). Each complex consists of either a single virus species having no known close relatives, e.g. EEE, VEE, Middelburg and Ndumu viruses, or several species, subtypes and varieties that are more closely related to each other than the other members of the genus, e.g. Semliki Forest virus and WEE virus. Often only plaque reduction or kinetic HI tests can distinguish these variants. Kinetic HI tests have also been used to differentiate between geographical variants of EEE virus (Casals, 1964). Studies utilising monoclonal antibodies have been able to define the alphavirus antigenic cross-reactivities more precisely and map the antigenic determinants.

A recent study sequenced one strain of each alphavirus species and this allowed for the classification of alphaviruses into six genotypes (as compared with seven antigenic complexes): Sindbis, Ndumu, VEE, WEE, Barmah Forest and Semliki Forest viruses. The authors included EEE and WEE in the same genotypic complex; this homology is to be expected, as WEE is thought to be a recombinant

Table 16.1 Antigenic classification of alphaviruses, global distribution, primary vertebrate hosts, primary and transmission vectors

Antigenic complex	Virus	Geographical distribution	Vertebrate host	Primary vector
Barmah Forest	Barmah Forest	Australia	Birds	*Cx. annulirostris*
Eastern equine encephalitis (EEE)	EEE	North and South America	Birds	Enzootic—*Culex* sp. Bridge vector—*Aedes* sp.
Middelburg	Middelburg	South, West and Central America	?	
Nduma	Nduma	South, West and Central America	?	
Semliki Forest	Semliki Forest	Africa and Asia	?	*Ae. abnormalis* *Ae. africanus*
	Chikungunya	Africa and Asia	Primates	*Ae. africanus* *Ae. aegypti* *Cx. tritaeniorhynchus*
	Getah	Asia and Australasia	Mammals	*Ae. aegypti*
	Mayaro	South America	?	
Western equine encephalitis (WEE)	WEE	Americas	Birds, mammals	*Cx. tarsalis*
	Aura	South America	?	*Ae. serratus*
	Fort Morgan	North America	Birds	
	Highlands J	North America	Birds	*Cs. melanura*
Venezuelan equine encephalitis (VEE)	VEE	The Americas	Mammals	Enzootic cycle—*Culex* sp. Epizootic cycle—*Aedes* sp.

virus which derives its non-structural genes from an EEE virus ancestor (Pfeffer *et al.*, 1997).

SPECTRUM OF DISEASE CAUSED BY ALPHAVIRUSES

Alphaviruses cause a wide range of disease in animals and humans, ranging from a clinically inapparent infection to a severe disease that may result in death. The main target organs are muscle, brain, reticuloendothelial system and the joints. This group of viruses may be clinically divided into those that are associated with fever, rash and polyarthritis found in the Old World and those that cause encephalitis, primarily found in the New World (Table 16.2). Middelburg and Ndumu viruses are not known to cause disease in humans. Some alphaviruses are also responsible for disease in animals, particularly Equidae (horses and related animals).

DIAGNOSIS OF ALPHAVIRUS INFECTIONS

The clinical features in a patient living or having recently travelled to an appropriate geographical region are the essential early components of establishing a differential diagnosis (Table 16.3). However, differentiation from other viral infections may be difficult, e.g., it is sometimes clinically difficult to differentiate infection with Ross River virus from rickettsial, rubella, parvovirus B19 or enterovirus infections. Laboratory confirmation may therefore be required to identify the causative agent.

Table 16.2 Range of human illness caused by alphaviruses

Clinical features	Virus
Fever, rash	Sindbis, Ockelbo
Fever, rash, polyarthritis	Ross River, Barmah Forest
Fever, rash, myalgia, arthralgia	Chikungunya, o'nyong-nyong, Mayaro, Sindbis, Ockelbo, Ross River, Barmah Forest, Igo Ora
Fever, encephalitis	Eastern equine encephalitis, Western equine encephalitis, Venezuelan equine encephalitis, Everglades, Semliki Forest

Table 16.3 Generalised alphavirus case definition

Clinical description	An illness with acute onset, with fever $\geqslant 38\,^{\circ}$C, including variations of the following: Rash Arthralgia Polyarthritis Myalgia, headache, nausea, vomiting Malaise and weakness Disorientation and drowsiness
Laboratory criteria for diagnosis in one or more areas	Isolation of virus from blood, CSF or synovial joint fluids Positive IgM serology or seroconversion (IgG) in paired serum Demonstration of virus antigen in autopsy tissue by immunocytochemistry or in serum by ELISA Positive PCR from serum, synovial joint fluid, CSF or autopsy tissue
Case classification	
Suspected	A case that meets the clinical case description
Probable	A case compatible with the clinical description with one or more of the following: Supportive serology (comparable IgG serology or positive IgM antibody test in acute or convalescent phase serum specimen) Occurrence at same location and time as other confirmed alphavirus cases
Confirmed	A suspected case that is laboratory-confirmed (National Reference Laboratory), that includes seroconversion and/or virus isolation or is PCR-positive or epidemiologically linked to a confirmed case or outbreak

Laboratory diagnosis includes viral culture, the detection of a specific antibody response and, more recently, the use of molecular techniques to detect the viral genome. In general, virus isolation is often only successful when acute-phase antibody-negative serum samples are used, particularly when the serum sample is taken in the first 48 h of illness. Thereafter, the amount of virus in serum reduces rapidly and isolation becomes increasingly difficult. Virus identification is facilitated by the use of murine monoclonal alphavirus-specific antibodies. Virus may be isolated by intracerebral inoculation of suckling mice as well as in a variety of cell culture systems, including monkey kidney (Vero) and mosquito (C6/36) cell lines. More recently methods have been developed to diagnose alphavirus infections using genomic detection methods. As these are RNA viruses, any polymerase chain reaction (PCR)-based assay must first transcribe the RNA into DNA. A reverse transcription-polymerase chain reaction (RT-PCR) has been developed for the genus-specific detection of alphaviruses. This utilises degenerate primers localised within a conserved region of the non-structural protein 1 and has become a routine sensitive and rapid alternative to virus isolation in the diagnosis of an acute infection (Pfeffer *et al.*, 1997).

Detection of an appropriate specific antibody response is frequently used to diagnose alphavirus infections. Class-specific IgM assays have been developed to diagnose an acute or recent infection with a particular alphavirus. However, care must be taken in the interpretation of the result, as cross-reactions may occur with other members of the same alphavirus antigenic complex (Table 16.1) (Calisher *et al.*, 1986). A serological diagnosis of a recent alphavirus infection is demonstrated by a rise in specific IgM or IgG antibodies, when acute and convalescent serum samples are tested in parallel. This is usually done using ELISA, IFA or neutralisation tests.

MANAGEMENT AND PREVENTION

Management of alphavirus infections is usually supportive and directed at symptomatic relief, e.g. the symptomatic relief of joint symptoms with non-steroidal antiinflammatory agents and aspirin. Prevention of alphavirus infections has focused on vector control and the protection of the individual against mosquito bites. A detailed knowledge of the vector and vertebrate host range is therefore essential to allow for a coordinated strategy to prevent and control alphavirus infections. Vaccines are also available against some of the individual alphaviruses infections, but are not generally available (see below).

ALPHAVIRUSES ASSOCIATED WITH FEVERS AND POLYARTHRITIS

Sindbis Virus

Sindbis virus is considered the prototype of the alphaviruses. It was originally isolated from *Culex* mosquitoes collected in the Egyptian village of Sindbis (Taylor *et al.*, 1955). In Sweden, symptomatic disease resulting from infection with a Sindbis-like agent has been termed Ockelbo disease. A Sindbis-related virus has also been described as the cause of Pogosta disease in Finland and as Karelian fever in the Karelian region of the former USSR. Babanki virus is a Sindbis-like agent that occurs in West and Central Africa; the clinical significance of the infection with this virus remains to be defined (Peters and Dalrymple, 1990).

Epidemiology and Host Range

Sindbis virus occurs in many parts of the world, including Europe, Asia, Africa and Australia. The virus is known to infect humans, domestic animals and birds, with birds forming the principal reservoir. Humans are not considered to be essential to the survival of the virus in nature. Sindbis virus is transmitted among birds by *Culex* mosquitoes. Infection in birds does not appear to result in disease. Where humans and birds exist in close proximity, e.g. in the Nile Valley, transmission to humans may occur (Peters and Dalrymple, 1990). Studies from South Africa have shown that the virus is distributed widely throughout the country. Transmission to the avian population, and probably to humans, occurs annually. Extensive human disease only occurs, however, during years of abundant rainfall and flooding (McIntosh *et al.*, 1964; Jupp *et al.*, 1986). In Europe, disease caused by Sindbis virus occurs after excursions into forested areas, e.g. by lumberjacks or berry pickers. Here the virus has been isolated from *Culiseta*, *Aedes* and *Culex* mosquitoes.

Clinical Disease

Sindbis virus is among the least virulent of the alphaviruses. Serological surveys suggest that infection with Sindbis virus is relatively common, but clinically apparent disease is unusual. When symptomatic, the spectrum of disease in humans varies from a mild illness to one consisting of a rash and arthralgia. The illness is usually characterised by a sudden onset of the rash, but occasionally prodromal symptoms may be present. The rash is usually macular or papular but may become vesicular or haemorrhagic. Malaise, fatigue and headache are frequently present (McIntosh *et al.*, 1964; Jupp *et al.*, 1986). The initial joint involvement is usually migratory, followed by a gradual resolution of symptoms.

Ockelbo disease was first described in the central part of Sweden in the 1960s in clusters of patients with fever, arthralgia and a rash (Niklasson and Vene, 1996). Some patients with Ockelbo disease have reported joint symptoms persisting for more than a year and recurrent joint problems were documented in one-third of a group of Swedish patients interviewed 2 or more years post-infection (Niklasson *et al.*, 1988). By contrast, reports from South Africa have emphasised the joint involvement less and have suggested that the involvement is of tendon and periarticular tissue, rather than a true arthritis (McIntosh *et al.*, 1964).

Pathogenesis

It is not clear whether the skin lesions are the result of a direct viral cytopathic effect or are immunopathological. Evidence to support the former hypothesis comes from Malherbe and Strickland-Cholmley (1963), who demonstrated the isolation of Sindbis virus from a vesicle in the absence of a serum viraemia. This was associated with a subsequent rise in specific antibody. However, other workers have failed to isolate Sindbis virus from skin lesions (McIntosh *et al.*, 1964). The pathogenesis of the joint complications, and whether they are articular or periarticular, is also unclear.

Diagnosis

Isolation of Sindbis virus from human sera has been reported, but this is frequently not successful, even using sera taken early on in the illness. This is because the viraemia associated with Sindbis virus infection is often of low level and transient. In addition, medical attention is frequently sought relatively late in the course of the illness. As mentioned above, Sindbis virus has also been isolated from a skin lesion. When inoculated into 3–5-day-old mice, either intracerebrally or intraperitoneally, Sindbis virus causes a fatal infection, which is preceded by a short period of paralysis. The virus has also been isolated *in vitro* in fibroblastic cell lines. Antibodies appear 7–10 days after the onset of illness and may be detected by HI, ELISA and immunofluorescence (IF) (McIntosh *et al.*,

1964; Doherty *et al.*, 1969; Espmark and Niklasson, 1984). Although the detection of Sindbis-specific IgM may be of use in diagnosis of an acute infection, this class of antibody may remain detectable 3–4 years after the initial infection. A positive IgM result must therefore be interpreted together with the available clinical information.

Ross River Virus

Infection with Ross River virus (RRV), also known as epidemic polyarthritis, is a major public health problem in Australia. It is the most common arboviral infection of humans in Australia. In the late 1970s and early 1980s, RRV also became endemic in the Pacific Islands (Table 16.4). In recent years it has also been increasingly identified in travellers returning to Europe.

Epidemiology and Host Range

Until 1979 the distribution of RRV infections was thought to be limited to Australia, Papua New Guinea and the Solomon Islands, all in the western half of the Pacific basin. In Australia both epidemic and sporadic transmission of RRV occurs. Epidemics are characteristically preceded by heavy rainfall and are located in river valleys and irrigated lands in coastal areas. However, other factors, such as temperature, are important—a sudden period of cold can delay the build-up of the vector and so abort an epidemic (Hawkes *et al.*, 1985). The virus was first isolated from *Aedes vigilax*, which is accepted as being the major vector in the coastal regions of Australia. Other mosquito species, including the salt marsh arthropod *Aedes comptorhynchus*, found in northern and southern coastal regions, and *Culex annulirostris*, which breeds in freshwater habitats, are also considered important vectors (Peters and Dalrymple, 1990). Besides humans, other possible vertebrate hosts include marsupials, domestic animals and rodents (Doherty, 1977).

In 1979 an explosive epidemic of RRV infection occurred in Fiji (Aaskov *et al.*, 1981). The virus spread to American Samoa and then to the Wallis and Futuna Islands and the Cook Islands. The mosquito vector in this region is unknown, although the virus has been isolated from *Aedes polynesiensis*, a mosquito that is found in many parts of the Eastern Pacific (Rosen *et al.*, 1981). Evidence suggests that humans are the most important vertebrate hosts in this region. A study from the Cook Islands showed that the incubation period could be as short as 3 days, and the explosive nature of this epidemic led to speculation that mechanical transmission of RRV may occur. This theory has been supported by laboratory evidence of mechanical transmission of RRV from viraemic donors to uninfected recipient suckling mice. In addition, it has also been suggested that transovarial transmission in mosquitoes is a potential survival mechanism for this virus (Kay, 1982).

The number of annual reported cases of RRV disease has increased during the past decade to 4000–6000. However, these figures represent a combination of improved laboratory diagnostic reagents, greater awareness by clinicians, housing developments on salt marshes and migration northwards to warmer climates in retirement (Mackenzie *et al.*, 2001).

Clinical Disease

Infection with RRV does not usually result in disease in humans and it has been estimated that 50 subclinical infections occur for each clinically recognised case (Table 16.2). The disease is not fatal. Adults are more

Table 16.4 Geographic distribution of the Semliki Forest virus complex

Virus species	Subtype	Main geographic distribution	Other features
Semliki Forest		Africa	Epidemic in Central African Republic
Chikungunya	Chikungunya	Africa, S.E. Asia, The Philippines	Epidemics in E. Africa, Asia
	O'nyong-nyong	West and East Africa, Zimbabwe	Epidemics in E. Africa, Zimbabwe
Getah	Getah	Malaysia, Japan, Australia, Cambodia, The Philippines	
	Bebaru	Malaysia	
	Ross River	Australasia, South Pacific	
	Sagiyama	Japan, Okinawa	One epizootic in Japan
Mayaro	Mayaro	Trinidad, Brazil	
	Una	Brazil, Colombia, Panama, Surinam, Trinidad, French Guyana	

likely to be symptomatic than children. The onset of clinical symptoms is characterised by joint pains (epidemic polyarthritis) accompanied by a rash and fever. In a recent postal survey of general practitioners in south Australia the complaint of 'pain in the joints' was the most important symptom for suspecting an infection with RRV, with joint effusion, rash and pyrexia being important signs (Stocks *et al.*, 1997; Flexman *et al.*, 1998). The rash may occur simultaneously with the joint pains or may follow 1–2 days later. Although the rash is usually macular, maculopapular or papular, vesiculation and petechiae have been described. The rash and joint pains are commonly accompanied by some degree of constitutional upset, including myalgia, headache, anorexia and nausea. The joint involvement is usually asymmetrical and migratory and most often affects the small joints of the hands and feet, together with the knees. In addition, there may also be periarticular swelling and a tenosynovitis (Clarke *et al.*, 1973; Hawkes *et al.*, 1985). The arthralgia and arthritis tend to run a relapsing course but with an overall gradual improvement. The symptoms of epidemic polyarthritis may last for 30–40 weeks, with some patients having symptoms for more than a year. While joint pain, rash and fever are the most common clinical features, a case of glomerulonephritis has also been reported in the acute phase of RRV disease (Fraser *et al.*, 1988). This report described a patient presenting with haematuria and proteinuria coincident with an acute RRV infection; the frequency of this complication has yet to be defined.

Pathogenesis

The pathogenesis of the disease is not completely understood. While virus has been isolated from the blood, it has not been isolated from either the skin or joints. However, RRV antigen has been detected by immunofluorescence at both of these sites. Histological examination of the skin lesions shows a mononuclear cell infiltration (Fraser *et al.*, 1983). It has also been shown that RRV is capable of infecting human synovial cells (Cunningham and Fraser, 1985). Serum complement is normal and circulating immune complexes do not usually exceed normal levels. It has therefore been suggested that RRV plays a direct role at these sites of inflammation.

Diagnosis

A key factor in diagnosis is knowledge of travel history. A differential diagnosis would also include rubella, other alphavirus-induced arthritis, dengue, rheumatoid arthritis and other chronic rheumatic diseases (Fraser, 1986).

Isolation of RRV is only successful using acute-phase antibody-negative serum samples. Both mosquitoes and mosquito cell lines have been used. The current method of choice for RRV isolation is the inoculation of the mosquito cell line, C6/36. As this virus does not display a cytopathic effect in C6/36 cells, viral antigen is detected using IF (Rosen *et al.*, 1981). RRV may also be isolated in Vero (E6) cells. More recently, methods have been developed to detect RRV RNA using RT-PCR. This methodology has potential application to virus surveillance programmes in mosquito populations (Sellner *et al.*, 1994).

The most sensitive and established serological assay involves the use of an IgM capture EIA. However, there is a complication in that the assay can remain positive for up to 2 years after the acute infection (Carter *et al.*, 1985). It should be noted that IgM antibody cross-reactions with Mayaro, chikungunya and Semliki Forest viruses occurs with sera from patients with RRV infections (Table 16.4). However, ratios of homologous to heterologous IgM titres are usually high and so, although this cross-reaction somewhat limits the diagnostic usefulness of this test, it can provide a reasonably specific and rapid diagnosis in an epidemic situation (Calisher *et al.*, 1986). The presence of RRV-specific IgA or low-avidity IgG can assist the diagnosis of a recent infection (Carter *et al.*, 1987). A more precise diagnosis can be made using neutralisation tests (Kanamitsu *et al.*, 1979).

Vaccine

An inactivated RRV vaccine is being developed. Preliminary studies have shown that antibodies to this candidate vaccine neutralised all strains of RRV tested, but to different degrees (Aaskov *et al.*, 1997). Further studies are awaited with interest as, while RRV does not usually cause a severe disease, it may result in considerable morbidity with an associated loss of productivity.

Barmah Forest Virus

This alphavirus has been recently reported to cause both clinical and subclinical infections in Australia. Clinical disease resulting from BFV infection was first reported in 1986. The first epidemic of human disease occurred in 1992 in the Northern Territory (Mackenzie *et al.*, 1994). To date, Australia is the only country in which this virus has been detected (Hills, 1996).

Barmah Forest virus (BFV) is the sole member of the seventh alphavirus serocomplex (Table 16.4). The nucleotide sequence of the BFV genome has recently been described and, from amino acid sequence comparisons with sequenced alphaviruses, BFV has been shown to be most closely related to RRV and Semliki Forest virus (Lee *et al.*, 1997). In recent years there has been an apparent increase in incidence of polyarthritis caused by BFV. This prompted a study on the molecular epidemiology of this alphavirus, which showed a high degree of sequence homology between BFV isolates with no evidence of geographical or temporal divergence (Poidinger *et al.*, 1997).

Epidemiology and Host Range

Barmah Forest virus is an alphavirus that is enzootic in Australia and has been isolated from the two most common vectors of RRV, *Culex annulirostris* and *Aedes vigilax*. It has been shown to circulate among mosquitoes and terrestrial animals, most noticeably marsupial species. Occupational and recreational exposure to these vectors is therefore an important risk factor for infection with this virus. A higher incidence of antibodies to BFV in RRV antibody-positive blood donors compared with RRV antibody-negative blood donors suggests a common ecology. Further information is required on the duration of viraemia in humans to determine whether the other vertebrate hosts are of importance in viral maintenance. Currently, human disease caused by BFV has not been recognised in southern Australia or Tasmania.

Clinical Disease

Human infections have been recognised since 1986 and its incidence has increased through greater clinical awareness and improved laboratory diagnostic methods. Currently, approximately 500 cases are recorded each year (Lindsey *et al.*, 1995). As mentioned above, both clinical and subclinical infections occur. The most common symptoms noted in a study from Queensland were arthritis, arthralgia, myalgia and fever, which were present in approximately 75% of patients (Table 16.2). In addition, half the patients in this study had a rash (Phillips *et al.*, 1990). A more recent study from New South Wales reported lethargy (89%), joint pain (82%) and rash (68%) as the most common symptoms. In the latter study, just over half of the

patients reported an illness lasting for more than 6 months. These authors also reported a possible association between the presence of a rash and an improved prognosis (Beard *et al.*, 1997). In general, the symptoms are similar to those associated with RRV infection; laboratory confirmation is therefore necessary to achieve a precise diagnosis. The wider availability of serological testing for BFV infections has also enabled their more unusual features to be described. Recently the first case of glomerulonephritis after BFV infection was diagnosed. The authors suggest that BFV infection should be considered as a possible aetiological agent for glomerulonephritis (Katz *et al.*, 1997).

Diagnosis

Clinical differentiation from RRV infection in patients living in endemic areas is difficult. Laboratory confirmation is therefore necessary for a precise diagnosis to be made. BFV has been isolated from a patient in the mosquito cell line, C6/36. The serological response to infection with this virus in humans remains to be defined precisely. However, in contrast to RRV infections, where the antibody response may be delayed for 7 days, a recent study demonstrated the presence of both HI and neutralising antibody titres in two patients with BFV infection at the onset of symptoms (Phillips *et al.*, 1990). This could be due to either a different serological response to these two viruses or, alternatively, BFV-associated disease may have a less clearly defined onset than that caused by RRV infections.

Chikungunya Virus

This virus was first isolated from patients and mosquitoes in the Newala district of Tanzania in 1952–1953. The name is derived from a local term for the illness and means 'that which bends up', referring to the crippling arthralgia and arthritis associated with infection with this virus. Chikungunya virus is found in the savannahs and forests of tropical Africa, as well as in many parts of Asia, including Thailand, Cambodia, Vietnam, Burma (now Myanmar), Sri Lanka and India (Table 16.4). The chikungunya strains from Africa and Asia have been shown to be closely related, using a panel of monoclonal antibodies prepared against strains from Africa and Asia (Blackburn *et al.*, 1995).

Epidemiology and Host Range

The epidemiology of chikungunya virus infections differs in Africa and Asia. In Africa this virus is transmitted in savannahs and forests by *Aedes* mosquitoes. The most important vertebrate host in the cycle of infection is the non-human primate, e.g. baboons and *Cercopithecus* monkeys. Bushbabies and certain species of bats may also be infected in nature, but their role in viral maintenance is likely to be of secondary importance. Humans may be infected in African villages and rural areas, particularly where *Aedes aegypti* is present in large numbers. In contrast to the situation in Africa, transmission in Asia is primarily from human to human by the vector *Aedes aegypti*. It has been suggested that infection with this virus may be common in certain parts of Africa, e.g. 47% of sera collected from 132 adults living in the Karamoja district of Uganda had antibodies to chikungunya virus detectable by HI (Rodhain *et al.* 1989).

Although the most important vector for chikungunya virus transmission to humans is the *Aedes* mosquito, transmission has also been described by *Mansonia africana*. The active replication of alphaviruses in the mosquito is essential for perpetuation in nature, but the explosive nature of the chikungunya epidemics has led to speculation that mechanical transmission of the virus may also occur from a viraemic host by an uninfected mosquito (Peters and Dalrymple, 1990).

Clinical Disease

The incubation period varies but is usually 2–4 days, with a range of 1–12 days. Chikungunya is an acute infection of abrupt onset of fever, headache and severe joint pains without prodromal symptoms. The joint pains are the dominant complaint and affect mainly the small joints of the hands, wrist and feet. This may be associated with an erythematous flush over the face and upper chest in approximately 80% of patients. A maculopapular rash, together with a generalised lymphadenopathy, appears 3–4 days later. Although the arthralgia may resolve within a few weeks, pain, swelling and morning stiffness may continue for months and even years after infection. Petechiae and bleeding from the gums does occur, but there are no significant haemorrhagic manifestations.

In contrast to the clinical presentation in adults, a study from Bangkok concentrating on a paediatric outpatient department showed that the most frequent presenting symptom of chikungunya virus infection in children was vomiting, which was present in 35% of patients. In addition, 18% had abdominal pain or anorexia. None of the patients in this study were noted to have joint symptoms; arthritis and arthralgia therefore appear to be less prominent features in children. On clinical examination of this paediatric population, the most frequent sign was a pharyngitis, which was present in 71% of patients, followed by facial flushing (24% of patients). None of these children had a rash. This study illustrates very clearly that the clinical presentation of chikungunya infections in adults and children differ (Halstead *et al.*, 1969). In Asia, several virus isolations have been made from severely ill children diagnosed as having haemorrhagic fever, similar to dengue haemorrhagic fever (DHF).

Haemorrhagic forms of chikungunya virus infection have been described in India and southeast Asia, but these are seldom as severe as dengue haemorrhagic fever. In a hospital-based study in Bangkok about 8% of children with suspected haemorrhagic fever had chikungunya virus infection (Nimmannitya *et al.*, 1969).

Pathogenesis

Chikungunya virus may be isolated from the blood early in the course of disease. As the disappearance of the viraemia correlates with the appearance of HI and neutralising antibodies, it would appear that recovery from infection correlates with the development of viral-specific antibody rather than cell-mediated immunity. This is further substantiated by the effect of serum antibody in mouse protection tests (Carey *et al.*, 1969). The haemostatic abnormality seen in both children and adult patients is possibly the result of an acquired platelet defect, as it has been shown that the association of chikungunya virus with human platelets *in vitro* promotes platelet clumping (Chernesky and Larke, 1977).

Diagnosis

The clinical features described above in a patient who has recently returned from, or is living in, sub-Saharan Africa or Asia enables a presumptive clinical diagnosis to be made. In addition, a minority of patients will have a leukopenia with a relative lymphocytosis. In most, however, the white cell count will be normal. The platelet count may be decreased, but this is usually not significant.

Chikungunya virus can be isolated by the intracerebral inoculation of suckling mice or by viral culture in either mosquito or mammalian cell culture systems (Peters and Dalrymple, 1990). Viraemia will be present in most patients during the first 48 h of disease and may be detected in sera as late as day 4 post-onset. Thereafter the amount of virus in serum drops rapidly and recovery becomes increasingly difficult. Both HI and neutralising antibodies appear on day 5–7 of the illness. The appearance of these antibodies is associated with a decrease in viraemia (Carey et al., 1969). HI antibodies rise rapidly and peak in the second week. Virus-specific IgM antibodies are readily detected by capture ELISA in patients recovering from infection and they persist in excess of 6 months. All patients will be serologically positive by day 5–7 post-onset of infection. However, cross-reaction occurs with other members of the same alphavirus antigenic complex, so the results obtained must be interpreted with caution (Table 16.3) (Calisher et al., 1986). The use of a specific IgM assay may be especially relevant in an epidemic situation. This was illustrated in an outbreak in Yangon in Burma (now Myanmar). Utilisation of a simple indirect ELISA was helpful in achieving an acute-phase diagnosis and results showed a strong concordance with HI (90% agreement), although ELISA was able to identify twice as many patients at initial hospital admission (Thein et al., 1992). The differential diagnosis within the laboratory should include Ross River, dengue, Sindbis and West Nile virus infections.

Vaccine

A formalin-inactivated chikungunya virus vaccine prepared in monkey kidney tissue culture has been described. Despite being apparently safe and immunogenic, its use has been limited to initial safety studies and laboratory workers (Harrison et al., 1971). More recently, a live-attenuated vaccine has been produced.

O'Nyong-Nyong Virus

'O'nyong-nyong' literally means 'weakening of the joints'. It was first described as an epidemic viral disease in East Africa (Haddow et al., 1960). Antigenically, o'nyong-nyong virus is a subtype of chikungunya virus (Table 16.1).

Epidemiology and Host Range

The initial epidemic began in 1959 in north-western Uganda and spread from there to Kenya, Tanzania, Mozambique, Malawi and Zaire (now Democratic Republic of Congo). It involved some 2 million people. Within an infected area spread was rapid, with an extremely high attack rate. In an affected village a high proportion of the population, regardless of age or sex, were incapacitated. This disease was also apparently unknown to the tribes who were affected. The origin of o'nyong-nyong virus is not clear. It might have existed unrecognised prior to the initial epidemic described above or, conversely, the epidemic may well have resulted from a mutant or recombinant virus. The vectors of this virus are *Anopheles funestus* and *Anopheles gambiae*. It is not known whether a non-human vertebrate host exists. After this initial epidemic very little further information on this virus was obtained until 1978 when it was isolated from *Anopheles funestus* mosquitoes in the Kao Plain in Kenya (Johnson et al., 1981). The re-emergence of epidemic o'nyong-nyong fever in south-western Uganda after an absence of 35 years has recently been described (Rwaguma et al., 1997).

Clinical Disease

The clinical features are similar to those of chikungunya virus infections, with a sudden onset of a 5 day fever often accompanied by a rigor. Characteristic features of the disease include joint pains followed by the development of a rash. Joint pain primarily affects the knees, although ankles, elbows or wrists also can be involved.

The morbilliform macupapular rash erupts on the face, extending to the trunk and extremities, 4–7 days post-onset of infection and is similar to that of chikungunya virus. Some fatalities have been described, but morbidity is substantial (Kiwanuka et al., 1999).

Diagnosis

Virus may be isolated in 1 day-old mice from serum samples taken during the acute stage of the infection. However, mouse passage or subinoculation into chick fibroblasts may be necessary. The mice demonstrate alopecia and runting. The virus may then be further identified using plaque inhibition, cross-neutralisation assays or HI (Williams and Woodall, 1961). Anti-bodies to o'nyong-nyong virus may be detected by CF, HI, ELISA, IF and neutralisation assays. Interpretation may be difficult, due to cross-reaction with chikungunya virus. However, the antibody titre to the homologous virus will be higher than that to the heterologous virus (Peters and Dalrymple, 1990).

Igbo Ora Virus

Igbo Ora virus is closely related to both chikungunya and o'nyong-nyong viruses. Human disease associated with infection with this virus is characterised by fever, arthritis and the development of a rash ('the disease that breaks your wings'). The virus was isolated from human sera from patients in Africa (Nigeria, central African Republic) in the latter part of the 1960s (Moore *et al.*, 1975) and was responsible for an epidemic that involved four villages in the Ivory Coast in 1984 (Peters and Dalrymple, 1990).

Mayaro Virus

Although infection with Mayaro virus was first recognised in Trinidad in 1954, it was an epidemic in Brazil in 1978 that permitted a detailed evaluation of human infections (LeDuc *et al.*, 1981; Pinheiro *et al.*, 1981).

Epidemiology and Host Range

During the extensive epidemic described by LeDuc and colleagues (1981), 20% of the entire population of approximately 4000 persons in the rural village of Belterra in Brazil were infected. The numbers infected were higher amongst those who lived near a plantation forest. The epidemic began with the onset of the wet season and ended with the onset of the dry season. This correlated with the abundance of the mosquito vector, *Haemagogus janthinomys*. In addition to humans, marmosets and other primates are susceptible to infection (Hoch *et al.*, 1981). It has therefore been suggested that non-human primates play an important role in the maintenance of this virus, as experimental infection of marmosets with Mayaro virus showed that a significant viraemia develops. The role of other vertebrates, e.g. birds, remains to be defined.

Clinical Disease

A detailed evaluation of the clinical features of infection with this virus in humans is available from studies done during the 1978 epidemic in Brazil. Fever, arthralgia and rash were the most frequently encountered clinical manifestations. Other symptoms included headache, myalgia and chills (Pinheiro *et al.*, 1981).

Diagnosis

Leukopenia, sometimes accompanied by a modest lymphocytosis, is a frequent finding. A mild thrombo-cytopenia may also be present. Mayaro virus may be isolated from acute-phase serum samples in an *in vitro* cell culture system using Vero cells. The virus may then be identified using HI or plaque reduction neutralisation tests. In addition, Mayaro virus is also pathogenic for infant mice on intracerebral inoculation. In the Belterra epidemic, virus was isolated from the serum in 97% of the patients bled in the first 24 h after the onset of symptoms. Thereafter, viral recovery rate decreased to only 7% on day 4. Serological evidence of a Mayaro virus infection can be achieved by demonstrating a seroconversion using HI in paired serum samples taken from a patient during the acute and convalescent phase of the illness (Pinheiro *et al.*, 1981). In addition, the use of a Mayaro virus-specific IgM assay has been described. Cross-reactivity of IgM antibody occurs with alphavirus infections by viruses belonging to the same antigenic complex (Table 16.1). However, the ratios of the homologous to heterologous IgM titres are high, allowing a reasonably specific and rapid diagnosis to be made. The IgM assay is therefore a useful diagnostic tool in an epidemic situation (Calisher *et al.*, 1986).

ALPHAVIRUSES ASSOCIATED WITH ENCEPHALITIS

The genus *Alphavirus* contains four viruses that produce encephalitis in humans; Eastern equine encephalitis (EEE) virus, Western equine encephalitis (WEE) virus, Venezuelan equine encephalitis (VEE) virus and Everglades virus. The EEE, WEE and VEE viruses were first isolated from the brains of dead horses in the 1930s. The severity of disease associated with infection with this group of viruses differs: EEE virus is the most neurovirulent, while infection with VEE virus is associated with a febrile illness, with encephalitis occurring infrequently. Focal epidemics of EEE virus have periodically occurred in eastern USA; WEE is endemic in western USA and Canada; and VEE virus in Central and South America and occasionally in North America. The Everglades virus is related to EEE but is restricted to the state of Florida, USA, and only five cases of encephalitis associated with it have been reported, despite a high seroprevalence (27%) in southern Florida.

Eastern Equine Encephalitis Virus

Eastern equine encephalitis virus is an important cause of human disease in the eastern states and some inland mid-western locations of the USA. Its distribution extends through Central America to Trinidad, Brazil, Guyana and as far south as Argentina (Weaver *et al.*, 1994). This virus is among the most virulent of the alphaviruses. It has been reported that there are two distinct antigenic variants (North American and South American), the former being genetically quite stable (Roehrig *et al.*, 1990). It causes severe disease in humans, certain species of birds such as the pheasant, as well as horses, all of whom have high fatality rates after infection.

Epidemiology and Host Range

The physical, biological and ecological factors associated with epizootic transmission are complex, but the abundance of EEE virus circulating in the enzootic cycle and the various characteristics of the epizootic vectors are important determinants of risk. In endemic areas birds are the most important vertebrate hosts and the natural cycle is between birds and the ornithophilic mosquito, *Culiseta melanura*. Birds vary in their susceptibility, with some, e.g. the pheasant, developing severe disease, while other avian species suffer no appreciable morbidity or mortality (Peters and Dalrymple, 1990). *Culiseta melanura* is thought to be the main endemic vector (Howard and Wallis, 1974). However, because of its ornithophilic nature, this mosquito is unlikely to play a major role in the transmission of EEE virus to horses or humans. However, the virus escapes from enzootic foci located in swamp areas through bridge vectors such as *Aedes sollicitans* and *Coquillettidia perturbans*, which are thought to be important in the transmission to these vertebrates. These species also feed on both mammals and birds and can transmit the virus to humans, horses and other hosts. Both humans and horses are 'dead-end' hosts for EEE virus infections; infected birds are therefore necessary for the epidemic spread of these species. In South and Central America the enzootic cycle is maintained in most forests where *Culex melanoconion* spp. are considered the primary vectors (Scott and Weaver, 1989). Disease in humans often follows an epizootic course in horses. Fewer than 10 cases of EEE are reported annually in the USA. Even during a major equine epizootic episode, EEE virus-associated disease in humans is rare. In addition to being limited to certain geographical regions, the prevailing climatic conditions, in the form of an unusually hot, wet summer, also play an important role, for this allows for an abundance of the vector *Culiseta melanura*. This, together with the presence of a susceptible bird population and an additional vector that can transmit virus from viraemic birds to susceptible horses and humans, are important predisposing factors for the occurrence of human and equine cases. Although the transmission cycles have not been well established, additional reservoirs of infection have been reported in forest-dwelling rodents, bats and marsupials (Ubico and McLean, 1995), reptiles and amphibians (Morris, 1988).

Clinical Disease

EEE virus infections may produce a severe, often fatal encephalitis in humans (Deresiewicz *et al.*, 1997; Farder *et al.*, 1940). The ratio of inapparent to apparent infections is approximately 23:1 in adults and 8:1 in children under the age of 4 (Goldfield *et al.*, 1968). The encephalitis associated with EEE virus infection tends to be fulminant; a recent study that reviewed all cases of EEE in the USA during 1988–1994 showed a mortality of 36%, with 35% of patients being left moderately or severely disabled. The remaining patients were left mildly disabled, with only one patient recovering fully. The most common clinical features were fever (83%), headache (75%), nausea and vomiting (61%) and malaise and weakness (58%). The incubation period for EEE virus is 4–10 days. However, the onset of neurological symptoms was associated with a rapid deterioration of the patient; 89% (32/36 patients) were or became stuporous or comatose, with about one-quarter having seizures. Interestingly, abdominal pain was present in 22% of cases, with two patients presenting with acute abdominal pain in the prodromal period (Deresiewicz *et al.*, 1997). Although it has been suggested that an age of 40 and a long prodromal course correlates with a good functional recovery (Przelomski *et al.*, 1988), others have found that these parameters do not significantly predict outcome (Deresiewicz et al., 1997). Deresiewicz et al. (1997) did, however, demonstrate that high initial cerebrospinal fluid white cell counts and the development of severe hyponatraemia were poor prognostic signs, possibly because both could be markers of intense cerebral inflammation.

Pathogenesis and Pathology

Post mortem histopathological studies have demonstrated necrotic foci together with arteriolar and venular inflammation and perivascular cuffing. An inflammatory meningeal infiltrate may be present. Although the distribution of the focal lesions may vary, involvement of the basal ganglia and thalami appears to be prominent (Deresiewicz et al., 1997). Viral particles have been visualised in the oligodendroglial cells by electron microscopy (Bastian et al., 1957). The neurological damage is probably due to a combination of a direct viral cytopathic effect, inflammatory damage and a vasculitis (Peters and Dalrymple, 1990).

Diagnosis

A diagnostic clue may be obtained from the prevailing climatic conditions (a hot wet summer), together with associated illness in the horse and pheasant populations. However, the symptoms are non-specific and confirmation needs to be obtained serologically, or by demonstration of virus in cerebrospinal fluid, or both. Neuroradiological imaging may be helpful, with focal lesions visible in the basal ganglia, thalami and brainstem (Deresiewicz et al., 1997).

Laboratory diagnosis is based on molecular detection of viral antigen, virus isolation or antibody detection. Samples for isolation can be CSF, blood or CNS tissue by inoculation into newborn mice or tissue culture using Vero cells or MRC-5 (Sotomayor and Josephson, 1999). As with all alphavirus infections, an acute serum sample should be taken as soon as possible after the onset of illness. EEE virus has been isolated from a laboratory worker on the second day of illness (Clarke, 1961). In this case, four of 25 1 day-old mice died after intracerebral inoculation with a serum sample taken from this patient. Further identification was done serologically. In addition, virus has also been isolated from post mortem brain tissue taken from a fatal case of EEE. More recently,

an RT-PCR-based assay has been developed to detect EEE virus RNA (Voskin et al., 1993).

Serology is an important diagnostic tool. Paired serum samples may be tested in parallel using ELISA (Scott and Weaver, 1989) or neutralisation tests. A class-specific IgM assay has also been described as a rapid and specific diagnostic tool. As EEE virus is the only species of virus belonging to the EEE complex (Table 16.1), cross-reaction with heterologous viruses belonging to the same antigenic complex does not pose a diagnostic problem (Calisher et al., 1986).

Prevention and Control

Protection against mosquito bites and control of the vector is important. An effective equine vaccine is licensed in the USA and is recommended for livestock in areas where EEE virus transmission is known to occur. Specific control measures to prevent human disease include a formalin-inactivated vaccine derived from a North American strain of EEEV (PE-6) is available for horses but not for general human use. The vaccine has been shown not to induce significant levels of neutralisation or anti-E″ antibody responses to South American strains of EEE virus (Strizki and Repik, 1995). However, as human disease is rare, even during an equine epizootic episode, this is only available to those considered to be at risk of exposure. Prompt notification of suspected cases of arboviral encephalitis to the local public health authority is also essential.

Western Equine Encephalitis Virus

The WEE complex in the New World contains three additional viruses in addition to WEE, named Highlands J (HJ), Fort Morgan (FM) and Aura. Only WEE is recognised as causing human disease (Calisher, 1994). Viruses in the WEE complex found in the Old World include Sindbis, Whataroa and Kyzlagach. Western equine encephalitis virus causes more human infections than the EEE virus, but the illness is less severe and mortality seldom exceeds 10%. Its distribution covers the Pacific coast of the USA, but also includes the great plains of the USA and Canada and extends into Central America and the northern parts of South America (Chamberlain, 1987; Reeves, 1987; Iversen, 1994). The WEE antigenic complex consists of six species (Table 16.5). It has been suggested that WEE virus arose through recombination between an

Table 16.5 Geographical distribution of the western equine encephalitis virus complex

Virus species	Subtype	Main geographic distribution	Other features
Western equine encephalitis (WEE)		N. America, Mexico, Guyana, Brazil, Argentina	Epizootics: N. America only
Aura		Brazil, Argentina	
Fort Morgan		Western USA	
Highland J		Florida, Eastern USA	
Sindbis	Sindbis	Africa, E. Mediterranean, Borneo, The Philippines, Australia, Sicily	
	Babinki	West and Central Africa	
	Whataroa	New Zealand	
	Kyzylagach	Azerbaijan	
	Ockelbo	Scandinavia, former USSR	

EEE virus-like virus and a Sindbis-like virus (Hahn *et al.*, 1988).

Epidemiology and Host Range

WEE virus is transmitted in the western USA by the mosquito *Culex tarsalis*. Birds are the most important vertebrate host. Endemic transmission results in a few human cases. In addition, major equine epidemics may result in a significant number of human cases. As with other arboviruses, climatic factors exert a major influence on the epidemiology and distribution of WEE virus.

In the eastern USA WEE virus is replaced by Highlands J virus, whose primary vector is *Culiseta melanura*, which is also the primary vector of EEE virus. The strictly ornithophilic nature of this vector explains the absence of significant disease outbreaks in the eastern USA. WEE virus and Highlands J viruses are closely related, both serologically and at a molecular level.

Clinical Disease

Most WEE infections of adults are asymptomatic, patients presenting with a sudden onset of fever, headache, nausea, vomiting, anorexia and malaise. This progresses in the most serious cases to restlessness, tremor, irritability, photophobia and altered mental status. Paralysis is not uncommon. The estimated case:infection ratio in adults is approximately 1:1000. This decreases to approximately 1:60 in children and 1:1 in babies (Peters and Dalrymple, 1990). Most cases of encephalitis occur in children, frequently under the age of 4 years, in whom the onset is marked by convulsions. This may

result in permanent neurological damage. Drowsiness, headache and mental confusion, sometimes leading to coma, may be seen in adults. *In utero* infection followed by an acute encephalitis has been documented (Shinefield and Townsend, 1953). Recovery from the acute illness may be slow and symptoms such as fatigability, irritability and headache may persist for up to 2 years (Earnest *et al.*, 1971).

Pathogenesis and Pathology

WEE virus is less neurovirulent than EEE virus in both humans and horses. Post mortem examination of the brain of fatal cases shows a perivascular mononuclear and polymorphonuclear infiltrate, together with parenchymal necrosis.

Diagnosis

During the acute phase of the illness, viral isolation may be attempted from blood, throat swabs or cerebrospinal fluid samples, using suckling mice, but this is frequently not successful. Virus may usually be isolated from brain biopsy material or post mortem brain tissue taken early on in the illness. However, serology, together with the appropriate clinical manifestations in a patient living in, or who has recently travelled to, an endemic area, forms the most important method of diagnosing of disease associated with infection with WEE virus. Classical serological techniques, e.g. HI, ELISA or neutralisation, can be used to demonstrate a rise in antibody titre between acute and convalescent serum samples. In addition, the detection of WEE virus-specific IgM can provide a rapid acute-phase diagnosis. However, cross-reaction may occur with other viruses within the complex (Table 16.1). Knowledge of the geographical distribution of the viruses within the complex allows interpretation of a positive IgM result, together with the appropriate patient details (Calisher *et al.*, 1986). Antigen detection using RT-PCR with patient serum or CSF is well established (Pfeffer *et al.*, 1997).

Prevention and Control

Vector control is an important aspect of the control of all mosquito-borne encephalitides. Outbreaks in humans and horses are associated with unusually high densities of mosquitoes. There is therefore a correlation between *Culex tarsalis* density and human cases of WEE virus infection. Besides vector control, changing behaviour patterns, e.g. air-conditioning houses and promoting indoor activities, may also protect from vector-borne diseases and are complementary to mosquito control programmes (Gahlinger *et al.*, 1986). An inactivated vaccine is available to those at risk. An inactivated vaccine is also available for horses.

Venezuelan Equine Encephalitis Virus

As the name suggests, Venezuelan equine encephalitis virus was first isolated in Venezuela, where it causes important epizootics in horses, but also infects humans. The geographical distribution includes Central and South America. VEE virus caused epidemics/epizootics among people and horses in Latin America from the 1920s to the 1970s. It reached the USA in 1971, but no further activity was reported until 1992–1993, when a small outbreak in Venezuela confirmed the re-emergence of VEE from its epizootic habitat to humans. This was followed by a major outbreak occurring in 1995, involving an estimated 75 000–100 000 people (Rico-Hesse *et al.*, 1995; Weaver *et al.*, 1996). A variant of the virus, known as Everglades

virus, is endemic in Florida and another variant, Mucambo virus, is found in Brazil, Trinidad and Surinam (Table 16.6).

Epidemiology and Host Range

Both epizootic and enzootic strains of VEE virus occur. Serotypes IAB and IC are equine virulent, while ID, IE and II, III and IV are equine avirulent (Table 16.6) (Weaver *et al.*, 1996). The principal vertebrate host for enzootic transmission is the rodent, although birds and other species may play a less important role. Horses may be infected by several subtypes or variants of VEE (Table 16.1) but they do not play an important role in enzootic transmission, which occurs primarily between small mammals and the *Culex* mosquitoes of the subgenus *Melanoconion* (Cupp *et al.*, 1986). In contrast, during equine epizootics horses do play an important role in viral spread. It has been suggested that epizootic strains of the VEE are maintained in other mammalian hosts and birds until the conditions are favourable for the development of an equine epizootic. A number of mosquito species have been implicated as likely vectors during epizootics. Human disease usually follows equine disease, but humans are not thought to be important in the maintenance of the epidemic, due to low-titre viraemia.

The major outbreak of VEE that occurred in Venezuela and Colombia in 1995 was remarkably similar to an outbreak occurring in 1962–1964. Both outbreaks followed unusually heavy rains, which led to an increase in the mosquito vector populations, and both occurred in the same geographic region. Phylogenetic analysis showed that isolates from the 1995 epidemic of VEE were closely related to the serotype IC viruses isolated during the 1962–1964 epidemic. As a similar virus was identified in mosquitoes in Venezuela in 1983, the authors raise the possibility of a serotype IC enzootic transmission cycle in northern Venezuela (Weaver *et al.*, 1996).

Table 16.6 Geographical distribution of the Venezuelan equine encephalitis virus complex

Virus species	Subtype	Variant	Main geographic distribution
Venezuelan equine encephalitis (VEE)	I	1 A–B, C, D, E, F	Venezuela, Colombia, South and Central America
	II	Everglades	Florida, USA
	IIIA	Mucambo	Brazil, Trinidad, Surinam
	IIIB	Tonte	South America
		Bijou Bridge	North America
	IV	Pixuna	Brazil
	V	Cabassou	South America
	VI	AG80-663	Africa

Clinical Disease

In horses, enzootic strains of VEE virus usually produce a fever and mild leukopenia. In contrast to this, horses infected with epizootic strains exhibit high fevers, severe leukopenia and signs of encephalitis. Infections in humans result in a range of symptoms. Natural human epidemics in Colombia in 1952 and 1995 and in Venezuela and Panama during 1962–1964, resulted in over 100 000 cases with 500 deaths, demonstrating the highly infectious nature and severity of the VEE virus.

These may be subclinical (usually caused by enzootic strains) or result in significant disease caused by epizootic strains of VEE (Table 16.3). Symptoms and signs in patients seeking medical care include fever, chills, severe headache, myalgia, vomiting and diarrhoea. Most patients will have an acute and self-limiting febrile illness; however, convulsions, disorientation and drowsiness may also be present (Weaver *et al.*, 1996). The proportion of cases that develop neurological sequelae appears to vary from outbreak to outbreak. A review of the medical records of patients with convulsions in the 1995 epidemic showed that, although the age varied greatly (2 months– 48 years), most were children; however, only approximately 20% of these were under 3 years of age. Of interest is that about half of these patients had their first seizure on days 6–10 after the onset of their illness and when their temperature had returned to normal (Weaver *et al.*, 1996). A further prospective study, which included a total of 13 patients, showed that six patients had a severe incapacitating febrile illness lasting 3–5 days, two others had a 'flu-like' illness, and the remaining five (38%) were asymptomatic (Martin *et al.*, 1972). The overall mortality is thought to be less than 1%. Fetal loss may occur in pregnant women with VEE.

Transmission can occur by the respiratory route as well as by mosquitoes. Accidental laboratory aerosol infection with epizootic strains of VEE has been reported to cause a febrile illness with abrupt onset of chills, headache, myalgia, vomiting and pharyngitis 2–5 days after exposure, without evidence of encephalitis (Erenkranz and Ventura, 1974).

Pathogenesis and Pathology

The disease caused by VEE virus in humans is relatively mild compared with that caused by either WEE or EEE viruses. In horses, as well as other species, there is a clear difference in the pathogenicity of the epizootic and the enzootic strains of VEE. Epizootic strains are generally more virulent, with infection in horses resulting in viral replication in the lymphoid tissue and bone marrow. This is associated with lymphoid necrosis and a lymphopenia and is accompanied by a high-titre viraemia. Spread to the central nervous system probably occurs in the bloodstream, resulting in a fatal encephalitis in horses, as well as rodents and some primates (Peters and Dalrymple, 1990).

Diagnosis

The diagnosis of VEE-associated disease should be suspected in patients presenting with a 'flu-like' illness in an appropriate geographical region when there is a concurrent equine epizootic. Material obtained from sick horses confirming an epizootic of VEE may therefore be an important indicator of human disease. Isolation of virus may be attempted from acute-phase serum and throat swabs, as well as from brain tissue obtained from aborted and stillborn fetuses (Weaver *et al.*, 1996). Culture of VEE virus has been achieved by inoculation into Vero or mosquito cells or suckling mice (Dietz *et al.*, 1979). Intracerebral inoculation of suckling mice may result in death within 72 h. Isolates identified in cell culture may be characterised further using VEE serotype-specific polyclonal sera. Alternatively, detection and genetic characterisation may be done using RT-PCR with sequencing of the products generated from the E3 and E4 genes (Weaver *et al.*, 1996; Brightwell *et al.*, 1998).

A number of serological assays (IFA, ELISA, HI) have been described. Acute and convalescent serum samples may be tested in parallel by HI. This may provide diagnostically useful information. More recently attention has been focused on the use of an IgG ELISA based on an antigen prepared from the attenuated VEE vaccine strain of virus. In experimentally infected guinea-pigs, VEE-specific IgG could be detected at 6 days post-inoculation, compared with 10 days for HI antibodies. However RRV, EEE and WEE virus-specific IgG exhibit a weak cross-reaction on the IgG ELISA, so results must be interpreted with caution. The appearance of IgG antibodies detectable by ELISA coincides with the development of antibodies detectable by plaque reduction neutralisation assay (PRN). While less sensitive than the IgG ELISA, PRN is more specific and therefore eliminates some of the problems of cross-reaction discussed above. It may therefore be used as a confirmatory test. VEE-specific

IgM antibody has been detected as early as 4 days post-inoculation in experimentally infected guinea-pigs (at a time at which infectious virus was present in the serum). In summary, suspected cases of VEE virus infection may be investigated serologically using a VEE-specific IgM and IgG ELISA, together with the more specific PRN as a confirmatory test (Coates *et al.*, 1992).

Prevention and Control

Personal protection against mosquito bites, together with vector control, as for other alphavirus infections, is important. Control of an equine epizootic by immunising horses is also important in the prevention of subsequent human disease. Two types of vaccine are currently available for the prevention of VEE in humans and horses. The first is a live attenuated vaccine, TC-83, produced by serial passage of wild virus in guinea-pig fetal heart cell culture. While this vaccine has been shown to be efficacious and relatively safe, 25% of individuals immunised develop a clinical illness with a low-grade viraemia. A formalin-inactivated vaccine, C-84, which is derived from the TC-83 strain of virus, has been shown to be safe and provides effective protection in experimental animals injected with virulent VEE virus, but only limited protection from aerosol challenge.

OTHER ALPHAVIRUSES

- *Semliki Forest virus* (SFV) is found in sub-Saharan Africa and has been used as a model virus for research. Although the disease potential for this virus remains to be elucidated, asymptomatic seroconversions have been described. However, the clinical features of infection with SFV have not been well defined. One scientist working with SFV developed an encephalitis—SFV was isolated from both cerebrospinal fluid and post mortem brain tissue (Peters and Dalrymple, 1990). This highlights the necessity for caution when working with any infectious agents of unknown pathogenic potential.
- *Getah virus* was originally isolated from *Culex gelidus* and *Culex tritaeniorhynchus* in Malaysia in 1955. The viruses Sagiyama, Bebaru and RRV are considered the subtypes of Getah. The virus is maintained in a cycle similar to Japanese encephalitis virus by *C. tritaeniorhynchus* and has the potential of being amplified in domestic pigs. The virus has been linked to disease in horses (fever,

rash and limb oedema). Although Getah virus has not been implicated in human disease, serological studies have demonstrated antibodies to Getah virus in sera taken from individuals from the Pacific Basin, Japan and Hanna Island in China (Johnson and Peters, 1996).

- *Una virus* was first isolated from *Psorophora ferox* mosquitoes originating from the Amazonian region of Brazil in 1959. The virus has also been isolated in Trinidad and is considered to be part of the SFV complex of viruses. As yet, this virus has not been recognised as causing human disease.

REFERENCES

Aaskov JG, Mataika JU, Lawrence GW *et al.* (1981) An epidemic of Ross River virus infection in Fiji, 1979. *Am J Trop Med Hyg*, **30**, 1053–1059.

Aaskov J, Williams L and Yu S (1997) A candidate Ross River virus vaccine: preclinical evaluation. *Vaccine*, **15**, 1396–1404.

Bastian FO, Wende RD, Singer DB *et al.* (1957) Eastern equine encephalomyelitis. Histopathological and ultrastructural change with isolation of the virus in a human case. *Am J Clin Pathol*, **64**, 10–13.

Beard JR, Trent M, Sam GA *et al.* (1997) Self-reported morbidity of Barmah Forest virus infection on the north coast of New South Wales. *Med J Aust*, **167**, 525–528.

Blackburn NK, Besselaar TG and Gibson G (1995) Antigenic relationship between chikungunya virus strains and o'nyong nyong virus using monoclonal antibodies. *Res Virol*, **146**, 69–73.

Brightwell G, Brown JM, Coates DM (1998) Genetic targets for the detection and identification of Venezuelan equine encephalitis viruses. *Arch Virol*, **143**, 731–742.

Calisher CH (1994) Medically important arboviruses of the United States and Canada. *Clin Microbiol Rev*, **7**, 89–116.

Calisher CH, El-Kafrawi AO, Mahmud MI *et al.* (1986) Complex-specific immunoglobulin M antibody patterns in humans infected with alphaviruses. *J Clin Microbiol*, **23**, 155–159.

Calisher CH, Shope RE, Brandt W *et al.* (1980) Proposed antigenic classification of registered arboviruses. 1. Togaviridae, Alphavirus. *Intervirology*, **14**, 229–232.

Carey DE, Myers RM, DeRainitz C *et al.* (1969) The 1964 chikungunya epidemic in Vellore, South India, including observations on concurrent dengue. *Trans R Soc Trop Med Hyg*, **63**, 434–445.

Carter IW, Smythe LD, Fraser JR *et al.* (1985) Detection of Ross River virus immunoglobulin M antibodies by enzyme-linked immunosorbent assay using antibody class capture and comparison with other methods. *Pathology*, **17**, 503–508.

Carter IWJ, Fraser JRE and Cloonan MJ (1987) Specific IgA response in Ross River virus infection. *Immunol Cell Biol*, **65**, 511–513.

Casals J (1964) Antigenic variants of eastern equine encephalitis virus. *J Exp Med*, **119**, 547–565.

Chamberlain RW (1987) Historical perspectives on the epidemiology and ecology of mosquito-borne virus encephalitides in the United States. *Am J Trop Med Hyg*, **37**, 8–178.

Chanas AC, Gould EA, Clegg JCS *et al.* (1982) Monoclonal antibodies to Sindbis virus glycoprotein E1 can neutralise, enhance infectivity and independently inhibit haemagglutination or haemolysis. *J Gen Virol*, **58**, 37–46.

Cheng RH, Kuhn RJ, Olson MG *et al.* (1995) Nucleocapsid and glycoprotein organisation in an envelope virus. *Cell*, **80**, 621–630.

Chernesky MA and Larke RPB (1977) Contrasting effects of rabbit and human platelets on chikungunya virus infectivity. *Can J Microbiol*, **23**, 1237–1244.

Clarke DH (1961) Two non-fatal human infections with the virus of Eastern equine encephalitis. *Am J Trop Med Hyg*, **10**, 67–70.

Clarke JA, Marshall ID and Gard G (1973) Annually recurrent epidemic polyarthritis and Ross River virus activity in a coastal area of New South Wales. I. Occurrence of the disease. *Am J Trop Med Hyg*, **22**, 543–550.

Coates DM, Makh SR, Jones N *et al.* (1992) Assessment of assays for the serodiagnosis of Venezuelan equine encephalitis. *J Infect*, **25**, 279–289.

Cunningham AL and Fraser JRE (1985) Ross River virus infection of human synovial cells *in vitro*. *Aust J Exp Biol Med Sci*, **63**, 197–204.

Cupp EW, Scherer JB, Bremner RJ *et al.* (1986) Entomological studies at an enzootic Venezuelan equine encephalitis virus focus in Guatemala, 1977–1980. *Am J Trop Med Hyg*, **35**, 851–859.

Deresiewicz RL, Thaler SJ, Hsu L *et al.* (1997) Clinical and neuroradiographic manifestations of eastern equine encephalitis. *N Engl J Med*, **336**, 1867–1874.

Dietz WH, Peralta PH and Johnson KM (1979) Ten clinical cases of human infection with Venezuelan equine encephalomyelitis virus subtype 1-D. *Am J Trop Med Hyg*, **28**, 329–334.

Doherty RL (1977) Arthropod-borne viruses in Australia, 1973–1976. *Aust J Exp Biol Med Sci*, **55**, 103–130.

Doherty RL, Bodey AS and Carew JS (1969) Sindbis infection in Australia. *Med J Aust*, **196**, 1016–1017.

Earnest MP, Goolishian HA, Calverley JR *et al.* (1971) Neurologic, intellectual and psychologic sequelae following western encephalitis. *Neurology*, **21**, 969–974.

Erenkranz NJ and Ventura AK (1974) Venezuelan equine encephalitis virus infection in man. *Ann Rev Med*, **25**, 9–14.

Espmark A and Niklasson B (1984) Ockelbo disease in Sweden: epidemiological, clinical and virological data from the 1982 outbreak. *Am J Trop Med Hyg*, **33**, 1203–1211.

Farder S, Hill A, Connerly ML, *et al.* (1940) Encephalitis in infants and children caused by the virus of the Eastern variety of equine encephalitis. *J Am Microbiol Assoc*, **114**, 1725–1731.

Flexman JP, Smith DW, Mackenzie JS *et al.* (1998) A comparison of the diseases caused by Ross River virus and Barmah Forest virus in Western Australia. *Emerg Infect Dis*, **169**, 90–92.

Fraser JR (1986) Epidemic polyarthritis and Ross River virus disease. *Clin Rheumat Dis*, **12**, 369–388.

Fraser JRE, Cunningham AL, Muller HK *et al.* (1988) Glomerulonephritis in the acute phase of Ross River virus disease. *Clin Nephrol*, **29**, 149–152.

Fraser JRE, Ratnamohan VM, Dowling JP *et al.* (1983) The exanthem of Ross River virus infection: histology, location

of virus antigen and nature of inflammatory infiltrate. *J Clin Pathol*, **36**, 1256–1263.

Gahlinger PM, Reeves WC and Milby MM (1986) Air conditioning and television as protective factors in arboviral encephalitis risk. *Am J Trop Med Hyg*, **35**, 601–610.

Garoff H, Simons H and Renkonen O (1974) Isolation and characterisation of the membrane proteins of Semliki Forest virus. *Virology*, **61**, 493–504.

Goldfield M, Welsh JN and Taylor BF (1968) The 1959 outbreak of eastern encephalitis in New Jersey. 5. The inapparent infection:disease ratio. *Am J Epidemiol*, **87**, 32–38.

Ha DQ, Calisher CH, Tien PH *et al.* (1995) Isolation of a newly recognised alphavirus from mosquitoes in Vietnam and evidence for human infection and disease. *Am J Trop Med Hyg*, **53**, 100–104.

Haddow AJ, Davies CW and Walker AJ (1960) O'nyong-nyong fever: an epidemic virus disease in East Africa. 1. Introduction. *Trans R Soc Trop Med Hyg*, **54**, 517–522.

Hahn CS, Lustig S, Strauss EG *et al.* (1988) Western equine encephalitis virus is a recombinant virus. *Proc Natl Acad Sci USA*, **85**, 5997–6001.

Halstead SB, Nimmannitya S and Margiotta MR (1969) Dengue and chikungunya virus infection in man in Thailand, 1962–1964. Observations on disease in outpatients. *Am J Trop Med Hyg*, **18**, 972–982.

Hardy JL (1987) The ecology of western equine encephalomyelitis virus in the central valley of California, 1945–1985. *Am J Trop Med Hyg*, **37**, 18–325.

Harrison SC (1986) Alphavirus structure. In *The Togaviridae and Flaviridae* (eds Schlesinger S and Schlesinger MJ), pp 21–34. Plenum, New York.

Harrison VR, Eckles KH, Bartelloni PJ *et al.* (1971) Production and evaluation of a formalin-killed chikungunya vaccine. *J Immunol*, **107**, 643–647.

Hawkes RA, Broughton CR, Naim HM *et al.* (1985) A major outbreak of epidemic polyarthritis in New South Wales during the summer of 1983–1984. *Med J Aust*, **143**, 330–333.

Hills S (1996) Ross River virus and Barmah Forest virus infection. Commonly asked questions. *Aust Fam Physic*, **25**, 1822–1824.

Hoch AL, Peterson NE, Le Duc J *et al.* (1981) An outbreak of Mayaro virus disease in Belterra, Brazil. III. Entomological and ecological studies. *Am J Trop Med Hyg*, **30**, 689–698.

Howard JJ and Wallis RC (1974) Infection and transmission of eastern equine encephalitis virus with colonized *Culiseta melanura* (Coquillett). *Am J Trop Med Hyg*, **23**, 522–525.

Iverson JO (1994) Western equine encephalomyelitis. In *Handbook of Zoonoses, Section B: Viral*, 2nd edn (eds Beran GW, Steele JH *et al.*), pp 25–31. CRC Press, Boca Raton, FL.

Johnson BK, Gichogo A, Gitau G *et al.* (1981) Recovery of O'nyong-nyong virus from *Anopheles funestus* in western Kenya. *Trans R Soc Trop Med Hyg*, **75**, 239–241.

Johnson RE and Peters CJ (1996) Alphaviruses. In *Field's Virology*, 3rd edn (eds Fields BN, Knipe DM, Howley PM *et al.*), pp 843–898. Lippincott-Raven, Philadelphia, PA.

Jupp PG, Blackburn NK, Thompson DL *et al.* (1986) Sindbis and West Nile infections in the Witwatersrand–Pretoria region. *S Afr Med J*, **70**, 218–220.

Kanamitsu M, Taniguchi K, Urasawa S *et al.* (1979) Geographic distribution of arbovirus antibodies in indigenous human populations in the Indo-Australian archipelago. *Am J Trop Med Hyg*, **28**, 351–363.

Katz IA, Hale GE, Hudson BJ *et al.* (1997) Glomerulonephritis secondary to Barmah Forest virus infection. *Med J Aust*, **167**, 21–23.

Kay BH (1982) The modes of transmission of Ross River Virus by *Aedes vigilax* (Skuse). *Aust J Exp Biol Med Sci*, **60**, 339–344.

Kiwanuka N, Sanders EJ, Rwaguma EB *et al.* (1999) O'nyong-nyong fever in south-central Uganda, 1996–1997: clinical features and validation of a clinical case definition for surveillance purposes. *Clin Infect Dis*, **29**, 1243–1250.

LeDuc JW, Pinheiro FP and Travassos da Rosa APA (1981) An outbreak of Mayaro disease in Belterra, Brazil. II. Epidemiology. *Am J Trop Med Hyg*, **30**, 682–688.

Lee E, Stocks C, Lobigs P *et al.* (1997) Nucleotide sequence of the Barmah Forest virus genome. *Virology*, **227**, 509–514.

Lindsey MDA, Johansen CA, Broom AK *et al.* (1995) Emergence of Barmah Forest virus in Western Australia. *Emerg Infect Dis*, **1**, 22–26.

Mackenzie JS, Chau KB, Daniels PW *et al.* (2001) Emerging viral diseases in South-east Asia and Western Pacific. *Emerg Infect Dis*, **7**, 497–504.

Mackenzie JS, Lindsay MD, Coelen RJ *et al.* (1994) Arboviruses causing human disease in the Australasian zoogeographic region. *Arch Virol*, **136**, 447–467.

Malherbe H and Strickland-Cholmley M (1963) Sindbis virus infection in man. Report of a case with recovery of virus from skin lesions. *S Afr Med J*, **36**, 547–552.

Mancini EJ, Clarke BE, Gowen T *et al.* (2000) Cryo-electron microscopy reveals the functional organization of an envelope virus, *Semliki Forest virus*. *Mol Biol*, **5**, 255–266.

Martin DH, Eddy GA, Sudia WD *et al.* (1972) An epidemiologic study of Venezuelan equine encephalomyelitis in Costa Rica, 1970. *Am J Epidemiol*, **95**, 565–577.

McIntosh BM, McGillivray GM, Dickinson DB *et al.* (1964) Illness caused by Sindbis and West Nile viruses in South Africa. *S Afr Med J*, **38**, 291–294.

Moore DL, Casey OR, Carey DE *et al.* (1975) Arthropod-borne viral infections of man in Nigeria, 1964–1970. *Ann Trop Med Parasitol*, **69**, 49–64.

Morris CD (1988) Eastern equine encephalitis. In *The Arboviruses: Epidemiology and Ecology*, vol. III (ed. Month TP), pp 2–20. CRC Press, Boca Raton, FL.

Niklasson B, Espmark A and Lundstrom J (1988) Occurrence of arthralgia and specific IgM antibodies three to four years after Ockelbo disease. *J Infect Dis*, **157**, 832–835.

Niklasson B and Vene S (1996) Vector-borne viral disease in Sweden: a short review. *Arch Virol* (suppl), **11**, 49–55.

Nimmannitya S, Halstead SB, Cohen SN *et al.* (1969) Dengue and chikungunya virus infection in man in Thailand 1962–1964. Observations on hospitalised patients with haemorrhagic fever. *Am J Trop Med Hyg*, **18**, 954–971.

Peters CJ and Dalrymple JM (1990) Alphaviruses. In *Field's Virology*, 3rd edn (eds Fields BN, Knipe DM, Howley PM *et al.*), pp 713–759. Lippincott-Raven, Philadelphia, PA.

Pfeffer M, Proebster B, Kinney RM *et al.* (1997) Genus-specific detection of alphaviruses by a semi-nested reverse transcription-polymerase chain reaction. *Am J Trop Med Hyg*, **57**, 709–718.

Phillips DA, Murray JR, Aaskov JG *et al.* (1990) Clinical and subclinical Barmah Forest virus infection in Queensland. *Med J Aust*, **152**, 463–466.

Pinheiro FP, Freitas RB, Travassos da Rosa JF *et al.* (1981) An outbreak of Mayaro virus disease in Belterra, Brazil. I. Clinical and virological findings. *Am J Trop Med Hyg*, **30**, 674–681.

Poidinger M, Roy S, Hall RA *et al.* (1997) Genetic stability among temporally and geographically diverse isolates of Barmah Forest virus. *Am J Trop Med Hyg*, **57**, 230–234.

Przelomski MM, O'Rourke E, Grady GF *et al.* (1988) Eastern equine encephalitis in Massachusetts: a report of 16 cases, 1970–1984. *Neurology*, **38**, 736–739.

Reeves HW (1987) The discovery decade of arbovirus research in western North America. *Am J Trop Med Hyg*, **37**, 94–100S.

Rico-Hesse R, Weaver SC, de Siger J *et al.* (1995) Emergence of a new epidemic of epizootic Venezuelan equine encephalitis virus in South America. *Proc Natl Acad Sci USA*, **92**, 5278–5281.

Rodhain F, Gonzalez JP, Mercier E *et al.* (1989) Arbovirus infections and viral haemorrhagic fevers in Uganda: a serological survey in Karamoja district, 1984. *Trans R Soc Trop Med Hyg*, **83**, 851–854.

Roehrig JT, Hunt AR, Change GJ *et al.* (1990) Identification of monoclonal antibodies capable of differentiating antigenic varieties of eastern equine encephalitis viruses. *Am J Trop Med Hyg*, **42**, 394–398.

Rosen L, Gubler DJ and Bennett PH (1981) Epidemic polyarthritis (Ross River) virus infection in the Cook Islands. *Am J Trop Med Hyg*, **30**, 1294–1302.

Rwaguma EB, Lutwama JJ, Sempala SD *et al.* (1997) Emergence of epidemic O'nyong-nyong fever in southwestern Uganda, after an absence of 35 years (Letter). *Emerg Infect Dis*, **3**, 77.

Scott TW and Weaver SC (1989) Eastern equine encephalomyelitis virus: epidemiology and evolution of mosquito transmission. *Adv Virus Res*, **37**, 277–328.

Sellner LN, Coelen RJ and Mackenzie JS (1994) Sensitive detection of Ross River virus: a one-tube nested RT-PCR. *J Virol Methods*, **49**, 47–58.

Shinefield HR and Townsend TE (1953) Transplacental transmission of Western equine encephalomyelitis. *J Pediatr*, **43**, 21–25.

Sotomayor EA and Josephson SL (1999) Isolation of eastern equine encephalitis virus in A549 and MRC-5 cell culture. *Clin Infect Dis*, **29**, 193–195.

Stocks N, Selden S and Cameron S (1997) Ross River virus infection. Diagnosis and treatment by general practitioners in South Australia. *Austr Fam Physic*, **26**, 710–717.

Strauss EG, Rice CM and Strauss JH (1984) Complete nucleotide sequence of the genomic RNA of Sindbis virus. *Virology*, **133**, 92–110.

Strauss EG and Strauss JH (1986) Structure and replication of the alphavirus genome. In *The Togaviridae and Flaviviridae* (eds Schlesinger S and Schlesinger MJ), pp 35–90. Plenum, New York.

Strizki JM and Repik PM (1995) Differential reactivity of immune sera from human vaccinees with field strains of eastern equine encephalitis virus. *Am J Trop Med Hyg*, **53**, 564–570.

Taylor RM, Hurlbut HS, Work TH *et al.* (1955) Sindbis virus: a newly recognised arthropod-transmitted virus. *Am J Trop Med Hyg*, **4**, 844–862.

Thein S, La-Linn M, Aaskov J *et al.* (1992) Development of a simple indirect enzyme-linked immunosorbent assay for the detection of immunoglobulin M antibody in serum from patients following an outbreak of chikungunya virus infection in Yangon. *Trans R Soc Trop Hyg,* **86**, 438–442.

Ubico SR and McLean RG (1995) Serological survey of neotropical bats in Guatemala for virus antibodies. *J Wildlife Dis,* **31**, 1–9.

Voskin MH, McLaughlin GL, Day JF *et al.* (1993) A rapid diagnostic assay for eastern equine encephalomyelitis viral RNA. *Am J Trop Med Hyg,* **49**, 772–776.

Wang KS, Kuhn RJ, Strauss EG *et al.* (1992) High-affinity laminin receptor is a receptor for Sindbis virus in mammalian cells. *J Virol,* **66**, 4992–5001.

Weaver SC, Dalgaro TK, Frey TK *et al.* (2000) Family *Togaviridae.* In *Virus Taxonomy: Classification and Nomenclature of Viruses. Seventh Report of the International Committee on Taxonomy of Viruses* (eds van Regenmortel MH, Fauquet CM, Bishop DHL *et al.*), pp 879–889. Academic Press, San Diego, CA.

Weaver SC, Hagenbaugh A, Bellew LA *et al.* (1994) Evolution of alphaviruses in the eastern equine encephalitis complex. *J Virol,* **68**(1), 158–169.

Weaver SC, Salas R, Rico-Hesse R *et al.* (1996) Re-emergence of epidemic Venezuelan equine encephalomyelitis in South America. VEE Study Group. *Lancet,* **348** 436–440.

WHO (1967) *Arboviruses and Human Disease.* WHO Technical Report Series No. 369. WHO, Geneva.

Williams MC and Woodall JP (1961) O'nyong-nyong fever: an epidemic virus disease in East Africa. II. Isolation and some properties of the virus. *Trans R Soc Trop Med Hyg,* **55**, 135–140.

17

Flaviviruses

Barry D. Schoub and Nigel K. Blackburn

National Institute for Communicable Diseases, Sandringham, South Africa

INTRODUCTION

The *Flaviviridae* are a family of viruses comprising over 70 members and are responsible for a major portion of disease and death in man and animals. The family is subdivided into three genera—*Flavivirus*, *Pestivirus* and *Hepatitis C virus*.

Flavivirus

The genus *Flavivirus* was formerly termed 'group B arboviruses' and prior to 1984 was placed together with the 'group A arboviruses' within the family *Togaviridae*. However, as knowledge of the flaviviruses increased, it became apparent that their features and properties, e.g. their replication strategies, structure and biochemistry, were sufficiently distinctive that they would need to be placed in a separate family, the *Flaviviridae*, with the two additional genera, *Pestivirus* and *Hepatitis C virus*, being added subsequently. More recently, GBV-C, also referred to as hepatitis G virus, has been tentatively added to the family *Flaviviridae*, although its taxonomic designation remains to be defined.

The majority of the genus *Flavivirus* are arboviruses, which are transmitted between a vertebrate host and an invertebrate (mosquito or tick) host. Replication and amplification of virus occurs in both the vertebrate and invertebrate hosts. With some of the flaviviruses man may be the major vertebrate host, e.g. in the viruses causing dengue and urban yellow fever, and the virus is maintained by being alternately transmitted from man to mosquito to man. In most of the flavivirus infections, the virus is maintained in nature by alternate infection of a variety of mammals or birds, or occasionally other vertebrate hosts, and their respective mosquito or tick vectors. Man is infected as an accidental event when he intrudes into this natural ecosystem. In these situations he is a dead-end host of no biological significance to the life-cycle of the virus. The non-arboviruses that are members of the genus *Flavivirus* may be found in either arthropods or in vertebrates, but not in both, and are of little medical importance.

Whether flaviviruses have a narrow or wide host range, their distribution is dependent on the ecology of their specific vertebrate and invertebrate hosts. Some flaviviruses have very restricted geographic distributions, such as *Kyasanur Forest virus*, found to date only in Karnataka (previously Mysore) State in India, *Omsk haemorrhagic fever virus*, found in the Omsk district of western Siberia, or *Rocio virus* in the Santista lowlands and the Ribeira valley of Sao Paulo state in south-east Brazil. By contrast, flaviviruses such as *West Nile virus* are distributed widely through Africa, Asia, large parts of Europe and, more recently, the USA and Canada. *Japanese encephalitis virus* is found in at least 16 countries in a wide belt stretching from eastern to south-eastern to southern Asia, affecting a combined population in excess of two billion. Dengue virus has moved over the past 20 years from south-east Asia into the Pacific, the Americas, Africa and Australia, progressively establishing itself in local populations of the widespread man-biting mosquito *Aedes aegypti*.

The clinical manifestations of the majority of flavivirus infections are relatively non-specific. In endemic areas, the diagnosis of infection is often

Principles and Practice of Clinical Virology, Fifth Edition. Edited by A. J. Zuckerman, J. E. Banatvala, J. R. Pattison, P. D. Griffiths and B. D. Schoub
© 2004 John Wiley & Sons Ltd   ISBN 0 470 84338 1

made on clinical suspicion, especially if the physician is alerted by epidemic activity in the region. Occasionally outbreaks of flavivirus infection may follow climatic events, e.g. heavy rains after a period of drought, which result in the formation of numerous stagnant pools, facilitating the breeding of mosquito vectors and also attracting bird life. Outbreaks may follow uncontrolled urbanisation and the breakdown of vector control measures, as has occurred in recent yellow fever outbreaks in West Africa. In some situations human cases may follow an extensive zoonosis in the vertebrate host, especially where birds or livestock are involved. Surveillance and epidemiological monitoring, which involve, amongst other things, the continual and sustained sampling of arthropod vectors and vertebrate hosts for arbovirus activity, is of critical importance in the prevention and management of outbreaks of flavivirus infections. Recently calls have been made for mobile units to be established and sent into the field to conduct clinical diagnosis and therapeutic research, as well as for epidemiological surveillance in endemic areas.

The diagnosis of infection due to flaviviruses becomes particularly difficult in individuals who have travelled from an endemic area and present themselves for medical management many thousands of miles away from their source of infection. In the modern era of jet travel, a history of travel and also a knowledge of the prevalent infections in different parts of the world, are now an important component of infectious diseases medicine. In addition, travellers should be educated to alert their attending physician should they become ill on returning home.

Pestivirus

The second genus in the family *Flaviviridae*, *Pestivirus*, is also referred to as the mucosal disease virus group. The viruses of this genus are the causes of important veterinary diseases worldwide, such as bovine viral diarrhoea, border disease of sheep and hot cholera. They are not known to be spread by arthropod vectors, transmission taking place by direct contact and also via faeces, urine and nasal secretions, as well as vertically. The pestiviruses are not able to infect humans, therefore will not be discussed further.

Hepatitis C Virus

The third and newest genus of the family *Flaviviridae*, is *Hepatitis C virus*. The biochemical and biophysical characteristics of the virus have been determined and have been shown to be characteristic of the family *Flaviviridae*. *Hepatitis C virus* is not an arbovirus and is not known to infect any non-human host in nature. Experimentally, the only animal able to be infected is the chimpanzee. Infection is transmitted by blood transfusion, penetrating injuries with blood-contaminated needles and instruments, sexually, and from mother to child during birth. Since the implementation of widespread screening for hepatitis B virus in blood, hepatitis C virus has become the major cause of post-transfusion hepatitis. Current screening programmes for hepatitis C have, in turn, reduced significantly the incidence of post-transfusion hepatitis due to this virus.

The most recent member of the family *Flaviviridae* is GBV-C virus. The virus was first detected in 1995 in laboratory tamarins experimentally inoculated with blood from a surgeon with clinical hepatitis. Three distinct agents were defined and called GBV-A, GBV-B and GBV-C, although it appeared that only GBV-C was a human virus (GBV-A and GBV-B were probably tamarin agents). Hepatitis G virus (HGV) was described a year later by a different laboratory, but subsequent analysis of HGV and GBV-C has suggested that they are identical viruses. Both are, however, distinct from HCV, having only 29% amino acid homology with it. The pathological role, if any, of GBV-C or HGV has not yet been established. Hepatitis C and GBV-C viruses are dealt with fully in Chapters 2 and 3.

PROPERTIES OF THE VIRUS

The type species of the genus *Flavivirus*, yellow fever virus, has been the most extensively studied member of the family.

Morphology and Morphogenesis

The virus particles are spherical, with a diameter of some 40–50 nm. The envelope is tightly applied to a 25–30 nm spherical core and surface peplomers are often visible. Replication of virus takes place in the cytoplasm of the cell in association with the rough and smooth endoplasmic reticulum. Accumulations of viral particles are seen within the lamellae and vesicles and replication is characteristically associated with the proliferation of intracellular membranes.

Biophysical and Biochemical Properties

The $S_{20}W$ of flaviviruses is 70–210, that of pestiviruses is 140 and that of hepatitis C virus is $\geqslant 150$. The buoyant density of the flaviviruses in CsCl is 1.22–1.24 g/cm^3 and 1.15–1.20 g/cm^3 in sucrose.

Flaviviruses

The nucleic acid of flaviviruses consists of a single molecule of positive-sense ssRNA. A single open reading frame (ORF) on the genomic RNA is translated directly into a polyprotein, which is further processed into the three structural proteins. In order from the N terminal, these are the internal RNA associated C protein and then the two envelope proteins, pre-M and E. The pre-M protein is a glycosylated precursor protein which is cleaved during or shortly after release from the cell into the non-glycosylated M membrane protein with no disulphide bridges (molecular weight 7–9 kDa). The E membrane protein is usually glycosylated and is considerably larger, with a molecular weight of 51–59 kDa and possessing six disulphide bridges formed by 12 conserved cysteine residues. The core protein C is rich in arginine and lysine, with a molecular weight of 14–16 kDa.

Following the translation of the three structural proteins, seven non-structural proteins are produced—the glycoproteins NS1, NS2A, NS2B, NS3, NS4A, NS4B and NS5. Two of these proteins, NS3 and NS5, are probably components of the RNA replicase.

The gene order is thus 5'-C–pre-M–E–NS1–NS2A–NS2B–NS3–NS4A–NS4B–NS5-3' (Figure 17.1).

The lipid content of the flavivirus envelope, which comprises some 17% of the viral weight, is derived from the host cell membrane. The E and M proteins are inserted into the envelope. The glycoprotein E is rich in mannose and complex glycans.

ANTIGENIC PROPERTIES

The antigenic properties of the genus *Flavivirus* are defined by serological tests, such as the highly cross-reactive pH-dependent haemagglutination-inhibition (HI) test, the less cross-reactive complement fixation (CF) test, and the much more specific neutralisation (NT) or plaque reduction neutralisation (PRNT) test. Other techniques mainly used for diagnostic serology are IgG and IgM detection by enzyme-linked immunosorbent assay (ELISA), and immunofluorescent (IF) assays, for antigen detection the polymerase chain reaction (PCR) or related molecular techniques are used. The antigenic features of the virus are characterised by reactivity with antigenic domains and epitopes on the membrane E protein of the virus.

The genus *Flavivirus* is subdivided further into subgroups on the basis of cross-neutralisation tests, using a polyclonal hyperimmune mouse ascitic fluid prepared against each member virus. The members of each subgroup give significant cross-neutralisation results against each other, whereas the 'unassigned' subgroup contains a miscellany of flaviviruses which will display only limited cross-reactivity with each other or with at least one other virus in any of the established subgroups. The antigenic classification of members of the genus *Flavivirus* of medical importance together with their respective vectors, disease manifestations, geographic distribution, vaccine availability

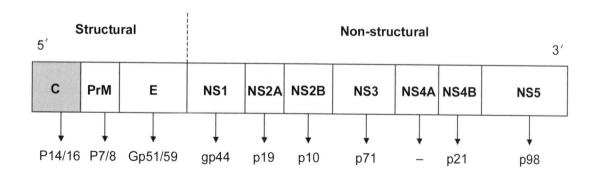

Figure 17.1 Schematic representation of the organisation of the gene of flavivirus

and frequency of reported cases, is given in Table 17.1. The flaviviruses which either cause no human disease or have only rarely been reported in association with illness will not be dealt with further here.

YELLOW FEVER

The yellow fever virus is the type species of the genus *Flavivirus* and also the source of its name—flavus is Latin for yellow. Yellow fever has been one of the classical diseases of antiquity, instilling dread and terror in the Americas, Europe and Africa from the seventeenth to the twentieth century. The disease has been romanticised in the classic works of Samuel Taylor Coleridge's *Rime of the Ancient Mariner* and Wagner's opera *The Flying Dutchman*. At the turn of the century, the disease almost put paid to the construction of the Panama Canal, and in West Africa yellow fever more than any other disease was responsible for the appellation 'the white man's grave'. As late as 1988, an estimated 44 000 cases with 25 000 deaths were estimated to have occurred in Nigeria in the 3 years 1986–1988.

History

The disease entity of yellow fever was first described in 1667 in Barbados, and in the following two centuries devastating epidemics raged on the continents of America and Africa and also, to some extent, in Europe. The panic and chaos was matched by the extravagance of the speculations as to the cause. The confusion was further aggravated by the difficulty in distinguishing it from the other tropical plagues of malaria and dengue. In 1848, Nott proposed that yellow fever was transmitted by the bite of a mosquito, a suggestion supported by Beauperthuy in 1854 and Carlos Finlay in 1881. In 1900 the US Army Yellow Fever Commission, under Major Walter Reed, demonstrated in historical experiments on human volunteers that the infection was indeed transmitted by mosquitoes. The following year, Walter Reed demonstrated that yellow fever was due to a filterable agent, the first human disease shown to be due to a filterable agent. The discovery of the aetiological agent of yellow fever, however, had to wait a further 26 years when workers of the Rockefeller Foundation's West Africa Yellow Fever Commission demonstrated the transmission of infection from a Ghanaian patient called Asibi to a rhesus monkey, and the subsequent passaging between

monkeys. The Asibi strain was later to be the parent strain of the 17D vaccine, developed by Nobel laureate Max Theiler at the Rockefeller Foundation in New York in 1937. The 17D vaccine strain was developed by serial passage through mouse embryo culture to chick embryo culture and then through minced chick embryo devoid of nervous tissue. The final vaccine virus, propagated through fertilised chicken eggs, is remarkably attenuated yet immunogenic, and the vaccine has proved to be very safe and effective, probably producing lifelong immunity after a single injection.

Epidemiology

Yellow fever occurs today in the tropics on both sides of the Atlantic. The endemic zone stretches between the latitudes of 10°N and 40°S in the Americas and 16°N to 10°S in Africa.

In the Americas, effective control of *Aedes aegypti* has resulted in the virtual disappearance of urban yellow fever from the western hemisphere. The last such epidemic of urban yellow fever occurred in Trinidad in 1954. However, jungle fever remains endemic in Bolivia, Brazil, Colombia, Ecuador, Peru, Panama, Venezuela and the Guyanas. The annual incidence by notification is 100 cases, although this is probably a substantially underestimated number. Remarkably, the infection has not extended to the heavy concentrations of *Aedes aegypti* which have built up in urban centres.

In Africa, recent epidemics of yellow fever have been far more extensive than those in the Americas. The features of jungle yellow fever differ in East and West Africa. In East Africa, endemic yellow fever activity is relatively quiet with few notified cases. However, two vast epidemics took place in 1940 in the Nuba mountains of Sudan, causing 40 000 infections with over 15 000 clinical cases and 1500 deaths. The second epidemic in 1960–1962, the largest epidemic of yellow fever ever recorded, took place in south-west Ethiopia, causing 30 000 deaths in 100 000 clinical cases in a rural population of some 1 million. In contrast to this, in West Africa, frequent outbreaks have occurred, usually on a considerably smaller scale than the two East African epidemics, with the exception of the Nigerian epidemic of 1986–1988, when an estimated 44 000 cases and 25 000 deaths may have occurred (WHO, 1991). Over the last two decades significant epidemics have been reported from several West African countries, both preceding the Nigerian

Table 17.1 Antigenic classification of flaviviruses of medical importance and their clinical and epidemiological features in man

Subgroup	Virus	Vector	Disease manifestations	Geographic distribution	Vaccine	Frequency of reported cases
Unassigned	Yellow Fever	M	Fever, HF, jaundice, etc.	Tropical Africa and South America	Yes	Numerous
	Rocio	M	Encephalitis	South-eastern Brazil	No	Uncommon
	Bussuquara*	M	Fever, arthralgia	South America	No	Rare
	Ilheus*	M	Fever, encephalitis	South America	No	Rare
	Sepik*	M	Fever	New Guinea	No	Rare
	Spondweni*	M	Fever	Africa	No	Rare
	Wesselsbron	M	Fever	Africa, Thailand	No	Uncommon
	Zika*	M	Fever, rash	Africa, Malaysia	No	Rare
Dengue	Dengue types 1–4	M	Fever, rash, myalgia, HF	Asia, Pacific, Americas, Africa	No	Numerous
Japanese encephalitis (mosquito-borne encephalitis)	Japanese encephalitis	M	Encephalitis	East Asia, Australasia	Yes	Numerous
	St Louis encephalitis	M	Encephalitis	North America, Jamaica, Haiti, South America	No	Numerous
	West Nile	M	Fever, rash, encephalitis	Africa, Asia, Europe, USA, Canada	No	Numerous
	Murray Valley encephalitis	M	Encephalitis	Australia, New Guinea	No	Uncommon
	Kokobera*	M	Arthritis	Australia	No	Rare
	Kunjin*	M	Fever, encephalitis	Australia, Borneo, Indonesia, Malaysia	No	Rare
	Usutu*	M	Fever, rash	Africa, Austria	No	Rare
Tick-borne encephalitis	TBE—European subtype (CEE)	T	Encephalitis	Central and Western Europe	Yes	Numerous
	TBE—far eastern subtype (RSSE)	T	Encephalitis	Asiatic Russia	Developmental	Numerous
	Omsk HF	T	Fever, HF	Western Siberia	CEE?	Numerous
	Kyasanur forest disease	T	Fever, encephalitis	Kanataka State, India	Yes	Uncommon
	Powassan	T	Encephalitis	North America	No	Uncommon
	Louping Ill*	T	Encephalitis	UK	No	Rare
	Negishi*	?	Encephalitis	Japan, Russia	No	Rare
	Kumlinge*	T	Encephalitis	Australasia	No	Rare
Rio Bravo	Rio Bravo*	?	Fever	USA, Mexico	No	Rare
	Dakar Bat*	?	Fever	Africa	No	Rare
Uganda S	Uganda S*	M		Africa, ?Far East	No	Rare
	Banzi*	M	Fever	Africa	No	Rare

*These viruses are of very little importance to clinical medicine and will not be discussed further.
**Numerous, >1000 cases reported, usually many thousands to millions; uncommon, 10–1000 cases reported; rare, <10 cases reported.
M, mosquito; T, tick; HF, haemorrhagic fever; TBE, tick-borne encephalitis; CEE, Central European encephalitis; RSSE, Russian spring-summer encephalitis.

epidemic, in the Ivory Coast (1982) and Burkina Faso (1983), as well as after it, Mali (1987), Angola (1988), Cameroon (1990) and Niger (1990). Yellow fever has expanded into Gabon, Liberia and Kenya, which reported their first cases since 1950 between 1992 and 1995 (WHO, 1996). Smaller, more recent outbreaks, e.g. in Guinea in 2000–2001, highlighted problems in the availability of yellow fever vaccine stocks for satisfactory outbreak response (Nathan *et al.*, 2001).

The transmission cycles of yellow fever and the ecological interrelationships of its vectors and reservoir hosts are complex. Essentially, three cycles of transmission are recognised:

1. *The enzootic forest cycle* represents the predominant maintenance of infection in its major vertebrate host, the monkey. In South America, *Alouatta*, *Cebus* and *Ateles* monkeys are the major primate reservoir hosts and they are infected by tree hole-breeding *Haemagogus* mosquitoes in the forest canopy. The monkey is, however, only a transient host because of the short-lived viraemia. The major amplification host is the mosquito, which remains infected for life and is also able to pass infection on transovarially. Occasionally a single or a few human cases may occur when man ventures into the forests. The cycle in Africa is similar and involves *Cercopithecus* and *Colobus* monkeys, with the *Aedes africanus* mosquito as the principal vector.
2. *The jungle yellow fever cycle* represents the most important epidemiological form of yellow fever with respect to human infection. Epizootic upsurges of yellow fever are frequent, both on the fringes of the rain forests and in the surrounding riverine gallery forests. Human infection occurs when forest mosquitoes invade adjacent plantations, clearings and villages. Once infection has been introduced into the human host, man-to-man transmission sustains the epidemics, resulting in the dramatic outbreaks reported in recent years. In South America, *Haemagogus* mosquitoes and possibly other mosquito species may establish epidemics in man. In East and Central Africa east of Cameroon, *Aedes simpsoni* will readily bite monkeys and man. In the East African epidemics in Sudan and Ethiopia, the anthropophilic *Aedes aegypti* was the most frequently responsible mosquito, as well as a number of 'wild' mosquitoes. In West Africa and Central Africa west of Cameroon, *Aedes simpsoni* does not bite man and *Aedes furcifer* is the major vector. In the Nigerian epidemic the major vector was *Aedes africanus*.
3. *The urban yellow fever cycle* is maintained by *Aedes aegypti* and was the dominant form of yellow fever before extensive mosquito control eliminated the disease from South American towns. Periodic reinfestations with *Aedes aegypti* have been observed in many South American countries and have revived fears of a resurgence of urban yellow fever. In West Africa, *Aedes aegypti* transmitted yellow fever is still responsible for outbreaks in towns and rural villages.

Clinical Features

The clinical presentation of yellow fever follows the general pattern of arbovirus disease—a short incubation period of 3–6 days followed by an acute biphasic illness. It is the severity and extent of the second phase of the acute illness which has imparted to this infection its classical awesomeness.

The initial phase of illness is characterised by a viraemia which renders the patient infectious to biting mosquitoes and is also responsible for the acute constitutional symptoms. These symptoms last about 3 days and are generally those of a non-specific febrile illness: headache, malaise, nausea, lassitude and widespread muscle pain, especially in the back. The differential diagnosis is wide and includes malaria, other arboviral infections including dengue, typhoid, rickettsial infections, influenza, enterovirus infections, acute HIV, etc. With more intensive and careful physical examination of patients, signs and symptoms more suggestive of yellow fever may be revealed, such as flushing of the head and neck, conjunctival injection, strawberry tongue and a relative bradycardia. Probably the majority of clinically manifest yellow fever infections are aborted at this phase of the illness, accounting for the underestimation of the true numbers of cases by up to 500-fold (WHO, 1991).

In cases of severe yellow fever, the early acute illness is followed by a brief period of remission before the onset of the haemorrhagic, hepatic and renal disease. The latter is heralded in by a return of fever, vomiting, abdominal pain, dehydration and prostration. The onset of the haemorrhagic diathesis is usually marked by coffee ground haematemesis, the classic 'black vomit', and bleeding from puncture sites where injections or drip needles have been inserted. This is accompanied by jaundice, albuminuria and oliguria. Deepening jaundice, massive haematemesis or haemoptysis or intra-abdominal bleeding, progressive renal failure, hypotension and shock may occur, followed by stupor, coma and death by the 7–10th day. Occasionally the illness may run a rapid fulminant course with death within a few days of onset. Mortality has been estimated to be of the order of 20–50% of cases entering the second phase of illness, although case fatality rates of up to 83% have been reported (WHO, 1990). These figures probably represent a marked overestimate of the fatality rate in the more severe cases which are likely to come to the attention of the health authorities. The differential diagnosis of severe yellow fever is usually that of the causes of viral haemorrhagic fever: Congo-Crimean haemorrhagic fever, Rift Valley fever, meningococcal septicaemia, Marburg and Ebola, generalised herpes simplex, as well as hepatitis B virus infection, leptospirosis and toxic hepatitis. During the severe second phase of illness, virus is usually absent from the blood and antibodies are present, suggesting that autoimmunity may well play a major role in the pathogenesis of severe yellow fever.

Patients who survive generally recover completely, although a chronic phase of illness lasting weeks or sometimes even months may occur in some individuals. This is characterised by prolonged jaundice and disturbances of liver function as well as prolonged renal failure. Occasionally sudden death may occur in the chronic phase as the result of myocardial damage or cardiac arrythmias.

A number of host factors may affect the clinical expression and severity of yellow fever virus infection. Age has played a significant role in South American epidemics, the majority of infections occurring in young adults, especially between the ages of 20–25. Age distribution has not, however, been a significant characteristic of African epidemics. In some epidemics gender has played a significant role in the distribution of cases, e.g. in the 1972–1973 Brazil epidemic there was a marked predominance of males affected: a 9:1 ratio, whereas in others there was only a slight male preponderance (e.g. 53% males in the 1986 Nigerian epidemic). More controversial has been the purported association of race and susceptibility to yellow fever, especially in the classical literature, which frequently made reference to the mildness of the disease in the indigenous inhabitants of the African jungle. There is, however, no evidence confirming any difference in susceptibility between races.

There are no known viral factors affecting either transmissibility or virulence. Although genomic heterogeneity has been demonstrated by fingerprinting and sequencing studies and also some antigenic heterogeneity has been observed between isolates, there has been no demonstrable clinical or epidemiological differences between American and African isolates.

Diagnosis

The development of reliable rapid tests for the urgent diagnosis of yellow fever has become a major public health priority in the management of the viral haemorrhagic fevers. The IgM antibody capture ELISA has become the test of choice for rapid serological diagnosis of yellow fever virus infection. Cross-reactions may occur but IgM antibody levels will normally be higher against yellow fever. Immunofluorescence tests using infected cells spotted onto microscope slides and then acetone-fixed can be used for detecting IgG and IgM in patients' sera. In the IF test, however, the rheumatoid factor may be a much greater problem than in the IgM antibody capture ELISA, and pre-treatment to remove IgG prior to IgM testing is necessary. The classical techniques, such as haemagglutination-inhibition (HI), complement fixation (CF) and neutralisation tests (NT), still have a place in yellow fever surveillance and diagnosis but a four-fold or greater rise in titre would have to be demonstrated before a definitive diagnosis could be made. Specific diagnosis still may be difficult, particularly if the patient has had previous experience of flavivirus infection. In these instances higher titres may appear against heterologous viruses, in keeping with the doctrine of original antigenic sin.

Isolation of virus may be performed in specialised reference laboratories, either by intracerebral or intraperitoneal inoculation of suckling mice or by the intrathoracic inoculation of male *Aedes aegypti* or *Toxorhynchites* mosquitoes. These techniques are particularly sensitive and are essential for epidemiological monitoring and research, but unfortunately take up to 3 weeks to provide an answer. More rapid viral isolation techniques using mosquito cell lines, such as the lines from *Aedes albopictus* (C6-36) and *Aedes pseudoscutellaris* (MOS 61), which are sensitive to infection and, combined with the IF test using monoclonal antibodies, may give a diagnosis within 3–4 days. It is recommended that early antibody is dissociated from viral antigen using dithiothreitol prior to isolation attempts in mosquito cell cultures. An antigen capture ELISA technique is available which is slightly less sensitive than virus isolation but is able to produce a specific result with the use of monoclonal antibodies in less than 24 h. A sensitive method for detecting and quantifying viral RNA has been developed using real-time reverse transcription PCR (RT-PCR).

Liver biopsy is contraindicated in acute yellow fever. However, liver tissue from post mortems may provide useful histopathological information. The classical liver pathology is that of a coagulative mid-zonal necrosis. The inclusion bodies which have been held to be pathognomonic of yellow fever are those in the cytoplasm due to eosinophilic degeneration (Councilman bodies) and intranuclear eosinophilic inclusion bodies (Torres bodies). Many of these features are, however, also found in fatal cases of viral haemorrhagic fever due to other viruses, and the histopathology is now no longer regarded as being diagnostic of yellow fever.

Control

The worldwide control of yellow fever has been achieved by immunisation and effective vector control, which have largely eliminated the urban yellow fever cycle due to *Aedes aegypti*. However, in recent times, poverty, war and competing health priorities have led to a reduction in immunisation and surveillance efforts, resulting in a resurgence of disease, especially in the endemic zone of Africa. In addition, reinfestation of towns and villages adjacent to forests with *Aedes aegypti*, aggravated by the massive uncontrolled urbanisation and population migrations to the towns of developing countries, also exacerbated particularly by severe drought, has renewed the spectre of urban yellow fever in Africa.

It is over 50 years since the development of the first yellow fever vaccine by Theiler, and the original method for the production of chick embryo-passaged 17D vaccine has undergone little modification over the years. The French neurotropic vaccine, developed by passage in mouse brain, is now no longer used because of the prohibitive danger of encephalitic complications. The vaccine is a live attenuated purified product produced by growing vaccine virus in chick embryos and is supplied as a lyophilised preparation, which should be stored frozen or at least kept at temperatures of not more than 5°C. After reconstitution it should be used immediately and any remnants discarded within an hour. A single dose of 0.5 ml given subcutaneously provides excellent, long-lasting immunity to 99% of vaccinees. Although international health regulations demand booster doses every 10 years, neutralising antibodies have been shown to persist for over 30 years and immunity is probably lifelong.

Side-effects to immunisation occur in less than 5% of recipients and are generally mild, low-grade fever, myalgia and headache. Occasionally, hypersensitivity reactions have been reported, especially in individuals allergic to egg protein. The most serious side-reaction, encephalitis, has been reported in 18 cases out of more than 35 million doses of vaccine which have been administered to date. Only two cases have occurred in children over the age of 7 months, although the only fatality was in a 3 year-old child. Regarding the latter case, it was postulated recently that a change identified in amino acid position 303 of the isolate P-16065 as compared to the parent vaccine virus 17D-204 USA may have affected the virulence of the vaccine virus (Jennings *et al.*, 1994).

The contraindications to immunisation are those determined by age, pregnancy, history of egg allergy and immunosuppression (Centers for Disease Control, 1990). The vaccine should not be given to children under the age of 9 months unless travel to an endemic area cannot be avoided but should, at any rate, never be given to infants less than 4 months of age. The effect of immunisation in pregnancy has not been determined; however, being a live attenuated vaccine, it should not routinely be given to pregnant women. However, if travel to an area with ongoing yellow fever cannot be avoided, the danger of infection would far outweigh the theoretical risk to a pregnant mother and her fetus. The vaccine should also be avoided in persons with a history of egg allergy or in immunosuppressed individuals, e.g. due to HIV infection, malignancy or immunosuppressive treatment. However, as in the case of pregnancy, the relative risks of travel to an endemic area vs. the slight or even theoretical risk of the vaccine, would need to be evaluated on an individual basis.

Immunisation policies with regard to yellow fever immunisation involve three aspects of the control of infection:

1. *International travellers* going to yellow fever endemic areas require prophylactic immunisation as a condition of entry to these countries, or exiting from endemic countries. There were two reports in 1996–1997 of travellers to the Amazon region of Brazil who died from yellow fever after returning to their respective countries. Neither had been vaccinated.
2. *Within endemic zones*, two kinds of immunisation policy have been practised. These are (a) the so-called 'fire-fighting' policy, where there is a response to an outbreak, or alternately (b) proactive routine immunisation to prevent outbreaks occurring.

(a) 'Fire-fighting' mass immunisation is usually put into operation in the early phases of an outbreak or in advance of an imminent epidemic, if effective surveillance is able to predict it. Although the 'fire-fighting' strategy may be cheaper than routine immunisation, it can often only be implemented after a considerable number of individuals have already been infected and the protective effect will be further delayed by another 7 days for antibodies to develop.

(b) A far more effective way of controlling yellow fever is proactive routine and sustained administration of vaccine. In Africa, 33 countries have been identified by the World Health Organization as endemic high-risk regions where yellow fever vaccine should be incorporated into the Expanded Programme on Immunization (EPI) schedule. However, only one of these countries, Gambia, has exceeded the target vaccine coverage of 80% (87% in 1994). In other countries coverage has ranged from 1% in Nigeria to 55% in Mauritania (WHO, 1996). Yellow fever vaccine should preferably be given together with measles vaccine at 9 months of age and can be administered simultaneously with measles vaccine with no reduction in efficacy of either vaccine. It can also be given simultaneously with other viral vaccines and also BCG, with no increase in reactivity or decrease in efficacy (however, yellow fever and cholera vaccines should preferably be separated by an interval of 3 weeks).

The current worldwide production of yellow fever vaccine is estimated to be of the order of 15 million doses/year. There are concerted efforts to improve on techniques for the production of yellow fever vaccine, e.g. by the use of tissue culture techniques and also the development of recombinant technology with reference to yellow fever immunisation.

Vector control strategies such as aerial spraying, domiciliary spraying and the enforcement of public health regulations to reduce collections of stagnant water and other breeding sites, have had successes in the past in eliminating *Aedes aegypti* and controlling urban yellow fever. Present-day socioeconomic difficulties have, however, hampered recent efforts to again control the reinfestation of villages and towns in Africa. Control of vectors responsible for the jungle yellow fever cycle is impractical.

There still remain many gaps in our knowledge of the epidemiology of the infection and the permanent control of the disease will probably need not only resources to implement what is already known, but also the elucidation of the remaining enigmas regarding the infection.

OTHER MEMBERS OF THE 'UNASSIGNED' SUBGROUP OF FLAVIVIRUSES

Rocio

Rocio virus is an arboviral cause of encephalitis localised to the Ribeira valley and Santista lowlands in the southern coastal region of Sao Paulo state in south-eastern Brazil. The virus was first isolated in 1975 from the brain of a fatal case of encephalitis diagnosed during an unusual epidemic of encephalitis in 1975–1976. No further cases have occurred since 1980, although two children from the Ribeira valley tested positive for IgM antibodies in 1989. A total of 821 cases were diagnosed during 1975–1978, twice as many in males and usually aged 15–30 years. The virus has been isolated from pools of mosquitoes, such as *Psorophora ferox*, and also from wild birds. The transmission cycle of the virus has not, however, been established.

Clinical and epidemiological features of the disease have been reviewed in 821 cases between 1975 and 1978 (Iversson, 1980). The disease commences with non-specific signs of pyrexia, headache and vomiting. This may then be followed by disturbances of consciousness and signs of encephalitis, including localising signs. Death may follow a prolonged coma or there may be a sudden fulminant course. Serious neurological sequelae occur in some 20% of clinical cases and the overall case fatality is found to be 10%. The IgM capture ELISA has been used to diagnose *Rocio virus* infection in children and is preferable to the HI test for identifying recent infection.

Wesselsbron

Wesselsbron virus was first isolated from a lamb in the village of Wesselsbron in South Africa in 1955. Virus has been isolated from 23 cases of infection, 11 of them resulting from laboratory infection or infection of laboratory field workers. The vertebrate host is chiefly livestock, especially sheep, and isolations have been made from throughout sub-Saharan Africa, especially South Africa. It has also been isolated from pools of wild-caught *Aedes* mosquitoes, such as *Aedes (neo) lineatopennis*. The major vector in sheep is *Aedes caballus-juppi*. Man is infected by mosquito bite or by direct contact in handling carcasses or tissues of animals that have died of the disease.

Human infection is characterised by a sudden onset of pyrexia, severe headache and retro-orbital pain associated with photophobia and hyperaesthesia of the skin, with an evanescent skin rash frequently present. Muscle and joint pains are also commonly seen. In severe cases signs of encephalitis, such as blurred vision and some mental impairment, may occur. Patients recover after a few days to a week and no permanent sequelae have been reported.

Diagnosis of infection may be achieved by isolation of the virus from blood or serological tests. The HI test is only useful in individuals with no previous flavivirus infection history, because of the extensive cross-reaction between Wesselsbron and other flaviviruses. The capture IgM assay is the test of choice for diagnosis of recent Wesselsbron infection.

DENGUE

Dengue is, at present, the most important arboviral cause of death and disease in man (Gubler and Costa-Valez, 1991). The infection has spread widely from south-east Asia to the Americas, the Pacific and Africa, now involving several million people annually. In all major tropical areas of the world the incidence of dengue fever (DF) and dengue haemorrhagic fever (DHF)/dengue shock syndrome (DSS) has increased dramatically over the past few years, with an ever-increasing frequency and extent of epidemics and a greater severity of cases. The spectre of the introduction of infection to *Aedes aegypti* populations in non-endemic countries is of great international concern.

History

Outbreaks of illnesses clinically resembling dengue fever have been recorded since 1779 and 1780 in Java (Indonesia), Cairo and Philadelphia. Similar epidemics of dengue-like illnesses occurred at 10–30 year intervals throughout tropical and subtropical regions of the world. Although the precise aetiology could not be established and infections such as chikungunya are clinically and epidemiologically very similar, the majority of these epidemics were probably dengue. The spread of the disease has been markedly accelerated by the advent of widespread air travel over the last three decades. Dengue fever was generally regarded as a relatively benign illness, affecting predominantly colonial expatriots living in tropical countries and, although responsible for severe and often incapacitating muscle pain, it was seldom lethal. However, the gravity of the dengue pandemic was really confirmed by the recognition in the 1950s of the severe complications of infection, viz. DHF/DSS affecting mainly children in the endemic areas. Epidemics of DHF/DSS ravaged south-east Asia and in the following 30 years was responsible for over 700 000 children being hospitalised and over 20 000 fatalities (Halstead, 1984).

In the western hemisphere, the first major epidemic of DHF/DSS struck Cuba in 1981 and was responsible for 24 000 cases of DHF and 10 000 of DSS (Gubler and Costa-Valez, 1991) (sporadic cases of suspected DHF had been reported from Central America since 1968). Only the energetic response of the Cuban health authorities, with intensive education and mass hospitalisation, kept the mortality down to only 158. Following on this epidemic, confirmed or suspected cases of DHF have been reported in the Americas almost every year, with the most severe outbreaks of dengue fever occurring in Peru in 1990, involving over 76 000 cases (Centers for Disease Control, 1991a). Dengue returned to Cuba in 1997. A summary of the present status of dengue worldwide is that there are 2.5 billion persons at risk, more than 20 million cases/year and 30 000 deaths. Imported cases of dengue in travellers returning to temperate countries are reported in the USA annually and DHF was reported in two cases in the UK in 1991 (Jacobs *et al.*, 1991). Blood donations collected during a dengue outbreak in Hong Kong were thought to have resulted in two cases of dengue from infected transfusion blood.

Virus Properties and Host Range

The dengue viruses form a subgroup of the genus *Flavivirus* and although extensive cross-reactivity is seen with serological tests such as haemagglutination inhibition (HI) which cannot reliably distinguish dengue from many other flaviviruses, neutralisation tests (NT) are able to define dengue virus as a distinct antigenic subgroup. There are four serotypes of dengue based on neutralisation tests. However, with all serological tests there is extensive cross-reactivity between the four serotypes, although they are distinguishable with the high specific plaque reduction neutralisation test. Following natural infection, protective immunity is homotypic. Dengue serotypes 1, 3 and 4 show a closer antigenic and genetic relationship to each other than dengue 2. However, within each of the serotypes, considerable heterogeneity and strain variation is demonstrable on nucleic acid sequence analysis and DNA/RNA hybridisation studies as well as by antigen signature analysis using monoclonal antibodies. The importance of these strain variations with respect to the epidemiology and virulence of the virus remains to be determined. Molecular analysis of isolates from the South Pacific suggested that the recent epidemics (1988–1989) were due to a new genotype, rather than a previously circulated DEN-1 strain.

The only vertebrate hosts of dengue virus in nature are man and several species of Asian and African subhuman primates. Other vertebrates can be infected experimentally only with difficulty, including baby mice, which usually require several blind passages of patient material to obtain an isolate. The invertebrate hosts of dengue are members of the genus *Aedes*, especially the subgenus *Stegomyia*. The most important mosquito hosts as far as human infection is concerned are *Aedes aegypti*, *A. albopictus* and *A. polynesiensis*. Other *Aedes* species, including *A. africanus*, *A. leuteocephalus* and the *A. furcifer* group, are involved in the maintenance of the forest cycle of dengue in Africa, whereas in Asia the mosquitoes concerned belong to the *A. niveus* complex.

EPIDEMIOLOGY

Dengue displays many epidemiological similarities to yellow fever and chikungunya viruses and there is considerable overlap in the ecologies of these three virus infections. Essentially there are three transmission cycles of dengue: a forest cycle in primates and involving forest species of *Aedes*; a rural or semi-rural cycle in humans, with the peri-domestic *Aedes* species being the vectors; and an urban cycle in humans involving domesticated *Aedes* species. By far the most important of these three for both endemic and epidemic human dengue is the urban cycle. It is, in fact, doubtful whether the forest cycle plays any significant direct role in human dengue.

The two major mosquito vectors of urban dengue are *A. aegypti* and *A. albopictus*. Although *A. albopictus* is considered more sensitive to oral infection with dengue viruses, *A. aegypti* is a more important vector for human disease and is especially responsible for explosive epidemics. The anthropophilic *A. aegypti* usually preferentially feeds on man and occasionally

also on domestic animals, while the purely domestic *A. albopictus* randomly feeds on man, domestic animals and feral animals and birds. To establish infection, *A. aegypti* would need to feed on individuals with high levels of viraemia, and this may select for viral strains of higher virulence, which are more likely to produce the severe epidemics associated with *A. aegypti*. In addition, the biting habits of *A. aegypti*, which characteristically takes interrupted blood meals and will thus feed on a number of individuals before becoming engorged, enhances its ability to spread the virus. It is thus not unusual for a single mosquito to spread infection amongst several individuals at a single feeding. In both mosquitoes, biting activities are maximal soon after daybreak and in late afternoon, and are related to human activities and movements. Outbreaks associated with both vectors are climatically influenced by heavy rainfall and high temperature.

The recent upsurge of dengue in existing endemic zones and the spread to new areas has been attributed to modern phenomena of human and social behaviour. Infestations of *A. aegypti* in tropical towns and villages, which were controlled by extensive spraying and other vector control measures in the 1950s and 1960s, have now resurged due to uncontrolled urbanisation and the mass migration of rural populations into informal housing settlements and squatter camps on the peripheries of cities and towns. These population movements have been accentuated by famine, poverty and war. Stagnant water pools and lack of reticulated water supplies have provided ample opportunities for mosquito breeding, coupled with the breakdown of vector control in many tropical countries. Overcrowding and grossly inadequate housing, which is so characteristic of the sprawling slums of the tropical world, greatly facilitate the spread of vector-borne diseases and is especially conducive to dengue transmission resulting from the interrupted feeding habits of *A. aegypti*. The spread of infection has also been enhanced by the modern era of jet travel, which facilitates the transportation of infected individuals to non-infected areas, creating the threat of the introduction of infection if infestations of *A. aegypti* are sufficiently high. Modern air travel has also been responsible for increasing the number of imported cases of dengue into countries where physicians are, in the main, ignorant of the infection, resulting in perplexing diagnostic difficulties until a history of travel to endemic zones is elicited. More recently, the influence of international trade in the spread of dengue has been observed. Motor vehicle tyres and casings from south-east Asia containing remnant pools of water where infected *A. albopictus* mosquito larvae have been found, have been shipped to various non-endemic areas of the world, posing a serious threat of introducing both the virus as well as its vector.

Clinical Features

The majority of infections with dengue virus, based on the extent of population seropositivity, are asymptomatic. Clinical manifestations of dengue occur in two forms—classical dengue fever and DHF/DSS. Classical dengue fever is an acute disease characterised by a sudden onset of fever, severe headache which is typically frontal in distribution, together with retro-orbital pain, nausea and vomiting. Severe muscle and bone pain and arthralgia are characteristic of dengue and usually more pronounced in the back, which led to it being termed 'break bone fever' by Dr Benjamin Rush in 1778. He also aptly described the associated severe depression as 'break heart fever'. There is frequently a diffuse, discrete maculopapular rash which usually heralds the recovery phase of the illness. In spite of the severity of symptoms, which may be incapacitating, the disease is temporary and full recovery takes place.

The grave complication of DHF/DSS is governed by two factors, prior infection and age. Thus, DHF and DSS occurs in approximately 0.18% and 0.007%, respectively, of cases of primary dengue fever compared to 2.0% and 1.1%, respectively, of dengue fever due to secondary infection (Halstead, 1981). It is also rare in individuals over the age of 15 years. DHF/DSS resembles yellow fever in its biphasic presentation. The first phase is not unlike uncomplicated dengue fever. This is followed by a brief remission of symptoms, when the fever subsides to normal or close to normal. There is then a sudden deterioration in the patient's condition, marked by profound prostration, hypotension, circulatory collapse and manifestations of bleeding and shock. Bleeding is seen commonly as petechiae in the skin and mucous membranes, especially in the oral cavity, ecchymoses, bleeding at injection and skin puncture sites, gastrointestinal bleeding and haemorrhagic pneumonia.

The cause of the haemorrhagic diathesis in DHF is complex. There is evidence of vascular injury with increased permeability and extravasation of fluid from the vascular into the interstitial fluid compartment, producing hypotension and DSS. Bleeding due to vascular damage is suggested by the presence of petechiae and a positive tourniquet test. In addition there is a marked thrombocytopaenia, although it is not yet clear what the relative contributions of impaired platelet formation due to direct suppression of megakaryocyte production in the bone marrow or excess destruction due to endothelial damage. Evidence exists for both. Thirdly, there is haematological evidence of a consumptive coagulopathy with a moderate increase in fibrin degradation products which, however, rarely reaches the stage of disseminated intravascular coagulation.

The definition of DHF is controversial. The WHO criteria for DHF are an acute onset of fever, haemorrhagic manifestations, which include at least a positive tourniquet test, a thrombocytopaenia of 100 000/ml or less and a haemoconcentration with a haematocrit increase by 20% or more. Manifestations of haemorrhagic fever, however, do differ from country to country and amendments to the criteria have been proposed to include, amongst others, references to the age of the patient (<16 years) (Halstead, 1989). The severity of DHF/DSS has also been graded by the WHO from I to IV (Anonymous, 1980):

Grade I   Fever with non-specific constitutional symptoms, the only haemorrhagic manifestations being a positive tourniquet test.

Grade II   As for Grade I, but with specific haemorrhagic manifestations.

Grade III Signs of circulatory failure or hypotension.

Grade IV   Profound shock with pulse and blood pressure undetectable.

Pathogenesis of DHF/DSS

The pathogenesis of DHF/DSS has been studied intensively for a number of decades. Nevertheless, the pathways to the development of severe dengue have not, as yet, been definitively established. Essentially, there are two hypotheses involving immunological or virological mechanisms.

The immunological theory of DHF/DSS is based on the phenomenon of antibody-mediated enhancement of infection. Investigations of antibody-mediated enhancement in dengue have been the hallmark studies of this phenomenon, which have since been shown to be important facets in the pathogenesis of a number of viral diseases, from rabies to HIV (Kurane et al., 1991). The major cell infected by dengue virus in vivo is the monocyte/macrophage (even though a number of cell lines from a variety of tissues may be infected in vitro). Three elements partake in the process of antibody-mediated enhancement: antibody, virus and the receptor for the Fc portion of IgG.

Evidence for the involvement of pre-existing antibodies comes from epidemiological observations that DHF/DSS is much more common in individuals with pre-existing antibodies. These pre-existing antibodies may be derived from passively acquired maternal antibodies in infants less than 1 year of age, or from previous infection in children over 1 year of age. This was particularly evident in the Cuban epidemic of 1981 when DHF/DSS due to type 2 virus was usually observed in individuals infected some 4 years previously with type 1 virus. Experimental work by Halstead and colleagues demonstrated enhancement of infection in experimental dengue in monkeys using human serum as well as sera from hyperimmunised animals. It was later demonstrated that only IgG antibody and not IgM, which has potent neutralising activity, was able to produce enhancement. Using monoclonal antibodies, enhancing epitopes on the E and pre-M proteins of dengue virus could be demonstrated, some of which could also be neutralising and others not (Kurane *et al.*, 1991).

The receptor on the monocyte/macrophage cells which form the third component of the enhancing complex is thought to be the FcγRI molecule which binds the Fc portion of IgG with great avidity and also, but probably to a lesser extent, the FcγRII molecule. The effect of the attachment of the virus–antibody complex to the FcγR receptor is both to enhance the binding of virus to its target cell and also to induce a signal to the cell facilitating internalisation of the complex. There remain, however, many unanswered questions with the antibody-mediated enhancement hypothesis. First, DHF/DSS may well occur in the absence of pre-existing antibodies, even though it is far more common for them to be there. It is also not clear whether binding of virus to its specific receptor is essential for infectivity. The mechanism by which enhanced infection of cells produces the components of a DHF/DSS syndrome is not known.

The alternative hypothesis of Rosen (1986) and colleagues holds that the severe complications of DHF/DSS are the direct results of properties of the virus, that is, the consequence of infection with unusually virulent strains of dengue circulating in a particular area and giving rise to outbreaks of DHF/DSS. However, as mentioned above, although nucleic acid sequencing techniques and antigen signature analysis have demonstrated strain variations within serotypes, no consistent relationship between strain variation and either virulence or heightened infectivity has been reliably demonstrated. There has also been no consistent association with serotype and DHF/DSS. Earlier observations, in both Thailand and the 1981 Cuban epidemic, suggested that dengue type 2 may be more frequently associated with DHF/DSS. Subsequent observations have now shown that all four serotypes may be responsible.

Neither of these two hypotheses is able to elucidate why the development of DHF/DSS is so dependent on age or why DHF/DSS is more likely to follow when dengue infection occurs in some areas but not in others.

Diagnosis

The clinical diagnosis of dengue, both the uncomplicated dengue fever form and DHF/DSS, if often unreliable. Dengue fever may resemble clinically a variety of acute febrile illnesses, although the severe muscle and bone pain is suggestive of dengue. Similarly, DHF may resemble other causes of haemorrhagic fever, although thrombocytopaenia with haemoconcentration and signs of a moderate consumptive coagulopathy is suggestive of dengue.

The most widely used serological test is the HI test, detecting antibodies as early as 4 days post-onset. A specific diagnosis of dengue can be made early in primary infections, but cross-reactions with other flaviviruses occur in late primary or secondary infections. The IgM antibody capture ELISA (MAC ELISA) is being used during outbreaks of dengue, and there are now rapid assays available for the detection of dengue IgG and IgM, although cross-reaction may occur with the IgG assay. The IgM antibodies may persist for over 3 months, so the test is also useful for retrospective studies, but this persistence may cause diagnostic problems in areas where dengue is endemic. A combined IgG and IgM assay, detecting high levels of IgG indicating secondary infection, is useful in dengue endemic areas. Immunofluorescent assays have been used successfully to detect dengue IgG and IgM antibodies. The CF test is more specific than the HI test, but the antibodies detected by this assay appear later and disappear earlier. The NT and PRNT tests are the most specific and sensitive but are difficult to perform and thus tend to be used only for specific purposes.

Virus isolation, the only definitive way of being able to type isolates, is difficult and if mice are used, a number of blind passages are usually required. Intracerebral inoculation of adult or larval *Toxorhynchites* spp. is a sensitive and rapid method for the isolation of dengue virus, giving results in 2–3 days.

The use of a rapid centrifugation method may increase sensitivity and reduce time scales. Intrathoracic inoculation of mosquitoes is easier and just as sensitive, but head squashes cannot be made or tested for specific dengue antigen for at least 7 days post-inoculation. The most commonly used system of virus isolation is the inoculation of mosquito cell lines, viz. *A. albopictus* (C6-36), *A. pseudoscutellaris* (AP-61) and *Toxorhynchites ambionensis* (TRA-248), which are almost as sensitive as mosquito inoculation, which allows specific results to be obtained within 2–3 days using fluorescent-labelled monoclonal antibodies. A combination of MAC ELISA and RT-PCR on peripheral blood leukocytes has been shown to give high levels of sensitivity and specificity.

Control

There is, at present, no licensed dengue vaccine. Current strategy is to develop a vaccine against all four serotypes. Successful trials of monovalent vaccines have been reported, but, as yet, not for experimental tetravalent vaccines. Because of the lack of availability of a vaccine, control of dengue depends on (a) surveillance to obtain early warning of epidemics or preferably to be able to predict impending epidemics, and (b) effective vector control.

Epidemiological surveillance may be of two types: first, proactive surveillance in interepidemic periods in endemic areas or in countries which are not yet infected but are vulnerable to the introduction of new infections because of high infestations of *A. aegypti*; second, reactive surveillance, where monitoring is instituted once suspected or confirmed cases of dengue have already occurred. This form of surveillance is very insensitive as numerous cases may occur which are not suspected to be dengue, before authorities are alerted to the outbreak. In the Comoros Islands, dengue type 1 was diagnosed in 62/116 clinical cases in 1993. However, an investigation to determine the prevalence of dengue infection in over-5 year-olds, using a dengue IgM assay, estimated that at least 60 000 recent cases had occurred at that time.

A number of instruments of surveillance may be used for proactive monitoring. Disease surveillance requires intensive educational efforts, especially at peripheral primary health care level, to alert health care workers as to the possibility of dengue. It is, however, very difficult to sustain interest, especially if no cases materialise. Viral and serological surveillance involves the active recruitment of specimens, e.g. as

carried out in Puerto Rico, where blood samples are collected by collaborating physicians on a regular basis and sent for analysis. Interest and cooperation is also difficult to sustain. The use of blood samples sent to laboratories for testing for acute febrile illnesses or 'viral syndromes' may be an easier way of recruiting specimens for serological testing. Surveillance may also utilise the routine investigation of all viral haemorrhagic fever cases, which should include tests for dengue. Vector surveillance may be of benefit to demonstrate low infestations (house index of <1%) or to look out for the introduction of exotic mosquito species, e.g. *A. albopictus*.

Vector control aims at the elimination of the main mosquito vector, *Aedes aegypti*. While this is technically feasible, with both adulticide campaigns using ultra-low-volume spraying with malathion and also larvicide treatment of stagnant water, the costs are high and the effects are temporary. In many tropical countries where *A. aegypti* eradication had been achieved, reinfestations have taken place to levels equalling, or even exceeding, those in pre-control times. However, long-term community-based programmes need to be implemented in endemic countries. In non-endemic countries there should be a vigilant monitoring for the possible importation of dengue, e.g. through motor car tyres, or travellers or migrants from endemic areas.

JAPANESE ENCEPHALITIS

Japanese encephalitis virus (JE) is the major arboviral cause of encephalitis worldwide. First described as a clinical entity in Japan in 1870, it is now thought to be responsible for about 50 000 cases annually, half of whom are left with permanent neurological or psychological handicap, and in a further quarter it is rapidly lethal. Infection has been demonstrated in 16 countries in south-east Asia, stretching to India in the west and to southern Russia in the north—a population of over 2 billion people.

Viral Features and Host Range

JE virus shows some cross-reactivity with *St Louis encephalitis virus*, *West Nile virus*, and *Murray Valley encephalitis virus*, and together they form the mosquito-borne encephalitis complex. The virus is antigenically relatively homogeneous and recovery from infection results in solid protection. Nucleic acid analysis, however, has revealed some significant heterogeneity. Using primer extension sequencing, isolates of JE virus could be separated into three distinct genotypic groups, each group found in separate geographic divisions (Chen *et al.*, 1990). The epidemiological significance of this remains to be established. In the early part of the year 2000, JE reappeared in the Australasian region and isolates were identified as genotype I, whereas all previous isolates were genotype II.

The vertebrate hosts of JE virus are man and his domestic animals and birds; no wild animals and birds are known to be infected to any significant extent. The major mosquito vector of the virus is *Culex tritaeniorhynchus*, although a number of other species of the genera *Culex*, *Monsonia*, *Aedes* and *Anopheles* have yielded isolates of JE virus.

Epidemiology

Nestling birds, particularly of the heron family, play an important epidemiological role in the dissemination of JE virus, with a second cycle involving domestic animals, particularly the pig. In seroprevalence studies, high NT antibodies were found in several other animal species, e.g. cattle, horses, dogs, monkeys and bats. As with the wild bird population, the high turnover of the domestic pig population resulting in a continuous supply of susceptible animals is a contributing factor to the pig being a major amplifying host for JE virus. JE rarely causes disease in domestic animals, although fatal encephalitis in horses and abortions in sows have been recorded. Studies on birds have implicated other species, whose main habitat is the rice paddies, as vertebrate hosts of JE virus—these water birds include water herons and bitterns. In India ardeid birds such as cattle egrets are implicated.

JE virus has been isolated from many species of mosquito but the principal vector in many areas is *Culex tritaeniorhynchus*. Other mosquitoes, mainly the *Culex* spp., are considered to be important in specific regions, e.g. *C. gelidus* in south-east Asia, for the transmission of JE virus.

Man is a dead-end host and plays little role in the amplification of the virus. JE is thus predominantly a rural problem, with disease closely related to rainfall and irrigation.

Clinical and Pathological Features

Infection with JE virus is considerably more widespread than the incidence of encephalitis would indicate. Infection may present non-specifically as a mild febrile illness or as an aseptic meningitis, or, rarely, as a variety of inflammatory manifestations in the viscera. The typical disease manifestations of acute meningomyeloencephaliis have been widely estimated to occur at between 1/20 (Rodrigues, 1984) to 1/600–800 persons infected (Halstead, 1981).

The major target cells for JE virus are the T lymphocyte and the peripheral blood mononuclear cells. In fatal cases of encephalitis, viral antigen is also demonstrable in the neurons. Factors determining the neuroinvasiveness of JE virus involve both viral and host factors. Nucleotide sequencing of non-neurovirulent mutants of JE virus have demonstrated single base changes in the coding region for E protein (Cecilia and Gould, 1991). Age is an important host factor determining neurovirulence, encephalitis being more common and more severe in the young as well as in elderly individuals. Experimental work in rats has shown a relationship between neurotropism and neuronal maturity in that the virus selectively infects immature neurons (Ogata *et al.*, 1991). The reason for greater neuroinvasiveness in the elderly is unknown, but is consistent with the features of the related St Louis encephalitis and West Nile virus, which similarly display greater neuroinvasiveness in the elderly.

The typical case of Japanese encephalitis commences after an incubation period of 1–2 weeks, with fever and headache, followed rapidly by depression of the level of consciousness, progressing from stupor to coma. Localising cranial nerve and other neurological signs occur in about 30% of cases and in children generalised seizures are common—the frequency of seizures in patients increases with the severity of the encephalitis. A quarter of cases of clinical encephalitis will recover with no permanent sequelae and a quarter will die rapidly. The remaining half will recover with varying degrees of permanent neuropsychiatric sequelae. In addition, especially in children, the virus may persist in lymphocytes and reactivate to give recurrent disease after recovery (Sharma *et al.*, 1991).

Grave prognostic signs include a short prodromal period, deep coma, decerebrate posture, breathing abnormalities and the ability to isolate virus from the CSF. Recently a reduction of serum iron levels has been demonstrated in patients due to the sequestering of iron in the spleen, and a direct relationship between low serum iron and prognosis has been shown (Bharadwaj *et al.*, 1991).

The pathology of the brain in fatal cases has revealed microfoci of necrosis scattered throughout the central nervous system, but especially involving the thalamus, the basal ganglia and the deep cerebral nuclei.

Diagnosis

Routine diagnosis is usually carried out by serology using HI, IF, CF or ELISA techniques. Test results should, however, be treated with caution because of extensive cross-reactivity with other flaviviruses and because up to a quarter of patients fail to demonstrate a serological rise in titre due to their late presentation to medical attention. A preferable serological test is the IgM antibody capture ELISA on serum or CSF, or a more recently developed particle agglutination assay, which detects JE specific IgM. The detection of specific IgM antibodies in CSF is diagnostic of acute Japanese encephalitis.

Virus isolation from blood is rarely successful during the acute illness because the viraemic phase is probably over by the time central nervous system symptoms appear. Virus isolation from the CSF is usually also unsuccessful and, if positive, indicates a poor prognosis, as mentioned above. A variety of isolation techniques are very sensitive to JE virus, including intracerebral inoculation of suckling mice, intrathoracic inoculation of live mosquitoes, the use of common mammalian cell lines such as Vero and LLC-MK2 and mosquito cell lines, especially those of *A. albopictus* and *A. pseudoscutellaris*.

Control

The major component of the control of Japanese encephalitis is widespread immunisation of both man and domestic animals, especially pigs. A number of human vaccines have been developed. A formalin-inactivated lyophilised vaccine of mouse brain origin, derived from the Nakayima-NIH strain of JE virus, is prepared by Biken, Japan, and widely used in Japan and Korea and also by travellers to endemic areas. In China, a BHK-prepared inactivated vaccine is used. Both vaccines are highly immunogenic and protection rates of over 90% are achieved. Experimental live attenuated vaccines are being developed and Chinese workers have successfully attenuated the SA14 strain by 100 passages in BHK cell culture (Stephenson, 1988). The live attenuated vaccine (SA14-14-2) is now widely used within the PRC. Recombinant DNA technology also holds promise for the future development of safe, effective JE vaccines (Konishi *et al.*, 1991), ChimeriVax-JE using YF 17D as a live vector for the envelope genes of SA14-14-2 is in the trial stage. Similarly, a number of veterinary vaccines have been used in pigs and horses. Vaccination thus holds

the potential to eliminate Japanese encephalitis. Reports of allergic reactions to the Biken vaccine have resulted in a cautionary warning being issued against routine administration of JE vaccine to travellers, except to those who are likely to be at high risk in endemic areas, particularly rural areas, for a month or longer during the season of vector activity (Nothdurft *et al.*, 1996).

Because man is only an incidental host, interruption of transmission of the virus would be independent of the extent of immunity in human populations, and eradication of infection would need to aim for the elimination of virus circulating in the vertebrate reservoir of domestic animals. At present, economic realities preclude anything approaching a sufficiently widespread programme of immunisation in domesticated pigs.

Vector control is difficult because of community resistance to mosquito control programmes, which need to include and may significantly tamper with subsistence agriculture of rural populations. Thus, methods which have been attempted include short-term drainage of rice fields and attempts to introduce more drought-resistant rice in order to reduce potential mosquito breeding sites. Ultra-low-volume insecticide spraying has had limited success, with increasing insecticide resistance, especially in *Culex tritaeniorhynchus*. Measures to prevent biting by mosquitoes, such as the use of insect repellents, mosquito netting, etc., should be encouraged. Most biting activity is concentrated at nightfall.

ST LOUIS ENCEPHALITIS

St Louis encephalitis virus (SLE) is the major cause of epidemic viral encephalitis in the USA. Although the distribution of the virus ranges from southern Canada to Argentina and a few sporadic cases have been reported in South and Central America, virtually all human disease has occurred in the USA.

Viral Features and Host Range

SLE is antigenically closely related to the other members of the Japanese encephalitis subgroup of flaviviruses. In addition, cross-immunity to other flaviviruses has also been demonstrated, including dengue virus type 2. Antigenic heterogeneity has been shown with monoclonal antibodies, although there is no evidence that this has any epidemiological implications. By means of T1 restriction mapping, a number of genotypes of SLE have been defined and have been used as epidemiological markers.

The major vertebrate hosts of SLE are birds, especially domesticated sparrows (*Passer domesticus*), which act as the main amplifying host (Centers for Disease Control, 1991b). In addition, small mammals such as racoons, opossums and rodents are also infected, as well as a variety of domestic animals. However, other than birds, there is no evidence that animals play any role as maintenance or amplifying hosts.

Invertebrate vectors of SLE are various species of *Culex* mosquitoes, depending on location. In the rural west it is *C. tarsalis*, in the northern and southern regions of the central USA it is mainly *C. pipiens* and *C. quinquefasciatus*, and in Florida *C. nigripalpus*.

Epidemiology

In all parts of the USA the transmission cycle of SLE involves birds and mosquitoes. Man and probably domestic animals are incidental and dead-end hosts. Epidemiological characteristics, however, differ in the three regions described above. Thus, in the central USA, where *C. pipiens* and *C. quinquefasciatus* are the major vectors, epidemic outbreaks result from the build-up of virus in domesticated house sparrows and mosquito larvae breeding in discarded containers and open house foundations, characteristic of older housing construction. Regular outbreaks have occurred at approximately 10 year intervals until 1977, followed by irregular, unpredictable outbreaks observed in large urban localities. In the western USA, SLE occurs as low-grade endemic activity transmitted by *C. tarsalis* and associated with agricultural irrigation, although there are exceptions, such as the large focal outbreak in Los Angeles in 1984, which was probably due to *C. pipiens* acting as an accessory vector.

Clinical Features

The majority (over 90%) of infections with SLE virus are asymptomatic. In clinically apparent cases, the disease is characterised by an abrupt onset of a febrile illness accompanied by constitutional symptoms of malaise, nausea, vomiting and headache. Occasionally there may be a more slow insidious onset. Central nervous system involvement may be in the form of aseptic meningitis or focal encephalitis. Encephalitis signs may be manifested as neck stiffness, dizziness,

ataxia, mental confusion and disorientation. Cranial nerve palsies may occur in about 20% of cases, but the absence of focal findings or seizures may be useful differential features to distinguish SLE from cases of focal encephalitis, such as herpes simplex. In more severe cases there may be midbrain involvement and progressively severe coma. Overall case fatality is approximately 9% of symptomatic cases, although in outbreaks it may reach 20%. The likelihood of encephalitis, and also its severity, is related directly to age, with case fatalities in the elderly during outbreaks reaching 30% (Monath, 1980).

Diagnosis

For rapid serological diagnosis of SLE infection, the IgM antibody capture ELISA is the method of choice, using either serum or CSF. Cross-reactions may occur if other flaviviruses are active in the area, but this is not a major factor in North America. The IF test on SLE-infected cells is a useful alternative to the IgM ELISA for testing sera, and the HI test may be used for surveys or diagnosis if acute and convalescent sera are available. In regions where flavivirus activity is confined mainly to one virus, the HI test would be a useful screening test, followed by the SLE IgM antibody capture ELISA test to determine recent SLE infection.

Control

Although Sabin developed an inactivated mouse-brain vaccine during the Second World War, no licensed vaccine is available at present because of the low priority accorded to the infection. Similarly, specific vector control programmes directed at SLE are either impractical or thought not to be of sufficient urgency. Secondary measures to protect against mosquito bites, such as insect repellent and screening, may be of some benefit during reported outbreaks.

WEST NILE VIRUS

West Nile virus (WN) is one of the most ubiquitous of human arbovirus infections, being found throughout Africa, in Asia, parts of Europe, USA and Canada. The virus was first isolated in the West Nile province of Uganda in 1937.

Viral Features and Host Range

WN is related by neutralisation tests to the other members of the JE subgroup of flaviviruses, particularly *Kunjin virus* which is believed to have evolved from, or is a variant of, WN virus.

The major vertebrate hosts of WN are birds, although in addition the virus is able to infect a variety of domesticated animals (particularly equines) and wild animals, as well as man and subhuman primates. There is a suggestion that WN is becoming more widespread throughout animal species, with isolates from dogs and around 100 species of birds. The death of a harbour seal due to WN has been recorded in the USA. The maintenance vectors of WN consist of a variety of mosquitoes, especially of the genus *Culex*. On the basis of a study of phylogenetic relationships of isolated viruses, WN can be broadly classified into two lineages, lineage I, consisting of isolates from Central and North Africa, Europe, Israel and North America. Isolates from Central and Southern Africa and Madagascar are classified as lineage II.

Epidemiology

The transmission cycle of WN consists mainly of wild birds as the vertebrate host and ornithophilic *Culex* mosquitoes as the maintenance vector. The major *Culex* mosquito vector in Africa and the Middle East is *C. univittatus*; in south-east Asia, *C. tritaeniorhynchus*; and in France, *C. modestus*. *Culex* species appear to be the main vectors in North America, with isolates having also been made from *Ochlerotatus* spp. and *Aedes* spp. Other vectors were also implicated with limited isolations.

Major epidemics of WN have been reported in Israel during the 1950s, in France in 1962 and the largest epidemic ever recorded took place in South Africa in 1974, which involved tens of thousands of individuals. Epidemics have occurred characteristically in relatively localised areas, e.g. close to Tel Aviv in the Israeli epidemic, in the Rhone delta in France and the semi-desert Karoo region and in and around major cities of the high veld of South Africa. The distribution of WN in South Africa is predominantly in the inland plateau region, where it shares the same geographical distribution and ecology as *Sindbis virus*, which also produces a disease which is usually clinically indistinguishable from WN. The presence of WN in the USA was first recognised in 1999, and had spread extensively to at least 43 states by October 2002, and to provinces of Canada.

Outbreaks of WN, as with many other arboviruses, have been governed by climatic conditions, such as heavy rainfall particularly in early summer, and high summer temperatures. During outbreaks high attack rates in humans have been observed, e.g. in some worst-affected towns in South Africa, 50–80% of the human population were infected due to the high rate of feeding by *C. univittatus*. This mosquito is probably also responsible for sporadic cases in interepidemic periods. In the early stages of the epidemic in the USA, WN virus infection was recognised in mid- to late summer. In 2002 the virus was detected as early as May. Because viraemia is low in man, epidemic activity is directly due to infection of mosquitoes from viraemic birds and human outbreaks are merely the 'spill-over' of extensive epizootic activity in birds—an important factor which facilitates epidemiological surveillance. Furthermore, no human-to-human transmission occurs, although there have been recent reports of transfusion and organ donor infection and a case of intrauterine transmission, and, as in the case of JE, human population immunity has no bearing on the suppression of epidemic activity itself, and susceptible individuals would remain vulnerable irrespective of the proportion of immune individuals in the population.

Clinical Features

In the majority of cases WN presents as a mild febrile illness. The onset of disease is characteristically sudden, following a short incubation period of 3–5 days. Fever is usually the first sign, followed by headache, nausea and vomiting. Ocular pain is frequently reported, as is pharyngitis. Muscle pain occurs diffusely and there may be arthralgia.

During the first few days after onset, a maculopapular rash usually appears, which is discrete, with each of the rash elements demarcated by a sharp halo. The rash usually first appears on the trunk and then spreads to the face and extremities, and may persist for a week. Unlike measles, there is no desquamation.

Convalescence is rapid in children but may be somewhat more prolonged in adults and characterised by weakness and malaise. The illness not infrequently recrudesces during the convalescent period. Up to October 2002, approximately 6% of reported cases in the USA were fatalities.

Although WN virus is classified virologically within the JE group of mosquito-borne encephalitides, involvement of the CNS was believed to be very rare. However, in the USA the incidence of CNS involvement was much more common, with approximately 0.7% of patients showing severe neurological illness and up to 69% of reported cases showing some clinical evidence of meningoencephalitis. Acute flaccid paralysis (AFP) attributed to Guillain–Barré syndrome has been associated with WN virus infection, several cases having been reported in the USA (Centers for Disease Control, 2002).

Rarely, cases of visceral involvement including severe hepatitis, occasionally with a haemorrhagic presentation, have been reported.

Diagnosis

The HI, CF or NT tests can be used for serological diagnosis of WN infection. The HI test detects antibodies within a few days after onset, but the IgM antibody capture ELISA is recommended as the diagnostic test of choice for WN virus infection. Cross-reactivity is not a problem in patients with no previous exposure to flavivirus infection or vaccination. The NT assay would be used to identify specific flavivirus antibodies.

Virus isolation may be readily achieved from blood from infected individuals, despite lower levels of viraemia. Suckling mice are particularly sensitive to intracerebral inoculation and, in addition, cell culture of mammalian origin as well as insect cell lines are commonly used for virus isolation. RT-PCR is a rapid method for the detection of WN viral RNA.

Control

With the impact of WN on human health in the USA, there has been increasing interest in the development of a vaccine. During outbreaks, vector control by insecticide spraying may be applied. Epidemiological surveillance makes use of sentinel animals, such as hamsters, goats, guinea-pigs or pigeons, to detect early warning signs of impending outbreaks.

MURRAY VALLEY ENCEPHALITIS

Murray Valley encephalitis virus (MVE) is a relatively uncommon cause of human disease—less than 1000 cases have been reported—all of them confined to Australia and New Guinea.

The disease was first recognised during two epidemics of a virulent encephalitis in Queensland and in the Murray Valley in 1917 and 1918. A number of epidemics were subsequently described until 1925, followed by an inexplicable gap until the 1950s. The last substantial epidemic took place in 1974 and since then only some individual sporadic cases have occurred.

The infection is found in a patchy distribution from New Guinea through Darwin to the northern parts of Western Australia and down the east coast as far south as Brisbane, and in the basin of the Murray Darling River. The virus was reintroduced to Central Australia in 2000 following a period of unusually high rainfall.

Viral Features and Host Range

The virus displays a close relationship with *Kunjin virus* and also JE. Two distinct strains can be demonstrated, a New Guinea and an Australian variant. Individual isolations within the two groups are, however, remarkably conserved.

Epidemiology

The major maintenance vector is *Culex annulirostris* and a number of vertebrate hosts, chiefly wild birds, are involved in the transmission cycle. Domestic animals are infected, but they probably do not play any significant role as amplifying hosts. Outbreaks have characteristically occurred in the summer months.

Clinical Features

As with most other arboviruses, the vast majority of infections are asymptomatic—only about 1/800–1000 infections being clinically manifest (Anderson, 1954). Once clinical disease occurs, however, high case fatality rates of 18–42% have characterised the various outbreaks. The clinical features in symptomatic patients are a sudden onset of high fever (up to 40.6°C), nausea, vomiting and severe frontal headache. Signs of encephalitis vary from mild neurological involvement with disturbances of consciousness and neck stiffness to rapid onset of coma with respiratory failure. Patients with severe neurological involvement and coma, who were kept alive on life-support systems and subsequently survived, have all had remaining permanent and severe sequelae.

Diagnosis

Serology is generally carried out by HI or ELISA tests. The RT-PCR assay may detect MVE early after onset of illness, providing a rapid and specific diagnosis.

TICK-BORNE ENCEPHALITIS

The tick-borne encephalitides (TBEs) are a closely related subgroup of viruses within the genus *Flavivirus*. Although serological tests such as HI and CF give considerable cross-reactivity with members of the flavivirus group, the tick-borne encephalitis (TBE) subgroup of flavivirus are far more closely antigenically related to each other. In contrast to many of their mosquito-borne arbovirus counterparts, the tick-borne encephalitis subgroup is found almost exclusively (with some exceptions, such as louping ill in the UK and Powassan in North America) in Asia and eastern and central Europe. Within the subgroup is the entity of TBE, which consists of two subtypes: TBE—Central European subtype, or *Central European encephalitis virus* (CEE), and TBE—Far Eastern subtype, or *Russian Spring-Summer encephalitis virus* (RSSE). Other viruses within the TBE subgroup are *Omsk haemorrhagic fever virus*, *Kyanasur forest disease virus* and *Powassan virus*, which will be considered separately.

Virological Features

CEE and RSSE viruses are particularly closely related to each other and are distinguishable only by monoclonal antibodies or specialised techniques such as antibody adsorption tests. However, monoclonal antibody studies of CEE, especially those directed against glycoprotein domains, demonstrate a degree of antigenic complexity. Also, studies of different isolates of RSSE from different geographical locations have shown a heterogeneity of biological characteristics, such as mouse pathogenicity and plaque size. The two viruses display clearly distinguishable biological differences from each other. The distribution of the two infections closely follows that of their arthropod vectors—*Ixodes ricinus* in the case of CEE and *Ixodes persulcatus* in the case of RSSE. The geographical distribution of CEE stretches from Russia in the east

through Finland and Sweden in the north, through Germany to France in the west and down to Italy, Greece and Yugoslavia in the south, encompassing the central European countries in between. RSSE is found predominantly in the taiga (the coniferous forest belt on the edge of the steppes and the tundra region of Siberia) and in western Siberia. Their pathogenic potentials are also different, CEE causing a very much milder disease in experimentally infected sheep and monkeys as compared to RSSE, and this is reflected also in the clinical expression of their respective infections in man. Domestic animals, such as sheep, goats and cows, infected with CEE excrete virus in their milk. The virus is also relatively stable to low pH and, experimentally, animals can rarely be infected by oral inoculation. In man, milk-borne transmission of CEE through ingestion of goat, sheep or cow's milk or dairy products made from them, such as cheese, is an important route of acquisition.

Epidemiology

Both CEE and RSSE are endemic diseases with an increased seasonal incidence in the summer months related to climatic conditions of temperature and humidity, which affect tick activity. Infections occur predominantly in rural populations, especially farmers and forest workers. In addition, some 10–20% of CEE infections are transmitted through ingestion of goat, sheep and cow's milk and dairy products. Seroprevalence studies of RSSE virus have shown population prevalences of up to 50% in inhabitants of the taiga. Seroprevalence to CEE depends on rural residence, occupation and age. Thus, in various studies in central Europe, seroprevalence figures of 11–20% have been found in hunters, 5% in farmers and 1% in children (Gresikova *et al.*, 1973).

Clinical Features

Disease due to CEE is relatively mild, with a low fatality of less than 5%. The incubation period is 1–2 weeks, followed by symptoms and signs of a non-specific febrile illness, headache, nausea, vomiting, lassitude and occasionally some signs of neurological disorders may appear, especially related to visual disturbances: blurring of vision and diplopia. This initial viraemic phase of the illness usually lasts some 4–6 days and is followed by a brief remission period.

The majority of individuals infected probably only experience a monophasic illness, which is rarely diagnosed specifically.

The second phase of the biphasic illness commences after a brief remission period, and is heralded in by a recrudescence of fever and signs of meningitis. The most important signs of encephalitis are extrapyramidal and cerebellar syndromes, which may often persist for months after recovery. Localising neurological signs, such as cranial nerve involvement, occur uncommonly and are usually mild. The mortality in various outbreaks which have been studied has varied (1–5%).

A more severe degree of encephalitis is usually seen with RSSE virus. The incubation period is similar but this is usually followed by sudden onset of fever and constitutional symptoms and, in the second phase of illness, a more intense meningitis. In some individuals an aseptic meningitis picture may be the sole clinical manifestation of disease. In others encephalitic signs and symptoms, such as disturbed consciousness, may lead to stupor, coma and death. A characteristic feature is lower motor neuron paralysis, which may resemble poliomyelitis but usually predominantly affects the upper limbs, spreading to the neck, and which may be followed by bulbar paralysis and death. The reported case fatality rates have varied (8–54%). In addition, residual paresis and atrophy of muscles of the upper limbs and neck may persist for long periods. Post-recovery epileptiform seizures may reflect permanent neural damage.

Diagnosis

The IgM antibody capture ELISA on serum or CSF is the serological test of choice for diagnosis of TBE virus infection. The HI test is useful but a significant rise in antibody level must be demonstrated before a diagnosis can be made. Virus can be isolated from blood or CSF but specimens must be taken early after onset of symptoms. The virus may also be readily isolated from post mortem tissues such as brain and also infected tick pools. The virus is readily isolated by intracerebral inoculation of suckling mice or cell cultures, such as Vero or chick embryo.

Control

Vaccines have been developed against both CEE and RSSE viruses. In the case of CEE, a number of candidate vaccines have undergone trials. The most commonly used human vaccine, FSME-Immun, has been administered extensively in central Europe with very few mild allergic-type side-effects (Stephenson, 1988). The seed virus was derived from an Austrian tick isolate cloned in chick embryo cells and the vaccine has proved to be highly effective. A non-pathogenic related virus isolated from a bank vole, the *Skalica virus*, is being investigated as a possible candidate for a live attenuated vaccine.

The development of vaccines for RSSE has been less successful. The original RSSE vaccine, developed by Silber soon after the recognition of the infection in 1937, consisted of an inactivated suspension of infected mouse brain. However, the presence of contaminating myelin posed an unacceptable risk of encephalitogenic side-effects and its use in man was withdrawn. Several attempts at developing a tissue culture-grown vaccine strain have not yielded a successful human vaccine. As with CEE, a surrogate non-pathogenic virus is being investigated as a possible live attenuated vaccine strain—the *Langat TP21 virus*, isolated in Malaya.

OMSK HAEMORRHAGIC FEVER

Viral Features and Host Range

Omsk haemorrhagic fever virus (OHF) is closely related to TBE and cannot be differentiated using polyclonal hyperimmune sera. They are differentiated on gel precipitation using cross-absorbed monospecific sera. The infection is conveyed by ixodid ticks, *Dermocenter reticulates* and *D. marginatus*. A number of animal species are susceptible and the virus has been isolated from wild rodents. However, the most important vertebrate host is the muskrat (*Ondatra zibethica*), which is highly susceptible to infection, the virus usually producing a rapidly fatal haemorrhagic disease. The virus is excreted in the urine and faeces of sick animals and horizontal infection as well as arthropod infection is thought to play a role in transmission. The majority of human infections (60%) have occurred in hunters of muskrats, with transmission occurring as a result of direct contact during the skinning of animals. A further 28% of infections occur in adult family contacts of hunters.

Epidemiology

Infection has been limited to the Omsk region in the forest-steppe landscape of western Siberia, adjacent to

TBE endemic zones. The majority of cases were recorded between 1945 and 1949. Between 1945 and 1958, a total of 1488 cases were recorded, with no typically transmitted cases occurring since then. Occasional laboratory-acquired infections have been reported (Jelinkova-Skalova et al., 1974).

Clinical Features

Clinically the disease presents with a sudden onset of fever, headache and myalgia. There is a recrudescence of fever followed by haemorrhagic manifestations, especially epistaxis, but also gastrointestinal bleeding and bleeding at other sites. Bronchopneumonia is a frequent complication and occasionally meningitis may occur with long-term complications, such as psychomotor retardation and depression.

Diagnosis and Control

Infection may be diagnosed by isolation of virus from patients' blood and intracerebral inoculation into suckling mice. Serological testing by ELISA, CF and NT are also available. Control measures to prevent infection involve the avoidance of ticks and care in handling muskrat carcasses in endemic areas, as well as laboratory safety measures. Because of extensive cross-reactivity, CEE vaccine would probably impart good protection.

KYASANUR FOREST DISEASE

Viral Features and Host Range

The first isolation of *Kyasanur forest disease virus* (KFD) was made in 1957 from a dead monkey found near the Kyasanur State forest in Kamataka (formerly Mysore) State in India. A few months previously a lethal epizootic amongst monkeys had been reported in the adjacent forested areas, with human cases termed 'monkey disease' by the villagers. So far all human cases have been limited to Kamataka State—on average, about 500/year, in addition to a number of laboratory-acquired infections in both India and the USA. There is no evidence of the disease having existed prior to 1957.

Epidemiology

In addition to monkeys, a number of rodents are known to be infected, such as rats and shrews, as well as bats and other animals. The main tick vector is *Haemophysalis spinigera*. Infection occurs predominantly in poor villagers working in forests.

Clinical Features

The disease is characterised by a sudden onset of fever after an incubation period of 3–8 days. The fever may rise rapidly to 40°C, associated with headache and severe myalgia reminiscent of dengue fever. Muscle pain is also predominantly found in the back and neck regions. A regular finding in patients in the acute stage is papulovesicular lesions on the soft palate. There is usually a cervical and axillary lymphadenopathy but occasionally this is generalised. Earlier reports of the disease laid great emphasis on the haemorrhagic manifestations, which occurred as early as the third day of illness. These consist of bleeding from the nose, gums and gastrointestinal tract. Associated with this there is a marked thrombocytopenia and neutropenia, but no evidence of bone marrow suppression or capillary damage. The cause of the haemorrhagic diathesis has more recently been thought to be auto-immune in nature (Pavri, 1989). Many of these earlier cases were reported in poor villagers, who were often infected with bacteria and parasites, and the associated raised interferon levels and IgE antibodies may also have contributed to the original clinical picture. Later studies of the disease, including those of laboratory-acquired infections, have rather put emphasis on neurological complications, such as severe headache, neck stiffness, coarse tremors, abnormal reflexes and mental disturbances. Mortality in KFD is approximately 5–10%.

Diagnosis and Control

The virus can be readily isolated from patients' blood using mice or cell culture and antibodies can be detected by HI, CF, NT or ELISA tests. Vector control programmes have been carried out in the forest, especially spraying in the vicinity of dead monkeys when these are encountered. A formalin-inactivated vaccine has been prepared in India and immunisation programmes of villages in the affected areas have been carried out.

POWASSAN VIRUS

Viral Features and Host Range

Powassan virus (POW) is named after the town of Powassan in northern Ontario, where the first human virus isolate was made from a fatal encephalitis case in a 5 year-old boy. The disease is rare, less than 50 cases having been reported worldwide. Case reports have come from Canada and the USA as well as Russia.

Epidemiology

A number of arthropod vectors have yielded isolates of the virus. In North America the major vector has been *Ixodes cookie*, with *Dermacentor andersoni*, *Ixodes marxi* and *I. spinipalpus* and, in Russia, *Haemaphysalis neumanni*, *Ixodes persulcatus* and *Dermacentor silvarum* occasionally being infected. In addition, infected mosquito species, *Aedes togoi* and *Anopheles hrycanus*, have also been reported. Vertebrates infected with POW have occurred mainly in mammals, but also birds, amphibians and reptiles.

Clinical Features

Clinical cases of POW have presented with encephalitis, meningoencephalitis and aseptic meningitis. In some cases focal encephalitic signs have occurred and in one case from Russia the patient died following bulbar paralysis. In a series of 19 cases in North America, two deaths occurred in the acute illness phase.

REFERENCES

Anderson SG (1954) Murray Valley encephalitis and Australian disease. *J Hyg*, **52**, 447.

Anonymous (1980) *Guide for Diagnosis, Treatment and Control of Dengue Haemorrhagic Fever*, 2nd edn. Technical Advisory Committee on DHF for the South-east Asian and Western Pacific Regions. World Health Organization, Geneva.

Bharadwaj M, Prakash V, Mathur A and Chaturvedi UC (1991) Prognostic significance of serum iron levels in cases of Japanese encephalitis. *Postgrad Med J*, **67**, 247–249.

Cecilia D and Gould EA (1991) Nucleotide changes responsible for loss of neuroinvasiveness in Japanese encephalitis virus neutralization-resistant mutants. *Virology*, **181**, 70–77.

Centers for Disease Control (1990) Yellow fever vaccine. Recommendations of the Immunization Practices Advisory Committee (ACIP). *Morbid Mortal Wkly Rep*, **39**, 1–6.

Centers for Disease Control (1991a) Dengue epidemic—Peru, 1990. *Morbid Mortal Wkly Rep*, **40**, 145–147.

Centers for Disease Control (1991b) St Louis encephalitis outbreak—Arkansas, 1991. *Morbid Mortal Wkly Rep*, **40**, 605–607.

Centers for Disease Control (2002) Acute flaccid paralysis syndrome associated with West Nile virus infection—Mississippi and Louisiana, July–August 2002. *Morbid Mortal Wkly Rep*, **51**, 825–827.

Chen WR, Tesh RB and Rico-Hesse R (1990) Genetic variation of Japanese encephalitis virus in nature. *J Gen Virol*, **71**, 2915–2922.

Gresikova M, Thiel W et al. (1973) Haemagglutinin-inhibition antibodies against arboviruses in human sera from different regions in Steiermark (Austria). *Zentralbl Bakteriol Parasit, Infektionsk Hyg*, **1**(224), 298.

Gubler DJ and Costa-Valez A (1991) A program for prevention and control of epidemic dengue and dengue haemorrhagic fever in Puerto Rico and the US Virgin Islands. *Bull PAHO*, **25**, 237–247.

Halstead SB (1981) Arboviruses of the Pacific and South-East Asia. In *Textbook of Paediatric Infectious Diseases* (eds Feigin RD and Cherry JD), p 1132. WB Saunders, Philadelphia, PA.

Halstead SB (1984) Selective primary health care: strategies for control of disease in the developing world. XI. Dengue. *Rev Infect Dis*, **6**, 251.

Halstead SB (1989) Antibody, macrophages, dengue virus infection, shock, and hemorrhage: a pathogenic cascade. *Rev Infect Dis*, **II**(suppl 4), S830–S839.

Iversson LB (1980) Aspects of the encephalitis epidemic caused by arbovirus in the Ribeira Velley, Sao Paulo, Brazil, during 1975–1978. *Rev Saude Publ*, **14**(1), 9–35.

Jacobs MG, Brook MG, Weir WRC and Bannister BA (1991) Dengue haemorrhagic fever: a risk of returning home. *Br Med J*, **302**, 828–829.

Jelinkova-Skalova E, Tesarova J, Buresova V et al. (1974) Laboratory infection with virus of Omsk haemorrhagic fever with neurological and psychiatric symptomatology. *Ceskoslovenska Epidemiol Microbiol Immunol* (*PRAHA*), **23**(4,5), 290–293.

Jennings AD, Gibson CA, Miller BR et al. (1994) Analysis of a yellow fever virus isolated from a fatal case of caccine-associated human encephalitis. *J Infect Dis*, **169**, 512–518.

Konishi E, Pincus S, Fonseca BAL et al. (1991) Comparison of protective immunity elicited by recombinant vaccinia viruses that synthesize E or NS1 of Japanese encephalitis virus. *Virology*, **185**, 401–410.

Kurane I, Mady BJ and Ennis FA (1991) Antibody-dependent enhancement of dengue virus infection. *Rev Med Virol*, **1**, 211–221.

Monath TP (1980) *Epidemiology in St Louis Encephalitis* (ed. Monath TP), chapter 6. American Public Health Association, Washington, DC.

Nathan N, Barry M, Van Herp M and Zeller H (2001) Shortage of vaccines during a yellow fever outbreak in Guinea. *Lancet*, **358**, 2129–2130.

Nothdurft HD, Jelinek T, Marschang A et al. (1996) Adverse reactions to Japanese encephalitis vaccine in travellers. *J Infect*, **32**, 119–122.

Ogata A, Nagashima K, Hall WW *et al.* (1991) Japanese encephalitis virus neurotropism is dependent on the degree of neuronal maturity. *J Virol*, **65**, 880–886.

Pavri K (1989) Clinical, clinicopathologic and hematologic features of Kyasanur forest disease. *Rev Infect Dis*, **II**, S854–S859.

Rodrigues RM (1984) Epidemiology of Japanese encephalitis in India. In *National Conference on Japanese Encephalitis, 1982*. Indian Council of Medical Research.

Rosen L (1986) The pathogenesis of dengue haemorrhagic fever. *S Afr Med J* (suppl), 40–42.

Sharma S, Mathur A, Prakash V *et al.* (1991) Japanese encephalitis virus latency in peripheral blood lymphocytes and recurrence of infection in children. *Clin Exp Immunol*, **85**, 85–89.

Stephenson JR (1988) Flavivirus vaccines. *Vaccine*, **6**, 471–482.

World Health Organization (1990) Yellow fever in 1988. *Wkly Epidemiol Rec*, **65**, 213–220.

World Health Organization (1991) Yellow fever—epidemic in Cameroon, 1990. *Wkly Epidemiol Rec*, **66**, 76–77.

World Health Organization (1996) Inclusion of yellow fever vaccine in the EPI. *Wkly Epidemiol Rec*, **71**, 181–185.

World Health Organization (1996) Yellow fever in 1994 and 1995. *Wkly Epidemiol Rec*, **71**, 313–318.

18

Bunyaviridae

Robert Swanepoel

National Institute for Communicable Diseases, Sandringham, South Africa

INTRODUCTION

At present the family *Bunyaviridae* comprises approximately 300 animal viruses assigned to four genera: *Orthobunyavirus* (named after *Bunyamwera virus*), *Phlebovirus* (named after phlebotomus/sandfly fever), *Nairovirus* (named after *Nairobi sheep disease virus*) and *Hantavirus* (named after *Hantaan virus*). A further 40 inadequately characterised animal viruses are considered possible members of the family and there is a genus of plant viruses (Karabatsos, 1985; Calisher and Karabatsos, 1989; Peters and LeDuc, 1991; Calisher, 1991; Murphy *et al.*, 1995). Most of the animal viruses were discovered in the course of surveys on haematophagous arthropods or wild vertebrates, and the fact that new members of the family are constantly being encountered has been interpreted to indicate that many remain to be discovered (Peters and LeDuc, 1991). Some of the viruses are important pathogens of humans or livestock, but the majority have no known medical or veterinary significance. Sometimes a pathogenic role is discovered for a virus years after its initial isolation. Although most members of the family are thought to be arthropod-borne (i.e. arboviruses), transmission by vectors has been demonstrated conclusively in comparatively few instances. Members of the rodent-associated genus *Hantavirus* are not considered to be arthropod-borne.

The origins of the family can be traced to the initial detection of close antigenic relationships within certain groups of viruses, including one containing *Bunyamwera virus* (named after a place in Uganda) (Casals, 1957, 1961; Casals and Whitman, 1960, 1961). Subse-quently the demonstration of weak serological cross-reactions between the groups resulted in the viruses being included in a Bunyamwera supergroup (Anonymous, 1967). The family *Bunyaviridae*, containing a single genus *Bunyavirus*, was erected when members of the supergroup and certain ungrouped viruses were found to have similar morphology (Murphy *et al.*, 1973; Porterfield *et al.*, 1974; Fenner, 1976) and later the genera *Phlebovirus*, *Uukuvirus*, *Nairovirus* and *Hantavirus* were added to the family as morphological and biochemical affinities between the viruses became evident (Bishop *et al.*, 1980; Matthews, 1981; Schmaljohn *et al.*, 1985). More recently, the uuku-viruses were reduced to a serogroup within the genus *Phlebovirus*, since they were found to share coding and replication strategies with the phleboviruses, while the genus *Bunyavirus* has been renamed as genus *Ortho-bunyavirus* (Simons *et al.*, 1990; Calisher, 1991; Murphy *et al.*, 1995). Within genera, members are still classified on the basis of antigenic affinities and they are arranged in serogroups, antigenic complexes, viruses (or serotypes), subtypes and varieties, in order of increasing relatedness, i.e. members of a genus may only exhibit distant antigenic relationship to each other, whereas differences between varieties of a virus are consistent but minimal. However, the concept of classification of viruses by serotype has had to be revised with respect to agents that fail to grow in laboratory culture systems, with greater emphasis being placed on the definition of genotypes through nucleotide sequencing of the genome. This applies particularly to recently discovered hantaviruses (Monroe *et al.*, 1999).

Principles and Practice of Clinical Virology, Fifth Edition. Edited by A. J. Zuckerman, J. E. Banatvala, J. R. Pattison, P. D. Griffiths and B. D. Schoub
© 2004 John Wiley & Sons Ltd   ISBN 0 470 84338 1

THE VIRUS

Structure

The viruses of the family are spherical, 80–120 nm in diameter, and have a host cell-derived bilipid-layer envelope through which virus-coded glycoprotein spikes or peplomers project (Figure 18.1). The virions contain three major structural proteins: two envelope glycoproteins, G1 and G2, and a nucleocapsid protein N, plus minor quantities of a large or L protein (145–259×10^3 Da), believed to be the viral transcriptase, an RNA-dependent RNA polymerase (Table 18.1) (Bishop, 1990; Schmaljohn and Patterson, 1990; Peters and LeDuc, 1991; Calisher, 1991) (*Hazara virus* of the genus *Nairovirus* is believed to have three glycoproteins). Members of the family have a three-segmented, single-stranded RNA genome and each of the segments, L (large), M (medium) and S (small), is contained in a separate nucleocapsid within the virion. The sizes of the structural proteins and RNA segments vary with genus (Table 18.1). The genomic RNA is in the negative-sense (complementary to mRNA), but the

S segment of the *Phlebovirus* genome consists of ambisense RNA, i.e. has bi-directional coding, a property which is shared only with the RNA of viruses of the family *Arenaviridae*. The first 8–13 nucleotide bases at the 3′ ends of the RNA segments tend to have a sequence which is conserved within the viruses of each genus, with a complementary (palindromic) consensus sequence occurring at the 5′ end; and the ends of the segments are non-covalently linked, so that the RNA occurs in a loosely bound circular configuration within the nucleocapsids. The segmented nature of the genome suggests that the potential exists for reassortment to occur in co-infections, and it is thought that this mechanism may have contributed to the evolution of diversity in the family, but experimental evidence indicates that there are genetic restraints and that reassortment occurs with facility only between closely related members of bunyavirus serogroups or different strains of an individual phlebovirus (Peters and LeDuc, 1991).

The L RNA segment of the genome codes for the viral transcriptase, and the M segment for the G proteins, as well as a non-structural protein NS_m in the

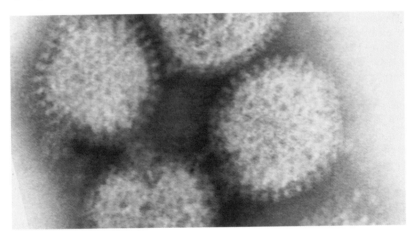

Figure 18.1

Table 18.1 Major biochemical properties of members of the *Bunyaviridae*. Information derived from sources cited in the text

Viruses	Molecular weights of major structural proteins ($\times 10^3$)			Molecular weights of RNA species ($\times 10^6$)		
	G1	G2	N	L	M	S
Bunyaviruses	108–120	29–41	19–26	2.7–3.1	1.8–2.3	0.3–0.5
Sandfly fever group	55–70	50–60	20–30	2.6–2.8	1.8–2.2	0.7–0.8
Uukuniemi group	70–75	65–70	20–25	2.0–2.5	1.0–1.3	0.4–0.7
Nairoviruses	72–84	30–40	48–54	4.1–4.9	1.5–2.3	0.6–0.7
Hantaviruses	64–76	52–58	48–54	2.2–2.9	1.2–2.9	0.6–0.75

genera *Orthobunyavirus* and *Phlebovirus*. The S segment RNA codes for the N protein, as well as a non-structural protein NS_S in the bunyaviruses and phleboviruses. Non-structural proteins have not as yet been demonstrated in the nairoviruses or hanta-viruses. The viral glycoproteins are responsible for recognition of receptor sites on susceptible cells, manifestation of viral haemagglutinating ability and for inducing protective immune response in the host. The N protein induces production of, and reacts with, complement-fixing antibody.

Biological Characteristics

Viruses which attach to receptors on susceptible cells are internalised by endocytosis and replication occurs in the cytoplasm. Virions mature primarily by budding through endoplasmic reticulum into cytoplasmic vesicles, which are presumed to fuse with the plasma membrane to release virus, but it appears that virus can also bud directly from the plasma membrane (Figure 18.2) (Anderson and Smith, 1987). Most of the viruses have been isolated and propagated by intra-cerebral inoculation of suckling mice, but the hantaviruses produce chronic and inapparent infection

of laboratory rodents. Members of the family can be grown in a variety of cell cultures (Vero cells have been most commonly used), but some of the viruses are non-cytolytic, so that their presence has to be demonstrated by immunofluorescence or similar means. Hanta-viruses are difficult to grow *in vitro*, and several of the more recently discovered members of the genus have not yet been adapted successfully to cell cultures (Monroe *et al.*, 1999).

An abridged classification of the family, showing selected members known to cause infection of humans and livestock in relation to their vectors and distribution, is presented in Tables 18.2–18.6 (Karabatsos, 1985; Calisher and Karabatsos, 1989; Peters and LeDuc, 1991; Calisher, 1991). In addition, high prevalences of antibody to many other viruses have been found in particular human populations, but conclusive evidence of infection or disease association is lacking: antigenic cross-reactivity between viruses can complicate the interpretation of survey findings or render it difficult to arrive at a serological diagnosis in individual cases of disease.

There is a broad tendency for antigenic grouping to correlate with geographic distribution and with the type of vector involved in transmission (Tables 18.2–18.4). Although a greater variety of arthropod-borne members occurs in tropical and subtropical countries

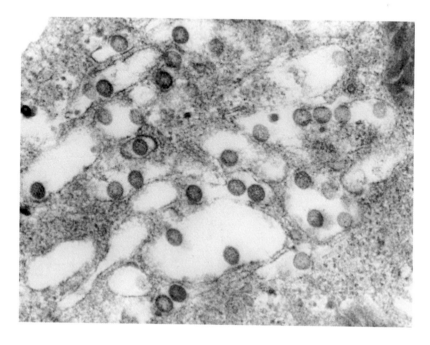

Figure 18.2

Table 18.2 Abridged classification of the genus *Orthobunyavirus* showing members known to cause infection of humans and domestic animals. Information derived from sources cited in the text

Serogroup ANTIGENIC COMPLEX Virus (synonym) Subtype Variety	Putative vectors	Human infection		Livestock disease	Distribution
		Natural	Laboratory		
Bunyamwera					
BUNYAMWERA (21)a					
Bunyamwera	Mosquitoes	+	+		Africa
Batai (Calovo)	Mosquitoes	+			Europe, Asia
Cache Valley	Mosquitoes	+		+	N. America
Maguari	Mosquitoes	+		?	S. America
Fort Sherman	Mosquitoes?	+			C. America
Germiston	Mosquitoes		+		Africa
Ilesha	Mosquitoes	+			Africa
Ngari	Mosquitoes	+	+		Africa, Madagascar
Shokwe	Mosquitoes	+			Africa
Tensaw	Mosquitoes	+			N. America
WYEOMYIA (8)					
Wyeomyia	Mosquitoes	+			C. and S. America
Three other complexes (3)					
Anopheles A					
TACAIUMA (6)					
Tacaiuma	Mosquitoes	+			S. America
One other complex (6)					
Anopheles B					
One complex (2)					
Bakau					
One complex (5)					
Bwamba					
BWAMBA (2)					
Bwamba	Mosquitoes	+			Africa
Pongola	Mosquitoes	+			Africa
Group C					
CARAPARU (5)					
Caraparu	Mosquitoes	+	+		C. and S. America
Ossa	Mosquitoes	+	+		C. America
Apeu	Mosquitoes	+	+		S. America
MADRID (1)					
Madrid	Mosquitoes	+			C. America
MARITUBA (6)					
Marituba	Mosquitoes	+	+		S. America
Murutucu	Mosquitoes	+	+		S. America
Restan	Mosquitoes	+			S. America
Nepuyo	Mosquitoes	+			C. and S. America
ORIBOCA (2)					
Oriboca	Mosquitoes	+	+		S. America
Itaqui	Mosquitoes	+			S. America
California					
CALIFORNIA ENCEPHALITIS (6)					
California encephalitis	Mosquitoes	+			N. America
Inkoo	Mosquitoes	+			Europe
La Crosse	Mosquitoes	+	+	+	N. America
Snowshoe hare	Mosquitoes	+			N. America
Tahyna (Lumbo)	Mosquitoes	+			Europe, Asia, Africa

(continued)

Table 18.2 *(continued)*

Serogroup
  ANTIGENIC COMPLEX
    Virus (synonym)
      Subtype
        Variety
	Putative vectors	Human infection		Livestock disease	Distribution

		Natural	Laboratory		
MELAO (7)					
Jamestown Canyon	Mosquitoes	+			N. America
Keystone	Mosquitoes		+		N. America
GUAROA (1)					
Guaroa	Mosquitoes	+			C. and S. America
One other complex (1)					
Capim					
Five complexes (10)					
Gamboa					
Two complexes (8)					
Guama					
GUAMA (4)					
Guama	Mosquitoes	+			C. and S. America
CATU (1)					
Catu	Mosquitoes	+	+		S. America
Three other complexes (7)					
Koongol					
One complex (2)					
Minatitlan					
One complex (2)					
Nyando					
NYANDO (2)					
Nyando	Mosquitoes	+			Africa
Olifantsvlei					
Two complexes (5)					
Patois					
Two complexes (7)					
Simbu					
AKABANE (2)					
Akabane	Ceratopogonids			+	Asia, Africa, Australasia
MANZANILLA (12)					
Oropouche	Ceratopogonids	+	+		S. America
Tinaroo	Ceratopogonids			+	Australasia
SHUNI (3)					
Shuni	Ceratopogonids	+		+	Africa
Aino	Ceratopogonids			+	Asia, Australasia
Four other complexes (8)					
Tete					
One complex (6)					
Turlock					
Two complexes (5)					
Ungrouped (4)					

[a]Figures in parentheses indicate the total numbers of recognised members of the relevant taxon.

of Latin America and Africa, many viruses, including several important pathogens, occur in temperate countries and the distribution of the family extends to the Arctic region. Moreover, there are many instances on record of residents of temperate countries, which lack indigenous disease, acquiring infection during travels abroad. Most of the viruses appear to be transmitted by culicine mosquitoes, including aedines, but some are transmitted by anopheline mosquitoes. Simbu serogroup viruses are associated particularly with ceratopogonid midges (*Culicoides* spp.), while the sandfly fever serogroup of phleboviruses (apart from Rift Valley fever and a few other mosquito-borne viruses), are associated with

Table 18.3 Abridged classification of the genus *Phlebovirus* showing members known to cause infection of humans and domestic animals. Information derived from sources cited in the text

Serogroup ANTIGENIC COMPLEX Virus (synonym)	Putative vectors	Human infection		Livestock disease	Distribution
		Natural	Laboratory		
Sandfly fever					
SANDFLY FEVER NAPLES (4)[a]					
Sandfly fever Naples	Phlebotomids	+			Europe, Africa, Asia
Toscana	Phlebotomids	+			Europe
CANDIRU (6)					
Alenquer	Phlebotomids?	+			S. America
Candiru	Phlebotomids?	+			S. America
PUNTA TORO (2)					
Punta Toro	Phlebotomids	+			C. America
RIFT VALLEY FEVER (3)					
Rift Valley fever (Zinga)	Mosquitoes	+	+	+	Africa
Four other complexes (8)					
Unassigned to complex (22)					
Sandfly fever Sicilian	Phlebotomids	+			Europe, Africa, Asia
Chagres	Phlebotomids	+			C. America
Uukuniemi					
UUKUNIEMI (13)					
Uukuniemi	Ixodids	+			Europe

[a]Figures in parentheses indicate the total numbers of members of the relevant taxon.

Table 18.4 Abridged classification of the genus *Nairovirus* showing members known to cause infection of humans and domestic animals. Information derived from sources cited in the text

Serogroup COMPLEX Virus (synonym)	Putative vectors	Human infection		Livestock disease	Distribution
		Natural	Laboratory		
Crimean-Congo haemorrhagic fever					
CRIMEAN-CONGO HAEMORRHAGIC FEVER (3)[a]					
Crimean-Congo haemorrhagic fever	Ixodids	+	+		E. Europe, Africa, Asia
Dera Ghazi Khan					
One complex (6)					
Hughes					
One complex (10)					
Nairobi sheep disease					
NAIROBI SHEEP DISEASE (2)					
Nairobi sheep disease (Ganjam)	Ixodids	+	+	+	Africa, Asia
Dugbe	Ixodids	+	+		Africa
Qalyub					
One complex (3)					
Sakhalin					
One complex (7)					
Thiafora					
One complex (2)					

[a]Figures in parentheses indicate the total numbers of members of the relevant taxon.

phlebotomids (sandflies). The Tete serogroup of bunyaviruses, the Uukuniemi serogroup of phleboviruses and the nairoviruses are associated with ixodid and argasid ticks. Some viruses have been isolated from more than one type of vector.

Transmission

It is characteristic of arthropod-borne viruses that they produce viraemia in at least one species of vertebrate to allow the infection to be acquired by biological vectors which take blood meals. During a so-called extrinsic incubation period, commonly lasting 1–2 weeks in dipterid vectors (mosquitoes, midges and sandflies), the virus replicates in the vector and spreads to produce infection of the salivary glands, thereby permitting transmission to occur to a second vertebrate host. Virus is thus maintained by circulation between the vector and a vertebrate host. The maintenance cycle may be cryptic, involving wild vertebrates which develop inapparent infection, with incidental spread of infection to susceptible domestic animals or humans which impinge on the cycle. It has been postulated that through selection pressure brought about by long association with the virus, natural maintenance hosts often develop transient viraemic infection without displaying susceptibility to the pathogenic effects of the virus concerned. Small mammals and birds, which occur in large numbers, breed prolifically to ensure a constant supply of non-immune individuals and are subject to periodic population explosions, constitute ideal maintenance hosts for arboviruses. Species susceptible to disease may themselves serve to amplify circulation of virus through infecting vectors, but humans serve this purpose for members of the *Bunyaviridae* in few instances only (Oropouche, sandfly fever) and are usually 'dead-end' hosts. Domestic animals which develop disease or undergo inapparent infection may serve as link hosts between the natural cycle and humans, which in turn gain infection from contact with infected tissues of livestock or products such as milk, or from vectors infected by feeding on livestock [Rift Valley fever, Crimean-Congo haemorrhagic fever (CCHF)].

Since the biting activity of arthropod vectors, and hence the infection of vertebrates, is seasonal, the fate of arthropod-borne viruses during winters or dry seasons of inactivity has long constituted a central enigma in the epidemiology of arbovirus diseases. Many plausible mechanisms for overwintering or hibernation of arboviruses have been described, including persistent infection of vertebrates, migration of infected birds or mammals, hibernation of infected adult vectors, and continuous vector activity in tropical locations (Reeves, 1974). Transovarial transmission of infection in arthropod vectors, however, theoretically constitutes an ideal mechanism for ensuring the perpetuation of the viruses, and comparatively early in the history of the investigation of arbovirus diseases convincing evidence was produced to indicate that the phenomenon occurs in phlebotomids and ixodid ticks (Tesh, 1984). The evidence for mosquito-borne viruses long remained in doubt, but in recent years many investigators have demonstrated transovarial transmission of bunyaviruses, particularly members of the California encephalitis serogroup, as well as *Rift Valley fever virus* and members of the families *Togaviridae* and *Flaviviridae* in mosquitoes (Tesh, 1984; Linthicum *et al.*, 1985; Peters and LeDuc, 1991; Swanepoel, 2003). Even in the absence of transovarial transmission of infection, the overwintering of viruses transmitted by ixodid ticks can be explained by the long intervals which occur between the feeding of successive instars of the vectors.

In general, viruses transmitted by dipterid flies (mosquitoes, midges and sandflies) may cause sporadic infections but are capable of causing explosive epidemics at irregular intervals of years, when climatic conditions are particularly favourable for the breeding of vectors, or human manipulation of the environment results in large-scale juxtaposition of susceptible persons or livestock and vectors. Viruses transmitted by ixodid ticks tend to cause sporadic disease in locations where there is occupational or recreational exposure of humans to ticks, but human intervention can precipitate the occurrence of larger outbreaks of disease.

Clinical syndromes associated with members of the *Bunyaviridae* range from inapparent infections known from routine monitoring of laboratory workers, through moderate to severe influenza-like illness with or without a maculopapular rash and characterised by fever (often biphasic), headache, myalgia, arthralgia and malaise, to encephalitis or haemorrhagic disease with necrotic hepatitis; while the hantaviruses of Asia and Europe are associated with a group of diseases known collectively as haemorrhagic fever with renal syndrome (HFRS), and the hantaviruses of the Americas are associated with an acutely fatal respiratory disease known as hantavirus pulmonary syndrome (HPS). The information presented below on the epidemiology and disease associations of individual viruses is derived from a few collated sources, except where indicated otherwise (Karabatsos, 1985; Calisher and Karabatsos, 1989; Porterfield, 1990; Gonzalez-Scarano and Nathanson, 1990; Peters and LeDuc, 1991; McKee *et al.*, 1991).

LABORATORY DIAGNOSIS

The appropriate specimens and laboratory methods required for confirming diagnoses of the more important diseases are indicated in the relevant sections dealing with the individual infections below.

Procedures developed and applied over decades for the isolation and identification of arthropod-borne members of the family, or for demonstrating immune responses, remain valid (Shope and Sather, 1979). However, there are residual problems concerning the sensitivity, specificity and rapidity with which certain infections can be diagnosed, and these are being solved through increasing utilisation of newer serological and molecular biological techniques. Isolation and identification of virus remains the definitive way of making a diagnosis, and this is especially true for what is perceived as a novel or as an undifferentiated febrile illness: it is easier to arrive at a serological diagnosis in diseases which are recognisable from their clinical presentation or from the circumstances under which patients become infected, such as Oropouche fever, sandfly fever, CCHF, Rift Valley fever, or HFRS. Sporadic undifferentiated febrile illnesses, in contrast, have usually been identified in the course of surveys, and the diagnosis of individual cases requires clinical acumen and recourse to the services of a specialised laboratory able to screen for a range of viruses known or considered likely to occur in the area where the infection was acquired.

Virus Detection and Identification

Most members of the family were discovered through intracerebral inoculation of suckling mice, and this method is still widely used for isolating the viruses. A few of the viruses are also pathogenic for weaned mice or hamsters, some even by a peripheral route, and this constitutes a useful screening method for preliminary identification of isolates, e.g. *Rift Valley fever virus*. Some viruses that are non-pathogenic for laboratory rodents, such as the hantaviruses (not known to be arthropod-borne), can nevertheless be isolated in rodents through demonstrating the presence of viral antigens in tissues. Many cytopathic and non-cytopathic viruses, such as CCHF, can be isolated in mammalian cell cultures and detected by immunofluorescence. The method has the advantage that it is usually rapid and therefore clinically useful, but it is not invariably more sensitive than the use of suckling mice for isolating viruses that are present in low concentrations in pathological specimens. Certain viruses which are non-pathogenic for laboratory mice, such as some of the neotropical phleboviruses, were only discovered because they proved to be cytopathic in mammalian cell cultures. Although it has not been proved for members of the *Bunyaviridae*,

some arboviruses can be isolated most successfully by inoculation of mosquito cell cultures, which do not manifest a cytopathic effect, or live mosquitoes, and in these instances the isolation of virus has to be demonstrated by immunological means.

In some diseases, such as Rift Valley fever or CCHF, rapid diagnoses can sometimes be achieved without culturing virus, by demonstrating the presence of viral antigens directly in infected blood or other tissues by enzyme-linked immunoassay, immunofluorescence or a variety of other immunological methods. This approach was used in the discovery of hantaviruses in rodent tissues. In certain diseases, such as La Crosse encephalitis, it appears that virus is seldom present in blood or other tissues in infective concentrations at the time that the disease is recognised, while other viruses, such as the hantaviruses, appear to be present but are extremely difficult to isolate and adapt to laboratory host systems. An alternative is to detect viral nucleic acids in tissue extracts or histological sections by hybridisation with specific radiolabelled nucleic acid probes. A more sensitive technique is to use reverse transcription and the polymerase chain reaction to detect viral nucleic acids, and this has been used with notable success on blood and other tissues of human patients and rodents infected with hantaviruses. A further advantage of the technique is that it may be possible to select consensus sequence primers which are specific for either individual viruses, groups of viruses or all potential members of a genus (Puthavathana *et al.*, 1992; Arthur *et al.*, 1992; Nichol *et al.*, 1993; Xiao *et al.*, 1994; Monroe *et al.*, 1999).

Isolates are generally identified by serological means, and by definition viruses react most specifically with antisera in neutralisation tests, but these are technically difficult to perform with some viruses, or may not yield results sufficiently rapidly to be clinically useful. Antisera tend to be more cross-reactive in the other serological tests commonly used for the investigation of the *Bunyaviridae* (viz. complement fixation, haemagglutination-inhibition, immunofluorescence and enzyme-linked immunoassay) and this is particularly true within serogroups of the genus *Bunyavirus*. The problem can be overcome, and the process accelerated, by using monoclonal antibodies to achieve simultaneous detection and identification of isolates, as in immunofluorescence tests on cell cultures. In instances where potentially new viruses, or viruses associated with undifferentiated illnesses, have to be identified, cross-reactivity can be useful. Unidentified isolates may have to be tested against antisera to all of the known viruses of the region involved, or even ultimately against antisera to hundreds of viruses which occur elsewhere in the world, and the process is facilitated by preliminary screening of the isolates with pools of antisera, or antisera that have deliberately been rendered cross-reactive by immunising laboratory animals sequentially with several viruses. Morphological or partial biochemical characterisation of isolates, e.g. by performance of electron microscopic examination or tests for sensitivity to ether and bile salts, may also facilitate the process of identifying a virus.

In instances where viral nucleic acids have been detected, these can be identified by hybridisation under stringent conditions with labelled probes that are specific for individual viruses, or by demonstrating specific endonuclease restriction enzyme digestion patterns with the products of a polymerase chain reaction. However, it is becoming more common to perform nucleotide sequencing on the products of polymerase chain reactions to obtain more exact information on the phylogenetic relationships of the aetiological agents concerned (Monroe *et al.*, 1999).

Serology

Serological diagnosis of infections is beset with the same problems of cross-reactivity that apply to antigenic identification of isolates, and the difficulties are compounded where patients have previously been infected with an antigenically-related virus: antibody response tends to be broadly cross-reactive within serogroups following sequential infections. Neutralising antibody, which reacts most specifically for individual viruses, usually becomes demonstrable by day 7–10 of illness (earlier in Rift Valley fever) and, after an initial post-convalescent decline in titre, tends to remain demonstrable for life, but the response is usually weak and difficult to demonstrate following *Nairovirus* infections. Complement-fixing antibody becomes demonstrable in the second or third week of illness, declines after several months, and tends to be group-specific with bunyaviruses and nairoviruses, but more specific among phleboviruses. Antibody demonstrable by haemagglutination-inhibition, indirect immunofluorescence or enzyme-linked immunoassay becomes detectable at about the same time as neutralising antibody and, after a post-convalescent decline in titre, remains demonstrable for a period of several years at least, and varies in specificity in different groups of viruses. Demonstration of IgM antibody activity in indirect immunofluorescence tests or enzyme-linked immunoassays is most useful for establishing a rapid diagnosis. Antibody titres tend to be highest against the homologous infecting virus, so that problems of cross-reactivity can sometimes be overcome by screening patients' sera with a range of antigens prepared from all members of the virus serogroup known to occur in the area concerned, as is done with members of the California encephalitis serogroup. An alternative is the preparation of purified antigens that contain virus proteins or peptides which react specifically with serotype antibody, and this includes preparation of antigens by recombinant DNA technology (Feldmann *et al.*, 1993). The same effect may be obtained by selective capture of viral proteins with monoclonal coating antibody in enzyme-linked immunoassays.

GENUS *ORTHOBUNYAVIRUS*

Serogroup Bunyamwera

Bunyamwera, Ilesha, Ngari, Germiston and Shokwe Viruses

Bunyamwera virus is widely distributed in Africa and has been isolated from aedines and other culicine mosquitoes, and/or human blood in Uganda, South Africa, Kenya, Nigeria, Central African Republic, Cameroon and Senegal. Antibody has been found in humans and/or domestic animals, rodents, bats and subhuman primates in the same countries as well as in Mozambique, Tanzania, Angola, Congo, Egypt and Tunisia. However, some of the antibody reactions recorded in surveys may have been due to infection with related viruses. Despite the widespread occurrence of antibody, human disease has seldom been recognised and the few cases which have been described include several laboratory infections. Clinical findings included fever, maculopapular rash, arthralgia, neck stiffness, vertigo and temporary loss of visual acuity. Severe encephalitis occurred in experimental infection of a tumour patient. Infection was confirmed in patients by isolation of virus from blood or demonstration of an immune response. It seems likely that disease may be more common than currently realised.

Ilesha virus has been isolated from the blood of febrile humans in Nigeria, Uganda, Cameroon and the Central African Republic, and from anopheline mosquitoes in the latter country. In addition, there is serological evidence that the virus occurs in Senegal and Ghana. Few cases of disease have been reported, and these consisted of undifferentiated febrile illness with a rash.

Ngari virus has been isolated from mosquitoes in Senegal, Burkina Faso, the Central Africa Republic and Madagascar, as well as from a sheep in Mauritania and the liver of a person who succumbed to cerebral malaria in Senegal. A virus isolated from the blood of a human patient during the 1997–1998 Rift Valley fever epidemic in north-east Kenya and adjacent Somalia was thought to be a new bunyavirus and given the name *Garissa virus*, but it has subsequently been found to be an isolate of *Ngari virus* (Bowen et al., 2001; Nichol, 2003). There were many deaths from haemorrhagic disease which could not all be confirmed as cases of Rift Valley fever, and antibody to *Ngari virus* was found in patients in both Kenya and Somalia, but the importance of *Ngari virus* as a human pathogen remains to be determined.

Shokwe virus has been isolated from mosquitoes, mainly aedines but also from other culicines in South Africa, Senegal, Ivory Coast and Kenya, and from rodents and the blood of a febrile human in Ivory Coast. Little is known of the pathogenic potential of the virus. *Germiston virus* has been isolated in South Africa, Zimbabwe, Mozambique, Kenya and Uganda from *Culex rubinotus*, a mosquito which selectively feeds on rodents, and from myomorph rodents (rats and mice) in Uganda. Antibody has been found in the sera of humans and/or cattle and rodents in South Africa, Botswana, Namibia and Angola. Two laboratory infections have been reported; one with undifferentiated febrile illness with rash, and the other with signs of mild encephalitis. Virus was isolated from the blood of the patients.

Batai Virus

Calovo virus, first isolated from anopheline mosquitoes in 1960 in what was then Czechoslovakia, is believed to be closely related or identical to *Batai virus*, which had previously been isolated from culicine mosquitoes in Malaysia in 1955. Furthermore, the name 'Olyka' was provisionally used for *Batai virus* isolated from mosquitoes in the Ukraine, and *Chittoor virus* isolated from anophelines in India is also considered to be closely related or identical to *Batai virus*. Altogether, this cluster of viruses has been isolated from anopheline and culicine mosquitoes in Malaysia, Thailand, Cambodia, India, Yugoslavia, Austria, the former USSR and Czechoslovakia. Antibody has been found in the same countries, as well as in Sri Lanka,

Romania, Hungary, Germany, Portugal and Finland, in the sera of humans and/or birds, rodents, domestic ruminants and deer. The findings in seroprevalence studies suggest that human infection is seldom accompanied by overt disease, but febrile illness with malaise, myalgia, anorexia and sometimes abdominal pain, tonsillitis, cough and dyspnoea (associated with lung infiltration), has been reported from Czechoslovakia and Malaysia on the basis of serological diagnoses.

Cache Valley, Maguari, Fort Sherman, Tensaw and Wyeomyia Viruses

Cache Valley virus has been isolated from culicine and anopheline mosquitoes from widely separated locations in the USA and from Jamaica, and antibody has been found in the sera of humans and/or horses, sheep, cattle, wild rodents, raccoons, deer and monkeys in the USA, Canada, Trinidad and Guyana. Despite the occurrence of high antibody prevalence rates, human disease has not been reported. Recently, however, the results of serological studies and pathogenicity trials, and the isolation of virus from a sentinel sheep, incriminated *Cache Valley virus* as the causative agent of an outbreak of congenital abnormalities (hydranencephaly–arthrogryposis syndrome) among sheep in Texas (Chung et al., 1990a, 1990b). *Maguari virus*, a subtype of *Cache Valley virus*, has been isolated from mosquitoes, mainly aedines, in Brazil, Argentina, French Guiana, Colombia and Trinidad, and from horse blood in Guyana and Colombia. Antibody has been found in the same countries, as well as in Peru, Surinam and Venezuela, in the sera of humans and/or horses, cattle, sheep, water buffalo and birds. Human disease has not been reported, but the virus is suspected of causing disease in horses. *Fort Sherman virus*, yet another subtype of *Cache Valley virus*, was isolated from the blood of a patient with fever, malaise, myalgia and sore throat in Panama, but no further information on the virus is available. *Tensaw virus* has been isolated from several species of anophelines in south-eastern USA, where antibody has been found in humans, dogs, cattle and raccoons. A single case of encephalitis was reported in 1973. *Wyeomyia virus* has been isolated from a range of culicine mosquitoes in Colombia, Panama, French Guiana and Trinidad, and antibody has been found in human sera in Panama and Trinidad. The virus has been isolated once from the blood of a patient with febrile illness in Panama.

Serogroup Anopheles A

Tacaiuma Virus

Tacaiuma virus was isolated from the blood of a sentinel monkey and from forest mosquitoes in the Amazon region of Brazil, as well as from mosquitoes in Argentina. Antibody has been found in humans in Brazil and French Guiana, and in horses, rodents, bats and birds in Brazil. The virus has been isolated once from the blood of a patient with febrile illness in Brazil.

Serogroup Bwamba

Bwamba and Pongola Viruses

Bwamba virus was originally isolated from blood samples from nine road workers with febrile illness in Uganda, and subsequently from eight febrile patients in Nigeria, three in the Central African Republic and one in Kenya, and from anopheline mosquitoes in Uganda, Nigeria and Senegal. Antibody was found in human sera in Uganda, Tanzania, Mozambique, South Africa, Botswana, Angola, Congo, Nigeria and Guinea; generally with very high prevalence, up to 97% in some populations, and including both children and adults. Antibody was also found in donkeys and a bird in South Africa. *Bwamba virus* appears to be an important pathogen and the eight isolations in the Nigerian series represented 5% of all arbovirus isolations from febrile patients over a 7 year period, while 18 diagnoses (virological and serological) made in similar patients in the Central African Republic represented 25% of arbovirus infections diagnosed over a 13 year period. The patients suffered prostrating illness with fever, headache, conjunctivitis, rash, epigastric pain and myalgia, and many had meningeal signs.

There have been numerous isolations of *Pongola virus* from mosquitoes, mainly aedines and other culicines, in South Africa, Mozambique, Kenya, Uganda, Ethiopia, Central African Republic and Ivory Coast. There has been one isolation of the virus from a febrile patient with headache and myalgia in Uganda (Kalunda *et al.*, 1985). Neutralising antibody has been found in humans in South Africa, Mozambique, Botswana, Namibia and Angola, and in cattle, sheep, goats and donkeys in South Africa, but interpretation of the findings is complicated by the fact that there is unidirectional cross-neutralisation of *Pongola virus* by antibody to its close relative, *Bwamba*

virus. Moreover, the fact that most human isolates have reacted as Bwamba serotype, while most mosquito isolates have reacted as Pongola serotype, merits further investigation, particularly in view of a report that passage of a Bwamba isolate in mosquitoes led to selection of virus reacting as Pongola serotype (Johnson *et al.*, 1978).

Serogroup C

Apeu, Caraparu, Ossa, Madrid, Marituba, Murutucu, Restan, Nepuyo, Itaqui and Oriboca Viruses

Apart from one virus, which occurs in Florida, USA, all of the known members of serogroup C occur in Central and South America and tend to be associated with tropical forests. The viruses named above have all been isolated from the blood of febrile humans, and variously from sentinel monkeys, rodents, occasional marsupials and fruit bats, and from a range of culicine mosquitoes in Brazil, Surinam, French Guiana, Guatamala, Honduras, Trinidad, Panama or Mexico. Serological evidence suggests that some of these viruses may also occur in Venezuela, Colombia and Peru. Pairs of the viruses which are closely related antigenically may circulate in the same geographic location yet occupy separate ecological niches, e.g. one virus circulates in arboreal monkeys and mosquitoes which feed in the canopy layer, while a closely related virus circulates in rodents and mosquitoes which feed at the level of the forest floor. Other pairs of closely related viruses coexist in the same habitat simply by utilising different vectors. Sporadic infections occur in persons who enter forests. No large outbreaks of disease have been reported, but disease is observed when susceptible outsiders, such as military personnel, enter endemic regions. Laboratory infections are relatively common. Disease, which lasts for up to a week and runs a benign course, is characterised by fever, rigors, headache, photophobia, conjunctivitis, tachycardia, myalgia, arthralgia, prostration, leukopenia and, occasionally, pain in the right upper quadrant of the abdomen and jaundice.

Serogroup California

California encephalitis, La Crosse, Snowshoe hare, Jamestown Canyon and Keystone Viruses

California encephalitis virus, which is distributed across the western USA and into Canada, was isolated from mosquitoes in the early 1940s and shortly thereafter serological evidence was produced to indicate that it causes encephalitis. However, from the mid-1960s onwards it became clear that most cases of what are loosely termed 'California encephalitis' are in fact due to infection with the *La Crosse* subtype of virus, and this agent is responsible for the majority of the approximately 100 cases of arbovirus encephalitis diagnosed in the USA annually, except in years when there are epidemics of St Louis encephalitis (a flavivirus). It must also be borne in mind that since its introduction into North America in 1999, the mosquito-borne flavivirus *West Nile virus* has been responsible for a proportion of cases of encephalitis recognised each year, particularly in elderly or immunocompromised patients.

Most cases of disease due to *La Crosse virus* are recorded in the mid-west states of Wisconsin, Iowa, Indiana, Minnesota and Ohio, but the virus is widely distributed and the infection is probably underdiagnosed elsewhere in the USA. The principal vector is *Aedes triseriatus*, a tree hole-breeding mosquito, and accordingly the virus tends to be focally distributed in woodlands, but also occurs in suburban situations where water that collects in discarded containers, such as motor vehicle tyres, affords mosquito breeding sites. The virus is passed transovarially in the vector and overwinters in mosquito eggs; infection is amplified in the succeeding spring and summer in small mammals such as chipmunks and squirrels. The vector is a diurnal feeder and the infection is seen most commonly in forest workers and children who enter woodlands for recreational purposes, but also occurs focally in rural and suburban residents. Males are more commonly infected than females, among both children and adults. Seroprevalence surveys and prospective studies indicate that most infections are inapparent or benign. Probably less than 1% of infected adults develop encephalitis, but the incidence may be up to four times greater in young children.

After an incubation period of 3–7 days there is sudden onset of fever, headache, lethargy, nausea and vomiting, pharyngitis and sometimes respiratory illness. There is seldom a cutaneous rash. In mild cases of overt disease there may be transient meningismus and disorientation and recovery within 1 week. In severe disease there may be greater disturbance of consciousness, aphasia, tremors, chorea, positive Babinski signs and other abnormal reflexes, and hemiparesis in about 20% of patients. Seizures may occur from the second day of illness onwards: in about half of severely ill patients there may be generalised, life-threatening convulsions, and in a further 25% there are focal convulsions associated with frontal or parietal brain lesions. Approximately one-third of severely ill patients become comatose. There may be marked leukocytosis, and examination of cerebrospinal fluid reveals elevated mononuclear and polymorphonuclear cell counts, but protein and glucose levels tend to remain normal. Electroencephalograms show generalized slow-wave activity or localised changes and sometimes epileptiform discharges. Treatment is symptomatic and includes monitoring and control of intracranial pressure and vigorous anticonvulsant therapy as indicated. Less than 1% of patients with severe disease succumb and most are discharged from hospital after about 2 weeks of illness, but may remain irritable and emotionally labile for a few weeks. There are seldom residua, but patients who suffer seizures in the acute illness may have recurrent convulsions over a period of 1 or more years, and lasting hemiparesis occurs in about 1% of patients. Virus has not been isolated from throat swabs, blood, stools or cerebrospinal fluid, and only with difficulty from brain specimens. Histopathological lesions are not pathognomonic and include cerebral oedema, perivascular cuffing and focal gliosis in grey matter. A variety of methods are used for making a serological diagnosis, but demonstration of IgM antibody activity by means of enzyme-linked immunoassay holds greatest promise as a rapid diagnostic technique. There is no vaccine.

Snowshoe hare virus is a mosquito-borne subtype of *California encephalitis virus* with a distribution extending from north-western USA across most of Canada to Alaska. The natural host appears to be the snowshoe hare, *Lepus americanus*, and serological evidence suggests that the virus is occasionally associated with encephalitis in children and adults.

Jamestown Canyon virus is a mosquito-borne virus which occurs widely in the USA, and high prevalence rates of antibody are found in white-tailed deer, and in humans where there are high concentrations of the deer. Serological evidence of an association with encephalitis in humans has been found from the early 1980s onwards (Grimstad *et al.*, 1986). Since antigens and tests commonly used for the serodiagnosis of 'California encephalitis' fail to allow response to *Jamestown Canyon virus* to be distinguished from response to other members of the serogroup, it is felt that the infection has probably been missed or underdiagnosed as a cause of encephalitis in the past, both in the mid-west states and elsewhere where the deer occurs. In contrast to *La Crosse virus*, *Jamestown Canyon virus* appears to cause encephalitis more frequently in adults than in children, and nervous disease is often preceded by respiratory illness.

Keystone virus is associated with swamp-breeding aedines and cotton rats and rabbits in south-eastern USA, and has been known to cause inapparent accidental infection in the laboratory.

Tahyna and Inkoo Viruses

Tahyna virus is widely distributed in countries of central Europe, including Yugoslavia, Germany and Italy, with antibody prevalence rates being particularly high in the Rhone Valley of France, the Danube basin in Austria and in the southern Moravia region of the former Czechoslovakia, where up to 95% of adults may be immune in some communities. Viruses described as being Tahyna-like have been isolated in the former USSR, while *Lumbo virus*, which was isolated from saltwater-breeding mosquitoes on the coast of Mozambique, is considered to be indistinguishable from *Tahyna virus*. Antibody to *Tahyna virus* has also been found in southern China and Sri Lanka. It is not yet clear whether a single virus occurs throughout this range or whether, as seems more likely, a cluster of closely related viruses, subtypes or varieties is involved.

The epidemiology of the disease has been studied most intensively in Moravia where seasonal flooding of level woodlands provides extensive breeding sites for mosquitoes. The virus is transmitted transovarially in *Aedes vexans*, which overwinters as eggs, and in *Culiseta annulata*, which overwinters as larvae. Amplification of infection in spring occurs in small mammals such as hedgehogs, hares and rabbits, as well as in domestic animals such as horses. Hedgehogs may themselves serve as reservoir hosts for overwintering of virus in instances where they undergo chronic infection during hibernation, with viraemia which persists for a few days after awakening. Once infection of vertebrates occurs in summer, other species of mosquito also become infected and serve as vectors for transmission of the virus.

Seroprevalence surveys indicate that infection is much more common than overt disease in rural residents of Moravia. Nevertheless, the infection accounts for up to 20% of patients hospitalised with febrile illness in the region, including both adults and children. Patients may present with undifferentiated febrile illness with leukocytosis, but pharyngitis, cough, and chest pain and infiltration (demonstrable by X-ray imaging) may predominate, or gastrointestinal symptoms such as nausea, vomiting and abdominal pain may be dominant. Aseptic meningitis occurs in a minority of patients but fatal disease is unknown. Virus can be isolated from blood early in the illness, but the infection is usually diagnosed by demonstration of an antibody response. There is no vaccine.

Inkoo virus was isolated from aedine mosquitoes in Finland. Distribution of the virus extends to the Lapland region in the north of the country, and antibody occurs in the sera of humans, cattle, deer and hares. Antibody prevalence rates of up to 25% have been recorded in humans, and a few cases of febrile illness have been confirmed serologically.

Guaroa Virus

Guaroa virus has been isolated from 12 febrile patients in Colombia and the Amazon region of Brazil, and from anopheline mosquitoes in Panama and Colombia. Antibody has been found in human sera in Colombia, Brazil, Argentina and Peru. Disease ascribed to infection with the virus was characterised by fever, headache, myalgia, arthralgia, prostration and leukopenia. Virus was isolated from the blood of the patients, and from a liver biopsy in one instance.

Serogroup Guama

Guama and Catu Viruses

Catu virus has been isolated from sentinel monkeys in Brazil, febrile humans and forest rodents in Brazil and Trinidad, and from culicine and anopheline mosquitoes in the same two countries plus French Guiana. *Guama virus* has been isolated from febrile humans and sentinel monkeys in Brazil, and from rodents and/or culicine mosquitoes in Brazil, Trinidad, Surinam, French Guiana and Panama. The two viruses cause isolated cases of benign disease characterised by fever, headache, myalgia and leukopenia, in persons who enter tropical forests. *Catu virus* has also been associated with laboratory infection.

Serogroup Nyando

Nyando Virus

Nyando virus has been isolated from anopheline and aedine mosquitoes in Kenya, Central African Republic and Senegal. Antibody has been found in human sera in Kenya and Uganda, and the virus was isolated from the blood of a single human patient with biphasic fever, myalgia and vomiting in the Central African Republic.

Serogroup Simbu

Oropouche Virus

Oropouche virus was originally isolated from the blood of a febrile patient in Trinidad, but large epidemics involving thousands of people have occurred exclusively in northern Brazil over the past 20 years. In addition to humans, the virus has been isolated from a sloth, a few species of culicine mosquitoes and the midge *Culicoides paraensis*. Antibody has been found in the sera of humans and/or monkeys and birds in Brazil, Trinidad and Colombia. Virus is thought to be maintained in nature by circulation in forest primates, sloths or birds and an unidentified vector, and is introduced into urban settings by infected travellers or by extension from the sylvatic cycle. Humans serve as amplifier hosts in the urban cycle, and the vector is the *Culicoides* midge, which breeds in decaying waste from tropical agricultural products. Epidemics occur when there are large concentrations of vectors and susceptible humans. Aerosol infection is suspected to have occurred in laboratory workers. The incubation period is 4–8 days, and there is sudden onset of fever, chills, headache, myalgia, arthralgia and prostration. There may be a rash, and occasionally signs of meningitis or encephalitis, but there are no deaths or sequelae. Viraemia lasts 2–5 days, as does illness, but myalgia persists for a further 3–5 days, and strenuous exertion in early convalescence can precipitate a relapse of symptoms.

Akabane, Aino, Tinaroo and Shuni Viruses

Most members of the Simbu serogroup do not occur in the Americas, but are widely distributed in Africa, Asia and Australasia. Of these latter viruses, only *Shuni virus* has been marginally implicated in causing human disease, but a few have been incriminated as causative agents in large outbreaks of abortion, stillbirth and congenital defects (hydranencephaly–arthrogryposis syndrome) in domestic ruminants, particularly sheep and cattle, and the suspicion exists that most members of the serogroup have the potential for producing this type of disease. *Akabane virus* has been incriminated in outbreaks of the disease in Japan, Australia and Israel, *Aino virus* in Japan and Australia, *Tinaroo virus* in

Australia and *Peaton virus* has been shown to be teratogenic in experimental infections in Australia. The viruses are transmitted by species of *Culicoides* midges which mostly breed in dung, independently of available surface water, but which are favoured by the humid conditions created by heavy rainfall. The natural hosts of the viruses are unknown, but antibodies have been found in wild herbivores. Infection is usually inapparent in domestic ruminants. However, if infection occurs in pregnant animals at critical stages of gestation, there may be embryonal or fetal death, or arrestation of brain development (hydranencephaly), and the consequent lack of trophic effect of nervous stimulation on skeletal muscles of the fetus results in postural defects of the limbs, with joints locked in flexion (arthrogryposis). Once the stage of organogenesis in gestation is past, fetuses are less susceptible to the harmful effects of infection (the timing varies with length of gestation in different species).

Shuni virus has been isolated from cattle, sheep, midges and once from the blood of a febrile human in Nigeria, and from cattle and mosquitoes in South Africa. It was also isolated from the brain of a horse with histopathological lesions of meningoencephalitis, which was submitted for laboratory examination for suspected rabies in Zimbabwe (Foggin and Swanepoel, 1977).

GENUS *PHLEBOVIRUS*

Serogroup Sandfly fever

Sandfly fever Naples, Sandfly fever Sicilian and Toscana Viruses

Sandfly fever (also known as phlebotomus fever or pappataci fever from the vector, *Phlebotomus papatasi*) has been known for at least two centuries as a febrile illness encountered by armies invading the Mediterranean basin. It was demonstrated shortly after the start of the twentieth century that the disease was caused by a virus transmitted by sandflies, but it was only during the Second World War that it was shown that there are in fact two distinct viruses and that there is no cross-immunity. Between them, the two viruses are known to occur in Morocco, Tunisia, Egypt, Sudan, Somalia, Italy, Greece, Yugoslavia, Turkey, the former USSR, Israel, Saudi Arabia, Iraq, Iran, Pakistan, India and Bangladesh, and are probably present in many intervening countries. Throughout this range, *Phlebotomus papatasi* is the vector and it breeds in moist soil in dark niches such as in rubble, drains, cracks in soil and in animal burrows, equally successfully in large cities and remote rural locations. The viruses are transmitted transovarially in the vector, which over-winters in the larval stage, and adult flies emerge to assume biting activity in summer. High infection rates have been recorded in newly emerged sandflies and it is not known whether amplification in vertebrates is essential to ensure perpetuation of the viruses, but humans develop sufficiently intense viraemia to serve as source for the infection of the vector. No wild vertebrate hosts of the viruses are known, but antibody has been found in gerbils (whose burrows are utilised by the vector). Sandflies are nocturnal feeders, but will feed in dark rooms where they rest during daylight hours. Human infection rates recorded in outbreaks range from 3–75% but the attack rate varies focally and is influenced by background immunity in the human population. Large epidemics have often occurred in association with socio-economic upheavals, wars or natural disasters, such as earthquakes, which create ideal breeding conditions for sandflies and/or lead to widespread exposure of susceptible humans to sandflies.

Experimental evidence suggests that most sandfly fever infections are symptomatic. Typically, there is sudden onset of fever of 2–4 days duration, severe headache, sore eyes and photophobia, myalgia, arthralgia, anorexia and malaise. Occasionally there may be sore throat, nausea and vomiting, abdominal pain and diarrhoea, epistaxis and dizziness. Patients may have injected conjunctivae and a flushed appearance, but there is seldom a rash and meningeal signs are rare. The disease may be milder in children. Treatment is symptomatic. Recovery is complete and no deaths have been recorded. There appears to be lifelong immunity to the homologous virus. The diagnosis can be confirmed by isolation of virus from blood taken in acute illness, or demonstration of IgM antibody activity, or rising antibody titres in convalescence. Prevention of infection includes the use of insect repellants, but the treatment of walls (sandfly resting sites) with residual insecticides is highly effective.

Toscana virus was first isolated in 1971 in Tuscany, Italy, from *Phlebotomus perniciosus*, a sandfly that breeds in forest litter. Antibody was found to be common in the sera of rural and suburban residents of the region, and an association was established between the occurrence of aseptic meningitis and serological evidence of infection with *Toscana virus*. Since then several cases of meningitis due to the infection have been encountered regularly each year in summer months in the endemic region, and these can sometimes be diagnosed by isolation of virus from cerebrospinal fluid in acute illness, but usually by demonstrating IgM antibody activity or rising antibody titres in sera taken during convalescence. The virus is transmitted transovarially in the vector, *P. perniciosus*, and no vertebrate maintenance host has been identified, but antibody has been found in rodent sera, and the virus has been isolated from an insectivorous bat. The vector is widely distributed in Europe and the virus has been isolated from cerebrospinal fluid from a meningitis patient in Portugal, so the disease may occur more widely than at present recognised.

Alenquer, Candiru, Punta Toro and Chagres Viruses

Alenquer virus and *Candiru virus* were isolated from the blood of febrile patients in the Amazon region of Brazil, but otherwise little is known of their biology, and it is surmised that they are transmitted by phlebotomid flies. *Punta Toro virus* and *Chagres virus* were isolated from febrile patients and from phlebotomids (*Lutzomyia* spp.) in Panama. These two viruses are known to be transmitted transovarially in phlebotomids, and antibodies to them have been found in primates, sloths, porcupines and other rodents. Disease thus far associated with all four viruses fits the description of classical sandfly fever, with the difference that epidemics are unknown and only isolated cases have been seen in persons who entered tropical forests for occupational or recreational purposes.

Rift Valley Fever Virus

The literature on Rift Valley fever has been reviewed extensively (Henning, 1956; Weiss, 1957; Easterday, 1965; Peters and Meegan, 1981; Shimshony and Barzilai, 1983; Meegan and Bailey, 1989; Swanepoel and Coetzer, 2003). It is an acute disease of domestic ruminants in mainland Africa and Madagascar, caused by a mosquito-borne virus and characterised by necrotic hepatitis and a haemorrhagic state, but infections are frequently inapparent or mild. Large outbreaks of the disease in sheep, cattle and goats are distinguished by heavy mortality among newborn animals and abortion in pregnant animals. Humans become infected from contact with tissues of infected animals or from mosquito bite, and usually develop mild to moderately severe febrile illness, but severe complications occur in a small proportion of patients.

The virus recently escaped from the African region to cause a major outbreak of disease on the Arabian Peninsula in 2000–2001.

The disease was first recognised in the Rift Valley in Kenya early in the twentieth century, but the causative agent was not isolated until 1930. Since then large outbreaks of the disease have been recorded in Kenya, South Africa, Namibia, Mozambique, Zimbabwe, Zambia, Sudan, Egypt, Mauritania and Senegal, while lesser outbreaks, periodic isolations of virus or serological evidence of infection have been recorded in Angola, Botswana, Burkina Faso, Cameroon, Central African Republic, Chad, Gabon, Guinea, Madagascar, Malawi, Mali, Nigeria, Somalia, Tanzania, Uganda and Zaire. Epidemics may be extremely severe and, for example, it is estimated that 500 000 ewes aborted and a further 100 000 sheep died in the first outbreak of the disease to be recognised in South Africa in 1950–1951.

Prior to the 1970s, epidemics were seen only in eastern and southern Africa, where they tend to occur at irregular intervals of 5–15 years or longer when above-average rainfall favours the breeding of the mosquito vectors. Meteorological conditions conducive to the occurrence of epidemics usually prevail over large tracts of Africa, so there has been some tendency for outbreaks in adjacent territories, such as Zimbabwe and Mozambique, Kenya and Tanzania or South Africa and Namibia, to coincide. The fate of the virus during inter-epidemic periods was unknown for decades, but on the basis of observations made in Uganda, Kenya and South Africa, it was widely accepted that the virus was endemic in indigenous forests, which extend in broken fashion from East Africa to the coastal regions of South Africa. The virus was thought to circulate in *Eretmapodites* spp. mosquitoes and unknown vertebrates in the forests, and to spread in seasons of exceptionally heavy rainfall to livestock-rearing areas, where the vectors were believed to be floodwater-breeding aedine mosquitoes of the sub-genera *Aedimorphus* and *Neomelaniconion*, which attach their eggs to vegetation at the edge of stagnant surface water. In contrast to other culicine mosquitoes, it is obligatory that the eggs of aedines be subjected to a period of drying as the water recedes before they will hatch on being wetted again when next the area floods. Thus, the aedine mosquitoes overwinter as eggs, which can survive for long periods in dried mud, possibly for several seasons if the area remains dry.

On the inland plateau of South Africa, where sheep rearing predominates, surface water gathers after heavy rains in undrained shallow depressions (pans) and farm dams which afford ideal breeding environments for aedines. On the watershed plateau of Zimbabwe, where cattle farming predominates, aedines breed in 'vleis', low-lying grassy areas which constitute drainage channels for surrounding high ground and which are flooded by seepage after heavy rains. Vleis correspond to what are termed 'dambos' in the livestock-rearing areas of central and eastern Africa. Sustained monitoring in Zimbabwe revealed that a low level of virus transmission to livestock occurred each year in the same areas where epidemics occurred. The generation of epidemics, therefore, was associated with the simultaneous intensification of virus activity over vast livestock-rearing areas where it was already present, rather than lateral spread from cryptic endemic foci. Comparison of the distributions of canopy forests and vleis in Zimbabwe, plotted from satellite images and aerial photographs, with the distribution determined for endemic Rift Valley fever, revealed remarkable overlap between the endemic areas and areas where vleis were common.

A major advance in the understanding of the epidemiology of the disease was made when the virus was isolated from unfed *Aedes mcintoshi* mosquitoes (= *Aedes lineatopennis* sensu lato) hatched in dambos on a ranch in Kenya during inter-epidemic periods in 1982 and 1984, confirming that the virus is endemic in livestock-rearing areas and indicating that it appears to be maintained by transovarial transmission in aedines. The available evidence suggests that in Zimbabwe, as in Kenya, *A. mcintoshi* is the most important maintenance vector of the virus, while *A. dentatus* is probably also a maintenance vector; the same two species, and possibly *A. unidentatus* and *A. juppi*, are maintenance vectors on the inland plateau of South Africa. Heavy rainfall and the humid conditions which prevail during epidemics favour the breeding of other biting insects besides aedine mosquitoes. Following extensive flooding of aedine breeding sites, significant numbers of livestock become infected and circulate high levels of virus in their blood during the acute stage of infection. Other culicines and anopheline mosquitoes then become infected and serve as epidemic vectors, particularly *Culex theileri* in southern Africa, and biting flies such as midges, phlebotomids, stomoxids and simulids serve as mechanical transmitters of infection. Although contagion has been demonstrated on occasion under artificial conditions, non-vectorial transmission is not considered to be important in livestock, as opposed to humans. Epidemics generally become evident in late summer, after there has been an initial increase in vector populations and in circulation of virus, and terminate in late autumn, when the onset of cold weather depresses vector activity, or when most animals are immune following natural infection, or after there has been successful intervention with vaccine.

Antibody surveys and laboratory studies have failed to prove that the virus is maintained in transmission cycles in rodents, birds, monkeys, baboons or other wild vertebrates, although it is felt that wild ruminants could play a role similar to their domestic counterparts in areas where they predominate. It is also believed that the possibility of endemicity of the virus in forests cannot be dismissed entirely, and merits further investigation.

It was recognised from the time of the original investigations in Kenya that febrile illness in humans accompanied outbreaks of disease in livestock, and that some patients experienced transient loss of visual acuity, but the occurrence of serious ocular sequelae was first reported in the 1950–1951 epidemic in South Africa. Human deaths following natural infection were first recorded in South Africa during the epidemic of 1974–1976, when seven patients are known to have died of encephalitis and haemorrhagic fever associated with necrotic hepatitis. Subsequently, deaths were also observed in Zimbabwe.

Outbreaks of Rift Valley fever were reported in the Sudan in 1973 and 1976. In 1977 and 1978 a major epidemic occurred along the Nile delta and valley in Egypt, causing an unprecedented number of human infections and deaths, as well as numerous deaths and abortions in sheep and cattle and some losses in goats, water buffaloes and camels. Estimates of the number of human cases of disease range from 18 000 to >200 000, with at least 598 deaths occurring from encephalitis and/or haemorrhagic fever. A severe epidemic occurred in 1987 in the Senegal River basin of southern Mauritania and northern Senegal. In Mauritania alone an estimated 224 human patients died of the disease, and there was a high rate of abortion in sheep and goats. Further outbreaks of Rift Valley fever occurred in Mauritania in 1993 and 1998, with smaller numbers of human casualties, while a minor outbreak of disease in livestock occurred in Senegal in 1994–1995.

The outbreaks of Rift Valley fever which occurred in North and West Africa differed in many respects from the pattern of disease which had hitherto been observed in sub-Saharan Africa; in particular, they occurred independently of rainfall in arid countries, apparently in association with vectors which breed in large rivers and dams. The presence of the virus in the Sudan and certain West African countries had long been known from antibody studies, and there had been periodic isolations of the virus in West Africa, where it was sometimes reported as *Zinga virus*, which is now known to be identical to *Rift Valley fever virus*. Various theories were advanced to account for the first known appearance of the virus in Egypt in 1977, including the carriage of infected mosquitoes from the Sudan at high altitude by prevailing winds associated with the inter-tropical convergence zone. The introduction of the virus through the transportation of infected sheep and cattle on the Nile or overland from northern Sudan to markets in southern Egypt was considered to have been the strongest possibility, and the movement of slaughter animals by sea could account for the evidence of infection detected in the northern and eastern coastal areas of Egypt. Although transportation on some routes would take a long time in relation to the course of the infection, Rift Valley fever virus has been shown to persist for prolonged periods in various organs of sheep, particularly the spleen, for up to 21 days after infection. The same could be true for goats and cattle, or even the camels brought in by overland caravan routes. It is believed that humans slaughtering or handling the tissues of such animals could have become infected and served as the amplifying hosts for the infection of mosquitoes since the main vector in the Egyptian epidemic, *Culex pipiens*, is known to be peridomestic and anthropophilic. In at least one instance there were indications that human infections centred on a location where introduced camels were slaughtered.

The occurrence of the epidemic in Egypt raised the spectre that Rift Valley fever could be introduced to the mainland of Eurasia, and the possibility was underscored by the fact that the virus is apparently capable of utilising a wide range of mosquitoes as vectors. Extensive preventive vaccination of livestock was undertaken at the time in the Sinai peninsula and Israel. However, only isolated outbreaks of Rift Valley fever were recorded in Egypt in 1979 and 1980, and thereafter the country remained free of the disease for 12 years, until ocular complications of the infection in humans and abortions in cattle and water buffalo were noted in the Aswan Governate in May 1993. On this occasion there was not the same tendency for an explosive outbreak of the disease to occur as in 1977–1978, but by October 1993 infections of humans and livestock, including sheep, had been recognised across the length of the country in Sharqiya, Giza and El Faiyum Governates, and further infections were observed in 1994 (Anonymous, 1993, 1994; Arthur *et al.*, 1993; Botros *et al.*, 1997).

From late October 1997 to February 1998, a large outbreak of Rift Valley fever occurred in north-eastern Kenya and adjoining southern Somalia, following the occurrence of heavy rains and extensive flooding in what is essentially an arid area, where people had been receiving food relief owing to the extreme drought conditions that had prevailed in the preceding 2 years (Anonymous, 1998; Woods *et al.*, 2002). There were heavy losses of livestock and an estimated 500 human deaths, but Rift Valley fever could not be confirmed in all instances. An agent isolated from human blood was thought to be a new bunyavirus and given the name *Garissa virus*, but was later found to be *Ngari virus*, originally isolated from mosquitoes in West Africa (Bowen *et al.*, 2001; Nichol, 2003). Antibody to *Ngari virus* was found in people in both Kenya and Somalia, but the importance of the virus as a human pathogen remains to be determined; many of the deaths could have been due to the appearance of malaria in an area not normally affected by this disease. It was subsequently established that extensive outbreaks of Rift Valley fever had also occurred elsewhere in Kenya and northern Tanzania following heavy rains in the region, and a few human deaths in southern Kenya were also ascribed to the disease.

In September 2000, Rift Valley fever broke out simultaneously in Jizan Province in south-west Saudi Arabia and in adjoining Yemen. The outbreaks lasted until early 2001, and resulted in 245 human deaths and the loss of thousands of sheep and goats. There had been heavy rains in the inland mountain range which runs parallel to the coast, with drainage from the mountains resulting in the creation of ideal mosquito-breeding habitats (Jupp *et al.*, 2002). There was speculation that the virus may have been imported from Africa with slaughter animals, or carried from Africa by wind-borne mosquitoes in 2000, but there were no known epidemics in the Horn of Africa at the time. It is much more likely that infected animals were imported during the 1997–1998 epidemic in East Africa, and that infection had smouldered on the Arabian Peninsula until ideal circumstances for an epidemic occurred following heavy rains in 2000. It remains to be determined whether the virus has become endemic on the Arabian Peninsula.

In contrast to the main vector in the Egyptian epidemic of 1977–1978, the principal mosquito vectors of *Rift Valley fever virus* in sub-Saharan Africa tend to be zoophilic and sylvatic, with the result that humans become infected mainly from contact with animal tissues, although there are instances where no such history can be obtained and it must be assumed that infection has resulted from mosquito bite. Occasional infections diagnosed in tourists from abroad who visited countries in Africa are also thought to have resulted from mosquito bites. Generally, persons who become infected are involved in the livestock industry, such as farmers who assist in dystocia of livestock, farm labourers who salvage carcases for human consumption, veterinarians and their assistants, and abattoir workers. There are numerous reports of humans becoming infected while investigating the disease in the field or laboratory, and the first known human fatality was recorded in 1934 in a laboratory worker, but since the infection was complicated by thrombophlebitis and the patient died from pulmonary embolism, the potential lethality of the virus for man was overlooked until fatal infections were recognised during the 1974–1976 epidemic in South Africa. The results of surveys following epidemics in southern Africa indicated that 9–15% of farm residents became infected, with a slight preponderance of adult males, although it appeared that housewives also gained infection from handling fresh meat.

No outbreaks of the disease have been recognised in urban consumer populations and it is surmised that the fall in pH associated with the maturation of meat in abattoirs is deleterious to the virus. Moreover, highest infection rates were found in workers in the by-products sections of abattoirs in Zimbabwe, and the implication is that the carcases of infected animals which reach abattoirs are generally recognised as being diseased and are condemned as unfit for human consumption.

Human infection presumably results from contact of virus with abraded skin, wounds or mucous membranes, but aerosol and intranasal infection have been demonstrated experimentally and circumstantial evidence suggests that aerosols have been involved in some human infections in the laboratory, and in the field during the Egyptian epidemic. Many infections in Egypt are thought to have resulted from the slaughter of infected animals outside of abattoirs, and the fact that the mosquito vector was anthropophilic is thought to explain the high incidence of infection which occurred in people of all ages and diverse occupations. Low concentrations of virus have been found in milk and body fluids, such as saliva and nasal discharges of sheep and cattle, and it appears that there may have been a connection between human infection and consumption of raw milk in Mauritania. In view of the intense viraemia which occurs in humans and the fact that virus has been isolated from throat washings, it is curious that there are no records of person-to-person transmission of infection.

Despite the sudden and dramatic change perceived in the nature of the human disease in the mid-1970s, it was deduced from the 598 reported deaths and 200 000 estimated cases of disease that Rift Valley fever had a case fatality rate of less than 1% in Egypt, where a high prevalence of schistosomiasis may have predisposed the population to severe liver disease. The fatality rate may even have been lower in relation to total infections, since an antibody prevalence rate of 30% was detected and the human population was estimated at 1–3 million in the areas affected by the epidemic. On the other hand, remarkably high estimates of 5% and 14% were made for case fatality rates in two separate populations in the 1987 epidemic in Mauritania, on the basis of the proportion of IgM antibody-positive persons who actually reported illness considered to be compatible with Rift Valley fever, but it can be deduced that the fatality rates in terms of total IgM antibody-positive persons are much closer to the corresponding fatality rate in Egypt.

The majority of Rift Valley fever infections in humans are inapparent or associated with moderate to severe, non-fatal, febrile illness. After an incubation period of 2–6 days, the onset of the benign illness is usually very sudden and the disease is characterised by rigor, fever that persists for several days and is often biphasic, headache with retro-orbital pain and photophobia, weakness, and muscle and joint pains. Sometimes there is nausea and vomiting, abdominal pain, vertigo, epistaxis and a petechial rash. Defervescence and symptomatic improvement occur in 4–7 days in benign disease and recovery is often complete in 2 weeks, but in a minority of patients the disease is complicated by the development of ocular lesions at the time of the initial illness or up to 4 weeks later. Estimates for the incidence of ocular complications range from <1% to 20% of human infections, and possibly the differences stem from failure to record mild cases in populations where illiterate persons are less likely to report minor disturbances of vision. The ocular disease usually presents as a loss of acuity of central vision, sometimes with development of scotomas. The essential lesion appears to be focal retinal ischaemia, generally in the macular or paramacular area, associated with thrombotic occlusion of arterioles and capillaries, and is characterised by retinal oedema and loss of transparency, caused by dense white exudate and haemorrhages. Sometimes there is severe haemorrhage and detachment of the retina. The lesions and the loss of visual acuity generally resolve over a period of months with variable residual scarring of the retina, but in instances of severe haemorrhage and detachment of the retina there may be permanent uni- or bilateral blindness.

Probably <1% of human patients develop the haemorrhagic and/or encephalitic forms of the disease. Underlying liver disease may predispose to the haemorrhagic form of the illness. The haemorrhagic syndrome starts with sudden onset of febrile illness similar to the benign disease, but within 2–4 days there may be development of a petechial rash, purpura, ecchymoses and extensive subcutaneous haemorrhages, bleeding from needle puncture sites, epistaxis, haematemesis, diarrhoea and melaena, sore and inflamed throat, gingival bleeding, epigastric pain, hepatomegaly or hepatosplenomegaly, tenderness of the right upper quadrant of the abdomen and deep jaundice. This is followed by pneumonitis, anaemia, shock with racing pulse and low blood pressure, hepatorenal failure, coma and cardiorespiratory arrest. Factors contributing to fatal outcome in the hepatic form of the disease include anaemia, shock and hepatorenal failure, with the kidney lesions possibly being as important as shock in producing anuria. A proportion of the less severely affected patients may make a protracted recovery without sequelae.

Encephalitis may occur in combination with the haemorrhagic syndrome. Otherwise, signs of encephalitis in humans may supervene during the acute illness or up to 4 weeks later and include severe headache, vertigo, confusion, disorientation, amnesia, meningismus, hallucinations, hypersalivation, grinding of teeth, choreiform movements, convulsions, hemiparesis, lethargy, decerebrate posturing, locked-in syndrome, coma and death. A proportion of patients may recover completely, but others may be left with sequelae, such as hemiparesis.

Abortion is the usual, if not invariable, outcome to infection of pregnant ruminants, but an attempt to relate the occurrence of abortion in humans to evidence of Rift Valley fever infection in Egypt produced inconclusive results.

By analogy with the course of events believed to follow natural infection with other arthropod-borne viruses, it can be surmised that the pathogenesis of the disease may involve some replication of virus at the site of inoculation, conveyance of infection by lymphatic drainage to regional lymph nodes, where there is further replication with spillover of virus into the circulation to produce primary viraemia, which in turn leads to systemic infection, and that intense viraemia then results from release of virus following replication in major target organs. Wild *Rift Valley fever virus*, which has not been subjected to serial passaging in laboratory host systems, is described as being hepato-, viscero- or pantropic, and immunofluorescence studies in laboratory animals indicate that replication occurs in littoral macrophages of lymph nodes, most areas of the spleen except T-dependent peri-arteriolar sheaths, foci of adrenocortical cells, virtually all cells of the liver, most renal glomeruli and some tubules, lung tissue and scattered small vessel walls, as well as in necrotic foci in the brains of individuals who develop the encephalitic form of the disease. These sites correspond to the lymphoid necrosis in lymph nodes and spleen, hepatic necrosis and adrenal, lung and glomerular lesions seen in humans and livestock, and the brain lesions in humans (encephalitis has not been described in natural disease of ruminants). Titration of infectivity in organ homogenates indicates that the liver and spleen are the major sites of virus replication. Cell damage is ascribed directly to the lytic effects of the virus, but the inflammatory response seen in human brain tissue suggests that there may also be an immunopathological element to the pathogenesis of encephalitis. The same may be true for ocular lesions. Recovery is mediated by non-specific and specific host responses, and the clearance of viraemia correlates with the appearance of neutralising antibody. No significant antigenic differences have been detected between isolates of the virus, although differences in pathogenicity for laboratory rodents have been demonstrated and immunity appears to be lifelong.

The haemostatic derangement which occurs in Rift Valley fever has been investigated in rhesus monkeys, but the mechanisms involved remain speculative. Impairment of coagulation occurs even in benign infection of monkeys, and moderate thrombocytopenia has been observed in benign infection in sheep, but haemostatic derangement is most severe in the fatal hepatic syndrome. It is postulated that the critical lesions are vasculitis and hepatic necrosis. Destruction of the antithrombotic properties of endothelial cells is thought to trigger intravascular coagulation, and the widespread necrosis of hepatocytes and other affected cells to result in the release of procoagulants into the circulation. Severe liver damage presumably limits or abolishes production of coagulation proteins and reduces clearance of activated coagulation factors, thereby further promoting the occurrence of disseminated intravascular coagulopathy, which in turn augments tissue injury by impairing blood flow. Vasculitis and haemostatic failure result in purpura and widespread haemorrhages.

Clinical pathology findings in humans are compatible with observations made in haematological and coagulation studies on monkeys, except that leukocytosis and anaemia may be more marked in severe human disease (Al Hazmi et al., 2003). In most species there is an initial leukopenia followed by leukocytosis, and the same may be true for humans. Monkeys may have prolonged activated partial thromboplastin times and prothrombin times even in benign infection, and in severe liver disease there may be depletion of

coagulation factors II, V, VII, IX, X and XII, thrombocytopenia and platelet dysfunction, increased schistocyte counts and depletion of fibrinogen, together with raised fibrin degradation product levels. Raised serum aspartate aminotransferase and alanine aminotransferase levels have been recorded even in benign disease in humans.

Treatment is essentially symptomatic, and supportive therapy in the haemorrhagic disease includes replacement of blood and coagulation factors. Results obtained in animal models suggest that the administration of immune plasma from recovered patients may be beneficial. The antiviral drug ribavirin inhibits virus replication in cell cultures and laboratory animals, and it has been suggested that it could be used even in benign disease in order to obviate the potentially serious complications which may occur in humans.

Specimens to be submitted for laboratory confirmation of the diagnosis include blood from live patients, and tissue samples, particularly liver, but also spleen, kidney, lymph nodes and heart blood of deceased patients. Tissue samples should be submitted in duplicate in a viral transport medium, and in 10% buffered formalin for histopathological examination.

Viral antigen can frequently be detected rapidly in tissues and/or blood by a variety of immunological methods, including immunodiffusion, complement-fixation, immunofluorescence and enzyme-linked immunoassay. Viraemia lasts for up to a week. The virus is cytopathic and can be isolated readily in almost all cell cultures commonly used in diagnostic laboratories, and identified rapidly by immunofluorescence. Virus can also be isolated in suckling or weaned mice, or hamsters, inoculated intracerebrally or intraperitoneally, and antigen can be identified in harvested brain or liver by the immunological methods mentioned above. Definitive identification of isolates is achieved by performing neutralisation tests with reference antiserum.

Histopathological lesions, particularly those in the liver, are considered to be pathognomonic, and are essentially similar in humans and domestic ruminants. The severity of the lesions varies from primary foci of coagulative necrosis, consisting of clusters of hepatocytes with acidophilic cytoplasms and pyknotic nuclei, multifocally scattered throughout the parenchyma, to massive liver destruction in which the primary foci comprising dense aggregates of cytoplasmic and nuclear debris, some fibrin and a few neutrophils and macrophages, can be discerned against a background of parenchyma reduced by nuclear pyknosis, karyorrhexis and cytolysis to scattered fragments of cytoplasm and chromatin, with only narrow rims of degenerate hepatocytes remaining reasonably intact close to portal triads. Intensely acidophilic cytoplasmic bodies, which resemble the Councilman bodies of yellow fever, are common, and rod-shaped or oval eosinophilic intranuclear inclusions may be seen in intact nuclei. Icterus may be evident.

Antibody to *Rift Valley fever virus* can be demonstrated in complement fixation, enzyme-linked immunoassay, indirect immunofluorescence, haemagglutination-inhibition or neutralisation tests. Diagnosis of recent infection is confirmed by demonstrating seroconversion or a four-fold or greater rise in titre of antibody in paired serum samples, or by demonstrating IgM antibody activity in an enzyme-linked immunoassay.

Benign Rift Valley fever in humans must be distinguished from other zoonotic diseases, such as brucellosis and Q fever, while the fulminant hepatic disease must be distinguished from the so-called formidable viral haemorrhagic fevers of Africa: Lassa fever, Crimean-Congo haemorrhagic fever, Marburg disease and Ebola fever. The occurrence of HFRS associated with hantavirus infections, is also a theoretical possibility in Africa.

An inactivated and a live attenuated vaccine are available for immunisation of livestock, but it is usually difficult to persuade farmers to vaccinate livestock during long inter-epidemic periods. The attenuated vaccine confers lifelong immunity in sheep, but is abortigenic and teratogenic in a small proportion of pregnant ewes. The attenuated vaccine is poorly immunogenic in cattle and they are immunised annually with the inactivated vaccine. A formalin-inactivated cell culture vaccine produced in the USA is used on an experimental basis to immunise persons, such as laboratory and field workers, who are regularly exposed to Rift Valley fever infection.

Serogroup Uukuniemi

Uukuniemi virus

Uukuniemi virus was originally isolated in Finland in 1960 from *Ixodes ricinus* ticks, which parasitise livestock but also bite humans. The virus has subsequently been isolated from ticks, birds and field mice in Finland, Norway, Poland, Lithuania and the former USSR and Czechoslovakia. Antibody to the virus has been found in human sera in Finland, Hungary and former Czechoslovakia, but no evidence has been presented to indicate that infection is associated with

disease. The remaining members of the serogroup have been isolated from ticks associated with passerine or sea birds, and have no known medical or veterinary significance.

GENUS NAIROVIRUS

Serogoup Crimean-Congo Haemorrhagic Fever

Crimean-Congo Haemorrhagic Fever Virus

The literature on CCHF is the subject of several comprehensive reviews (Chumakov, 1974; Hoogstraal, 1979, 1981; Watts *et al.*, 1989). A disease given the name 'Crimean haemorrhagic fever' was first observed on the Crimean peninsula in 1944, and it was demonstrated through the inoculation of human subjects that the disease was caused by a tick-transmitted virus, but the virus itself was only isolated in laboratory hosts (mice) in 1967. In 1969, it was shown that the agent of Crimean haemorrhagic fever was identical to a virus named 'Congo' which had been isolated in 1956 from the blood of a febrile child in Stanleyville (now Kisangani) in what was then the Belgian Congo (now Zaire), and since that time the two names have been used in combination.

The distribution of CCHF virus extends over eastern Europe, Asia and Africa: the presence of the virus or antibody to it has been demonstrated in the former USSR, Bulgaria, Greece, Turkey, Hungary, Yugoslavia, France, Portugal, Kuwait, Dubai, Sharjah, Iraq, Iran, Afghanistan, Pakistan, India, China, Egypt, Ethiopia, Mauritania, Senegal, Burkina Faso, Benin, Nigeria, Central African Republic, Zaire, Kenya, Uganda, Tanzania, Zimbabwe, Namibia, South Africa and Madagascar. However, the evidence for France and Portugal is based on limited observations and needs to be confirmed.

In many instances virus or antibody was discovered in deliberate surveys, but in some countries of eastern Europe and Asia the presence of CCHF first became evident in nosocomial outbreaks of disease, or in epidemics which arose in circumstances where humans were exposed to ticks and livestock on a large scale, such as in major land reclamation or resettlement schemes in Bulgaria and parts of the former USSR. Notable outbreaks of the disease in Eurasia during recent years have resulted from the exposure of people to blood and ticks from slaughter stock imported from Africa and Asia to Saudi Arabia in 1990, the United Arab Emirates in 1994–1995, and Oman in 1995, plus large-scale exposure of war refugees to outdoor conditions in Kosovo in 2000 and Albania in 2001 (El Azazy and Scrimgeour, 1997; Khan *et al.*, 1997; Papa *et al.*, 2002a, 2002b; Scrimgeour *et al.*, 1996; Williams *et al.*, 2000). Prior to 1981, a total of 15 cases of the disease had been reported in Africa, eight of them laboratory infections, and only one patient had developed haemorrhagic manifestations and died. Since then sporadic cases of haemorrhagic disease and deaths have been diagnosed regularly each year in southern Africa, probably as a result of increased awareness among clinicians, and severe disease has also been recorded elsewhere in Africa.

The virus has been isolated from at least 29 species of ixodid ticks, but for most species there is no definitive evidence that they are capable of serving as vectors, and in some instances the virus recovered from engorged ticks may merely have been present in the bloodmeal imbibed from a viraemic host. Members of three genera of ixodid ticks, *Hyalomma*, *Dermacentor* and *Rhipicephalus*, have been shown to be capable of transmitting infection trans-stadially and transovarially, but *Hyalomma* ticks are considered to be the principal vectors, and with the exception of Madagascar the known distribution of CCHF virus coincides with the world distribution of members of this genus of ticks. Moreover, the prevalence of antibody to CCHF virus detected in the sera of wild vertebrates in southern Africa was highest in large herbivores, known to be the preferred hosts of adult *Hyalomma* ticks, and in small mammals such as hares, which are the preferred hosts of immature *Hyalomma*. Mammals of intermediate size, and passerine and water birds, generally lacked evidence of infection, but antibody was found in ostriches, which are known to be parasitised by adult *Hyalomma* ticks. Virus or antibody has also been demonstrated elsewhere in the sera of small mammals of Eurasia and Africa, such as little susliks, hedgehogs, hares and certain myomorph rodents, and in some instances it has been shown that these hosts develop viraemia of sufficient intensity to infect ticks.

High prevalences of antibody occur in domestic ruminants in areas infested by *Hyalomma* ticks and the virus causes inapparent infection or mild fever in cattle, sheep and goats, with viraemia of sufficient intensity to infect ticks. It is doubtful whether transovarial transmission occurs with sufficient frequency in ticks to ensure indefinite perpetuation of the virus in the absence of amplification of infection in vertebrate hosts, and in particular, it is believed that the infection of small vertebrates constitutes an important amplifying mechanism, which facilitates trans-stadial transmission of virus by adult ticks to large vertebrates.

Young ruminants generally acquire natural infection early in life and are viraemic for about a week. Humans become infected when they come into contact with the viraemic blood of young animals in the course of performing procedures such as castrations, vaccinations, inserting ear tags or slaughtering the animals. Animals which are raised under tick-free conditions and moved to infested locations later in life may acquire tick-borne diseases of livestock at the same time that they become infected with CCHF virus, and consequently humans become infected from contact with viraemic blood in the course of treating sick animals or butchering those that die. The available evidence suggests that the infection in humans is acquired through contact of viraemic blood with broken skin, and this accords with the fact that nosocomial infection in medical personnel usually results from accidental pricks with needles contaminated with the blood of patients, or similar mishaps. Common source outbreaks involving more than one case of the disease can occur when several people are exposed to infected tissues. Infection appears to be limited to those who have contact with fresh blood or other tissues, probably because infectivity is destroyed by the fall in pH which occurs in tissues after death, and there has been no indication that CCHF virus constitutes a public health hazard in meat processed and matured according to normal health regulations. Many human infections result directly from tick bite, and it has been observed that people can also become infected from merely squashing ticks between the fingers. Some patients are unable to recall contact with blood or other tissues of livestock, or having been bitten by ticks, but live in or have visited a rural environment where such exposure to infection is possible. Town dwellers sometimes acquire infection from contact with animal tissues or tick bite while on hunting or hiking trips.

The majority of patients tend to be adult males engaged in the livestock industry, such as farmers, herdsmen, slaughtermen and veterinarians. Seroprevalence studies indicate that infection of humans is uncommon despite the widespread evidence of infection in livestock, and this may be explained by the facts that viraemia in livestock is short-lived, and of low intensity compared to that in other zoonotic diseases, such as Rift Valley fever, and that humans are not the preferred hosts of *Hyalomma* ticks. The low prevalences of antibody generally found in populations at risk, and the paucity of evidence of inapparent infection encountered among the cohorts of cases of the disease, suggests that infection is frequently symptomatic.

Incubation periods are generally short, usually 1–3 days (maximum 9) following infection by tick bite, and are usually 5 or 6 days (maximum 13) in persons exposed to infected blood or other tissues of livestock or human patients. Onset of the disease is usually very sudden. Patients develop fever, rigors, chills, severe headache, dizziness, neck pain and stiffness, sore eyes, photophobia, myalgia and malaise, with intense backache or leg pains. Nausea, sore throat and vomiting commonly occur early in the illness and patients may experience non-localised abdominal pain and diarrhoea at this stage. Fever is often intermittent and patients may undergo sharp changes of mood over the next 2 days, with feelings of confusion and aggression. By day 2–4 of illness, patients may exhibit lassitude, depression and somnolence, and have a flushed appearance with injected conjunctivae or chemosis. By this time, tenderness may be localised in the right upper quadrant of the abdomen, and hepatomegaly may be discernible. Tachycardia is common and patients may be slightly hypotensive. There may be lymphadenopathy, and enanthem and petechiae of the throat, tonsils and buccal mucosa.

A petechial rash appears on the trunk and limbs on day 3–6 of illness, and this may be followed rapidly by the appearance of large bruises and ecchymoses, especially in the anticubital fossae, upper arms, axillae and groin. Epistaxis, haematemesis, haematuria, melaena, gingival bleeding and bleeding from the vagina or other orifices may commence on day 4 or 5 of illness, or even earlier. Sometimes a haemorrhagic tendency is evident only from the oozing of blood from injection or venepuncture sites. There may be internal bleeding, including retroperitoneal and intracranial haemorrhage. Severely ill patients may enter a state of hepatorenal and pulmonary failure from about day 5 onwards and progressively become drowsy, stuporous and comatose. Jaundice may become apparent during the second week of illness. The mortality rate is approximately 30% and deaths generally occur on days 5–14 of illness. Patients who recover usually begin to improve on day 9 or 10 of illness, but asthenia, conjunctivitis, slight confusion and amnesia may continue for a month or longer.

Changes in clinical pathology values recorded during the first few days of illness include leukocytosis or leukopenia, and elevated aspartate transaminase, alanine transaminase, γ-glutamyl transferase, lactic dehydrogenase, alkaline phosphatase and creatine kinase levels, while bilirubin, creatinine and urea levels increase and serum protein levels decline during the second week. Thrombocytopenia, elevation of prothrombin ratio, activated partial thromboplastin time, thrombin time and fibrin degradation products, and depression of fibrinogen and haemoglobin values are also evident during the first few days of illness, indicating that the occurrence of disseminated intravascular coagulopathy is probably an early and central event in the pathogenesis of the disease. Changes are more severe in fatal than in non-fatal infections, and the occurrence of certain markedly abnormal clinical pathology values during the first 5 days of illness are predictive of fatal outcome (Swanepoel et al., 1987, 1989).

It is surmised that peripherally introduced CCHF virus undergoes some replication at the site of inoculation, and that haematogenous and lymphborne spread of infection occurs to organs such as the liver, which are major sites of replication. Although it has not been shown conclusively that there is infection of endothelium, capillary fragility is a feature of the disease and there is evidence of formation of circulating immune complexes with complement activation, and this would contribute to damage of the capillary bed and the genesis of renal and pulmonary failure. Endothelial damage would account for the occurrence of a rash and would contribute to haemostatic failure through stimulating platelet aggregation and degranulation, with consequent activation of the intrinsic coagulation cascade. It is clear from the results of therapeutic administration of platelets to patients that they are consumed, and evidence of depression of thrombopoiesis in bone marrow has been reported. Widespread tissue damage in organs such as the liver would result in further release of procoagulants, such as tumour necrosis factor, into the bloodstream and impairment of the circulation through the occurrence of a disseminated intravascular coagulopathy would contribute to further tissue damage. Damage to the liver would also impair synthesis of coagulation factors to replace those which are consumed.

Lesions in the liver vary from disseminated foci of coagulative necrosis, mainly mid-zonal in distribution, to massive necrosis involving over 75% of hepatocytes, and a variable degree of haemorrhage, with little or no inflammatory cell response. Lesions in other organs include congestion, haemorrhage and focal necrosis in the central nervous system, kidneys and adrenals, and general depletion of lymphoid tissues. Fibrin deposits may be seen in small blood vessels in parenchymatous organs including the liver, and thrombus formation and infarction may contribute to the pathogenesis of the necrotic lesions in these organs.

Where possible, patients are treated by specially trained staff in institutions equipped for handling formidable viral haemorrhagic fevers, and barrier-nursing techniques are used for the protection of medical personnel. Therapy appropriate for disseminated intravascular coagulopathy, such as the use of heparin, may be contemplated early in the course of the disease by clinicians well versed in the treatment of haemostatic failure, but the procedure is considered to be risky, and generally only patients who acquire nosocomial infection come to medical attention at a sufficiently early stage. Standard treatment consists of replacement of red blood cells, platelets, other coagulation factors, protein (albumin) and intravenous feeding, as indicated by clinical pathology findings. Immune plasma from recovered patients has been used in therapy, but there is no firm evidence from controlled trials of the value of the treatment, and there has been a lack of a uniform product with proven virus-neutralising activity. Ribavirin has been found to inhibit virus replication in cell cultures and in suckling mice, and preliminary results of a trial in human patients are promising.

On account of the propensity of the virus to cause laboratory infections, and the severity of the human disease, investigation of CCHF is generally undertaken in maximum-security laboratories in countries which have biosafety regulations. Specimens to be submitted for laboratory confirmation of the diagnosis include blood from live patients and, in order to avoid performing full autopsies, heart blood and liver samples taken with a biopsy needle from deceased patients. Virus can be isolated from blood and organ suspensions in a wide variety of primary and line cell cultures, including Vero, CER and BHK$_{21}$ cells, and identified by immunofluorescence. Isolation and identification can be achieved in 1–5 days, but cell cultures lack sensitivity and usually only detect high concentrations of virus present in the blood of severely ill patients during the first 5 days or so of illness. Intracerebral inoculation of suckling mice is more sensitive and can be used to demonstrate low concentrations of virus present in blood up to 13 days after the onset of illness. Virus antigen can sometimes be demonstrated in the blood of severely ill patients with intense viraemia, or in liver suspensions, by enzyme-linked immunoassay.

Antibodies, both IgG and IgM, become demonstrable by indirect immunofluorescence from about day 7 of illness (slightly earlier by enzyme-linked immunoassay), and are present in the sera of all survivors of the disease by day 9 at the latest. The IgM antibody activity declines to undetectable levels by 4 months after infection, and IgG titres may begin to decline gradually at this stage, but remain demonstrable for at least 5 years. Recent or current infection is confirmed by demonstrating seroconversion, or a four-fold or greater increase in antibody titre in paired serum samples, or IgM antibody activity in a single sample. Patients who succumb rarely develop a demonstrable antibody response and the diagnosis is confirmed by isolation of virus from serum, or from liver specimens. Observation of necrotic lesions compatible with CCHF infection in sections of liver provides presumptive evidence in support of the diagnosis.

The disease must be distinguished from the other so-called formidable viral haemorrhagic fevers: Lassa fever, Marburg disease, Ebola fever and HFRS (hantavirus infections), other febrile illnesses such as Rift Valley fever, Q fever and brucellosis, which can be acquired from contact with animal tissues, as well as tick-borne typhus (*Rickettsia conorii* infection, commonly known as tickbite fever), but many other conditions including bacterial septicaemias may resemble CCHF.

The control of CCHF through the application of acaricides to livestock is impractical, particularly under the extensive farming conditions which prevail in the arid areas where *Hyalomma* ticks are most prevalent. Pyrethroid preparations are available which can be used to kill ticks which come into contact with human clothing. Veterinarians, slaughtermen and others involved with livestock should be aware of the disease and take practical steps, such as the wearing of gloves, to limit or avoid exposure of naked skin to fresh blood and other tissues of animals. Inactivated mouse brain vaccine for the prevention of human infection has been used on a limited scale in eastern Europe and the former USSR. Development of a safe and effective modern vaccine is inhibited by the limited potential demand for such a vaccine.

Serogroup Nairobi Sheep Disease

Nairobi Sheep Disease Virus

Nairobi sheep disease virus was first isolated from sheep blood in Kenya in 1910 and is known to be associated with disease of small ruminants, specifically sheep and goats, in a narrow band straddling the equator from Kenya in the east to Congo in the west. Antibody, but not disease, has also been found to the north of Kenya in Ethiopia and Somalia, and southwards along the east of the continent to Mozambique and Botswana. The virus can be transmitted trans-stadially by a range of ixodid ticks, including *Amblyomma variegatum*, but the endemic vector appears to be *Rhipicephalus appendiculatus*, in which transovarial transmission occurs. The disease in sheep and goats is characterised by fever, haemorrhagic gastroenteritis and abortion in pregnant animals. High mortality occurs when susceptible sheep or goats are introduced into an endemic area, but within such areas young animals appear to undergo benign infection as maternal immunity wanes, and there is a high prevalence of immunity in adult animals. Attenuated live and killed vaccines for sheep and goats are available in East Africa. Small antelope are susceptible to the disease, and rodents develop viraemic infection, but seroprevalence studies have failed to identify wild maintenance hosts of the virus. Larger ruminants, such as cattle and buffalo, are not susceptible to the disease. The virus has been isolated from human blood in association with febrile illness with arthralgia and malaise in Uganda, and laboratory infection has been recorded. Antibody prevalence rates of up to 20% have been found in humans in endemic areas.

Ganjam virus, first isolated from ixodid ticks in India in 1954, is considered to be identical to *Nairobi sheep disease virus*. It has been isolated from the blood of sheep and humans with febrile illness in India, where it is associated with ticks of the genus *Haemaphysalis*. There is speculation that the virus may have been translocated from India to Africa with ectoparasites on sheep and goats, which have been traded along sea routes for centuries.

Dugbe Virus

There have been approximately 600 isolations of *Dugbe virus* from ixodid ticks, mainly *Amblyomma variegatum*, in Nigeria, Central African Republic and Ethiopia. The virus has also been isolated frequently from cattle blood in surveys, and from a giant rat (*Cricetomys gambianus*), aedine mosquitoes and *Culicoides* midges in Nigeria, and there is serological evidence of the occurrence of the virus in Senegal and Uganda. There have been seven isolations of the virus from the blood of persons with benign febrile illness in Nigeria and Central African Republic (including a laboratory infection). One patient had mild meningitis and virus was isolated from cerebrospinal fluid. Surprisingly, serosurveys have not revealed widespread human infection.

GENUS *HANTAVIRUS*

Hantaan, Dobrava, Seoul, Puumala, Sin Nombre and Related Viruses

Hantaviruses are associated with a range of nephrotic diseases in Asia and Europe, known variously as haemorrhagic nephrosonephritis, Korean haemorrhagic fever, Songo fever, epidemic haemorrhagic fever and nephropathia epidemica, but use of the generic term 'haemorrhagic fever with renal syndrome' (HFRS) is advocated, while the term 'hantavirus pulmonary syndrome' (HPS) is preferred for respiratory disease associated with hantaviruses in the Americas.

The existence of a febrile disease with haemorrhagic and renal manifestations has been recognised in Eurasia at least since the early years of the twentieth century and, in fact, descriptions of similar disease can be traced back to antiquity. A disease known by various names, including haemorrhagic nephrosonephritis, and which caused outbreaks among civilians and soldiers, was investigated independently in the far eastern region of the former USSR and in Manchuria prior to the Second World War, and by the early 1940s it was established that the condition could be transmitted to human volunteers by inoculation of filtrates of patients' blood or urine, or tissue extracts from *Apodemus* field mice (it had been observed that the incidence of disease was greatest at the end of summer, when the mice were most numerous). At the same time a febrile syndrome with abdominal pain, backache and renal manifestations was recognised in Scandinavia and numerous cases of this disease, later named nephropathia epidemica (NE), were observed in soldiers during the Second World War.

Thousands of cases of a disease named Korean haemorrhagic fever were observed in soldiers and civilians during the Korean war of the early 1950s, and the disease continued to be seen after the war. In 1976 it was found that convalescent sera from patients in Korea could be used to demonstrate the presence of an antigen by immunofluorescence in the tissues of *Apodemus agrarius* field mice caught near the Hantaan river. The antigen was shown to be associated with a virus that could be subcultured in field mice. Named *Hantaan virus*, it was successfully grown in cell cultures in 1981, and shortly thereafter characterised as a member of the family *Bunyaviridae* and placed in a new genus, *Hantavirus*. The virus is widely distributed as the causative agent of HFRS in Asia, particularly in the eastern portion of the former USSR, China and

Korea. Virus associated with a severe form of HFRS in the Balkans (Albania, Greece, former Yugoslavia and Bulgaria) was found to be distinct from *Hantaan virus*, and was named *Dobrava virus*. It is associated with the yellow-necked field mouse, *A. flavicollis*. More recently, a second virus has been found in association with *A. agrarius*, the reservoir host of *Hantaan virus*, and named *Saaremaa virus*; it causes milder disease than *Hantaan virus*.

In 1980 the presence of the causative agent of nephropathia epidemica was demonstrated by immunofluorescence in the tissues of *Clethrionomys glareolus* voles in Finland, and subsequently the agent, named *Puumala virus*, was grown in cell cultures and shown to be related to *Hantaan virus*. Although evidence obtained in former Yugoslavia, Germany, Belgium, France and Britain suggests that *Puumala virus* occurs widely in Europe, it is most prevalent at northerly latitudes, extending into the Arctic circle in Scandinavia and the adjoining western portion of the former USSR, where highest concentrations of the bank vole occur.

Seoul virus was isolated in 1980 in Korea from the tissues of peridomestic rats, *Rattus rattus* and *R. norvegicus*, in association with human disease which occurred in urban as opposed to rural environments. It has been incriminated of causing human disease in Japan, China and Korea, but has been isolated from rats in Egypt, the USA and elsewhere, and probably has a worldwide distribution. Isolation of the virus from rats led to speculation that hantaviruses in general may have been disseminated worldwide with ship-borne rodents. However, the distribution patterns of most hantaviruses within the interiors of continents, and the evolution of particular host relationships, constitute evidence against recent spread of the viruses.

The findings in Asia and Europe prompted interest elsewhere and, as a result, *Prospect Hill virus* was isolated from *Microtus pennsylvanicus* voles in the USA, but no disease associations have been described for this virus.

In May 1993, an outbreak of an acute respiratory disease in adults, with a high fatality rate, was recognised in the Four Corners region of south-western USA, where the borders of the states of Utah, Colorado, Arizona and New Mexico meet, but the initial occurrence of cases could be traced back to late 1992. Antibody cross-reactive with the antigens of known hantaviruses was found in the sera of patients, and by means of reverse transcription and the polymerase chain reaction with consensus sequence hantavirus primers, it was possible to demonstrate the presence of nucleic acid of a novel hantavirus in the tissues of patients. The nucleotide sequence of the entire genome of the virus was determined even before it could be isolated and grown in cell cultures. The outbreak was apparently associated with a population explosion of the deer mouse, *Peromyscus maniculatus*, incriminated as the natural host of the virus. Sporadic cases of similar disease were recognised elsewhere in the USA, some retrospectively, and by the end of 1993 a total of 53 cases had been confirmed (Nichol *et al.*, 1993; Bremner, 1994; Duchin *et al.*, 1994). After objections were raised to various names proposed for the new virus, the name *Sin Nombre* (Spanish for 'without name') *virus* was adopted and the disease was referred to as HPS (for hantavirus pulmonary syndrome).

Isolated cases and outbreaks of HPS were subsequently recognised beyond the distribution range of *Peromyscus maniculatus* in the USA, in Canada, and in several countries of South America. A succession of new hantaviruses was discovered in association with HPS, or in rodents tested speculatively in surveys, and many of these have been associated with HPS (Table 18.5). Several new viruses were also discovered in rodents in Europe and Asia, and unidentified viruses which had previously been isolated from bandicoots in Thailand and from suncid shrews in India were found to be hantaviruses. In general, the new viruses were discovered through the detection of cross-reactive antibody activity to hantavirus antigens, followed by the application of the polymerase chain reaction to detect viral nucleic acid, and genetic characterisation. Adaptation to cell cultures followed the initial identification of the viruses, but *in vitro* culture has not yet been achieved in all instances. It is suspected that, in addition to the hantaviruses currently known to be human pathogens, some of the remaining viruses may also prove to be associated with disease (Table 18.5) (Schmaljohn and Hjelle, 1997; Kanerva *et al.*, 1998; Monroe *et al.*, 1999; Schmaljohn *et al.*, 2002).

Serological classification of hantaviruses has lagged behind genetic characterisation, primarily because the lack of *in vitro* culture systems for some of the viruses has prevented the performance of definitive cross-neutralisation tests, but the extant information on antigenic affinities is in agreement with the genetic clustering of the viruses, which in itself conforms with the phylogeny of the rodent hosts (Table 18.5) (Puthavathana *et al.*, 1992; Arthur *et al.*, 1992; Chu *et al.*, 1994, 1995; Schmaljohn and Hjelle, 1997; Kanerva *et al.*, 1998; Monroe *et al.*, 1999). In brief, all hantaviruses are antigenically related, with the greatest affinities existing within clusters designated as Hantaan-like, Puumala-Prospect Hill-like, and Sin Nombre-like, while *Thottapalayam virus* from shrews

Table 18.5 Abridged list of members of the genus *Hantavirus*. Information derived for sources cited in the text

Vertebrate host Order: Subfamily (Virus genotype) *Subtype/variety*	Known/suspected host	Disease	Distribution
Rodentia: Murinae			
(Hantaan-like viruses)			
Hantaan	*Apodemus agrarius*	HFRS	Asia
Dobrava	*Apodemus flavicollis*	HFRS	Europe
Saaremaa	*Apodemus agrarius*	HFRS	Europe
Amur	*Apodemus peninsulae*	HFRS	Asia
Seoul	*Rattus rattus*; *R. norvegicus*	HFRS	Worldwide
Thailand	*Bandicota indica*		Asia
Rodentia: Arvicolinae			
(Puumala-Prospect Hill-like viruses)			
Puumala	*Clethrionomys glareolus*	HFRS (NE)	Europe
Tobetsu	*Clethrionomys rufocanus*		Japan
Topografov	*Lemmus sibiricus*		Siberia
Khabarovsk	*Microtus fortis*		Siberia
Tula	*Microtus arvalis*; *M. rissiaemeridionalis*	HFRS	Europe
Prospect Hill	*Microtus pennsylvanicus*		N. America
Bloodland Lake	*Microtus ochrogaster*		N. America
Isla Vista	*Microtus californicus*		W. USA, Mexico
Rodentia: Sigmodontinae			
(Sin Nombre-like viruses)			
Sin Nombre	*Peromyscus maniculatus* (Grassland form)	HPS	W. and C. USA, Canada
Monongahela	*Peromyscus maniculatus nubiterrae* (Forest form)	HPS	E. USA, Canada
New York	*Peromyscus leucopus* (Eastern haplotype)	HPS	E. USA
Blue River	*Peromyscus leucopus* (S.W./N.W. haplotypes)	HPS	C. USA
Limestone Canyon	*Peromyscus boylii*		S.W. USA, central Mexico
Bayou	*Oryzomys palustris*	HPS	S.W. USA
Black Creek Canal	*Sigmodon hispidus* (Eastern form)	HPS	S.E. USA
Muleshoe	*Sigmodon hispidus* (Western form)		S. USA
Caño Delgadito	*Sigmodon alstoni*		Venezuela
Andes	*Oligoryzomys longicaudatus*	HPS	Argentina, Chile
Oran	*Oligoryzomys longicaudatus*	HPS	N.W. Argentina
Lechiguanas	*Oligoryzomys flavescens*	HPS	C. Argentina
Bermejo	*Oligoryzomys chacoensis*		N.W. Argentina
Hu 39694[a]	Unknown	HPS	C. Argentina
Pergamino	*Akadon azarae*		C. Argentina
Maciel	*Necromys benefactus*		C. Argentina
Laguna Negra	*Calomys laucha*	HPS	Paraguay, Bolivia
Juquitiba	Unknown	HPS	Brazil
Castelo dos Sonhos	Unknown	HPS	Brazil
Araraquara	Unknown	HPS	Brazil
Rio Mamore	*Oligoryzomys microtis*	HPS	Bolivia, Peru
El Moro Canyon	*Reithrodontomys megalotis*		W. USA, Mexico
Rio Segundo	*Reithrodontomys mexicanus*		Costa Rica
Choclo	*Oligoryzomys fulvescens*	HPS	Panama
Calabazo	*Zygodontomys brevicauda*		Panama
Insectivora: Crocidurinae			
Thottapalyam	*Suncus murinus*		India

[a]Virus will be named when the rodent host or distribution is identified.
HFRS, haemorrhagic fever with renal syndrome; HPS, hantavirus pulmonary syndrome.

in India is more distantly related to the others. Viruses of the Hantaan-like group are associated with rodent hosts of the subfamily Murinae and with HFRS; Puumala-Prospect Hill-like viruses are associated with the subfamily Arvicolinae (voles and lemmings) and with NE, and Sin Nombre-like viruses with the subfamily Sigmodontinae and with HPS (Table 18.5). Despite the fact that *Seoul virus* appears to be very widely distributed, incontrovertible evidence of disease associated with hantaviruses (detection of virus) has been obtained only for Asia, Europe and the Americas, while elsewhere there has only been inconclusive serological evidence of infection. However, *Seoul virus*, *Hantaan virus* and *Puumala virus* have been encountered as contaminants of laboratory rodent colonies and are known to have caused infections in laboratory workers in the former USSR, Korea, Japan, Belgium, France and England. In one instance virus was inadvertently preserved for years in rat tissues kept in frozen storage. Hence, the potential exists for inadvertent dissemination of the viruses.

The distributions of the hantaviruses, insofar as they are known, tend to overlap, but conform to the distributions of the rodent hosts. Individual viruses have been isolated from more than one type of rodent, but each tends to have a particular association with a single species of rodent. The viruses appear to be apathogenic for their reservoir hosts. After the rodents become infected there is an initial viraemia followed by the persistence of infection, probably for life, in lungs, kidneys and possibly other organs, with chronic excretion of virus in urine, faeces and saliva, despite the occurrence of a demonstrable immune response. There does not appear to be intrauterine transfer of infection, and transmission between rodents is thought to occur by bite, aerosol or contamination of dust, food and other fomites with excreted virus. Gamasid mite parasites of rodents are suspected to be capable of transmitting infection, but transmission occurs in the laboratory in the absence of mites. Foci with very high infection rates are observed among rodents in nature.

Humans become infected by the same means as rodents, but airborne infection from dust contaminated with rodent urine and faeces appears to be the principal mechanism, and has been observed to occur even in persons who briefly visited infected colonies of laboratory rodents. Infection occurs in three main situations: rural or sylvatic infection with Hantaan-like, Puumala-like or Sin Nombre-like viruses occurs in persons who have occupational, residential or recreational exposure to rodent-infested buildings or to the outdoors, urban infection with *Seoul virus* occurs indoors in association with rat infestations,

while all of the viruses may cause infections associated with laboratory rodents. Rodents are subject to periodic population explosions and crashes, and the incidence of human infection with Hantaan-like, Puumala-like and Sin Nombre-like viruses increases in years when the rodents are most numerous. Person-to-person spread of hantavirus infection has been observed in outbreaks of HPS caused by *Andes virus* in Argentina, but it has not been established whether transmission is associated with direct contact, droplets, aerosols or contaminated fomites (Wells *et al.*, 1997). Numerous cases of HPS have been reported in the Americas, and up to 200 000 hospitalised cases of HFRS are recorded in Eurasia each year, with more than half occurring in China (Schmaljohn and Hjelle, 1997; Monroe *et al.*, 1999).

Four clinical forms of HFRS are recognised and these vary in order of increasing severity from nephropathia epidemica associated with *Puumala virus* infection, through mild or rat-borne HFRS associated with *Seoul virus* infection, to Far Eastern HFRS associated with *Hantaan virus* carried by *A. agrarius* fieldmice, and so-called Balkan HFRS associated with *Dobrava virus* carried by *A. flavicollis* mice.

Far Eastern HFRS occurs in China, the eastern part of the former USSR and Korea, mainly in adult males with occupational exposure to the outdoors, such as farmers, forest workers and soldiers stationed in the field, and seldom occurs in persons under 10 years of age. Most cases are seen in autumn and early winter when crops are harvested and the rodents are most numerous, and subsequently when the agricultural products are stored in proximity to homesteads. The incidence of asymptomatic infection is unknown, but it was noted that American soldiers participating in an exercise in Korea who seroconverted had all been ill, while in parts of Korea high antibody prevalence rates without corresponding levels of disease have been observed.

The classical form of Far Eastern HFRS described in Korea has well marked phases, but these may overlap and be obscured in mild cases (Lee, 1982). An incubation period of 2–3 weeks is followed by the abrupt onset of a febrile phase, which lasts 3–7 days and is marked by high fever, chills, malaise, myalgia, anorexia, headache, dizziness, ocular pain and abdominal and back pain, which is felt particularly in the renal area as a result of peritoneal and retroperitoneal oedema. Proteinuria is marked during this phase. Towards the end of the phase there is characteristic flushing of the face, neck and anterior chest, with the conjunctivae, palate and pharynx assuming an injected appearance, followed by the emergence of fine petechiae on the face, neck, soft palate and chest, together with conjunctival haemorrhages. Patients next enter a hypotensive phase which lasts hours to 2 days, and is marked by classical shock: tachycardia, narrowed blood pressure, cold and clammy skin, dulled senses and confusion. One-third of fatal cases enter irreversible shock at this stage. There is marked proteinuria, microscopic haematuria, raised haematocrit levels (haemoconcentration), leukaemoid reaction and thrombocytopenia. Capillary haemorrhages are prominent. The patients then enter an oliguric phase which lasts 3–7 days. Blood urea and creatinine levels increase, blood pressure begins to normalise, but hypertension may result from a hypervolaemic state. Bleeding tendencies increase markedly, and there may be epistaxis, conjunctival, cerebral and gastrointestinal haemorrhages and extensive purpura. There may be severe nausea and vomiting, lung oedema and symptoms referable to the central nervous system. Most deaths occur at this stage. A diuretic phase which follows may last days or weeks, and marks the start of clinical recovery. Diuresis of 3–6 L/day is common, but is influenced by dehydration, electrolyte imbalance or secondary infections. Severely ill patients are at risk in this phase and may lapse into shock. A convalescent phase with progressive recovery of glomerular filtration rate, renal blood flow and urine-concentrating ability, may last 2–3 months. Mortality has been reduced from the 10–15% observed during the Korean war to 5%, with intensive supportive therapy and renal dialysis.

Balkan HFRS, associated with *Dobrava virus*, is also seen mainly in adult males, including woodcutters, shepherds and military personnel, but cases generally occur in spring and summer, possibly because there is not the same type of cereal crop farming as in the Far East, and the reservoir host is encountered in outdoor activities and at campsites during the warmer months of the year. The disease is essentially similar to Far Eastern HFRS, but is more severe, with a higher proportion of patients requiring renal dialysis, and with a greater tendency for the development of disseminated intravascular coagulopathy and haemorrhages. Reported death rates range from 5% to 35%.

Natural outbreaks of mild or rat-borne HFRS, as opposed to outbreaks associated with laboratory rodent colonies, have been recorded in cities in Japan, China and Korea. The disease occurs in urban residents who have no contact with field rodents, and most cases are seen in spring and early summer. The disease is less severe and runs a shorter course than disease associated with *Hantaan virus*

infections, and has less distinct clinical phases. There is also less tendency for haemorrhages and renal failure to occur, and frequently signs of liver involvement are dominant: abdominal pain, hepatomegaly and hepatic dysfunction. There are few deaths and mortality has been estimated at 1% or less.

Infection with Puumala-type virus occurs widely in Europe, but the disease, nephropathia epidemica, is recognised most frequently in Scandinavia and the neighbouring western region of the former USSR. The disease affects mainly adult males and infection appears to be associated principally with outdoor activities. Disease is seen most commonly in late autumn and early winter, but many cases occur in late summer following the traditional vacation season. Cases seen during the colder months are ascribed to the invasion of homes and barns by voles at the onset of winter. The incubation period is thought to be about 1 month, but a range of 3 days to 6 weeks has been reported. There is abrupt onset of fever, headache and malaise. By the third or fourth day of illness there is nausea, vomiting and abdominal and lumbar pain. At this stage there may be azotemia, oliguria and proteinuria, which peaks 1 week after the onset of illness and declines over the next 3–6 days. Patients are extremely ill during the oliguric phase, and may manifest somnolence, restlessness, confusion and meningismus. Transient myopia or blurred vision is regarded as pathognomonic. Facial flushing and maculopapular rash of the neck and trunk are seen occasionally, as are hepatomegaly, cervical lymphadenopathy and haemorrhages, such as epistaxis and gastrointestinal bleeding. Patients seldom require renal dialysis. The oliguria is followed by polyuria of 3–4 L daily for 7–10 days. At one stage it was thought that HFRS/NE and HPS were entirely distinct syndromes, but it is now recognised that there is some overlap, and in particular a proportion of NE patients may develop pulmonary infiltration similar to HPS, and some may even exhibit respiratory distress. Clinical improvement begins with the onset of polyuria, and 2 weeks after the onset of fever patients are subjectively well, but backache and lassitude may recur over weeks, and hyposthenuria may persist for months. Recovery is usually complete, and mortality is consistently <1%. The relatively high prevalence of antibody found in surveys suggests that inapparent infections may outnumber cases of overt disease by up to 20-fold.

It should be stressed that the hantaviruses overlap in distribution and in the severity of HFRS which they induce and for instance, neither rural or urban domicile of patients nor season of occurrence of disease, allow *Hantaan virus* and *Seoul virus* infections to be distinguished with certainty in Asia. Infections with *Dobrava*- and *Puumala*-type viruses in the Balkans may be equally difficult to distinguish on occasion.

Persons who develop HPS are often healthy young adults, but may be of any age and either sex, although the disease occurs infrequently in children. Infection is acquired in similar manner to HFRS from occupational, residential or recreational exposure to the outdoors or rodent-infested buildings, and in many instances infected rodents have been found in the homes of victims. Incubation periods are similar to HFRS, generally falling into the range 2–3 weeks, but the disease is characterised by severe cardiopulmonary dysfunction rather than renal failure and haemorrhage, despite the fact that there is similar underlying capillary permeability and marked thrombocytopenia. Onset of the prodromal phase of the disease is marked by sudden development of fever, headache, severe myalgia and a cough which may be productive in some instances. Gastrointestinal manifestations in some patients include abdominal pain, nausea, vomiting and diarrhoea. After 3–6 days of illness there is progressive tachypnoea, tachycardia and hypotension preceding the onset of acute respiratory distress with pulmonary oedema. Patients are generally hospitalised at this stage, but some may die before they can be admitted. In addition to tachypnoea, tachycardia and hypotension, on admission patients may be found to have proteinuria, leukocytosis with neutrophilia, plus increased myeloid precursors and atypical lymphocytes, haemoconcentration, and thrombocytopenia, plus increased prothrombin and partial-thromboplastin times, although there is no rash and seldom a tendency towards overt or internal bleeding. Within 2 days of being admitted to hospital most patients develop diffuse bilateral interstitial and alveolar pulmonary infiltration and pleural effusions demonstrable on radiographs, with hypoxaemia which has necessitated intubation, mechanical ventilation and oxygen supplementation in up to 88% of patients in some outbreaks. Renal insufficiency can occasionally follow prolonged hypoperfusion, but early renal insufficiency and increased serum creatine kinase levels (evidence of skeletal muscle inflammation) are not uncommon in infection with *Andes virus*, *Bayou virus* and *Black Creek Canal virus*. Death generally occurs 6–8 days after the onset of illness, often within 48 h of admission to hospital, but can range from 2 days after the observed onset of illness to more than 2 weeks. Fatality rates often exceed 40%, and incurable shock and myocardial dysfunction may contribute to the high mortality. Autopsies reveal non-cardiogenic pulmonary oedema and serous pleural effusions, with scant lymphoid infiltration of the lung tissue. Some survivors manifested transient diuresis, but otherwise they make an uneventful recovery without sequelae (Nichol *et al.*, 1993; Bremner, 1994; Duchin *et al.*, 1994; Schmaljohn and Hjelle, 1997; Kanerva *et al.*, 1998).

The underlying lesion in the pathogenesis of hantavirus syndromes appears to be vascular damage, and this is thought to be mediated by both viral invasion of endothelial cells and immunopathological mechanisms. Capillaries and small blood vessels dilate and there is extravasation of plasma and cellular elements into tissues, and the pathological changes observed in multiple systems all appear to be referable to the vascular damage (Kanerva *et al.*, 1998).

Treatment of HFRS involves complex, phase-specific monitoring and support of homeostasis, including fluid and electrolyte balances. Trials of ribavirin for the treatment of the disease in China have been complicated by difficulties such as lack of uniformity of clinical status of patients at the time of protocol entry, but there are indications that use of the drug reduces mortality and leads to improvement of objective markers of patient well-being and clinical pathology values. Epidemiological evidence suggests that there is lifelong immunity to hantaviruses, at least to the homologous serotype. There has been research on recombinant vaccines, but these are likely to find application only in Asia where suitable populations at risk can be identified.

Investigation of hantavirus infections is usually undertaken in high-security laboratories to minimise the exposure of staff to infection. Isolation and identification of hantaviruses is a notoriously difficult and time-consuming procedure, and is rarely successful on serum and urine specimens from patients. Demonstration of viral antigens in sera and urine is equally unsuccessful. Viral nucleic acids of hantaviruses can be detected in the tissues of human patients and experimentally and naturally infected rodents by means of reverse transcription and the polymerase chain reaction with appropriate primers (Xiao *et al.*, 1992; Arthur *et al.*, 1992; Grankvist *et al.*, 1992; Nichol *et al.*, 1993; Monroe *et al.*, 1999). Detection of IgM antibody by enzyme-linked immunoassay holds greatest promise as a rapid diagnostic technique. Antibody activity appears to be present in the sera of HFRS patients from the time of hospitalisation, and titres increase rapidly over the next 2 weeks. Owing to the antigenic cross-reactivity between hantaviruses, it may be difficult to determine the serotype of the virus responsible for the infection from antibody tests, but this can sometimes be inferred by using a range of antigens in enzyme-linked immunoassays (Feldmann *et al.*, 1993) or by performing neutralisation tests with the full range of serotypes: antibody titres tend to be highest against the homologous infecting serotype. In attempts to diagnose infection by an unknown hantavirus, particularly in an locations where local viruses are unknown, it is advisable that antigens representative of all four antigenic types be included in the tests: Hantaan-like, Puumala-Prospect Hill-like, Sin Nombre-like and Thottapalyam viruses.

POSSIBLE MEMBERS OF THE FAMILY *BUNYAVIRIDAE*

Bhanja, Kasokero, Bangui, Issyk-Kul, Tataguine and Wanowrie Viruses

Bhanja virus has been isolated from ixodid ticks of five genera—*Haemaphysalis*, *Amblyomma*, *Dermacentor*, *Boophilus* and *Hyalomma*—variously in India, the former USSR, Yugoslavia, Bulgaria, Slovakia, Somalia, Central African Republic, Nigeria and Senegal. It has been suggested that the wide distribution of the virus could have resulted from the carriage of immature ticks on migrating birds, although birds do not themselves appear to be susceptible to the virus. Isolations of the virus have also been made from a hedgehog, ground squirrel and blood samples from cattle and sheep in Nigeria. Antibody has been found in cattle, sheep and goats parasitised by the ticks, and in human sera in Slovakia, Yugoslavia, Italy and the

Central African Republic. Mild febrile illness was observed in two human patients who acquired laboratory infection, and serological evidence of infection was obtained in a patient who suffered meningoencephalitis in Yugoslavia.

Kasokero virus was isolated from fruit bats in Uganda and caused four laboratory infections marked by febrile illness, headache, myalgia, arthralgia, abdominal pain, diarrhoea, chest pain, cough, as well as hyperactive reflexes in one patient. *Bangui virus* was isolated from the blood of a patient with febrile illness, headache and rash in the Central African Republic, and antibody was found in the sera of local residents.

Issyk-Kul virus was isolated from several species of insectivorous bat and from argasid tick parasites of bats, birds and anopheline and aedine mosquitoes in the Central Asian Republics of the former USSR. It was demonstrated that aedine mosquitoes and argasid ticks are able to transmit the virus. Antibody was found in human sera and virus was isolated on at least 19 occasions from the blood of persons suffering from febrile illness with headache, dizziness, cough, nausea and vomiting. The cases included laboratory infections. *Keterah virus*, isolated from argasid tick parasites of bats and from bat blood in Malaysia, has been shown to be closely related or identical to *Issyk-Kul virus*. It is difficult to be certain whether the natural vectors of *Issyk-Kul/Keterah virus* are argasid ticks or mosquitoes.

Tataguine virus has been isolated from anopheline mosquitoes in Senegal, Nigeria, Cameroon and Central African Republic. It appears to be a potentially important pathogen: antibody has been found in human sera in Senegal and Nigeria, and there have

Table 18.6 Abridged classification of possible members of the family *Bunyaviridae*. Information derived from sources cited in the text

Serogroup ANTIGENIC COMPLEX *Virus*	Putative vectors	Human infection		Distribution
		Natural	Laboratory	
Bhanja				
BHANJA (3)[a]				
Bhanja	Ixodids	+	+	Europe, Africa, Asia
Yogue				
YOGUE (2)				
Kasokero	Unknown		+	Africa
Six other serogroups (17)				
Ungrouped (22)				
Bangui	Unknown	+		Africa
Issyk-Kul (Keterah)	Mosquitoes?	+	+	Asia
Tataguine	Mosquitoes	+		Africa
Wanowrie	Ixodids	+		Africa, Asia

[a]Figures in parentheses indicate the total numbers of recognised members of the relevant taxon.

been at least 31 isolations of the virus from the blood of febrile humans in Senegal, Nigeria, Central African Republic and Cameroon. The infections were characterised by febrile illness with headache, rash and arthralgia.

Wanowrie virus has been isolated from *Hyalomma* ticks in India, Iran and Egypt. Little else is known about the virus except that it was isolated in Sri Lanka from the brain of a human patient who succumbed to febrile illness with abdominal pain, vomiting, haematemesis and passing of blood per rectum.

REFERENCES

Al Hazmi M, Ayoola EA, Abdurahman M *et al.* (2003) Epidemic Rift Valley fever in Saudi Arabia: a clinical study of severe illness in humans. *Clin Infect Dis*, **36**, 245–252.

Anderson GW Jr and Smith JF (1987) Immunoelectron microscopy of Rift Valley fever viral morphogenesis in primary rat hepatocytes. *Virology*, **161**, 91–100.

Anonymous (1967) *Arboviruses and Human Disease*. Technical Report Series No. 369. World Health Organization, Geneva.

Anonymous (1993) Rift Valley fever. *Wkly Epidemiol Rec*, **68**, 300–301.

Anonymous (1994) Rift Valley fever. *Wkly Epidemiol Rec*, **69**, 74–75.

Anonymous (1998) An outbreak of Rift Valley fever, Eastern Africa, 1997–1998. *Wkly Epidemiol Rec*, **73**, 105–109.

Arthur RR, El-Sharkawy MS, Cope SE *et al.* (1993) Recurrence of Rift Valley fever in Egypt. *Lancet*, **342**, 1149–1150.

Arthur RR, Lofts RS, Gomez J *et al.* (1992) Grouping of hantaviruses by small (S) genome segment polymerase chain reaction and amplification of viral RNA from wild-caught rodents. *Am J Trop Med Hyg*, **47**, 210–224.

Bishop DHL (1990) *Bunyaviridae* and their replication. Part I: *Bunyaviridae*. In *Virology*, 2nd edn (eds Fields BN and Knipe DM), pp 1155–1173. Raven, New York.

Bishop DHL, Calisher CH, Casals J *et al.* (1980) Bunyaviridae. *Intervirology*, **14**, 125–143.

Botros BA, Swanepoel R, Graham RR *et al.* (1997) Genetic characterization of Rift Valley fever isolates from the 1997 and 1993–1994 outbreaks in Egypt. Abstracts of the 46th Annual Meeting of the American Society of Tropical Medicine and Hygiene, Colorado Springs Resort, Lake Buena Vista, FL, 7–11 December.

Bowen MD, Trappier SG, Sanchez AJ *et al.* (2001) A reassortant bunyavirus isolated from acute hemorrhagic fever cases in Kenya and Somalia. *Virology*, **291**, 185–190.

Bremner JAG (1994) Hantavirus infections and outbreaks in 1993. *Commun Dis Rep*, **4**, R5–9.

Calisher CH (1991) *Bunyaviridae*. *Arch Virol*, **121**(suppl 2), 273–283.

Calisher CH and Karabatsos N (1989) Arbovirus serogroups: definition and geographic distribution. In *The Arboviruses: Epidemiology and Ecology*, vol I (ed. Monath TP), pp 19–57. CRC Press, Boca Raton, FL.

Casals J (1957) The arthropod-borne group of animal viruses. *Trans NY Acad Sci*, **19**, 219–235.

Casals J (1961) Procedures for identification of arthropod-borne viruses. *Bull WHO*, **24**, 727–734.

Casals J and Whitman L (1960) A new antigenic group of arthropod-borne viruses. The Bunyamwera group. *Am J Trop Med Hyg*, **9**, 73–77.

Casals J and Whitman L (1961) Group C. A new serological group of hitherto undescribed arthropod-borne viruses. Immunological studies. *Am J Trop Med Hyg*, **10**, 250–258.

Chu Y-K, Jennings G, Schmaljohn C *et al.* (1995) Cross-neutralization of hantaviruses with immune sera from experimentally infected animals and from hemorrhagic fever with renal syndrome and hantavirus pulmonary syndrome patients. *J Infect Dis*, **172**, 1581–1584.

Chu Y-K, Rossi C, LeDuc J *et al.* (1994) Serological relationships among viruses in the in the Hantavirus genus, family Bunyaviridae. *Virology*, **198**, 196–204.

Chumakov MP (1974) [Contribution to 30 years of investigation of Crimean haemorrhagic fever]. In *Medical Virology*, vol 22 (ed. Chumakov MP), pp 5–18. *Trudy Inst Polio Virus Entsef Akad Med Nauk SSSR* [In Russian. English translation: NAMRU3-T950].

Chung SI, Livingston CW Jr, Edwards JF *et al.* (1990a) Evidence that Cache Valley virus induces congenital malformations in sheep. *Vet Microbiol*, **21**, 297–307.

Chung SI, Livingston CW Jr, Edwards JF *et al.* (1990b) Congenital malformations in sheep resulting from in utero inoculation of Cache valley virus. *Am J Vet Res*, **51**, 1645–1648.

Duchin JS, Koster FT, Peters CJ *et al.* (1994) Hantavirus pulmonary syndrome: a clinical description of 17 patients with a newly recognized disease. *N Engl J Med*, **330**, 949–955.

Easterday BC (1965) Rift Valley fever. *Adv Vet Sc*, **10**, 65–127.

El Azazy OM and Scrimgeour EM (1997) Crimean-Congo haemorrhagic fever virus infection in the western province of Saudi Arabia. *Trans R Soc Trop Med Hyg*, **91**, 275–278.

Feldmann H, Sanchez A, Morzunov S *et al.* (1993) Utilization of autopsy RNA for the synthesis of the nucleocapsid antigen of a newly recognized virus associated with hantavirus pulmonary syndrome. *Virus Res*, **30**, 351–367.

Fenner F (1976) Classification and nomenclature of viruses. Second Report of the International Committee on Taxonomy of Viruses. *Intervirology*, **7**, 1–116.

Foggin CM and Swanepoel R (1977) Unpublished observations. Veterinary Research Laboratory, Causeway, Harare, Zimbabwe.

Gonzalez-Scarano F and Nathanson N (1990) Bunyaviruses. In *Virology*, 2nd edn (eds Fields BN and Knipe DM), pp 1195–1228. Raven, New York.

Grankvist O, Juto P, Settergren B *et al.* (1992) Detection of nephropathia epidemica virus RNA in patient samples using a nested primer-based polymerase chain reaction. *J Infect Dis*, **165**, 934–937.

Grimstad PR, Calisher CH, Harroff RN and Wentworth BB (1986) Jamestown Canyon virus (California serogroup) is the etiologic agent of widespread infection of Michigan humans. *Am J Trop Med Hyg*, **35**, 376–386.

Henning MW (ed.) (1956) Rift Valley fever. In *Animal Diseases in South Africa*, 3rd edn, pp 1105–1121. Central News Agency Ltd, Cape Town.

Hoogstraal H (1979) The epidemiology of tick-borne Crimean-Congo haemorrhagic fever in Asia, Europe and Africa. *J Med Entomol*, **15**, 307–417.

Hoogstraal H (1981) Changing patterns of tick-borne diseases in modern society. *Ann Rev Entomol*, **26**, 75–99.

Johnson BK, Chanas AC, Squires EJ *et al.* (1978) The isolation of a Bwamba virus variant from man in western Kenya. *J Med Virol*, **2**, 15–20.

Jupp PG, Kemp A, Grobbelaar A *et al.* (2002) The 2000 epidemic of Rift Valley fever in Saudi Arabia: mosquito vector studies. *Med Vet Entomol*, **16**, 245–252.

Kalunda M, Lwanga-Ssozi C, Lule M and Mukuye A (1985) Isolation of Chikungunya and Pongola viruses from patients in Uganda. *Trans R Soc Trop Med Hyg*, **79**, 567.

Kanerva M, Mustonen J and Vaheri A (1998) Pathogenesis of Puumala and other hantavirus infections. *Rev Med Virol*, **8**, 67–86.

Karabatsos N (ed.) (1985) *International Catalogue of Arboviruses, Including Certain Other Viruses of Vertebrates*, 3rd edn. American Society of Tropical Medicine and Hygiene, San Antonio.

Khan AS, Maupin GO, Rollin PE *et al.* (1997) An outbreak of Crimean-Congo hemorrhagic fever in the United Arab Emirates, 1994–1995. *Am J Trop Med Hyg*, **57**, 519–525.

Lee HW (1982) Korean haemorrhagic fever. *Progr Med Virol*, **28**, 96–113.

Linthicum KJ, Davies FG and Kaairo A (1985) Rift Valley fever virus (family *Bunyaviridae*, genus *Phlebovirus*). Isolations from Diptera collected during an inter-epizootic period in Kenya. *J Hyg*, **95**, 197–209.

Matthews REF (1981) The classification and nomenclature of viruses: summary of results of meetings of the International Committee on Taxonomy of Viruses in Strasbourg, August 1981. *Intervirology*, **16**, 53–60.

McKee KT Jr, LeDuc JW and Peters CJ (1991) Hantaviruses. In *Textbook of Human Virology*, 2nd edn (ed. Belshe RB), pp 615–632. Mosby Year Book, St Louis, MO.

Meegan JM and Bailey CL (1989) Rift Valley fever. In *The Arboviruses: Epidemiology and Ecology*, vol IV (ed. Monath TP), pp 51–76. CRC Press, Boca Raton, FL.

Monroe MC, Morzunov SP, Johnson AM *et al.* (1999) Genetic diversity and distribution of *Peromyscus*-borne hantaviruses in North America. *Emerg Infect Dis*, **5**, 75–86.

Murphy FA, Harrison AK and Whitfield SG (1973) *Bunyaviridae*: morphological and morphogenetic similarities of Bunyamwera serologic supergroup viruses and several other arthropod-borne viruses. *Intervirology*, **1**, 297–316.

Murphy FA, Fauquet CM, Bishop DHL *et al.* (1995) Sixth Report of the International Committee on Taxonomy of Viruses. *Archiv. Virol.*, Supplement 10, 1–586.

Nichol ST (2003) Centers for Disease Control and Prevention, Atlanta, GA, USA (personal communication).

Nichol ST, Spiropoulou CF, Morzunov S *et al.* (1993) Genetic identification of a hantavirus associated with an outbreak of acute respiratory illness. *Science*, **262**, 914–917.

Papa A, Bino S, Llagami A *et al.* (2002a) Crimean-Congo hemorrhagic fever in Albania, 2001. *Eur J Clin Microbiol Infect Dis*, **8**, 603–606.

Papa A, Bosovic B, Pavlidou V *et al.* (2002b) Genetic detection and isolation of Crimean-Congo hemorrhagic fever virus, Kosovo, Yugoslavia. *Emerg Infect Dis*, **8**, 852–854.

Peters CJ and LeDuc JW (1991) Bunyaviridae: bunyaviruses, phleboviruses and related viruses. In *Textbook of Human Virology*, 2nd edn (ed. Belshe RB), pp 571–614. Mosby Year Book, St Louis, MO.

Peters CJ and Meegan JM (1981) Rift Valley fever. In *CRC Handbook Series in Zoonoses*, sect B, vol I (ed. Beran G), pp 403–419. CRC Press, Boca Raton, FL.

Porterfield JS (1990) Alphaviruses, Flaviviruses and Bunyaviridae. In *Principles and Practice of Clinical Virology*, 2nd edn (eds Zuckerman AJ, Banatvala JE and Pattison JR), pp 434–448. Wiley, Chichester.

Porterfield JS, Casals J, Chumakov MP *et al.* (1974) Bunyaviruses and Bunyaviridae. *Intervirology*, **2**, 270–272.

Puthavathana P, Lee HW and Yong Kang C (1992) Typing of hantaviruses from five continents by polymerase chain reaction. *Virus Res*, **26**, 1–14.

Reeves WC (1974) Overwintering of arboviruses. *Progr Med Virol*, **17**, 193–220.

Schmaljohn CS, Beaty BJ, Calisher CH *et al.* (2002) In *ICTVdB—The Universal Virus Database*, version 3 (ed. Büchen-Osmond C), http://www.ncbi.nlm.nih.gov/ICTVdB, Oracle, Arizona: ICTVdB Management, Columbia University, The Earth Institute, Biosphere 2 Center.

Schmaljohn CS, Hasty SE, Dalrymple JM and LeDuc JW (1985) Antigenic and genetic properties place viruses linked to hemorrhagic fever with renal syndrome into a newly-defined genus of Bunyaviridae. *Science*, **227**, 1041–1044.

Schmaljohn C and Hjelle B (1997) Hantaviruses: a global disease problem. *Emerg Infect Dis*, **2**, 95–104.

Schmaljohn CS and Patterson JL (1990) Bunyaviridae and their replication. Part II: Replication of Bunyaviridae. In *Virology*, 2nd edn (eds Fields BN and Knipe DM), pp 1175–1194. Raven, New York.

Scrimgeour EM, Zaki A, Mehta FR *et al.* (1996) Crimean-Congo haemorrhagic fever in Oman. *Trans R Soc Trop Med Hyg*, **90**, 290–291.

Shimshony A and Barzilai R (1983) Rift Valley fever. *Adv Vet Sci Comp Med*, **27**, 347–425.

Shope E and Sather GE (1979) Arboviruses. In *Diagnostic Procedures for Viral, Rickettsial and Chlamydial Infections*, 5th edn (eds Lennette EH and Schmidt NJ), pp 767–814. American Public Health Association, Washington, DC.

Simons JF, Hellmann U and Petterson RF (1990) Uukuniemi virus S RNA segment: ambisense coding strategy, packaging of complementary strands into virions, and homology to members of the genus *Phlebovirus*. *J Virol*, **64**, 247–255.

Swanepoel R (2003) Classification, epidemiology and control of arthropod-borne viruses. In *Infectious Diseases of Livestock*, 2nd edn (eds Coetzer JAW and Tustin RC). Oxford University Press Southern Africa, Cape Town.

Swanepoel R and Coetzer JAW (2003) Rift Valley fever. In *Infectious Diseases of Livestock*, 2nd edn (eds Coetzer JAW and Tustin RC). Oxford University Press Southern Africa, Cape Town.

Swanepoel R, Gill DE, Shepherd AJ and Leman PA (1989) The clinical pathology of Crimean-Congo hemorrhagic fever. *Rev Infect Dis*, **11**, S794–800.

Swanepoel R, Shepherd AJ, Leman PA *et al.* (1987) Epidemiologic and clinical features of Crimean-Congo haemorrhagic fever in southern Africa. *Am J Trop Med Hyg*, **36**, 120–132.

Tesh RB (1984) Transovarial transmission of arboviruses in their invertebrate vectors. In *Current Topics in Vector Research*, vol II (ed. Harris KF), pp 57–76. Praeger, New York.

Watts DM, Ksiazek TG, Linthicum KJ and Hoogstraal H (1989) Crimean-Congo haemorrhagic fever. In *The Arboviruses: Epidemiology and Ecology*, vol II (ed. Monath TP), pp 177–222. CRC Press, Boca Raton, FL.

Weiss KE (1957) Rift Valley fever—a review. *Bull Epizoot Dis Africa*, **5**, 431–458.

Wells RM, Estani SS, Yadon ZE *et al.* (1997) An unusual hantavirus outbreak in southern Argentina: person-to-person transmission? *Emerg Infect Dis*, **2**, 171–174.

Williams RJ, Al Busaidy S, Mehta FR *et al.* (2000) Crimean-Congo haemorrhagic fever: a seroepidemiological and tick survey in the Sultanate of Oman. *Trop Med Int Hlth*, **5**, 99–106.

Woods CW, Karpati AM, Grein T *et al.* (2002) An outbreak of Rift Valley fever in north-eastern Kenya, 1997–98. *Emerg Infect Dis*, **8**, 138–144.

Xiao S-Y, Chu Y-K, Knauert FK *et al.* (1992) Comparison of hantavirus isolates using a genus-reactive primer pair polymerase chain reaction. *J Gen Virol*, **73**, 567–573.

Xiao S-Y, LeDuc JW, Chu YK and Schmaljohn CS (1994) Phylogenetic analyses of of virus isolates in the genus *Hantavirus*, family *Bunyaviridae*. *Virology*, **198**, 205–217.

19

Arenaviruses

Colin R. Howard

Royal Veterinary College, University of London, UK

INTRODUCTION

The arenaviruses are a group of enveloped, single-stranded RNA viruses, the study of which has been pursued for two quite separate reasons. First, lymphocytic choriomeningitis virus (LCM) has been used as a model of persistent virus infections for over half a century; its study has contributed a number of cardinal concepts to our present understanding of interactions between viruses and the host immune system. Although LCM infections of humans are rare, this virus remains the prototype of the *Arenaviridae* and is a common infection of laboratory mice, rats and hamsters. Second, certain arenaviruses cause severe haemorrhagic diseases in man, notably Lassa fever in Africa, and Argentinian haemorrhagic fever in South America. More recently, several new arenaviruses have been described from South America, two of which are associated with human infections. In common with LCM, the natural reservoir of these infections is a limited number of rodent species (Howard, 1986). Although the initial isolates from South America were at first erroneously designated as newly defined arboviruses, there is no evidence to implicate arthropod transmission for any arenavirus. However, similar methods of isolation and the necessity of trapping small animals have meant historically that the majority of arenaviruses have been isolated by workers in the arbovirus field. A good example of this is Guanarito virus, which emerged during investigation of a dengue virus outbreak in Venezuela (Salas *et al.*, 1991). The discovery of Sin Nombre virus as a cause of hantavirus pulmonary syndrome has led to a resurgence of interest in the link between zoonoses and persistent virus infections of rodents (see Chapter 18 for a description of the hantaviruses). The Four Corners outbreak of hantavirus pulmonary syndrome in 1993 served to heighten awareness that fevers of hitherto unknown origin might equally be the result of infection with agents normally maintained in rodent reservoirs. This is particularly so in Argentina, where virologists and clinicians specialising in Argentinian haemorrhagic fever have been in the vanguard of national efforts linking respiratory disease with the discovery of new hantaviruses that can coexist with arenaviruses in the same rodent populations.

With the current concern about the so-called 'emerging viruses', the arenaviruses are a good illustration of how environmental changes may result in an altered balance between man and natural animal hosts, leading to unexpected diseases which can severely challenge local and national public health resources. In addition, there is a wide spectrum of pathological processes associated with these viruses that give useful insights into other zoonotic infections. All the evidence is that the morbidity of Lassa fever and South American haemorrhagic fevers due to arenavirus infection results from the direct cytopathic action of these agents. This is in sharp contrast to the immunopathological basis of 'classic' lymphocytic choriomeningitis disease seen in adult mice infected with LCM virus.

For a general overview of the arenaviruses, see Oldstone (2002a, 2002b). A comprehensive overview of the arenaviruses causing human disease can be found on http://www.cdc.gov/ncidad/dvrd/spb and http://www.who.int/health-topics/index

Principles and Practice of Clinical Virology, Fifth Edition. Edited by A. J. Zuckerman, J. E. Banatvala, J. R. Pattison, P. D. Griffiths and B. D. Schoub
© 2004 John Wiley & Sons Ltd   ISBN 0 470 84338 1

Table 19.1 The arenaviruses: host and geographical distribution

Virus	Natural host	Human disease	Distribution
Worldwide			
Lymphocytic choriomeningitis	*Mus musculus, Mus domesticus*	Aseptic meningitis	Europe, North and South America
Old World			
Ippy	*Arvicanthus* sp.	Not recorded	Central African Republic
Lassa	*Mastomys natalensis*	Lassa fever	West Africa
Mobala	*Praomys jacksoni*	Infection possible	Central African Republic
Mopeia	*Mastomys natalensis*	Infection possible	Mozambique, Zimbabwe
New World			
Allpahuayo	*Oecomys* sp.	Not recorded	Peru
Amapari	*Oryzomys gaedi, Neocomys guianae*	Not recorded	Brazil
Bear Canyon	*Peromyscus californicus*	Infection possible	USA
Flexal	*Neocomys* spp.	Not recorded	Brazil
Guanarito	*Sigmodon alstoni Zygodontomys brevicuda*	Venezuelan haemorrhagic fever	Venezuela
Junín	*Calomys musculinus, C. laucha, Akadon azarae*	Argentinian haemorrhagic fever	Argentina
Latino	*Calomys callosus*	Not recorded	Bolivia
Machupo	*Calomys callosus*	Bolivian haemorrhagic fever	Bolivia
Paraná	*Oryzomys buccinatus*	Not recorded	Paraguay
Pichinde	*Oryzomys albigularis*	Not recorded	Colombia
Pirital	*Sigmodon alstoni*	Not recorded	Venezuela
Oliveros	*Bolomys obscurus*	Not recorded	Argentina
Sabiá	Unknown	Brazilian haemorrhagic fever	Brazil
Tacaribe	*Artibeus literatus* (bat)	Infection possible	Trinidad
Tamiami	*Sigmodon hispidus*	Not recorded	Florida, USA
Whitewater Arroyo	*Neotoma albigula*	Not recorded	New Mexico, USA

PROPERTIES OF THE VIRUS

Nomenclature and Natural History

The morphological, physicochemical and serological properties of the arenaviruses were first summarised by Pfau (1974). The members of the family currently identified are listed in Table 19.1. The various strains and isolates of LCM are now considered to be a genus within the family *Arenaviridae*. A close serological relationship exists between LCM, Lassa virus and other arenaviruses from Africa. For this reason, they are loosely referred to as the 'Old World' arenaviruses, in contrast to those from the Americas, although now LCM can be found worldwide except in Australia. The 'New World' arenaviruses show varying degrees of serological relationships with Tacaribe virus, first isolated in Trinidad. For this reason, viruses from the Americas are frequently regarded as members of the Tacaribe complex.

The *Arenaviridae* take their name from the sand-sprinkled appearance when viewed in the electron microscope (Latin *arena* = sand). With the exception of LCM, all are referred to by names that reflect the geographical area in which they were isolated (Figure 19.1). Various strain designations are also commonly used, in particular for LCM and arenaviruses isolated from man. Multiple isolations of non-pathogenic viruses that infect New World rodents are made less frequently, with the exception of Pichinde virus, in which a large number of field isolates from Colombia have been characterised. However, the recent resurgence of interest in these viruses has uncovered a number of new arenaviruses that have tentatively been described as new members of the *Arenaviridae*. Several of these may be new variants of existing family members.

All but one of the 21[1] members of the *Arenaviridae* so far described have rodents as their natural reservoir hosts. Although rodents are divided into over 30

---

[1]At the time of writing (January 2003), two further putative arenaviruses have been recorded (Cupixi and Rio Carcarana viruses).

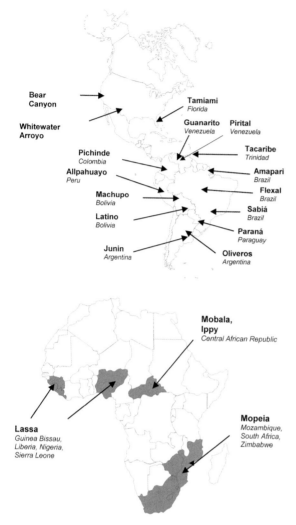

Figure 19.1 Geographical distribution of Old World (a) and New World (b) arenaviruses. *Lymphocytic choriomeningitis virus* (LCM) can be found on all continents except Australasia

families distributed worldwide, arenaviruses are predominantly found within two major families: Muridae (e.g. mice and rats) and Cricetidae (e.g. voles, lemmings, gerbils). The nature of the original reservoir for LCM virus remains obscure, but it appears to be mainly in species of the Muridae which evolved in the Old World and subsequently spread to most parts of the globe. Interestingly, there is a wide range of tropism and virulence among those strains of LCM virus originally isolated from laboratory mouse colonies.

The natural reservoirs of Lassa virus and the remaining Old World arenaviruses are members of the genus *Mastomys*. This is also a member of the Muridae and, in common with the host of LCM, frequents human dwellings and food stores. In contrast, nearly all arenaviruses isolated from the South American continent are associated with cricetid rodents, whose members frequent open grasslands and forest. The exception is Tacaribe virus, which was originally isolated from the fruit bat, *Artibeus literatus*.

ULTRASTRUCTURE OF ARENAVIRUSES AND INFECTED CELLS

Negative-staining electron microscopy of extracellular virus shows pleomorphic particles, of diameter 80–150 nm (Figure 19.2). The virus envelope is formed from the plasma membrane of infected cells. A significant thickening of both bilayers of the membrane together with an increase in the width of the electron-translucent intermediate layer is characteristic of arenavirus maturation. Little is known about the internal structure of the arenavirus particle, although thin sections of mature and budding viruses clearly show the ordered, and often circular, arrangements of host ribosomes that are typical of this virus group and confer the 'sandy' appearance from which its name is derived. Distinct well-dispersed filaments 5–10 nm in diameter are released from detergent-treated virus. Two predominant size classes are present, with average lengths of 649 nm and 1300 nm, respectively; these lengths do not show a close relationship with the two virus-specific L and S RNA species. Each is circular and beaded in appearance. Convoluted filamentous strands up to 15 nm in diameter can be seen in preparations of spontaneously disrupted Pichinde virus. These appear to represent globular condensations which arise from an association between neighbouring turns of the underlying helix. The basic configuration of the filaments shows a linear array of globular units up to 5 nm in diameter, probably representing single molecules of the viral polypeptide. These filaments progressively fold through a number of intermediate helical structures to produce the stable 15 nm diameter forms (Young, 1987).

Arenaviruses replicate in experimental animals in the absence of any gross pathological effect. However, cellular necrosis may accompany virus production, not unlike that seen in virus-infected cell cultures. The variable pathological changes associated with arenavirus infections are further complicated by the occasional appearance of particles in tissue sections

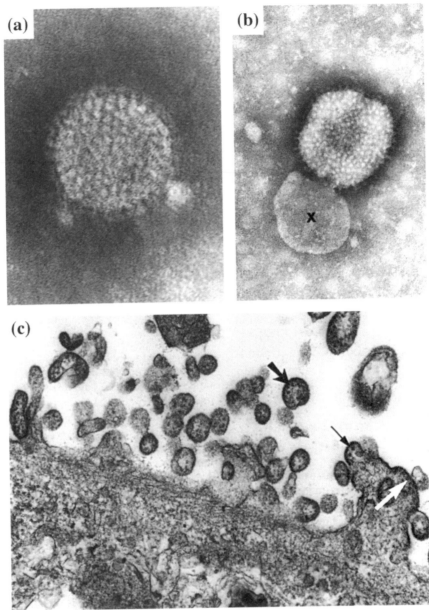

Figure 19.2 Electron microscopy of arenaviruses. (a) Negatively stained Lassa fever particle showing the whole surface covered in projections. Few particles are less than 100 nm, and many are twice this size (× 300 000). (b) Mopeia virus from southern Africa. Here the negative stain has disrupted the particle, the contents of which (X) have been extruded. × 150 000. (c) Lassa fever particles budding from an infected Vero cell. The thick arrow shows a mature particle, the thin arrow a maturing particle at the plasmalemma. Nucleocapsids and ribosomes line up immediately below the thickened membrane (white arrow) (× 39 000). Micrographs courtesy of Dr D. S. Ellis

that react strongly with fluorescein-conjugated anti-sera. Granular fluorescence with convalescent serum in the perinuclear region of acutely infected Vero cells is often seen. In addition, intracytoplasmic inclusion bodies are a prominent feature in virus-infected cells, both *in vitro* and *in vivo*. These usually appear early in the replication cycle and consist largely of single ribosomes which later become condensed in an electron-dense matrix, sometimes together with fine filaments (Murphy and Whitfield, 1975).

CHEMICAL COMPOSITION

Proteins

All arenaviruses contain a major nucleocapsid associated protein of molecular weight 60–68 kDa with two glycoproteins in the outer viral envelope. These envelope glycoproteins are not primary gene products but arise by proteolytic cleavage of a larger, 75 kDa glycoprotein precursor polypeptide (GPC). Maturation and release of virus do not seem to be markedly inhibited in the presence of tunicamycin, an inhibitor of glycosylation but glycoprotein processing is essential for infectivity.

The major glycoprotein species (GP2) in the molecular weight range of 34–42 kDa represents the C-terminal cleavage product of the GPC envelope glycoprotein precursor. The first 59 amino acids at the N-terminus of GPC act as a signal sequence, containing two distinct hydrophobic domains that could function during glycoprotein transport and virus assembly. GP1 is cleaved from the N-terminus at a unique cleavage site that is conserved among all arenaviruses except Tacaribe. GP1 assembles into tetramers linked by disulphide bonds. GP2 is also thought to form tetrameric structures proximal to GP1 in the glycoprotein peplomer, penetrating the viral membrane to form electrovalent bonds with the underlying N-RNA nucleocapsids.

A major antigenic site recognised by antibodies has been located between amino acids 390 and 405, and cross-reactive monoclonal antibodies bind epitopes in this region. The corresponding N-terminal product of GPC cleavage (GP1) is probably highly glycosylated with at least four antigenic domains. Neutralising monoclonal antibodies to LCM virus map to two of these regions and there is less sequence homology between the GP1 than between the GP2 molecules of different arenaviruses. Polyclonal neutralising antibody appears to react predominantly with conformation-dependent structures within one of these domains.

The internal nucleocapsid-associated (N) protein accounts for over 70% of the protein present in purified virus and infected cells, and remains bound to the virus genome after solubilisation of the virus to form structures resembling a string of beads seen by electron microscopy. Cleavage products of the N protein are a consistent feature of both virus and virus-infected cells. Cleavage is not noticeable in Vero cells; yields of arenaviruses are lower in these cells, perhaps due to reduced availability of N for packaging. N protein accumulates in the cytoplasm of infected cells, with a fragment of the N protein often seen in the nuclei, the exact function of which is not clear. Molecular cloning studies have shown a surprisingly high degree of homology between the 558–570 amino acid N proteins of Old and New World arenaviruses, with structural motifs and RNA-binding domains particularly conserved. This would account for the serological cross-reactions seen using certain monoclonal antibodies raised against such epidemiologically distinct viruses and may indicate precise functional roles in virus replication for certain domains of the N polypeptide.

A minor component with a molecular weight in excess of 150 kDa is often observed in infected cells and is found with purified nucleocapsids. This L protein is coded by the larger RNA genome segment as shown by the study of reassortment viruses and represents the virus-specific RNA polymerase (Fuller-Pace and Southern, 1989; Lukashevich et al., 1997). Amino acid sequences common to all RNA-dependent RNA polymerases are present along the open reading frame coding for the L protein, which suggest the conservation of certain functional domains. An additional two sequences are shared with the RNA polymerases of bunyaviruses. A small, 11 kDa viral polypeptide, the Z protein, is considered to play a role in controlling the replication and expression of the genome owing to its zinc-binding properties. The Z protein may also modulate the interferon response to infection in vivo by binding to the nuclear oncoprotein PML (Djavani et al., 2001).

Nucleic Acid

The genome of arenaviruses consists of two single-stranded RNA segments of different sizes, designated L and S, with S RNA being more abundant. Analysis of RNA is complicated by the presence of ribosomal 18S and 28S RNA, although these cellular RNA species are not essential for virus replication. The total ribosomal RNA content may in turn be influenced by the varying proportions of infectious to non-infectious particles present in virus stocks, particularly if cells are infected at a multiplicity above 0.1. In addition, there are small quantities of both cell and viral low molecular weight RNA. One of these species, mRNA coding for the viral Z protein, may have a role in the initial stages of infection. There is no obvious role for these host RNA molecules in either replication or the establishment of persistent infections (see Replication, below).

Extracted virion RNA is not infectious and the detection of a viral RNA polymerase led to the belief that arenaviruses adopt a negative-strand coding strategy with respect to viral protein synthesis. However, the actual coding strategy from the L and S RNA strands is not entirely in accord with all negative-strand RNA viruses, as some genetic information can only be expressed by a genomic sense mRNA. This 'ambisense' strategy is also a characteristic of some bunyavirus genomes (see Chapter 18). Such a coding strategy allows for the independent regulation of arenavirus envelope and nucleocapsid proteins.

The S strand codes for the nucleoprotein (N) and the envelope glycoprotein precursor (GPC) in two main open reading frames located on RNA molecules of opposite polarity. The 3' half of the S RNA codes for the N protein by production of an mRNA with a viral-sense sequence specific for the GPC protein. Thus, expression of the genome is by synthesis of subgenomic RNA from full-length templates of opposite polarities. The reading frames for the two major gene products are separated by a hairpin structure of approximately 20 paired nucleotides. This intergenic region may act as a control mechanism for genome expression by forming stable stem–loop structures that in turn regulate transcription. The S RNA of Tacaribe and Junín viruses are thought to form a second stem–loop structure.

The L RNA strand represents about 70% of the viral genome; reassortment studies with virulent and avirulent strains of LCM virus have shown that the lethality of the disease in guinea-pigs is associated with the properties of the L RNA. The L protein is encoded by a large open reading frame covering 70% of the L RNA strand: it is expressed via mRNA complementary in sense to the viral genome. The mRNA for the Z protein is also expressed from the L RNA strand.

All arenavirus genomes have a conserved 3'-terminus at the ends of the L and S RNA; this sequence is inversely complementary to the 5'-terminus of the same RNA strand. There is some evidence by electron microscopy of intramolecular and intramolecular complexes promoted by this arrangement of 3'- and 5'-termini nucleotide complentarity.

Phylogenetic Analysis

Sequencing of PCR products can give useful quantitative comparisons between newly discovered isolates and those already characterised, providing caution is exercised both in the choice of primer sets and the method of analysis. Bowen et al. (1997) analysed at least one strain of all arenaviruses known at that time, using maximum parsimony to generate an unrooted phylogenetic tree (reviewed by Clegg, 2002; Figure 19.3). The results confirmed that the distant relationship between Old World and New World arenaviruses are broadly consistent with the previously determined serological relationships, using polyclonal and monoclonal antibodies. The New World arenaviruses are divisible into three lineages: clade A contains the viruses Pichinde, Tamiami, Paraná and Flexal; clade B the viruses Sabiá, Tacaribe, Amaparí, Guanarito and the human pathogens Machupo and Junín; and clade C consists of Oliveros and Latino viruses. Interestingly, Whitewater Arroyo virus, isolated in the USA, appears closely related to Tamiami, until recently the only arenavirus found in North America. However, full-length analysis of Whitewater Arroyo virus S RNA strand has shown a quite separate ancestry for the nucleocapsid (N) and envelope (GP1, GP2) proteins, almost certainly the result of recombination between two ancestral arenaviruses. There is less variability among the Old World members. As may be expected from their natural history, Mopeia and Mobala viruses are closely related to Lassa Fever virus. LCM virus occupies the distinctive position of being closely related to the probable ancestral virus.

The propensity to cause serious human illness appears to have evolved on two distinct occasions. The South American pathogens are all confined to clade B, suggesting these viruses have acquired the capacity to infect humans as a result of a common mutational event. Lassa fever virus, by contrast, has likely acquired its ability to cause serious haemorrhagic disease in humans by a separate evolutionary event.

For a thorough discussion of the phylogenetic relationships among the arenaviruses, the reader is referred to Clegg (2002).

REPLICATION

Arenaviruses replicate in a wide variety of mammalian cells, although either BHK-21 cells or monkey kidney cell lines are preferred for molecular studies (Howard, 1986). Arenaviruses can also infect a number of primary human cell lines and macrophages, including some members of the family that do not otherwise cause human infections. Most arenaviruses also grow well in mouse L cells but the simultaneous production of C-type retroviruses restricts the usefulness of such cells. The widely conserved cell protein α-dystroglycan has been identified as the cellular receptor for Old

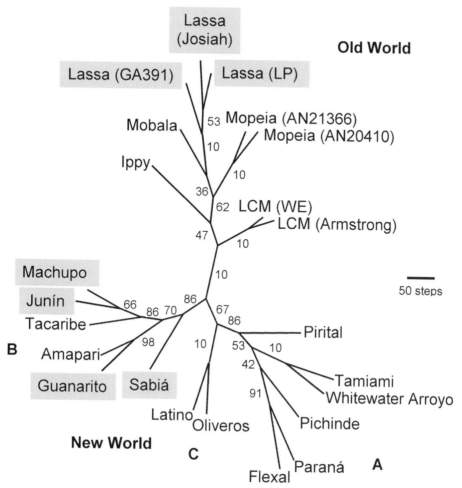

Figure 19.3 Phyogenetic analysis of Old and New World arenaviruses using nucleocapsid (N) gene sequences. The New World viruses are divisable into at least three clades (A–C). Reproduced from Clegg (2002) by permission of Springer-Verlag GmbH & Co. KG

World arenaviruses, such as Lassa fever and Mobala, and those New World arenaviruses Latino and Oliveros in clade C (Cao *et al.*, 1998). However, other cell surface proteins and co-factors may also be involved.

At low multiplicities of infection (i.e. below 0.1) the latent period is approximately 6–8 h, after which cell-associated virus increases exponentially. The titre of extracellular virus reaches a maximum 36–48 h after infection. The passage history of any particular virus stock is probably one of the most critical factors in determining the kinetics of arenavirus replication.

Infected cells undergo only limited cytopathic changes in the cell lines commonly employed, with little or no change in the total level of host cell protein synthesis; virus yields vary in different susceptible cell types. Plaque assays are possible, but only under well-defined conditions. Cultures of persistently infected cells are readily established, with morphology and growth kinetics similar to those of uninfected cells.

The major feature of an ambisense coding strategy is that it allows for independent expression and regulation of the N and GPC genes from the S RNA segment. The N protein is expressed late in acute infection and continues to be expressed in persistently infected cells in the absence of glycoprotein production. This is explained by the production of a subgenomic mRNA from a negative polarity, virus-sense template. A control mechanism must therefore exist which determines the fate of nascent RNA of negative polarity, destined either for encapsidation or as a template for N protein-specific mRNA. In contrast, the template for glycoprotein-specific mRNA is of complementary sense to viral RNA and, as such, would not be required for nascent virus production. The lack of glycoprotein late in the replicative cycle or in persistently infected cells would therefore imply selective transcriptional or translational control of this gene product.

Both viral RNA and its complementary strand contain at least one hairpin sequence, which may provide recognition points for termination of transcription by viral RNA polymerase. The nucleotide sequence in the hairpin region is of coding sense and may be transcribed, either as a discrete mRNA species or as a result of extended transcription of N or GPC messengers through this region. The reading frames for viral gene products transcribed from LCM and Pichinde viral genomes would fit this hypothesis. In addition, a sequence for ribosomal 18S subunit binding is present on both mRNA molecules, although its significance remains uncertain.

DIAGNOSIS OF HUMAN ARENAVIRUS INFECTIONS

The diagnosis of arenavirus infections may be made by demonstration of a four-fold rise in specific antibody titre, the presence of specific IgM antibodies, or isolation of the virus. Although arenaviruses can easily be grown in a variety of mammalian cell cultures, it must be remembered that clinical specimens from patients suspected as having a viral haemorrhagic fever should always be handled in biologically secure containment facilities. For this reason tests for antibody are more useful, since inactivated viral antigens for serology can prepared easily. For routine isolation, the E6 clone of Vero cells is the cell line of choice, although all arenaviruses grow well in primate and rodent-derived fibroblast cell lines. However, a cytopathic effect (CPE) is often difficult to see, and inoculated cultures often require examination by immunofluorescence (IF) or immunoperoxidase assay in order to detect viral antigens.

IF-based specific viral antibody tests are often the preferred method for the diagnosis of human arenavirus infections. In the case of Lassa fever, infected cell substrates are used that have been treated by ultraviolet (UV) light, acetone and cobalt irradiation to ensure safety. Drops of cell cultures dried onto glass slides can be prepared in a central laboratory and these preparations remain stable for many months. Most of the antigen detected within acetone-fixed infected cells represents cytoplasmic nucleocapsid protein. In the

case of the New World arenaviruses, serological cross-reactions in the IF test, e.g. with sera from patients with Bolivian (Machupo) and Argentinian (Junín) haemorrhagic fevers, are found with fixed cultures. Substrates prepared from other members of the Tacaribe complex, which includes Junín and Machupo viruses, also react with sera taken from these patients during the acute phase and into early convalescence. Greatest cross-reactivity is seen between the closely related Junín and Machupo antigens, closely followed by Tacaribe virus-infected cells. ELISA has been used as an alternative to IF for early and rapid diagnosis; its use was restricted by the small amounts of antigen available for coating the solid phase but this has changed with the availability of recombinant antigens.

As a first step towards diagnosis, the use of PCR can be considered, provided that primer sets have been rigorously tested beforehand and the temperature cycling conditions optimised. The need is often to give a first indication as to which of the various causes of viral haemorrhagic fever may be present, and thus it is often the case that PCR reactions need to be conducted in parallel using a range of primer sets specific for as many as six different agents, whether these be arenaviruses or other suspected causes, e.g. filoviruses. Drosten et al. (2002) have shown that this is possible; overcoming the common problems of low sensitivity and non-specific amplification often associated with such multiplex PCR tests. The advantages of PCR include the opportunity to obtain sequence information, of increasing relevance to the identification of new family members. Also PCR is useful for diagnosis in the early stages of disease when antibodies have yet to develop. The drawback, however, is that PCR does not discriminate between the presence of RNA fragments and infectious virus. Thus, isolation of virus using cell cultures in a high-security facility should be attempted whenever possible.

ANTIGENIC RELATIONSHIPS

Monoclonal antibodies are used to distinguish between virus strains because they can be prepared against epitopes which go unrecognised when polyclonal antisera are used. Buchmeier et al. (1981) summarised the patterns of reactivity with a panel of monoclonal antibodies directed against laboratory strains of the homologous LCM virus, and Lassa and Mopeia viruses. Antibodies directed against the smaller, GPC envelope glycoprotein cross-reacted by immunofluorescence with all substrates examined, whereas antibodies directed against the larger GP1 glycoprotein were either strain-specific or reacted with a subset only of the strains examined, presumably by binding to previously unrecognised epitopes. The observation that certain of these broadly cross-reactive antibodies also reacted with Pichinde virus suggests that epitopes on surface envelope structures among Old World and New World arenaviruses are conserved. A similar comparison has also been undertaken with monoclonal antibodies to Lassa tested against the Mopeia and Mobala viruses from Africa. Again, various degrees of cross-reactivity were observed with reagents specific for the GP2 external glycoprotein. Mobala virus from the Central African Republic, however, appears to be distinct, as several cross-reactive monoclonal antibodies originally prepared against LCM virus failed to recognise Mobala-infected substrates. Clegg and Lloyd (1984) analysed an extensive range of different determinants common to all strains of both viruses on the internal nucleocapsid and on at least one of the two glycoproteins.

The plaque reduction neutralisation test is highly specific for all members of the *Arenaviridae*; it is notable that the few examples of cross-reactivity were obtained with high-titre animal antisera raised against Junín, Tacaribe and Machupo viruses. However, the ease with which neutralising antibodies can be quantified varies greatly. No cross-reactions have been observed between Junín and Machupo viruses in plaque reduction tests with human convalescent sera despite sharing a close antigenic relationship. A similar marked specificity of neutralisation has been demonstrated with LCM and Lassa sera, although neutralising antibodies to Lassa virus can be detected only with great difficulty. The sensitivity of the neutralisation test for LCM virus can be increased by incorporating either complement or anti-γ-globulin into the test system.

CLINICAL AND PATHOLOGICAL ASPECTS

Immune Response

The classic example of virus-induced immunopathological disease is LCM virus infection of adult mice (Casals, 1975) in which intracerebral inoculation causes severe disease and death. In contrast, if mice are infected before or shortly after birth they develop a non-pathogenic lifelong carrier state. The newborn mouse is immunologically immature and the virus does stimulate an immune response; in these circumstances the virus causes no illness. The immunologically mature mouse mounts an immune response following

LCM virus infection and a fatal choriomeningitis results, but without evidence of neuronal damage (Lehmann-Grube, 1971). Immunosuppression, either by neonatal thymectomy or by use of antilymphocytic serum, protects adult mice against fatal LCM infection; the pathological damage thus appears to be immune-mediated.

The immune responses are best understood in acute infection of mice. Intraperitoneal injection of adults gives rise to an asymptomatic acute infection of 2–3 weeks' duration. Studies of such infections have resulted in a number of findings with implications beyond the field of arenavirus research. First, the description by Rowe (1954) of the immune-mediated pathology of acute LCM infection was the first demonstration that the pathogenicity of the viruses may not be solely related to their cytolytic effects. The observation that LCM virus infected cells were lysed by cytotoxic T cells led to the concept that recognition of a target cell requires the presence of both viral antigen and class I antigen of the host's major histocompatibility complex (Zinkernagel and Doherty, 1979). Second, the persistence of virus in mice infected shortly after birth has provided a model for both host and viral factors involved in the establishment and maintenance of chronic infection. The finding of virus antigen–antibody complexes in persistently infected animals shows that B cell tolerance is not involved. Finally, activation of natural killer cell activity early in acute infection, which coincides with the production of interferon, has helped increase our knowledge of innate immunity against virus infection.

The direct demonstration of virus replication in lymphocytes is of substantial importance for understanding arenavirus pathogenesis, as these cells provide a continuing source of virus that enters the circulation and play a key role in the temporal and quantitative control of the immune response (Murphy and Whitfield, 1975). Viral antigen is present in the cells of the lymphatic system in mice persistently infected with LCM virus. Most of the virus in the blood of carrier mice is associated with approximately 2% of the total circulating lymphocyte population. Precursor or immature lymphocytes may support the replication *in vitro* of LCM virus when they are stimulated to proliferate by phytohaemagglutinin, in agreement with the general finding that arenaviruses grow best in actively dividing cells. Such clonal expansion may be triggered *in vivo* by viral antigen binding to appropriate lymphocyte receptors.

Arenaviruses can replicate in peritoneal and tissue macrophages. Virus can be recovered from mononuclear cells and macrophages of adult mice infected with LCM virus when these cells become activated as a result of the uptake of heterologous antigens. This does not occur in athymic mice, suggesting that infection of macrophages requires T cell activity.

Interferon

Interferon is induced early in acute LCM virus infection of mice, and its appearance correlates with the appearance of infectious virus in the blood. There have been few studies of the levels of α-interferon in acute arenavirus infection of man. Elevated levels can be detected in the early stages of Argentinian haemorrhagic fever, and these coincide with the onset of fever and backache. Although there is no correlation between the titres of interferon and circulating virus, Levis and Saavedra (1984) have suggested that at least some of the clinical signs may be directly attributable to interferon, particularly the depression of platelet and lymphocyte numbers that result from Junín virus infection of leukocytes and macrophages.

The role of natural killer cells in controlling arenavirus infection is not clear, although many are found in the blood and spleen of LCM virus-infected mice as early as 1 day after infection. This response declines rapidly, however, until by the fourth day almost all the cytolytic immune activity is H-2-restricted.

Antibodies

Antibodies against the nucleocapsid can be detected by complement fixation (CF) and immunofluorescence early in the acute phase of most arenavirus infections. Infectious virus–antibody complexes can be detected 4 days after LCM virus infection of mice but there is no evidence that B cell responses play a role in the pathology of the acute infection. Immunity to arenaviruses appears in general to be type-specific; an infection with one member of the family does not necessarily confer protective humoral or cellular immunity against arenaviruses that can be distinguished by neutralisation tests *in vitro*. However, cross-reactive antibodies may confer some degree of protection in some instances, e.g. immunisation of guinea-pigs with Tacaribe virus protects against subsequent challenge with the normally virulent Junín virus. These responses are clearly different from the anamnestic responses that may be induced as a result of antigenic similarities between the nucleocapsid proteins of the two viruses concerned.

Cellular Immunity

The role of cellular immunity during acute LCM infection is manifested by a cytotoxic T cell response associated with the clearing of virus; e.g. CD8$^+$ T cells cultured and cloned *in vitro* and injected intravenously reduce the amount of virus 100-fold in the spleens of acutely infected mice. Cytotoxic T cell responses are restricted by the need for activated T cells to recognise both viral antigen and host cell proteins encoded by the H-2 region, a concept developed in LCM-infected mice which as referred to above has radically altered our concept of the mechanisms by which the infected host clears virus from infected tissues. The generation of specific cellular toxicity is related to the replication of the virus in target organs; inoculation with live virus appears necessary as a primary cytotoxic T cell response is not seen if the virus is inactivated. This has implications for the development of inactivated arenavirus vaccines should the stimulation of cellular immunity prove essential for protection, as many workers believe. T cell clones from mice infected with the Armstrong strain of LCM virus lyse a wide range of LCM virus strains. This finding demonstrates that cytotoxic responses to arenaviruses are haplotype-restricted but show a broad cross-reactivity for conserved viral determinants. Some of these determinants have now been mapped to an immunodominant domain of GP2 (amino acids 278–286; Whitton *et al.*, 1988). Such T cell clones can discriminate between cells infected with a given strain of virus containing only a single amino acid substitution in this region; this implies that mutations in this region of the genome may lead to selection of a virus variant with altered pathogenicity.

In contrast to LCM virus, the role of cellular immunity in Lassa virus infection seems to play only a minor role. The human host is clearly restricted in its ability to clear the virus and prevent virus replication in tissues, possibly because of an impaired cytotoxic T cell response. The poor neutralising antibody response and the high degree of viraemia contrast sharply with those in patients with South American haemorrhagic fevers, in whom there is little viraemia and neutralising antibodies develop rapidly during acute infection. The prospects of immunotherapy thus seem poor and greater emphasis has, therefore, been placed on the use of antiviral agents (see below).

PERSISTENT INFECTION

Antibodies

Mice persistently infected with LCM virus produce antibodies to all the major structural proteins. This finding was contrary to the view previously held that viral persistence is established or maintained *in vivo* as a result of an absence of specific B cell responses to some or all viral antigens. As viral proteins continue to be produced in the tissues of such animals, circulating antigen–antibody complexes are formed which can be detected by binding Clq. It is worth noting that, despite the existence of antibody to all LCM virus structural polypeptides, sera from persistently infected mice are negative by CF tests; this was the original basis for the belief that carrier animals do not produce a humoral response to this virus. Antibodies in the sera of such animals bind to the surface of virus infected cells, but are unable to mediate complement-dependent cytolysis, suggesting that viral antigens at the plasma membrane may be either masked, thereby preventing further immune reactions, or removed by antigenic modulation. This notion would imply that persistently infected mice are deficient in viral antibody of the complement fixing subclass of IgG, but this has not been proven.

Cell-mediated Immunity

Mice persistently infected with LCM virus should mount a normal T cell response to unrelated immunogens, indicating a state of tolerance only to specific antigens. However, it has been difficult to distinguish T cell suppression from an absence of virus-specific T cell clones. Here it is pertinent to mention that persistence of LCM virus in mice infected at birth or *in utero* was one of the important observations made by Burnet and Fenner to support the concept of tolerance to 'self' antigens. The time of infection is critical, as LCM infection induced 24 h after birth results in a cytotoxic T cell response typical of acute disease. The failure of mice infected before this time to mount an adequate cytotoxic response is presumably related to maturation of T cell function; it appears to be virus specific because adult carrier mice challenged with other unrelated arenaviruses mount normal cytotoxic T cell responses. Thus, the block appears to be either in recognition of infected cells or in their expression of type-specific antigenic determinants. The relationship between the virus and the host immune response may be more complex than hitherto believed, however, as

there is evidence for arenaviral RNA being transcribed into complementary DNA, presumably mediated by endogenous retroviral reverse transcriptase (Klenerman *et al.*, 1997). This would imply that long-term persistence of viral gene sequences as retroviral elements results in continual low-level expression of viral proteins. Thus immune responsiveness is maintained by the continued presentation of viral sequences as MHC–peptide complexes.

PATHOLOGY OF ARENAVIRUS INFECTIONS: GENERAL FEATURES

The mechanisms by which arenaviruses cause disease in man are not fully understood. There is no evidence that either immunopathological or allergenic processes play any part in causing disease; it appears to be more likely that disease is caused by direct damage of cells by the virus. Post mortem studies on patients who died from Junín virus infection have shown generalised lymphadenopathy, endothelial swelling in the capillaries and arterioles of almost every organ, accompanied by a depletion of lymphocytes in the spleen. The virus first replicates in lymphoid tissue, whence it invades the reticuloendothelial system and those cells concerned in the humoral and cellular immune responses; the host's defence mechanisms are thus impaired. Fatal illness is invariably associated with capillary damage leading to capillary fragility, haemorrhages and irreversible shock (Johnson *et al.*, 1973). Disseminated intravascular coagulation is not a typical feature. Although Lassa fever is often regarded as being hepatotropic, the extent of hepatic damage is insufficient to account for the severity of the clinical disease and serum transaminase values often remain within normal limits except in severe cases. Studies of Lassa virus-infected rhesus monkeys have shown that changes in vascular function may play a much greater role in pathogenesis, as a result either of viral replication in the vascular epithelium or secondary effects of virus activity in different organs. Platelet and epithelial cell functions fail immediately before death and are accompanied by a drop in the level of prostacyclin; these functions rapidly return to normal in animals surviving infection (Fisher-Hoch *et al.*, 1987). Impairment of the functions of vascular epithelium in the absence of histological changes appears to be a common feature of the final stages of viral haemorrhagic diseases in general and suggests that hypovolaemic shock may be amenable to treatment with prostacyclin.

The pathogenesis of Argentinian haemorrhagic fever has been studied in guinea-pigs infected with Junín virus, this being a suitable model of human disease. There is a pronounced thrombocytopenia and leukopenia characteristic of human infections, and animals die of severe haemorrhagic lesions. Bone marrow cells are destroyed with release of proteases and acid and alkaline phosphatases into the blood; this leads to consumption of the C4 complement component. These effects may lead in turn to progressive alterations in vascular permeability and platelet function (Rimoldi and de Bracco, 1980). The most extensive histopathological studies have been made on tissues from patients with Lassa fever (Walker and Murphy, 1987). However, there are many similarities in the pathological lesions found in man following Junín and Machupo virus infections. Focal non-zonal necrosis in the liver has been described in all three conditions, with hyperplasia of Kupffer cells, erythrophagocytosis and acidophilic necrosis of hepatocytes. Councilman-like bodies can be observed together with cytoplasmic vacuolations and nuclear pyknosis or lysis. As with other organs, there is little evidence of cellular inflammation. Lesions in other organs have been described, including interstitial pneumonitis, tubular necrosis in the kidney, lymphocytic infiltration of the spleen and minimal inflammation of the central nervous system and myocardium (Walker and Murphy, 1987). The hepatic changes may range from mild, focal necrosis to extensive zonal necrosis, involving up to 50% of hepatocytes. These changes are consistent with a direct cytolytic action of the virus; nevertheless, the simultaneous presence of Lassa virus and specific antibodies during the later stages of the acute disease suggests that antibody-dependent cellular immune reactions may also occur. Microscopic changes in the kidneys are minimal, although it is not clear whether the functional impairment is due to the deposition of antigen–antibody complexes.

Lymphocytic Choriomeningitis

Clinical and Pathological Features

Infection is often inapparent but may present as an influenza-like febrile illness, as aseptic meningitis or as severe meningoencephalomyelitis. The great majority of LCM infections are, however, benign. The incubation period is 6–13 days. In the influenza-like illness there is fever, malaise, muscular pains and bronchitis. An early leukopenia followed by lymphocytosis is a constant finding. Generally, the mean value of mono-

nuclear cells is approximately 600 cells/mm^3, although counts of up to 3000/mm^3 have been recorded. A coryza, together with retro-orbital pain, anorexia and nausea are common. During the acute phase a large number of mononuclear cells are present in the cerebrospinal fluid as part of a pleocytosis, although the absolute number varies with time after onset.

As with all central nervous system diseases, the cerebrospinal fluid (CSF) is at increased pressure, with a slight rise in protein concentration, normal or slightly reduced sugar concentration, and a moderate number of cells, mainly lymphocytes (150–400/mm^3). It has been noted that the majority of such patients have a history of influenza-like illness immediately prior to the onset of meningitis. The meningeal form is more common; the same symptoms may remain mild and be of short duration and patients recover within a few days, but there can be a more pronounced illness with severe prostration lasting 2 weeks or more. Chronic sequelae have been reported on occasion, including parotitis and orchitis. Other symptoms include continuing headache, paralysis and personality changes. The few deaths reported have followed severe meningoencephalomyelitis. In this most severe form, patients may rapidly develop a bilateral papilloedema, confusion and paralysis of the extremities over a 1 week period. An erythematous rash followed by haemorrhage and death has also been reported. Virus can be isolated from blood, CSF and, in fatal cases, from brain tissue. However, the preferred method of diagnosis is antibody detection by immunofluorescence, although the test is not readily available in most clinical virology laboratories. Because of the possible diagnosis of related, more hazardous arenaviruses, samples should be referred to a national reference laboratory.

Epidemiology

Man is usually infected through contact with rodents. In the past, these have been acquired in laboratories, where LCM may be a contaminant in laboratory colonies of mice and hamsters. In particular, virus is shed from the urine of persistently infected animals, resulting in contamination of skin and working surfaces. Hamsters kept as pet animals have also played a role in human infection. The mechanism of transmission of the virus to man is not fully understood but is likely to involve dust contaminated by urine, the contamination of food and drink, or via skin abrasions.

A variant of LCM virus has been isolated from captive New World primates. The histopathology in infected marmosets and tamarins is remarkably similar to that seen in Lassa virus infection in humans. It is suspected that these animals acquired the virus from infected *Mus musculus* rodents (Montali *et al.*, 1995; Stephensen *et al.*, 1991).

Diagnosis of Bolivian and Argentinian Haemorrhagic Fevers

Although the clinical features of Bolivian and Argentinian haemorrhagic fevers are similar, the laboratory diagnosis of these diseases is approached in a somewhat different manner. In the case of Junín, virus can be recovered consistently from the blood from the 3rd to the 8th day of illness; in contrast, direct recovery of Machupo virus from acutely ill patients is much more difficult. In both instances, serological methods are more useful.

Complement-fixing antibodies may be detected sufficiently early in both cases, provided that suitable paired sera are available. Although this technique has now largely been superseded by the use of more sensitive immunofluorescence methods and ELISA, the appearance of CF antibodies may still provide useful information as to the course of the infection and signal the onset of convalescence. Early use of immunofluorescence techniques for the diagnosis of Argentinian haemorrhagic fever showed that specific antibodies could be detected by the indirect method approximately 30 days after onset of symptoms. Specific staining is generally seen as a bright, granular fluorescence evenly distributed over the cytoplasm of the fixed infected cell substrate. The titre of immunofluorescent antibodies increases from the 12th to the 20th day of illness and is a mixture of IgG and IgM antibodies.

Neutralising antibodies to both Machupo and Junín viruses persist for many years at high titre, appearing simultaneously with CF antibodies. The sensitivity and specificity of neutralisation tests for detecting immunity to Junín virus has proved to be of value retrospectively in the detection of subclinically infected individuals. The test may be carried out in Vero cell monolayers by varying virus dilution in the presence of a fixed concentration of serum. Antibody titres are then expressed as an index calculated by subtracting the logarithmic differences between the virus titre in control and experimental reactions. Inapparent infections have been shown in approximately 20% of laboratory workers handling known or presumptively positive specimens by this method.

Argentinian Haemorrhagic Fever (Junín Virus)

Clinical and Pathological Features

Argentinian haemorrhagic fever has been known since 1943 and Junín virus, the causative agent, was first isolated in 1958. The virus causes annual outbreaks of severe illness, with between 100 and 3500 cases, in an area of intensive agriculture known as the wet pampas in Argentina. Mortality in some outbreaks has been in the range of 10–20%, although the overall mortality is generally 3–15%. After an incubation period of 7–16 days, the onset of illness is insidious, with chills, headache, malaise, myalgia, retro-orbital pain and nausea; these are followed by fever, conjunctival injection and suffusion, a pharyngeal enanthema and erythema and oedema of the face, neck and upper thorax. A few petechiae may be seen, mostly in the axilla. There is hypervascularity and occasional ulceration of the soft palate. Generalised lymphadenopathy is common. Tongue tremor is an early sign, and some patients present with pneumonitis. In the more severe cases the patient's condition becomes appreciably worse after a few days, with the development of hypotension, oliguria, haemorrhages from the nose and gums (Figure 19.4), haematemesis, haematuria and melaena. Oliguria may progress to anuria and pronounced neurological manifestations may develop. Laboratory findings have included leukopenia with a decrease in the number of CD4$^+$ cells, thrombocytopenia and urinary casts containing viral antigen. Patients recover when the fever falls, followed by diuresis and rapid improvement. Death may result from hypovolaemic shock. Subclinical infections also occur. Man-to-man transmission has not been observed.

Epidemiology

Argentinian haemorrhagic fever has a marked seasonal incidence, coinciding with the maize harvest between April and July, when rodent populations reach their peak. Agricultural workers, particularly those harvesting maize, are, not surprisingly, the most commonly affected. The main reservoir hosts of Junín virus are *Calomys* field voles that live and breed in burrows under the maize fields and in the surrounding grass banks (Figure 19.5). Other rodent species may also be

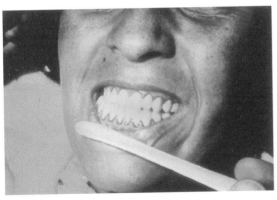

Figure 19.4 Bleeding from the gum margin in a case of Argentinian haemorrhagic fever. Reproduced from Howard (1986)

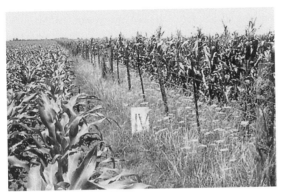

Figure 19.5 The habitat for the rodent *Calomys* sp. in the wet pampas of Argentina. Reproduced from Howard (1986)

infected. *Calomys* spp. have a persistent viraemia and viruria, and virus is also present in considerable quantities in the saliva. The mode of transmission of Junín virus to man has not been conclusively established. The virus may be carried in the air from dust contaminated by rodent excreta or may enter by ingestion of contaminated foodstuffs.

Therapy

In contrast to Lassa fever, antibodies play a major role in recovery from Junín infection. Controlled trials of immune plasma collected from patients at least 6 months into convalescence have shown a dramatic reduction in mortality if plasma is given within the first 8 days of illness (Maiztegui *et al.*, 1979). The efficacy of

this therapy is directly related to the titre of neutralising antibody in the plasma; as a result a dose of no less than 3000 'therapeutic units'/kg body weight has been recommended (Enria *et al.*, 1984). The late development of a neurological syndrome is seen in up to 10% of patients treated with immune plasma; it is often benign and self-limiting but points to the possible persistence of viral antigens on cells of the central nervous system well into convalescence. Treatment with immune plasma also restores the response of peripheral blood lymphocytes to antigenic stimuli, suggesting that administration of plasma also results in the modulation of cellular immunity.

Prophylaxis

There have been attempts to produce a vaccine against Argentinian haemorrhagic fever. The XJC1$_3$ strain of virus grown in the brains of suckling mice is relatively non-pathogenic and was administered to 636 volunteers between 1968 and 1970. Over a period of 3 years, 70 cases of Junín virus infection occurred among the population but there were no cases amongst those immunised. However, the vaccine often induced a mild febrile reaction or a subclinical infection and its use was discontinued, despite the fact that over 90% of vaccinees maintained neutralising antibody for up to 9 years. There have been renewed attempts during recent years to develop a new vaccine strain sufficiently attenuated for human use and meeting modern day requirements as to derivation, manufacture and potency. Several clones have been prepared from the original XJ isolate, one of which exhibits less neurovirulence than the XJCl$_3$ strain, yet protected rhesus monkeys against challenge with wild-type Junín virus (McKee *et al.*, 1993). This 'Candidate 1' vaccine has been tested in a double-blind study in volunteers.

Bolivian Haemorrhagic Fever (Machupo Virus)

Clinical Features

Bolivian haemorrhagic fever was first recognised in 1959 in the Beni region in north-eastern Bolivia, with 470 reported cases in the years up to 1962. The disease continued in that region more or less annually for a number of years in the form of sharply localised epidemics. Its incidence has decreased considerably since the late 1960s and human infections are now rarely reported. It is worth noting that the discovery of a common morphology and serological cross-reaction between Machupo and LCM virus led to the concept of the family *Arenaviridae*. The mortality in individual outbreaks varied (5–30%). The most notable outbreak affected 700 people in the San Joaquin township between late 1962 and the middle of 1964. The mortality was 18%. In July 1994, a fresh outbreak occurred in north-eastern Bolivia, with at least seven deaths. These were the first recorded since 1971; for reasons that are obscure, this outbreak did not appear linked to any major changes in rodent numbers or behaviour.

The clinical disease is similar to Argentinian haemorrhagic fever. The incubation period ranges from 7 to 14 days and the onset is insidious, beginning with an influenza-like illness accompanied by malaise and fatigue. This is followed by abdominal pain, anorexia, tremors, prostration and severe limb pain. About one-third of patients show a tendency to bleed, with petechiae on the trunk and palate, and bleeding from the gastrointestinal tract, nose, gums and uterus. Almost half the patients develop a fine tremor of the tongue and hands, and some may have more pronounced neurological systems. The acute disease may last 2–3 weeks and convalescence may be protracted, generalised weakness being the most common complaint. Clinically inapparent infections are rare. Machupo virus, the responsible agent, is readily isolated from lymph nodes and spleen taken at necropsy. Isolation of the virus from acutely ill patients has proved difficult, however, the best results being obtained from specimens taken 7–12 days after the onset of illness.

Epidemiology

The rodent reservoir of Machupo virus is the field vole, *Calomys callosus*; over 60% of animals caught during the San Joaquin epidemic were found to be infected. The distribution of cases in the township was associated with certain houses and *C. callosus* was trapped in all households where cases occurred. Transmission to man is probably by contamination of food and water or by infection through skin abrasions. Transmission from man to man is unusual but a small episode took place in 1971, well outside the endemic zone. The index case, infected in Beni, carried the infection to Cochabamba and, by direct transmission, caused five secondary cases, of which four were fatal.

Abnormally low rainfall, combined with an increase in the use of insecticide, led to a rapid decline in the numbers of cats, with the result that the population of Machupo-infected rodents increased dramatically, thus increasing the opportunity for human contact with contaminated soil and foodstuffs. This balance has since been restored, consistent with the decline in the number of reported cases over the past two decades.

Treatment

As with AHF, treatment is largely supportive. Although attempts have been made to use convalescent immune plasma from survivors of Machupo infection, a combination of a lack of facilities in Bolivia suitable for treating collected plasma and the absence of a controlled trial as to the efficacy of its use means that the treatment of patients with immunoglobulin remains speculative. Ribavirin has been administered during the 1994 outbreak, but again there is no certain indication that ribavirin is effective against Machupo infection.

Lassa Fever

History. In 1969 Lassa virus made a dramatic appearance in Nigeria as a lethal, highly transmissible disease. The first victim was an American nurse, who was infected in a small mission station in the Lassa township in north-eastern Nigeria, whence the virus and the disease derive their names. The origin of the infection was never determined, although it is thought to have been acquired through direct contact with an infected patient in Lassa. When the nurse's condition steadily deteriorated, she was flown to the Evangel Hospital in Jos, where she died the following day. While she was in hospital she was cared for by two other American nurses, one of whom also became infected by direct contact, probably through skin abrasion. This nurse became unwell after an 8 day incubation period and died following an illness lasting 11 days. The head nurse of the hospital, who had assisted at the post mortem of the first patient, fell ill 7 days after the death of the second patient for whom she had cared, and from whom she probably acquired the infection. This third case was evacuated to the USA by air. After a severe illness under intensive care she slowly recovered. A virus, subsequently named Lassa, was isolated from her blood by workers at the Yale Arbovirus Unit. One of these virologists became ill but improved after an immune plasma transfusion donated by the third case. Five months after this infection, a laboratory technician in the Yale laboratories, who had not been working with Lassa virus, fell ill and died. The manner in which this infection was acquired has never been determined. This trail of events not unnaturally earned for Lassa virus a formidable notoriety, which was sharply enhanced by two more devastating hospital outbreaks—one in Nigeria, the other in Liberia.

The fourth outbreak was seen in Sierra Leone in October 1972. In sharp contrast to the previous outbreaks, this one was not confined to hospitals, although hospital staff were at considerable risk and several became infected. Most of the patients acquired their illness in the community and there were several intrafamilial transmissions. This led to a revision of the initial view, formed from experience of nosocomial infections, that Lassa fever has a high mortality.

Lassa fever has since continued to occur in west Africa, usually as sporadic cases (Monath, 1987). Between 1969 and 1978 there were 17 reported outbreaks affecting 386 patients, in whom the mortality was 27%. Eleven of the episodes were in hospitals, where the case fatality rate reached 44%; two were laboratory infections, two were community-acquired outbreaks, and two were prolonged community outbreaks. Eight patients were flown to Europe or North America. One of them was evacuated with full isolation precautions and the remainder, of whom five were infectious, travelled on scheduled commercial flights as fare-paying passengers. Fortunately, no contact cases resulted.

Clinical features. Lassa virus causes a spectrum of disease ranging from subclinical to fulminating fatal infection. Studies in Sierra Leone show that most patients present with only a mild form of the disease and this is resolved by good primary health care. The incubation period ranges from 3 to 16 days and the illness usually begins insidiously. The disease is difficult to distinguish in the early stages from other systematic febrile illnesses, most notably malaria, septicaemia and yellow fever. The most reliable clinical signs on presentation are a sore throat, myalgia, abdominal and lower back pains, accompanied by vomiting. Occasionally a faint maculopapular rash may be seen during the second week of illness on the face, neck, trunk and arms. Cough is a common symptom, and light-headedness, vertigo and tinnitus appear in a few patients. The fever generally lasts 7–17 days and is variable. Convalescence begins in the second to fourth weeks, when the temperature returns to normal and the symptoms improve. Most patients complain of extreme fatigue for several weeks. Loss of hair is common and deafness afflicts one in four patients, and there may be brief bouts of fever.

In a significant number of cases, the symptoms suddenly worsen after the first week, with continuing high fever, severe prostration, chest and abdominal pains, conjunctival injection, diarrhoea, dysphagia and vomiting. One important physical finding is a distinct pharyngitis; yellow-white exudative spots may be seen on the tonsillar pillars together with small vesicles and ulcers. The patient appears toxic, lethargic and dehydrated; the blood pressure is low and there is sometimes a bradycardia relative to the body temperature. Patients in whom the disease is eventually fatal not uncommonly have a high sustained fever. There may be cervical lymphadenopathy, an encephalopathy, coated tongue, puffiness of the face and neck, and blurred vision. In approximately 25% of cases there is marked involvement of the CNS, manifested by disorientation, ataxia and seizures. Progression to severe haemorrhaging occurs in around one-fifth of patients and it is among such patients that mortality exceeds 50%. Death is due to shock, anoxia, respiratory insufficiency and cardiac arrest. Lassa fever is particularly severe in pregnant women. A study of 75 women in Sierra Leone showed that 11/14 deaths were the result of infection during the third trimester; a further 23 patients suffered abortion in the first and second trimesters.

Epidemiology. Lassa virus has been repeatedly isolated from the multimammate rat *Mastomys natalensis* in Sierra Leone and Nigeria. This rodent is a common domestic and peridomestic species, and large populations are widely distributed in Africa south of the Sahara. During the rainy season it may desert the open fields and seek shelter indoors. Some genetic variation has been shown in *Mastomys* populations inhabiting different ecological niches; however, there appears to be no difference in the prevalence of antibody and virus in at least two of the karotypes found in West Africa. The animals are infected at birth or during the perinatal period. Like other arenaviruses, Lassa virus produces a persistent, tolerant infection in its rodent reservoir host with no ill effects and without any detectable immune response. The animals remain infectious during their lifetime, freely excreting Lassa virus in urine and other body fluids. The correlation between the prevalence of antibody in a community and the degree of infestation by infected rodents, however, is poor.

Studies of the ratio of clinical illness to infections have recently confirmed that Lassa fever is endemic in several regions of West Africa. It has been estimated that only 1–2% of infections are fatal—substantially less than the figures of 30–50% originally associated with the early nosocomial outbreaks. However, there may still be up to 300 000 infections per year, with as many as 5000 deaths (McCormick *et al.*, 1986b). The seroconversion rates among villagers in Sierra Leone vary from 4 to 22 per 100 susceptible individuals per year; up to 14% of febrile illness in such population groups is due to Lassa virus infection. There is a marked variation as to the severity of the disease according to different geographical regions. This may in part be due to genotypic variation of Lassa virus, or dose and route of infection, or a combination of these factors (Fisher-Hoch, 1993). There is a relatively high rate of asymptomatic and mild infections in endemic areas. One reason for this may be the frequency of reinfections; although about 6% of the population lose antibody annually, rises in antibody titre are also often observed. It is not clear whether reinfection results in clinical disease. A frequent finding of incomplete immunity after infection would have profound implications for the use of a vaccine.

There may be secondary spread from person to person in conditions of overcrowded housing and particularly in rural hospitals. There is a particularly high risk to staff and patients on maternity wards, as Lassa fever is a major cause of spontaneous abortion. Medical attendants or relatives who provide direct personal care are most likely to contract the infection; as noted above, accidental inoculation with a sharp instrument and contact with blood have caused infection in a few cases. Airborne spread may take place, as well as mechanical transmission. Although in Sierra Leone there has been no evidence of airborne spread in hospital outbreaks, one of the 1970 outbreaks in Nigeria is believed to have been caused by airborne transmission from a woman with severe pulmonary infection.

Lassa fever is a major cause of spontaneous abortion in West Africa. The virus is readily recovered from the blood and placenta of aborted fetuses. Women generally recover quickly after such abortions, showing a dramatic decline in viraemia, partially due to massive bleeding at the time of abortion (A. Demby, personal communication). Paediatric Lassa fever is known to occur more commonly in male children, for unknown reasons. Presenting as an acute febrile illness, the case fatality rate may approach 30% in children with widespread oedema, abdominal distension and bleeding.

Diagnosis. It is important to note that serodiagnosis and virus isolation should be attempted only in

Table 19.2 Differential diagnosis of arenavirus fevers

Yellow fever
Malaria
Bacterial septicaemia
Enteric fevers (typhoid, paratyphoid)
Streptococcal pharyngitis
Typhus
Trypanosomiasis
Leptospirosis
Other viral haemorrhagic fevers

laboratories equipped (Biosafety level P4) to provide maximum containment to protect the investigator. Suspected cases should be reported immediately to local and national public health authorities prior to any attempt to handle specimens.

The diagnosis of Lassa fever is confirmed by isolation of the virus or demonstration of a specific serological response. Infection in the early stages can be confused clinically with a number of other infectious diseases, particularly malignant malaria (Table 19.2) (Woodruff, 1975). The two most reliable prognostic markers of fatal infections are the titres of circulating virus and of aspartate aminotransferase (AST). Patients in whom the titre of virus exceeds 10^4 $TCID_{50}$/ml accompanied by AST levels above 150 IU have a poor prognosis, and fatality rates approach 80%. In contrast, patients with virus and enzyme levels below these values have a greater than 85% chance of survival (Johnson *et al.*, 1987). This demonstration of an association between the degree of viraemia and mortality is unique for virus infections and contrasts with the difficulty in predicting the outcome in patients with Argentinian and Bolivian haemorrhagic fevers. Although Lassa fever can be diagnosed accurately from the presence of IgM antibodies on admission, there is no correlation between the time of appearance, the titre of specific antibodies and clinical outcome.

Lassa virus grows readily in Vero cell culture and virus can usually be isolated within 4 days. Virus can be cultured from serum, throat washings, pleural fluid and urine; it is excreted from the pharynx for up to 14 days after the onset of illness and in urine for up to 67 days after onset. Lassa infection can be diagnosed early by detection of virus-specific antigens in conjunctival cells using indirect immunofluorescence. The use of RT-PCR method is possible, although these techniques are of limited practical use in endemic areas.

The most sensitive serological test for the detection of Lassa antibodies is indirect immunofluorescence; antibodies can be detected by this method in the second week of illness. Complement-fixing antibodies develop more slowly and are rarely detectable before the third week after onset. On occasion, complement-fixing antibodies failed to develop in patients from whom Lassa virus has been isolated. Neutralising antibodies are difficult to measure *in vitro*, in sharp contrast to infections by the South American arenaviruses, for reasons that are unclear.

Therapy. Although the passive administration of Lassa immune plasma may suppress viraemia and favourably alter the clinical outcome, it does not always do so, particularly if the patient has a high virus burden (McCormick *et al.*, 1986b). Failure may be due to the difficulty in assessing accurately the titre of viral neutralising antibodies in the plasma, the late and non-uniform nature of this response in convalescence, and antigenic variation. The widespread occurrence of human immunodeficiency virus (HIV) infections in West Africa precludes at present the use of immune plasma from convalescent individuals in this region. This is in marked contrast to the benefit of immune plasma in the treatment of Junín infections. This may be due either to the high titre of neutralising antibodies that develops soon after the acute phase or to the lesser importance of antibody in the resolution of Lassa virus.

Greater success has been achieved with antivirals. In one study of patients with a poor prognosis, treatment for 10 days with intravenous ribavirin (60–70 mg/kg/day) within 6 days after the onset of fever showed a reduced case fatality rate of 5% (McCormick *et al.*, 1986a). In contrast, patients treated 7 or more days after the onset of fever had a case fatality rate of 26%. In the Sierra Leone study, viraemia of greater than $10^{3.6}$ TCID$_{50}$/ml on admission was associated with a case fatality rate of 76%. Patients with this risk factor who were treated with intravenous ribavirin within 6 days of the onset of fever had a case fatality rate of 9% compared with 47% in those treated 7 days or more after the onset of illness. Oral ribavirin is less effective. A difficulty with its use, however, is that ribavirin can induce haemolytic anaemia in over 40% of patients.

The introduction of vaccines against Junín virus has stimulated the expectation that a vaccine could also be developed for the prevention of Lassa virus infections. However, the perceived necessity for a strong cell-mediated response would dictate the development of an attenuated vaccine; this raises concerns, however, as to a possible reversion to virulence of any attenuated Lassa virus vaccine. Given these technological difficulties and the limited numbers globally at risk of infection, it is unlikely that such a vaccine will be developed in the near future.

Control. Containment of Lassa fever depends upon the strict isolation of cases, rigorous disinfection, rodent control and effective surveillance. Nosocomial transmission presents a considerable risk and patient isolation—in isolators if available—is an absolute must. Strict procedures for dealing with body fluids and excreta need to be enforced. Disinfection with 0.5% sodium hyperchlorite or 0.5% phenol in detergent is recommended for instruments and surfaces. Given the higher virus burden in cases of Lassa fever compared to patients with Junín or Machupo infections, surveillance of those having been in contact with Lassa fever patients is also a high public health priority. WHO recommends that those who have been in non-casual contact with cases should be observed for 3 months after their last contact with the patient. This follow-up should consist of taking body temperature measurements twice daily. Infection should be suspected if the body temperature exceeds 38.3°C (101°F) and the contact hospitalised immediately.

Rodent control is frequently difficult, although much can be done to minimise contact by isolating foodstuffs, preventing rodent entry into dwellings, and reducing the chance of inhabitants coming into contact with rodent excreta.

EMERGING ARENAVIRUS INFECTIONS

Brazilian Haemorrhagic Fever (Sabiá Virus)

This arenavirus was isolated in 1990 from human cases at autopsy (Lisieux *et al.*, 1994). The source of this infection was uncertain but is likely to have been acquired by exposure to infected rodents in an agricultural setting in an area immediately outside São Paulo. As a continuing reminder of the potential severity of these infections, a laboratory worker became critically ill after having been accidentally exposed to an aerosol containing Sabiá virus. The virus was first isolated from a fatal case of haemorrhagic fever. A laboratory-acquired infection was characterised by a febrile illness accompanied by leukopenia and thrombocytopenia. There is little information regarding the epidemiology of this virus, although the extensive liver necrosis seen in the first case is a warning that this and other haemophagic fevers may on first examination be mistaken for yellow fever.

Venezuela Haemorrhagic Fever (Guanarito Virus)

Between May 1990 and March 1991 an outbreak occurred among residents of Guanarito municipality on the central plains of Venezuela. Originally mistaken as dengue fever, a total of 104 cases were recorded with a mortality rate of around 25%. The Guanarito virus was subsequently isolated from the spleens of such cases at autopsy. The principal rodent hosts of this virus have been identified (Table 19.1) (Tesh *et al.*, 1994).

The disease has a clinical profile similar to that of Argentinian haemorrhagic fever, with patients manifesting a thrombocytopenia, haemorrhaging and neurological signs. Pharyngitis has been observed and deafness reported in convalescent patients. Although initial reports suggest a high mortality for this infection, antibody prevalence rates of up to 3% have been found among healthy individuals and up to 10% of household contacts have anti-Guanarito virus antibodies.

Oliveros Virus

This new agent has been isolated from a small rodent, *Bolomys obscurus*, within the endemic region of Argentinian haemorrhagic fever (Bowen *et al.*, 1997). With a rodent host distinct from that of Junín virus, approximately 25% of captured *B. obscurus* have been found to contain antibodies to this virus. At present, there are no indications that this virus causes significant numbers of human infections (Mills *et al.*, 1996).

Whitewater Arroyo Virus and Other Isolates from the USA

As a consequence of the 1993 hantavirus outbreak on the Colorado Plateau, there has been intensive study of rodent populations in order to gauge the extent of Sin Nombre virus distribution and the risk that infected rodents present to rural populations in the USA. During one such study, Kosoy *et al.* (1996) found an unexpectedly high level of arenavirus antibodies in pack rats (*Neotoma* spp.) caught in the Whitewater Arroyo of New Mexico. Members of the family to which *Neotoma* belongs are ubiquitous throughout the south-western part of the USA. Independently Fulhorst and colleagues (1996) described the isolation of a hitherto unknown arenavirus from trapped examples of *N. albigula*. The importance of these findings became evident when in 1999 and 2000 three female patients residing in California presented with symptoms subsequently ascribed to infection with the same arenavirus. Although there was no obvious link between the three cases, each presented with non-specific febrile symptoms and acute respiratory distress. Two developed a lymphopenia and thrombocytopenia, and two also showed signs of liver failure and haemorrhage. All three died within 1–8 weeks of onset. Virus was recovered in one and all three gave PCR products that were 87% identical with Whitewater Arroyo virus.

Yet further new isolations have been made recently. A virus closely related, but distinct from, Whitewater Arroyo virus has been isolated from the California mouse *Peromyscus californicus*. Infectious virus was recovered from 5/27 animals caught in the Santa Ana mountains of southern California, close to the Bear Canyon trailhead. It cannot be ruled out that the tentatively dubbed Bear Canyon virus represents an additional arenavirus that has yet to be associated with human disease.

SUMMARY

The increasing numbers of human infections due to arenaviruses is beginning to require a greater vigilance on the part of public health workers. Arenavirus aetiology for febrile illnesses in individuals residing in endemic areas should be considered, particularly those who are likely to have come into regular contact with rodents by virtue of their lifestyle or occupation.

Although until recently there has been little or no evidence for human arenavirus infection in north America, Europe and Asia, this situation has changed considerably since a greater awareness of the potential for emerging infections has developed among clinicians and microbiologists, particularly in geographical areas where the last decades have seen clearance of woodland, forest and scrub in advance of extensive changes in agricultural practices. This potential has been augmented by changing or abnormal weather patterns, these serving to promote behavioural, if not also numerical, changes in rodent populations. Particularly in the Americas, arenavirus investigations have progressively become interleaved with studies on hantavirus distribution, especially in endemic zones where a particular species of rodent may be infected with either a hantavirus or an arenavirus. The only certainty is that the number of arenaviruses identified hitherto will increase as more becomes known regarding the natural history of these agents.

REFERENCES

Bowen MD, Peters CJ, Mills JN and Nichol ST (1996) Oliveros virus: a novel arenavirus from Argentina. *Virology*, **217**(1), 362–366.

Bowen MD, Peters CJ and Nichol ST (1997) Phylogenetic analysis of the Arenaviridae: patterns of virus evolution and evidence for co-speciation between arenaviruses and their rodent hosts. *Mol Phylogenet Evol*, **8**(3), 301–316.

Buchmeier MJ, Lewicki HA, Tomori O and Oldstone MB (1981) Monoclonal antibodies to lymphocytic choriomeningitis and pichinde viruses: generation, characterization, and cross-reactivity with other arenaviruses. *Virology*, **113**(1), 73–85.

Cao W, Henry MD, Borrow P et al. (1998) Identification of alpha-dystroglycan as a receptor for lymphocytic choriomeningitis virus and Lassa fever virus. *Science*, **282**(5396), 2079–2081.

Casals J (1975) Arenaviruses. *Yale J Biol Med*, **48**(2), 115–140.

Clegg JC (2002) Molecular phylogeny of the arenaviruses. *Curr Top Microbiol Immunol*, **262**, 1–24.

Clegg JCS and Lloyd G (1984) The African arenaviruses Lassa and Mopeia: biological and immunochemical comparisons. In *Segmented Negative Strand Viruses*, pp 341–347. Academic Press, Orlando, FL.

Djavani M, Yin C, Lukashevich IS et al. (2001) Mucosal immunization with *Salmonella typhimurium* expressing Lassa virus nucleocapsid protein cross-protects mice from lethal challenge with lymphocytic choriomeningitis virus. *J Hum Virol*, **4**(2), 103–108.

Drosten C, Gottig S, Schilling S et al. (2002) Rapid detection and quantification of RNA of Ebola and Marburg viruses, Lassa virus, Crimean-Congo hemorrhagic fever virus, Rift Valley fever virus, dengue virus, and yellow fever virus by real-time reverse transcription-PCR. *J Clin Microbiol*, **40**(7), 2323–2330.

Enria DA, Briggiler AM, Fernandez NJ et al. (1984) Importance of dose of neutralising antibodies in treatment of Argentine haemorrhagic fever with immune plasma. *Lancet*, **ii**, 255–256.

Fisher-Hoch SP (1993) Arenavirus pathophysiology. In *The Arenaviridae* (ed. Salvato MS), pp 299–323. Plenum, New York.

Fisher-Hoch SP, Mitchell SW, Sasso DR et al. (1987) Physiological and immunologic disturbances associated with shock in a primate model of Lassa fever. *J Infect Dis*, **155**(3), 465–474.

Fulhorst CF, Bowen MD, Ksiazek TG et al. (1996) Isolation and characterization of Whitewater Arroyo virus, a novel North American arenavirus. *Virology*, **224**(1), 114–120.

Fuller-Pace F and Southern P (1989) Detection of virus-specific RNA-dependent RNA polymerase activity in extracts from cells infected with lymphocytic choriomeningitis virus: *in vitro* synthesis of full-length viral RNA species. *J Virol*, **63**, 1938–1944.

Howard CR (1986) Arenaviruses. In *Perspectives in Medical Virology*, vol. 2 (ed. Zuckerman AJ). Elsevier, Amsterdam.

Johnson KM, McCormick JB, Webb PA et al. (1987) Clinical virology of Lassa fever in hospitalized patients. *J Infect Dis*, **155**(3), 456–464.

Johnson KM, Webb PA and Justines G (1973) Biology of Tacaribe-complex virus. In *Lymphocytic Choriomeningitis virus and other Arenaviruses* (ed. Lehmann-Grube F), pp 241–258. Springer-Verlag, Vienna.

Klenerman P, Hengartner H and Zinkernagel RM (1997) A non-retroviral RNA virus persists in DNA form. *Nature*, **390**, 298–301.

Kosoy MY, Elliott LH, Ksiazek TG et al. (1996) Prevalence of antibodies to arenaviruses in rodents from the southern and western United States: evidence for an arenavirus associated with the genus *Neotoma*. *Am J Trop Med Hyg*, **54**(6), 570–576.

Lehmann-Grube F (1971) Lymphocytic choriomeningitis virus. *Virol Monogr*, **10**, 1.

Levis SC and Saavedra MC (1984) Endogenous interferon in Argentine haemorrhagic fever. *J Infect Dis*, **149**, 428–433.

Lisieux T, Coimbra M, Nassar ES et al. (1994) New arenavirus isolated in Brazil. *Lancet*, **343**(8894), 391–392.

Lukashevich IS, Djavani M, Shapiro K et al. (1997) The Lassa fever virus L gene: nucleotide sequence, comparison, and precipitation of a predicted 250 kDa protein with monospecific antiserum. *J Gen Virol*, **78**(3), 547–551.

Maiztegui JI, Fernandez JM and de Damilano AJ (1979) Efficacy of immune plasma in treatment of Argentine haemorrhagic fever and association between infection and a late neurological syndrome. *Lancet*, **ii**, 1216–1217.

McCormick JB, King IJ, Webb PA et al. (1986a) Lassa fever. Effective therapy with ribavirin. *N Engl J Med*, **314**(1), 20–26.

McCormick JB, Walker DH, King IJ et al. (1986b) Lassa virus hepatitis: a study of fatal Lassa fever in humans. *Am J Trop Med Hyg*, **35**(2), 401–407.

McKee KT Jr, Oro JG, Kuehne AI et al. (1993) Safety and immunogenicity of a live-attenuated Junin (Argentine hemorrhagic fever) vaccine in rhesus macaques. *Am J Trop Med Hyg*, **48**(3), 403–411.

Mills JN, Barrera Oro JG, Bressler DS et al. (1996) Characterization of Oliveros virus, a new member of the Tacaribe complex (*Arenaviridae*: *Arenavirus*). *Am J Trop Med Hyg*, **54**(4), 399–404.

Monath TP (1987) Lassa fever—new issues raised by field studies in West Africa. *J Infect Dis*, **155**(3), 433–436.

Montali RJ, Connolly BM, Armstrong DL et al. (1995) Pathology and immunohistochemistry of callitrichid hepatitis, and emerging disease of captive New World primates caused by lymphocytic choriomeningitis virus. *Am J Pathol*, **147**(5), 1441–1449.

Murphy FA and Whitfield SG (1975) Morphology and morphogenesis of arenaviruses. *Bull WHO*, **52**(4–6), 409–419.

Oldstone MB (2002a) Arenaviruses. I. The epidemiology molecular and cell biology of arenaviruses. Introduction. *Curr Top Microbiol Immunol*, **262**, V–XII.

Oldstone MB (2002b) Arenaviruses. II. The molecular pathogenesis of arenavirus infections. Introduction. *Curr Top Microbiol Immunol*, **263**, V–XII.

Pfau CJ (1974) Biochemical and biophysical properties of the arenaviruses. *Prog Med Virol*, **18**, 64–80.

Rimoldi MT and de Bracco MM (1980) *In vitro* inactivation of complement by a serum factor present in Junin-virus infected guinea-pigs. *Immunology*, **39**(2), 159–164.

Rowe WP (1954) *Studies on Pathogenesis and Immunity in Lymphocytic Choriomeningitis Virus of the Mouse*. nm 005.048.14.01. US Naval Medical Research Institute, Department of Defense, Washington, DC.

Salas R, Manzione W, de Tesh RB et al. (1991) Venezuelan haemorrhagic fever. *Lancet*, **338**, 1033–1036.

Stephensen CB, Jacob JR, Montali RJ *et al.* (1991) Isolation of an arenavirus from a marmoset with callitrichid hepatitis and its serologic association with disease. *J Virol,* **65**(8), 3995–4000.

Tesh RB, Jahrling PB, Salas R and Shope RE (1994) Description of Guanarito virus (*Arenaviridae: Arenavirus*), the etiologic agent of Venezuelan hemorrhagic fever. *Am J Trop Med Hyg,* **50**(4), 452–459.

Walker DH and Murphy FA (1987) Pathology and pathogenesis of arenavirus infections. *Curr Top Microbiol Immunol,* **133**, 89–113.

Whitton JL, Gebhard JR, Lewicki H *et al.* (1988) Molecular definition of a major cytotoxic T lymphocyte epitope in the glycoprotein of lymphocytic choriomeningitis virus. *J Virol,* **62**(3), 687–695.

Woodruff AW (1975) Handling patients with suspected Lassa fever entering Great Britain. *Bull WHO,* **52**(4–6), 717–721.

Young PR (1987) *Arenaviridae.* In *Animal Virus Structures* (eds Nermut MV and Steven AC), pp 185–198. Elsevier, Amsterdam.

Zinkernagel RM and Doherty PC (1979) MHC-restricted cytotoxic T cells: studies on the biological role of polymorphic major transplantation antigens determining T cell restriction-specificity, function and responsiveness. *Adv Immunol,* **27**, 151–177.

20

Filoviruses

Susan P. Fisher-Hoch

University of Texas, Brownsville, TX, USA

INTRODUCTION

Human infections with filoviruses are rare, but their occurrence has invariably been dramatic and mysterious. Their first appearance was in Marburg, Germany, in 1967 (Martini, 1971). Thirty-one people were infected: laboratory technicians, medical personnel, animal care personnel and their relatives. Seven of them died. Primary cases had been exposed to tissues and blood from African green monkeys imported into Germany and Yugoslavia from Uganda. A virus isolated from these patients was found by electron microscopy to be unique among mammalian pathogens, having a strange, looped and branched filamentous form, hence the name 'filovirus' (Figure 20.1a) (Johnson *et al.*, 1977). No more was heard of these viruses until 1976 and 1979 when epidemics of a haemorrhagic disease with very high mortality in northern Zaire (now the Democratic Republic of Congo; DRC) and in southern Sudan were found to be due to two strains of a related, yet distinct filovirus (Bowen *et al.*, 1980; Richman *et al.*, 1983; Johnson *et al.*, 1977) This was named Ebola virus, after a river in Zaire (World Health Organization, 1978a, 1978b; Baron *et al.*, 1983). Over the next 10 years rare, sporadic cases of filovirus infections in Africa were the only continuing evidence of the existence of these viruses. Their natural host and ecology remained elusive, but they were thought to be exclusively African, occurring principally in Zaire, Sudan, Uganda and Kenya (Figure 20.2). The mystery deepened when in 1989 a filovirus was isolated near Washington, DC, from dying cynomolgus monkeys shipped to the USA from the Philippines (Jahrling *et al.*, 1990). No epidemiological link with Africa could be found, and when laboratory-confirmed human infections were documented during this epizootic, all were asymptomatic. The new virus was the closest relative of Ebola virus yet seen, serologically even more closely related than Marburg virus, and appeared to be Asian in origin. Ideas about the epidemiology and clinical spectrum of filoviruses had to be drastically revised.

This was the position in 1994 when news came from Zaire (DRC) of a fresh outbreak of the original Zaire strain of filovirus. Following this outbreak, relatively frequent epidemics of Ebola Zaire in Gabon and the Congo, Ebola Sudan in Uganda and Marburg in eastern Congo have been reported, and several outbreaks of Ebola Zaire are ongoing and apparently closely linked to a major epizootic in great apes. This epizootic, combined with hunting and loss of habitat, is now thought to threaten chimpanzees and gorillas in the area with extinction.

VIROLOGY

Despite intensive efforts, the natural history of filoviruses remains one of the mysteries of virology. At first they were thought to be related to rhabdoviruses, but it has become clear that they form a family of their own, designated *Filoviridae* on account of their filamentous appearance (Kiley *et al.*, 1982). Nucleotide sequence analyses place the family in the order *Mononegavirales*, which also includes the *Paramyxoviridae* and *Rhabdoviridae* (Table 20.1) (Kiley *et al.*, 1988; Pringle, 1991).

Principles and Practice of Clinical Virology, Fifth Edition. Edited by A. J. Zuckerman, J. E. Banatvala, J. R. Pattison, P. D. Griffiths and B. D. Schoub
© 2004 John Wiley & Sons Ltd   ISBN 0 470 84338 1

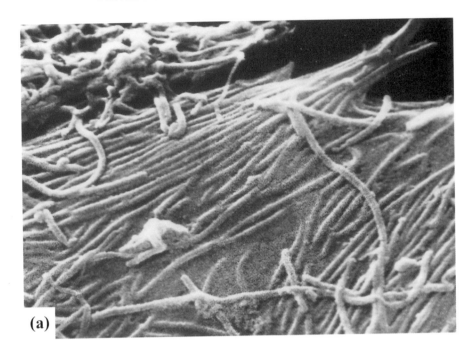

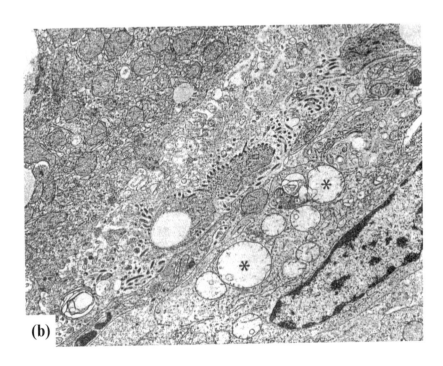

Figure 20.1   Electron micrographs of filoviruses (a) Scanning electron micrograph of Ebola virus (× 500). (b) Liver section from a cynomolgus monkey that died of Ebola (Reston) infection, showing extruding particles from cells in hepatic sinuses. Stars are in vacuoles also seen in Ebola-infected liver (× 8400). Both courtesy of C. Goldsmith

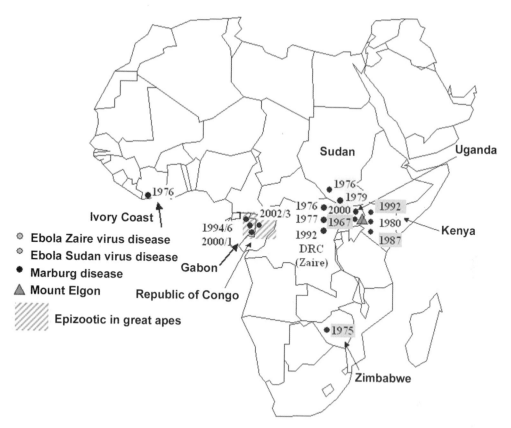

Figure 20.2 Map of Africa showing approximate locations and dates of Ebola and Marburg epidemics and origins of known index cases. Note the equatorial rain forest distribution of the outbreaks.

Table 20.1 Tree of the order *Mononegavirales* showing the suggested relationship of the *Filoviridae* to paramyxo- and rhabdoviruses, based on nucleic acid sequencing of the nucleic protein gene

Family	Genus	Virus
Rhabdoviridae	*Vesiculovirus*	Chandipura virus
		Vesicular stomatitits virus
	Lyssavirus	Rabies
Paramyxoviridae	*Morbillivirus*	Measles
	Paramyxovirus	Newcastle disease virus
		Mumps
		Parainfluenza type 3
	Pneumovirus	Respiratory syncytial virus
		Pneumonia virus of mice
Filoviridae	—	Ebola
		Marburg

Filoviruses undergo rapid, lytic replication in the cytoplasm of a wide range of host cells. The nucleocapsids acquire the envelope with its surface projections by a process of extrusion of cell membrane rather than a discrete orderly budding, which may account for the striking pleomorphism of these viruses (Johnson *et al.*, 1977). Filoviruses are among the largest known viruses, with highly variable length (up to 14 000 nm), apparently due to concatamerisation (Regnery *et al.*, 1980). The virions are of uniform 80 nm diameter, with a helical nucleocapsid, consisting of a central axis 20–30 nm in diameter, surrounded by a helical capsid 40–50 nm in diameter, with 5 nm cross-striations. A host cell membrane-derived layer with 10 nm projections in regular array surrounds the nucleocapsid and the terminal windings of nucleocapsid found at one end of the particle. The virions contain a single negative-strand RNA genome ranging from 4×106 (Marburg virus) to 4.5×106 Da (Ebola virus) (Regnery *et al.*, 1980). The RNA is a template for at least seven polypeptides, a nucleoprotein (NP), a glycoprotein (GP), a polymerase (L) and four other undesignated proteins (VP40, VP35, VP30 and VP24), two of which are associated with the nucleocapsid (Elliott *et al.*, 1985). The Ebola virus glycoprotein gene produces two molecular species, one a soluble truncated protein (sGP), which is secreted from infected cells, and the other the full-length glycoprotein consisting of two subunits, GP1 and GP2, the latter being anchored in the membrane. GP1 and GP2 are heavily glycosylated, and together provide the surface spikes seen by electron microscopy, and these proteins are responsible for viral entry. Marburg virus differs in that it does not possess a sGP (Feldmann *et al.*, 1999). An abundant but poorly glycosylated protein, VP40, and the nucleoprotein (N) are associated with the nucleocapsid. The VP40 has been shown to be able to bud from mammalian cells as lipid-bound virus-like particles, which are probably able to interact with cellular proteins, specifically a ligase (Licata *et al.*, 2003). The importance of lipids is further illustrated by the observation that Ebola and Marburg viruses' proteins compartmentalise within lipid rafts during viral assembly, and both entry and exit of the virus may be through these rafts (Bavari *et al.*, 2002). The VP24 protein is believed to be a secondary matrix protein which appears to localise to the plasma membrane and the perinuclear region and may play a role in assembly and budding (Han *et al.*, 2003).

Oligonucleotide restriction mapping of viral RNA has shown that there are about 60 differences between the Ebola (Zaire) and Ebola (Sudan) strains, whereas the 1976 and 1979 Ebola (Sudan) strains were almost identical (Cox *et al.*, 1983). The Ebola viruses are genetically stable, with about 50–60% of their oligonucleotides distinct from those of Marburg virus (McCormick *et al.*, 1983). Nucleotide and amino acid sequence analyses of Ebola (Zaire) and Marburg viruses show similar organisation and structure, with the nucleoprotein gene positioned at the extreme 3' end of the genome (Sanchez *et al.*, 1992). Homology in the N-terminal 400 residues of the nucleoprotein gene is strongest from positions 130–392 of the Marburg sequence, containing 34 identical amino acids, and having in turn a high degree of identity with paramyxovirus nucleoprotein sequences and, to a lesser extent, with corresponding rhabdovirus sequences. Computer-generated dendrogram analysis of this region among the *Mononegavirales* shows the closest relationship between Marburg and Ebola, suggesting common ancestral origin. The next nearest relative is respiratory syncytial virus, which in turn is related to the other paramyxo- and myxoviruses. Most distant are the rhabdoviruses.

Radioimmunoprecipitation studies of antibody responses in monkeys infected with different Ebola viruses show that though there was cross-reaction between Asian and African filovirus nucleoproteins. No cross-reacting antibody to the glycoprotein between Asian and African filoviruses is observed (Fisher-Hoch *et al.*, 1992a). There is, however, apparently close identity at the glycoprotein level among Asian filoviruses, but not African filoviruses. The Asian viruses so far isolated are probably related very closely to each other, and may indeed be variants of the same strain.

EPIDEMIOLOGY

Epidemics: Marburg Virus Disease

In 1967, a fulminating haemorrhagic fever struck a number of laboratory workers in Marburg and Frankfurt, Germany, and Belgrade, Yugoslavia (Martini, 1971). The virus name was taken from the German city where most of the cases occurred. There were 31 human cases, 25 of which were primary infections with seven deaths (Table 20.2). None of six secondary cases died. Twenty primary cases were in Marburg, four in Frankfurt and one in Belgrade. All primary cases had handled blood or tissues from shipments of African green monkeys (*Cercopithecus aethiops*) soon after being imported from Uganda, via London. Epidemiological investigations revealed that 20/29 persons with blood contact became infected, and 4/13 exposed to tissue culture. Among the primary human cases in Marburg, 10 had assisted in autopsies and three had trephined monkey skulls. One of the laboratory staff had dissected kidneys, one had handled tissue culture from the monkeys, one broke a test tube which had contained contaminated material, and five had merely cleaned contaminated glassware. None of the animal attendants not in contact with blood, or laboratory personnel who used precautions, such as protective gloves and clothing, were infected. There were no further primary cases upon institution of compulsory wearing of protective clothing with gloves and masks for work with monkeys and cleaning procedures, and use of disinfectants. Five of the secondary cases resulted from person-to-person contact at home or in hospital. The sixth was the wife of a veterinarian who became ill several weeks after recovery of her husband, from whose semen Marburg virus was later recovered. One physician inoculated herself accidentally with a needle through a rubber glove. In Belgrade, the single primary

Table 20.2 Table of the reported human cases and deaths from filovirus infections in Africa

Virus/year	Place of infection	Total cases	Deaths	Mortality (%)
Marburg				
1967	Marburg, Germany	31	7	31
1967	Belgrade, Yugoslavia	2	0	
1975	Zimbabwe	2	1	
1980	Mount Elgon, Kenya	1	1	
1999	Durba, DRC (Zaire)	76	52	68
Total		*112*	*61*	*54*
Ebola Zaire				
1976	Yambuku, Zaire	318	280	88
1976	UK	1	0	
1977	Tandala, Zaire	1	1	
1980	Nzoia, Kenya	1	0	
1994	Kikwit, Zaire	315	242	77
1994–1995	Gabon	49	30	61
1996	Gabon	60	45	75
2000–2002	Gabon	30*	22*	73
2000–2002	Republic of Congo	92*	80*	87
Total		*745*	*598*	*80*
Ebola Sudan				
1976	Maridi, Sudan	284	151	53
1979	Maridi, Sudan	34	22	65
1999	Uganda (Gula district)	425	224	53
Total		*743*	*995*	*54*
Ebola Reston				
1990	Richmond, Virginia	4	0	
1990	Manila, Philippines	12	0	
Total		*16*	*0*	
Total cases		3120	2649	

*Provisional figures, since these current outbreaks are ongoing, few cases have been laboratory confirmed and data are difficult to confirm. In these circumstances mortality may be artificially high, since only the most severe cases will be recorded.

case, a veterinarian, performed autopsies towards the end of the monkeys' 6 week quarantine. His wife fell ill 10 days after nursing him at home. Despite the death of a total of 99 animals during quarantine in Belgrade, these were the only two human infections.

About 400–600 animals originating from four shipments reached Europe from Uganda over a 3 week period. Frankfurt received only 40–60 animals from two shipments, and Belgrade about 300 animals from three shipments. The remainder went to Marburg. All spent 60–87 days in a holding facility in Uganda before being shipped to London, Heathrow, where they spent 6–36 h in an animal hostel prior to being forwarded to Germany. In Marburg, the monkeys were housed in separate rooms with no recirculation of 'air-conditioned' ventilated air. Published data are unclear as to whether ongoing enzootics were observed inside Germany or the details of animal movements. Data on the Belgrade enzootics are,

however, better recorded. Three shipments of monkeys from the same source in Uganda were received, two of which were in transit at Heathrow airport, London. The third arrived directly via Munich. Unusually high mortality during 6 weeks' quarantine was noted in all three shipments; 46/99 animals died from the first, and 20 and 30 from the second two. The Belgrade epizootic was clearly characterised by ongoing transmission with daily death of one or more animals (Figure 20.3) (Martini, 1971).

Epidemiological studies after the 1967 epidemics concluded that two or three infected monkeys would have been sufficient to initiate the epizootic and all three outbreaks of human disease. It was stated at the time that evidence clearly pointed to transmission between monkeys in quarantine facilities by direct contact with equipment. Direct contact with blood and tissues was documented for all human cases and there was significant evidence against transmission to

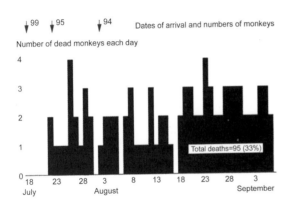

Figure 20.3 A histogram of the epizootic of Marburg virus infections in monkeys imported into Belgrade in 1967. Derived from Stojkovic *et al.* (1971)

humans by air. No evidence was ever produced that supported the hypothesis that the monkeys were infected in transit in London from any number of a wide range of mammals and birds also temporarily lodging at the airport hostel. Furthermore, no evidence could be found of epizootics in Uganda, but later some indirect, controversial information emerged that there had at that time of the outbreak been excess deaths in monkey colonies in islands near Lake Kyoga, north of Lake Victoria, to the east of Mount Elgon in Kenya. In Uganda monkeys were captured in this area and placed in holding facilities, reportedly in single cages. They were then transported to Entebbe. Here they were held for at least 3 days before shipment. At the time of the outbreak the trade had expanded considerably and holding times had been reduced, and it may be imagined that some crowding may have ensued. During July and August 1967, 1772 *C. aethiops* were housed in Entebbe and 1290 exported, the majority to Germany and Yugoslavia (Henderson *et al.*, 1971).

For two decades only three further, isolated primary human Marburg infections and only two secondary cases were observed. These were adventurous tourists or expatriate residents: one a traveller in Zimbabwe and two others from the Mount Elgon region of western Kenya, not far from the shores of Lake Victoria (Gear *et al.*, 1975; Teepe *et al.*, 1983; Smith *et al.*, 1982). Extensive epidemiological investigations in Zimbabwe and on Mount Elgon revealed no clues to the origin of these infections. Medical facilities are limited in these areas, and isolated cases in local residents may go unnoticed unless dramatic epidemics supervene.

In 1999, Marburg re-emerged in the east of the Democratic Republic of the Congo, in the community of Durba. There were an estimated 76 cases and 52 deaths. A very difficult investigation was conducted in what was essentially a war zone in a state of anarchy. Cases were found to be associated with illegal working of a partially flooded gold mine infested with all manner of wildlife. There appeared to have been a series of primary cases among these illegal miners, rather than a point source epidemic, with secondary cases in their households. The investigating team had to leave for security reasons, and it is unclear what happened subsequently. It is possible that sporadic Marburg disease continues in the area, which is a region of continuing civil unrest.

Epidemics: Ebola Virus Disease

It was not until nearly a decade after the Marburg outbreak that simultaneous outbreaks of another lethal haemorrhagic fever struck suddenly in northern Zaire and Sudan in 1976 (Figure 20.2) (World Health Organization, 1978a, 1978b). Two more filoviruses were isolated: Ebola (Zaire) and Ebola (Sudan) (Johnson *et al.*, 1977). In 1976 the largest outbreak recorded took place in equatorial rain-forest areas of northern Zaire. In retrospective case-searching exercises the case definition of probable Ebola haemorrhagic fever used was a person living in the epidemic area who died after 1 or more days with two or more symptoms and signs (headache, fever, abdominal pain, nausea and/or vomiting and bleeding) and who had received an injection or had had contact with a probable or proven case in the 3 preceding weeks. Virus isolation, visualisation of the virus by electron microscopy, or an Ebola virus-specific immunofluorescent antibody (IFA) titre of 64 or more was required in addition to confirm a case. Using these definitions, 280 deaths in 318 probable or confirmed cases were identified: case fatality 88%. The index case may have been a recent traveller in the northern Equateur region of Zaire, who attended the outpatient clinic of a mission hospital in Yambuku apparently for treatment of acute malaria, where he received an injection of chloroquine. It remains unclear whether this man was the source of the epidemic or whether he was infected by his injection, since another patient with a similar illness was admitted to the hospital at about the same time. The subsequent nine cases, however, had all received treatment for other diseases at the hospital. Although all ages and sexes were affected, the highest incidence was in women aged 15–29 years, but these were frequently patients attending antenatal and outpatient clinics at the hospital, and the major risk factor was receiving an injection at this hospital. Needles were in short supply, and were not sterilised between use. Eleven of the 17 staff members of the hospital died, and the outbreak only terminated 4 weeks after it began, when the hospital was closed. Although transmission was focused in the outpatient clinics of the hospital, there was subsequent dissemination in surrounding villages to people caring for sick relatives or attending childbirths. The overall secondary attack rate was about 5%, but nearer 20% in close relatives of a case. Illness:infection ratios in one village exceeded 10:1. Ebola virus antibody in persons not ill and without contact with cases during the epidemic was only conclusively identified in four individuals. However, the following year, 1977, a single fatal case was identified in Tandala, also in northern Zaire (Table 20.2). There was no ensuing epidemic, but serological and epidemiological investigations uncovered two possible cases dating back to 1972, and 7% prevalence of IFA antibody in the local population (Heymann et al., 1980). Unfortunately, non-specific reactions to the Ebola virus antigens used at that time make interpretation of much of these serological data uncertain.

At the same time as the 1976 Yambuku epidemic, an outbreak of a similar disease occurred in southern Sudan (Figure 20.2) (World Health Organization, 1978b). This outbreak was strongly associated with index cases in a single cotton weaving factory. There were 151 deaths in 284 cases identified (case fatality about 53% case definition not stated). The focus of the infection was in the town of Nzara, where the factory was located, and spread was to close relatives (67 cases). The epidemic was augmented by high levels of transmission at nearby Maridi hospital, following transfer of one of the Nzara patients, and further cases were transferred to Juba and Khartoum. There were 203 cases in Maridi, 93 of which were probably infected in the hospital, and 105 in the community. Forty-one staff members died, and at the height of the epidemic all wards contained patients with overt haemorrhage. The highest attack rates were associated with nursing a patient, but not with sleeping in the same room. In 1979 there was a similar outbreak, when 22/34 infections (65%) were fatal (Baron et al., 1983). Although closely related, the viruses from Zaire and Sudan were found to be distinct, confirming the conclusions of epidemiological investigations that the two 1976 epidemics were

independent. The two virus strains isolated in Sudan in 1976 and 1979, however, are identical (Cox et al., 1983).

Between 1979 and 1994 the disease fell silent, with only one case of human Ebola infection recorded (Teepe et al., 1983). In 1994 all this changed. A large, hospital-based outbreak in Kikwit resulted in the deaths of 242/315 cases. This outbreak resembled those that had gone before, in that a hospital was the amplifying focus of the outbreak, with many needle-borne transmissions, and the virus then spilled over into the community, with cases among close contacts of the sick (Reiter et al., 1999). The original source was traced to a single forest worker, but intensive studies still failed to reveal the primary host. Soon afterwards the first of three epidemics appeared in Gabon. The index cases were apparently gold panners or hunters in the forest, one outbreak resulting from finding and handling the carcass of a dead chimpanzee in the forest. All the primary cases handled the uncooked meat at some stage. People who ate the cooked meat did not get sick.

Ebola Sudan did not reappear until October 2000, and when it did it was by way of a massive epidemic in Uganda. The origins of the outbreak are obscure, but it appeared to originate in the northern part of the country where rebel fighting was ongoing. The epidemic was centred in the Gulu district and was not brought under control until mid-January 2001. There were a total of 425 cases and 224 deaths (case fatality 53%). Attack rates were calculated to be between 4.5 and 12.6/10 000 depending on the case definition (Okware et al., 2002).

Infections with Ebola Zaire re-emerged in Gabon and the neighbouring Republic of Congo in 2000 and continue to date. As of 30 December 2002, WHO reported 30 confirmed cases (14 laboratory confirmed and 16 epidemiologically linked), including 22 deaths, in Gabon and neighbouring villages across the Congolese border. Epidemics in the Congo are ongoing in 2003, and appear to be closely associated with the epizootics in great apes, described in the section on ecology. As of 27 February 2003, there were five confirmed and 92 probable cases of Ebola, with 80 deaths in the Cuvette Ouest Region of the Congo. These outbreaks are proving difficult to control because of the remoteness of the area, the association with the ongoing great ape epizootic and the fears and resistance of the communities which are affected. These fears were sufficient in one community for a schoolteacher to be attacked and killed for accusations of being the cause of the epidemic.

Epizootics: Reston Virus

In 1989 and early 1990, a filovirus closely related to Ebola virus was isolated from *Cynomolgus* monkeys in quarantine facilities in Reston, Virginia, in Texas and in Pennsylvania (Jahrling *et al.*, 1990; Centers for Disease Control, 1989). The monkeys had recently been imported into the USA from the Philippines. The first shipment arrived via Amsterdam, and exhaustive enquiries ruled out a link with African animals during transit. Early the following year more shipments of monkeys from the same source arrived, this time directly from the Philippines over the Pacific Ocean, and several more filovirus isolations were made from sick and dying monkeys (Centers for Disease Control, 1990a). No link with Africa or African animals could be identified in the Philippines, and in the absence of such evidence this must be considered at present the first Asian filovirus. Pathogenicity for cynomolgus monkeys was uncertain because of a high rate of concurrent infection with simian haemorrhagic fever virus (SHFV), a DNA virus which is a known severe simian pathogen unrelated to the *Filoviridae*. This co-infection added enormously to the complexity of this episode (SHFV also produces haemorrhagic disease, although it does not apparently infect humans). In the first reported epizootic, 223/1050 exposed animals died, with increased handling a risk factor for disease and death. The natural host and geographical distribution are also unknown, although the infected monkeys (*Macaca mulatta*) apparently originated in India (Palmer *et al.*, 1968).

In 1990, concern about the risk to humans led to a temporary ban on importation into the USA of cynomolgus, rhesus and African green monkeys. Evidence for ongoing epizootics and transmission was sought in the Philippine export facilities which had provided the monkeys (Hayes *et al.*, 1992). Antigen detection enzyme-linked immunosorbent assays (ELISAs) on liver homogenates revealed that 85/161 (52.8%) of monkeys that died there over a period of less than 3 months were positive for filovirus antigen, as were 6.7% of monkeys tested in an initial serological survey. Incidence was calculated to be 24.4/100 animals, or 0.6/100 monkeys/day of follow-up. Documented case fatality at this institution was 82.4%, and survivors developed high-titre IFA antibody. Average duration of viraemia was 5.6–2.4 days. Diarrhoea and respiratory problems were the most frequently recorded manifestations. In the 73% of monkeys positive for filovirus by IFA at this facility the geometric mean antibody titre was 145. A protective factor was the presence of antibody to filovirus at the time of entry to the facility (Hayes *et al.*, 1992). As in the USA, many of the filovirus-infected monkeys were co-infected with SHFV, which means that all data from these epizootics are difficult to interpret and conclusions are open to question.

Epidemiology: Reston Virus

In the Philippines, 186 people were studied who lived in wildlife collection areas or worked in four primate export facilities in Manila (Miranda *et al.*, 1991). Twelve (6%) were filovirus antibody-positive by IFA and in the facility experiencing the epizootic 22% were positive, significantly higher than the other export facilities [relative risk 5.6; 95% confidence interval (CI) 1.09–24.14] (Hayes *et al.*, 1992). In that facility the workers in the animal hospital had the highest titres: 3/5 had titres of >256. However, there was no illness in any of the positive individuals, and no association between seropositivity and other risk factors, such as bites, scratches or eating monkey meat. In the facility at Reston, Virginia, five animal handlers had a high level of daily exposure to infected and dying animals (Centers for Disease Control, 1990b, 1990c). Four of these had serological evidence of recent infection by IFA, and three were observed to seroconvert during the period of the epizootic. One cut his finger while performing a necropsy on an infected animal. Daily monitoring of this individual revealed transient viraemia and seroconversion, but neither he nor his colleagues had any illness attributable to filovirus infection.

Serological Surveys of Humans

Serosurveys of village populations in epidemic areas have shown the presence of low-titred Ebola and Marburg antibodies. If these reactions can be confirmed by other methods and in prospective studies, then infection without a serious clinical disease is more common than realised at present. In serosurveys in Zaire, antibody prevalence to Ebola virus has been 37%. Serosurveys in individuals not in contact with patients in Sudan have had antibody prevalence of 1–4% to an Ebola-related virus. Unfortunately, the IFA test used for these studies is unreliable at low titre or in the absence of a history of clinical disease, and serological reports need to be interpreted with considerable caution. Antibody, sometimes with high prevalence, has been reported in monkeys and humans from many geographical locations, including unlikely populations such as Cona Indians from Central America (Heymann *et al.*, 1980) and Alaskans. Specificity is not improved by the use of Western blot techniques, since non-specific antibody to some of the Ebola virus proteins can also be seen in this test. This problem appears to be unique to Ebola virus (Zaire, Sudan and Reston strains), and is not encountered with Marburg serology. Lack of correlation of serology with Ebola disease supports the conclusion that the titres are non-specific, although it remains possible that they may reflect past infection with unrecognised non-pathogenic filoviruses. ELISA and other techniques for antibody assays under development may allow some of these issues to be settled.

ECOLOGY

Until the early 1990s, outbreaks of human disease may have been unusual, because transmission from the natural reservoir to humans is rare. Searches for evidence of virus infection in many species of animals captured in central African countries have failed to provide any clues as to the possible reservoir. The original ecological setting of Marburg and Ebola appeared to centre around central and south central Africa (Figure 20.2), particularly the Mount Elgon area of western Kenya and Uganda. Surveys of wild monkeys from the Lake Kyoga area in northern Uganda in the 1970s, where the original Marburg-infected group originated, failed to yield virus but about 10% of sera reacted with crude Marburg antigen in a complement fixation test, and in at least three animals neutralising antibody could be demonstrated. The 1987 case was a boy who had spent considerable time in Kitum Cave on Mount Elgon, collecting minerals and other items, near to the sugar cane factory where the 1980 case had worked. Extensive searches for the reservoir in the area around the sugar cane-processing factory and around Kitum Cave were unsuccessful. The cave contained large numbers of bats, and was visited by a wide range of mammals, birds, reptiles and insects. Sentinel animals and other means of searching for the virus failed to identify bats (or any of a number of wild mammals) as the ultimate source. Similarly, a thorough study of insects and mammals along the trail of the 1975 traveller in Zimbabwe did not produce evidence of the source of infection.

Bats remain highly suspect, since they were implicated directly in the Kitum Cave case, which contains enormous colonies of bats. In Sudan in 1976 and 1979 both index cases had been from a cotton factory, where the roof was heavily infested with bats, concentrated over the store room where both index cases worked. Antibody could not be detected in bat sera, and no virus was isolated from bat tissues in either investigation, but limited sampling, particularly in the Sudan studies, could have missed infected animals (serological studies in bats and other exotic species present a serious challenge in terms of species-specific reagents). An animal study showed that Ebola virus can replicate in bats without causing disease (Swanepoel *et al.*, 1996). This is strong evidence that bats can carry the silent infection, which is a prerequisite for maintaining the virus in a wild population over time. Other suggestions, such as rodents and even plants as primary hosts have never been substantiated. If this were a rodent virus, the ubiquity of most rodents would mean that primary infections in humans would be much more frequent, as is the case with Lassa fever, so rodents are unlikely as hosts. There is no precedent for a plant virus infecting humans.

Given the insensitivity and lack of specificity of the original tests, early data on animal surveys, including bat studies, probably do not reflect the real situation. What we do know is that things changed in the 1990s, and that large apes, specifically chimpanzees and gorillas, have become increasingly implicated in transmission to humans. The first indication of the significance of chimpanzees in the chain of transmission came with the report of an outbreak in Gabon in 1996, resulting from the handling and butchering of a dead chimpanzee found in the forest by some villagers (Georges *et al.*, 1999). Since 1994, four human epidemics have occurred in north-east Gabon, and ape carcasses have been found near the sites of three of these. That the great apes are not the natural host is made clear by the fact that mortality in both species is as high as in humans. From 2000 on, repeated epidemics in Gabon and in bordering DRC and the Republic of Congo have been linked with the epizootic in great apes. This epizootic has contributed in large part to a catastrophic decline in great ape populations, threatening them with extinction. The populations have been reduced by more than a half between 1983 and 2000. A great ape nest group survey in Gabon near Minkébé, an area where there had been a human epidemic, recorded a 99% fall in nest groups over the study period (Walsh *et al.*, 2003). In Mekambo in neighbouring Congo, many ape carcasses have been found, and in Lossi, a population of 143 individually identified gorillas has been reduced to seven. The epizootic is gradually making its way south and west. Logging and a booming commercial bush meat trade also contributes to the declines, but Ebola is thought to have been responsible at least equally. Of further concern is that handling of dead carcasses, with the potential of commerce in infected bushmeat, increases the probability of human epidemics, which is exactly what is being seen in the same areas. Extermination of the great apes would certainly reduce the possibility of human Ebola epidemics, but that seems too high a price to pay. Furthermore, the natural host, be it bat or other occult species, will remain as the primary source. Efforts to control the epizootic are called for, particularly as it threatens the great wildlife refuges, but given the remoteness of the area and the lack of a vaccine and a means of delivery, it is difficult to know what measures might be effective.

TRANSMISSION AND RISK FACTORS

Person-to-person spread has been the major mode of transmission in epidemics. Contact with patients ill with Ebola is the most important factor in determining risk of illness. Other risk factors associated with human-to-human transmission are infection from contaminated materials such as needles, contact with blood or secretions, preparation of a body for burial or, occasionally, sexual contact. Close contact with blood or tissues of infected monkeys is also important. The virus enters through mucous membranes or skin lesions, and outbreaks have been abruptly terminated when blood and needle transmission were interrupted (Fisher-Hoch, 1993). In later sporadic outbreaks, one secondary Marburg case nursed the index patient with no protective clothing, and later assisted with resuscitation procedures. She also handled wet tissues from the companion of the index case, who was also infected (Gear et al., 1975). In 1980, a patient died 5 h after being admitted to a Nairobi hospital and the attending doctor subsequently became ill with, but survived, Marburg infection. Furthermore, epidemiological studies in Zaire and Sudan do not suggest spread through casual contact or by aerosol transmission. A formal study of risk factors for virus transmission in the Sudan epidemic in 1979 showed that caring for an ill patient carried a relative risk five times greater than persons with a lesser degree of physical contact, and no cases occurred in persons who entered the room of an ill patient but had no physical contact. These data confirm that Ebola is not an airborne disease and depends on close contact, probably with infected blood or secretions, for its propagation. The mode of acquisition of primary infection is totally unknown.

The most significant risk factor for the monkeys infected in the epizootic in the Philippines was being an occupant of a gang cage (six-fold increase of risk; $p < 0.001$; OR 5.96; 95% CI 2.87–12.38) (Hayes et al., 1992). Although one infected monkey was identified at a second exporting facility, no transmission could be documented. Significantly, this second facility routinely housed their animals in single cages. Ebola (Reston) has been identified at high titre in respiratory secretions in monkeys, and respiratory transmission at close quarters may be a factor in epizootics with this virus. This last hypothesis is supported in part by the genetic relationship between the filoviruses and known respiratory pathogens. However, there was strong evidence for monkey-to-monkey transmission by re-use of needles for routine procedures, such as tuberculin testing or antibiotic administration.

Laboratory Infections

The outbreak of Marburg virus in 1967 was caused by infection of individuals handling fresh monkey tissues or contaminated equipment without gloves or other protective clothing. Otherwise there has only been one reported laboratory-acquired infection (needlestick) with Ebola virus, in 1976 (Emond et al., 1977).

Because of its lethal potential, Ebola has been a candidate for biological warfare. Little information is available, but it has been handled extensively in biological research, and further accidental infections may have occurred, specifically in the former Soviet bloc. The key to safe laboratory handling of this virus is extreme care in avoiding accidental inoculation.

DISEASE

Clinical Spectrum

The incubation period for Marburg virus disease is 3–9 days (Martini, 1971) and for Ebola virus about 10 days; 5–7 days for needle transmission and 6–12 days for person-to-person spread (World Health Organization, 1978a, 1978b; Baron et al., 1983). The incubation period for the Ebola-related virus from Sudan may be slightly longer than for the more lethal Ebola (Zaire) strain, and appears to be dose-dependent. The illness-to-infection ratio for Marburg and Ebola viruses approaches unity, since few if any asymptomatic infections have ever been observed. In contrast, Ebola (Reston) virus, in all individuals documented to have been infected, was uniformly asymptomatic (Table 20.2) (Centers for Disease Control, 1990b, 1990c; Miranda et al., 1991).

The human disease caused by the African viruses is dramatic (Figure 20.4). The onset is abrupt, with fever, severe headache (usually periorbital and frontal), myalgia, arthralgia, conjunctivitis and extreme malaise. Sore throat is a common symptom, often associated with severe swelling and dysphagia, but no exudative pharyngitis. A papular, eventually desquamating rash may occur in some patients, especially on the trunk and back, and morbilliform rash has been observed on white skins. In non-human primates petechiae are striking. Gastrointestinal symptoms develop in most patients on the second or third day of illness, with abdominal pain, and cramping followed by diarrhoea and vomiting. Jaundice is not a feature of Marburg or Ebola disease. The bleeding begins on about the fifth day of illness and is most commonly from the mucous membranes: gastrointestinal tract, gingiva, nasopharynx and vagina. Death occurs in a large proportion of patients, and is associated with hypovolaemic shock and severe bleeding. Infection in pregnancy results in high maternal fatality and virtually 100% fetal death. The persistence of vomiting and the onset of any signs of mucosal bleeding carry a high risk of fatal outcome. Central nervous system involvement has led to hemiplegia and disorientation, and sometimes frank psychosis. Even in convalescence patients show prolonged weakness, severe weight loss, and in a few survivors serious but reversible personality changes are recorded, namely confusion, anxiety and aggressive behaviour.

Mortality

The death-to-infection ratio is related to virus strain (Table 20.2). Of the 29 known primary Marburg infections, 10 died (35%). No fatalities occurred among the 10 secondary cases (overall mortality 25.6%). The mortality ratios during the two epidemics of Ebola disease in Sudan were 55% and 65%, while that during the Zaire epidemic in 1976 was 88%. Patients in these epidemics received little or no medical care, and mortality might be substantially lowered with modern intensive care. Reduction in case fatality with human transmission has also been observed in Ebola infections, where human-to-human transmission was followed-up to six generations (Figure 20.5). This may represent some degree of viral attenuation with human passage.

ANIMAL MODELS

African green monkeys that had been recently imported from Uganda were the source of the Marburg outbreak (Henderson *et al.*, 1971), and cynomolgus monkeys were the source of the newly described Asian filovirus (Jahrling *et al.*, 1990; Centers for Disease Control, 1989). Both are important species for importation and medical research, and the monkey has been the most successful animal used for the study of the pathogenesis of filoviruses (Bowen *et al.*, 1980; Fisher-Hoch *et al.*, 1983; Baskerville *et al.*, 1978). The ability of any of the viruses to kill guinea-pigs is variable. Ebola (Zaire) kills guinea-pigs consistently

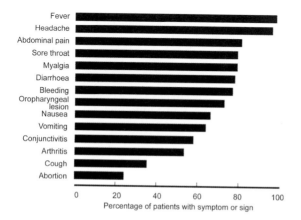

Figure 20.4 Frequency of symptoms and signs in Ebola haemorrhagic fever in Zaire in 1976

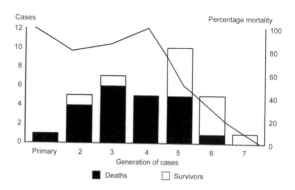

Figure 20.5 Mortality of cases of Ebola haemorrhagic fever in Sudan in 1979 showing the effect of successive human-to-human transmission

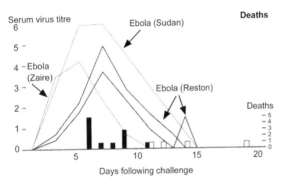

Figure 20.6 Comparison of the outcome and viraemia in 31 monkeys challenged with filoviruses. Dotted lines denote mean viraemia in monkeys infected with African filoviruses and solid lines mean viraemia in monkeys infected with Asian filoviruses. Numbers of deaths are shown by bars, dark bars are from African virus infections, and light bars from Asia virus infections

after several adaptive passages; the Sudan strain and Marburg virus do not. Only the Zaire virus was found to be lethal for suckling mice (McCormick *et al.*, 1983).

Rhesus monkeys inoculated intraperitoneally with 103–104 guinea-pig infectious units of Ebola (Zaire) virus become febrile 3–5 days after inoculation, and develop a petechial rash on the forehead, face, limbs and chest on day 4–5. Severe prostration with diarrhoea and bleeding leads to rapid death in almost all animals. Although similar in onset, the disease caused by the filovirus from Sudan is characterised by lower incidence of viraemia, enzyme and immune disturbances and some survivors, in keeping with the 53% case fatality reported from the 1976 human Sudan outbreak (Figure 20.6), and lack of pathogenicity in suckling mice (Baron *et al.*, 1983; World Health Organization, 1978b; McCormick *et al.*, 1983). Petechiae are rarely seen, and then only in dying monkeys. Viraemias and liver enzymes do not reach the levels seen in Ebola (Zaire) filovirus infections, but as the illness progresses severe thrombocytopenia, neutrophilia and lymphopenia developed, with very high aspartate transaminase (AST) and lactate dehydrogenase (LDH) levels. The monkeys are obviously very sick, including the survivors, but haematological and biochemical parameters return essentially to normal by day 20, and recovery is rapid and complete. Although systematic comparisons have not been made, Marburg virus infection in monkeys apparently resembles Ebola (Sudan) infection. However, African green monkeys inoculated experimentally with the virus soon after the 1967 outbreak all died, regardless of route of inocula-

tion, but progression to death was slowed if the inoculum titre was reduced.

Ebola (Reston) was first identified in an epizootic in an animal-handling facility, where transmission and a high death rate were observed in cynomolgus monkeys (Centers for Disease Control, 1989). However, the disease is characterised by slower development of viraemia, delayed onset of enzyme and immune disturbances, and lower mortality than in the African viruses (Figure 20.6). However, since these animals were co-infected with SHFV, the observations on filovirus pathogenesis are inconclusive (Jahrling *et al.*, 1990). Viraemia rises and peaks later than in Sudan infection. There was also histologically less evidence of extracellular distribution of filovirus antigen. When disease is severe or fatal, peak liver enzyme levels may be very high. It is clear that the host genetics also contribute, in that African green monkeys are less susceptible to severe or fatal disease due to Ebola (Sudan) or Ebola (Reston) than cynomolgus monkeys. Ebola (Zaire) infection, however, seems uniformly fatal in all species so far challenged.

PATHOGENESIS AND IMMUNOLOGY

Pathogenesis and immunology need to be discussed together, since they are inextricably linked, and some of the major manifestations of disease may be immunopathological in origin. The processes are clearly complex, reflecting a host–parasite relationship which is in no way adapted, and which may result from chance similarities in viral and host proteins favouring a wide range of events, including viral entry, replication and induction of host proteins, which damage rather than protect. Other factors, such as infecting dose, route of infection and host genetics, also undoubtedly play major roles. Indeed, the more we learn, the more we understand the complexity of the processes involved and how little we yet understand them.

Among the long-established facts are that high titres of virus are found in serum and tissues taken at autopsy, and particles may be seen in large numbers, with some obvious tropism for reticuloendothelial cells (Figure 20.1b) (Baskerville *et al.*, 1985; Fisher-Hoch *et al.*, 1992a). The most profound physiological alteration, and that which is invariably associated with death, is shock, manifested by hypotension, effusions and facial oedema. Severe, acute fluid loss, often with frank bleeding into the tissue and into the gut, is characteristic and results in dehydration and electrolyte and acid–base imbalance. Several years before the discovery of cytokines and other cellular messengers, it was observed that aortic endothelial cells from experimentally infected primates, although intact by histology and electron microscopy, had markedly reduced *in vitro* ability to produce prostacyclin compared with endothelium from normal uninfected control animals (Fisher-Hoch *et al.*, 1985). Thus, profound disruption of biochemical integrity of the endothelial cell was proposed, and subsequent data show that this is probably the case. Since there is no evidence for extensive destruction of endothelial cells by virus by histology or electron microscopy, it must be assumed that the fluid losses are due to these functional changes rather than lytic destruction of the endothelium by replicating virus. Nevertheless, profuse extracellular antigen suggests that overwhelming viral replication may be the underlying process causing the rapid multi-system collapse seen in Ebola (Zaire) infections (Baskerville *et al.*, 1985).

Bleeding is prominent, manifested as petechiae, uncontrolled bleeding from venepuncture sites and haemorrhagic effusions. Thrombocytopenia is invariable, but bleeding is not usually of sufficient volume to account for the shock, neither is it associated with solid evidence of significant disseminated intravascular coagulation (DIC) in the small number of animals or humans studied. As in Lassa fever, platelet dysfunction has been described in experimentally infected primates, in which there is a decline in *in vitro* platelet aggregation, beginning 1–3 days prior to the onset of bleeding and shock and progressing to virtually no aggregation at death. This leads to an increase in platelet factor 4 (PF4) levels in plasma, and concomitant decrease in platelet-derived PF4, suggesting that the platelets are being stimulated but are unable to aggregate (Fisher-Hoch *et al.*, 1985). In primates, profound lymphopenia early in disease is followed by marked neutrophilia. Laboratory evidence of only moderate DIC appears late in disease and is probably a consequence of the process, rather than the underlying primary pathology. Liver enzymes, aspartate (AST) and alanine transaminases (ALT) are raised, but the rise in AST is disproportionately higher than ALT, as was described in the early Marburg cases (Martini, 1971; Fisher-Hoch *et al.*, 1985).

At autopsy both Marburg- and Ebola-infected humans and primates show widespread haemorrhagic diathesis into skin, membranes and soft tissue. There is focal necrosis in liver, lymph nodes, ovaries and testis. Most prominent are eosinophilic inclusion bodies in hepatocytes (Councilman-like), without significant inflammatory response (Baskerville *et al.*, 1985). Focal necrosis is observed in many organs, including liver, lymphatic organs, kidney, testes and ovaries, but usually not sufficient to produce organ failure, and there is little infiltration of inflammatory cells in areas of tissue damage.

That the Asian filoviruses have a lesser pathogenic potential in primates is consistent with observations in accidental human infection. Other biological properties, such as the speed of replication in tissue culture, support the contention that there are clear differences in virulence between African and Asian filovirus. In a Reston-infected monkey, virus particles were observed embedded in the basement membrane of lung alveoli, and replication in the lung may occur with this filovirus, with which respiratory manifestations have been a feature in epizootics. The possibility of pulmonary involvement needs further study.

Past Infection and Persistence

Humans and non-human primates with documented acute infection with Ebola (Zaire), Sudan or Reston filoviruses seroconvert promptly to high-titre IFA to antigens prepared from all three viruses. Low-titre antibody may be associated with filovirus infection in the past, and also with immunity, but this remains to be demonstrated. Although Marburg virus has been isolated from semen 7 months after acute infection (Martini, 1971) and from the anterior chamber of the eye 2 months after acute infection (Gear *et al.*, 1975), human infections have been few, survivors scarce, and most experimentally infected non-human primates have not survived (Heymann *et al.*, 1980; World Health Organization, 1978a, 1978b; Fisher-Hoch *et al.*, 1985). A systematic study of the potential of the Ebola filovirus strains to persist in non-human primates failed to detect persistent filovirus. This was despite intensive efforts, including laparotomy to obtain serial specimens, co-cultivation and use of polymerase chain reaction (PCR). It cannot at present be excluded that passage in animals, specifically into additional non-human primates, or use of a more sensitive, or more broadly reactive PCR primer system, might not identify a few virions in tissues of recovered animals, perhaps in immunologically privileged sites such as the eye. However, these are likely to be at such low titre as to present an insignificant risk to people. Immunosuppression of such animals might also lead to reactivation, but filovirus disease in monkeys after release from quarantine has never been reported, and since many have been experimentally immunosuppressed for many years, reactivation of disease should have been observed by now, were it occurring.

Very little is understood about the immunology of Ebola virus infections except for the observation, made many years ago, that neutralising antibodies are difficult to demonstrate in both humans and primates, and that like many zoonotic viruses, notably Lassa virus and now the SARS HCoV, appear to be able to circulate in humans in the presence of detectable antibody and to show varying ability to persist at least for short periods following acute infection. Recent studies using specimens from patients in Gabon have shown that the innate immune system plays a very important role in the disease (Baize et al., 1999). Evidence from these studies and from animal studies suggest that the proinflammatory response is a central figure in both pathogenesis of severe disease and protection from disease, in that an early, orderly innate immune response was observed in infected individuals who never developed disease (Leroy et al., 2000). Conversely, primate studies have shown that infection of monoculear phagocytes is critical, that this triggers a cascade of cytokines/chemokines and oxygen free radicals, and that it is this process, not direct viral replication destroying critical cells, which leads to the manifestations of disease. These manifestations are associated with massive intravascular apoptosis (Baize et al., 1999; Hensley et al., 2002).

LABORATORY OBSERVATIONS

General Laboratory Findings

Clinical laboratory observations are limited to the Marburg outbreak. No acute-phase investigations were undertaken during the care of the one laboratory infection. There is invariably biochemical evidence of hepatic disease, with elevated AST levels maximal by day 7 of illness. Bilirubin is not elevated, and ALT is disproportionately low. These findings are reproducible in non-human primates experimentally infected with Ebola virus (AST:ALT ratio, 7:1) and the prothrombin time is relatively normal until the final stages of disease. Marked wasting in these diseases is dramatic and due to actual loss of muscle mass. The pathophysiology of this is not understood, although the raised AST may reflect some associated extra-hepatic process. Lymphopenia and thrombocytopenia are marked. As soon as 24 h after infection a marked lymphopenia is observed in experimentally infected animals. The lymphocytes disappear rapidly at the same time as a significant neutrophilia develops, with absolute counts as high as $20 \times 10^9/l$, in the absence of concurrent bacterial infection.

Laboratory Diagnosis

Care should be taken in both drawing and handling blood specimens, since virus titre may be extremely high and the virus is stable for long periods even at room temperature (Elliott et al., 1982). Gloves should be worn at all times, and discarded into disinfectant. All sharp instruments, needles, syringes, etc. should be discarded to a puncture-resistant container with a lid, as is recommended for HIV-infected specimens (Centers for Disease Control and National Institutes of Health, 1988; Centers for Disease Control, 1988a). A blood specimen should be taken without anticoagulant and serum separated. All procedures should be carried out by the most experienced staff under the most stringent safety facilities available at the admitting hospital or clinic (Biological Safety Level 3 if possible) (Centers for Disease Control, 1988b). Serum should be transferred to a leak-proof plastic container and double wrapped in further leak-proof containers in which it may be transported to a suitable reference laboratory. Sera may be safely handled for immunological tests by inactivating with γ-irradiation, or, if this is unavailable, heating to 60°C for 30 min. High or rising titre filovirus-specific IgG is diagnostic, as is the presence of IgM by IFA. Virus may be isolated and identified within 2–3 days if suitable facilities are available.

Although morphologically similar, Marburg and Ebola viruses are immunologically distinct. The indirect immunofluorescent assay for Marburg and Ebola viruses was the original basic diagnostic serological test for these viruses evaluated for the diagnosis of human Ebola virus disease (Wulff and Johnson, 1979). In acute infections, a rising filovirus-specific IFA titre (four-fold) in paired serum, or a high IgG titre (> 64) and presence of IgM antibody with a clinical illness compatible with haemorrhagic fever are consistent with the diagnosis (Ksiazek et al., 1992). Marburg virus antibody is usually specific, but Ebola virus serology in the absence of a history of recent disease was consistently plagued by low-titre, non-specific reactions using the IFA. This problem appears to be related to the use of native antigens. Newer systems using ELISA technology based on recombinant antigens have superior specificity and have replaced the older assays. ELISAs using recombinant nucleoprotein (NP) are the most broadly reactive and the most sensitive (Groen et al., 2003). Use of other proteins as antigens, e.g. recombinant VP35, results in a strain-specific assay but is less sensitive (Ksiazek et al., 1992). False positives are also seen in Western blot and radioimmunoprecipitation assays using native proteins.

Most filoviruses may easily be isolated from serum, blood or tissue specimens stored at minus 70°C in Vero E-6 cells, but biological safety level 4 containment facilities are recommended for isolation. Blood specimens unrefrigerated for up to 10 days have yielded virus strains. Marburg and the Zaire variant of Ebola virus are readily isolated from blood specimens taken in the first week of illness, by inoculation of Vero or other mammalian cell cultures and identified by IFA within 2–5 days after inoculation of cells. The Sudan variant of Ebola virus, however, may be more difficult to recover from blood or tissues of patients and success may depend on blind passage of cultured cells in guinea-pigs monitored for febrile response. Specimens, including throat washings, urine, various soft tissue exudates, semen and anterior eye fluid, may also contain virus. Virus identification is made generally by direct immunofluorescence of the tissue culture using monoclonal antibodies. Impression preparations made from a postmortem liver biopsy may be probed with monoclonal antibodies by IFA for presence of virus antigen which is abundant in liver and spleen. Using this system, sensitivity for the Reston virus in liver is 0.96 and specificity 0.98 compared with viral culture.

An antigen-detection ELISA system in serum has been used extensively, employing monoclonal antibodies (Ksiazek et al., 1992; Hayes et al., 1992). This assay has been used extensively in human and epizootic outbreaks. One study showed that a positive antigen test was obtained in symptomatic patients, but once symptoms had resolved in survivors, the test became negative (Baize et al., 1999). More sensitive is PCR, which may still be positive after symptoms have resolved.

PATIENT MANAGEMENT

General Patient Management

Fluid, electrolyte, respiratory and osmotic imbalances should be managed carefully. Patients may require full intensive care support, including mechanical ventilation, along with blood, plasma or platelet replacement. The maintenance of intravascular volume is a particular challenge but every effort is justified, since the crisis is short-lived and complete recovery can be expected in survivors. Pregnant patients may present with absent fetal movements, and maternal survival may depend on aggressive obstetric intervention.

Although much has been written about disseminated intravascular coagulation (DIC), particularly the use of heparin, there is little evidence for the role of DIC in pathogenesis, and this drug remains controversial and potentially dangerous. The only experience has been the therapy of two individuals with Marburg disease in South Africa. However, both of these patients were secondary Marburg infections, and none of 10 known secondary patients with Marburg infection have died.

Specific Therapy

No antiviral therapy, including convalescent plasma, ribavirin or related compounds have been shown to be effective against either Marburg or Ebola virus infection in patients or in experimentally infected non-human primates, although some compounds are currently under investigation. An undefined 'rapid response', recorded after administration of passive antibodies and interferon to the laboratory worker who suffered accidental inoculation of Ebola virus, led to early optimism that convalescent plasma might be effective, and this approach was used in the Kikwit outbreak, with uncertain outcome since all those treated were infected later in the outbreak, and it may be that subsequent generations of infections show some attenuation of the virus. Certainly blood or plasma transfusion might be effective in symptomatic support of a patient with Ebola infection. However, its value as specific therapy is doubtful, since it does not protect animals from simultaneous challenge with homologous virus. Suitably screened and stored human plasma is, in any event, unavailable. Human interferon is ineffective in vitro.

Efforts continue to seek antiviral agents effective against filoviruses. A product isolated from a cyanobacterium, Nostoc elliposporum, named cyanovirin-N (CV-N), has shown some potential to prevent transmission of human immunodeficiency virus (HIV) by binding to surface glycoproteins specifically through oligosaccharides. Since Ebola glycoproteins are heavily glycosylated, CV-N was studied for its ability to do the same with Ebola virus and it was found to bind with considerably affinity to carbohydrates on GP1 and GP2 (Barrientos et al., 2003). Studies of this kind give hope that eventually we will be able to develop effective antiviral therapy.

CONTROL

Containment

Since the reservoir(s) of the viruses are not known, no specific precautions can be identified which would avoid infections from the natural source of the viruses. The obvious exception to this generality is containment of monkeys which might be infected with one of these viruses. Prompt identification of active cases is critical, and is in great part dependent on an accurate and detailed history (Centers for Disease Control, 1988b). Interruption of person-to-person spread of the virus is essential to control. The most important issue is that of awareness in the medical community that these diseases exist, and they may result in extensive nosocomial spread if not recognised early and if appropriate isolation of the patient is not achieved. Thus, early institution of safe and orderly care of the ill can be set up, with effective surveillance of high-risk contacts and prompt isolation of further cases. This has been shown to ensure rapid control of an epidemic.

The experience in Uganda provided the only unique data showing the value of a national approach to control combined with strong community participation (Okware *et al.*, 2002). This extensive outbreak presented major logistic problems, threatening to spread throughout the country. The Ugandans set up a series of Task Forces at different administrative levels, including a District Talk Force in each district of the country. Programmes included public education, mobilisation of communities, training for health care workers and village volunteers, and timely dissemination of information using radio, mobile phones and foot and motor patrols. Scouts were recruited for active case finding. Isolation wards and a temporary field laboratory were set up. One of the major obstacles was lack of laboratory facilities. Burial teams were established for safe burial, since it soon became clear that the preponderance of female cases was associated with ritual cleansing of the dead.

Contacts

High-risk contact is associated with direct contact with blood or body fluids from acutely infected humans or animals, or sexual contact with a convalescent case. Laboratory accidents must be treated seriously, with careful review of level of risk. If this is thought to be high, isolation for the incubation period (17 days is adequate) and tracing and surveillance of any further potential contacts, such as family members, are necessary. If the risk is low, simple surveillance of the individual by daily telephone contact for fever during the incubation period suffices. It must be remembered that biocontainment facilities do not protect against injury with needles or other sharps. There is no evidence for or against the use of passive antibody in prophylaxis. Suitably screened and stored material is in any event unavailable.

Hospital Containment

The key to prevention of transmission in both endemic and non-endemic areas has consistently been good hospital and laboratory practice, with strict isolation of febrile patients and rigorous use of gloves and disinfection. Intensive care, surgery and air transport should not be denied. Patient isolators are not recommended, since the hazard to contacts is not via aerosols, but by direct inoculation of virus in blood or other material. Isolators induce loss of manual dexterity and fatigue, inhibit intensive care procedures and communication, do not protect against sharp instrument injury and have no provision for resuscitation. The 1988 CDC Guidelines for the Management of Patients with VHFs recommends routine patient isolation in a single room, preferably but not necessarily with negative air pressure gradient from the hallway, through an anteroom to the patient room (Centers for Disease Control, 1988b). Staff education and strict supervision, use of gloves, gowns and masks, and rigorous disinfection with fresh liquids are mandatory. The recommendations issued for management of AIDS patients are also adequate for containment of filoviruses (Centers for Disease Control, 1987).

Vaccine

There is no candidate vaccine for filoviruses. Fears that this agent might be used in biological warfare have stimulated studies to develop suitable candidates, primarily by genetic engineering of constructs in vaccinia virus or other vectors. The potential target population for a vaccine, however, military interests apart, is vanishingly small, and it is therefore unlikely that resources for vaccine development will be available in the near future. Simple challenge studies with Ebola (Zaire) in a very small number of animals surviving less pathogenic filovirus infections—Ebola (Sudan or Reston strains)—showed variable protection (Figure 20.7) (Fisher-Hoch *et al.*, 1992a). Filoviruses do not induce classical neutralising antibodies, and reliable protection may be difficult to achieve, particularly with a killed vaccine. The acceptability of an attenuated live virus is difficult to conceive, but the apparently benign course of Ebola (Reston) infection in humans is an interesting possibility. Presumably, safety testing (phases I and II) would

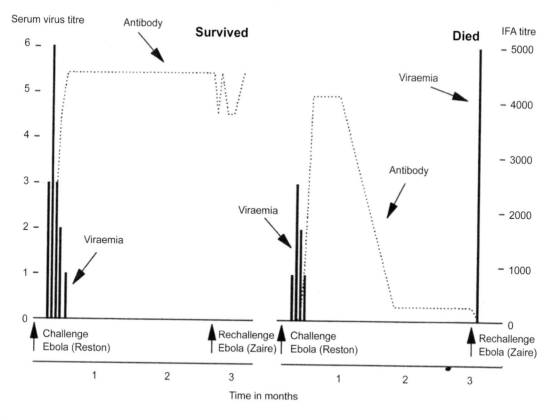

Figure 20.7 Outcome, antibody profile and viraemia in two of four cynomolgus monkeys that survived Ebola (Reston) challenge and that were subsequently challenged with Ebola (Zaire). In this experiment, one of the monkeys died on rechallenge. A further monkey that survived Ebola (Sudan) survived rechallenge with Ebola (Zaire). Reproduced from Fisher-Hoch *et al.* (1992a) by permission of The University of Chicago Press

be difficult if not impossible. Nevertheless, a live homologous vaccine may be effective, since an association was observed between protection and possession of pre-existing antibody to filovirus at the facility in Manila during the epizootic of Ebola (Reston), and protection correlated with antibody titre. Even then, a small number of animals (six) with pre-existing antibody were infected (Hayes *et al.*, 1992).

Efforts to produce newer generation vaccines such as Venezuelan equine encephalitis virus (VEE) replicons, liposomes containing inactivated vaccine and DNA vaccines have had mixed results. A highly acclaimed report of an effective DNA vaccine turned out to be a disappointment. Although effective in rodents (guinea-pigs), the efficacy claimed in primates was against a six-virion challenge (Sullivan *et al.*, 2000). Other flaws in the design of the animal studies also invalidate the claims of the authors. Subsequently, careful animal studies have shown that vaccines developed and tested

for efficacy in rodents (guinea-pigs mostly) consistently failed to protect primates (Geisbert *et al.*, 2002). Development of an effective vaccine requires a better understanding of the pathophysiological and immunological differences between rodents and primates infected with filoviruses, and this presents a significant scientific challenge.

REFERENCES

Baize S, Leroy EM, Georges-Courbot MC *et al.* (1999) Defective humoral responses and extensive intravascular apoptosis are associated with fatal outcome in Ebola virus-infected patients. *Nature Med*, **5**, 423–426.

Baron RC, McCorrnick JB and Zubeir OA (1983) Ebola virus disease in southern Sudan: hospital dissemination and intrafamilial spread. *Bull WHO*, **61**, 997–1003.

Barrientos LG, O'Keefe BR, Bray M et al. (2003) Cyanovirin-N binds to the viral surface glycoprotein, GP(1,2) and inhibits infectivity of Ebola virus. Antiviral Res, **58**, 47–56.

Baskerville A, Bowen ET, Platt GS et al. (1978) The pathology of experimental Ebola virus infection in monkeys. J Pathol, **125**, 131–138.

Baskerville A, Fisher-Hoch SP, Neild GH and Dowsett AB (1985) Ultrastructural pathology of experimental Ebola haemorrhagic fever virus infection. J Pathol, **147**, 199–209.

Bavari S, Bosio CM, Wiegand E et al. (2002). Lipid raft microdomains: a gateway for compartmentalized trafficking of Ebola and Marburg viruses. J Exp Med, **195**, 593–602.

Bowen ET, Lloyd G, Harris WJ et al. (1977) Viral haemorrhagic fever in southern Sudan and northern Zaire: preliminary studies on the aetiological agent. Lancet, **i**, 571–573.

Bowen ET, Platt GS, Lloyd G et al. (1980) A comparative study of strains of Ebola virus isolated from southern Sudan and northern Zaire in 1976. J Med Virol, **6**, 129–138.

Centers for Disease Control (1987) Recommendations for prevention of HIV transmission in health-care settings. Morbid Mortal Wkly Rep, **36**, 3S–18S.

Centers for Disease Control (1988a) Update: universal precautions for prevention of transmission of human immunodeficiency virus, hepatitis B virus and other blood-borne pathogens in health-care settings. Morbid Mortal Wkly Rep, **37**, 377–388.

Centers for Disease Control (1988b) Management of patients with suspected viral hemorrhagic fever. Morbid Mortal Wkly Rep.

Centers for Disease Control (1989) Ebola virus infection in imported primates—Virginia, 1989. Morbid Mortal Wkly Rep, **38**, 831–838.

Centers for Disease Control (1990a) Ebola-related filovirus infection in non-human primates and interim guidelines for handling non-human primates during transit and quarantine. Morbid Mortal Wkly Rep, **39**, 22–30.

Centers for Disease Control (1990b) Update: filovirus infection in animal handlers. Morbid Mortal Wkly Rep, **39**, 221.

Centers for Disease Control (1990c) Update: evidence of filovirus infection in an animal caretaker in a research/service facility. Morbid Mortal Wkly Rep, **39**, 296–297.

Centers for Disease Control, and National Institutes of Health (1988) Biosafety in Microbiological and Biomedical Laboratories. US Government Printing Office, Washington, DC.

Cox NJ, McCormick JB, Johnson KM and Kiley MP (1983) Evidence for two subtypes of Ebola virus based on oligonucleotide mapping of RNA. J Infect Dis, **147**, 272–275.

Elliott LH, Kiley MP and. McCormick JB (1985) Descriptive analysis of Ebola virus proteins. Virology, **147**, 169–176.

Elliott LH, McCormick JB and Johnson KM (1982) Inactivation of Lassa, Marburg, and Ebola viruses by gamma irradiation. J Clin Microbiol, **16**, 704–708.

Emond RTD, Evans B, Bowen ETW and Lloyd G (1977) A case of Ebola virus infection. Br Med J, **ii**, 541–544.

Feldmann H, Volchkov VE, Volchkova VA and Klenk HD (1999) The glycoproteins of Marburg and Ebola virus and their potential roles in pathogenesis. Arch Virol **15** (suppl), 159–169.

Fisher-Hoch SP (1993) Stringent precautions are not advisable when caring for patients with viral haemorrhagic fevers. Rev Med Virol, **3**, 713.

Fisher-Hoch SP, Brammer TL, Trappier SG et al. (1992a) Pathogenic potential of filoviruses: role of geographic origin of primate host and virus strain. J Infect Dis, **166**, 753–763.

Fisher-Hoch SP, Perez-Oronoz GI, Jackson EL et al. (1992b) Filovirus clearance in non-human primates. Lancet, **340**, 451–453.

Fisher-Hoch SP, Platt GS, Lloyd G et al. (1983) Haematological and biochemical monitoring of Ebola infection in rhesus monkeys: implications for patient management. Lancet, **ii**, 1055–1058.

Fisher-Hoch SP, Platt GS, Neild GH et al. (1985) Pathophysiology of shock and hemorrhage in a fulminating viral infection (Ebola). J Infect Dis, **152**, 887–894.

Gear JS, Cassel GA, Gear AJ et al. (1975) Outbreak of Marburg virus disease in Johannesburg. Br Med J, **4**, 489–493.

Geisbert TW, Pushko P, Anderson K et al. (2002) Evaluation in nonhuman primates of vaccines against Ebola virus. Emerg Infect Dis, **8**, 503–507.

Georges AJ, Leroy EM, Renaut AA et al. (1999) Ebola hemorrhagic fever outbreaks in Gabon, 1994–1997: epidemiologic and health control issues. J Infect Dis, **179** (suppl 1), S65–S75.

Groen J, van den Hoogen BG, Burghoorn-Maas CP et al. (2003) Serological reactivity of baculovirus-expressed Ebola virus VP35 and nucleoproteins. Microbes Infect, **5**, 379–385.

Han Z, Boshra H, Sunyer JO et al. (2003) Biochemical and functional characterization of the Ebola virus VP24 protein: implications for a role in virus assembly and budding. J Virol, **77**, 1793–1800.

Hayes CG, Burans JP, Ksiazek TG et al. (1992) Outbreak of fatal illness among captive macaques in the Philippines caused by an Ebola-related filovirus. Am J Trop Med Hyg, **46**, 664–671.

Henderson BE, Kissling RE, Williams MC et al. (1971) Epidemiological studies in Uganda relating to the 'Marburg' agent. In Marburg Virus Disease (eds Martini GA and Siegert R), pp 166–176. Springer-Verlag, Berlin.

Hensley LE, Young HA, Jahrling PB and Geisbert TW (2002) Proinflammatory response during Ebola virus infection of primate models: possible involvement of the tumor necrosis factor receptor superfamily. Immunol Lett, **80**, 169–179.

Heymann DL, Weisfeld JS, Webb PA et al. (1980) Ebola hemorrhagic fever: Tandala, Zaire, 1977–1978. J Infect Dis, **142**, 372–376.

Jahrling PH, Geisbert TW, Dalgard DW et al. (1990) Preliminary report: isolation of Ebola virus from monkeys imported to USA. Lancet, **335**, 502–505.

Johnson KM, Lange JV, Webb PA and Murphy FA (1977) Isolation and partial characterisation of a new virus causing acute haemorrhagic fever in Zaire. Lancet, **i**, 569–571.

Kiley MP, Bowen ET, Eddy GA et al. (1982) Filoviridae: a taxonomic home for Marburg and Ebola viruses? Intervirology, **18**, 24–32.

Kiley MP, Cox NJ, Elliott LH et al. (1988) Physicochemical properties of Marburg virus: evidence for three distinct virus strains and their relationship to Ebola virus. J Gen Virol, **69**, 1957–1967.

Ksiazek TG, Rollin PE, Jahrling PB *et al.* (1992) Enzyme immunosorbent assay for Ebola virus antigens in tissues of infected primates. *J Clin Microbiol*, **30**, 947–950.

Leroy EM, Baize S, Volchkov VE *et al.* (2000) Human asymptomatic Ebola infection and strong inflammatory response. *Lancet*, **355**, 2210–2215.

Licata JM, Simpson-Holley M, Wright NT *et al.* (2003) Overlapping motifs (PTAP and PPEY) within the Ebola virus VP40 protein function independently as late budding domains: involvement of host proteins TSG101 and VPS-4. *J Virol*, **77**, 1812–1819.

Martini GA (1971) Marburg virus disease, clinical syndrome. In *Marburg Virus Disease* (eds Martini GA and Siegert R), pp 1–9. Springer-Verlag, Berlin.

McCormick JB, Bauer SP, Elliott LH *et al.* (1983) Biologic differences between strains of Ebola virus from Zaire and Sudan. *J Infect Dis*, **147**, 264–267.

Miranda ME, White ME, Dayrit MM *et al.* (1991) Seroepidemiological study of filovirus related to Ebola in the Philippines (letter). *Lancet*, **337**, 425–426.

Okware SI, Omaswa FG, Zaramba S *et al.* (2002) An outbreak of Ebola in Uganda. *Trop Med Int Health*, **7**, 1068–1075.

Palmer AE, Allen AM, Taaso NM and Sholokov A (1968) Simian hemorrhagic fever I. Clinical and epizootiologic aspects of an outbreak among quarantine monkeys. *Am J Trop Med Hyg*, **17**, 404–412.

Pringle CR (1991) The order Mononegavirales. *Arch Virol*, **117**, 137–140.

Regnery RL, Johnson KM and Kiley MP (1980) Virion nucleic acid of Ebola virus. *J Virol*, **36**, 465–469.

Reiter P, Turell M, Coleman R *et al.* (1999) Field investigations of an outbreak of Ebola hemorrhagic fever, Kikwit, Democratic Republic of the Congo, 1995: arthropod studies. *J Infect Dis*, **179** (suppl 1), S148–S154.

Richman DD, Cleveland PH, McCormick JB and Johnson KM (1983) Antigenic analysis of strains of Ebola virus: identification of two Ebola virus serotypes. *J Infect Dis*, **147**, 268–271.

Sanchez A, Kiley MP, Klenk HD and Feldmann H (1992) Sequence analysis of the Marburg virus nucleoprotein gene: comparison to Ebola virus and other non-segmented negative-strand RNA viruses. *J Gen Virol*, **73**, 347–357.

Smith DH, Johnson BK, Isaacson M *et al.* (1982) Marburg-virus disease in Kenya. *Lancet*, **i**, 816–820.

Stojkovic LJ, Bordjoski M, Gligic A and Stefanovic Z (1971) Two cases of cercopithecus monkeys-associated haemorrhagic fever. In *Marburg Virus Disease* (eds Martini GA and Siegert R), pp 24–33. Springer-Verlag, Berlin.

Sullivan NJ, Sanchez A, Rollin PE *et al.* (2000) Development of a preventive vaccine for Ebola virus infection in primates. *Nature*, **408**, 605–609.

Swanepoel R, Leman PA, Burt FJ *et al.* (1996) Experimental inoculation of plants and animals with Ebola virus. *Emerg Infect Dis*, **2**, 321–325.

Teepe RG, Johnson BK, Ocheng D *et al.* (1983) A probable case of Ebola virus haemorrhagic fever in Kenya. *E Afr Med J*, **60**, 718–722.

Walsh PD, Abernethy KA, Bermejo M *et al.* (2003) Catastrophic ape decline in western equatorial Africa. *Nature*, **422**, 611–614.

World Health Organization (1978a) Ebola haemorrhagic fever in Zaire, 1976: report of an International Commission. *Bull WHO*, **56**, 271–293.

World Health Organization (1978b) Ebola haemorrhagic fever in Sudan, 1976: report of a WHO/International Study Team. *Bull WHO*, **56**, 247–270.

Wulff H and Johnson KM (1979) Immunoglobulin M and G responses measured by immunofluorescence in patients with Lassa or Marburg virus infections. *Bull WHO*, **57**, 631–635.

Rabies and Other Lyssavirus Infections

Mary J. Warrell

John Radcliffe Hospital, Oxford, UK

INTRODUCTION

Rabies is a zoonosis infecting a variety of mammal species in different areas of the world. The domestic dog is the most important vector, mainly in Asia and Africa, and is responsible for >90% of human infections. Sylvatic or wildlife rabies is endemic in Asia, Africa, the Americas, Australia and most of Europe. Almost all infections are due to classical rabies, genotype I, viruses. The remainder are due to the six genotypes of rabies-related viruses. In humans the disease is invariably fatal in unvaccinated people; during the last 25 years, the very few previously vaccinated survivors have had profound neurological deficits. Prevention with pre- or post-exposure rabies immunisation is therefore crucial to prevent fatal infection.

In English, rabies is also known as 'hydrophobia', 'lyssa' and 'mad dog bite': in French, *la rage* or *l'hydrophobie*; in Italian, *la rabbia*; in Spanish *la rabia*; in Portuguese, *a raiva* or *hidrofobia*, and in German, *die Tollwut*.

HISTORY

Rabies in dogs and the importance of saliva in its transmission may have been recognised in pharaonic times and in China in the seventh century BC (Théodoridès, 1986). Aristotle (322 BC) described rabies in animals but seemed to deny that humans could be infected or could die from the disease. Celsus, in *De medicina* (first century AD), described hydrophobia in afflicted humans and recognised that the disease was spread by saliva. In the sixteenth century, Fracastoro strengthened the concept of rabies as a contagious disease. A scientific or experimental approach to rabies was delayed until 1793, when John Hunter suggested that the transmission of rabies should be studied by inoculating saliva from rabid animals and humans into dogs and that attempts should be made to inactivate the 'poison' in the saliva. These ideas may have inspired the animal experiments on transmission by Zinke and Magendie and Breschet (Théodoridès, 1986).

Galtier found that rabbits could be infected with rabies and were more convenient experimental animals than dogs. In 1881, he first demonstrated specific immunisation against the disease (Théodoridès, 1986). Pasteur adopted the use of rabbits in his studies of rabies beginning in 1880. He was the first to recognise that the major site of infection was the central nervous system. Pasteur was able to protect dogs from challenge by immunising them with a virus attenuated in desiccated rabbit spinal cord and in 1885 he used this as a vaccine successfully for the first time in Joseph Meister and Jean-Baptiste Jupille, boys who had been severely bitten by rabid dogs. The reputation of modified forms of Pasteur's vaccine increased during the first half of the twentieth century, but its efficacy remained uncertain. The bite of a mad dog then caused rabies in only about 30% of untreated patients, although with wolf bites the risk was higher. In Iran, treatment of bites by rabid wolves with classical Semple brain tissue vaccine only reduced the case fatality about 10% compared with unvaccinated patients. A dramatic natural experiment in 1954, when a rabid wolf invaded a village and bit 29 people,

Principles and Practice of Clinical Virology, Fifth Edition. Edited by A. J. Zuckerman, J. E. Banatvala, J. R. Pattison, P. D. Griffiths and B. D. Schoub
© 2004 John Wiley & Sons Ltd   ISBN 0 470 84338 1

demonstrated the protective value of passive immunisation in patients with severe bites (Baltazard and Bahmanyar, 1955). This led to a general recommendation that, in addition to the vaccine, this should be included in rabies post-exposure prophylaxis.

Negri described his diagnostic inclusion body which allowed the laboratory diagnosis of rabies in 1903. The introduction of the more specific and sensitive immunofluorescence method in 1958 has now replaced the Seller's stain for Negri bodies. Remlinger, in 1903, showed that rabies was caused by a filterable agent. It was not until 1936 that the size of the virus was established and it was first seen by electron microscopy in 1962 (Théodoridès, 1986).

Improvements in Pasteur's vaccine were achieved by Semple and Fermi, who killed the virus rather than attenuated it, and by Fuenzalida and Palacios, who developed a suckling mouse brain vaccine which carried a lower risk of neuroparalytic complications. Growth of rabies virus in tissue culture was achieved by the 1930s, leading to the development, by Wiktor and his colleagues, of the first tissue culture vaccine for human use.

CLASSIFICATION

The family *Rhabdoviridae* (*rhabdos* = rod; Greek) includes several genera of viruses found in plants, arthropods, fish, birds, reptiles and mammals. Almost all of those known to infect man belong to two morphologically similar genera, *Lyssavirus* and *Vesiculovirus*. Members of the genus *Vesiculovirus* cause vesiculostomatitis of cattle and horses. In man,

influenza-like symptoms occur occasionally, and two cases of encephalitis have been reported (Quiroz *et al.*, 1988). The genus *Lyssavirus* (*lyssa* = rage, frenzy; Greek) comprises seven genotypes: genotype 1, classical rabies; genotype 2, *Lagos bat virus*; genotype 3, *Mokola virus* in shrews and cats; genotype 4, *Duvenhage virus* in bats; genotypes 5 and 6, *European bat lyssavirus*, found in insectivorous bats; and genotype 7, *Australian bat lyssavirus* in flying foxes (fruit bats). All these rabies-related viruses have been associated with human disease except for *Lagos Bat virus* (see Table 21.1, and section on Human Infections with Rabies-related Viruses, below). The recently identified bat lyssaviruses from Eastern Europe: Aravan, Khujand, Irkut and West Caucasian bat virus have yet to be classified.

The genus *Lyssavirus* has been divided into two phylogroups as a result of serological and genetic analyses (Badrane *et al.*, 2001). Phylogroup I comprises all genotypes except *Mokola virus* and *Lagos bat virus*, which form phylogroup II. All phylogroup I genotypes have caused fatal rabies-like encephalitis in man, whereas *Mokola virus* probably caused three known human infections, one of which was a fatal encephalitis without typical features of rabies. Experimentally, phylogroup II viruses are less pathogenic and there is little if any cross-neutralisation with the phylogroup I lyssaviruses.

VIRUS STRUCTURE (Wunner, 2002)

The bullet-shaped rabies virions measure 180×75 nm (Figure 21.1). The genome is a single non-segmented

Table 21.1 The genus *Lyssavirus*

Genotype	Source	Known distribution
Phylogroup I		
1 Rabies virus	Dog, fox, raccoon, skunk, bat, etc.	Widespread
4 Duvenhage	Insectivorous bat (e.g. *Nycteris thebaica*)	South Africa, Zimbabwe (very rarely identified)
5 European bat lyssavirus	1a. Bats, e.g. *Eptesicus serotinus*	Northern and Eastern Europe
	1b. Bats, e.g. *Eptesicus serotinus*	Western Europe
6 European bat lyssavirus	2a. *Myotis dasycneme* bat	The Netherlands (rare)
	Myotis daubentonii bat	UK (and Ukraine in other bat spp.)
	2b. *Myotis daubentonii* bat	Switzerland (very rare)
7 Australian bat lyssavirus	Flying foxes (*Pteropus* spp.)	Australia
	Insectivorous bats	
Phylogroup II		
3 Mokola	Shrews (*Crocidura* spp.), cats	South Africa, Nigeria, Cameroon, Ethiopia (rare)
2 Lagos bat virus	Bats, cats	Africa (rare)
	Has *not* been detected in man	

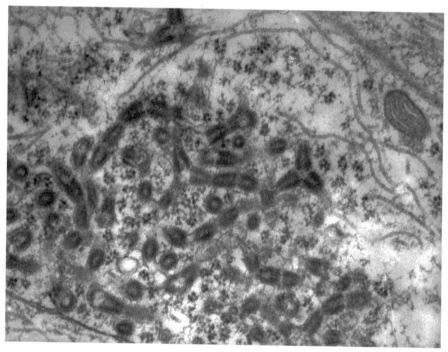

Figure 21.1   Negatively stained electron micrograph of Högyes strain of fixed rabies virus in mouse cerebral cortex. Courtesy of G. Gosztonyi

strand of negative-sense non-infectious RNA of 11.9 kb which bears coding sequences for five polypeptides. This RNA is associated with a nucleoprotein (N) a phosphoprotein (P) and an RNA-dependent RNA polymerase (L) to form a tight helical coil, the ribonucleoprotein (RNP) complex core of the virion. A layer of matrix (M) protein covers this cylindrical structure. The outermost lipoprotein envelope is composed of a host-derived lipid bilayer and the virion-encoded glycoprotein (G) bearing spikes projecting 8–10 nm above the virion surface. Each projection is a trimer of G molecules with a distal knob. The envelope covers all except the flat end of the virion, resulting in the characteristic bullet shape.

The viral nucleoprotein has 450 amino acids, ($\sim$57 kDa) and is an integral component of the RNP complex. It is the most conserved protein throughout the genus *Lyssavirus*, and so its antigens are employed both for genus-specific simple immunofluorescent antibody techniques and genotype-specific monoclonal antibody and PCR assays for diagnosis. N protein encapsidates viral RNA, protecting it from ribonucleases, and has a role in regulating RNA transcription. The lyssavirus N is phosphorylated, unlike all other rhabdovirus nucleoproteins. Nascent N molecules rapidly aggregate together or combine with molecules

of viral P protein, often in large accumulations of filamentous matrix, forming the diagnostic Negri bodies (Figure 21.2), which may also include other proteins.

The phosphoprotein has 297 amino acids ($\sim$40 kDa), and exists in at least two forms. It has previously been known as membrane-associated 1 (M1) protein and non-structural (NS) protein. Its functions include binding to nascent N, so preventing its polymerisation, and non-specific binding to cellular RNA. P also forms a complex with L protein and so has roles in genome transcription and replication. P has been shown to attach to dyenin light chain (LC8) molecules, which suggests an involvement in the transport of rabies virus components intracellularly, including by the dyenin microtubular system which effects retrograde axonal transport (see section on Pathogenesis, page 638).

The viral RNA polymerase is the largest protein (hence the designation L), containing approx 2142 amino acids ($\sim$190 kDa). The action of this RNA-dependent RNA polymerase is essential early in infection of a cell, to transcribe the primary genomic RNA. The many functions of L include transcription, replication, polyadenylation and protein kinase activities. The P protein is an essential enzymic co-factor.

The matrix protein has 202 amino acids ($\sim$25 kDa) and covers the RNP complex. It has several functions,

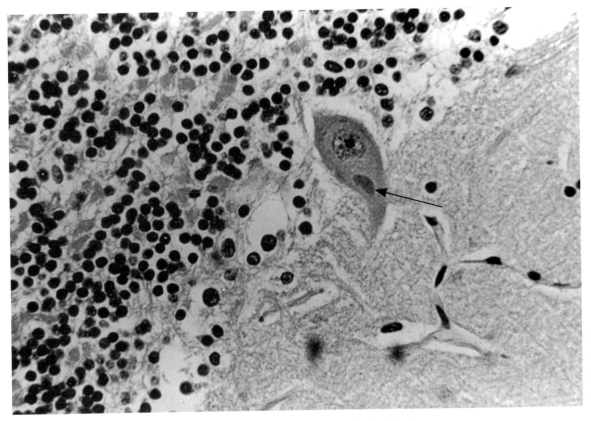

Figure 21.2 A Negri body (arrow) in a cerebellar Purkinje cell. Courtesy of F. A. Murphy

including the compacting of the loose helical core structure, regulation of viral RNA transcription and interaction with the lipid bilayer and the G protein to enable budding of virus from the cell membrane.

The surface glycoprotein is N-glycosylated with branched chain oligosaccharides, which show micro-heterogeneity within the virion. It has 505 amino acids ($\sim 65\,kDa$). The external domain of the G molecule is a trimeric spike connecting via a transmembrane anchor to a cytoplasmic domain, which is closely associated with the M protein. The distal knob on the surface projection is important in pathogenesis, as it bears binding sites for cellular receptors and effects pH-dependent fusion with endosomal membranes. A reversible change in conformation of the protein into an activated hydrophobic state initiates membrane fusion. A single amino acid replacement at arginine 333, at antigenic site III on the ectodomain, can radically reduce the virulence of the virus (Dietzschold et al., 1983). The G also promotes the passage of virus from cell to cell, is involved in axonal transport and it is essential for trans-synaptic spread (see section on Pathogenesis, below). G epitopes are most important

as they are the only inducers of rabies neutralising antibodies, which are protective. They can also induce helper and minimal cytotoxic T cell responses.

REPLICATION (Wunner, 2002)

Entry of virus into a cell occurs by cell receptor-mediated adsorptive endocytosis into an endosome (see section on Pathogenesis, below). If this is acid containing, the surface viral glycoprotein enables low pH-dependent fusion with the endosomal membrane, uncoating and liberating the nucleocapsid (or RNP complex) into the cytoplasm. Catalysed by the viral L protein, the primary genomic negative-strand RNA is transcribed, starting with a short leader RNA and followed by 5' monocistronic positive-strand mRNAs, and later the full-length antigenome replicative RNA. The amount of mRNA produced is greatest from the 5' end, in the order of N, P, M, G and L. Protein synthesis proceeds in the cytoplasm on host cell ribosomes. The unstable nascent nucleoprotein and phosphoprotein encapsidate and stabilise the progeny negative-strand genomic RNA by binding to its 5' end, or they may aggregate to form localised masses, which accumulate and become inclusions. The viral polymerase is incorporated into the strand of nucleoprotein, which forms a tight helical coil aided by the action of the viral matrix protein. The resulting RNP complex migrates to the cell membrane, where the nascent viral glycoprotein has become concentrated and inserted into the lipid membrane. The matrix protein interacts with the cytoplasmic domain of the glycoprotein, and promotes budding of the bullet-shaped virion. The membrane at the flat-ended base bears no G protein. Viral maturation can occur intracellularly by budding through endoplasmic reticulum, as seen especially in neurons (Iwasaki et al., 1985; Gosztonyi, 1994). Unlike vesicular stomatitis virus, rabies virus replication requires the presence of the nucleus in the host cell.

INACTIVATION OF VIRUS AND STABILITY OF VACCINE ANTIGEN

Rabies virus in a PBS buffer solution is rapidly inactivated by heat: at 56°C the half-life is <1 min; at 37°C the half-life is prolonged to about 3 h in moist conditions and at 4°C to 3–4 days experimentally. The stabilising presence of serum or other buffer solutions enhances survival. The lipid coat of the virion renders it vulnerable to disruption by detergents and simple 1% soap solution. Ethanol (45%), iodine solutions (with 1/10 000 available iodine), 3% sodium hydroxide, 1% benzalkonium chloride, 3% formalin, neat chloroform and acetone all inactivate the virus (Kaplan et al., 1966). Hypochlorite and glutaraldehyde solutions are suitable for laboratory use with the normal precautions, but phenol is not an effective virucidal compound.

Although benzylkonium chloride and other quaternary ammonium compounds are virucidal experimentally, they are not recommended for cleaning rabies-infected wounds at the concentrations in normal clinical use because they are inactivated by the presence of soap (Kaplan et al., 1966), which is recommended as first aid treatment of animal bites.

The potency and immunogenicity of lyophilised cell culture vaccine is retained after tropical ambient temperatures for 11 weeks (Nicholson et al., 1983). In reconstituted liquid form, the potency may fall significantly after a week or two, and it is unwise to keep an open vial for several days because of the risk of microbial contamination causing denaturing of antigen, loss of potency and possible infection of the recipient.

EPIZOOTIOLOGY AND EPIDEMIOLOGY

Rabies is transmitted within populations of relatively few species of mammals, principally within the domestic dog population, causing urban rabies. The vectors of sylvatic, or wildlife, rabies vary in different parts of the world and the virus circulates within the species group, maintaining infection with a constant virus type. As a result of the geographical compartmentalisation of rabies within a mammalian species, there has been a tendency for adaptation and divergence of virus strains, which can be identified by monoclonal antibody tests and genetic analysis (Smith, 2002). There is occasional overspill between these intraspecies cycles, e.g. when a rabid raccoon bites a fox in North America. Transmission occurs more commonly to non-vector mammalian species, e.g. when a cow or sheep is bitten by a rabid red fox in Europe.

Rabies is enzootic in terrestrial mammal species in most of the world, but rabies-related lyssaviruses alone are found in bats in a few countries (Figure 21.3). Areas of the world which have been reported to be free of rabies include: Ireland, Iceland, Finland, Sweden, mainland Norway, Portugal, Italy, Greece, the Mediterranean islands, New Zealand, Papua New Guinea, Japan, Taiwan, Hong Kong Islands (but not the New Territories), Singapore, Sabah, Sarawak, some islands of Indonesia (e.g. Bali), many islands of the Indian Ocean and Oceania (e.g. Solomon Islands, Fiji, Samoa and Cook Islands), Uruguay, some Caribbean islands (e.g. Barbados, Bahamas, Jamaica, St Lucia, Antigua and others), Antarctica and, until recently, the UK. Some countries are generally free but infected animals occasionally cross land borders. The epizootiology is constantly changing, so local advice should be sought for detailed information.

Rabies is spread between mammals by bites; by contamination of intact and abraded mucosal membranes by virus-laden saliva; by ingestion of infected prey; transplacentally and possibly by inhalation of aerosols (in heavily populated bat caves). The principal reservoir or vector species in different geographical areas are as follows:

Europe (World Health Organization; www.who-rabies-bulletin.org)

- Red fox (*Vulpes vulpes*)—from Poland to Slovenia and then eastwards to include the Russian Federation.
- Arctic fox (*Alopex lagopus*)—northern USSR.

- Raccoon dog (*Nyctereutes procyonoides*)—The Baltic States, Poland, Belarus, Ukraine and the Russian Federation.
- Wolf (*Lupus lupus*)—Lithuania, Belarus, Ukraine, Turkey and the Russian Federation.
- Domestic dog (*Canis familiaris*)—Dominant vector in Turkey. Cases also found from the Baltic States south to Croatia and eastwards to the Russian Federation, which are likely to be due to infection from foxes or other wildlife.
- Insectivorous bats harbour the rabies-related European bat lyssaviruses (Amengual *et al.*, 1997). Transmission to terrestrial mammals has very rarely been found, to date only in four sheep in Denmark and a stone marten in Germany.

  - *Genotype 5, EBL 1a* is found mainly in *Eptesicus serotinus* (serotine bats), in The Netherlands, Denmark, Germany, Poland, Hungary and the Russian Federation (isolates also from the Slovak Republic and Czech Republic, but typing not available).
  - *EBL 1b* is also found in *Eptesicus serotinus* in The Netherlands and in France and in several species in Spain.
  - *Genotype 6, EBL 2a* is rarely identified in *M. dasycneme* (pond bat), in The Netherlands but three isolations were made in the UK: two from *Myotis daubentonii* (Daubenton's bat) in New-haven in 1996, in Lancashire in 2002 and from the Scottish patient in 2002. Single infected bats were found in the Ukraine and Germany (Johnson *et al.*, 2003).
  - *EBL 2b* was isolated from a *M. daubentonii* in Switzerland and from the Swiss or Finnish human case (see section on Human Infections with Rabies-related Viruses, page 647).

Middle East

- Dominant vectors are the fox and the wolf. Dogs may be infected from wildlife.
- Other vectors include jackals, e.g. in Israel, and hyenas, e.g. in Jordan.

Asia

- Domestic dog (*Canis familiaris*) is the dominant vector.
- Frugivorous and insectivorous bats in the Philippines are seropositive for lyssavirus (see section on Recovery from Infection in Animals, p 641).

Africa (King *et al.*, 1994)

- Domestic dog (*Canis familiaris*)—rabies is predominant throughout the continent and in Madagascar.
- Black-backed jackals (*Canis mesomelas*)—Southern Africa.
- Yellow mongoose (*Cynictis penicillata*)—Southern Africa.
- Bat-eared fox (*Otocyon megalotis*)—Southern and East Africa.
- Frugivorous and insectivorous bats—*Duvenhage virus* very rarely found (see section on Human Infections with Rabies-related Viruses, p 647).

North America (Centers for Disease Control: http://www.cdc.gov/ncidod/dvrd/rabies/ Epidemiology/Epidemiology.htm)

- Arctic fox (*Alopex lagopus*)—Alaska, north-west Canada.
- Red fox (*Vulpes fulva*)—Ontario, Quebec and north-east USA, but many are infected here by raccoons.
- Grey fox (*Urocyon cinereoargenteus*)—Arizona, Texas.
- Striped skunk (*Mephitis mephitis*) and other species—Saskatchewan, Manitoba, (central Canada) California, Central USA and probably infected by raccoons in north-eastern coastal states.
- Raccoon (*Procyon lotor*)—Eastern coastal states of USA from Florida to the Canadian border, and adjacent regions of Canada.
- Insectivorous bats—widespread throughout continental USA, e.g. Mexican free-tailed bat (*Tadarida braziliensis mexicana*), red bat (*Lasiurus borealis*), big brown bat (*Eptesicus fuscus*), hoary bat (*Lasirus cinereus*), silver-haired bat (*Lasionycteris noctivagans*) and eastern pipistrelle (*Pipistrellus subflavus*).
- Coyote (*Canis latrans*)—a few cases persist in Southern USA.

Caribbean

- Vampire bat (*Desmodus rotundus*)—Trinidad, Tobago.
- Mongoose (*Herpestes* spp.)—Granada, Puerto Rico, Cuba, Dominican Republic.

Central and South America

- Domestic dog rabies in Mexico and some areas of Central and South America.
- Vampire bat (*Desmodus* spp.) causing bovine paralytic rabies from Mexico south to the northern parts of Argentina and Chile (McColl *et al.*, 2000).

Australia

- Flying foxes or fruit bats (*Pteropus* spp.) and occasionally insectivorous bats in Eastern coastal regions harbour Australian bat lyssavirus (McColl *et al.*, 2000) (see section on Human Infections with Rabies-related Viruses, p 648; Table 21.1).

Vampire bat rabies has serious economic effects on farmers. The bats feed on the blood of large mammals, particularly cattle, transmitting, in the process, a form of paralytic bovine rabies. This disease causes an estimated loss of 50 000 head of cattle each year in Brazil. Recent outbreaks have been reported from Ecuador. **Bat rabies** in the Americas is all due to genotype 1 virus, whereas bats in the rest of the world harbour only the rabies-related lyssaviruses: *European bat lyssavirus*, *Australian bat lyssavirus* or *Duvenhage virus* (McColl *et al.*, 2000).

Cyclical epizootics of rabies, such as the **fox epizootic** *in Europe*, result from an uncontrolled increase in the population of the key reservoir species. This epizootic started in Poland at the end of the Second World War and spread to France, but has now been controlled by vaccination in Western Europe (see control).

Many other species of domestic and wild mammals have been found to be infected with rabies. These are thought to be infected by local known vector species.

INCIDENCE OF HUMAN RABIES

The true global incidence of human rabies has been obscured by under-reporting and is not reflected in official figures. The areas of highest known incidence are where dog rabies is endemic, as dogs are the cause of more than 95% of human infections, e.g. in India, Bangladesh and Pakistan an estimated total of 40 000 deaths occur annually, according to the World Health Organization (2001). There are very few data from Africa. In Latin America, the highest mortalities are reported from Brazil, Mexico, Bolivia and Peru.

Most indigenous human rabies in the USA is associated with insectivorous bat rabies virus, usually the silver-haired bat or the eastern pipistrelle. In the last 10 years, a total of 28 deaths from rabies were reported, of which six (21%) were imported during the incubation period in patients infected by dogs abroad. All 22 indigenous patients were infected with bat virus but only one had recognised a bat bite. It has been suggested that rabies is under-diagnosed in the USA (Messenger *et al.*, 2002).

In the UK nine people have died of rabies since 1980, eight of whom were infected abroad. Four were infected in the Indian subcontinent, three in Africa and one in the Philippines. After a century of freedom from indigenous rabies, a man died of EBL 2a infection in Scotland in 2002 (see p 648). In continental Europe about 10 rabies deaths are now reported annually in the Russian Federation or in Turkey.

PATHOGENESIS

Entry of Virus into the Nervous System

Bites by rabid animals usually inoculate virus-laden saliva through the skin into muscle. Local replication of virus in striated muscle may occur and account for the long incubation periods often observed (Charlton *et al.*, 1997); then virus becomes detectable experimentally at local motor or sensory nerve endings (Murphy, 1977). Direct invasion of neurons has also been shown after peripheral inoculation.

The rabies virus infects a great variety of cell types *in vitro* and *in vivo*, and viral attachment has been demonstrated to several types of cell surface receptors, including carbohydrates, phospholipids and sialylated gangliosides. This binding is not specific and there is no evidence yet that these receptors are important *in vivo*, but it might explain the diversity of tissue culture cell lines which will support rabies infection.

Specific binding occurs at neuromuscular junctions, where it co-localises with the nicotinic acetylcholine receptor (Lentz *et al.*, 1982; Jackson, 2002b). Binding at this postsynaptic site is competitive with cholinergic ligands, including the snake venom neurotoxin, α-bungarotoxin, which shows sequence homology with rabies virus glycoprotein. This may explain the varied susceptibility of different species to rabies infection. The muscle cells of the susceptible fox bear more nicotinic acetylcholine receptors than those of the resistant opossum, and rabies virus binds well to fox muscle membranes *in vitro*, but not to opossum membranes (Baer *et al.*, 1990). Furthermore, there is now evidence that the virus attaches specifically to the neural cell adhesion molecule NCAM, or CD 56, which is present on susceptible cell lines (Thoulouze et al., 1998) and also the neurotrophin receptor p75 (Langevin et al., 2002) on neuron cell membranes and in axons.

Entry of virus into a cell can occur by endocytosis into a vesicle and pH-dependent fusion of the viral glycoprotein with the endosomal membrane, releasing the ribonucleoprotein complex into the cytosol.

Transport of Virus to the Brain

Rabies antigen can be found along the nervous pathways from a peripheral site of infection towards the brain during the incubation period. The migration of virus from a wound in a peripheral nerve to the CNS occurs within motor axons via the retrograde fast axonal transport system. Its progress can be blocked by sectioning nerves or by metabolic inhibition with locally applied colchicine, which disrupts the axon microtubular system. The rate varies experimentally but in human neurons it is estimated at 50–100 mm/day. Viral movement is not affected by the presence of extracellular neutralising antibody (Tsiang, 1993). Since rabies has strictly retrograde axonal movement, it has been used as a tracer to identify neural pathways. The rabies P protein associates with LC8, a component of a cytoplasmic dynein light chain, suggesting a means of attachment of the viral RNP complex to the retrograde dyenin axonal motor (Raux et al., 2000; Jacob et al., 2000). Further studies show that binding of viral proteins to the LC8 molecule is not essential for pathogenesis (Mebatsion, 2001), and that the viral G protein alone can take advantage of the retrograde microtubular transport (Mazarakis et al., 2001). Viral replication is intraneuronal, but the mechanism of interneuronal spread is unknown. The fact that budding of virus is very rarely seen at synapses by EM suggests that infectious naked nucleocapsids may be transferred trans-synaptically (Gosztonyi, 1994). However, interneuronal infection has been shown to be dependent on the presence of viral G protein (Etessami et al., 2000). Although rabies infection downregulates host cell gene expression overall, a few genes are upregulated, including ones associated with synaptic vesicle function (Prosniak et al., 2001).

Effect of Infection on the Brain

Rabies progresses rapidly through the spinal cord and brain, with massive intraneuronal viral replication and accumulation of viral proteins, resulting in inclusion formation and eventually Negri bodies (see section on Virus Structure, above). Virus has been observed emerging from post-synaptic membranes with viral pinocytosis at axon terminals in animals. Contact with the extracellular environment is thereby avoided. Infected glial cells have rarely been observed in man, and they are not a significant route of dissemination of virus. Infection of the limbic system affects the behaviour of the host which, in a vector species, increases the chance of transmitting the disease.

The areas of maximum inflammatory change in the human brain do not correlate with the distribution of Negri bodies. EEG evidence of pathology is greater in infections with attenuated virus than virulent street strains (Tsiang, 1993) and neuronal death is not a prominent feature at post mortem. Pathogenic strains of virus cause less neuronal apoptosis than avirulent ones; indeed, rabies infection may have surprisingly little visible pathological effect on the brain. The level of viral glycoprotein expression on the neuron surface correlates with the degree of apoptosis and there is downregulation of glycoprotein expression in virulent strains, and so apoptosis only appears at a terminal stage of infection (Dietzschold et al., 2001) The cause of the gross neuronal dysfunction of living cells remains elusive but it may be associated with altered activity at a variety of neurotransmitter binding sites (Tsiang, 1993; Jackson, 2002b). Rabies infection of neurons alters cellular gene expression, not only in infected cells but probably also in uninfected neurons (Prosniak, 2001). The depletion of metabolic pools may limit cell survival (Dietzschold et al., 2001). Changes in the functional expression of some channels, and attenuation of inhibition of others, have been shown in vitro (Iwata et al., 2000). The suggestion that nitric oxide might cause pathogenic neurotoxicity in rabies remains unproven (Jackson, 2002b).

Centrifugal Spread of Virus from the Brain

Finally, there is a phase of diffuse centrifugal spread by axonal transport of virus from the brain by many nerve pathways, including the autonomic nervous system. Virus has been isolated from human tissues such as peripheral nerve, skeletal and cardiac muscle, kidney, lung, skin, salivary, lacrimal and adrenal glands (Helmick et al., 1987). Rabies antigen has been detected in nerves and ganglia adjacent to these organs and the gastrointestinal tract, and extraneurally in tongue tissues, often without an inflammatory reaction (Jackson et al., 1999). Viraemia is not thought to occur (Helmick *et al.*, 1987). Virus is shed from human salivary and lacrimal glands, the respiratory tract, rarely in urine (Helmick *et al.*, 1987) and possibly in milk.

The predominant site of replication changes as the virus reaches the salivary gland. In contrast to neural cells, there is profuse production of extracellular virus from acinar cells. Viral budding occurs into the gland lumen or intercellular canniculae. Virus is secreted into the saliva, from which it is available to infect a new host.

IMMUNOLOGY

Immune Responses to Rabies Virus

Following a rabid bite, no immune response can be detected until after the development of symptomatic rabies encephalitis, suggesting that the virus can evade or suppress the immune system while in transit into and out of the brain, during the entire incubation period. An immunosuppressive effect of rabies infection has been shown experimentally to rabies antigens and also unrelated viral antigens (Camelo *et al.*, 2001). Rabies neutralising antibody, which is only induced by antigens on the glycoprotein envelope (Wunner, 2002), is protective against rabies following challenge in animals. *In vitro*, this antibody impairs viral attachment and penetration of cells, and reduces cell to cell spread of virus. Although the presence of neutralising antibody is the best available indicator of protective immunity, the level does not correlate with protection in all experiments, showing that other immune mechanisms are also effective (Lodmell *et al.*, 2001). RNP antigens can confer protection from death experimentally, in the absence of neutralising antibody. T and B cell specific epitopes have been identified on the N molecule, and N can prime the immune system to enhance the neutralising antibody response to G protein. This RNP-induced immunity is more cross-reactive with other strains, including rabies-related viruses, than that stimulated by G protein. There is evidence that N acts as a weak superantigen by directly inducing proliferation of human CD4 Th2 cells bearing the Vβ8 TCR (Lafon, 1997) but the effect of this unexpected finding on disease or the host immune response remains elusive.

Survival of infection in animals is associated with a strong immune response, including neutralising antibody, and upregulation of MHC class II mRNA expression in the CNS early in infection (Irwin *et al.*, 1999). The activity of CD4$^+$ T lymphocytes and B cells are crucial. Clearance of rabies virus infection from the central nervous system has only been demonstrated in rodents by treatment with a single rabies virus-neutralising monoclonal antibody before the onset of clinical signs (Dietzschold *et al.*, 2001). Although rabies G and N proteins bear epitopes which can induce activation of CD8$^+$ T cells, virulent strains do not do so. The role of cytotoxicity in rabies encephalitis is not clear. Infected human brains show remarkably little pathology, so apoptosis is unlikely to be a significant cause of death, which is in keeping with experimental findings.

Response in Human Encephalitis

In unvaccinated humans with encephalitis, neutralising and other antibodies appear in serum about 7 days after the first symptom, later in the cerebrospinal fluid (CSF) (Anderson *et al.*, 1984). In patients whose lives are prolonged by intensive care, antibody titres may rise to very high levels. A low level of rabies-specific IgM is sometimes detectable in serum and CSF, but there is no evidence to date that it precedes the IgG response (Warrell *et al.*, 1988).

A minimal lymphocyte response is detected histologically in brain, blood and CSF (Warrell *et al.*, 1976) and there is no pleocytosis in 40% of patients in the first week of illness, or in 13% in the second week (Anderson *et al.*, 1984). Evidence of cell-mediated immunity, by specific lymphocyte transformation tests, was found in 6/9 furious encephalitis patients, but not in seven with paralytic disease (Hemachudha *et al.*, 1988).

It has long been recognised that the rabies incubation period is shorter than average in patients who were inadequately vaccinated and develop rabies. Although high levels of neutralising antibody are protective, low levels can accelerate the terminal phase of the illness, resulting in the 'early death' phenomenon (Prabhakar and Nathanson, 1981). The effect can be produced in mice by adoptive transfer of antibody or immune B lymphocytes during the incubation period.

Interferon-α (IFN-α) prevents rabies viral replication *in vitro*, but only very low levels have been found in the serum and CSF of one-third of patients with encephalitis (Merigan *et al.*, 1984). Mice die of rabies despite high levels of IFN-α and IFN-β in the brain, and high doses of intravenous and intrathecal IFN-α after the onset of symptoms of human rabies encephalitis have not proved effective therapy in man (Merigan *et al.*, 1984; Warrell *et al.*, 1989). In contrast, the early appearance of IFN-γ in infected rodent brain was associated with survival or delayed mortality (Koprowski and Dietzschold, 1997).

Immune Response to Rabies Vaccine

Despite the anergy seen in patients with encephalitis, rabies virus proteins are highly immunogenic when given as vaccine. Neutralising antibody usually becomes detectable in serum 7–14 days after starting a primary course of vaccine. Antibody production is accelerated if the dose of tissue culture vaccine is given in multiple sites, either by increasing the dose of intramuscular treatment or by dividing a single dose between several intradermal sites (Suntharasamai et al., 1987; Turner et al., 1976). The early IgM component of the antibody response does not protect against rabies experimentally, has low affinity for viral antigens and is confined to the vascular system, so it is unlikely to be important in immediate post-exposure prophylaxis (Turner, 1985).

No antibody or T lymphocyte function test predicts protection against disease, but the level of neutralising antibody, induced by rabies G protein, gives the best correlation available, and should be used to evaluate vaccines. The standard mouse serum neutralisation test is cumbersome and takes 2–3 weeks, but is now replaced by tissue culture methods: the rapid immuno-fluorescent focus inhibition test (RIFFIT; Smith et al., 1996), which takes 24 h, or the similar fluorescent antibody virus neutralisation (FAVN) test (Cliquet et al., 1998), which is easier to read and automate, but takes 40 h. The results are expressed in International Units (IU/ml), compared with an International Standard serum. An arbitrary minimum neutralising antibody level of 0.5 IU/ml indicates unequivocal seroconversion and is taken to be the minimum adequate response after a pre- or post-exposure course of vaccine.

Other antibody tests employing killed virus antigen are more convenient but detect a variety of non-neutralising antibodies, whose titres show less correlation with protection from disease. Refinements in the ELISA methodology have led to increasing specificity. Following vaccination, human peripheral blood lymphocytes were transformed in response to a variety of rabies and rabies-related virus antigens. The neutralising antibody level did not correlate with the proliferative indices.

The amount of antibody induced by vaccine is partly determined by the host. Lower titres were found in people over 50 years old. Kuwert observed that in a population of vaccinees 10% had poor, relatively delayed antibody induction (Kuwert et al., 1981). Immunosuppression due to drugs, HIV, cirrhosis or other disease can also impair the response to vaccine.

ROUTES OF INFECTION

Human infections usually result from inoculation of virus-laden saliva through the skin by the bite of a rabid dog or other mammal. Broken skin and intact mucosae can admit the virus, and scratches, abrasions and previous open skin lesions can be contaminated with infected saliva. Intact skin is an adequate barrier to the infection. The following are very unusual routes of human infection:

1. *Human-to-human* transmission has only been documented in recipients of corneal transplant grafts. Six virologically proven cases have been reported in which infected corneae were transplanted from donors who had died of unsuspected rabies. The one patient who survived received high-dose post-exposure treatment and IFN (Sureau et al., 1981). Two further cases resulted in clinically diagnosed rabies in India. Rare reports of infection by human bite or kissing (Fekadu et al., 1996) have been persuasive, but infection from another source could not be excluded. Despite this, thousands of people dying of rabies have been nursed in poverty-stricken homes, yet their relatives in intimate contact with saliva and tears have not developed rabies. This indicates that the infection is not easily transmitted from man to man.

2. *Inhalation* has been reported from the USA, where there were two laboratory accidents involving the inhalation of fixed virus during vaccine preparation (Centers for Disease Control, 1977; Winkler et al., 1973). Airborne rabies virus was assumed to be the cause of death of two people 50 years ago who had recently visited caves in Texas that were very densely populated with insectivorous Mexican free-tailed bats. Aerosol transmission of rabies virus was demonstrated in caves experimentally, presumably from infected bats' nasal secretions and possibly urine (Winkler, 1975). However, no further human cases have been reported. Infection could also be due to unnoticed physical contact with a bat (Messenger et al., 2002; Gibbons, 2002).

3. *Vaccine-induced rabies* (Rage de laboratoire). Incomplete inactivation of virus in human vaccine should no longer be a problem, but in the worst incident 18 people developed paralytic rabies in

Fortaleza, Brazil, in 1960. The incubation period was 4–13 days after receiving the vaccine (Pará, 1965).

4. *Transplancental infection* has occurred in animals, but only once documented virologically by antigen detection in the brain tissue of a mother and infant in Turkey. Several women with rabies encephalitis have been delivered of healthy babies.

5. *Oral infection* has been shown in animals, although high titres are needed. The transmission of rabies from mother to suckling infant via the breast milk has been suspected in at least one human case and is said to occur in animals. However, there have been no documented cases of transmission of rabies by ingestion of milk from an infected animal. Boiling and pasteurisation inactivate rabies virus. Transmission of virus is theoretically possible from ingestion of raw milk, but it is not a criterion for post-exposure immunisation. Nevertheless, in the US people who had drunk milk from rabid cows were given rabies prophylaxis (Centers for Disease Control, 1999b).

CLINICAL FEATURES OF RABIES IN ANIMALS

In domestic dogs, the incubation period ranges from 5 days to 14 months, but is usually 3–12 weeks. It is under 4 months in 80% of cases. Prodromal symptoms include change in temperament, fever and, as in many humans, intense irritation at the site of the infecting bite. The familiar picture of a 'mad dog' with furious rabies is seen in only 25% of infected animals. The commoner paralytic or dumb presentation is less dramatic and more dangerous, as it may not be recognised. The clinical features of furious canine rabies include irritability, convulsions, dysphagia, laryngeal paralysis causing an altered bark, hypersalivation, trembling, snapping and extreme restlessness, causing the animal to wander for miles. Dogs with furious rabies attack and swallow inanimate objects, often breaking their teeth and injuring their mouths in the process. Dogs with paralytic rabies may be reclusive and exhibit paralysis of the jaw, neck and hind limbs, dysphagia and drooling of saliva. Virus may be excreted in the saliva 7 days before the appearance of symptoms and the animal usually dies within 7–10 days of onset. Among other species, signs are usually furious in horses, cats, mustelids and viverrids, and usually paralytic in foxes and bovines. Although rabid animals are commonly unable to swallow, they do not exhibit hydrophobia.

Recovery from Infection and Chronic Rabies in Dogs, Vampire Bats and other Mammals

Rabies is not a universally fatal disease in mammals. The pathogenicity of rabies viruses can vary greatly when tested in another mammal species. Dogs, cats, bats and, most often, mice have recovered from experimental infection with street rabies virus. It is conceivable that a low dose of virus inoculated in the wild could immunise without causing disease. Although the fox is one of the most susceptible species to rabies, about 3% of animals survive the infection and become immune. Animals of several species have been found to be seropositive and so are assumed to have recovered from rabies. These include the natural rabies vectors: mongooses in Granada; foxes and raccoons in Alabama; hyenas in Tanzania; bats in Europe, the Philippines (Arguin *et al.*, 2002) and Australia; and, very rarely, stray or unvaccinated dogs in Ethiopia and Nigeria (Sérié and Andral, 1962; Ogunkoya *et al.*, 1990).

Vampire bats have long been considered chronic carriers of rabies virus, and some bats were reported to have carried rabies in their saliva for more than 2 months before death, but there is now doubt about the validity of these reports (Jackson, 2002b). Some bats recover from infection but there is no evidence of excretion of virus following recovery, and experimental inoculation has failed to induce a carrier state.

The repeated shedding of rabies virus in the saliva of apparently healthy dogs is a cause for great concern. This chronic infection is exceptionally rare (Jackson, 2002b) but has been reported in an Indian dog, and in Ethiopian and Nigerian dogs. Thorough searching in other areas has not revealed any chronically infected animals. The incidence of chronic rabies is presumed to be so low that it has not influenced the recommendations for post-exposure treatment.

In Tanzania recently 37% of hyenas were found to be seropositive and rabies was detected by PCR techniques in 13% of saliva samples from seropositive animals, although all attempts at virus culture failed. Infection was not associated with disease or decreased survival. The virus strain was distinct from those of other local species and may be of low virulence. It is assumed that prolonged and perhaps repeated infection occurred with a strain of low virulence (East *et al.*, 2001).

Infection of apparently healthy bats by *European bat lyssavirus* (genotype 5, EBL 1), has been found in wild *Myotis* and other species of Spanish insectivorous bats and bats in a Dutch zoo, with an antibody prevalence in up to 20% of some populations (Serra-Cobo *et al.*,

2002). Wellenberg *et al.* (2002) found rabies RNA in brain and other tissues of healthy-looking bats (Wellenberg *et al.*, 2002). Sublethal EBL 1 infection of bats in Seville similarly was revealed by PCR in oropharyngeal swabs of live bats (Echevarria *et al.*, 2001). To date there has been no isolation of live virus from these asymptomatic persistently infected bats in Europe.

CLINICAL FEATURES IN HUMANS

Incubation Period

The extreme range is from 4 days to 19 years or more. A Thai patient was savagely bitten on the shoulder by a rabid dog, but received no active or passive immunisation against rabies. This unusually deep and damaging bite may have inoculated virus directly into the brachial plexus, explaining the shortest reported incubation period of 4 days after naturally occurring infection with street virus; it is 20–90 days in more than 60% of cases. The incubation period is reported to be more than 1 year in 1–7% of cases. It tends to be shortest with severe bites on the face, head and neck, especially in children, and in experimental animals injected with larger doses of virus. Average incubation periods for bites on the head and neck are 25–48 days; for the extremities 66–69 days; for the upper limb 46 and for the lower 78 days. Some of the very long incubation periods mentioned in the literature may have been explained by a second more recent, but forgotten, exposure. Alternatively, the virus may remain quiescent until activated by some kind of stress, which has been shown experimentally and suspected in immigrants to the USA with incubation periods up to 6 years (Smith *et al.*, 1991). The incubation appears to be shorter in patients who have received (unsuccessful) post-exposure treatment than in those who have not (Hattwick, 1974).

Prodromal Symptoms

A vague feverish illness associated with a change in mood may precede, by up to about a week, the appearance of definite signs of rabies encephalomyelitis. The patient becomes anxious, agitated, apprehensive, restless, irritable and tense and may suffer from nightmares, insomnia, loss of concentration and depression. Physical symptoms include vague malaise, anorexia, headache, other aches and pains, weakness, tiredness, fever, chills, sore throat and other symptoms suggestive of upper respiratory tract infection, influenza or gastroenteritis. This wide range of misleading symptoms has encouraged inappropriate referral to psychiatrists, otolaryngologists, gastroenterologists and other specialists. Itching, tingling, burning, pain, numbness or some other paraesthesia at the site of the healed bite wound is experienced by about half the patients and may be associated with trembling, fasciculations, muscle contractures or weakness of the bitten limb. Most of the patients infected by corneal transplants noticed pain behind the grafted eye. Although local paraesthesia is suggestive of imminent rabies encephalomyelitis, this symptom is also surprisingly common in healthy victims of animal bites who fear that they are developing rabies. It might be the result of trauma by the bite or by vigorous local infiltration of rabies immunoglobulin. Pruritis is, in our experience, by far the commonest local prodromal symptom; neuritic pain is also reported. Itching may be so intense that the patient excoriates large areas of skin by scratching.

Clinical Presentations of Rabies Encephalomyelitis

Rabies can take two clinical forms. In the more familiar type, furious or agitated rabies, the brainstem, cranial nerves, limbic system and higher centres bear the brunt of the infection, while in dumb or paralytic rabies the medulla, spinal cord and spinal nerves are principally involved. The predominantly but not exclusively paralytic picture seen in human victims of vampire bat transmitted rabies and other evidence from experimental rabies infection in animals suggests that the virus strain or size of infecting inoculum may contribute to the pattern of central nervous system infection. Host factors may also modify the pattern of the disease; the apparent frequency of the dumb form of rabies varies from species to species (it is common in bovines but rare in cats) and there is a widely quoted impression that dumb rabies is more likely to develop in those who have received antirabies vaccine (Hattwick, 1974). Many different clinical features and patterns of presentation of human rabies have been described over the past 100 years and, since the recognition of strains of classical rabies *Lyssavirus* genotype I and rabies-related viruses, clinicians have been interested in attempting to associate distinctive clinical patterns with these various viruses. This is premature. Even the use of the term 'classical rabies' for a clinical presentation has become misleading, as it has been applied to the furious form of the disease (Jackson,

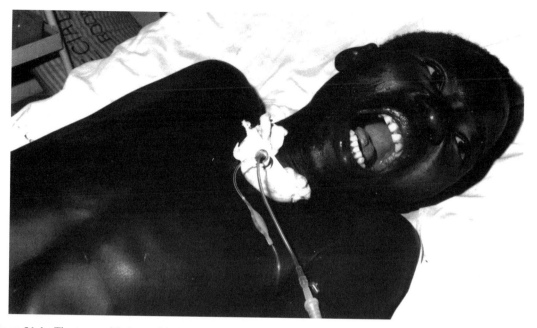

Figure 21.4 The terror of furious rabies in an 18 year-old Nigerian, bitten on the temple by a dog. After 13 days he developed classical hydrophobic spasms. Periods of lucidity were interspersed with episodes of extreme agitiation, violent struggling, shouting and terrifying hallucinations. Courtesy of D. A. Warrell

2002a) and also to both furious and paralytic forms, to distinguish them from hypothetical atypical patterns (Hemachudha *et al.*, 2002).

Furious (Agitated) Rabies

This is the more familiar and probably the commoner presentation in humans, except in those infected by bats. Without intensive care, most patients with furious rabies die within a week of their first prodromal symptom and within a few days of developing hydrophobia. This short and hectic clinical course is characterised initially by hydrophobia, aerophobia and periods of extreme excitement, alternating with lucid intervals, features of autonomic system dysfunction and finally by unconsciousness and complete paralysis. Hydrophobia (from the Greek, 'dread of water') is a reflex series of forceful jerky inspiratory muscle spasms provoked by attempts to drink water and associated with an inexplicable terror (Figure 21.4). Driven by thirst to confront this terror, the patients attempt to drink but, even before the liquid has reached their lips, a rapid succession of violent inspiratory gasps is provoked. Forcible contractions of the diaphragm depress the xiphisternum and contractions of the accessory muscles of

inspiration, particularly the sternocleidomastoids, are visible during these spasms. There is usually no evidence of laryngospasm and most patients deny pain in the neck or retrosternal region. There is no difference between provoked 'phobic' spasms and inspiratory spasms. A draught of air on the skin produces a similar reflex response, 'aerophobia'. Initially, the spasms affect mainly the inspiratory muscles, but a generalised extension response may be produced, not infrequently ending in opisthotonos and generalised convulsions with cardiac or respiratory arrest. The hydrophobic response may be reinforced by unpleasant consequences of the inspiratory spasms, such as aspiration of water up the nose or into the trachea. However, the first attack may occur without preceding difficulty in swallowing and with no opportunity for the establishment of a conditioned reflex. The hydrophobic response may eventually be produced merely by the sight, sound, mention or thought of water, touching the palatal mucosa, splashing water on the skin, loud noises, bright lights and by the patient's attempting to speak. There may be associated excitement, agitation and aggression and many patients develop generalised convulsions and die during a hydrophobic spasm.

Cardiac tachyarrhythmias and ECG evidence of myocarditis may be observed during this phase of the disease (Warrell *et al.*, 1976; Jackson *et al.*, 1999). There is transient hypertension during the hydrophobic spasms and the violent inspiratory spasms may result in pneumothorax (Warrell *et al.*, 1989). Pneumomediastinum may result from alveolar rupture or tears in the lower oesophagus. If the patient survives this phase of the disease and sinks into coma, hydrophobia is replaced by a variety of respiratory arrhythmias (cluster or Biot's breathing and Cheyne–Stokes respiration), with long apnoeic periods.

Pathophysiology of Hydrophobia
(Warrell *et al.*, 1976)

There is some clinical evidence that the inspiratory spasms of hydrophobia may be an exaggeration of reflexes which normally protect the respiratory tract from foreign bodies. These include sneezing, coughing, the neonate's aspiration reflex and perhaps the immersion reflex, all of which have a powerful inspiratory contraction as their main motor effect. In furious rabies there is a selective brainstem encephalitis which damages cells in the region of the nucleus para-ambigualis (where the inspiratory motor neurons are situated) and in the limbic system. These lesions could disinhibit the respiratory tract protective reflexes and explain the associated terror of hydrophobia. The responses could be reinforced by conditioning, resulting in the heightened reaction to a variety of sensory stimuli which provoke spasms.

Other Features of Furious Rabies

Alternating phases of extreme arousal and calm, lucid intervals are typical of furious rabies. Physical findings include meningism, cranial nerve lesions (especially III, VII, VIII), upper motor neuron lesions, muscle fasciculations and involuntary movements. However, conventional neurological examination may fail to disclose any abnormality unless a hydrophobic spasm is observed. Evidence of autonomic stimulation includes lacrimation, hypersalivation and excessive sweating, piloerection, high fluctuating body temperature and blood pressure, pupillary abnormalities and Horner's syndrome. Involvement of the amygdaloid nuclei and limbic system may explain the increased libido, priapism and spontaneous orgasms/ejaculations in a small minority of patients. These symptoms are reminiscent of Klüver–Bucy syndrome, which can be induced experimentally in rhesus monkeys and by surgical treatment for temporal lobe epilepsy in

Table 21.2 Complications of rabies encephalitis

Cardiovascular	Arrhythmias, hypotension, cardiac failure
Respiratory	Asphyxiation (hydrophobic spasm)
	Pneumonia
	Respiratory failure
	Pneumothorax, pneumomediastinum
	Adult respiratory distress syndrome
Neurological	Convulsions
	Diabetes insipidus
	Syndrome of inappropriate anti-diuretic hormone
	Hypo- or hyperpyrexia
	Cerebral oedema
Gastrointestinal	Stress ulcers
	Mallory–Weiss syndrome
	Haemorrhage

humans following bilateral temporal lobectomy. Evidence of an extensive axonal neuropathy was found in two patients with furious rabies in the second week of intensive care. The normal progression of furious rabies is to coma and death within a week of the first symptom, but some patients have been kept alive for several months in intensive care units. In these cases a variety of other complications can develop (see Table 21.2).

Paralytic Rabies

This form is less likely to be recognised as rabies than furious disease, which has contributed to its being apparently less common in humans. The patients may become literally dumb ('*rage muette*'), because their laryngeal muscles are paralysed, but the term 'dumb rabies' also describes the quieter symptoms and more insidious and protracted clinical course exemplified by its other French name, '*rage tranquille*'. There was a famous outbreak of paralytic rabies in Trinidad, involving 20 people, mostly children, between 1929 and 1931. After prodromal fever and headache, burning, tingling, numbness, cramp or weakness developed in one foot, followed by a gradually ascending paralysis and hypoaesthesia, eventually affecting the respiratory and deglutitive muscles. Constipation, urinary retention, high fever and profuse sweating were common. Some patients survived for 3 weeks and only one showed terminal hydrophobic spasms. Vampire bats were eventually implicated. Paralytic rabies was also seen in patients with post-vaccinal rabies (due to defective inactivation of vaccine) and in two patients who inhaled a vaccine strain of virus. Neurological signs include quadriparesis with predominant involvement of proximal muscles, loss of deep tendon reflexes and progressive paralysis. In most patients sensation is intact, but in some there is evidence of ascending myelitis with loss of pinprick and joint position sense and fasciculations. Myxoedema has been claimed to be a distinguishing feature of paralytic rabies (Hemachudha et al., 2002). However, this transient local mounding of muscle in response to percussion, which was used historically to lateralise pulmonary tuberculosis, is unlikely to be a helpful sign as it is associated with a variety of pathological conditions (wasting, myxoedema, hyponatraemia) and may also be found in healthy people (Jackson, 2002a). Fasciculation in the muscles becoming involved in the ascending paralysis was mentioned in the original description of paralytic rabies, by Gamaleia in 1887. Cranial nerve involvement may result in ptosis, external ophthalmoplegia, paralysis of the tongue and deafness. Most patients with paralytic rabies do not experience hydrophobia, but in a few, it may be represented by some terminal respiratory spasms. The course of the disease is less acute and stormy than furious rabies. Even without intensive care, patients may survive for up to 30 days before they succumb to bulbar and respiratory paralysis.

Differential Diagnosis of Rabies and Infections by Rabies-related Viruses

In a rabies endemic area, the diagnosis of furious rabies may be obvious in a patient with hydrophobic spasms who has a history of being bitten by a dog within the previous few weeks or months. However, exposure to a mammal bite or scratch may not be remembered, as in the majority of cases of Genotype 1 insectivorous bat-transmitted rabies in the USA (Noah et al., 1998). Although hydrophobia is a pathognomonic sign of furious rabies, it may be misdiagnosed as a laryngopharyngeal or even a psychiatric problem. Some of the reported misdiagnoses and differential diagnoses of furious and paralytic rabies are listed in Table 21.3. Rabies phobia, an hysterical response to the fear of rabies, differs from true rabies in its shorter incubation period, which may be only a few hours after the bite, exaggerated aggressive and dramatic symptoms and its excellent prognosis. Severe (cephalic) tetanus, involving the cranial nerves, is distinguished by its shorter incubation period, the presence of trismus, the persistence of muscular rigidity between spasms and the absence of pleocytosis.

Table 21.3 Differential diagnosis of rabies

Furious rabies
  Hysterical pseudo-hydrophobia
  (Cephalic) tetanus
  Other brainstem encephalitides (e.g. complicating serum sickness)
  Other causes of muscle spasms (e.g. phenothiazine dystonia, tetany, strychnine poisoning)
  Delirium tremens
  Porphyria
  Cerebrovascular accident, epilepsy

Paralytic rabies
  Post-vaccinal encephalomyelitis
  Paralytic poliomyelitis
  Other causes of acute ascending paralysis (e.g. acute idiopathic inflammatory polyneuropathy—Guillain–Barré syndrome)
  Herpes simiae (B virus) encephalomyelitis (after monkey bites)

In those countries where nervous tissue vaccines are still used, post-vaccinal encephalomyelitis (PVE) is the commonest differential diagnosis of paralytic rabies. In PVE, symptoms usually develop within 2 weeks of the first dose of vaccine, but no clinical or laboratory features reliably distinguish the two conditions while the patient is still alive, save for the absence of demonstrable rabies virus in skin biopsies, saliva or CSF. Herpes simiae (B virus) encephalomyelitis, transmitted by monkey bites, has a much shorter incubation period than rabies (3–4 days). Vesicles may be found in the monkey's mouth and at the site of the bite. The diagnosis can be confirmed virologically and the patients treated with aciclovir.

Clinical Diagnostic Methods in Human Rabies

Haematological and Biochemical Tests

Routine haematological and biochemical tests are initially normal, apart from neutrophil leukocytosis. Later, hypernatraemia or hyponatraemia may reflect diabetes insipidus or the syndrome of inappropriate ADH secretion, respectively. In a majority of patients, there is a lymphocytic pleocytosis and sometimes an elevated protein concentration in the CSF. Hypoglycorrhachia has been reported (Roine et al., 1988).

Neurological Investigations

The electroencephalogram (EEG) may be normal or may show the expected wide range of non-specific changes, including evidence of seizure activity. Electromyography has revealed evidence of primary axonal neuropathy.

Most reported computed tomographic (CT) scans in rabies have been normal, especially in the early stages. Hypodensities of the basal ganglia and of cortical lesions have been described.

Reports of magnetic resonance imaging (MRI) have mainly been in patients with paralytic rabies, although, surprisingly, both paralytic and encephalitic rabies patients are said to show a similar distribution of ill-defined, mildly T2-weighted hyperintensity of the brainstem, hippocampus, hypothalamus, deep and subcortical white matter and deep and cortical grey matter (Haemachudha et al., 2002). Minimal gadolinium enhancement, indicating mild inflammation, may be seen in the later stages of the clinical course. Similar changes in the spinal cord, suggestive of myelitis, might indicate a diagnosis of paralytic rabies. The non-specific changes reported to date would not be diagnostic of rabies infection.

Recovery from Rabies Encephalitis

Animals of several species have recovered from rabies (see above) and humans with paralytic rabies can survive for several weeks, especially with intensive care, but the illness progresses relentlessly. Five patients over the last 30 years have been claimed as survivors of encephalitis. All had received some rabies vaccine before the onset of symptoms. No virus or viral antigen was detected in any patient and so the diagnoses were based on finding high rabies neutralising antibody levels in the CSF.

Two of the patients were treated post-exposure with rabies vaccines of nervous tissue origin. In Argentina in 1972, a 45 year-old woman was bitten by her clinically rabid dog, began a course of suckling mouse brain vaccine 10 days later (Porras et al., 1976). Three weeks after the bite she had parasthesiae of the bitten arm, with tremors, myoclonic spasms, ataxia and other signs of cerebellar dysfunction. She recovered but relapsed twice following booster doses of rabies vaccine. Clinical features included hypertonia, tetraparesis, dysphonia, dysphagia, varying levels of consciousness and a cardiac conduction defect, with slow resolution over a year. The CSF and serum neutralising antibody levels were very high. The clinical features typical of rabies were the apparently subjective parasthesiae of the bitten limb, the cardiac conduction defect (if it was a new finding) and the high antibody level. Cerebellar signs have rarely been reported in rabies. The rabies antibody response to nervous tissue vaccines are higher than usual in patients with severe post-vaccinal encephalitis (Hemachudha et al., 1989).

The second patient was a 9 year-old boy in Ohio, USA in 1970, who was bitten by a proven rabid big brown bat (Eptesicus fuscus) on the thumb, and began treatment with duck embryo vaccine the next day (Hattwick et al., 1972). After 20 days he developed a meningitic illness progressing to encephalitis, with unilateral weakness maximal in the bitten arm. Focal seizures, paralysis, cerebral oedema and coma ensued, lasting more than a week. He also had an atrial arrhythmia. Prolonged intensive care resulted in complete recovery in 6 months. The CSF and serum rabies antibody levels were high. Features suggesting rabies were the dominant signs in the bitten limb, a cardiac arrhythmia and the high antibody level. Now, 30 years later, the patient lives a normal life.

The third case was a 32 year-old laboratory worker in New York in 1977 who was thought to have inhaled an aerosol of a fixed strain of rabies (SAD) virus (Centers for Disease Control, 1977). He had had pre-exposure prophylaxis with duck embryo rabies vaccine with a neutralising antibody titre of 1:32 6 months before exposure. Fever, encephalitic symptoms, spastic hemiparesis, myoclonus, impaired conciousness and respiratory arrest developed over 2 weeks, and the rabies neutralising antibody titres were high in the serum and CSF. A gradual improvement was followed by onset of a personality disorder and dementia. Two and a half years later he still had profound neurological deficits.

A Mexican boy severely bitten on the head by a proven rabid dog was given a course of vero cell vaccine (see section on Prophylaxis, below), starting the following day, but no rabies immune globulin (RIG) treatment (Alvarez et al., 1994). Nineteen days later he developed encephalitis with fever and convulsions. Intracranial hypertension and coma ensued. He improved over 3 weeks, and reacted to painful stimuli, but quadriplegia persisted, he became blind and deaf and eventually died after 2 years and 10 months. High titres of rabies antibody appeared in the CSF and the serum. A second boy with similar clinical features survived at least 9 months.

The most recent case of survival was reported from India (Madhusudana et al., 2002). A 6 year-old girl was severely bitten by a stray dog, which died 4 days later. The wound was not cleaned but she was given purified chick embryo cell rabies vaccine (see section on Prophylaxis, below) on days 0, 3 and 7 after the bite. Sixteen days later she would not drink and developed fever, hallucinations and impaired consciousness, which progressed to coma with excessive salivation and focal seizures. Rabies antibody titres rose to very high levels in serum and CSF. After 3 months of coma, improvement began very slowly but after 18 months she had spasticity, tremors and involuntary limb movements.

Neurological illnesses following human diploid cell rabies vaccine has been reported rarely (see below; Side Effects of Tissue Culture Vaccine) but have been relatively mild.

Rabies virus was not isolated, nor was antigen identified, in these patients thought to have recovered from rabies, but false negative results may have been obtained because samples were taken late, when there was already a high titre of antibody neutralising the virus or covering the epitopes of the antigens. The diagnosis of rabies in such cases might more readily be confirmed in future, with the development of sensitive RT-PCR techniques for detecting viral RNA. The diagnosis may remain in some doubt in those patients given vaccines of nervous tissue origin, as post-vaccinal encephalitis can produce similar signs and symptoms (Label and Batts, 1982).

The term 'survival' is more appropriate than 'recovery' in the three patients given tissue culture vaccines, as all had profound residual neurological deficits. Severe impairment of nervous function was irreversible before the infection was controlled, presumably by the immune response.

Human Infections with Rabies-related Viruses
(see section on Classification, above)

Mokola (Lyssavirus Genotype 3)

Two cases of *Mokola virus* infection occurred in girls admitted to University College Hospital, Ibadan, in 1968 and 1971. The first was a 3½ year-old child who presented with a febrile convulsion, and had a temperature of 105°F and a sore throat. She recovered. Virus was isolated from her cerebrospinal fluid, but no specific complement-fixing antibodies were detected. A similar strain of *Mokola virus*, isolated from a shrew, was being handled in the laboratory at the same time (Familusi and Moore, 1972). The second case, was a 6 year-old, admitted after 6 days of feverish illness.

Initially she had a cough and vomited but later became drowsy, confused and weak. She died 3 days after admission. *Mokola virus* was isolated from brain tissue, and a *Coxsackie A virus* isolated from a rectal swab (Familusi *et al.*, 1972). A laboratory worker recovered from a mild *Mokola virus* infection (Crick, 1981).

Duvenhage (Lyssavirus Genotype 4)

This virus was named after a 31 year-old white South African man who had been bitten on the lip by a bat of unknown species (Meredith *et al.*, 1971). One month later he noticed headache, dizziness and aching in the neck and back. He began to sweat profusely and suffered involuntary spasms of the face and limbs. During the next 3 days he became progressively more confused, irritable and aggressive, had nightmares and noticed difficulty in swallowing. He showed typical hydrophobia. He was agitated, and had involuntary spasms of the neck and back. Touch provoked spasms of the face, arms and trunk and aggressive episodes. These features became more marked before he died 24 h after admission.

European Bat Lyssaviruses

Genotype 5, EBL 1. Two human deaths from rabies have been reported from Russia in 1977 and 1985, following bat bites (Selimov *et al.*, 1989) One month after being bitten on the hand, a 15 year-old girl became unwell with fever, anxiety and paraesthesia of the bitten hand. She developed an acute ascending paralysis, encephalitis and myocarditis and died 5 days later. An 11 year-old girl was bitten on the lip by a bat in Belgorod. Three weeks later she became unwell with pain in the bitten cheek, weakness and drowsiness. She developed typical furious rabies and died 6 days later. No rabies antigen was detected in brain impression smears by the immunofluorescent test, but virus was isolated in suckling mice and proved to be an EBL 1.

Genotype 6, EBL 2. Two human infections due to EBL 2 virus have been documented. An unvaccinated 30 year-old Swiss zoologist in Finland who studied bats had been bitten several times by bats in Malaysia and Switzerland during the previous 5 years. Most recently, in southern Finland he had been bitten by a sick Daubenton's bat (*Myotis daubentonii*) 51 days before the first symptoms, which were numbness of the palm of his right hand and pain in the neck radiating to his right cheek. Next day, he became unable to walk, was feverish and generally weak, with numbness of the right arm and neck and retrosternal pain. The following day, 4 days after the first symptom, there was myoclonic twitching of the feet, trismus and typical hydrophobic symptoms of furious rabies. Delirium, muscle spasms, convulsions and respiratory failure followed. He developed diabetes insipidus and fluctuations in blood pressure and heart rate and finally died 23 days after his first symptom (Roine *et al.*, 1988). As no EBL virus has been isolated from a Finnish bat, but EBL 2b has been found in Switzerland, it is possible that his infection originated from there.

The second patient, a 55 year-old unvaccinated bat conservationist, had been bitten by bats on several occasions in Scotland, most recently in Angus in 2002 on the left hand about 4 months before his illness. He developed pain, paraesthesiae and diminished sensation in the left arm. He was prescribed non-steroidal antiinflammatory drugs and, 5 days later, presented to a hospital in Dundee, Scotland with acute haematemesis attributable to these drugs. He was feverish, disinhibited, dysarthric and had gaze-evoked nystagmus. His upper limbs were areflexic but the lower limb tendon reflexes were brisk. He showed truncal, upper limb and gait ataxia. Sensation to touch was decreased over the left arm. There was no meningism and CSF was normal, apart from a mildly raised protein concentration. Five days after admission, he became suddenly confused, aggressive and agitated and, the next day, deteriorated with a collapsed lung and respiratory failure, decreased consciousness and hypersalivation. Neither aerophobia or hydrophobia was observed. He was mechanically ventilated in the intensive care unit but he became comatose and generally flaccid with extensor plantar responses. There was electrophysiological evidence of a peripheral, predominantly motor axonal neuropathy. He died 19 days after the first prodromal symptom (Nathwani *et al.*, 2003). EBL RNA was identified ante mortem in saliva by RT-PCR. Post mortem IF and RT-PCR tests were positive on brain samples and EBL 2a was isolated.

Australian Bat Lyssavirus (Lyssavirus Genotype 7)

There have been two reported human fatalities from *Australian bat lyssavirus* infection in Queensland, Australia. A 39 year-old woman, who cared for bats, had been scratched by bats during the previous 30 days. She was admitted to hospital with a history of a few days of left shoulder pain, dizziness, vomiting,

headache, fevers and chills. Her left arm became progressively weaker, she became ataxic with cerebellar signs, slurred speech, diplopia and dysphagia. Over the next few days she developed bilateral facial palsies, progressive quadriplegia with asymmetrical reduction of deep tendon reflexes and fluctuating level of consciousness. She continued to deteriorate and died 20 days after the start of her illness. Rabies antibody was detected and viral RNA was identified by PCR in the CSF (Samaratunga *et al.*, 1998). The virus isolated from post mortem brain was the insectivorous bat (*Saccolaimus* sp.) variant of *Australian bat lyssavirus*.

The second case was a 37 year-old woman who had been bitten on her left hand by a flying fox or fruit bat (*Pteropus* sp.) (Hanna *et al.*, 2000). 27 months later she presented to hospital with a 5 day history of fever, vomiting, anorexia, pain around the left shoulder girdle, paraesthesiae of the dorsum of the left hand, sore throat and difficulty in swallowing. She was feverish, unable fully to open her mouth, was drooling saliva and had difficulty speaking. There was increased muscle tone, painful spasms provoked by examination and spasmodic attempts to swallow provoked by examination of the throat. She had a neutrophil leukocytosis. She deteriorated over the next 12 h, becoming agitated with dysphagia, dysphonia and increasingly severe and frequent muscle spasms, which were uncontrollable by medication. She was mechanically ventilated but died 19 days after the first symptom. *Australian bat lyssavirus* was detected by PCR in saliva. A post mortem revealed diffuse pancarditis, and virus was isolated from the brain.

DIAGNOSIS

Intravitam Diagnosis of Human Rabies Encephalitis
(Table 21.4)

The laboratory diagnosis of rabies is rarely attempted in developing countries, but confirmation of infection will be useful to guide the appropriate management of the patient, relatives and staff, prevent unnecessary investigations and allow characterisation of the virus. Routine haematological and biochemical tests are likely to be normal initially, but a plasma neutrophil leukocytosis may be present. A mild pleocytosis is only seen in 60% of patients in the first week (Anderson *et al.*, 1984). The diagnosis can be made by virus isolation, identification of antigen or, in unvaccinated

Table 21.4 Human rabies diagnosis

Sample	Aim	Test
Intravitam		
REPEAT until a diagnosis is made:		
Skin punch biopsy*	Antigen detection	IFA test on frozen section
	RNA detection	PCR
Saliva, tears, CSF	Virus isolation	Tissue culture
		Mouse inoculation test
	RNA detection	PCR
Serum	Serology	Antibody test
		Unvaccinated, test immediately
		Vaccinated, save for comparison later
CSF	Antibody detection	Test immediately with serum
Post mortem		
Brain.* Needle biopsy (see text) or	Antigen detection	IFA test on impression smear
brainstem and cerebellum	RNA detection	PCR
	Virus isolation	Tissue culture
		Mouse inoculation test
Serum	Serology	Antibody test

*Collect in small dry container, well sealed, keep cool during transport. *Do not freeze.*

people, antibody detection, and taking serial samples for all tests will enable rapid detection of the infection.

Isolation of Rabies Virus

Culture of the virus from saliva, throat, tracheal or eye swabs, brain biopsy samples and, rarely, the CSF is most successful during the first week of illness (Anderson *et al.*, 1984) and in seronegative patients. The isolation of virus is best attempted in murine neuroblastoma cells, which can be performed in microtitre plates in 4 days (Webster and Casey, 1996), whereas the inoculation of suckling mice yields results in 1–3 weeks.

Antigen Detection

The most rapid diagnosis of rabies during life can be made by direct immunofluorescent antibody (IFA) identification of antigen in a skin biopsy (Noah *et al.*, 1998). A full-thickness biopsy, preferably taken with a disposable biopsy punch, must include the bases of hair follicles. It is taken from a hairy area, usually the nape of the neck, and in addition near the original bite wound, if there is an adjacent proximal hairy area. Tissue is collected in a small dry container and kept cool but not frozen. Vertical frozen sections through hair follicles indicate rabies antigen in the nerve twiglets around the base of the follicles, in a

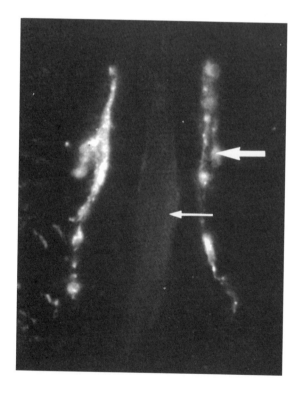

Figure 21.5 Vertical section through a skin biopsy, showing a hair (small arrow) surrounded by its follicle. The bright fluorescence (large arrow) indicates rabies antigen in neurones surrounding the follicle, and is a rapid means of diagnosing rabies during life. (Courtesy of M. J. Warrell)

characteristic pattern (Bryceson *et al.*, 1975) (Figure 21.5). Careful controls of specificity are needed. For a reliable result, more than 20 sections including hair follicles are compared with sections stained with an adsorbed negative control conjugate. The method is 60–100% sensitive (Blenden *et al.*, 1986; Warrell *et al.*, 1988), and false positives have not been reported. This test requires a cryostat being available for use with infected tissue. Antigen detection by IFA in the corneal smear test is too insensitive to be useful (Anderson *et al.*, 1984; Warrell *et al.*, 1988) and false positives have occurred. Brain biopsy samples are ideal for antigen detection (see animal diagnosis) or culture, but biopsy is very rarely indicated.

PCR techniques now seem to be a reliable means of identifying and genotyping rabies strains (Noah *et al.*, 1998). The RT-PCR test has given positive results using RNA extracted from saliva samples, and also from CSF, skin biopsy tissue and urine. Nested PCR techniques enhance the sensitivity still further (Trimarchi and Smith, 2002).

Antibody Detection

In unvaccinated patients, the diagnostic appearance of rabies antibody often occurs during the second week of illness, but it may not happen until after the third week. Antibody may be detectable in the CSF a few days later (see section on Immunology, above). A low level of rabies-specific IgM has been detected in the serum and occasionally in the CSF of rabies patients, but it did not appear earlier than IgG, and IgM has also been found in post-vaccinal encephalitis patients (Warrell *et al.*, 1988). In vaccinated people, very high levels of antibody in the serum, and especially in the CSF, have been considered diagnostic (Hattwick *et al.*, 1972).

Post Mortem Diagnosis in Humans

Post mortem diagnosis can be made by any of the above tests, but rabies virus is most readily detected in the brainstem and cerebellum. Brain tissue can, however, be obtained without a full post mortem examination. Needle necropsies are taken with a Vim–Silverman or other long biopsy needle via the medial canthus of the eye, through the superior orbital fissure; via the nose through the ethmoid bone; by an occipital approach through the foramen magnum; or through burr holes or open fontanelles in children. Tissue is collected in small dry containers and kept cool but not frozen. The IFA test for antigen takes about 3 h to perform on brain impression smears (Trimarchi and Smith, 2002). Viral isolation from brain by inoculation of murine neuroblastoma cells or of suckling mice might be successful even if the IFA staining is negative. A retrospective diagnosis using formalin-fixed brain specimens is possible by protein digestion and antigen detection by IFA or enzymatic techniques. Genomic and mRNAs can also be analysed by *in situ* hybridisation (Warner *et al.*, 1997; Trimarchi and Smith, 2002). Rabies-related viruses may give a weak or negative reaction in the IFA test.

Diagnosis in the Biting Mammal
(Trimarchi and Smith, 2002)

Suspect rabid animals should be euthanised immediately and their brains tested for rabies infection (World Health Organization, 1997). In practice this is often impossible if the animal escapes, or if laboratory facilities are not available. Observation in captivity is potentially dangerous and uncertain. Animal brain samples should include brainstem and cerebellum, but tissue can be obtained without craniotomy, via the occipital foramen. Tissue is collected in small dry containers and kept cool but not frozen. The diagnosis can be confirmed by a direct IFA test on acetone-fixed brain impression smears. A rapid enzyme immuno-diagnosis kit will detect rabies antigen in a suspension of brain tissue. This is useful for laboratories without a fluorescence microscope, although the method is up to 3% less sensitive than the IFA test. No single laboratory method is sufficiently accurate for this crucial diagnosis. The IFA test has been found to be about 2% less sensitive than virus isolation in tropical dog rabies endemic areas, while false positive results are rare. Culture of virus should be attempted in antigen-negative samples. The sensitivity of detection, especially on decomposing samples, can be further increased using PCR methods, which can also identify genetic sequences in the viral G or N proteins characteristic of the vector species and geographical origin of the rabies or rabies-related virus. The diagnosis can also be made on formalin-fixed brain specimens (see section on Diagnosis in Humans, above).

MANAGEMENT OF HUMAN RABIES ENCEPHALOMYELITIS

The undisputed mortality from human rabies is 100% in unvaccinated patients. All five of the patients reported to have 'survived' had received some rabies vaccine before the onset of symptoms. Despite many attempts at intensive care treatment over 30 years, no patient has recovered mentally or physically (see section on Recovery, above). Life can be prolonged by this treatment, but many complications arise (see Table 21.2). Heavy sedation and analgesia should be given to relieve the agonising symptoms. Ketamine, an anaesthetic agent and a non-competitive antagonist of the N-methyl-D-aspartate (NMDA) receptor, has specific anti-rabies activity (Lockhart *et al.*, 1992), but the human therapeutic dosage is unlikely to give an adequate concentration for an antiviral effect in the brain (Jackson *et al.*, 2003). Immunosuppressive drugs, including corticosteroids, rabies hyperimmune serum antiviral agents, such as vidarabine, cytosine arabinoside, ribavirin (Centres for Disease Control, 1984; Warrell *et al.*, 1989) and IFN-α (Merigan *et al.*, 1984; Warrell *et al.*, 1989) have not proved useful.

Until a new specific therapy is available, palliative care is recommended. Patients and their relatives should be advised that although intensive care therapy may prolong life, there can be no expectation of survival without severe permanent neurological disabilities (Jackson *et al.*, 2003).

PATHOLOGY

Rabies causes an acute non-suppurative meningo-encephalomyelitis, usually accompanied by diagnostic intracellular inclusions known as Negri bodies (Figure 21.2). These are masses of dense eosinophilic material in neuronal cytoplasm. Electron microscopy shows they are composed of disorganised filaments in an amorphous matrix, largely consisting of rabies ribonucleoprotein. The inclusions described by Negri contained a basophilic inner body, which may include fragments of cellular organelles and occasional virions, probably mechanically trapped by the fusion of smaller inclusions. Negri bodies are found in about 75% of patients and are most numerous in the hippocampus, Purkinje cells, medulla and ganglia (Perl, 1975). Inclusions with no internal structure were called 'lyssa bodies' by Goodpasture. These contain the nucleoprotein alone and are usually smaller than Negri bodies.

By the time the patient dies, cerebral congestion with some petechial haemorrhages is usual, but without gross oedema (Tangchai *et al.*, 1970). Inflammation with perivascular mononuclear cell infiltrate is common, with neutrophils seen only at an early stage. Neuronophagia, microglial reaction, ganglion cell degeneration, foci of demyelination and perineural

infiltrates (Babes' nodules) are less frequent. All changes may be widespread and are most pronounced in the grey matter of the brainstem and spinal cord, and in paralytic rabies spinal cord pathology may predominate. Children often show meningeal inflammation (Perl, 1975). The degree of histopathological change in rabies encephalitis varies from absence of any inflammation (Tangchai *et al.*, 1970; Iwasaki *et al.*, 1985) to complete disruption of neuron structure in a patient treated with intensive care for several weeks. Peripheral nerve changes include axonal degeneration of myelinated and unmyelinated nerve fibres with leukocyte infiltration and degeneration in dorsal root ganglia, especially in the region of the site of the bite.

Extra-neural changes include focal degeneration of salivary and lacrimal glands, liver, pancreas, adrenal medulla, lymph nodes and ocular tissues. An interstitial myocarditis with round cell infiltration has been described (Warrell *et al.*, 1976; Metze and Feiden, 1991) and tissue in the myocardium is also affected, which may account for associated cardiac arrhythmias.

HUMAN RABIES PROPHYLAXIS

Rabies Vaccines

Two rabies vaccines are now licensed for use in the UK and USA: human diploid cell vaccine (HDCV) (Aventis Pasteur) and purified chick embryo cell (PCEC) vaccine (Rabipur™, Chiron Behring). Both are in 1 ml dose vials. PCEC is cheaper to produce. Elsewhere, purified vero cell vaccine (PVRV) (Verorab™, Aventis Pasteur) is widely available, but the single dose vial contains 0.5 ml.

Pre-exposure Prophylaxis
(World Health Organization, 1997;
Centers for Disease Control, 1999a)

No rabies deaths have been reported in those given pre-exposure prophylaxis with post-exposure boosting. Pre-exposure immunisation is indicated for residents of, or visitors to, areas where dog rabies is endemic and all those at occupational risk of contact with a rabid animal or rabies virus in quarantine facilities, customs departments, zoos, laboratories or hospitals. Those staying in rural areas of foreign countries where rabies is enzootic in other mammals (foxes, jackals, wolves, coyotes, mongooses, bats, etc.) should seek advice about the risk.

Subsequent post-exposure treatment will be simplified and much cheaper after a prophylactic course. Immunisation is especially important for children. The high cost of vaccine is the only constraint to widespread pre-exposure immunisation. Official recommendations on the need for pre-exposure rabies vaccine use a risk assessment analysis to define a length of stay in the endemic area, but as rabies is a fatal disease, and a primary vaccine course is only required once, treatment should be encouraged for all visiting endemic areas.

Pre-exposure Vaccine Regimens
(Figure 21.6)

One dose of HDCV, PCEC or PVRV is given i.m. into the deltoid on days 0, 7 and 28 (or 21). An economical but effective alternative is to give the vaccine intradermally (i.d.) if more than one person is to be immunised. The dose of 0.1 ml of any of the these vaccines is injected i.d. over the deltoid to raise a papule. If the injection is too deep, the needle should be withdrawn and the procedure repeated. Opened ampoules should be stored in the fridge and used the same day. The ampoules do not contain preservatives and so cannot be sanctioned pharmaceutically as multi-dose vials, hence the need to use or discard after 1 day. The level of antibody may

be lower following i.d. vaccine, but the quality of the secondary immune response to a booster dose is similar for i.d. and i.m. injections. Chloroquine antimalarial chemoprophylaxis may inhibit the induction of rabies antibody after i.d. vaccination, so the larger dose must be given i.m.

Booster Doses of Vaccine

A booster dose i.m. or i.d. 1 year later enhances and prolongs the immune response, which lasts more than 10 years in 96% of people (Strady et al., 1998). The neutralising antibody level after 3 years has been used to decide whether to give a booster dose every 3 years or every 10 years (Strady et al., 2000). If no serology is available or affordable, doses may be given every 5–10 years to those at continued risk of infection. In the USA, frequent serology and boosters are recommended only for those at high risk, but no boosters are given after the primary course for travellers (Centers for Disease Control, 1999a). An antibody test should be performed 6 monthly for rabies laboratory staff and all those at continued high risk and a booster dose given if the titre is < 0.5 IU/ml.

Pre-exposure rabies prophylaxis

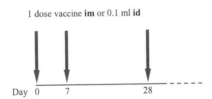

Standard im post-exposure vaccine regimen

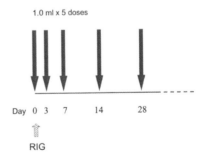

Post-exposure treatment when previously vaccinated

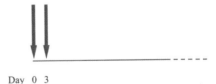

Figure 21.6 Intramuscular rabies vaccine regimens. Each arrow represents one dose (whole ampoule) of vaccine. RIG = rabies immune globulin

Measurement of neutralising antibody levels after treatment is necessary only if immunosuppression is suspected, e.g. in patients with AIDS. Those with low CD4$^+$ counts may fail to mount any antibody response to repeated doses of vaccine.

Post-exposure Treatment

Post-exposure treatment is in great demand, especially where dog rabies is endemic. According to WHO data, about 5 million people in China, 1 million in India and 500 000 in Vietnam are treated with vaccine annually.

Any bite or close contact with an animal in a rabies endemic area is a potential exposure to rabies virus. Evaluation of the risk of infection depends on the history and clinical features of both the patient and the biting animal, and also knowledge of the local vectors and epidemiology of rabies.

The Site of Infection?

The virus gains access through any bite, scratch or contamination of broken skin or mucous membrane by animal's saliva, but intact skin is an adequate barrier against infection. The risk of infection is greatest from bites on the head, neck and hands and multiple bites carry a higher risk than single bites. Other routes of infection are very rare (see section on Route of Infection, above).

The Animal Species and Behaviour?

An unprovoked attack by a known local rabies vector (see section on Epidemiology, above), or an animal which may have been in contact with a vector species, suggests a high risk of exposure. Abnormal behaviour, either excitable or with partial paralysis, is typical of rabies and wild animals can appear unusually tame. Vaccination of domestic animals is not always protective; 20% of proven rabid dogs in Bangkok had been vaccinated (Mitmoonpitak and Tepsumethanon, 2002).

To Confirm Exposure

Every effort should be made to obtain a virological diagnosis, by examining the animal's brain for rabies antigen and other tests if appropriate (see section on Diagnosis of Biting Animal, above).

If rabies exposure is suspected or proven, post-exposure prophylaxis must be started as soon as possible. The greater the delay in starting treatment, the greater the risk of virus entering a peripheral nerve, where it becomes inaccessible to immune attack. If in doubt, vaccinate; it is worth giving prophylaxis even if several weeks have elapsed. The recommended criteria for treatment are shown in Table 21.5.

Primary Post-exposure Treatment

For those who have not had a previous course of vaccine, the treatment consists of three parts: wound treatment, active immunisation with vaccine, and passive immunisation with rabies immune globulin.

Treatment of wounds. Immediate vigorous washing, scrubbing and flushing with soap and water, detergent or water alone are recommended for all animal bite wounds, including those without risk of rabies. Kaplan showed that this first aid treatment can be 50% effective in preventing rabies experimentally (Kaplan and Cohen, 1962). He also suggested local infiltration, proximal to the wound, with procaine hydrochloride 1% in saline for pain, as this may also have some antiviral action, followed by application of either 70% ethanol or povidone iodine. Suturing the wound should be avoided or postponed. Tetanus prophylaxis may be required. Giving a prophylactic antimicrobial agent should be considered for serious bites or those on the hands (co-amoxyclav, doxycycline or erythromycin for dog or cat bites).

Vaccine regimens (Figure 21.6). A course of five i.m. injections of HDCV or PCEC vaccine are given into the deltoid on days 0, 3, 7, 14 and 28 (World Health Organization, 1997; Centers for Disease Control, 1999a). Economical intradermal (i.d.) post-exposure treatment has been used for 15 years in Asia (see below). Although an i.d. regimen may have some advantages, it is not officially recommended in Europe and North America, where full i.m. treatment is freely available. If immunosuppression is suspected, due to diseases such as AIDS or drugs, the antigenic stimulus can be increased by doubling the initial dose of i.m. vaccine (one i.m. dose into each deltoid) or by dividing a whole single dose between multiple sites intradermally (see below). A shortened course of i.m. treatment, requiring four instead of five doses of tissue culture vaccine, is used occasionally outside the UK. Two doses are injected on the first occasion, one into each deltoid muscle. A single dose is given on days 7

Table 21.5 The decision to give post-exposure treatment

Category	Type of contact with a suspect or confirmed rabid domestic or wild* animal, or animal unavailable for observation	Recommended treatment
I	Touching or feeding of animals Licks on intact skin	None, if reliable case history is available
II	Nibbling of uncovered skin Minor scratches or abrasions without bleeding Licks on broken skin	Administer vaccine immediately. Stop treatment if animal remains healthy throughout an observation period[†] of 10 days or if animal is killed humanely and found to be negative for rabies by appropriate laboratory tests
III	Single or multiple transdermal bites or scratches Contamination of mucous membrane by animals' saliva	Administer rabies immmunoglobulin and vaccine immediately. Stop treatment if animal remains healthy throughout an observation period[†] of 10 days or if animal is killed humanely and found to be negative for rabies by appropriate laboratory tests

This table is a simplification of the WHO recommendations (1997).
*Exposure to rodents, rabbits and hares seldom, if ever, requires specific anti-rabies treatment.
[†]This observation period applies only to dogs and cats. Other domestic and wild animals suspected as rabid should be killed humanely and their tissues examined using appropriate laboratory tests. An exception may be made for animals of threatened or endangered species.

and 21 (Vodopija *et al.*, 1988). Multisite injections might accelerate the antibody response (Anderson *et al.*, 1981; Suntharasamai *et al.*, 1987) but the antibody titre wanes more rapidly than with the conventional regimen. Pregnancy is not a contraindication to rabies vaccination.

Rabies immune globulin (RIG). RIG should be given with every primary post-exposure treatment. It is most important for severe exposure to infection—bites on the head, neck or hands or multiple bites. Passive immunisation provides some protection for the 7–10 days before vaccine-induced immunity appears. RIG apparently neutralises virus in the wound and enhances the T lymphocyte response to rabies (Celis *et al.*, 1985). The dose of 20 units/kg body weight of human RIG (or 40 units/kg equine RIG, outside Europe and North America) should be infiltrated deep under and around the wound. If this is anatomically impossible, e.g. in a bitten finger, give the rest by i.m. injection at a site remote from the vaccine, but not into the gluteal region. For multiple bites the RIG can be diluted two- or three-fold in saline to ensure infiltration of all wounds. The recommended dose of RIG must not be exceeded, as this will impair the immune response to the vaccine. Serum sickness has not been reported with human RIG. As there are problems of production and supply of RIG worldwide, efforts to find alternative products continue, including the use of a collection of monoclonal antibodies and novel strategies to manufacture immune globulins *in vitro*.

Post-exposure Treatment in Previously Vaccinated Patients

Treatment of animal bites, including immediate wound cleaning, is always urgent. Provided that a complete pre- or post-exposure course of a tissue culture vaccine has been given previously, or if a serum rabies neutralising antibody level of $>0.5\,IU/ml$ has been recorded, an abbreviated course of only two doses of vaccine may be used. It is injected i.m. into the deltoid on days 0 and 3. RIG treatment is not necessary (World Health Organization, 1997; Centers for Disease Control, 1999a). If there is any uncertainty about past treatment, the full post-exposure regimen and RIG must be used.

How Effective is Post-exposure Treatment?

The untreated mortality from proven rabid dog bites in India was 35% and 57% in separate studies more than 35 years ago. Optimal modern post-exposure treatment, started on the day of the bite, in healthy recipients is practically 100% effective. 'Failures of treatment' to date are due to failure to deliver the three components correctly and promptly, or failure of the patients' immune response, e.g. if there is delay in starting treatment; failure to clean the wound; failure to complete the course of vaccine; injections of vaccine or RIG into the buttock; failure to infiltrate the wound with RIG; or immunosuppression by drugs, HIV, cirrhosis or other illness. There has been no suggestion that treatment has failed because the potency of the recommended vaccines was low, or that the vaccine virus strain did not protect against the infecting virus. Only two people are known to have died despite complete prompt treatment with modern products (Hemachudha *et al.*, 1999). Nevertheless, if wounds are extensive and severe, especially from wolf bites, primary post-exposure treatment cannot ensure survival.

Efficacy Against Rabies-related Viruses
(see pp 632, 636)

Tissue culture vaccines do afford some protection against *European bat lyssavirus* (genotypes 5 and 6) but they are probably less effective than they are against the genotype 1 rabies strains and *Australian bat lyssavirus* (genotype 7). Vaccine is less protective against *Duvenhage virus* (lyssavirus genotype 4) and gives little or no protection against *Mokola virus* (genotype 3) (King and Turner, 1993; Badrane *et al.*, 2001).

Side-effects of Tissue Culture Vaccines

There is very wide variation in the incidence of side-effects in different groups of recipients. Mild erythema and pain at injection sites are reported in 7–64% of HDCV recipients, and local irritation is more common (13–92%) after i.d. injections. Generalised symptoms of headache, malaise and fever occur in 3–14% (World Health Organization, 1997) and up to 3% reported a 'rash' distant from the injection site. There are similar data for PCEC and PVRV vaccine.

Rare case reports of neurological illness temporally associated with tissue culture vaccine treatment have described a Guillian–Barré-like syndrome (Bøe and Nyland, 1980; Bernard *et al.*, 1982; Knittel *et al.*, 1989; Chackravarty, 2001), a relapsing mild hemiplegia (Tornatore and Richert, 1990) or symptoms restricted to an arm in two patients (Gardner, 1983). The incidence of neurological disease after these rabies vaccines is no more than after other commonly used vaccines.

Late booster doses of HDCV were followed, 3–13 days later, by a systemic allergic reaction in 6% of vaccinees in the USA (however, reaction rates were not evenly distributed between the groups of volunteers) (Dreesen *et al.*, 1986). The urticarial rash, angioedema and arthralgia respond to symptomatic therapy. It is possibly caused by an IgE-mediated reaction to β-propiolactone-modified vaccine

components (Warrington *et al.*, 1987). Repeated booster doses of vaccine for people at continued high risk of infection can be avoided by serological testing to confirm the need for further treatment.

What to Do if Bitten in a Rabies Endemic Area

If bitten by a mammal in a rabies endemic country (or if any direct contact with a bat in the Americas), immediately wash the wound thoroughly (see above). Seek advice on the local epidemiology from a doctor. If there is a risk of rabies infection, start post-exposure treatment without delay. Tissue culture vaccines are too expensive for worldwide use, and so nervous tissue vaccines are still produced in many developing countries. The potency of Semple (sheep brain) or suckling mouse brain vaccines is variable and they are associated with neurological reactions; the incidence is estimated at 1/200 for Semple vaccine (Bahri *et al.*, 1996). Suckling mouse brain vaccine carries a lower risk; estimates vary between 1/8000 and 1/27 000 courses. Nevertheless, if only locally produced animal brain vaccine is available it might be reasonable to begin treatment immediately, despite the risk of allergic encephalomyelitis, and change to one of the European vaccines as soon as possible. If RIG is not available initially, it should be given up to 7 days after starting vaccine. Equine RIG is widely used in Asia and Africa, and there is a 1–6% incidence of serum sickness, but anaphylaxis is rare. If the risk of rabies exposure seems high, it is worth curtailing a holiday to seek a recommended vaccine and RIG.

Two other post-exposure treatment regimens are recommended by the World Health Organization (1997) (Figure 21.7). They are economical multisite intradermal regimens which use only 40% of the amount of vaccine needed for the standard i.m. course. The eight-site regimen gives an accelerated antibody response: on day 0 use a whole 1 ml vial to inject about 0.1 ml PCECV or HDCV i.d. at eight sites (deltoids, thighs, suprascapular, lower anterior abdominal wall); on day 7 give 0.1 ml i.d. at four sites (deltoids, thighs); and on days 28 and 91, 0.1 ml i.d. at 1 site (Warrell *et al.*, 1985). There is no report of the use of PVRV, which contains 0.5 ml/ampoule, with this schedule, but the equivalent dose would be 0.05 ml/site.

The two-site intradermal post-exposure regimen has been used widely in Asia accompanied by RIG. It was designed for use with PVRV (Chutivongse *et al.*, 1990), with an i.d. dose of 0.1 ml/site. If other (1.0 ml) vaccines are used, each i.d. dose must be 0.2 ml. On

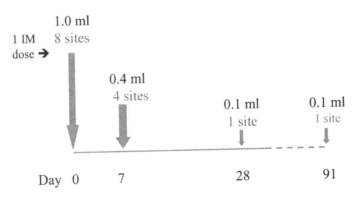

Eight-site id post-exposure vaccine regimen

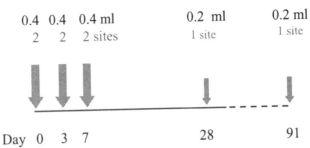

Two-site id post-exposure vaccine regimen

Figure 21.7 Intradermal post-exposure rabies vaccine regimens. The height of the arrows indicates the amount of vaccine used. 1 ml here represents one ampoule of vaccine = one i.m. dose = usually 1 ml, but 0.5 ml for PVRV

days 0, 3 and 7, give one i.d. dose at two sites (deltoids); on days 28 and 91, give one i.d. dose at one site (deltoid).

The two i.d. regimens use a similar total amount of vaccine, and aseptic techniques are essential when sharing ampoules. Opened ampoules should be used within 24 h. A comparative study showed that the eight-site method induces neutralising antibody more rapidly and to higher levels than the two-site regimen, which is important when RIG is not available (Madhusudana *et al.*, 2001).

CONTROL OF ANIMAL RABIES

The ability to control animal rabies depends on: the prevalence and host range of rabies in wild and domestic mammals in the region; the effectiveness of the local rabies surveillance network; the mode of

transmission of infection; the suitability of animal rabies vaccines; the social and cultural attitudes of the population to the vector species; and the financial resources to implement a control programme.

Urban Rabies

This is an epizootic of infection in domestic and stray dogs. Muzzling, vaccinating and restricting the movement of owned dogs and reducing the number of strays was effective in eradicating rabies from some islands and peninsulas. In several large cities in South America, intense mass vaccination programmes were dramatically effective in reducing the incidence of canine rabies and eliminating human disease. The size of urban dog populations, as with wild species, is determined by availability of food, water and shelter. Attempts to eliminate stray dogs by shooting and poisoning are difficult, unpopular and inefficient as fertility increases, restoring the numbers. Oral rabies vaccines for stray dogs have not proved very effective or easy to distribute; but methods of clearing rubbish to reduce the food supply, with parenteral vaccination and fertility control of strays, can be successful in localised areas. The involvement of the residents is essential. The role and influence of traditional methods of rabies prophylaxis must be taken into account and overcome tactfully by discussion and education.

Vaccination of owned dogs and cats should be mandatory in these areas. Facilities for viral diagnosis, disease surveillance and pre- and post-exposure vaccination of humans are also necessary. Countries free of rabies should prevent reinvasion by controlling the importation of mammals and by enforcing strict quarantine regulations from areas with urban rabies.

Wildlife Rabies

Attempts to reduce populations of vector species such as foxes and skunks have not been effective in the long term. Live attenuated rabies virus vaccine and a live vaccinia recombinant vaccine expressing rabies glyco-protein proved immunogenic by the oral route in foxes and apathogenic in other local species. Since 1978, these oral rabies vaccines, disguised in baits, have been distributed over the countryside by hand or by aeroplane (Brochier et al., 1996). The massive control campaigns have proved very successful in Western Europe. Fox rabies has been virtually eliminated in Switzerland, France, Luxembourg, Belgium and parts of other European countries. Long-term surveillance is planned to prevent resurgence. Vaccinia recombinant vaccines have also been used to control coyote, raccoon and fox rabies in North America. Raccoon rabies has been spreading North along the Eastern coastal States of the USA and the infection has reached Ontario, despite an intensive campaign of oral vaccination. New vaccines are being developed for skunks, mongooses and jackals. A single human infection by vaccinia recombinant rabies vaccine has been reported in a pregnant woman with a chronic skin condition, epidermolytic hyperkeratosis (Rupprecht et al., 2001).

Despite much work on developing DNA vaccines for rabies, none has yet proved suitable for use in animals or man.

In Latin America vampire bat rabies is a major cause of death in cattle, with disastrous economic consequences. Specific control methods include vaccination of cattle or treatment with anticoagulants, to

which bats, but not cattle, are highly sensitive. Vaccination of bats is being investigated.

No attempts have been made to control rabies in some vector species despite their potential to infect man. Insectivorous bats in North America and Europe are examples, due to their inaccessibility. Practical measures to avoid contact with bats and a low threshold for giving post-exposure treatment are the only means of preventing human infection (Centers for Disease Control, 1999a). In rabies endemic areas, people should be educated to avoid unnecessary contacts with wild and domestic carnivores and to seek medical advice immediately if they are bitten or scratched.

REFERENCES

Alvarez L, Fajardo R, Lopez E et al. (1994) Partial recovery from rabies in a nine-year-old boy. Pediatr Infect Dis J, 13, 1154–1155.

Amengual B, Whitby JE, King A et al. (1997) Evolution of European bat lyssaviruses. J Gen Virol, 78, 2319–2328.

Anderson LJ, Baer GM, Smith JS et al. (1981) Rapid antibody response to human diploid rabies vaccine. Am J Epidemiol, 113, 270–275.

Anderson LJ, Nicholson KG, Tauxe RV and Winkler WG (1984) Human rabies in the United States, 1960 to 1979: epidemiology, diagnosis, and prevention. Ann Intern Med, 100, 728–735.

Arguin PM, Murray-Lillibridge K, Miranda ME et al. (2002) Serologic evidence of Lyssavirus infections among bats: the Philippines. Emerg Infect Dis, 8, 258–262.

Badrane H, Bahloul C, Perrin P and Tordo N (2001) Evidence of two Lyssavirus phylogroups with distinct pathogenicity and immunogenicity. J Virol, 75, 3268–3276.

Baer GM, Shaddock JH, Quirion R et al. (1990) Rabies susceptibility and acetylcholine receptor. Lancet, 335, 664–665.

Bahri F, Letaief A, Ernez M et al. (1996) [Neurological complications in adults following rabies vaccine prepared from animal brains.] Presse Med, 25, 491–493.

Baltazard M and Bahmanyar M (1955) Practical trial of antirabies serum in people bitten by rabid wolves. Bull WHO, 13, 747–772.

Bernard KW, Smith PW, Kader FJ and Moran MJ (1982) Neuroparalytic illness and human diploid cell rabies vaccine. J Am Med Assoc, 248, 3136–3138.

Blenden DC, Creech W and Torres-Anjel MJ (1986) Use of immunofluorescence examination to detect rabies virus antigen in the skin of humans with clinical encephalitis. J Infect Dis, 154, 698–701.

Bøe E and Nyland H (1980) Guillain–Barré syndrome after vaccination with human diploid cell rabies vaccine. Scand J Infect Dis, 12, 231–232.

Brochier B, Aubert MF, Pastoret PP et al. (1996) Field use of a vaccinia-rabies recombinant vaccine for the control of sylvatic rabies in Europe and North America. Rev Sci Technol, 15, 947–970.

Bryceson AD, Greenwood BM, Warrell DA *et al.* (1975) Demonstration during life of rabies antigen in humans. *J Infect Dis*, **131**, 71–74.

Camelo S, Lafage M, Galelli A and Lafon M (2001) Selective role for the p55 Kd TNF-α receptor in immune unresponsiveness induced by an acute viral encephalitis. *J Neuroimmunol*, **113**, 95–108.

Celis E, Wiktor TJ, Dietzschold B and Koprowski H (1985) Amplification of rabies virus-induced stimulation of human T-cell lines and clones by antigen-specific antibodies. *J Virol*, **56**, 426–433.

Centers for Disease Control (10 Feb 2004) http://www.cdc.gov/ncidod/dvrd/rabies/Epidemiology/Epidemiology.htm

Centers for Disease Control (1977) Rabies in a laboratory worker—New York. *Morbid Mortal Wkly Rep*, **26**, 183–184 and 249–250.

Centers for Disease Control (1984) Human rabies—Texas. *Morbid Mortal Wkly Rep*, **33**, 469–470.

Centers for Disease Control (1999a) Human rabies prevention—United States, 1999. Recommendations of the Advisory Committee on Immunization Practices (ACIP). *Morbid Mortal Wkly Rep*, **48**, 1–21.

Centers for Disease Control (1999b) Mass treatment of humans who drank unpasteurized milk from rabid cows—Massachusetts, 1996–1998. *Morbid Mortal Wkly Rep*, **48**, 228–229.

Chakravarty A (2001) Neurologic illness following post-exposure prophylaxis with purified chick embryo cell antirabies vaccine. *J Assoc Physicians India*, **49**, 927–928.

Charlton KM, Nadin-Davis S, Casey GA and Wandeler AI (1997) The long incubation period in rabies: delayed progression of infection in muscle at the site of exposure. *Acta Neuropathol (Berl)*, **94**, 73–77.

Chutivongse S, Wilde H, Supich C *et al.* (1990) Postexposure prophylaxis for rabies with antiserum and intradermal vaccination. *Lancet*, **335**, 896–898.

Cliquet F, Aubert M and Sagne L (1998) Development of a fluorescent antibody virus neutralisation test (FAVN test) for the quantitation of rabies-neutralising antibody. *J Immunol Meth*, **212**, 79–87.

Crick J (1981) Rabies. In *Virus Diseases of Food Animals* (ed. Gibbs EPJ), pp 469–516. Academic Press, London.

Dietzschold B, Morimoto K and Hooper DC (2001) Mechanisms of virus-induced neuronal damage and the clearance of viruses from the CNS. *Curr Top Microbiol Immunol*, **253**, 145–155.

Dietzschold B, Wunner WH, Wiktor TJ *et al.* (1983) Characterization of an antigenic determinant of the glycoprotein that correlates with pathogenicity of rabies virus. *Proc Natl Acad Sci USA*, **80**, 70–74.

Dreesen DW, Bernard KW, Parker RA *et al.* (1986) Immune complex-like disease in 23 persons following a booster dose of rabies human diploid cell vaccine. *Vaccine*, **4**, 45–49.

East ML, Hofer H, Cox JH *et al.* (2001) Regular exposure to rabies virus and lack of symptomatic disease in Serengeti spotted hyenas. *Proc Natl Acad Sci USA*, **98**, 15026–15031.

Echevarria JE, Avellon A, Juste J *et al.* (2001) Screening of active lyssavirus infection in wild bat populations by viral RNA detection on oropharyngeal swabs. *J Clin Microbiol*, **39**, 3678–3683.

Etessami R, Conzelmann KK, Fadai-Ghotbi B *et al.* (2000) Spread and pathogenic characteristics of a G-deficient rabies virus recombinant: an *in vitro* and *in vivo* study. *J Gen Virol*, **81**, 2147–2153.

Familusi JB and Moore DL (1972) Isolation of a rabies related virus from the CSF of a child with 'aseptic meningitis'. *Afr J Med Sci*, **3**, 93–96.

Familusi JB, Osunkoya BO, Moore DL *et al.* (1972) A fatal human infection with Mokola virus. *Am J Trop Med Hyg*, **21**, 959–963.

Fekadu M, Endeshaw T, Alemu W *et al.* (1996) Possible human-to-human transmission of rabies in Ethiopia. *Ethiop Med J*, **34**, 123–127.

Gardner SD (1983) Prevention of rabies in man in England and Wales. In *Rabies: A Growing Threat* (ed. Pattison JR), pp 39–49, Van Nostrand Reinhold, Wokingham.

Gibbons RV (2002) Cryptogenic rabies, bats, and the question of aerosol transmission. *Ann Emerg Med*, **39**, 528–536.

Gosztonyi G (1994) Reproduction of *Lyssavirus* and functional aspects of pathogenisis. In *Lyssaviruses* (eds Rupprecht CE, Dietzschold B and Koprowski H), pp 43–68. Springer-Verlag, Berlin.

Hanna JN, Carney IK, Smith GA *et al.* (2000) Australian bat lyssavirus infection: a second human case, with a long incubation period. *Med J Aust*, **172**, 597–599.

Hattwick MA (1974) Human Rabies. *Publ Health Rev*, **3**, 229–274.

Hattwick MA, Weis TT, Stechschulte CJ *et al.* (1972) Recovery from rabies. A case report. *Ann Intern Med*, **76**, 931–942.

Helmick CG, Tauxe RV and Vernon AA (1987) Is there a risk to contacts of patients with rabies? *Rev Infect Dis*, **9**, 511–518.

Hemachudha T, Khawplod P, Phanuphak P and Griffin DE (1989) Enhanced antibody response to rabies virus in patients with neurologic complications following brain tissue-derived rabies vaccination. *Asian Pac J Allergy Immunol*, **7**, 47–50.

Hemachudha T, Laothamatas J and Rupprecht CE (2002) Human rabies: a disease of complex neuropathogenetic mechanisms and diagnostic challenges. *Lancet Neurol*, **1**, 101–109.

Hemachudha T, Mitrabhakdi E, Wilde H *et al.* (1999) Additional reports of failure to respond to treatment after rabies exposure in Thailand. *Clin Infect Dis*, **28**, 143–144.

Hemachudha T, Phanuphak P, Sriwanthana B *et al.* (1988) Immunologic study of human encephalitic and paralytic rabies. Preliminary report of 16 patients. *Am J Med*, **84**, 673–677.

Irwin DJ, Wunner WH, Ertl HC and Jackson AC (1999) Basis of rabies virus neurovirulence in mice: expression of major histocompatibility complex class I and class II mRNAs. *J Neurovirol*, **5**, 485–494.

Iwasaki Y, Liu DS, Yamamoto T and Konno H (1985) On the replication and spread of rabies virus in the human central nervous system. *J Neuropathol Exp Neurol*, **44**, 185–195.

Iwata M, Unno T, Minamoto N *et al.* (2000) Rabies virus infection prevents the modulation by α(2)-adrenoceptors, but not muscarinic receptors, of Ca(2+) channels in NG108-15 cells. *Eur J Pharmacol*, **404**, 79–88.

Jackson AC (2002a) Human disease. In *Rabies* (eds Jackson AC and Wunner AH), pp 219–244. Elsevier Science/Academic Press, San Diego, CA.

Jackson AC (2002b) Pathogenesis. In *Rabies* (eds Jackson AC and Wunner AH), pp 245–282. Elsevier Science/Academic Press, San Diego, CA.

Jackson AC, Warrell MJ, Rupprecht CE *et al.* (2003) Management of rabies in humans. *Clin Infect Dis*, **36**, 60–63.

Jackson AC, Ye H, Phelan CC *et al.* (1999) Extraneural organ involvement in human rabies. *Lab Invest*, **79**, 945–951.

Jacob Y, Badrane H, Ceccaldi PE and Tordo N (2000) Cytoplasmic dynein LC8 interacts with lyssavirus phosphoprotein. *J Virol*, **74**, 10217–10222.

Kaplan MM and Cohen D (1962) Studies on the local treatment of wounds for the prevention of rabies. *Bull WHO*, **26**, 765–775.

Kaplan MM, Wiktor T and Koprowski H (1966) An intracerebral assay procedure in mice for chemical inactivation of rabies virus. *Bull WHO*, **34**, 293–297.

King AA, Meridith CD and Thomson GR (1994) The biology of Southern African lyssavirus variants. In *Lyssaviruses* (eds Rupprecht CE, Dietzschold B and Koprowski H), pp 267–295. Springer-Verlag, Berlin.

King AA and Turner GS (1993) Rabies: a review. *J Comp Pathol*, **108**, 1–39.

Knittel T, Ramadori G, Mayet WJ *et al.* (1989) Guillain–Barré syndrome and human diploid cell rabies vaccine. *Lancet*, **1**, 1334–1335.

Koprowski H and Dietzschold B (1997) Rabies: lessons from the past and a glimpse into the future. In *In Defense of the Brain: Current Concepts in the Immunopathogenesis and Clinical Aspects of CNS Infections* (eds Peterson P and Remington JS), pp 329–357. Blackwell, Malden, MA.

Kuwert EK, Barsenbach C, Werner J *et al.* (1981) Early/high and late/low responders among HDCS vaccines? In *Cell Culture Rabies Vaccines and Their Protective Effect in Man* (eds Kuwert EK, Wiktor TJ and Koprowski H), pp 160–167. International Green Cross, Geneva.

Label L and Batts DH (1982) Transverse myelitis caused by duck embryo rabies vaccine. *Arch Neurol*, **39**, 426–430.

Lafon M (1997) Rabies virus superantigen. In *Viral Superantigens* (ed. Tomonari K), pp 151–170. CRC Press, Boca Raton, FL.

Lancet (1991) Human rabies: strain identification reveals lengthy incubation. *Lancet*, **337**, 822–823.

Langevin C, Jaaro H, Bressanelli S *et al.* (2002) Rabies virus glycoprotein (RVG) is a trimeric ligand for the N-terminal cysteine-rich domain of the mammalian p75 neurotrophin receptor. *J Biol Chem*, **277**, 37655–37662.

Lentz TL, Burrage TG, Smith AL *et al.* (1982) Is the acetylcholine receptor a rabies virus receptor? *Science*, **215**, 182–184.

Lockhart BP, Tordo N and Tsiang H (1992) Inhibition of rabies virus transcription in rat cortical neurons with the dissociative anesthetic ketamine. *Antimicrob Agents Chemother*, **36**, 1750–1755.

Lodmell DL, Parnell MJ, Bailey JR *et al.* (2001) One-time gene gun or intramuscular rabies DNA vaccination of non-human primates: comparison of neutralizing antibody responses and protection against rabies virus 1 year after vaccination. *Vaccine*, **20**, 838–844.

Madhusudana SN, Anand NP and Shamsundar R (2001) Evaluation of two intradermal vaccination regimens using purified chick embryo cell vaccine for post-exposure prophylaxis of rabies. *Natl Med J India*, **14**, 145–147.

Madhusudana SN, Nagaraj D, Uday M *et al.* (2002) Partial recovery from rabies in a six-year-old girl. *Int J Infect Dis*, **6**, 85–86.

Mazarakis ND, Azzouz M, Rohll JB *et al.* (2001) Rabies virus glycoprotein pseudotyping of lentiviral vectors enables retrograde axonal transport and access to the nervous system after peripheral delivery. *Hum Mol Genet*, **10**, 2109–2121.

McColl KA, Tordo N and Aguilar Setien AA (2000) Bat lyssavirus infections. *Rev Sci Technol*, **19**, 177–196.

Mebatsion T (2001) Extensive attenuation of rabies virus by simultaneously modifying the dynein light chain binding site in the P protein and replacing Arg333 in the G protein. *J Virol*, **75**, 11496–11502.

Meredith CD, Rossouw AP and van Praag Koch H (1971) An unusual case of human rabies thought to be of chiropteran origin. *S Afr Med J*, **45**, 767–769.

Merigan TC, Baer GM, Winkler WG *et al.* (1984) Human leukocyte interferon administration to patients with symptomatic and suspected rabies. *Ann Neurol*, **16**, 82–87.

Messenger SL, Smith JS and Rupprecht CE (2002) Emerging epidemiology of bat-associated cryptic cases of rabies in humans in the United States. *Clin Infect Dis*, **35**, 738–747.

Metze K and Feiden W (1991) Rabies virus ribonucleoprotein in the heart. *N Engl J Med*, **324**, 1814–1815.

Mitmoonpitak C and Tepsumethanon V (2002) Dog rabies in Bangkok. *J Med Assoc Thai*, **85**, 71–76.

Murphy FA (1977) Rabies pathogenesis. *Arch Virol*, **54**, 279–297.

Nathwani D, McIntyre PG, White K *et al.* (2003) Fatal human rabies caused by European bat *Lyssavirus* type 2a infection in Scotland. *Clin Infect Dis*, **37**, 598–601.

Nicholson KG, Burney MI, Ali S and Perkins FT (1983) Stability of human diploid-cell-strain rabies vaccine at high ambient temperatures. *Lancet*, **i**, 916–918.

Noah DL, Drenzek CL, Smith JS *et al.* (1998) Epidemiology of human rabies in the United States, 1980 to 1996. *Ann Intern Med*, **128**, 922–930.

Ogunkoya AB, Beran GW and Umoh JU (1990) Serological evidence of infection of dogs and man in Nigeria by lyssaviruses (family *Rhabdoviridae*). *Trans R Soc Trop Med*, **84**, 842–845.

Pará M (1965) An outbreak of post-vaccinal rabies (rage de laboratoire) in Fortaleza, Brazil, in 1960. Residual fixed virus as the etiological agent. *Bull WHO*, **33**, 177–182.

Perl DP (1975) The pathology of rabies in the central nervous system. In *The Natural History of Rabies* (ed. Baer GM), vol I, pp 235–272. Academic Press, New York.

Porras C, Barboza JJ, Fuenzalida E *et al.* (1976) Recovery from rabies in man. *Ann Intern Med*, **85**, 44–48.

Prabhakar BS and Nathanson N (1981) Acute rabies death mediated by antibody. *Nature*, **290**, 590–591.

Prosniak M, Hooper DC, Dietzschold B and Koprowski H (2001) Effect of rabies virus infection on gene expression in mouse brain. *Proc Natl Acad Sci USA*, **98**, 2758–2763.

Quiroz E, Moreno N, Peralta PH and Tesh RB (1988) A human case of encephalitis associated with vesicular stomatitis virus (Indiana serotype) infection. *Am J Trop Med Hyg*, **39**, 312–314.

Raux H, Flamand A and Blondel D (2000) Interaction of the rabies virus P protein with the LC8 dynein light chain. *J Virol*, **74**, 10212–10216.

Roine RO, Hillbom M, Valle M *et al.* (1988) Fatal encephalitis caused by a bat-borne rabies-related virus. Clinical findings. *Brain*, **111**, 1505–1516.

Rupprecht CE, Blass L, Smith K *et al.* (2001) Human infection due to recombinant vaccinia-rabies glycoprotein virus. *N Engl J Med*, **345**, 582–586.

Samaratunga H, Searle JW and Hudson N (1998) Non-rabies *Lyssavirus* human encephalitis from fruit bats: Australian bat Lyssavirus (pteropid lyssavirus) infection. *Neuropathol Appl Neurobiol*, **24**, 331–335.

Selimov MA, Tatarov AG, Botvinkin AD *et al.* (1989) Rabies-related Yulivirus: identification with a panel of monoclonal antibodies. *Acta Virol (Praha)*, **33**, 542–546.

Série C and Andral L (1962) Études expérimentales sur la rage en Éthiopie. II. Pouvoir virulicide du sérum des chiens errants. *Ann Inst Pasteur*, **98**, 688–693.

Serra-Cobo J, Amengual B, Abellan C and Bourhy H (2002) European bat lyssavirus infection in Spanish bat populations. *Emerging Infectious Diseases*, **8**, 413–420.

Smith JS (2002) Molecular epidemiology. In *Rabies* (eds Jackson AC and Wunner WH), pp 79–111. Elsevier Science/Academic Press, San Diego, CA.

Smith JS, Fishbein DB, Rupprecht CE and Clark K (1991) Unexplained rabies in three immigrants in the United States. A virologic investigation. *N Engl J Med*, **324**, 205–211.

Smith JS, Yager PA and Baer GM (1996) A rapid fluorescent focus inhibition test (RFFIT) for determining rabies virus-neutralising antibody. In *Laboratory Techniques in Rabies* (eds Meslin F-X, Kaplan MM and Koprowski H), pp 181–192. World Health Organization, Geneva.

Strady A, Lang J, Lienard M *et al.* (1998) Antibody persistence following preexposure regimens of cell-culture rabies vaccines: 10-year follow-up and proposal for a new booster policy. *J Infect Dis*, **177**, 1290–1295.

Strady C, Jaussaud R, Beguinot I *et al.* (2000) Predictive factors for the neutralizing antibody response following pre-exposure rabies immunization: validation of a new booster dose strategy. *Vaccine*, **18**, 2661–2667.

Suntharasamai P, Warrell MJ, Viravan C *et al.* (1987) Purified chick embryo cell rabies vaccine: economical multisite intradermal regimen for post-exposure prophylaxis. *Epidemiol Infect*, **99**, 755–765.

Sureau P, Portnoi D, Rollin P *et al.* (1981) Prévention de la transmission inter-humaine de la rage après greffe de cornée. *CR Acad Sci Paris*, **293**, 689–692.

Tangchai P, Yenbutr D and Vejjajiva A (1970) Central nervous system lesions in human rabies. A study of twenty-four cases. *J Med Assoc Thailand*, **53**, 471–486.

Théodoridès J (1986) *Histoire de la Rage*. Cave Canem, Masson, Paris.

Thoulouze MI, Lafage M, Schachner M *et al.* (1998) The neural cell adhesion molecule is a receptor for rabies virus. *J Virol*, **72**, 7181–7190.

Tornatore CS and Richert JR (1990) CNS demyelination associated with diploid cell rabies vaccine. *Lancet*, **335**, 1346–1347.

Trimarchi CV and Smith JS (2002) Diagnostic evaluation. In *Rabies* (eds Jackson AC and Wunner AH), pp 307–349. Elsevier Science/Academic Press, San Diego, CA.

Tsiang H (1993) Pathophysiology of rabies virus infection of the nervous system. *Adv Virus Res*, **42**, 375–412.

Turner GS (1985) Immune response after rabies vaccination: basic aspects. *Ann Inst Pasteur/Virol*, **126E**, 453–460.

Turner GS, Aoki FY, Nicholson KG *et al.* (1976) Human diploid cell strain rabies vaccine. Rapid prophylactic immunisation of volunteers with small doses. *Lancet*, **1**, 1379–1381.

Vodopija I, Sureau P, Smerdel S *et al.* (1988) Interaction of rabies vaccine with human rabies immunoglobulin and reliability of a 2–1–1 schedule application for postexposure treatment. *Vaccine*, **6**, 283–286.

Warner CK, Whitfield SG, Fekadu M and Ho H (1997) Procedures for reproducible detection of rabies virus antigen mRNA and genome *in situ* in formalin-fixed tissues. *J Virol Meth*, **67**, 5–12.

Warrell DA, Davidson NM, Pope HM *et al.* (1976) Pathophysiologic studies in human rabies. *Am J Med*, **60**, 180–190.

Warrell MJ, Looareesuwan S, Manatsathit S *et al.* (1988) Rapid diagnosis of rabies and post-vaccinal encephalitides. *Clin Exp Immunol*, **71**, 229–234.

Warrell MJ, Nicholson KG, Warrell DA *et al.* (1985) Economical multiple-site intradermal immunisation with human diploid-cell-strain vaccine is effective for post-exposure rabies prophylaxis. *Lancet*, **i**, 1059–1062.

Warrell MJ, White NJ, Looareesuwan S *et al.* (1989) Failure of interferon alfa and tribavirin in rabies encephalitis. *Br Med J*, **299**, 830–833.

Warrington RJ, Martens CJ, Rubin M *et al.* (1987) Immunologic studies in subjects with a serum sickness-like illness after immunization with human diploid cell rabies vaccine. *J Allergy Clin Immunol*, **79**, 605–610.

Webster WA and Casey GA (1996) Virus isolation in neuroblastoma cell culture. In *Laboratory Techniques in Rabies* (eds Meslin F-X, Kaplan MM and Koprowski H), pp 96–104. World Health Organization, Geneva.

Wellenberg GJ, Audry L, Rønsholt L *et al.* (2002) Presence of European bat lyssavirus RNAs in apparently healthy *Rousettus aegyptiacus* bats. *Arch Virol*, **147**, 349–361.

Winkler WG (1975) Airborne rabies. In *The Natural History of Rabies* (ed. Baer GM), pp 115–121. Academic Press, New York.

Winkler WG, Fashinell TR, Leffingwell L *et al.* (1973) Airborne rabies transmission in a laboratory worker. *J Am Med Assoc*, **226**, 1219–1221.

World Health Organization (10 Feb 2004) *Rabies Bulletin Europe. Rabies Surveillance Report*. www.who-rabies-bulletin.org

World Health Organization (1997) WHO Recommendations on rabies post-exposure treatment and the correct technique of intradermal immunization against rabies. WHO/EMC/ZOO.96.6 http://www.who.int/emc-documents/rabies/docs/whoemczoo966.pdf (10 Feb 2004).

World Health Organization (2001) Strategies for the control and elimination of rabies in Asia. Geneva July 2001. WHO/CDS/CSR/EPH/2002.8

Wunner WH (2002) Rabies virus. In *Rabies* (eds Jackson AC and Wunner WH), pp 23–77. Elsevier Science/Academic Press, San Diego, CA.

22

Papillomaviruses

Dennis McCance

University of Rochester, Rochester, NY, USA

INTRODUCTION

Papillomavirus is one of the two genera of the family *Papovaviridae*. However, as will be seen, the viruses belonging to this group are quite different from the other genera, both in genome size and organisation as well as pathogenesis.

The papillomaviruses (Latin: *papilla* = nipple; *oma* = tumour) produce in their host benign skin tumours (papillomas), containing variable amounts of infectious virus, and have been a recognised lesion since the fifth century BC. Common hand and plantar warts are the most frequent skin papillomas of man and until recently these viruses generated little clinical or scientific interest, since the typical lesions were a cosmetic nuisance and the viruses were not thought to be involved in serious disease. However, 20 years ago the first papillomavirus isolated from invasive carcinoma of the cervix was described (Durst *et al.*, 1983). Since then papillomaviruses have been linked with other squamous cell carcinomas (SCCs) of mucosal and cutaneous epithelia and interest in these viruses has been stimulated, resulting in significant advances in our understanding of the natural history and pathogenic process.

CLASSIFICATION

At present papillomaviruses are classified into five super-groups: A, genital human papillomaviruses, (HPV); B (associated with epidermodysplasia verruciformis); C (ungulate fibropapillomaviruses); D (bovine papillomaviruses, causing true papillomas); and E (animal and human cutaneous PVs). There are 11 groups under super-group A, two under B and C and one group under each of D and E. The classification results from the deduced evolutionary relationships amongst the papillomaviruses as judged by the sequence similarity of their genomes. For example, A9 contains the commonly isolated virus HPV-16 and the related viruses HPV-31, -33, -35, -52 and -58. Table 22.1 has a breakdown on the classification. Note that two of the animal viruses, rhesus monkey and pygmy chimpanzee papillomaviruses, are grouped with the human genital isolates in groups A9 and 10, respectively.

PHYSICAL AND CHEMICAL PROPERTIES

Structure

The capsids of the papillomaviruses have icosahedral symmetry containing 72 capsomeres with a diameter of 52–55 nm (Figure 22.1).

Genome

The human papillomavirus (HPV) virion contains a double-stranded DNA molecule of 5×10^6 Da molecular weight with an average of 7900 base pairs. The DNA, when in the virion, has a supercoiled circular configuration.

The molecular organisation of the papillomavirus genome is well conserved between viruses of various species and an example of one of the common genital isolates is shown in Figure 22.2A. In this figure the

Principles and Practice of Clinical Virology, Fifth Edition. Edited by A. J. Zuckerman, J. E. Banatvala, J. R. Pattison, P. D. Griffiths and B. D. Schoub
© 2004 John Wiley & Sons Ltd   ISBN 0 470 84338 1

Table 22.1   Classification of the *Papillomavirus* subfamily

Super-groups																
Group A											B		C		D	E
1	2	3	4	5	6	7	8	9	10	11	1	2	1	2	1	1
32	3	61	2a	26	30	18	7	16	6b	34	5	4	B1	E1	B3	1a
42	10		27	51	45	40	43	31	11		8	48	B2	D1	B4	41
	28		57	69	53	39		33	13		9	50			B6	63
	29				56	59		35	44		12	60				Co
					66	68		52	55		14d	65				Ro
						70		58	P1		15					Cr
								67			17					
								R1*			19					
											20					
											21					
											22					
											23					
											24					
											25					
											36					
											37					
											38					
											47					
											49					

*R, rhesus monkey papillomavirus; P, pygmy chimpanzee papillomavirus; B, bovine papillomavirus; Cr, cottontail rabbit papillomavirus; Co, canine oral papillomavirus; D, deer papillomavirus; E, elk papillomavirus; Ro, rabbit oral papillomavirus.
Adapted from the Los Alamos National Laboratory HPV database: http://hpv-web.lanl.gov/

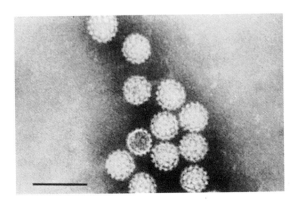

Figure 22.1   Electron micrograph of human papillomavirus from a genital wart (negative stain; × 154 000; bar = 100 nm). Courtesy of Dr J. D. Oriel

so are read in the same direction, remembering that transcription is in the 5′ to 3′ direction. HPV-16 codes for five early and three late proteins. There is an upstream regulatory region (URR), which contains the major early promoter at base 97 and enhancer elements for transcription of early genes and also contains the origin of replication. A late promoter for the transcription of the capsid protein mRNA has been identified and lies in the E7 ORF at 670, although some of the late transcripts may initiate around this nucleotide.

Viral Coded Proteins

There are five proteins coded for by the early region of the HPV genome and three late proteins. Because there are differences in the pathogenesis of various HPV types, this is reflected in some of the functions of the early proteins. Therefore, for brevity a short summary of the functions of HPV-16 (Figure 22.2) early (E prefix) and late (L prefix) proteins is presented and their molecular weights are shown in Table 22.2.

Three of the early proteins, E6, E7 and E5, have properties which are consistent with the virus having to stimulate the infected cells into S-phase, so the viral

genome is represented as a linear molecule with the boxed areas indicating the open reading frames (ORFs) and for convention is divided into two areas, coding for early (E) and late (L) proteins. Because of the overlapping nature of the ORFs, the mRNAs transcribed are complex and it is not always clear which proteins each transcript codes (Figure 22.2B). All the ORFs are transcribed from the same strand and

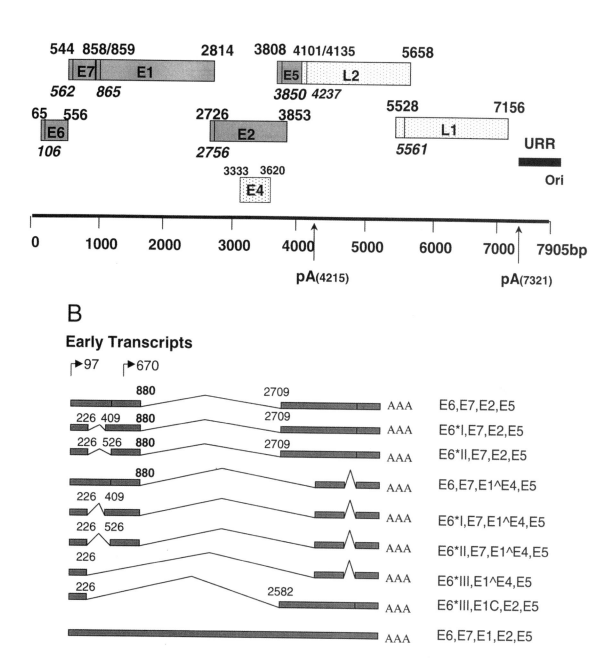

Figure 22.2 (A) Schematic of the HPV-16 genome organisation. The early genes are solid grey and the late genes are speckled. The base pairs of the open reading frames are shown and the ATG start codon is shown in italics. E4 is spliced to the N-terminal of E1 (E1^E4) since it has no ATG of its own. The poly A + signals for the early and late mRNA are shown (pA). The origin (Ori) of replication and the upstream regulatory region (URR) or the main early promoter region are indicated. (B) Determination of mRNA species detected in many cases by RT-PCR, so some of the 5′ and 3′ ends are uncertain. E4 is always expressed as a fusion of E1^E4

Table 22.2 Molecular weights of HPV-16 proteins

Protein	Molecular weight (kDa)[a]
E1	70
E2	45
E4	17
E5	8
E6	16
E7	11
L1	55
L2	50

[a]Molecular weight on SDS-PAGE gels may be different, e.g. E7 runs at 15–16 kDa because of charged amino acids in the N-terminus of the protein, but codes for a protein of 11 kDa and L1 runs at 75 kDa.

DNA has the cell's replicative machinery available for propagation of the genome. It has to be remembered that the virus is attempting to replicate in cells that are programmed to differentiate and so will have little or no replicative enzymes available to the virus. Both E6 and E7 are important for the efficient immortalisation of human keratinocytes and have functions which disrupt the normal control of G_1 to S phase progression. E6 has been shown to bind the human p53 protein and cause its rapid degradation through the ubiquitin proteolysis pathway (Scheffner et al., 1990). It has been shown to bind a number of other cellular proteins (McMurray et al., 2001), but the biological consequences of the binding are unclear. For instance, E6 has also been shown to bind to a Ca^{2+} binding protein called E6BP, which has homology to a cellular protein, ERC-55, of unknown function (Chen et al., 1995) and also binds to proteins with a PDZ domain, such as membrane-associated guanylate kinase homologues (MAGUKs), which are found at the membrane and are thought to be involved in intra- and intercellular interactions (Thomas et al., 2001). The biological consequences of these interactions have not been delineated, although it appears that binding to MAGUK proteins may correlate with the ability of E6 to cooperate with E7 for immortalisation. E7 binds another cellular protein, the retinoblastoma gene product (pRB; Dyson et al., 1989), and derepresses the inhibitory activity of Rb for transcription factors that are important for expression of genes, whose products are essential for DNA synthesis. Repression of transcription may be due to the binding by Rb of a histone deacetylase protein (Brehm et al., 1998), which functions to condense chromatin and restrict the access of transcription factors to DNA. E7 appears to compete for the binding site of the deacetylase on Rb. Both these cellular proteins are negative regulators of the cell cycle and so interference with their normal function may allow cells to divide in an uncontrolled manner. E7 has also been shown to bind to other cellular proteins, such as various members of the AP-1 family of transcription factors, and to upregulate their activity (Antinore et al., 1996) and also some members of the basal transcription machinery, such as TATA-binding protein (TBP; Phillips and Vousden, 1997).

E1 and E2 are involved in the replication of the HPV genome (see section on Viral Replication, below). E2 has additional functions in that it can positively and negatively regulate transcription from the early promoter. The full-length E2 protein contains a transactivation domain at the 5′ end and a DNA binding domain in the 3′ half, and the active complex is a dimer. Negative regulation of the HPV early promoter is due to the fact that one of the E2 binding sites lies next to the TATA box of this promoter and so E2 binding sterically inhibits binding of the TATA-binding protein and therefore inhibits initiation of the early transcripts.

E5 is a membrane-associated hydrophobic protein with transforming activity for rodent fibroblasts. The E5 protein inhibits the acidification of endosomes (Straight et al., 1995) by binding to the smallest subunit (16 kDa) of the vacuolar ATPase, a multi-component proton pump (Conrad et al., 1993). In human keratinocytes this results in the delay of the epidermal growth factor receptor (EGFR) degradation and a hyperstimulated cell. Since the EGFR is the major growth factor receptor on keratinocytes, this activity may be important for stimulating cells into S phase for viral DNA replication. E5 can transform rodent fibroblasts and in the presence of the epidermal growth factor there is an increase in the efficiency of transformation (Leechanachai et al., 1992).

The late proteins L1 and L2 are the major and minor capsid proteins, respectively, of the virion. The DNA and amino acid sequences are highly conserved between HPV types, especially in the L1 protein. The amino acid homology can be as high as 76% between HPV 16 and 33 (group A9). However, even within groups of PVs type-specific epitopes predominate, although some weak cross-reactivity has been observed, so it is possible to differentiate between types on a serological basis (see next section).

The mRNA for the E4 protein is spliced, with the 5′ portion coded for by the first few base pairs of E1, spliced to the E4 open reading frame. The message is detected late in infection, although it has the prefix of an early gene. E4 interacts with cellular microfilaments, causing them to collapse (Doorbar et al., 1991), but the motive for this interaction is not clear, although it has been suggested that this might allow the virions to be more easily released from the differentiated keratinocyte after transfer to a new susceptible host.

There are host-coded histone proteins, H2a, H2b, H3 and H4, associated with the viral DNA within the virion.

SEROLOGY

The expression of the major capsid protein, L1, in yeast and insect cells resulting in the folding and production of virus-like particles (VLPs) has permitted serological studies on the relatedness of HPVs and to determine serological responses in infected patients. VLPs of human papillomaviruses consisting of L1, were synthesised using baculovirus vectors and insect cells, allowing the formation of an icosahedral structure similar to that of the virion (Kirnbauer et al., 1992). VLPs can also be produced which contain both the major (L1) and minor (L2) capsid proteins, and the latter appears to stabilise the icosahedral structure and also has been shown to possess neutralising epitopes. Antiviral antibodies have been produced to virions of HPV-11 and -16 and these antibodies recognise VLPs of the L1 protein from HPV-11 and -16, respectively (Rose et al., 1994) but do not cross-react. Therefore, VLPs are recognised by antibodies raised to infectious virus particles, and vice versa. The antibodies to VLPs or virions detect conformational epitopes, unlike earlier serological studies, where disrupted particles, or fusion proteins of L1 or peptides of regions of L1 were used either as targets or to raise antibodies to the L1 protein, and produced extensive cross-reactivity. This cross-reactivity was so complete that antibodies to disrupted BPV-1 particles recognised linear epitopes in most HPV types. Therefore, it was only with the production of VLPs that the serological differences between HPVs, even those closely related, became apparent, e.g. within one group, say A9 containing HPV-16, -31 and -33, polyclonal antibodies only react well with the type to which the antibodies were raised, although some cross-reactivity has been observed. The level of cross-reactivity is very low and is probably not biologically relevant in cross-protection. Monoclonal antibodies to virions or VLPs have shown that there are predominantly type-specific epitopes, although in closely related viruses such as HPV-6 and -11, where L1 is over 80% homologous at the amino acid level, cross-reactive epitopes have been observed. While there is little cross-reactivity at the antibody level, there appears to be more at the T cell receptor level, as lymphoproliferative assays show some cross-reactivity between types such as HPV-6 and -16.

VIRAL REPLICATION

Infection of tissue culture cells with papillomavirus particles and subsequent propagation of infectious virus has not been achieved. The major problem is that HPV virion production depends on differentiating epithelial cells and by their nature these cells do not grow in vitro. However, recently (Frattini et al., 1996) it has been possible to transfect human keratinocytes, the natural host cell, with HPV-31 DNA, select stable cell lines containing episomal copies of HPV-31 DNA, and then differentiate the cells using the raft culture system and show that virus particle production occurs in a few cells in the uppermost part of the differentiated epithelium. HPV-11 DNA has also been replicated in keratinocytes by the same laboratory, although because HPV-11 is unable to immortalise human keratinocytes, the cells senesce and so the replicating DNA is lost. The distribution of the virus particles is the same as that observed in infected epithelium (Figure 22.3). The level of virus production is very low and not enough to produce virus particles for serology or infectivity studies. However, propagation of HPV types has been successful in a nude mouse kidney capsule system (Kreider et al., 1985) and in human skin grafts onto the epithelium of SCID mice (Bonnez et al., 1998). In the former system human foreskin tissue fragments are mixed with a viral suspension of HPV and then the tissue is transplanted under the kidney capsule of a nude mouse. Over the next 60 days the tissue fragments grow and produce infectious HPV virus. Both HPV-11 and -16 have been propagated in this animal model; however, the system is obviously complex, requiring skills and animal facilities not available to all. In the alternative method, the tissue fragments are placed under the skin of the immunocompromised SCID mouse and so the growth of the tissue can be monitored and, while the surgical skills are less demanding, the model is not routine.

The origin of replication of HPV-11 and -31 (Frattini and Laimins, 1994; Lu et al., 1993) has been mapped extensively and the region is conserved in other HPV types. The mapping has been achieved by cloning the origin region into a bacterial vector and transfecting mammalian cells, along with plasmids expressing the E1 and E2 proteins of the respective virus. The E1 and E2 proteins are the only HPV-specific products necessary for the replication of the origin-containing plasmid. The origin region of the

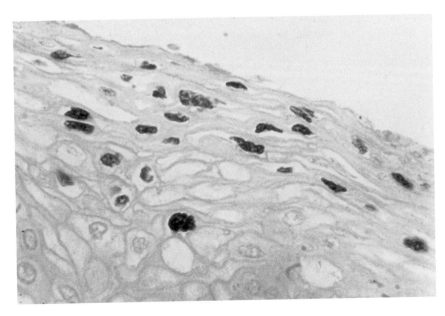

Figure 22.3 A section of biopsy containing CIN 1, showing nuclear staining of HPV-16 L1 antigen using a monoclonal antibody, followed by alkaline phosphatase-tagged antimouse secondary antibodies. Note that the dark-staining nuclei are found in the outer, differentiated part of the epithelium

DNA has been mapped to a region at the 3' end of the URR (Figure 22.2a) and both E1 and E2 have specific DNA binding sites at the origin. In addition to binding at the origin, E1 and E2 can bind together and E1 has been shown to have ATPase and helicase activities, which are typical of viral proteins, such as SV_{40} large that are involved in the initiation of viral T DNA replication.

NATURAL HISTORY OF HPV INFECTIONS

HPVs infect and replicate in squamous epithelium on both keratinised and mucosal surfaces. Most people are infected with certain cutaneous viruses, such as the ones causing hand and foot warts (HPV types 1, 2, 3, 4), during childhood and adolescence. A small group of individuals with the rare autosomal recessive disease epidermodysplasia verruciformis (EV) harbour a number of virus types not often isolated from normal people (Table 22.1, groups B1 and 2). Two common presentations in EV patients are multiple warts, which may be so numerous as to produce coalescent areas and dry, scaly flat lesions, which may be red or heavily pigmented. These latter skin lesions, although not having a wart-like appearance, contain many of the unusual types of HPV in groups B1 and B2. Squamous

cell carcinomas develop in nearly one-third of patients with EV, usually in areas of skin exposed to the sun (face, neck and hands being most commonly affected); HPV-5 and -8 are commonly found in these lesions

Table 22.3 HPV types isolated from patients with the genetic disease epidermodysplasia verruciformis (EV) and associated diseases

HPV type	Lesions
5	Warts/SCC
8	SCC
9	Warts
12	Warts
14	SCC
15	Warts
17	Warts/SCC
19	Warts
20	Warts/SCC
21	Warts
22	Warts
23	Warts
24	Warts
25	Warts
36	Warts
46	Warts
47	Warts

SCC, squamous cell carcinoma. HPV types -38 (melanoma), -41 (SCC) and -48 (SCC) were isolated from immunosuppressed patients. This table was assembled with the help of Dr C. Wheeler.

while types -14, -17 and -20 (Table 22.3) account for a smaller number. While the viruses found in EV patients are not isolated from normal individuals, some types, such as -5 and -8, have been detected in squamous cell carcinomas in allograft recipients. Because the disease EV is rare, and with the isolation of some of the EV-associated HPVs from transplant patients, it suggests that these viruses must be circulating in the community, infecting normal individuals perhaps without any associated clinical lesions.

As discussed above, there are mucotropic HPVs which mostly infect the genito-urinary tract. Common isolates like HPV-6 and -11, which cause benign condyloma, can also infect the oral cavity, particularly the larynx. Infection of the larynx is rare, but usually requires several episodes of surgery or laser treatment for removal of recurrent lesions. Frequent recurrences may be due to the fact that only the visible lesions are treated, although healthy-looking areas of mucosal tissue may harbour HPV genomes. The oral cavity is also infected with other HPV types associated with oral warts and hyperkeratosis.

Transmission is thought to occur from one epithelial surface to another in exfoliated cells containing infectious virus, rather than free virus particles. Therefore, direct contact is the most efficient way to transmit infection. Direct contact through sexual intercourse is the most important mode of transmission of genital viruses. However, an infected mother may transmit virus to her neonate during delivery through the birth canal. This route of infection is thought to be a major cause of larynx warts in babies and young children. It is possible that other modes of transmission occur for the genital viruses, since a number of studies have detected DNA in the genital and perianal regions of young children. However, the route of transmission, apart from those mentioned above, is unclear.

Infection of the genital mucosa is common and involves hundreds of thousands of new cases each year, usually among sexually active individuals, with 18–30 year-olds having the highest incidence (cf. common hand warts). The transmission rate was first described back in the 1970s when Oriel (1971) showed that 64% of partners of individuals with genital warts also developed warts. Subsequent studies have shown that up to 90% of male partners have shared common HPV types with their partner's cervical isolates. Therefore, transmission of HPV types is common in the relatively stable setting of partners, although the frequency of transmission during casual sex with different partners is still unclear.

Infection with certain of the genital HPV types increases the risk of malignant disease, especially of the cervix, and in the next section there will be a discussion of the pathogenesis of the genital HPV types.

PATHOGENESIS

HPVs cause benign and malignant changes in epithelial cells. It is the latter property that will be dealt with in this section, since certain HPV types are the most important component of the aetiology of genital cancers and cervical cancer is one of the most common causes of cancer-related death in women worldwide.

Oncogenic Potential of Papillomaviruses

Until recent epidemiological and laboratory-based studies, most of the evidence for an oncogenic potential of HPVs came from research with animal papillomaviruses. Work in the 1930s showed that the cottontail rabbit papillomavirus (CRPV) produced benign tumours in this animal, its natural host, and that these benign tumours in 25% of cases would become malignant after 12 months. Benign tumours produced in domestic rabbits became malignant more frequently and within a shorter time. Also, application of hydrocarbons or tar produced in both animal species a higher and more rapid malignant conversion. The viral DNA was detected in both the benign and the malignant lesions. These results suggested that the CRPV produced the benign lesion, but other factors, genetic and environmental, may be necessary for production of malignant disease. More recently, oesophageal, intestinal and bladder papillomas produced by bovine papillomavirus type 4 (BPV 4) were shown to become malignant when cattle were fed on a diet of bracken. In this case the BPV 4 DNA was detected only in the benign lesion and was not detectable after malignant conversion. Recently a rhesus monkey papillomavirus type 1 has been isolated from a lymph node metastasis of a penile carcinoma. This virus is sexually transmitted and is associated with both penile and cervical cancers. This animal virus may serve as a good, if expensive, model to investigate the natural history of papillomavirus infections.

In humans, one-third of patients with EV develop squamous cell carcinoma, usually in sun-exposed areas. Over 30% of these lesions contain HPV DNA, most commonly types -5 or -8. This suggests that, given the right environmental or genetic conditions, benign lesions may develop into carcinoma with the help of HPVs. Other evidence of a helper function associated with malignant conversion concerns laryngeal papillomas, where a high rate of malignant disease was observed in patients who were treated with X-irradiation some 40 years ago. With the increase in the number of allograft recipients there has been an increase in reports of squamous cell carcinomas at many different sites. The cutaneous cancers are associated with those viruses isolated from similar lesions in EV patients and the genital cancers harbour the viruses found in similar cancers in immunocompetent individuals. The increased incidence of disease in immunosuppressed individuals, suggests that the immune response is important in controlling infectious and tumour development.

It is the genital papillomaviruses that are responsible for the most common HPV-associated cancers and these types will be discussed in more detail in the following sections.

Genital Cancers Associated with HPVs

The association between the genital cancers, especially cervical cancer, is now known to be causal rather than casual, but not everyone infected with an oncogenic HPV type will develop cancer. In fact, it appears that people can be infected and have transitory disease, which spontaneously regresses, or perhaps have no obvious lesions resulting from infection. It is not clear why the outcome from infection can be so varied, but the immune response may play an important role, as well as other less well-described factors, such as genetic background and response of the epithelial cells to infection.

HPV Infection and the Normal Cervix

It has been observed for some time that HPV DNA could be detected in cervical cells from women with a normal cervix, as assessed by normal cytology, and no visible lesion upon colposcopic examination. What is not clear, however, is whether the cervix epithelium is really normal, or whether there are micro-lesions present which harbour the virus. So far no histologically normal cervix has been shown to harbour oncogenic HPV DNA. The rate of detection of HPV DNA in cervical cells varies dramatically, depending on the method used to detect the DNA, the age and demographics of the group studied. The most sensitive technique, the polymerase chain reaction (PCR; see section on Diagnosis, below), which is prone to cross-contamination, has recorded levels of 80% positivity in women with a normal cervix in cross-sectional studies. These results are high and were carried out on a very

small number of individuals; they have not been reproduced in studies using much larger numbers. However, HPV infection of the genital tract is common, although there is variation in isolation rate, depending on the age and lifestyle of the individuals studied. In studies of young women aged 18–25 years, up to 46% had detectable HPV DNA by PCR (Bauer et al., 1991) in epithelial cells from a normal cervix. HPV types -16 and -18, which are commonly found in malignant disease, account for about one-third of the viruses detected. This infection rate has been observed in other populations of young sexually active women. While similar studies on large populations of males have not been carried out, it is clear from smaller studies that males are infected at similar rates, a finding that would be expected with a sexually transmitted disease. Therefore, a large number of young women may be infected with HPV types, which cause malignant disease. It is clear that while many individuals will develop transitory premalignant disease, only a small number will ever develop malignant disease, but recognising those at risk is not possible at present. HPV detection decreases in older women aged >40 years and is usually in the 5–10% range. While the level of infection is lower in older women, it has been shown that they are more likely to have underlying disease (see next section).

HPVs Infection and the Abnormal Cervix

The most common genital lesion caused by HPV infection is the benign genital wart (condylomata acuminata). HPV-6 and -11 are the predominant types associated with these lesions, which are benign and where the rare malignant conversion has only been documented in patients with an underlying immune deficiency. These warts are distributed throughout the female genital tract on the cervix, vaginal wall, vulva and perianal region. In males the lesions are found on the penis, scrotum and perianal region.

The premalignant lesions associated with HPV can occur on the same sites as described above for warts, although the cervix is the site where malignant conversion is most often observed. The premalignant lesions of the cervix are called intraepithelial neoplasia and are graded, according to the Bethesda system (Kurman et al., 1994), as low-grade squamous

Table 22.4 Genital HPVs and their associated risk of cancer

Low risk	6, 11, 40, 42–45, 53–55, 57, 59, 61, 67, 71, 74, 82
High risk	16, 18, 31–35, 51–52, 56, 58, 61, 66, 68, 70, 73

intraepithelial lesions (LSILs) or high-grade squamous intraepithelial lesions (HSILs). HPV-6 and -11 are found in LSILs, while the oncogenic types, HPV-16 and -18, are found in all grades and in malignant disease. Table 22.4 gives a breakdown of the high- and low-risk HPV types. The premalignant cervical lesions occur almost entirely on the transformation zone, the metaplastic zone between native squamous epithelium of the exocervix and the columnar epithelium of the endocervical canal, and are white in appearance after the addition of 5% acetic acid to the surface of the epithelium. Invasive cancer arises from these areas of HSILs and malignant cells migrate up into the uterus and out to local lymph nodes. HPV-16 is the most common virus found in intraepithelial and malignant disease. It has been found in 70% of cases of HSILs in Germany and the UK and worldwide has been isolated in 50–60% of cases of invasive cancer of the cervix.

HPV-6 and -11 have not been found in malignant disease of the cervix, but have been isolated from local invading lesions of the vulva, such as verrucous carcinoma. However, when the genomes of the viruses were sequenced, it was found that there were duplications in the long control region, which may be associated with the change in pathogenesis. The HPV types and associated lesions are shown in Table 22.5.

Table 22.5 Genital human papillomavirus types and the site of associated lesions[a]

HPV type	Associated lesion	Site	HPV type	Associated lesion	Site
HPV-6a–f	Condylomata acuminata	Vulva	39	LSIL/HSIL	Cervix and penis
		Vagina		PIN	
		Cervix		Malignant carcinoma	
		Penis	40	LSIL/HSIL	Cervix and penis
		Shaft	42	LSIL/HSIL/VIN	Cervix and vulva
		Prepuce	43	LSIL/HSIL	Cervix
		Urethral meatus	44	LSIL/HSIL	Cervix
		Perianal	45	LSIL/HSIL	Cervix
		Larynx		Malignant carcinoma	
	LSIL/HSIL[b]	Cervix	51	LSIL/HSIL	Cervix
	VIN I–III[c]	Vulva		Malignant carcinoma	
	PIN I–III[d]	Penis	52	LSIL/HSIL	Cervix
HPV-11a, b	Condylomata acuminata	Vulva		Malignant carcinoma	
		Cervix	53		Normal cervix
		Perinanal	54	Condyloma	Penis
		Larynx	55	Bowenoid papulosis	Penis
	LSIL/HSIL	Cervix	56	LSIL/HSIL	Cervix
	PIN I–III	Penis		Malignant carcinoma	
16	Condylomata acuminata	Vulva, cervix and penis	57	Intraepithelial neoplasia	Oral cavity, cervix
	LSIL/HSIL	Cervix	58	LSIL/HSIL	Cervix
	VIN I–III	Vulva		Malignant carcinoma	
	PIN I–III	Penis	59	VIN	Vulva
	Bowenoid papulosis	Vulva and penis	61	VIN	Vulva
	Malignant carcinoma	Cervix, vulva and penis	66	LSIL/HSIL	Cervix
18	LSIL/HSIL	Cervix and penis		Malignant carcinoma	
	Malignant carcinoma		67	Intraepithelial neoplasia	Cervix
31	LSIL/HSIL	Cervix			Vulva
	Malignant carcinoma		68	LSIL/HSIL	Cervix
30	LSIL/HSIL	Cervix		Malignant carcinoma	Cervix
33	LSIL/HSIL	Cervix	69	Intraepithelial neoplasia	Cervix
	Malignant carcinoma		70	Condyloma	Vulva
34	LSIL/HSIL	Cervix		Malignant carcinoma	Cervix
35	LSIL/HSIL	Cervix	71	VAIN[e]	Vagina
	Malignant carcinoma		74	VAIN	Vagina
			82	HSIL	Cervix

[a]Adapted from De Villiers (1989) and updated with the help of Dr C. Wheeler.
[b]Low-grade squamous intraepithelial lesion and high-grade squamous intraepithelial lesion of the cervix.
[c]Vulvar intraepithelial neoplasia.
[d]Penile intraepithelial neoplasia.
[e]Vaginal intraepithelial neoplasia.

There is a difference in the state of the HPV-16 DNA in premalignant and malignant lesions. In LSILs and HSILs the HPV DNA is free and unintegrated, while in the majority of malignant cells the DNA is integrated. While integration is random within the chromosomes, the cells, which acquire malignant potential, contain the HPV genome integrated in the E1 or E2 regions of the DNA, resulting in the retention of the expression of the E6 and E7 proteins, which appear essential for the malignant phenotype. It is not clear how important integration is for the development of invasive cancer, since in a minority of cases the viral DNA is episomal in malignant cells, but continued expression of E6 and E7 appears necessary.

Malignant disease of the penis while rare in developed countries is much more common in developing parts of the world. HPV-16 and -18 were detected in over 50% of penile cancers in Brazil (McCance et al., 1986), where in one area of the northeast of the country the incidence of penile cancer is 10 times the frequency seen in Europe. Again, in malignant disease of the penis the viral DNA is integrated into the host cell chromosomes in the majority of cases.

While HPV types have a role in the aetiology of cervical cancer, there are certainly other factors involved that act with the virus to produce invasive disease, since not everyone infected and exhibiting premalignant lesions will develop cancer. It is estimated that up to 25% of women with LSILs will progress to HSILs if not treated, while most will regress over a 3 year period. However, in older women (>40 years of age) infection and persistence are associated with more serious underlying disease and so they are a group to be closely monitored (McCance, 1998). The co-factors involved have not been delineated, although smoking and use of oral contraceptives (>5 years) may be such components.

Persistent Infections

Epidemiological evidence suggests that HPVs can persist in squamous epithelium without producing clinically obvious lesions. Up to 50% of allograft recipients develop cutaneous warts within a year after transplant, this proportion being high when compared with the incidence in age-matched controls. This suggests that transplanted patients experience either new infections or reactivation of persistent virus, the latter being supported by the finding of HPV DNA sequences in biopsies of normal areas of larynx from individuals who have had episodes of laryngeal papillomas. As the recurrence rate of laryngeal warts is high, this suggests that the virus is capable of persisting somewhere in the larynx, respiratory tract or oral cavity without producing recognisable lesions—an inapparent infection.

Also, the viruses associated with the lesions in EV patients are not normally found in lesions from immunocompetent individuals, yet EV is such a rare disease that these patients cannot circulate the viruses amongst themselves. It would seem that these viruses are circulating in the normal population, causing inapparent infections. This is supported by the fact that viruses isolated from warts and SCC in immunosuppressed individuals, are often the same types observed in EV patients.

In addition, during pregnancy genital warts can appear on the vulvar epithelium and then disappear postpartum. It is not known if this is an hormonal effect or due to pertubations in the immune response that may accompany pregnancy, or the result of acquiring a recent infection from her partner. In none of the above situations is there any direct evidence as to which cells harbour the virus. The basal epithelial cells are the most likely site, although there is a considerable turnover of cells. However, not all cells in the basal epithelium have the same capacity to divide, so the viral DNA may be sequestered in quiescent basal cells which, when they subsequently divide, may activate replication and produce lesions.

DIAGNOSIS

Apart from the familiar hand and verruca warts found on the hands and feet, respectively, the clinical appearance of papillomavirus infections varies considerably, from the scaly flat lesions on cutaneous epithelium of individuals with EV to the aceto-white flat lesions on the cervix. The reader is referred to specific papers for details of the clinical presentation of genital lesions (Walker et al., 1983). This section will deal with the laboratory diagnosis of HPV, in particular the genital isolates.

Culture Methods

Although several efforts have been made, no easily amenable cell type has been capable of supporting replication, with production of infectious papillomavirus particles. The nude mice kidney capsule model, or the SCID mouse subcutaneous system has been used to propagate some HPV types, but they cannot be considered *in vitro* systems and are not amenable to most virus laboratories. Also, the raft system (McCance *et al.*, 1989) produces low amounts of infectious virus and the technique itself is rather cumbersome. Therefore, there is no readily available culture system for HPV propagation.

Serological Methods

Recently, with the advent of yeast and baculovirus produced virus-like particles (VLPs), it is now possible to detect antibodies by an ELISA technique in the serum of patients infected with HPV. At present there is a limited number of HPV types that have been used in these assays, but the initial results suggest that antibodies are detected in approximately 50% of infected individuals, which is less sensitive than DNA-based detection methods. These assays have only been carried out for some of the genital isolates. The reasons for the low positivity rates in infected people are unclear, but it has to be remembered that the virus is confined to the stratified epithelium of the genital tract and few cells in a lesion support viral particle production. In addition, the mature viral particles are only produced in the outer layers of the epithelium, where the immune response is at its least effective. Therefore, serological assays may not be very sensitive for diagnosis or screening purposes. However, the serological data and the natural history of the virus suggest that either the virus is not very immunogenic, or possibly induces an inappropriate response.

Polymerase Chain Reaction (PCR)

The most sensitive method for the detection of HPV infection is by PCR. This is a powerful technique, which amplifies a specific piece of DNA from a small amount of template. The advantages of this method are: (a) the extreme sensitivity; (b) the versatility, in that it can be used to detect more than one type of HPV when degenerate primers are used—in fact, it is possible to detect even unknown HPV types (ones that have not been cloned and sequenced); (c) it is possible to test large populations. The major disadvantage is that, because of the sensitivity of the method, it is possible to amplify contaminating sequences and so have false positives. This was a major problem in earlier studies but, now that this is recognised, investigators have been more careful and included strict controls.

Several sets of partially degenerative or degenerative primers have been used to detect HPV types in the

DNA extracted from lesions, and are directed to the L1 open reading frame. The first described, MY09/MY11 (Bauer *et al.*, 1991), has been improved (PGMY09/PGMY11) and used with a filter containing 27 HPV types (Gravitt *et al.*, 1998), meaning that the PCR products can be directly hybridised to the filter, allowing for a quick method to detect specific HPV types. Other sets, such as GP5$^+$/GP6$^+$ (de Roda Husman *et al.*, 1995) and SPF-10 (Kleter *et al.*, 1998), have also been used successfully to detect multiple HPV types in clinical samples. The main difference between the sets of primers is that some detect certain HPV types better than others, but since these types are of low frequency in the populations studied, in reality there is little difference in the sensitivity of detection between the sets (van Doorn *et al.*, 2002). None of the PCR sets have been licensed for use as diagnostic tools, although the Hybrid Capture Method described next has been approved for diagnostic use in the USA.

Hybrid Capture Method

This method is commercially available as a kit from Digene Diagnostics, MD, USA, and uses type-specific RNA probes to detect viral DNA in samples. This method is not as sensitive as PCR, but does not have the problems of false positives associated with PCR, since it does not rely on the PCR-type amplification of the signal. In practice, although not as sensitive as PCR, the method is sufficiently sensitive to detect HPV DNA and has been shown to be superior to one cytologic test in detecting HPV from lesions diagnosed as atypical squamous cells of unknown significance (ASCUS) or above. Cytological smears diagnosed as ASCUS are difficult to interpret, since after biopsy more serious disease may be detected. HPV typing has been shown to be helpful in these situations. This test detects 16 mucosal types, whereas PCR can theoretically detect all HPV types.

TREATMENT

Although in most cases warts are a cosmetic nuisance and will eventually disappear spontaneously, they are notoriously difficult to treat. However, since premalignant lesions, especially on the cervix, may lead to malignant disease, treatment to eliminate disease is important. This section will concentrate on the treatment of genital areas, as others (Bunney, 1982) have dealt extensively with common hand and plantar warts.

Podophyllin

Podophyllin is a resin mixture obtained from the roots of *Podophyllum* (American mandrake) and is an irritant on cutaneous and mucous surfaces. It is an antimitotic agent and should be used with care. It is painted carefully onto the surface of warts and should remain for no longer than 6 h and then be washed off. It is poorly adsorbed by cutaneous surfaces and so has a limited effect. Several treatments are required and the continual inflammation produced can lead to fibrosis of the areas treated without getting rid of the lesions. Podophyllin is even less effective in treatment of plantar warts and should never be used for treatment of hand warts.

Cryotherapy

Liquid nitrogen ($-190°C$) and dry ice (solid carbon dioxide, $-50°C$) can be applied to warts to produce local destruction of the lesion. Care should be taken to limit application to the lesion and not surrounding areas, as this will lead to pain and blistering of the healthy area. Cryoprobes are used to apply these cryogens to the cervix.

Electrodiathermy

This is used in treating mucosal lesions, such as those on the cervix, to destroy the diseased tissue by heat.

Laser Evaporation

The carbon dioxide laser has been used to treat lesions on mucosal surfaces (cervix and vaginal wall) (Singer and Walker, 1985) as well as cutaneous lesions. The success rate of laser treatment of the cervix is very good, with cure rates of 85–90%. However, its efficacy with cutaneous lesions has not as yet been assessed adequately. The difficulty with these lesions is knowing how deep to vaporise to eliminate diseased tissue.

Loop Electrosurgical Excision Procedure (LEEP)

This is a relatively new procedure for the removal of cervical lesions and makes use of a heated loop, which very precisely removes the complete lesion. One advantage over laser evaporation is that the lesion is removed intact and the tissue can be used for pathological staging without having to biopsy the lesion first. In addition, the margins of the lesion are intact and so the extent of lesion removal can be assessed. Also it allows the lesion to be used for other studies, such as HPV typing.

Surgery

Curettage of common warts is not a common mode of treatment. In any case, not all warts are suitably sited for surgical removal. Furthermore, if all the abnormal tissue is not moved, small islands of warts can recur around the site of the initial lesion.

Interferon

Interferon has been used to treat recurrent laryngeal warts and cervical neoplasias. In the former cases, tumour load was first reduced by surgery or by CO_2 laser, interferon then being given parenterally. Although recurrences were rare within 2 years after starting the interferon course, it was necessary to maintain patients on interferon to prevent new lesions. The expense of this regime and possible side-effects associated with interferon administration provide drawbacks to this method of treatment. Cervical premalignant lesions have also been treated with interferon, but variable results have been reported.

Prevention by Vaccination

There is now a major thrust to develop a vaccine to try and protect against infection. The major capsid protein of papillomaviruses, L1 can be produced in yeast or insect cells and folds into an icosahedral structure, called a virus-like particle (VLP), since it is similar in structure to the complete infectious virion. In animal studies, the antibodies raised to the VLPs are conformational and recognise the virion and can neutralise infection. Vaccine trials have taken place to immunise dogs against oral papillomavirus infection (Suzich *et al.*, 1995). The dogs were immunised intramuscularly with VLPs of canine oral papillomavirus and then challenged with live virus placed on scarified areas of the oral cavity. Protection was 100%, indicating that it is possible to immunise against infection with intramuscular inoculations. Phase 1 trials have been carried out in humans using VLPs from HPV-6 and -11 and good antibody responses were detected in all patients at all doses used. These responses were to conformational epitopes on L1, as was the case in the study using dogs.

At the time of writing there are Phase II trials investigating the response to VLPs of the virus types - 16 and -18. There are also plans for Phase III trials to test the efficacy of these vaccines. At the time of writing it is not clear what will be considered a successful outcome. Will the end-point be protection against infection or disease? Normally it is protection against disease that is the end-point, but since it may take years for HPV-associated lesions to be obvious, protection against infection would be a faster way to determine efficacy. If absence of disease is the end-point, then it will need to be a long trial (5 years or more) and will need a large number of participants (perhaps 20 000). No matter, these are exciting times for HPV vaccine biology, and other possible vaccines are being developed and may be in trial before the next edition of this book.

REFERENCES

Antinore MJ, Birrer MJ, Patel D et al. (1996) The human papillomavirus type 16 E7 gene product interacts with and transactivates the API family of transcription factors. EMBO J, 15, 1950–1960.

Bauer HM, Ting Y, Greer CE et al. (1991) Genital human papillomavirus infection in female university students as determined by a PCR-based method. J Am Med Assoc, 265, 472–477.

Bonnez W, DaRin C, Borkhuis C et al. (1998) Isolation and propagation of human papillomavirus type 16 in human xenografts implanted in the severe combined immunodeficiency mouse. J Virol, 72, 5256–5261.

Brehm A, Miska EA, McCance DJ et al. (1998) Retinoblastoma protein recruits histone deacetylase to repress transcription. Nature, 391, 597–601.

Bunney M (1982) Viral Warts: Their Biology and Treatment. Oxford University Press, Oxford.

Chen, JJ, Reid CE, Band V and Androphy EJ (1995) Interaction of papillomavirus E6 oncoproteins with a putative calcium binding protein. Science, 269, 529–531.

Conrad M, Bubb VJ and Schlegel R (1993) The human papillomavirus type 6 and 16 E5 proteins are membrane-associated proteins which associate with the 16 kDa pore-forming protein. J Virol, 67, 6170–6178.

de Roda Husman AM, Walboomers JM, van de Brule AJ et al. (1995) The use of general primers GP5 and GP6 elongated at their 3′ ends with adjacent highly conserved sequences improves human papillomavirus detection by PCR. J Gen Virol, 76, 1057–1062.

De Villiers E-M (1989) Heterogeneity of the human papillomavirus group. J Virol, 63, 4898–4903.

Doorbar J, Ely S, Sterling J et al. (1991) Specific interaction between HPV-16 E1–E4 and cytokeratins results in collapse of the epithelial cell intermediate filament network. Nature, 352, 824–826.

Durst M, Gissmann L, Ikenberg H and zur Hausen H (1983) A papillomavirus DNA from a cervical carcinoma and its prevalence in cancer biopsy samples from different geographic regions. Proc Nat Acad Sci USA, 80, 3812–3815.

Dyson N, Howley PM, Munger K and Harlow E (1989) The human papillomavirus 16 E7 oncoprotein is able to bind to the retinoblastoma gene product. Science, 243, 934–937.

Frattini M, Lim H and Laimins LA (1996) In vitro synthesis of oncogenic human papillomaviruses requires episomal templates for differentiation-dependent late expression. Proc Nat Acad Sci USA, 91, 3062–3067.

Frattini MG and Laimins LA (1994) Binding of the human papillomavirus E1 origin-recognition protein is regulated through complex formation with the E2 enhancer-binding protein. Proc Natl Acad Sci USA, 91, 12398–12402.

Gravitt PE, Peyton CL, Apple RJ and Wheeler CM (1998) Genotyping of 27 human papillomavirus types by using L1 consensus PCR products by a single-hybridization, reverse line blot detection method. J Clin Microbiol, 36, 3020–3027.

Kirnbauer R, Booy F, Cheng N et al. (1992) Papillomavirus L1 major capsid protein self-assembles into virus-like particles that are highly immunogenic. Proc Natl Acad Sci USA, 89, 12180–12184.

Kleter B, van Doorn LJ, ter Schegget J et al. (1998) Novel short-fragment PCR assay for highly sensitive broad-spectrum detection of anogenital human papillomaviruses. Am J Pathol, 153, 1731–1739.

Kreider JW, Howett MK, Wolfe SA et al. (1985) Morphological transformation in vivo of human uterine cervix with papillomavirus from condylomata acuminata. Nature, 317, 639–641.

Kurman RJ, Henson DE, Herbst AL et al. (1994) Interim guidelines for management of abnormal cervical cytology. The 1992 National Cancer Institute Workshop. J Am Med Assoc, 271, 1866–1869.

Leechanachai P, Banks L, Moreau F and Matlashewski G (1992) The E5 gene from human papillomavirus type 16 is an oncogene which enhances growth factor-mediated signal transduction to the nucleus. Oncogene, 7, 19–25.

Lu JZ, Sun YN, Rose RC et al. (1993) Two E2 binding sites (E2BS) alone or one E2BS plus an A/T-rich region are minimal requirements for the replication of the human papillomavirus type 11 origin. J Virol, 67, 7131–7139.

McCance DJ (1998) Human papillomaviruses and cervical cancer [editorial]. J Med Microbiol, 47, 371–373.

McCance DJ, Kalache A, Ashdown K et al. (1986) Human papillomavirus types 16 and 18 in carcinomas of the penis from Brazil. Int J Cancer, 37, 55–59.

McCance DJ, Kopan R, Fuchs E and Laimins LA (1988) Human papillomavirus type 16 alters human epithelial cell differentiation in vitro. Proc Natl Acad Sci USA, 85, 7169–7173.

McMurray HR, Nguyen D, Westbrook TF and McCance DJ (2001) Biology of human papillomaviruses. Int J Exp Pathol, 82, 15–33.

Oriel JD (1971) Natural history of genital warts. Br J Vener Dis, 47, 1–13.

Phillips AC and Vousden KH (1997) Analysis of the interaction between human papillomavirus type 16 E7 and the TATA-binding protein, TBP. J Gen Virol, 78, 905–909.

Rose RC, Bonnez W, Da Rin C et al. (1994) Serological differentiation of human papillomavirus types 11, 16 and 18 using recombinant virus-like particles. *J Gen Virol*, **75**, 2445–2449.

Scheffner M, Werness BA, Huibregtse JM *et al.* (1990) The E6 oncoprotein encoded by human papillomavirus types 16 and 18 promotes the degradation of p53. *Cell*, **63**, 1129–1136.

Singer A and Walker P (1985) The treatment of CIN: conservative methods. *Clin Obstet Gynecol*, **12**, 121–132.

Straight SW, Herman B and McCance DJ (1995) The E5 oncoprotein of human papillomavirus type 16 inhibits the acidification of endosomes in human keratinocytes. *J Virol*, **69**, 3185–3192.

Suzich JA, Ghim SJ, Palmer-Hill FJ *et al.* (1995) Systemic immunization with papillomavirus L1 protein completely prevents the development of viral mucosal papillomas. *Proc Natl Acad Sci USA*, **92**: 11553–11557.

Thomas M, Glaunsinger B, Pim D *et al.* (2001) HPV E6 and MAGUK protein interactions: determination of the molecular basis for specific protein recognition and degradation. *Oncogene*, **20**, 5431–5439.

van Doorn L-J, Quint W, Kleter B *et al.* (2002) Genotyping of human papillomavirus in liquid cytology cervical specimens by the PGMY line blot assay and the SPF10 line probe assay. *J Clin Microbiol*, **40**, 979–983.

Walker PG, Singer A, Dyson JL *et al.* (1983) Colposcopy in the diagnosis of papillomavirus infection of the uterine cervix. *Br J Obstet Gynaecol*, **90**, 1082–1086.

23

Human Polyomaviruses

Kristina Dörries

Julius-Maximilians University, Würzburg, Germany

CLASSIFICATION AND DETECTION

The human polyomaviruses were previously grouped in the large group *Papovaviridae* with papillomaviruses, polyomaviruses and SV40, the so-called vacuolising agent. However, molecular studies showed that *Simian virus 40* (SV40) is closely related to the other polyomaviruses and, with growing knowledge on the genomic structure and function of proteins, the previous subfamily is now classified as independent family, *Polyomaviridae*. The classical human viruses are now grouped as *Polyomavirus hominis* (huPyV), type 1 (BKV) and type 2 (JCV). For both viruses, different genotypes have been described. The small non-enveloped viruses of about 40 nm in diameter contain single genomes of covalently closed superhelical double-stranded DNA. Although *Murine polyomavirus* was detected almost 50 years ago, the existence of primate polyomaviruses was not realised until the 1960s, with the detection of SV40 in monkeys. 10 years later, JCV and BKV were described. JCV was isolated from brain tissue of a patient with progressive multifocal leukoencephalopathy (PML), employing human fetal brain spongioblast cultures. BKV grew in cell cultures after inoculation with urine from a renal transplant recipient (Padgett and Walker, 1976; Zu Rhein, 1969).

VIRION STRUCTURE AND COMPOSITION

Polyomaviruses are non-enveloped viruses with icosahedral capsids containing three virus-encoded proteins, VP1, VP2 and VP3. The shell surrounds a DNA molecule that is stabilised by cellular histones in chromatin structure. From studies on SV40 and *Murine polyomavirus* it has been established that 360 molecules of the major capsid protein VP1 are associated with approximately 30–60 molecules of each of the minor capsid proteins, VP2 and VP3. The icosahedron is composed of 72 pentamers. Each consists of five VP1 molecules and one molecule of VP2 or VP3. VP1 is the most related capsid protein among the three primate viruses. This complicates the development of highly specific serologic assays, which are important for addressing a possible involvement of polyomaviruses in cancer, as well as spread of SV40 in the human population.

Virus preparations contain at least two kinds of particles. *In vitro* passage of polyomaviruses at high multiplicity is accompanied by the generation of considerable amounts of empty capsids. In addition, defective viral genomes containing deletions, duplications and rearrangements of viral genetic information can be encapsidated, if they are within the appropriate size limits. *In vivo*, the amount of empty shells is considerably lower, indicating highly effective virus growth under natural conditions. Complete virus particles form a band at a density of 1.34 g/ml in $CsCl_2$ equilibrium density gradients, whereas empty capsids have a density of about 1.29 g/ml (Figure 23.1).

Although the structure of the huPyV capsid has not been completely established, it has been reported that recombinant JCV VP1 self-assembles into pentameric capsomeres and, under appropriate conditions, these molecules will further assemble into virus-like empty capsids (Chang *et al.*, 1997). Calcium ions are required

Principles and Practice of Clinical Virology, Fifth Edition. Edited by A. J. Zuckerman, J. E. Banatvala, J. R. Pattison, P. D. Griffiths and B. D. Schoub
© 2004 John Wiley & Sons Ltd   ISBN 0 470 84338 1

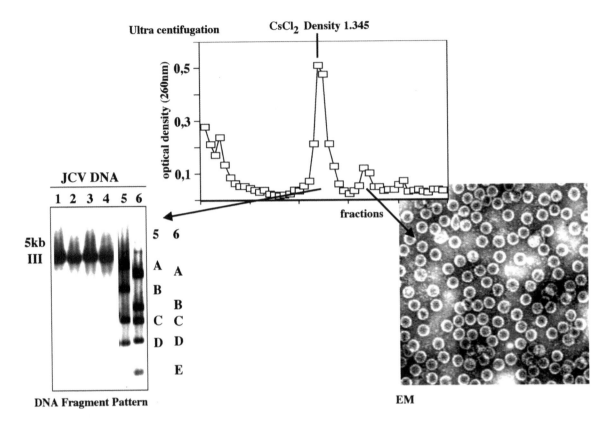

Figure 23.1 JCV purification out of PML brain tissue. Middle: Optical profile of the centrifugation with localisation of virus particles in two bands; intact virus particles at a density of 1.345 g/ml CsCl$_2$. Left: Restriction endonuclease cleavage of DNA extracted from the major peak of the gradient followed by Southern blotting and JCV-specific radioactive hybridisation. 1–4 cleavage with single cut enzymes *Eco*RI, *Bam*HI, *Hpa*I, *Pst*I generating linearised form III DNA of about 5 kb in length; 5,6 cleavage with single and more cut enzymes in combination (*Bam*HI/*Pvu*II, *Bam*HI/*Hind*III, respectively) generating DNA fragments 5: A–D and 6: A–E. Right: Electron micrograph of negatively stained JCV icosahedral virus particles of the small virus peak representing empty shells without encapsidated viral DNA

for capsid stability and disulphide bonds may exist between capsid proteins, as reducing agents are required to disassemble virus particles. The human polyomaviruses are able to haemagglutinate erythrocytes at high virus concentrations. Each virus also has distinct antigenic epitopes and can be distinguished by neutralisation and haemagglutination-inhibition assays (Pass and Shah, 1982).

VIRUS LIFE CYCLE

Polyomavirus expression is essentially divided into three major phases. After expression of the regulatory early protein large T antigen (TAg) early post-infection, TAg initiates replication of viral DNA. Shortly after the onset of DNA replication, virus multiplication enters the late phase, which includes expression of late mRNAs. Translation of the late regulatory agnoprotein and the production of viral capsid proteins are followed by virion assembly. Regulated by complex interactions of viral promoter elements with cellular factors and the viral regulatory proteins, late genes are expressed efficiently only after DNA replication. In contrast, early genes continue to be expressed at late stages of infection, then serving as viral transcription factors. The functions of TAg and agnoprotein are controlled by consecutive phosphorylation events. However, the tropism of huPyV is predominantly to resting, differentiated cells. In order to produce enzymes necessary for virus growth, they have evolved mechanisms to overcome cell cycle growth arrest. A majority of the cell cycle-stimulating activities are induced by TAg. Consequently, expression of TAg can lead to transformation of a cell from a normal to a growth-deregulated state. The best studied cellular growth-promoting and -inhibitory proteins interacting with TAg are the tumour suppressor proteins, retinoblastoma binding protein (pRB), p53 and their downstream factors (Del Valle *et al.*, 2001; Sullivan and Pipas, 2002).

In comparison to other polyomaviruses, JCV has a long lytic life cycle with an early transcription and DNA replication phase lasting about 5 days followed by continuing initiation of late RNAs for 15–20 days. The virus has a stringent cell specificity and replicates efficiently *in vitro* only in primary human fetal glial cell cultures, rich in spongioblasts, a precursor cell of oligodendrocytes (Walker and Padgett, 1983). In such other cell lines as embryonic kidney, amnion or urine-derived epithelium virus growth is rather limited. In contrast, BKV has broader cell specificity and can be grown in a wide range of human cell types.

Molecular Structure of the Genome

The genomic structure is closely related among the primate polyomaviruses. The supercoiled, circular, double-stranded DNA of the human viruses is about 5100 bp in length. The genome is divided into two regions, encoding multiple overlapping genes. Each DNA strand carries about half of the genetic information. Early and late mRNAs are synthesised bidirectionally from opposite strands of the genome. Protein coding sequences consist of open reading frames for the early and late proteins. The non-coding region directs the activity and specificity of virus multiplication. It is divided into two regulatory segments with a single origin of DNA replication (ORI) and the transcriptional control elements (TCR) within the promoter region (Dörries, 1997; Kim *et al.*, 2001; Raj and Khalili, 1995) (Figure 23.2).

The coding sequences exhibit high DNA sequence homology. Homology between the human viruses is greater in all proteins than between JCV and SV40 (69%). JCV DNA shares 83 and 59% amino acid homology with BKV in the case of large TAg and agnogene, respectively. The rates are even higher in functionally active regions of the virus genes. The early region codes for the tumour or TAgs. Both human polyomaviruses encode two major proteins, small t (tAg) and large TAg, based on size. The multifunctional TAg directly controls the virus life cycle and interacts with key cellular regulatory circuits. The huPyV proteins have not been studied to the same extent as those of SV40, but extensive sequence homology points to similar functional activities. This includes effects on nuclear localisation, viral DNA replication by direct DNA binding, helicase activities and binding to DNA polymerase-α, which initiates DNA replication. Interaction with cellular tumour suppressor proteins is associated with cellular transformation and TAg as a transcription factor is known to be crucial for the regulation of early and late gene transcription. Many of the activities depend on the TAg viral chaperone domain, which interacts with cellular chaperones to orchestrate functions that require the rearrangement of multiprotein complexes (Sullivan and Pipas, 2002).

The tumour antigens are generated from a common pre-mRNA molecule by one alternative splicing event leading to identical N-termini and different C-terminal DNA sequences. Recently, three additional early virus proteins, T'135, T'136, and T'165 were characterised in JCV-infected cells. All T proteins use the first alternative splice donor site leading to the same 132 N-terminal amino acids (AA). For T' proteins, a second splice donor site is combined with alternate acceptor sites. Whereas T'165 shares the C-terminus with TAg, T'135 and T'136 have unique ends encoded by an alternative reading frame. Expression of the proteins is modulated during the virus life cycle and appears to be related to TAg-mediated DNA replication and transcriptional control. T' proteins may utilise the shared tumour suppressor and chaperone binding domains to enhance DNA replication by differential interaction with pRB and related proteins or the transcription factor Tst-1. Significant differences in the splicing patterns of JCV-infected and JCV-transformed cells and increased expression of the '17 kDa' species suggest correlation with the transforming activity of JCV. Additionally, it has been proposed that the apoptotic function of TAg might be negatively influenced by T' proteins (Kim *et al.*, 2001).

The late region of the viral genome encodes two minor (VP2 and VP3) and a major (VP1) capsid protein. Late mRNAs are generated from a common precursor by alternative splicing. The sequences of the minor proteins VP2 and VP3 overlap. VP2 contains the entire VP3 sequence at its C-terminus and an additional sequence of approximately 400 AAs at its N-terminus. In contrast, the major protein VP1 is

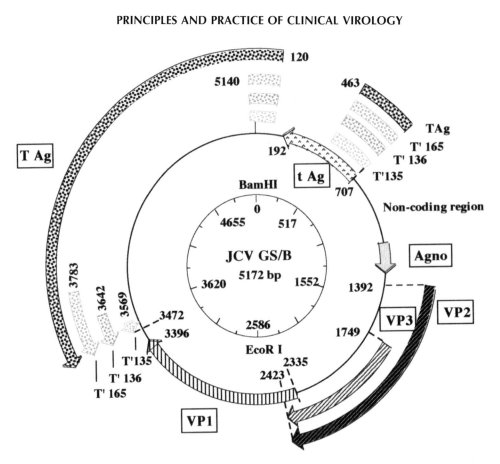

Figure 23.2 Circular map of the human polyomavirus JC subtype GS/B genome. Coding DNA segments are represented by shaded arrows. Numbers designate the first nucleotide of the start and stop codons for early (large T Antigen, small t Antigen, T prime proteins T′ 165, T′ 135, T′ 136) and late proteins (agnogene, virus capsid proteins VP1, VP2, VP3). Position of splice donor and acceptor sites are indicated by nucleotide numbers. The position of the unique *Bam*HI and *Eco*RI restriction sites are indicated on the inner circle

generated by an alternative reading frame. The three primate polyomaviruses all encode the non-structural regulatory agnoprotein in an open reading frame in the late leader region. The sequences are homologous in the first two-thirds of the amino-terminus but divergent in the carboxy-terminal one-third. The protein is probably not necessary for virus multiplication but rather takes part in the orchestration of efficient progeny virus production. It is produced late in the virus lytic cycle and physically and functionally interacts with the early key regulator TAg and the cellular transcription factor YB-1. Recently, it became obvious that agnoprotein plays an important role in the viral life cycle by modulating viral gene transcription and DNA replication. Likewise, it is suspected to be involved in the morphogenesis of virus particles, the localisation of the major capsid protein to the nucleus, may regulate intracellular vesicular transport by

interaction with cytoskeletal proteins, and appears to deregulate cell proliferation by association with the tumour suppressor p53. Although studies on agnoprotein function are only at the beginning, the protein is obviously a central regulator of the late virus life cycle (Table 23.1).

The non-coding part of the genome is framed by the start codons for early and late genes. The ORI is located between the TATA box and the initiation codon for the early genes. This segment includes the conserved binding sites for large TAg. Corresponding to similar DNA replication strategies, the polyomavirus ORI DNA segment is highly conserved in sequence and structure. In contrast, the promoter region to the late side of the control region reveals extensive differences. Heterogeneity of structure and sequence of individual transcription factor binding sites is reflected in the divergent cell type specificity and

Table 23.1 Human polyomavirus early and late proteins

Protein	BKV		JCV	
	Size (aa)	Mol wt (kDa)	Size (aa)	Mol wt (kDa)
Early				
t Ag	172	20	172	20.2
T Ag	695	90	688	79.3
T′ 135	NR	NR	135	17
T′ 136	NR	NR	136	22
T′ 165	NR	NR	165	23
Late				
Agno	66	8	71	8
VP1	362	46[a]	354	39.6
VP2	351	40.5[a]	344	37.4
VP3	232	30.5[a]	225	25.7

[a]Molecular weight varies considerably between laboratories.
aa, amino acids; NR, not reported.

activity of transcription among the huPyV types (Dörries, 1997).

Control of Viral Gene Expression

DNA Replication

Regulatory mechanisms leading to DNA replication are closely related among the primate polyomaviruses. This is reflected in an ORI that is constructed by protein binding elements with comparable sequence and spacing requirements. Bidirectional replication takes place in the presence of the core ORI and TAg, proceeding from the ORI elements with the TAg binding sites terminating at a site about 180° from the initiation site. The features shared by all ORI regions are an inverted repeat on the early side, a GC-rich palindrome in the centre and an AT sequence on the late side of ORI. All core ORIs contain these elements and replication studies on the human polyomaviruses have confirmed that, besides TAg binding, site II and the inverted repeat are essential for DNA replication. Whereas the presence of flanking sequences stimulates DNA replication, the TCR does not affect DNA replication activity directly. Interestingly, the efficiency of DNA replication directed from the JCV ORI is substantially lower than from the SV40 and BKV ORIs. TAg produced in each of the viruses considerably varies in its ability to support replication from the homologous or heterogeneous origins. This became clear as BKV TAg was found to activate replication from the JCV ORI, but JCV TAg failed to drive replication from the heterogeneous BKV ORI. It is likely that

differences of ORI sequences or spacing among the primate polyomaviruses are responsible for these observations (Kim *et al.*, 2001) (Figure 23.3).

Transcriptional Expression

The transcriptional control region (TCR) of the human polyomaviruses is composed of a great number of different regulatory protein-binding motifs. Promoter activity is mediated bidirectionally, and often independently from the binding motifs, by multiple interactions of transcription factors and associated cellular and viral proteins stimulating basal, cell type-specific and, in response of external stimuli, induced functions of the viral promoter (Raj and Khalili, 1995; Sweet *et al.*, 2002). The JCV early (JCVE) and late (JCVL) promoters have been intensively examined in recent years, and it can be assumed that the mechanisms leading to huPyV expression are highly related. For better understanding of the complicated regulatory pathways controlling huPyV growth and pathogenicity, the function of the JCV promoter is more closely examined. The JCV control region has been artificially dissected in the ORI domain and following four TCR subdomains (A–D), in each of which a clustering of early and late interactive promoter sites is observed (Figure 23.4).

Outside of the TCR domain, on the early site of ORI, a binding sequence is located for the potent transcriptional enhancer nuclear factor κB (NF-κB). The site bidirectionally increases transcription from the late and to a lesser extent from the early promoter in glial cells. NF-κB is constitutively expressed in B lymphocytes, one of the sites of JCV persistence. NF-κB can be retained in the cytoplasm by an inhibitor κB protein. This binding can be released through stimulation by a number of agents as tumour promoters, such as phorbol–myristate–acetate or inflammatory cytokines. It results in the transport of NF-κB to the nucleus, where the binding to the consensus DNA sites exerts activity. Upon PMA treatment, both JCV promoters are responsive to NF-κB induction, leading to increased JCV activity. In addition, tumour necrosis factor α (TNFα) is able to enhance binding of NF-κB to the JCV κB site. This stimulated the idea that activation of the transcriptional control *in vivo* is dependent on the expression of immunological active factors involved in immunologically regulated signalling pathways to modulate JCV expression.

It had been shown that interference with κB function in late gene expression decreased activity but did not

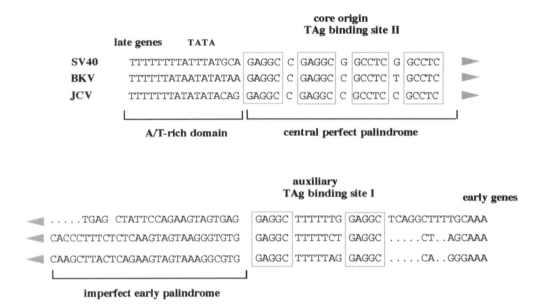

Figure 23.3 Alignment of the DNA sequence encompassing the origin of DNA replication in the non-coding genomic region of the primate polyomaviruses SV40, BKV and JCV. All sequences are given in the sense of the early coding strand. TAg consensus pentanucleotide recognition sites common to all virus strains are in boxes

abolish it. This suggested that additional TCR elements might confer inducibility to the JCVL promoter. At present, it is thought that cross-communication between motifs is mediated by a 40 kDa protein complex distinct from the classical NF-κB subunits. In the presence of classical NF-κB binding proteins, this complex may not effectively interact with the κB sequence. However, if the NF-κB activators are not expressed, the 40 kDa protein may bind and downregulate JCVL gene transcription. This may come into effect during the persistent state of infection.

Additionally, the GRS motif within ORI might interact with the κB motif. GRS is similarly inducible by PMA and inflammatory cytokines. The responsive region interacts with the protein GBP-i, which is induced in a wide range of cell types; thus, it could play a role in mediating JCV activation at all suspected sites of persistence. Comparable to the NF-κB-class of proteins, the GBP-i complexes probably represent a combinatorial assembly of various protein species, which is changed upon induction. Duality of function could involve the basal transcriptional machinery and other transcription proteins associated with late promoter activity. One potential factor is transforming growth factor β (TGFβ), acting through the GRS and the NF-1 sites. In such a model, the status of the viral promoter could be modulated through the GRS and variable interaction of cytokine-induced proteins.

Although these cytokines may use different signal transduction pathways for protein activation, the nuclear milieu will in consequence contain the factors leading to expression by interaction with a promoter containing the respective contact sites.

Most JCV TCR subtypes contain SP1 binding site one (SP1-I), just upstream from the TATA box. It appears to activate early promoter activity. SP1-II and III are located downstream from the TATA box. SP1-II is important for TAg-mediated transactivation of the early promoter, but is not involved in the regulation of basal expression. Interestingly, SP1 associates with Pur α and regulates myelin basic protein expression during brain development, whereas TAg downregulates its transcription by interacting with Pur α in an animal model; thus, a close association of these proteins with SP-1 can be assumed (Kim *et al.*, 2001).

Domain C contains the JCV early minimal core promoter (MCP), which is constituted by the TATA box region and the immediately adjacent binding site for the transcription factor Tst-1/SCIP/Oct-6, a member of the POU-domain protein family. In glial cells, Tst-1 was found to be one of the permanently produced cell type selective transcriptional regulators. Both JCV promoter orientations are stimulated by DNA binding of Tst-1 in glial cells to sequence motifs involving the TATA box and overlapping in part with adjacent OP-1 and YB-1 binding sites.

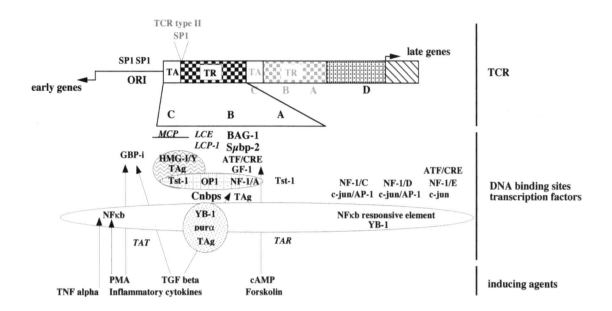

Figure 23.4 JCV transcriptional control region with most prominent protein binding sites and respective interaction of cellular and viral transcription factors. Transcriptional control region (TCR) structure of prototype JCV Mad-1 is shown between the start codons (arrows) for early and late genes (agnogene). ORI origin of DNA replication; TA TATA box; TR tandemly repeated promoter elements; similar shading represents identical DNA sequences; A–D, dissected promoter domains; MCP, minimal core promoter; LCE, lytic control element. Binding sites and the respective proteins are indicated below the promoter domains. Filled circles indicate interaction of transcription factors. *TAT, TAR* HIV-1-related transactivation domains. Arrows indicate interaction of inducing agents with the respective proteins. **V**, position of SP1 binding site in JCV TCR type II genomes

Like most POU proteins, Tst-1/SCIP/Oct-6 is an intrinsically weak transcriptional regulator. To compensate for this weakness, Tst-1 has to rely on viral or glial specific co-activators. TAg has been identified as the viral co-activator that stimulates the function of Tst-1 synergistically by direct interaction. The modular synergism of the two proteins does not require DNA binding of JCV TAg in presence of a functional binding site of Tst-1. In addition, TAg can activate the high mobility group proteins HMG-I/Y as cellular co-activators. Although not a transcriptional regulator by itself, HMG is believed to serve as a promoter-specific accessory factor, modifying the transcriptional function. The JCV AT-rich region with the Tst-1 site provides a binding site for HMG proteins, and HMG binding substantially stimulates Tst-1 binding to the Tst-1-responsive element.

Although Tst-1 and HMG are able to synergistically activate JCV gene expression, the TST-1 site alone is not enough to mediate efficient cooperativity. It is assumed that additional cross-talk occurs with the glial cell-specific late transcriptional silencer OP-1, which,

downstream of the Tst-1 binding site at the poly(dA) stretch, contacts with an overlapping pentanucleotide motif (penta). Recently, another cellular nucleic acid binding protein Cnbps has been identified that negatively regulates the JCV early promoter, and TAg binding protein p53 is discussed as a transcriptional silencer. The OP-1 motif also interacts with the adjacent NF-1 site. OP-1 and NF-1 form a composite element that increases JCV early activity and reduces JCV late activity (Kim *et al.*, 2001; Raj and Khalili, 1995).

The penta motif also differentially binds members of the lytic control element binding protein family, LCP-1, recognising alternative DNA structures. This factor bears remarkable similarity to Pur α and influences early and late promoter functions. Therefore, the region is designated the JCV lytic control element (LCE). Subsequent studies have demonstrated that this element interacts with Pur α and YB-1. YB-1 is a member of a gene family, originally isolated from a human B cell expression library, which is responsive to a wide variety of stimuli, including stress signals drug and interleukin-2 treatment in T cells. The essential contact site is located in the C/T-rich sequence on the early strand of the LCE without affecting the adjacent NF-1 binding site. YB-1 binds to double-stranded and single-stranded DNA and activates transcription from both the early and late viral promoters. The function is attributed to both its interactions with DNA and its ability to interact with other proteins.

The single-stranded DNA- and RNA-binding protein Pur α binds to penta on the late LCE strand. Cross-communication with the proteins on the LCE mediates reduced or increased binding to YB-1, thereby influencing early activation. Although TAg has no binding capacities to LCE sequences, close association of YB-1, Pur α and TAg and the complexity of binding events suggests that the interplay is important for a broad spectrum of different functions during the JCV life cycle. The model of Pur α and YB-1 interaction in TAg-mediated transition of JCV early-to-late promoter activity is based on the following findings: Pur α increases early promoter activity with minor effects on the late sequences; TAg increases late activity considerably; and YB-1 elevates basal activity on the early and late promoter, with a higher rate in the late phase. Increasing concentrations of TAg results in a gradual decrease in Pur α early enhancement.

In contrast to early expression, cooperative action of Pur α and TAg leads to interference of Pur α with the TAg late stimulatory effect, thus suggesting that Pur α and TAg each exert antagonistic effects on the other's transcriptional activity. The mechanism by which the two regulators influence each other's activities is not yet clear; however, TAg may indirectly destabilise the association of Pur α with the LCE. In this respect, TAg might cause dissociation of Pur α from the LCE by increasing the rate of YB-1 binding.

From these findings it was proposed that at the initial phase of infection strong binding of Pur α to the LCE preferentially stimulates transcription of the early genome. As the lytic cycle proceeds, the composition of DNA–protein complexes in the LCE is altered. The increasing level of TAg facilitates YB-1-mediated dissociation of Pur α from the pentanucleotide repeat by stabilising the association of YB-1 with DNA. Removal of Pur α from the LCE results in a substantial decrease in early promoter activity. At the same time, YB-1-associated Pur α release of the late promoter allows TAg to enhance the expression during the late phase of infection. Thus, it appears likely that Pur α, YB-1 and TAg are involved in the transition from early to late gene expression.

The B domain in the early orientation positively contributes to expression in glial cells and is also important for transcriptional activation of JCVL genes. The central motif responds to glial factor 1 (GF-1) and appears to be part of the human SμbP-2 factor (Kim et al., 2001). GF-1 protein expression is most abundant in brain tissue. Interestingly, the amount of GF-1 is higher in kidney cells than in other cell types. Therefore it is suggested that the level of GF-1 in kidney cells could be responsible for the ability of JCV to replicate in urogenital tissue. Binding to the GF-1 site stimulates transcription from the JCVL promoter and to a lesser degree from the JCVE promoter.

As mentioned above, pronounced high-affinity NF-1 binding sites, NF-1 A/B, are located just upstream from the A/T rich region. Three more NF-1 sites, C, D and E, are found in domain A and further into the late region. Closely associated are three overlapping binding sites for the nuclear factor Jun. A consensus sequence similar to that of activation transcription factor ATF or cyclic AMP-responsive element (CRE) is localised on the latter half of NF-1 site A/B. A sequence with partial homology to ATF/CRE sites overlaps NF-1 site E. NF-1 site D coincides with a site resembling the sequence for the activator protein AP-1. Interaction at the binding sites involves NF-1 or NF-1-like factors, ATF/CRE-related factors and Jun-related (AP-1-like) factors. Isolated binding sites do not mediate activity, suggesting an essential role of the surrounding binding sites and interactions of related proteins for the activation process.

It was reported that NF-1 sites A/B are involved in basal as well as in glial cell-specific modulation. This discrepancy was recently explained by the detection of an activating glial cell-specific NF-1 form. It became clear that the level of transcriptional activity and specificity of the NF-1 sites is due to the homodimeric–heterodimeric nature of different NF-1 molecules, and to the combinatorial interaction of NF-1 with adjacent proteins (Monaco et al., 2001). Apart from the prominent activity conveyed by NF-1 onto the JCVE, the sites are additionally involved in JCVL cell-specific activation by TAg transactivation. BAG-1, a novel factor, interacts with anti-apoptotic Bcl-2 protein. Binding to the NF-1 site activates the JCVE and JCVL promoters. As BAG-1 is ubiquitously expressed, this might be an important regulator in persistence (Devireddy et al., 2000).

Cell-specific activity in glial cells include the cyclic AMP (cAMP)-responsive element (CRE) overlapping with the AP1 site. The second messenger cAMP and forskolin substantially increase JCVE expression.

Activity is mediated by a CRE-binding protein (CREB) and is not influenced by the NF-1 site. However, this does not exclude the possibility that the binding of other proteins to CRE may modulate expression without directly interacting with JCVE sites. Additionally, a glial cell-specific modification of CREB might be responsible for activation. Thus, it is likely that a significant contribution to the enhanced glial cell-specific expression of JCV comes from inducible transcription factors interacting with unique motifs on the JCV promoter. Importantly, the mechanisms of induction for the factors are through different signal transduction pathways. This combination allows a highly flexible JCV transcriptional response to a large number of environmental signals.

At present, in domain A two potential promoter elements have been identified, a transactivator element associated to HIV-1 TAR homologous sequences and Tst-1 binding sites. The D domain is located close to the start codon of the late proteins in the leader of the late RNAs. It spans binding sites for cellular proteins NF-1, c-Jun, YB-1 and a NF-κB-responsive region (Raj et al., 1995). YB-1 exhibits the ability to modulate basal and activated levels of transcription of JCVL through its influence on p65 on the NF-κB site. This points to a potential role for YB-1 as a transcriptional co-activator for regulation from the NF-κB site. The YB-1 site on the B domain does not account for such pronounced effects, thus the D domain probably represents the optimal site for interaction of YB-1 and NF-κB/rel subunits.

NF-κB/rel subunits modulate JCV late promoter activity from the D domain, revealing an extensive duality of NF-κB/rel-mediated effects. The subunits appear to function mutually antagonistically in terms of their transcriptional activity from either the D domain or the NF-κB site. Basal uninduced transcription appears to be positively regulated by p50/52 from the D domain, whereas induced transcription is positively regulated by p65 from the NF-κB site. At present, it appears likely that the interplay between NF-κB subunits and the D domain is dependent on direct and specific interaction of YB-1 and the NF-κB/rel subunits, influencing each other's binding capacity to their respective target DNAs. Since each of the NF-κB dimers can potentially interact with the NF-κB site, multiple levels of regulation can be mediated by the complex interactions of NF-κB/rel subunits. This provides an exquisite control mechanism over constitutive and induced NF-κB activity. However, the importance of the motif in the viral life cycle and in association

with immunomodulators has not yet been clarified (Sweet et al., 2002).

Heterologous Transactivation of Virus Transcription

Additional to activating effects of cellular transcription factors, viruses are considered to influence JCV expression through the direct or indirect interaction of a heterogeneous gene product. In general, transactivation can occur at any step of protein synthesis, beginning with the initiation of transcription and ending with posttranslational modifications. In the case of JCV, promoter activity and DNA replication were affected.

The question of whether HIV-1 may transactivate JCV is discussed, since it has become clear that PML is one of the most prevalent opportunistic infections in AIDS patients. The HIV-1-encoded transregulatory protein Tat has been found to be a potent activator of the JCVL promoter. Tat is a transcriptional activator and an essential component for the establishment of a productive HIV-1 infection. The transacting responsive region (TAR) mediates activation of the HIV-1 promoter. In the JCV promoter, at least two responsive elements, the TAT element in the ORI domain and the TAR element, have been identified. Transactivation occurs in vitro at the level of transcription by HIV-Tat induction of the JCVL promoter. Correspondingly, BKV TAg is able to transactivate the HIV-1 long terminal repeat (LTR). Although HIV-1 expression in oligodendrocytes is regularly low, Tat protein appears to be secreted by the HIV-1-infected cell. Localised to the JCV-infected oligodendrocyte, it could induce transcription on Tat-responsive genes. Recently, co-infection with another retrovirus, HTLV-1, in PML tissue raised the question of whether HTLV-1 could activate JCV expression. It was found that the JCV promoter is modulated by interaction with the regulatory protein Tax. Thus, a transactivating effect comparable to that of HIV-1 Tat protein is conceivable.

Transactivation is also postulated for herpes viruses. Human cytomegalovirus (CMV) is highly prevalent in men. CMV infection is often activated in immuno-impaired patients, and common target tissues are kidney, lung, the CNS and lymphoid organs. Molecular interaction of CMV with JCV is mediated in vitro by the HCMV immediate-early transactivator 2 (IE2). Stimulation of the JCVE promoter by IE2 leads to increased JCV DNA replication. Similarly, it was found that BKV TAg is able to induce the expression of CMV early gene expression (Dörries, 2001).

Although co-localisation of HCMV and the human polyomaviruses appears to be possible, neither in AIDS patients nor after kidney transplantation with a high incidence of CMV infection has a correlation of polyomavirus and CMV viruria been observed. Lack of interaction among CMV and the human polyomaviruses was confirmed by treatment of haemorrhagic cystitis with aciclovir. Although CMV replication decreased, no influence on BKV-associated HC was reported. In contrast, aciclovir therapy was beneficial in single PML cases. Therefore, at present it cannot be decided whether transactivation of CMV contributes to the pathogenesis of polyomavirus-associated disease.

Human herpesvirus 6 (HHV6) infection was co-localised with JCV in oligodendrocytes of PML lesions by *in situ* PCR. HHV6 has a high prevalence in the adult population, establishing persistent infection in the brain, urogenital tract, lung, liver and peripheral blood cells. HHV6 activation often occurs after transplantation. Obviously, huPyV and HHV6 have a wide range of target organs in common. Due to putative transactivation mechanisms of other herpesviruses, a comparable interaction of HHV6 with the human polyomaviruses is thinkable.

Although the mechanisms of huPyV transactivation by heterogeneous viruses *in vivo* are at present not understood, the increasing number of HIV-1 patients with active polyomavirus infections argues for a potential role of concomitantly infecting viruses for the activation of polyomavirus infections in men.

Genomic Heterogeneity of Viral Subtypes

In early studies, JCV DNA populations from PML brain tissue exhibited a remarkable genomic homogeneity within one patient. In contrast, analysis of JCV isolates from different individuals revealed that a large number of JCV subtypes exist. Comparable variations in the BKV and the SV40 genome pointed to a general role of genomic heterogeneity among the polyomaviruses (Dörries, 1997; Knowles, 2001). Throughout JCV genomes, numerous single-base changes have been observed and the TCRs exhibit extensive structural differences. Single base mutations in coding genes do not affect the reading frames and most are silent, having no effect on the amino acid composition of the proteins. In contrast to BKV, JCV DNA does not exhibit sufficient sequence variation to generate different serotypes. Therefore genotypes are exclusively

defined by their DNA sequence. The biological significance of the changes remains uncertain, as the role of protein alterations for the viability or cell specificity of viral subtypes is not yet clarified (Pfister *et al.*, 2001; Sala *et al.*, 2001). Among all viral genes, VP1 shows the greatest degree of variation, whereas the agnogene is the most conserved part. The clustering of mutations on the terminal end of VP1 and TAg proteins provides the tool for V-T subtyping of JCV genotypes in different regions of the world. It is used for virus transmission studies and as a marker for early population migration.

At present, major V-T genotypes are assigned to different geographic regions by creation of a phylogenetic tree from isolates all over the world. Three separate JCV genotypes 1 were found in individuals of European origin. Type 2, the so-called European/Asian type, was traced in a wide region extending from Europe to western and eastern Asia. Additional types (3, 6) were dominantly found in African states and in Afro-Americans. Type 7 is located in the south-east Asia and southern China populations. Although prevalent subtypes vary considerably in the Asian region, most territories are dominated by type 2A, which is closely related to the Japanese types Cy and My. Type 8 is a related JCV clade in the South Pacific region (Agostini *et al.*, 2001; Hatwell and Sharp, 2000). The relationship among genotypes is still under debate and it can be assumed that the number of true genotypes will increase with more populations tested for their JCV strains.

Changes within the non-coding region of JCV are used for classification of three major TCR subtypes: class I, class II and the archetype. All major JCV variants isolated so far can be grouped into those basic types. The extensive heterogeneity of the JCV TCR gave rise to the hypothesis that the rearrangements might be involved as a virulence factor in the pathogenic process. It was assumed that JCV TCRs may change from a basic persisting subtype in peripheral organs to a virulent type growing efficiently in glial cells (Dörries, 1997) (Figure 23.5).

The variable TCR elements are constructed of conserved segments with a high degree of sequence conservation that can be deleted or duplicated and rejoined to new units in individual subtypes. The junctions between these domains are variable in length and are preferentially used as breaking regions, thus serving as a source of rearranged sequence pattern. Type I DNA contains two TATA sequences by inclusion of the TATA box in the repeated element; type II DNA has only one TATA sequence and a 23 bp insertion, which includes a potential enhancer

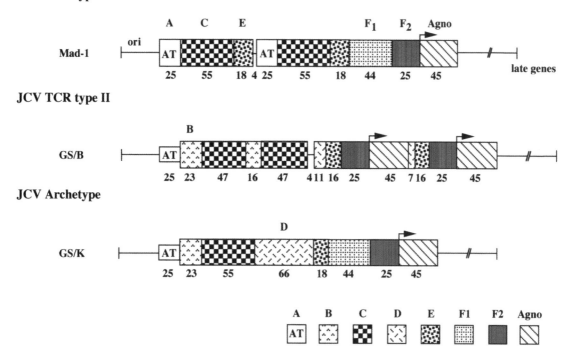

Figure 23.5 Structure of the major JCV TCR subtypes. JCV TCR subtype I, American JCV prototype Mad-1; TCR type II, European JCV prototype GS/B; archetype, European isolate JCV GS/K. The sequence is divided into seven boxed segments of identical nucleotide sequence (A, B, C, D, E, F1, F2), differing in nucleotide length. Identical shading represents the same DNA sequence. A represents the TATA box. The initiation codon for the putative agnogene (Agno) is indicated by an arrow. Segment length is given in base pairs; AT, TATA box; Ori, origin of DNA replication

core sequence followed by extensively rearranged repeats. The archetype, with a single promoter element and a 66 bp insertion, does not exhibit any major repetitions.

Genomic comparison of JCV populations in affected CNS tissue and persistently infected renal tissue of the same PML patient revealed the presence of homogeneous populations of highly related subtypes at both sites of infection. However, in contrast to the brain-derived virus type with duplicated promoter elements, the kidney-derived virus exhibited an archetypal control region. This provided evidence that a peripheral virus type may invade the CNS during persistence, and that duplicated promoter elements may subsequently be generated anew in each host. The assumption was evaluated by analysis of JCV DNA populations in PML patients. Heterogeneous genome populations could only be found at a low rate in the active stage of disease. As a possible explanation, it

was suggested that TCR rearrangements (a) might be a rather isolated event or (b) could be preferentially associated with early stages of disease; alternatively (c) rearrangements might be generated at activated states during persistent infection. In this case, more virulent subtypes in heterogeneous TCR populations might outgrow others, leading to the homogeneous populations found in PML tissue. Recently, in the active disease process of a long-term PML survivor, only one prominent variant was detected. In contrast, at autopsy additional subtypes were found, which were not related to the first sequence. This indicates that some virus types may outgrow others in the active disease process, but it also suggests that JCV TCR subtypes can be disseminated to the brain during persistent infection from the periphery.

Activation of polyomavirus infection is frequently observed under impairment of the immune system. JCV genomes in such individuals revealed mostly homogeneous TCR populations of single promoter elements. Only a minor group carried virus populations with duplicated rearranged TCR forms. Obviously, immune impairment does not play a major role in the induction of rearrangements from the archetypal structure. However, analysis of JCV TCR types in non-immunosuppressed and healthy individuals from different countries in the world revealed that human populations with JCV types of dominantly single promoter elements exist alongside others discerning JCV PML-type TCRs in persistent infection. Comparison of TCR types in persistently infected organs revealed comparable distribution patterns of TCR types in kidney, brain and peripheral blood cells. From this finding it can be assumed that the TCR rearrangements are not associated with a specific cell type. The low prevalence of variant TCR types in almost all patient groups points rather to the existence of a number of stable TCR subtypes that might be less sensitive to rearrangements than to a high rate of rearrangements in each individual (Elsner and Dörries, 1998).

On the basis of these findings, the question for the transcriptional activity of subtype control regions is essential to answer (Ault, 1997). Initial experiments point to a more complicated situation than assumed by the DNA sequence of JCV promoter elements alone. In contrast to all assumptions, it was recently found that the rate of early transcriptional activity mediated by duplicated TCRs can be similar to that of single promoter structures. Additionally, it was confirmed that the overall cell type-specificity of individual subtypes is not affected by structural changes (author's observations). In contrast to these findings, JCV TCR type 2 was recently detected at increased frequency in PML patients. Therefore, it remains open whether TCR heterogeneity is a determining factor in virus growth rate or is related to pathogenicity (Ferrante *et al.*, 2001; Pfister *et al.*, 2001; Sala *et al.*, 2001).

Interestingly, JCV European/American genotype 2 genomes linked to PML type TCRs were described in a number of PML patients. In consequence, it was asked whether a specific genotype might constitute a pathogenic strain. As a possible molecular basis for altered neurovirulence, mutations were discussed, which lead to alternative splicing of early mRNA transcripts with expression of T' proteins. Functional changes in the zinc finger motif of TAg, changes in the late regions of the genome that could be involved in protein folding, virion assembly or virus-receptor binding could also influence pathogenicity (Agostini *et al.*, 2001). However, genotypes 1 and 2 can be linked to both archetypal and PML-type TCR elements, and both

were isolated from PML and persistently infected individuals. Although at present no archetypal genome was described as the only variant in a PML case, from the relationship of archetypal and PML-type regulatory regions, it is conceivable that PML-type JCV TCRs have been generated from single promoter elements. Since geographic clustering of JCV TCR type II genomes cannot be excluded, whether a specific type of JCV genotype/TCR subtype combination is dominantly associated with PML remains to be further evaluated.

Although genomic analysis of BKV remains rather limited, diverging sequences have been observed, including the TCR and the coding sequences. A geographic association of BKV subtypes has not been performed and attempts to associate BKV subtypes with clinical conditions have not yet been successful. In contrast to JCV, serological groups corresponding to BKV genotypes have been detected. Sequence variation was located to the amino-terminal quarter of the VP1 major capsid protein, with changes in the amino acid sequence and potential implications for the secondary and tertiary structure of the protein. Interestingly, genotypes are often not stable in an individual, but change in multiple or serial samples. The genetic instability appears to be extraordinary; however, the significance of this finding is not certain (Knowles, 2001).

State of Human Polyomavirus Infection in Target Organs

Primary Infection

Primary contact with the human polyomaviruses is generally asymptomatic. It usually occurs during childhood or early in adulthood, leading to lifelong infection in the immunocompetent host. Viruses normally undergo an initial replication cycle in cells proximal to the site of entry and prior to viraemia. The route of infection has not yet been defined, although BKV seroconversion has been associated with tonsillitis, upper respiratory tract disease, mild pyrexia and transient cystitis. Investigation of nasopharyngeal aspirates and saliva by PCR occasionally demonstrated the presence of BKV DNA, but subsequent virus isolation often was not successful. BKV-specific IgM antibody in umbilical cord blood or in the sera of children aged <2 weeks suggested prenatal infection. This was supported recently by PCR detection of BKV DNA in maternal and fetal material. In addition, BKV DNA in male and female genital tissue against a background of a low prevalence of JCV DNA pointed to possible sexual transmission. However, as the detection of BKV DNA was exclusively dependent on PCR findings, it remains open whether the oropharyngeal tract or alternative routes of transmission are involved in primary infection. Therefore, the alimentary tract was proposed as the more likely port of entry (Moens and Rekvig, 2001; Stoner and Hübner, 2001) (Figure 23.6).

Similarly, the site of JCV entry has not yet been localised, although direct infection of B lymphocytes and tonsillar stroma favours the respiratory tract (Monaco *et al.*, 1996). In contrast, recent detection of JCV in the colon (Ricciardiello *et al.*, 2000) suggests the lower gastrointestinal tract as a possible entry site. Irrespective of the site of entry, viraemia is thought to occur, based on the finding that virus reaches sites of persistence very early in infection.

Despite the knowledge that JCV infection is widespread in the population, almost nothing is known about how JCV is transmitted in humans. Studies on sewage in Europe revealed that human polyomaviruses are distributed to fresh waters by faecal contamination (Bofill-Mas and Girones, 2001). Genome analyses in and around Tokyo suggest that population density and environmental conditions may affect the transmission of JCV. One route of transmission was elucidated by tracing JCV subtypes in Japanese families, in which both parents and children excreted JCV in their urine. Typing of JCV genomes in individual family members revealed the presence of different viral subtypes (Agostini *et al.*, 2001). In about 50% of persons, the JCV strains originated from infection outside families. Children have many opportunities to come into contact with urinary JCV infection; therefore, urinary excretion can

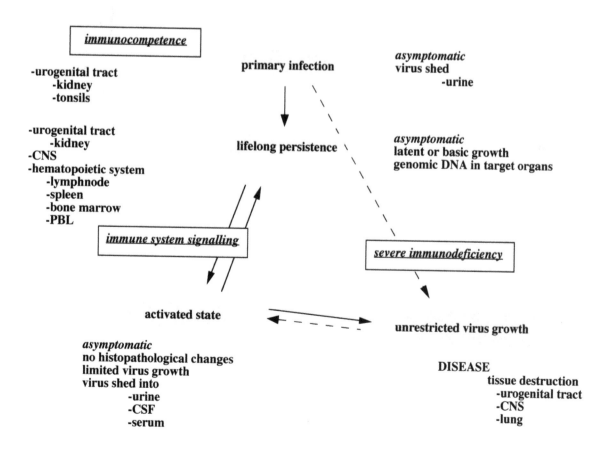

Figure 23.6 Course of human polyomavirus infection

be a prominent source of JCV in the human population.

Persistent Infection

The discovery of BKV came from the observation of cytological abnormalities in the urinary sediment of a kidney transplant patient. Later it became clear that BKV is a urotheliotropic virus affecting the epithelia of the renal calyces, renal pelvis, ureter and urinary bladder. Analyses of prostate biopsies revealed virus infection in 60% of asymptomatic tissue, comparable to the rate of infection in the bladder. Sperm gave an incidence of 95% and cervix and vulvar tissue an incidence of 70%. In contrast, glandular tissue was free of JCV virus and in sperm 21% of the samples were positive for JCV DNA. The high rate of BKV DNA in asymptomatic tissue and semen suggests that these sites might be involved in polyomavirus persistence (Knowles, 2001; Moens and Rekvig, 2001).

Similarly, JCV was detected in the urinary tract of immunosuppressed individuals and pregnant women. PCR analysis suggests that the number of affected individuals closely parallels the percentage of persons with serological evidence for contact with JCV. Thus, the kidney is one site of huPyV infection (Arthur and Shah, 1989). JCV DNA was detected in the kidneys of two children with combined immunodeficiency disease who developed PML during primary JCV infection. Additional presence of JCV DNA in spleen, lymph node and lung cells support the thesis that JCV persistence in individual organs is most likely established during primary infection. Repeated detection of JCV DNA in the ureters of non-immunosuppressed patients characterised the renal tract as a site of persistence. The higher detection frequency in the renal medulla indicates that epithelial cells lining collective tubules are the major targets. The presence of JCV in urothelial sediments suggests that they are more often subject to activation processes than other cells in the renal tract. In a study of the presence of JCV DNA in colorectal cancers, JCV DNA was additionally detected by PCR in the colon mucosa of 76% of normal patients, suggesting that the virus is highly prevalent in the human upper and lower gastrointestinal tract of immunocompetent individuals (Ricciardiello et al., 2000).

The dissemination of the human polyomaviruses to a wide range of organs led to the hypothesis of a possible haematogeneous spread in the host. This was supported by an early report on polyomavirus particles in lymphocytes of immunocompetent children and induced studies on a general role of lymphoid cells in the establishment of polyomavirus persistence. In tonsils, BKV DNA was associated with the lymphoid tissue of Waldeyer's ring, thus indicating the involvement of lymphocytes in polyomavirus infection. Lymphoid interaction of BKV was further supported by a stimulatory effect of virus infection on human lymphocytes in cell culture, and the demonstration of specific BKV receptors on the surface of peripheral blood cells. Interestingly, only a small number of cells carried receptors for BKV, which were described as B lymphocytes. Nevertheless, virus protein expression was restricted to less than 1% of the cells, thus indicating attenuated replication in lymphocytes. Although the virus is able to attach to and penetrate into monocytes, expression remained negative. However, the treatment of monocyte cultures with BKV antisera was followed by antibody-dependent enhancement of virus replication. Therefore, it can be assumed that circulating monocytes or tissue-resident macrophages in the normal individual might be permissive for polyomavirus infection. The presence of full-length BKV DNA in the leukocytes of persistently infected individuals confirmed involvement of BKV in peripheral blood infection, similar to that in kidney and brain tissue (Dörries, 1997). A large body of analyses has been performed, concentrating on the search of virus DNA in peripheral blood cells (PBMC) by PCR. The results were highly variable, rendering incidences of no BKV DNA present to 60% of BMT patients, 10–100% of HIV-1 patients or no virus in a group of SLE patients. Similarly, in healthy individuals 53%, 71% and 94% contrasted a finding of no virus DNA, respectively. Even two recent reports with advanced PCR techniques including excessive precautions against contamination demonstrated BKV DNA at rates of 26% vs. 55% (Knowles, 2001). This might be due to geographical differences; however, comparison of selected groups, sample preparation and primer pairs revealed major differences. Most of the studies on the presence of BKV DNA in PBL were performed by nested PCR techniques, often at the limits of detection. The amount of BKV DNA was estimated to be very low, as compared with that of JCV in peripheral blood cells. Taken together the high variability in the detection rate of BKV DNA in haematopoietic cells makes a decision on the role of BKV in blood cell infection difficult. However, there is a body of evidence for a regular lymphotropism of BK virus in the host. This includes detection of BKV-specific DNA and mRNA in PBMC, as well as indirect evidence for BKV susceptibility of monocytes.

Haematogeneous spread of JCV to the CNS had been suspected in early reports because of the exceptional multifocal distribution of JCV foci in PML. Occasional involvement of the spleen and lymph nodes led to the concept that lymphoid cells might be regularly involved in virus spread. This was confirmed by demonstrating JCV DNA and capsid protein in a small number of mononuclear cells of bone marrow and spleen in PML/AIDS patients. These cells were characterised as B lymphocytes by cellular markers, whereas CD4/CD8$^+$ T lymphocytes were not affected. The presence of JCV infected mononuclear cells in perivascular parenchyma and in Virchow–Robin spaces further supported the haematogeneous route of entry into the brain for JCV. Although JCV DNA could not be detected in the spleens of HIV-1 patients and controls, the detection rate of 40% in PML patients suggests that virus DNA may accumulate in lymphoid organs.

The thesis of lymphocytes as a reservoir for JCV closed a gap in the understanding of viral pathogenesis. It was conceivable that JCV-infected lymphoid cells may act as a vector for JCV dissemination. The role of JCV infection in lymphoid cells was further clarified by the detection of tonsillar B lymphocytes and tonsillar stromal cells as host cells for JCV infection (Monaco et al., 1996). Cultivation of tonsillar cells followed by demonstration of JCV DNA established the susceptibility of tonsillar cells. These findings not only strongly suggest the involvement of the tonsils in primary infection but also argue for a persistent polyomavirus infection in tonsillar cell types.

The role of lymphoid cells in JCV persistence and pathogenesis was studied more intensively by asking whether JCV DNA is present in circulating peripheral blood cells during periods of immunocompromise. The infection rates in peripheral lymphocytes of PML patients were the highest (30–100%), irrespective of the underlying disease or the affected cell type, the virus load or the number of infected cells (Andreoletti et al., 1999; Dörries, 2001; Dubois et al., 1997; Koralnik et al., 1999). This pointed to a regular involvement of lymphoid cells in the disease process. The association of JCV with PBMC from the bone marrow and blood of leukaemia patients added further support to the idea that polyomaviruses might be lymphotropic.

The question of whether peripheral blood cells play a role in the dissemination of JCV during persistence was addressed by studies on risk group patients without evidence of PML. Detection of JCV DNA in leukaemia patients at a rate of 10–60% prior to and past BMT revealed that these patients are at a high risk for JCV association with peripheral blood cells.

Interestingly, the amount of virus DNA detected was highly variable and did not correspond to the timespan after BMT. This pointed to an intermittent rather than a continuous course of virus replication. In HIV-1 infected patients, as the most prominent risk group, comparable detection rates were reported. This allows the assumption that virus replication leading to the detection of JCV DNA in PBMC is independent of the type of immune impairment (Andreoletti et al., 1999; Lafon et al., 1998).

Regular association of JCV with PBMC at a rate of more than 80% was further confirmed by amplification of JCV DNA in PBMC of healthy persons. In situ hybridisation added support to the idea that the human polyomaviruses are associated with peripheral blood cells (Dörries et al., 1994). Experimental evidence was added by interaction of JCV with human B lymphocyte cell lines. Susceptibility of haematopoietic precursor cells for virus infection was mediated by enhanced expression of the transcription protein nuclear binding factor NF-1. This additionally argued for the involvement of those cell types in natural JCV infection (Dörries, 1997; Monaco et al., 2001). However, PCR studies in different laboratories produced markedly divergent results. Incidence rates ranged from none detected to 59%. In most PBMC samples the concentration of virus-specific DNA was estimated to be in the range of less than one genome equivalent in 20 cells, this probably being the reason for the low rates of detection or even failure to amplify JCV DNA by PCR, as loss of targets by DNA extraction methods appears to be a critical step in the detection of persisting virus genomes.

Further characterisation of the virus–cell interaction addressed the question of the cellular target of JCV in lymphoid tissue or peripheral blood. The first reports pointed to the B lymphocyte in bone marrow and spleen as the only target cell. However, in B lymphocyte-depleted PBMC JCV-specific amplification was similarly reported (Dubois et al., 1997). Subsequent studies suggested that JCV could be associated with several haematopoietic cell types (Dörries et al., 2003; Koralnik et al., 1999). Generally, the detection rate in PML patients was higher than in those with HIV-1 infection alone, and healthy individuals had the lowest incidence for JCV in blood cells. Although unsorted cells from normal persons were negative for JCV, virus DNA could be detected in sorted populations from the same patient. This corresponds to reports of a low virus load in PBMC. Virus–cell association could either be detected in all of B and T lymphocytes, in granulocytes and in monocytes of a given blood sample, or only in a single population or any combination of cell types. Interestingly, the most prominent cell affected was the granulocyte, a cell type that may not only be specifically associated with JCV infection, but can also be involved in phagocytosis (Dörries *et al.*, 2003). These results suggest that JCV DNA molecules are regularly associated with cell types of different lineages; however, the type of association remains to be elucidated. Similarly, investigations on JCV expression in haematopoietic cells rendered controversial results. JCV mRNA was detected in PBMC and in B lymphocytes of PML patients. In contrast, no expression could be found in HIV-1 patients and blood donors (Andreoletti *et al.*, 1999; Dubois *et al.*, 1997; Lafon *et al.*, 1998). This discrepancy could be explained by a preferential latent state of virus infection in PBMC that might be activated in PML. Clearly, more experiments are necessary to understand the role of JCV DNA in PBMC for viral persistence and possible consequences for the disease process.

Although the suggestion that haematopoietic cells are a reservoir for the virion in the diseased brain might be questionable, it is conceivable that JCV-infected lymphoid cells may act as a vector for JCV CNS invasion and dissemination during persistent infection (Gallia *et al.*, 1997). Apart from how the virus might be disseminated to the CNS, the pathogenic question, of whether PML results from cytolytic invasion of the CNS under severe immunosuppression or as a consequence of a preceding persistent infection, is controversially discussed (Dörries, 1997). Although JCV can easily be demonstrated in disseminated areas of PML autopsy material virus DNA or protein, it has not been detected in the healthy CNS by classical methods. However, application of PCR revealed frequent JCV infection in the brain of patients without evidence for PML. In contrast to fetal brain tissue, JCV DNA sequences were present in about 30–70% of adults, depending on the experimental groups. JCV obviously has no topographical preference, because dissemination patterns are comparable to those in PML. Cloning of genomic JCV DNA molecules in brain tissue resulted exclusively in unique, full-length, episomal JCV genomes. Compared to thousands of genome equivalents present in affected PML samples, the amount of virus-specific DNA in asymptomatic individuals is much lower, with an estimated range of 1–100 genome equivalents/20 cells, and even less. Thus, persistent polyomavirus infection in the CNS is probably restricted to isolated cells and most likely represents chronic infection and not the early stage of disease (Elsner and Dörries, 1998).

The findings prove that human peripheral polyomavirus infection is associated with subclinical virus entry into the CNS, probably long before the development of clinically overt PML. Which cell type is targeted by the virus is not yet known; however, virus activation may lead to an increased number of infected cells and a higher detection frequency in cases of severe immunosuppression, in patients with malignant diseases and in the elderly, this being in line with the assumption that impairment of immune competence favours involvement of the CNS in polyomavirus infection.

Concomitant JCV and BKV Infection

Double infection of JCV and BKV was particularly established after organ transplantation, in HIV-1 infected patients, in pregnancy and in a small number of immunocompetent individuals by urinary excretion or antibody rise against both viruses. Molecular detection of JCV- and BKV-specific DNA confirmed that concomitant persistence frequently occurs in kidney tissue. Extensive homologies of the genomic structure, similarities of virus spread and state of infection very early started the discussion on possible other sites of dual JCV and BKV infection. After PBMC were found to be a target of polyomavirus infection, the presence of JCV and BKV DNA in blood cells of the same individuals was not astonishing. A high rate of concomitant infection was evidenced molecularly in both healthy and immunosuppressed individuals. As JCV protein expression was detected in lymphoid cells of immunosuppressed patients, and BKV virus is able to replicate in lymphocytes *in vitro*, it is likely that both huPyV infections are periodically activated in persistently infected PBMC.

Although BKV was not expected to invade the CNS at a high rate, the cell specificity of BKV is less stringent than that of JCV, therefore several laboratories searched for double infection in the CNS. Cloning from CNS gene libraries and PCR revealed frequent BKV dissemination to the brain. Indirectly, BKV infection of the human CNS was confirmed by the report of a subacute BKV-associated meningoencephalitis in an AIDS patient. The physical state and genetic complexity of BKV genomes was comparable to that of JCV DNA; however, a low concentration of brain-derived BKV-specific PCR products suggests a considerably lower activity of BKV in the CNS than that of JCV. The detection of amplification products belonging to both polyomavirus species gives strong evidence for concomitant polyomavirus infection in the CNS. Additionally, it demonstrates that not only JCV but also BKV is neurotropic in the human host, and frequently establishes persistent CNS infection.

The rate of adult healthy individuals found positive for concomitant infection was astounding, but the data correspond to recently discussed rates of infection with BKV of almost 100% by the age of 10 and JCV reaching more than 90% in adulthood. Therefore, the number of positive cases probably reflects the true incidence of polyomavirus infection in the European population.

Asymptomatic Activation of Infection

Transient polyomavirus viruria probably occurs at the time of primary infection; however, in most instances the presence of virus in the urine is due to activation processes. It was assumed that activation of infection in healthy individuals was predominantly related to alterations of immunocompetence in the older age groups. Recently, PCR was used to show that JCV DNA was present in urine of about 30% of American and 60% of Japanese and European healthy individuals. The incidence of excretion depended on age, with lower rates in the young, then a gradual increase with age. Because of the high frequency of JCV excretion throughout adulthood, the authors suggest that JCV infection may regularly not be in a latent persistent state but in a productive one. Since all other data were accumulated by less sensitive methods, it is conceivable that virus expression is permanently maintained at a basic level.

Pregnancy is among the most common conditions that have been linked to viral activation. The incidence of viruria, as detected by periodic cytological examination, was about 3–7% in the case of JCV and 15% in the case of BKV. The onset of viruria was late in the second trimester and during the third trimester of pregnancy. In excreters, virus shedding, once it was established, continued intermittently to term and then ceased in the *postpartum* period. The detection rates parallel high or rising antibody titres in a comparable study population, and therefore represent probably the true rate of activated persistent infections.

Renal transplant recipients experienced viruria at a higher rate (9–19%), compared to a rate of 2.4% in pregnant women with similar detection sensitivities. Duration periods may be months or even years. In bone marrow transplant recipients, almost all viruria

was due to BKV, with an incidence of up to 50% in the post-transplant period. Although these findings point to a significant role of the immune state for the level of polyomavirus expression in the kidney, an enhancement of urinary excretion by HIV-1-induced immunosuppression was not detectable. Similarly, PML patients do not necessarily have concomitant JCV viruria. Aggressive chemotherapy does not increase virus frequency, and in other immunosuppressive diseases viruria can be intermittent, with sparsely distributed infected cells in cytologically positive urine, similarly pointing to a rather low rate of virus production (Arthur and Shah, 1989).

Activation at other sites of persistent infection has been less intensively examined. This is due to reduced virus expression in asymptomatic transient activation states and to the low virus load in persistently infected healthy individuals. Although the presence of JCV DNA in PBMC appears to be a common event, activation can so far only be deduced from the presence of higher amounts of virus DNA in immunologically impaired individuals. Additionally, in HIV/ PML patients mononuclear cells expressing JCV-specific proteins were characterised in PML tissue. Thus, it appears likely that a possible JCV infection in lymphocytes is activated under as-yet unknown circumstances (Gallia et al., 1997).

The presence of JCV DNA in the brain tissue of immunocompetent patients in a distribution comparable to that in PML, and increasing incidence of detection with age and in patients with malignancies, point to viral activation in the CNS. The detection of virus-specific protein in a limited number of glial cells in non-PML brain, and PCR amplification of JCV-specific products in the CSF of the same patients' groups, argues for asymptomatic JCV activation in persistently infected brain tissue (Dörries, 1997).

If the current knowledge is summarised, it must be assumed that activation of BKV and JCV infection occurs species-specifically and as a result of immune system alterations induced by pregnancy, older age, malignant tumour growth or AIDS. Some of those individuals may undergo sporadic activation as a consequence of their genotypes or of incidental transactivation events by other viruses. In general, however, virus growth appears to be dependent on the impairment of immunological control, resulting in a differentially regulated activation pattern in the target organs. Although related mechanisms are so far unknown, the higher frequency of deficiencies correlated with T cell function in PML patients points to deficient cellular immunity as a major virulence factor.

Polyomavirus-associated Diseases

Activation of huPyV infection may either represent transient asymptomatic events or pathological processes. The induction of fatal disorders, however, is almost exclusively observed under long-lasting severe impairment of the immune system. BKV is a urotheliotropic virus, almost exclusively linked to urogenital tract diseases (Arthur and Shah, 1989). Mild courses are reported in primary BKV infection, whereas BKV disease is rather associated with persistent BKV infection, often diagnosed in lymphoma and AIDS patients (Moens and Rekvig, 2001). Virus-associated pathogenic effects are observed in BKV-associated nephropathy (BKN) and ureteral stenosis as complications of renal transplantation (RT), as well as in haemorrhagic cystitis in bone marrow transplant (BMT) patients. After BMT, BK viruria is detected often during episodes of cystitis, leading to severe haemorrhage in about 25% of BMT patients. Haemorrhage and viruria are most likely due to viral activation in the uroepithelium. Recent studies suggest that interstitial tubular nephritis is the most frequent disease after RT. Clinical features may mimic graft rejection or drug toxicity, but histopathological examination almost always demonstrates BKV infection. Immunosuppressive therapies increase the incidence of BKV-associated disease, thereby confirming a close relationship of virus growth and immunomodulation (Table 23.2).

Strong evidence for BKV-induced systemic and CNS disease came from AIDS patients. Histopathological evaluation revealed association of BKV with affected lung, kidney, and CNS tissue. The major pathological findings were tubulointerstitial nephropathy, interstitial desquamative pneumonitis and subacute meningoencephalitis. In the kidney alterations principally consisted of focally accentuated tubular necroses. Virus products were detected in epithelial cells along the entire nephron. Alterations in the lung were characterised by intra-alveolar aggregates of desquamated pneumocytes. Virus products were detected in exfoliated pneumocytes, epithelial cells and smooth muscle cells of the bronchioli. Occasionally, isolated endothelial cells in the lung carried virus protein. A common feature in both organs was focal interstitial fibrosis with a mild inflammatory response. Whereas fibrocytes were infected, inflammatory cells were free of virus products.

In the CNS, no pathological changes apart from mild inner atrophy were described. Mononuclear cells indicating chronic inflammation loosely infiltrated thickened fibrotic leptomeninges. In the cortex and adjoining white matter, endematous tissue alterations were found. Reactive astrocytes were localised in the outer layers of the cerebral cortex. The ventricular system exhibited focal degeneration of its ependyma and spongiform destruction of subjacent brain tissue. The choroid plexus showed fibrosis of the stroma and atypical epithelial cells. In some areas, necrosis

Table 23.2 Human polyomavirus-associated diseases

Patients	JCV infection		BKV infection	
	Disease	Cell type involved	Disease	Cell type involved
Immunocompetent	None observed	–	Mild respiratory disease Mild pyrexia Transient cystitis	–
Immunocompromised Urogenital system	None observed	–	Ureteral stenosis Haemorrhagic cystitis Tubulonephritis	Epithelial cells Fibrocytes
Lung	None observed	–	Interstitial pneumonitis	Epithelial cells Pneumocytes Endothelial cells Fibrocytes

CNS	Progressive multifocal leukoencephalopathy (PML)	Oligodendrocytes
		Astrocytes
		Peripheral blood
		  mononuclear cells
		B lymphocytes
			Subacute meningoencephalitis	Epithelial cells
				Fibrocytes
				Endothelial cells
				Astrocytes
				Ependymal cells
				Peripheral blood
				  mononuclear cells

and exfoliation of the plexus epithelium occurred. Small infiltrates were seen in association with the lesions.

The dominant target cells of BKV infection were fibroblasts of the loose reticular connective tissue, endothelial and smooth muscle cells of blood vessels, astrocytes and infiltrating macrophages in pons and medulla oblongata. Epithelial cells in the choroid plexus and astrocytes of the subependymal brain tissue were additionally infected. The only glial cell type involved in BKV-associated CNS disease was the astrocyte, whereas oligodendrocytes and nerve cells were not affected. The high number of cell types involved in BKV infection *in vivo* demonstrates the broad BKV cell specificity and points to a higher relationship of BKV to SV40 than to JCV. The detection of a BKV-associated disease affecting the kidney, lung and CNS is in line with the involvement of those organs in BKV persistence.

In contrast to BKV, JCV was never observed as an aetiologic agent in urogenital tract or lung disease. The most prominent disease associated with JCV is the CNS disorder PML (Berger and Major, 1999; Walker and Padgett, 1983; Zu Rhein, 1969). Although SV40 was described as the cause of PML in three American and Japanese patients, it later became clear that most probably JCV was the only agent responsible for the disease.

PML is a demyelinating disorder occurring as a late complication of pre-existing systemic diseases that impair immunological competence. Several years of treatment precede PML in diseases such as rheumatoid arthritis, chronic asthma, sarcoidosis, lupus erythematosus and chronic polymyositis. Prior to the AIDS era, malignant proliferative diseases were the dominant basic disorders in PML in about half of the cases. In HIV-1-infected patients, a steadily increasing number of cases was associated with AIDS prior to the highly active antiretroviral therapy (HAART). Although longer PML survival times can be observed under HAART, the rate of PML patients remains stable at about 5% of AIDS patients (Antinori *et al.*, 2001). Additionally, a higher frequency of PML can be observed in correlation with immunomodulatory therapies and is probably due to higher JCV activation rates (Table 23.3).

The onset of PML is often insidious. In the earliest manifestation, multiple pinhead-sized demyelinating lesions are described beneath the cortical ribbon. New small foci are continuously being added in neighbouring tissue as the growth centres of new lesions. This concept of the histological evolution of the disease is supported by the clinical evolution: the onset might be

Table 23.3 Causes for JCV activation and induction of PML prior to the AIDS epidemic

Conditions associated with activation of persistent infection	PML (% of cases* except AIDS)
Age	None
Pregnancy	None
Inflammation	None
Transplantation	Rare
Diabetes	Rare
Lymphoproliferative disease	62.2
Myeloproliferative disease	6.5
Carcinomatous disease	2.2
Immune deficiency states	16.1
Granulomatous/inflammatory disease	7.4

*Brooks and Walker (1984).

gradual, but each new functional impairment becomes progressively more severe. Once clinical signs appear, the disease usually progresses steadily. Early neurological symptoms regularly indicate multiple disseminated lesions in the brain. The extent and topography of the lesions correlate well with the duration and symptomatology of the illness (Table 23.4).

The pathognomonic feature of the disease is the striking alteration of oligodendrocytes in all lesions. Oligodendrocytes are located in the peripheral rim surrounding the zone of myelin loss. The central area is composed of reactive astrocytes, including giant cells in mitosis and astrocytes resembling the malignant cells of pleomorphic glioblastomas. Infection of

Table 23.4 Development of PML lesions

Early Lesion
  Altered oligodendrocytes in areas of demyelination
    Nuclei enlarged (two- to three-fold)
    Regular chromatin pattern is lost
    Nuclei tint deeply with basophilic dyes
    Irregular basophilic nucleic inclusions
  Seldomly activated pleomorphic microglia
  Pinhead size (mm) lined up the cortical ribbon

Aging Lesion
  Reduced number of altered oligodendrocytes in the centre of demyelination
  Shrinkage of nuclei at the rim of lesions
  Widely distributed larger foci with coherent tissue

Late Lesion
  Altered oligodendrocytes at the peripheral advancing zone surrounding the area of myelin loss in the centre
  Very sparse or absent oligodendrocytes
  Singly scattered reactive hypertrophic astrocytes
  Giant astrocytes in mitosis
  Astrocytes resembling cells in pleomorphic glioblastomas forming irregular necrotic patches (cm)

ependymal or endothelial cells has never been convincingly demonstrated.

The basic cause of tissue destruction is a cytolytic JCV infection of the oligodendrocyte. Destruction of these cells results in loss of myelin, tissue breakdown and impairment of brain function. Infected oligodendrocytes mediate highly effective virus growth in the range of $> 10^{10}$ virus particles/g tissue. Viral expression products and virions are found in the nuclei and cytoplasm of the oligodendrocytes. Bizarre astrocytes may contain JCV; however, the question of whether astrocytes may actively support infection has not yet been answered. On the grounds of morphological changes and occasional reports of intracellular virus particles, it is suggested that astrocytes may represent a semipermissive cell type, mediating reduced JCV expression or, alternatively, being sensitive to virus transformation.

In contrast to classic PML, in the AIDS patient frontoparietal and grey matter involvement increases and inflammatory reaction with perivascular mononuclear cell infiltrates is often observed. Mononuclear cells in the Virchow–Robin spaces occasionally contain JCV-specific DNA and capsid antigen, and in the subcortical white matter adjacent to blood vessels the density of infected cells appears to be increased. In addition, beneath the ependymal layers, JCV-infected cells are detected. This indicates a close topographical association of infected cells and the ventricular system. These findings might be explained by an essentially faster progress of the disease, or by differences in the immunological control of JCV infection in HIV/PML (Mazlo *et al.*, 2001).

The duration of disease after the onset of neurological symptoms is reported to be 4–6 months on average (Berger and Major, 1999). However, there are cases of > 12 months duration, with an intermittently progressive or a subclinical course over years. These cases are most often found in combination with HIV-1 infection in patients receiving HAART. Since the introduction of HAART, the definition of HIV/PML cases has had to be adapted to changes in the disease pattern, probably resulting from HAART-induced immune reconstitution, in about half of the patients. For these two groups a terminology is newly proposed for disease outcome. It is based on diagnostic criteria for definitive, probable and possible PML, with a definition of PML outcome based on disease activity. Disease progression can be classified as 'active' or 'inactive', based on clinical, radiological, virological and pathological criteria. Patients in 'active PML' have high diagnostic evidence of disease activity through the course of illness. The great majority of these patients die within a few months. Patients with 'inactive PML' lack evidence for disease activity. Stabilisation of PML may occur at any time during disease progression; however, usually it is achieved in a few months after first diagnosis. There is virtually no progression over years of follow-up, even after withdrawal of HAART (Cinque *et al.*, 2003). Use of these criteria as standard terminology in the description of clinical and biological studies would greatly assist understanding of the mechanisms of pathogenesis and therapeutic intervention.

Oncogenicity of the Human Polyomaviruses

Cancer is thought to progress through multiple stages, and with each step cells with an increasingly malignant phenotype may arise. Progression can be driven by mutations in tumour suppressor genes or oncogenes; it can also be dependent on newly acquired transforming proteins. These genes encode proteins regulating genome stability, cell cycle proliferation or apoptosis. The polyomaviruses with the large TAg provide a prototype of viral oncogenes targeting cellular regulatory proteins, thereby interfering with cellular functions. The first 121 AA comprise the shortest fragment to induce transformation. Here it binds to the retinoblastoma family of tumour suppressors and a number of other cellular proteins believed to ultimately activate the p53 tumour suppressor pathway. Activation leads to elevated steady-state levels of p53, ending in a block of the cell cycle. In addition apoptotic genes are induced. Association of TAg with or binding to p53 results in inactivation of its transcriptional activation potency, preventing the growth-inhibitory functions of genes downstream from p53. In cases where TAg expression is followed by malignant transformation, a general correlation is observed between production of higher levels of TAg and the appearance of tumours. Animal models are useful tools to ascertain molecular markers as indicators for tumour induction and progression. In contrast, in humans these markers can be used to prove hypotheses on polyomavirus oncogenicity, even in the absence of viral protein expression (Sullivan and Pipas, 2002).

The discussion of a possible oncogenicity of a huPyV in humans had its origin not only in the oncogenic potential of large TAg but also in the bizarre pleomorphism of astrocytes within lesions of PML. This was described as a hallmark of PML in the initial description of the disease and later oligodendroglioma and multifocal glioblastoma were reported, corresponding topographically to the demyelinated lesions in PML. Thus, oncogenicity of JCV and BKV was examined almost from the beginning in experimental animal systems. Developing tumour types reflected the cell type specificity of the viruses. Corresponding to the specificity of JCV for glial cells, predominantly brain tumours were observed. The highest yield was found after intracerebral inoculation of newborn Syrian hamsters, whereas peripheral nervous system tumours are prominent after intraocular virus administration. Central nervous system tumours are located in the cerebrum, cerebellum, brainstem and spinal cord. Mesenchymal tumours within the cerebral meninges are classified as malignant meningiomas. Ependymomas are the dominant type of intraventricular tumours, and occasionally choroid plexus tumours develop. The most common neoplasms were medulloblastomas at a rate of 95% in newborn hamsters. These are followed by malignant astrocytomas, glioblastoma multiforme, neuroectodermal tumours and pineocytomas. The neuro-oncogenic potential in primates was confirmed by the occurrence of malignant glial brain tumours in about 50% of adult monkeys after intracranial infection. The predominant type was characterised as astrocytoma grade 4. JCV TAg expression in tumour cells suggests that the early region of JCV DNA was present in most tumours, and rescue of JCV from tumour tissue was occasionally successful. The virus genome was regularly integrated in tandem copies at single or multiple sites, comparable to the pattern seen in hamster tumours.

The majority of JCV-induced CNS tumour types in hamsters have their human counterpart in tumours of infants, older children or young adults. In view of the giant glial cells being key features in PML, the tendency to form malignant astrocytomas and giant cells appears to be more a characteristic of JCV than that of the animal species inoculated. Although the course of PML does not allow extensive tumour growth, it can therefore be hypothesised that a semipermissive persistent JCV infection might provide the cellular background for transformation and tumour induction in the human host.

The oncogenic potential of BKV appears to be less pronounced, as it only induces tumours in rodents but not in non-human primates. The most prominent cell types affected by BKV infection in men—epithelial cells, fibrocytes, ependymal cells, astrocytes and endothelial cells—are reflected by different tumour types induced in experimental animal models. The type essentially depends on the route of infection, on the amount of virus inoculated and on the BKV isolate used. In addition, as co-factors the age and immunocompetence of the host influences the rate of malignancy.

After intraperitoneal inoculation tumours are rarely observed; subcutaneous infection yielded sarcomas with an incidence of 2–12%. Intravenous application results in ependymomas. They are sometimes associated with peripheral tumours, insulinomas, osteosarcomas and tumours of the intestine. In contrast, intracerebral inoculation resulted in choroid plexus papillomas and papillary ependymomas without a sign of peripheral tumours in 88% of the animals. The disseminated localisation of tumours demonstrates a marked tissue tropism and multioncogenicity of BKV in hamsters. Genetic differences of virus stocks with high transforming capacities and predilection for specific tumour types could be mapped to the BKV transcriptional promoter elements, suggesting that the transforming capacity might depend on TCR function.

In the tumours BKV DNA is either tandemly integrated in the cellular genome or in a free episomal state. In most tumours complex integration patterns of multiclonal origin were observed. Most cells express nuclear TAg, virus often can be rescued by cell fusion with permissive cells and tumour-derived cell lines grow permanently, maintaining their tumour-inducting potential. Selection of defined integration pattern and decrease in the amount of BKV DNA during prolonged tumour cell culture may point to rearrangements of integrated BKV DNA in the course of tumour growth. This could give rise to cells with simpler integration patterns and loss of viral DNA. Even an intact TAg gene is not necessarily needed for maintenance of cell growth, once the transformed state is established.

The spectrum of BKV-induced tumour types is comparable in all sensitive animal species. Thus, specificity of viral transcription might be one of the major selection criteria for huPyV-associated transforming activity in animal systems. In view of this assumption, it is discussed that human polyomaviruses might also be responsible for the respective tumour types in their natural host. Consequently, a large number of laboratories have evaluated the role of huPyVs in the aetiology of human tumours with most virological and molecular methods available. Despite the oncogenicity of these viruses in animal systems, association with human tumours remains controversial (Del Valle et al, 2001; Dörries, 1997; Major et al, 1992; Stoner and Hübner, 2001). However, with the introduction of PCR and the better understanding of molecular steps leading to malignant transformation, human tumour induction by polyomaviruses finds more and more arguments.

TAg expression was analysed immunohistologically in medulloblastomas, oligodendrogliomas, astrocytomas, glioblastomas, ependymomas, choroid plexus and urinary tract tumours. The results were inconsistent. Antibody titres to TAg in sera from tumour-bearing patients exhibited no significant difference to sera of normal people. From these findings the conclusion can be drawn that TAg is not regularly expressed in human tumours. Since TAg must not be expressed necessarily at all stages of tumour growth, the presence of huPyV-related DNA sequences was analysed repeatedly in a large number of tumours. So far, in one laboratory JCV DNA sequences were detected in 57% of oligodendrogliomas, about 75% of various astrocytomas, 60% of glioblastomas, 83% of ependymomas and 87% of medulloblastomas. Examination of the p53 level in tumours expressing TAg revealed that the number of tumour samples often closely paralleled those with p53 immunoreactivity. In addition, double labelling suggested close association of both proteins within the tumour cell (Del Valle et al., 2001). JCV DNA sequences have also been detected in colorectal tumours. Although this does not represent a known site of persistence, the demonstration of JCV DNA in normal mucosa adjacent to these tumours points to the colonic epithelial cell as a new target for JCV infection (Laghi et al, 1999; Ricciardiello et al., 2000).

BKV DNA was only occasionally detected by classical methods in series of human tumour types that were frequently described in animal models. This included brain tumours, osteosarcomas, insulinomas and Kaposi's sarcoma. Analyses of the state of BKV DNA revealed mostly episomal virus DNA, even if virus was rescued, this being rather more indicative of a persistent state of infection than of an association with transforming activities. After the introduction of PCR, BKV DNA was demonstrated in a variety of human tumours, including brain, pancreas and various urinary tract neoplasms (Corallini et al., 2001; Moens and Rekvig, 2001). There are studies accumulating that are not solely based on PCR results, viz. demonstration of DNA sequences using Southern blot analysis and DNA sequencing indicate that BKV DNA can be present in the integrated state. Interestingly, rearrangements of the respective viral DNA sequence probably interfere with BKV DNA replication and productive infection. This may lead to accumulation of TAg and transformation events. Presence of TAg in neuroblastomas and its interaction with cellular proteins was confirmed by immunohistochemistry and by immunoprecipitation of TAg/p53 complexes.

In contrast to these findings, the presence of JCV or BKV DNA or protein in tumour tissue could not be confirmed by others (Moens and Rekvig, 2001). This may be explained either by technical differences among laboratories or by different handling of samples. However, even detection of virus DNA in tumour tissue makes a differentiation of persistent infection and transformation difficult. First, it cannot be excluded that blood-derived virus may be found by highly sensitive detection methods in tumour tissue. Since the state of DNA in tumour cells is not yet unequivocally characterised, the presence of episomal DNA does not exclude persistent infection.

Furthermore, it cannot be ruled out, that polyomaviruses interact synergistically with other factors to induce malignant growth in human cells. In that case, the presence of virus DNA in tumour tissue could be a consequence of an event occurring early in the natural history of the tumour, when the cell cycle might be deregulated by TAg and its interaction with cellular factors. After genetic alterations are established, the virus genome and transcription products might be dispensable. In such a setting, the role of huPyV remains uncertain and a more detailed analysis of tumour tissues and the steps leading to transforming events in the animal models will be required to answer the question of whether or not JCV and BKV are involved in human tumorigenesis.

DIAGNOSTIC EVALUATION OF POLYOMAVIRUS-ASSOCIATED DISEASE

Diagnosis of PML by Biopsy

The most important disease linked to the human polyomaviruses is PML. The classic method of PML diagnosis involves neurological evaluation and neuroimaging of the brain followed by definitive laboratory diagnosis on biopsy material (Dörries et al., 1998b). Open surgery for PML diagnosis has been almost completely replaced by stereotactic biopsy. Topographical selection of samples at the outer rim of the lesions provides the best material for virus detection. Diagnosis is based on the identification of virus products and typical cellular changes in glial cells. The extraordinary multiplication rate of the virus in diseased tissue allows detection of viral nucleic acids and proteins by classical immunohistological methods. Molecular detection of JCV by PCR in biopsy samples is usually confirmed by histopathology. As pathological criteria for the term 'active PML' in AIDS, the presence of JCV-infected glial cells, bizarre astrocytes and lipid-laden macrophages in the context of demyelination are essential. In contrast, 'inactive PML' is characterised by the presence of demyelinated areas without JCV proteins, detected by immunohistochemistry. Regression of astrocytic and oligodendroglial changes and the disappearance of macrophages and JCV proteins was already described in one case of biopsy-proven PML in the pre-AIDS era (Cinque *et al.*, 2003).

It is accepted that polyomavirus DNA is present in the CNS of adults with former virus contact (Dörries, 1997; Major *et al.*, 1992; Weber and Major, 1997). In the asymptomatic state of infection virus DNA is regularly not detectable by diagnostic PCR analysis of single brain samples. If the infection is activated in immunoimpaired individuals, the virus load might increase and could then be detectable. However, compared to the thousands of genome equivalents present in PML tissue, the amount of virus is considerably lower. Consequently, in cases with doubtful results quantitative PCR analysis of any type differentiates a persistently activated and a PML-associated JCV infection. At present, a combination of stereotactic biopsy and PCR techniques ensures a rapid diagnosis of PML with the highest sensitivity and specificity available.

Demonstration of Polyomavirus DNA in CSF

In view of the high frequency of PML in AIDS patients and the future development of immunomodulatory therapies, introduction of less invasive methods with a comparable detection rate in early diagnosis is urgently required (Dörries *et al.*, 1998b; Major *et al.*, 1992; Weber and Major, 1997). Although the concentration of JCV in affected tissue is extraordinarily high, virus load in CSF is considerably lower and PCR is the only technique available for virus detection, although undoubtedly the most sensitive method, PCR on CSF, often causes divergent diagnostic results. Reports on the test specificity vary (10–80%). Since polyomavirus PCR has not yet been standardised, variable specificity rates are in part caused by technical differences. With the increasing number of reports, factors such as primer quality, sensitivity of the detection system, extraction methods and sample volume are eliminated. Even the sensitivity of the test systems was enhanced by a second nested PCR amplification of the primary products with internal primer pairs, providing detection limits in the range of about 10 genomes. However, nested PCR on the CSF

of a high-risk HIV-1 patient without PML similarly revealed positive JCV amplification. Thus, increase of the detection limits by nested PCR may lead to an increasing number of false-positive PML diagnoses and reduces the prognostic significance of the technique. This finding is explained by asymptomatic activation of JCV CNS infection in states of immunocompromise. Whether this is indicative for an early state of disease or might represent a timely restricted activation is not yet known.

In addition, even in nested PCR reactions, CSF samples remained negative in autopsy-verified PML cases. Serial sampling revealed that the virus load is low, often almost not detectable early after first diagnosis and may increase at late stages of disease. In these cases repeated CSF sampling at time intervals depending on clinical and radiological progression of disease appear to be an essential factor for virus detection. Nevertheless, there are cases remaining negative even at late stages of the disease. Concentration of virus, destruction of tissue, therapy and disease history is comparable to that of patients shedding JCV either continuously or intermittently into the CSF (Eggers *et al.*, 1999). At present, an explanation for the absence of JCV in those cases cannot be given.

PCR diagnosis is the most sensitive method for the detection of virus in body fluids; however, in view of asymptomatic activation of JCV, persistent infection under immunosuppression, differential diagnosis of PML and subclinical infection by PCR analysis alone cannot, at present, be recommended for routine diagnosis. Further data on the amount of JCV shed into the CSF in the course of PML in comparison to that in CSF of non-PML patients have to be accumulated and the techniques used among laboratories have to be standardised. None of the presently available clinical, radiological and virological parameters can be used as a stand-alone criterion for the diagnosis of PML. Thus, to date, PCR can only be understood as a supporting diagnostic tool. The new definition scheme for PML is based on criteria for 'definite PML' involving: (a) progressive uni- or multifocal neurological disease; (b) typical magnetic resonance imaging (MRI) lesions; associated with (c) typical brain biopsy features with confirmation of JCV specific products. 'Probable PML' represents cases with typical clinical and imaging findings, with amplification of JCV DNA in CSF but without bioptic diagnosis. Absence of histological confirmation and JCV demonstration in CSF in a setting of typical PML clinical and radiological findings leads to a diagnosis of 'possible PML'. If either pathological diagnosis can be performed or JCV can be detected in

CSF in serial CSF samples, this may later classify for a 'definite PML' diagnosis. Incidentally discovered white matter lesions or JCV amplification in CSF without active clinical or radiological findings should not be considered as representative for PML (Cinque et al., 2003).

Polyomavirus-specific Humoral Immune Response

Attempts to establish additional diagnostic procedures concentrate on the virus-specific humoral immune response. Reports focus on the determination of virus-specific antibodies and their dynamic titre changes in acute disease. The predominant polyomavirus subgroup-specific antigenic sites on the major capsid protein VP1 are accessible only after disruption of virions, in virus-infected cells or on purified VP1 protein. Consequently, virus-specific antisera risen against intact virus particles are species-specific. Species-specific antibodies can be distinguished from one another by neutralisation and haemagglutination-inhibition (HAI) tests, with a good correlation of virus-specific HAI and neutralising antibody titres (Pass and Shah, 1982).

The prevalence of BKV-specific antibodies in sera is about 50% by the age of 3 years and nearly all individuals are seroconverted by the age of 10 years (Knowles, 2001). The incidence of JCV antibodies is about 50% during adolescence and more than 80% by adulthood. The rates differ slightly according to demographic data and geographical distribution. Further discrepancies can probably be explained by differential sensitivity of the detection techniques.

The range of polyomavirus-specific HAI antibody titres is not dependent on age or sex, but in pregnant women rising titres indicate an incidence of active infection of more than 25%. Since virus-specific antibodies in normal persons and age-matched patients with various tumours and lymphomas exhibited similar geometric mean titres, this is believed to be the result of activation processes mediated by pregnancy. Titres in patients with malignancies remain stable even under multidrug- or immunotherapy, thus demonstrating that JCV antibody titres in sera are not markedly influenced by these diseases or associated therapies. Equally, under PML, the range of JCV-specific serum and HAI titres cannot be distinguished from those in the general population. This is explained by the severe basic illnesses abrogating a normal antibody increase, but it cannot be excluded that the low sensitivity of the HAI test may not pick up modest titre changes. Use of the enzyme immunoassay (EIA) for the detection of huPyV-specific antibodies reveals a better sensitivity, with geometric mean titres 10 times higher than that of HAI; however, the quality of the results is identical to that of preceding studies (Weber et al., 2001). Although recombinant proteins as antigens are a prerequisite for the diagnostic EIA, it is not yet clear whether species-specific huPyV Ig class G antibodies can be differentiated from group-specific antibodies with recombinant virus capsids. Extensive studies on possible cross-reactions among the recombinant primate polyomavirus antigens are under way.

The first polyomavirus-specific IgM assays were performed with BKV antigen. Cross-reactivity of BKV with JCV IgM was not evaluated, and whether virus-specific IgM can be distinguished in double infections remains unresolved. However, the prevalence of BKV-specific IgM in children was consistent with age distribution of primary BKV infection. The occurrence of BKV IgM at approximately 5% in sera from healthy blood donors is consistent with the finding that BKV activation is uncommon in healthy adults. Thus, possible cross-reactive IgM antibodies might be in the minority. JCV-specific IgM sero-antibodies were detected in 15% of healthy blood donors. In the same group almost all sera contained HAI antibodies, suggesting that blood donors harbour the virus in a persistent state. The high prevalence of JCV infections in adults led to the assumption that the presence of IgM is frequently associated with JCV activation in the healthy. In about half of PML patients, a rise of IgM antibodies with increasing levels was observed under progression of the neurological illness. At present, the high prevalence of IgM-positive sera in healthy persons does not allow a correlation of IgM presence with acute disease (Knowles et al., 1995).

In early studies the CSF was usually found to be unremarkable in PML, and JCV HAI titres were only rarely detected. Thus, in the past the humoral immune response was regarded as essentially unhelpful for diagnosis and studies on JCV antibodies and their dynamic changes in the CSF of PML patients were limited to single cases. However, recently a slight increase in CSF protein was reported in about one-quarter of PML patients, an elevated IgG albumin index in about one-fifth, and a slight pleocytosis in other patients (Berger and Major, 1999). Further analyses revealed moderate blood–brain barrier impairment in PML patients. JCV-specific intrathecally synthesised HAI antibodies and oligoclonal bands were detected in the CSF of 67% confirmed PML cases. Additionally, changes of HAI titre in the

CSF were observed under PML treatment, suggesting that JCV-specific antibody titres might be responsive to therapeutic intervention. Thus, JCV intrathecally produced HAI antibodies appear to be suggestive of active JCV multiplication within the CNS. This was further confirmed by EIA analyses with recombinant JCV VP1 capsid protein as antigen. An intrathecal immune response was detected in 78% of PML patients vs. 3% of controls. Detection of JCV-specific oligoclonal bands was slightly less sensitive. Interestingly, a JCV-specific intrathecal immune response against JCV VP1 evolved in HIV-1 patients during therapy. At present, it appears likely that a response evolves over time in the majority of PML patients (Weber et al., 2001).

The range of titres in individual PML patients appears to be highly dependent on the state of the disease and may additionally reflect the type of underlying disease, with characteristics differently affecting parameters of the immune system. Analyses of virus-specific, intrathecally produced antibodies and oligoclonal bands are well matched in PML vs. non-immunosuppressed cases. It can be assumed that a mild intrathecal immune response with presence of oligoclonal JCV-specific antibodies indicates intraCNS growth of JCV. It remains to be determined whether the finding of intrathecally produced JCV-specific antibodies and oligoclonal bands is indicative for acute disease and PML only, or might also be characteristic for a persistent activated state under immune impairment of other diseases. A thorough examination of the humoral immune response to JCV in the high-risk groups has to be performed in order to define specificity and frequency of intrathecal JCV-specific antibodies, prior to a decision on the usefulness of these assays as a diagnostic tool in PML.

Polyomavirus-specific Cellular Immune Response

JCV activation occurs in the context of immune impairment, and humoral immunity obviously is not able to control JCV spread. Therefore, from the early beginnings breakdown of cellular immunity was suspected to play a major role in the pathogenesis of polyomavirus diseases. However, studies on the immune responses are limited and did not contribute to a general understanding of polyomavirus-associated mechanisms of immune control. Recently, it was found that the major histocompatibility complex (MHC) classes II and I were expressed at high levels in PML

lesions, thus indicating an intact antigen presentation. In HIV/PML patients, immune reconstitution by HAART is related to a rise in helper $CD4^+$ T lymphocyte counts as well as a drop of HIV-1 load and clinical improvement of JCV-related neurological symptoms. However, about 50% of HIV/PML patients do not respond to HAART, despite reduction of HIV-1 load and rise in $CD4^+$ counts. Therefore it appears likely that the $CD4^+$ T cell subset does not play an important role in PML development.

Studies on cytotoxic T lymphocytes revealed the presence of JCV-specific circulating cells directed against the early TAg and the capsid protein VP1 in survivors of PML. Comparison of the CTL response demonstrated that a strong JCV-specific CTL response is related to the outcome of disease. Recently, a cytotoxic epitope of JCV VP1 was used to characterise the CTL in PML patients and control subjects. A CTL response was detected in patients with a prolonged disease course but in none of the classic PML patients, or in non-PML HIV-1 patients, or healthy controls. These data confirm that the JCV-specific cellular immune response plays an important role in PML. In addition, it is conceivable that the JCV-specific CTL response may provide a useful diagnostic and prognostic tool in the therapeutic management of these patients (Du Pasquier et al., 2001; Koralnik et al., 2001).

TREATMENT OF POLYOMAVIRUS-ASSOCIATED DISEASES

Treatment of huPyV infections concentrated for years on PML. Different treatment regimens have been proposed on the basis of molecular findings and small series of patients. However, randomised therapeutic trials were introduced only recently and the observation of stabilised PML or even remission highlights the inadequacies of early anecdotal reports suggesting the value of a specific therapy (Berger and Major, 1999; Major et al., 1992; Weber and Major, 1997).

Nucleoside analogues have been found to interfere with viral DNA synthesis in virus infections, and several compounds have been tried in the treatment of PML. Cytosine arabinoside (ARA-C, cytarabine) has been used from the early beginnings, with various degrees of improvement being reported. Recently acquired molecular data showed that cytosine-β-D-arabinofuranoside suppressed JCV replication in tissue culture, thus supporting the potential interference of ARA-C with PML. However, the study on efficacy of

ARA-C by the AIDS Clinical Trials Group, trial 243, showed no benefit (Hall *et al.*, 1998). In contrast, in a small group of non-AIDS PML patients the treatment stabilised PML in 36% of the patients for 1 year (Aksamit, 2001). However, in the presence of a demonstrable *in vitro* effect of ARA-C, it was hypothesised that the failure of the drug might be due to insufficient delivery of the drug through conventional intravenous and intrathecal routes. The so-called 'convection-enhanced intraparenchymal delivery' was developed which may enhance the efficacy of ARA-C (Levy *et al.*, 2001). Other analogues, such as adenosine arabinoside (ARA-A, vidarabine), iodo-desoxyuridine or zidovudine, similarly do not appear to have an effect in the treatment of PML.

The use of highly active antiretroviral therapy (HAART) in patients with HIV-related PML is associated with disease stabilisation. Prolonged survival in about 50% of the patients is associated with decrease of JC viral load in the CSF. The survival rate significantly increased in patients receiving a protease inhibitor-containing regimen. The effect of HAART on PML is believed to be the result of improved immune defence. However, in half of the patients PML progressed despite virological and immunological response to HAART. Failure to respond to HAART, as demonstrated by high plasma viral loads, has been associated with poor PML prognosis and a course of disease similar to that in absence of antiretroviral therapy. Nevertheless, the use of HAART has significantly improved survival time, although the prognosis of HIV/PML patients is still severe (Antinori *et al.*, 2001; Cinque *et al.*, 2003).

Cidofovir diphosphate, a structural analogue of deoxycytidine triphosphate, is known as a potent inhibitor of human herpes and papillomaviruses. It demonstrated a significant inhibitory effect on replication activity *in vitro* and was therefore introduced as a potential drug in PML treatment. Anecdotal reports pointed to clinical improvement and following studies reported beneficial effects, either alone or in combination with HAART, in AIDS-associated PML. However, new pilot studies did not report a beneficial effect in patients receiving potent antiretroviral agents, therefore the efficacy of the drug remains controversial.

The use of immune modulatory agents in PML therapy is based on the findings of extended survival in patients with improvement of the immunological competence. α-Interferon has established efficacy in the treatment of other polyomavirus-associated diseases, and prolonged survival was reported. In contradiction to these results, other studies reported no significant enhancement in survival time. Similar discrepancies were found with the combination of adenine arabinoside and β-interferon or transfer factor revealing no efficacy, whereas interferon alone was associated with modest improvement in the clinical picture and on MRI. Recently, an effect on survival after interleukin-2 treatment of a lymphoma patient after bone marrow transplantation was contradicted in another patient. In addition, treatment with low-dose heparin sulphate was suggested to prevent seeding of JCV to the CNS by activated lymphocytes. Other agents have been tried, either alone or in combination. No effect has been found with corticosteroid therapy or tilorone, an immune enhancer. The use of antisense oligonucleotides to prevent virus-specific protein expression has been proposed, but awaits development of the respective drugs. Thus, unequivocal effective therapy of PML as yet remains elusive, and further investigations and collaborative efforts are desperately needed to decide which of the different approaches might be effective for the treatment of PML.

In recent years the incidence of BKV-associated diseases has increased. Diseases of the urothelia are predominantly found in a setting of therapeutic immunosuppression schemes, states which also favour transient asymptomatic BKV activation. Among renal transplant patients, up to 60% have BKV reactivation, as shown by the presence of infected cells in the urine, whereas BKV has been implicated as a cause for BKV-associated nephropathy (BKN) in about 5%. Careful reduction of the doses of immunosuppressive therapy helped to stabilise or improve the disease. It has been suggested that the new immunosuppressive drugs, such as tacrolimus or mycophenolate mofetil, played an active role in promoting BKV infection. Remission could be achieved by decrease of high-dose therapy or replacement by cyclosporin A. Similarly, BKV was more frequent in patients with quadruple therapy than in those with double therapy. A reduction of immunosuppressive therapy in renal transplant patients was also successful in ureteric stenosis. Cidofovir has been successfully used in bone marrow (BMT) recipients with BK viruria and concomitant cystitis. Treatment with vidarabine appears to have some benefit in BKV-associated haemorrhagic cystitis but, as with prostaglandin E2 treatment, gave variable results (Moens and Rekvig, 2001).

Although for the treatment of polyomavirus diseases a number of drugs and therapeutic regimens were associated with some beneficial effect, an established antiviral therapy is not available. The high prevalence of these viruses in humans and the pathogenic potential makes intensive analyses of viral activation mechanisms and following development of specific drugs an essential aim for the near future.

ACKNOWLEDGEMENTS

Work in the author's laboratory was supported by Graduate College 520, Immunomodulation, of the Deutsche Forschungsgesellschaft and by Grant 1999.061 of the Wilhelm Sander-Stiftung.

REFERENCES

Agostini HT, Jobes DV and Stoner GL (2001) Molecular evolution and epidemiology of JC virus. In *Human Polyomaviruses. Molecular and Clinical Perspectives* (eds Khalili K and Stoner GL), pp 491–526. Wiley-Liss, New York.

Aksamit AJ (2001) Treatment of non-AIDS progressive multifocal leukoencephalopathy with cytosine arabinoside. *J Neurovirol*, **7**, 386–390.

Andreoletti L, Dubois V, Lescieux A *et al.* (1999) Human polyomavirus JC latency and reactivation status in blood of HIV-1-positive immunocompromised patients with and without progressive multifocal leukoencephalopathy. *AIDS*, **13**, 1469–1475.

Antinori A, Ammassari A, Giancola ML *et al.* (2001) Epidemiology and prognosis of AIDS-associated progressive multifocal leukoencephalopathy in the HAART era. *J Neurovirol*, **7**, 323–328.

Arthur RR and Shah KV (1989) Occurrence and significance of papovaviruses BK and JC in the urine. *Prog Med Virol*, **36**, 42–61.

Ault GS (1997) Activity of JC virus archetype and PML-type regulatory regions in glial cells. *J Gen Virol*, **78**, 163–169.

Berger JR and Major EO (1999) Progressive multifocal leukoencephalopathy. *Semin Neurol*, **19**, 193–200.

Bofill-Mas S and Girones R (2001) Excretion and transmission of JCV in human populations. *J Neurovirol*, **7**, 345–349.

Brooks BR and Walker DL (1984) Progressive multifocal leukoencephalopathy. *Neurol Clin*, **2**, 299–313.

Chang D, Fung CY, Ou W *et al.* (1997) Self-assembly of the JC virus major capsid protein, VP1, expressed in insect cells. *J Gen Virol*, **78**, 1435–1439.

Cinque P, Koralnik IJ and Clifford DB (2003) The evolving face of HIV-related progressive multifocal leukoencephalopathy: defining a consensus terminology. *J Neurovirol* (in press).

Corallini A, Tognon M, Negrini M and Barbanti-Brodano G (2001) Evidence for BK virus as a human tumor virus. In *Polyomaviruses. Molecular and Clinical Perspectives* (eds Khalili K and Stoner GL), pp 431–460. Wiley-Liss, New York.

Del Valle L, Gordon J, Ferrante P and Khalili K (2001) JC virus in experimental and clinical brain tumorigenesis. In *Human Polyomaviruses. Molecular and Clinical Perspectives*

(eds Khalili K and Stoner GL), pp 409–430. Wiley-Liss, New York.

Devireddy LR, Kumar KU, Pater MM and Pater A (2000) BAG-1, a novel Bcl-2-interacting protein, activates expression of human JC virus. *J Gen Virol*, **2**, 351–357.

Dörries K (1997) New aspects in the pathogenesis of polyomavirus-induced disease. *Adv Virus Res*, **48**, 205–261.

Dörries K (2001) Latent and persistent human polyomavirus infection. In *Human Polyomaviruses. Molecular and Clinical Perspectives* (eds Khalili K and Stoner GL), pp 197–237. Wiley-Liss, New York.

Dörries K, Arendt G, Eggers C *et al.* (1998b) Nucleic acid detection as a diagnostic tool in polyomavirus JC-induced progressive multifocal leukoencephalopathy. *J Med Virol*, **54**, 196–203.

Dörries K, Sbiera S, Drews K *et al.* (2003) Association of human polyomavirus JC with peripheral blood of immunoimpaired and healthy individuals. *J Neurovirol* (in press).

Dörries K, Vogel E, Günther S and Czub S (1994) Infection of human polyomavirus JC and BK in peripheral blood leukocytes from immunocompetent individuals. *Virology*, **198**, 59–70.

Dubois V, Dutronc H, Lafon M *et al.* (1997) Latency and reactivation of JC virus in peripheral blood of human immunodeficiency virus type 1-infected patients. *J Clin Microbiol*, **35**, 2288–2292.

Du Pasquier RA, Clark KW, Smith PS *et al.* (2001) JCV-specific cellular immune response correlates with a favorable clinical outcome in HIV-infected individuals with progressive multifocal leukoencephalopathy. *J Neurovirol*, **7**, 318–322.

Eggers C, Stellbrink HJ, Buhk T and Dörries K (1999) Quantification of JC virus DNA in the cerebrospinal fluid of patients with human immunodeficiency virus-associated progressive multifocal leukoencephalopathy—a longitudinal study. *J Infect Dis*, **180**, 1690–1694.

Elsner C and Dörries K (1998) Human polyomavirus JC control region variants in persistently infected CNS and kidney tissues. *J Gen Virol*, **4**, 789–799.

Ferrante P, Mediati M, Caldarelli-Stefano R *et al.* (2001) Increased frequency of JC virus type 2 and of dual infection with JC virus type 1 and 2 in Italian progressive multifocal leukoencephalopathy patients. *J Neurovirol*, **7**, 35–42.

Gallia GL, Houff SA, Major EO and Khalili K (1997) Review: JC virus infection of lymphocytes-revisited. *J Infect Dis*, **176**, 1603–1609.

Hall CD, Dafni U, Simpson D *et al.* (1998) Failure of cytarabine in progressive multifocal leukoencephalopathy associated with human immunodeficiency virus infection. AIDS Clinical Trials Group 243 Team. *N Engl J Med*, **338**, 1345–1351.

Hatwell JN and Sharp PM (2000) Evolution of human polyomavirus JC. *J Gen Virol*, **5**, 1191–1200.

Kim H-S, Henson JW and Frisque RJ (2001) Transcription and replication in the human polyomaviruses. In *Human Polyomaviruses. Molecular and Clinical Perspectives* (eds Khalili K and Stoner GL), pp 73–126. Wiley-Liss, New York.

Knowles WA (2001) The epidemiology of BK virus and the occurrence of antigenic and genomic subtypes. In *Human Polyomaviruses. Molecular and Clinical Perspectives* (eds Khalili K and Stoner GL), pp 527–559. Wiley-Liss, New York.

Knowles WA, Luxton RW, Hand JF *et al.* (1995) The JC virus antibody response in serum and cerebrospinal fluid in progressive multifocal leucoencephalopathy. *Clin Diag Virol*, **4**, 183–194.

Koralnik IJ, Du Pasquier RA and Letvin NL (2001) JC virus-specific cytotoxic T lymphocytes in individuals with progressive multifocal leukoencephalopathy. *J Virol*, **75**, 3483–3487.

Koralnik IJ, Schmitz JE, Lifton MA *et al.* (1999) Detection of JC virus DNA in peripheral blood cell subpopulations of HIV-1-infected individuals. *J Neurovirol*, **5**, 430–435.

Lafon ME, Dutronc H, Dubois V *et al.* (1998) JC virus remains latent in peripheral blood B lymphocytes but replicates actively in urine from AIDS patients. *J Infect Dis*, **177**, 1502–1505.

Laghi L, Randolph AE, Chauhan DP *et al.* (1999) JC virus DNA is present in the mucosa of the human colon and in colorectal cancers. *Proc Natl Acad Sci USA*, **96**, 7484–7489.

Levy RM, Major E, Ali MJ *et al.* (2001) Convection-enhanced intraparenchymal delivery (CEID) of cytosine arabinoside (AraC) for the treatment of HIV-related progressive multifocal leukoencephalopathy (PML). *J Neurovirol*, **7**, 382–385.

Major EO, Amemiya K, Tornatore CS *et al.* (1992) Pathogenesis and molecular biology of progressive multifocal leukoencephalopathy, the JC virus-induced demyelinating disease of the human brain. *Clin Microbiol Rev*, **5**, 49–73.

Mazlo M, Ressetar HG and Stoner GL (2001) The neuropathology and pathogenesis of progressive multifocal leukoencephalopathy. In *Human Polyomaviruses. Molecular and Clinical Perspectives* (eds Khalili K and Stoner GL), pp 257–336. Wiley-Liss, New York.

Moens U and Rekvig OP (2001) Molecular biology of BK virus and clinical and basic aspects of BK virus renal infection. In *Human Polyomaviruses. Molecular and Clinical Perspectives* (eds Khalili K and Stoner GL), pp 359–408. Wiley-Liss, New York.

Monaco MC, Sabath BF, Durham LC and Major EO (2001) JC virus multiplication in human hematopoietic progenitor cells requires the NF-1 class D transcription factor. *J Virol*, **75**, 9687–9695.

Monaco MCG, Atwood WJ, Gravell M *et al.* (1996) JC virus infection of hematopoietic progenitor cells, primary B lymphocytes, and tonsillar stromal cells: implications for viral latency. *J Virol*, **70**, 7004–7012.

Padgett BL and Walker DL (1976) New human papovaviruses. *Prog Med Virol*, **22**, 1–35.

Pass F and Shah KV (1982) Immunology of human papovaviruses. In *Immunology of Human Infection. Part II, Viruses and Parasites; Immunodiagnosis and Prevention of Infectious Disease* (eds Nahmias AJ and O'Reilly RJ), pp 225–241. Plenum Medical, New York.

Pfister LA, Letvin NL and Koralnik IJ (2001) JC virus regulatory region tandem repeats in plasma and central nervous system isolates correlate with poor clinical outcome in patients with progressive multifocal leukoencephalopathy. *J Virol*, **75**, 5672–5676.

Raj GV and Khalili K (1995) Transcriptional regulation: lessons from the human neurotropic polyomavirus, JCV. *Virology*, **213**, 283–291.

Ricciardiello L, Laghi L, Ramamirtham P (2000) JC virus DNA sequences are frequently present in the human upper and lower gastrointestinal tract. *Gastroenterology*, **119**, 1228–1235.

Sala M, Vartanian JP, Kousignian P *et al.* (2001) Progressive multifocal leukoencephalopathy in human immunodeficiency virus type 1-infected patients: absence of correlation between JC virus neurovirulence and polymorphisms in the transcriptional control region and the major capsid protein loci. *J Gen Virol*, **82**, 899–907.

Stoner GL and Hübner R (2001) The human polyomaviruses: past, present and future. In *Human Polyomaviruses. Molecular and Clinical Perspectives* (eds Khalili K and Stoner GL), pp 611–663. Wiley-Liss, New York.

Sullivan CS and Pipas JM (2002) T antigens of simian virus 40: molecular chaperones for viral replication and tumorigenesis. *Microbiol Mol Biol Rev*, **66**, 179–202.

Sweet TM, Valle LD and Khalili K (2002) Molecular biology and immunoregulation of human neurotropic JC virus in CNS. *J Cell Physiol*, **191**, 249–256.

Walker DL and Padgett BL (1983) Progressive multifocal leukoencephalopathy. *Comp Virol*, **18**, 161–193.

Weber T and Major EO (1997) Progressive multifocal leukoencephalopathy: molecular biology, pathogenesis and clinical impact. *Intervirology*, **40**, 98–111.

Weber T, Weber F, Petry H and Luke W (2001) Immune response in progressive multifocal leukoencephalopathy: an overview. *J Neurovirol*, **7**, 311–317.

Zu Rhein GM (1969) Association of papova-virions with a human demyelinating disease (progressive multifocal leukoencephalopathy). *Prog Med Virol*, **11**, 185–247.

24

Human Parvoviruses

Kevin E. Brown

National Heart, Lung and Blood Institute, Bethesda, MD, USA

INTRODUCTION

Parvoviruses are, as their name suggests, small viruses (from the Latin, *parvum* meaning small), with a single-stranded DNA genome. To date there is only one known human pathogen (parvovirus B19) in this entire family of viruses. The family *Parvoviridae* consists of two subfamilies, the *Densovirinae* and the *Parvovirinae*: the *Densovirinae* are all viruses of insects, and the *Parvovirinae* are viruses of vertebrates (Berns *et al.*, 1995; Table 24.1). The *Parvovirinae* is further subdivided into three genera, based on the transcription map and their ability to replicate efficiently, either autonomously (*Parvovirus*), with helper virus (*Dependovirus*) or in erythroid progenitor cells (*Erythrovirus*).

The genus *Parvovirus* contains a wide range of viruses of mammals and birds, some of which cause major diseases in their animal hosts, but some, first isolated as contaminants of cell cultures, have unknown primary hosts. No member of this family is known to infect humans. *Dependovirus* spp. have been described in a number of mammalian and avian species. To date at least eight different primate dependoviruses have been described (Gao *et al.*, 2002) and adeno-associated viruses -2, -3 and -5 are common human infections. Although AAV DNA has been detected in some fetal abortion tissues (Friedman-Einat *et al.*, 1997; Tobiasch *et al.*, 1994), none of the dependoviruses have been linked definitively with disease in either humans or animals.

Parvovirus B19 was discovered initially in the serum of an asymptomatic blood donor (coded 19 in panel B) as a cause of false positive results in counter-immunoelectrophoresis tests for the detection of hepatitis B virus surface antigen (Cossart *et al.*, 1975). In 1983 the chemical nature of the agent was described (Summers *et al.*, 1983) and the virus was classified initially with the autonomous parvoviruses. However, more recently B19 parvovirus was reclassified as the first member and type species of the genus *Erythrovirus*. Subsequently, three simian parvoviruses have been identified in cynomolgus monkeys, pigtailed macaques and rhesus macaques (Green *et al.*, 2000; O'Sullivan *et al.*, 1994). These erythroviruses share with B19 up to 60% homology, similar genome organisation and similar biological behaviour in natural hosts. Interestingly, among the Parvovirinae in general, the sequence homology suggests that B19 parvovirus (genus *Erythrovirus*), minute virus of mice (genus *Parvovirus*) and adeno-associated virus (genus *Dependovirus*) are equally different from each other, suggesting that they diverged at about the same evolutionary point in time.

Although parvovirus-like particles have been described in human stool specimens (Paver *et al.*, 1973), these particles have not yet been fully characterised and so their classification must await definitive molecular studies. Moreover, similar particles may on occasion be found in the faeces of asymptomatic individuals, so the precise pathogenic role of these agents remains unclear. More recently, workers in Japan found evidence of single-stranded DNA virus in the serum of a patient with hepatitis of unknown aetiology (Nishizawa *et al.*, 1997). Although thought originally to be a parvovirus, subsequent studies have shown that this virus, named TTV, is a member of a large group of related circoviruses (small DNA viruses with a single-stranded circular genome).

Principles and Practice of Clinical Virology, Fifth Edition. Edited by A. J. Zuckerman, J. E. Banatvala, J. R. Pattison, P. D. Griffiths and B. D. Schoub

Table 24.1 The *Parvovirinae*

Subfamily	Genus	Virus	Host
Parvovirinae	*Parvovirus*	Aleutian mink disease virus	Minks
		Canine parvovivus (CPV)	Dogs, foxes
		Mice minute virus (MVM)	Mice
		Porcine parvovirus (PPV)	Pigs
		Feline parvovirus (FPV)	Cats
	Dependovirus	Adeno-associated virus 1–6 (AAV)	Humans, primates
		Avian adeno-associated virus (AAAV)	Birds
		Canine adeno-associated virus (CAAV)	Dogs
		Bovine adeno-associated virus (BAAV)	Cattle
	Erythrovirus	Parvovirus B19 (B19)	Humans
		Simian parvovirus (SPV)	Primates
		Rhesus parvovirus (RhPV)	Primates
		Pigtailed macaque parvovirus (PtPV)	Primates

As with the human adeno-associated viruses, infection with these TTV-like viruses is common, and has not been associated with any disease.

PARVOVIRUS B19

Structure

In electron micrographs of negatively stained preparations, parvovirus B19 appear as non-enveloped, icosahedral particles with a diameter of 18–25 nm, and often both 'full' and 'empty' capsids are visible (Figure 24.1). The infectious particles have a buoyant density of ~1.41 g/ml in caesium chloride gradients, whereas the empty particles have a density of 1.31 g/ml. The particles do not contain lipids or carbohydrates. As with all parvovirus particles, the infectious particle is stable over a wide range of pH and resistant to lipid solvents. It is not quite as resistant to heat as other parvoviruses (Blumel *et al.*, 2002), but still only shows a 2.5 log reduction in infectivity when heat-treated at 50°C for 8 h (Miyagawa *et al.*, 1999). At high concentrations, infectious virus is still present after 80°C treatment for 72 h (Bartolomei Corsi *et al.*, 1988). B19 can be inactivated by formalin, β-propiolactone, oxidising agents and γ-irradiation.

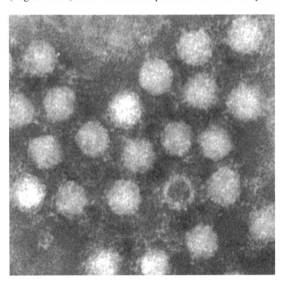

Figure 24.1 The appearance of B19 virus particles by immune electron microscopy showing the icosahedral structure

Genome Organisation

Parvovirus virions consist of a linear single strand of DNA with a molecular weight of approximately 1.8×10^6. In contrast to the autonomous parvoviruses, which preferentially encapsidate single-stranded DNA of negative polarity, parvovirus B19 encapsidates both positive and negative strands with equal frequency. The genome of B19 virus is one of the largest among the parvoviruses, with ~5500 nucleotides. All parvovirus genomes have palindromic sequences at both 5′ and 3′ termini. These segments of the DNA fold back on themselves to form hairpin loops, which are stabilised by hydrogen bonding. The hairpin termini of B19 virus are identical at the 5′ and 3′ end, and substantially longer than those of most parvoviruses, with terminal repeat sequences of 365 nucleotides in length. There is some mismatching in the middle of the hairpin, leading to the occurrence of two different sequence configurations referred to as 'flip' and 'flop', which is typical of parvovirus genomes (Deiss *et al.*, 1990).

The transcription map of B19 distinguishes it from other *Parvovirinae*. There is a single strong promoter at the far left side of the genome (map point 6, or p6) and unusual polyadenylation signals in the middle of the genome. As is usual with parvoviruses, the 5' end of the genome codes for the non-structural protein and the 3' end of the genome for the capsid proteins. There are nine RNA transcripts in infected erythroid cells, and the three major viral proteins, one non-structural protein and two capsid proteins, are produced by alternative splicing from the promoter and its accompanying leader sequence (Figure 24.2; Ozawa *et al.*, 1987). The relative quantities of the major and minor capsid proteins are in part regulated by the presence of multiple upstream AUG codons situated before the authentic transcription initiation codon (Ozawa *et al.*, 1988). In addition, there are transcripts for several smaller peptides of 7.5 and 11 kDa (Luo and Astell, 1993; St Amand and Astell, 1993) of unknown function.

Viral Proteins

The only unspliced transcript encodes the non-structural protein, a 78 kDa phosphoprotein (Ozawa and Young, 1987). Consistent with its role in viral propagation, the protein has DNA-binding properties (Leruez-Ville *et al.*, 1997), adenosine and guanosine triphosphatase activity (Momoeda *et al.*, 1994) and nuclear localisation signals (Momoeda, Young and Kajigaya, unpublished observations). Expression of the non-structural protein causes host cell death through induction of apoptosis (Moffatt *et al.*, 1998; Ozawa *et al.*, 1988).

There are two structural proteins in B19 virus, VP1 (84 kDa) and VP2 (58 kDa), which differ only in that VP1 has an additional 227 amino acids at the amino-terminus (Shade *et al.*, 1986). The capsid of B19 is composed of 60 capsomeres: VP2 is the major capsid protein, with only ~5% VP1 in the infectious particle. Expression of VP2 capsomeres alone will self-assemble to form recombinant empty capsids that resemble B19 particles morphologically and antigenically (Kajigaya

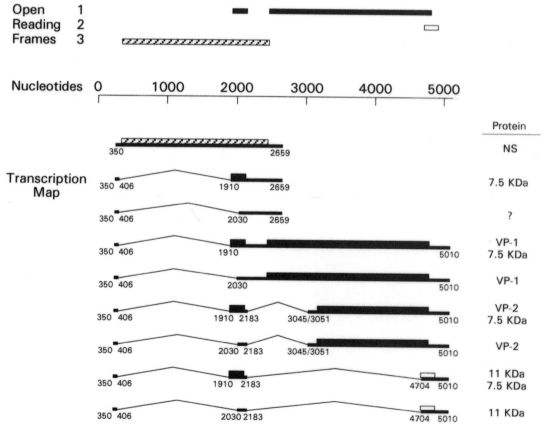

Figure 24.2 Transcription map of parvovirus B19

et al., 1991). The VP1 unique region is known to be important in generating neutralising antibodies (Saikawa *et al.*, 1993) and has phospholipase activity (Zadori *et al.*, 2001).

Structural studies of B19 have been undertaken for B19 using both crystal diffraction and cryo-EM studies. They indicate that, as seen for the autonomous parvovirus, B9 has the central structural core of eight antiparallel β-sheets, but the prominent spikes on the three-fold axis of canine and feline parvoviruses are absent from B19 capsids (Agbandje *et al.*, 1994; Chipman *et al.*, 1996).

Virus Variation

No antigenic variation in B19 has been demonstrated, and there appears to be a single, stable antigenic type of B19 virus. Infection is followed by lifelong immunity, which also indicates a single neutralisable type. Minor variation between different isolates of the virus in their reactivity with mouse monoclonal antibodies has been detected but this has so far not proved to be of epidemiological or diagnostic significance.

Similarly, the genome of B19 virus shows a constancy that is typical of viruses with DNA genomes, with $\sim 2\%$ sequence variability between isolates. Small changes of nucleotide sequence have been detected by several investigators using restriction enzyme analysis or direct sequence analysis, but there is no correlation to specific disease presentation. In a study of 12 viruses isolated in Japan at two different times, 1981 and 1986–1987, the genome type differed during each time period, but B19 viruses with similar genome types disseminated widely in Japan during each time period (Umene and Nunoue, 1990).

In 1998, a B19 isolate, tentatively termed V9 was identified in a French child with transient aplastic crisis, which on sequence analysis was seen to be markedly different ($> 10\%$ nucleotide difference) from other B19 sequences (Nguyen *et al.*, 1999). Subsequent studies have identified both similar sequences, and a third group of B19 isolates with 10% sequence difference from both classical B19 sequences and V9 sequences (Nguyen *et al.*, 2002; Servant *et al.*, 2002). It is unknown whether these different genotypes will have different disease characteristics. The prevalence of these viruses in the general population is also unknown currently, with no variant B19 sequences detected in plasma pools from more than 120 000 Danish blood donors (Nguyen *et al.*, 2002). In addition, despite the differences in the DNA sequences, the capsid proteins sequence is conserved, and V9 capsids show serological cross-reactivity with B19 capsids (Heegaard *et al.*, 2002).

PATHOGENESIS

For a number of years following its discovery, B19 virus appeared to be associated with, at most, a mild, non-specific, febrile illness accompanied by self-limiting leukopenia. In the early 1980s the central role of B19 virus in the aetiology of aplastic crisis in chronic haemolytic anaemias (Pattison *et al.*, 1981) was identified and then, in 1983, erythema infectiosum (fifth disease) began to emerge as the common manifestation of B19 virus infection (Anderson *et al.*, 1983). Subsequently the virus has been shown to be responsible for a significant percentage of cases of hydrops fetalis (Anand *et al.*, 1987) and to cause chronic infection in the immunocompromised (Kurtzman *et al.*, 1988, 1989a). It is now clear that the pathogenesis of B19 virus-associated disease involves two components. The first is due to the lytic infection of susceptible dividing cells and the second is dependent upon interaction with the immune response.

Volunteer Studies

Two studies of volunteers infected experimentally have allowed the kinetics of infection to be elucidated (Anderson *et al.*, 1985a; Potter *et al.*, 1987). In both cases volunteers (nine and three, respectively) were infected by intranasal inoculation of a saline solution containing approximately 10^8 virus particles. The volunteers were followed daily and clinical, biochemical, haematological and viral studies undertaken (Figure 24.3).

Viraemia was first detected from day 6 and reached a peak at days 8–9 at about 10^{11} particles/ml, a level comparable to that seen in natural infections in blood donors and patients with aplastic crisis (Anderson *et al.*, 1985b). Virus was also detected in throat swabs and gargles at the time of viraemia only. Virus was not found in urine or faeces. On days 6–8 the volunteers showed the typical symptoms of a viraemia, with headache, myalgia and chills, associated with pyrexia. These features are generally thought to be due to the production of inflammatory cytokines. During the viraemia reticulocyte numbers fell to undetectable levels, recovering 7–10 days later, and there was a consequent temporary fall in haemoglobin of about 1 g/dl in a normal individual. Lymphopenia, neutropenia and thrombocytopenia also occurred, although slightly later, with the lowest numbers being recorded 6–10 days after inoculation and not so consistently as the changes in reticulocyte numbers and haemoglobin concentration.

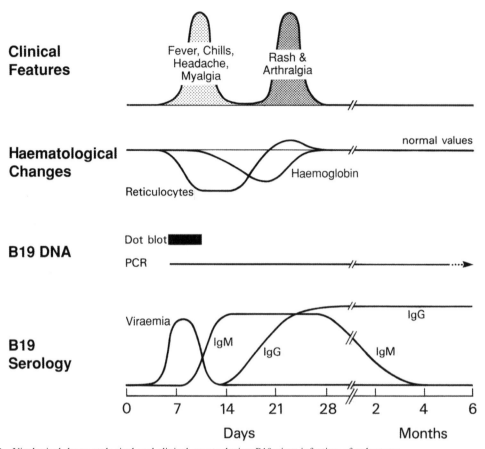

Clinical Features — Fever, Chills, Headache, Myalgia / Rash & Arthralgia

Haematological Changes — normal values / Reticulocytes / Haemoglobin

B19 DNA — Dot blot / PCR

B19 Serology — Viraemia / IgM / IgG / IgG / IgM / IgG

Days: 0 7 14 21 28 Months: 2 4 6

Figure 24.3 Virological, haematological and clinical events during B19 virus infection of volunteers

In the second study, bone marrow morphology was examined at intervals (Potter *et al.*, 1987). On day 6 post-inoculation the marrow appeared normal. However, at day 10 there was an almost total loss of erythroid precursors at all stages of development. The erythroid progenitor cells (BFU-E) from bone marrow and peripheral blood were reduced at this time. The myeloid compartment of the bone marrow appeared normal, but myeloid precursors from peripheral blood were reduced as soon as 2 days from the onset of the viraemia.

The viraemia resolved as the patients developed a detectable antibody response (Figure 24.3) and a second phase of the illness began in most of the volunteers at day 15–17 (Anderson *et al.*, 1985a), as the IgM response peaked and IgG became detectable, characterised by pruritis followed by the development of a fine maculopapular cutaneous eruption. The rash extended over the limbs and was accompanied by arthralgia and a mild arthritis. The rash was present

for 2–4 days and the joint symptoms for 4–6 days. In the second study none of the patients developed the second phase symptoms. It may be significant that in the second study all (3/3) the volunteers were male and that joint symptoms in natural B19 infection appear to be much less frequent in male patients.

All the volunteers who received $< 10^6$ virus particles in the inoculum and were B19 antibody-negative (IgG < 0.3 au) developed viraemia and an antibody response to the virus. Volunteers with a positive B19 IgG (IgG < 2 au) did not become infected. One of the pilot volunteer patients had 'equivocal' levels of IgG and appeared to develop a modified infection, with minimal viraemia and a boosting of his immune response.

In both studies, viraemia was monitored by the relatively insensitive dot–blot hybridisation technique. Studies with PCR, especially nested PCR, indicate that B19 DNA can be detected for many weeks or months following acute infection (Clewley, 1989; Musiani *et al.*, 1995; Patou *et al.*, 1993).

Cell Tropism

Parvovirus B19, like the autonomous parvoviruses, depends on certain host cell factors or functions only present in cells transiting the late S or early G_2 phase of mitosis for replication. However, B19 also has a very narrow target cell range and can only be propagated in human erythroid precursor cells. When bone marrow or peripheral blood cells are cultured to develop erythroid colonies in the presence of B19 virus, the formation of colonies is inhibited. For erythroid cells from bone marrow, susceptibility to parvovirus B19 increases with differentiation; the pluripotent stem cell appears to be spared and the main target cells are the BFU-E and CFU-E cells (cells capable of giving rise to erythroid colonies *in vitro*) and erythroblasts (Takahashi *et al.*, 1990).

Erythroid progenitors from a variety of sources have been used to study *in vitro* viral replication, including human bone marrow (Ozawa *et al.*, 1987), fetal liver (Brown *et al.*, 1991b; Yaegashi *et al.*, 1989) and peripheral blood. B19 will also replicate in a limited number of erythropoietin-dependent cell lines, including UT7/Epo (Shimomura *et al.*, 1993) and KU812Ep6 (Miyagawa *et al.*, 1999). However, the yield of virus from all these cultures is poor, and they cannot be used as a source of antigen for diagnostic tests.

Erythroid specificity of parvovirus B19 is due to the tissue distribution of the virus' cellular receptor, globoside, also known as blood group P antigen (Brown *et al.*, 1993). P antigen is found on erythroid progenitors, erythroblasts and megakaryocytes. Purified P antigen (globoside) blocks the binding of virus to erythroid cells and these cells can be protected from infection by preincubation with monoclonal antibody to globoside. P antigen is also present on endothelial cells, which may be targets of viral infection involved in the pathogenesis of transplacental transmission, possibly vasculitis and the rash of fifth disease, and on fetal myocardial cells (Rouger *et al.*, 1987). Rare individuals who genetically lack P antigen on erythrocytes are resistant to B19 infection, and their bone marrow cannot be infected with B19 *in vitro* (Brown *et al.*, 1994b). However, erythroid specificity may also be modulated by specific erythroid cell transcription factors (Liu *et al.*, 1992).

The virus is cytotoxic, producing a cytopathic effect with characteristic light and electron microscopic (Young *et al.*, 1984) changes. Infected cultures are characterised by the presence of giant pronormoblasts (Figure 24.4), 25–32 μm in diameter, with cytoplasmic vacuolisation, immature chromatin and large eosino-philic nuclear inclusion bodies. These cells have been recognised for more than 50 years and were originally observed in patients with haemolytic anaemia and aplastic crisis (Owren, 1948). By electron microscopy virus particles are seen in the nucleus and lining cytoplasmic membranes, and infected cells show marginated chromatin, pseudopod formation and cytoplasmic vacuolation, all typical of cells undergoing apoptosis (Morey *et al.*, 1993). However, not all the giant pronormoblasts contain virus particles, and part of the cytopathy probably reflects the expression of the non-structural protein. Megakaryocytopoiesis is also inhibited by B19 parvovirus *in vitro* but this is in the absence of virus replication and almost certainly due to the cytotoxic effect of non-structural protein (Srivastava *et al.*, 1990).

Immune Response

The pattern of parvovirus disease is strongly influenced by the immune response. Bone marrow depression in parvovirus infection occurs during the early viraemic phase and under normal conditions is terminated by a neutralising antibody response. The pathogenesis of the rash in erythema infectiosum and polyarthropathy is almost certainly immune complex-mediated. In volunteer studies, the rash and joint symptoms appeared when the high titre of viraemia had dropped significantly and coincident with a detectable immune response (Anderson *et al.*, 1985a).

Persistent B19 parvovirus infection is the result of failure to produce effective neutralising antibodies by the immunosuppressed host. Antibodies to parvovirus, as determined in immunoassays or ELISA, are not present in most patients, but a pattern of antibody response suggestive of early infection (weak IgM antibody and IgG antibody directed to the major capsid protein) may be found in patients with congenital immunodeficiency (Kurtzman *et al.*, 1989b). A poor reaction on immunoblot testing is a consistent finding and correlates with poor neutralising activity for the virus in erythroid colony assays (Kurtzman *et al.*, 1989b). Confirming that the role of the humoral response appears to be dominant in controlling human parvovirus infection, administration of commercial immunoglobulins can cure or ameliorate persistent parvovirus infection in immunodeficient patients: fifth disease symptoms can be precipitated by treatment of persistent infection with immunoglobulin (Frickhofen *et al.*, 1990).

The infected fetus may suffer severe effects because red blood cell turnover is high and the immune response deficient. During the second trimester there is a great increase in red cell mass. Parvovirus particles can be detected by electron microscopy within the haematopoietic tissues of liver and thymus (Field *et al.*, 1991). B19 DNA and capsid antigen have been detected in the myocardium of infected fetuses (Porter *et al.*, 1990), and there is evidence that the fetus may develop myocarditis (Naides and Weiner, 1989), compounding the severe anaemia and secondary cardiac failure. By the third trimester, a more effective fetal immune response to the virus may account for the decrease in fetal loss at this stage of pregnancy.

EPIDEMIOLOGY

Parvovirus B19 is a common infection in humans, and serological studies indicate that infection is worldwide, with infections occurring in all populations, apart from some isolated groups in Africa (Schwarz *et al.*, 1989) and Brazil (de Freitas *et al.*, 1990). In temperate climates infection occurs throughout the year but outbreaks are more common in late winter, spring and the early summer months. These outbreaks of infection are often centred on primary schools, where up to 40% of the school may be clinically affected by the rash illness of erythema infectiosum. If one includes subclinical infection then the attack rates may be as high as 60% of the susceptible population in a school (Plummer *et al.*, 1985). During these outbreaks, susceptible adults (parents and teachers of cases) frequently become infected.

In addition to seasonality, the virus exhibits longer-term cycles: in Jamaica, peaks of incidence (monitored as cases of aplastic crisis) occur every 3–4 years. In the UK, the cycle seems somewhat longer, with peaks occurring every 4–5 years.

Clinical observations of the frequency of cases of erythema infectiosum among different age groups reflect the serological profile of the population; antibodies are most commonly acquired between ages 4–10 years, after which the frequency continues to rise, but more slowly. By age 15 years approximately 50% of children have detectable IgG. Infection also occurs in adult life, so that more than 90% of the elderly have detectable antibody (Cohen and Buckley, 1988). Women of child-bearing age show an annual seroconversion rate of 1.5% (Koch and Adler, 1989). Studies in different countries (USA, France, Germany, Japan) show similar patterns.

Case-to-case intervals, determined by the time elapsing between acquisition and excretion of the virus, are independent of the type of disease. Volunteer studies predict case-to-case intervals of 6–11 days, which accords well with case-to-case intervals observed both in outbreaks of erythema infectiosum and in aplastic crisis. Transmission between siblings is common, and in families where more than one child is affected by chronic haemolytic anaemia all susceptibles should be monitored for 2 weeks if one develops an aplastic crisis.

Transmission

Although spread from respiratory tract to respiratory tract is the common route of transmission of B19 virus, the high-titre viraemia which occurs during infection can lead to transmission by blood and blood products. Virus is found in donated units of blood, although the incidence of high titre is low (1/20 000–40 000 in epidemic periods; Cohen *et al.*, 1990), as would be expected of an acute infection circulating mainly among children. However, testing donated blood samples by more sensitive PCR technique suggests that B19 can be detected in ~1/3000 units (McOmish *et al.*, 1993) and perhaps in >1/150 samples in one study (Yoto *et al.*, 1995). Blood-borne transmission has been shown to occur in recipients of whole blood and of factor VIII concentrates (Mortimer *et al.*, 1983). The frequency of B19 seropositivity among haemophiliacs is significantly higher than in normals, except for those haemophiliacs who have received factor VIII concentrates that have been heated to 80°C for 72 h (Williams *et al.*, 1990). Even so, B19 virus can be transmitted by treated blood products (Lyon *et al.*, 1989).

Table 24.2 Disease manifestations and persistence of parvovirus B19 infection in different host populations

Disease	Acute/ chronic	Host
Fifth disease	Acute	Normal children
Polyarthropathy syndrome	Acute/ chronic	Normal adults
Transient aplastic crisis	Acute	Patients with increased erythropoiesis
Persistent anaemia	Chronic	Immunodeficient /immunocompromised patients
Hydrops fetalis/ congenital anaemia	Acute/ chronic	Fetus (<20 weeks)

CLINICAL FEATURES

The consequences of B19 virus infection range from the wholly asymptomatic to serious and potentially fatal conditions in a minority of the population that is particularly predisposed. The spectrum of clinical consequences of infection depends in part on the natural variation in symptomatology that occurs, and in part on recognisable host factors (Table 24.2).

Minor Illness

Combined clinical and laboratory studies of infection in children, in whom B19 infection is most common, have indicated that about half of all infections are asymptomatic. Non-specific respiratory tract illness is the next most common consequence of infection, at least in boys (Grilli et al., 1989). This can be mild or severe enough to mimic influenza and these respiratory tract illnesses coincide with the viraemic phase of the illness.

Rash Illness/Erythema Infectiosum

Erythema infectiosum is most common in children aged 4–11 years and was probably first described by Robert Willan in 1799 and illustrated subsequently in his 1808 textbook (van Elsacker-Niele and Anderson, 1987). In 1905, Cheinisse classified it as the 'fifth rash disease' of the classical exanthema of childhood (Cheinisse, 1905), and this name, 'fifth disease', remains in use to this day. The link between B19 virus infection and erythema infectiosum was made in 1983 (Anderson et al., 1984). During the last 10 years the use of specific laboratory tests for the diagnosis of B19 virus infection has revealed a spectrum of rash illness, due to B19 infection, in which the classic features of erythema infectiosum occupy a central position and parvovirus B19 is now known to be the only aetiological agent for erythema infectiosum (Anderson et al., 1984).

Fifth disease was well described by clinical investigators prior to the discovery of B19 (Ager et al., 1966; Balfour, 1969; Brass et al., 1982). Infection is characterised by a non-specific prodromal illness which often goes unrecognised. Fifth disease may be associated with symptoms of fever, coryza, headache and mild gastrointestinal symptoms (nausea, diarrhoea). The exanthem occurs in three stages. Approximately 18 days after acquisition of the virus, and 2–5 days following the prodromal stage of the infection, the classic 'slapped-cheek' eruption appears, a fiery red rash on the cheek, accompanied by relative circumoral pallor (Figure 24.5). The edges of the involved areas may be slightly raised. At this stage the appearance may be suggestive of scarlet fever, drug sensitivity or other allergic reactions, or collagen vascular diseases. The second stage appears 1–4 days later, an erythematous maculopapular rash on the trunk and limbs. This rash is initially discrete but spreads to involve large areas. As this eruption fades it produces a typical lacy or reticular pattern. This third stage of the exanthem is highly variable in duration and may be transient or recurrent over 1–3 or more weeks, with periodic evanescence and recrudescence. The rash can be exacerbated by exercise, emotion, hot baths or sunlight. In addition, there may be great variation in the eruption's appearance, from a very faint erythema that is easily missed to a florid exanthema, and it is often pruritic in adults, especially on the soles of the feet (Woolf et al., 1989). While classic cases of erythema infectiosum are easy to recognise clinically, especially during outbreaks, the wide variation in the form of the rash may make individual cases hard to distinguish from other viral exanthema, including rubella.

Erythema infectiosum is essentially a benign disease in which the major complication is joint involvement (see below). Other reported complications include cases of transient haemolytic anaemia, encephalitis with recovery without residua, and encephalopathy in a 9 month-old boy, resulting in permanent sequelae. Each of these cases occurred prior to the appreciation of B19 virus as the causative agent for erythema infectiosum; in view of the difficulty in diagnosing sporadic cases of erythema infectiosum on clinical grounds, it cannot be certain that these cases were due to B19 virus infection.

There have been occasional cases of B19 infection associated with a purpuric rash. In most B19 infections the platelet count is normal (Lefrère et al., 1985) but thrombocytopenia has been recorded (Mortimer et al., 1985b; Saunders et al., 1986). Although the purpura in most cases of B19 infection is transient, some patients diagnosed with idiopathic thrombocytopenic purpura do have evidence of recent B19 infection (Murray et al., 1994). Similarly some B19 infections may resemble clinical Henoch–Schonlein purpura, but it is unclear what percentage of cases of this condition are caused by B19 (Heegaard and Taaning, 2002). Rarely, other dermatological presentations are seen; vesicopustular rash (Naides et al., 1988), glove and stocking syndrome (Halasz et al., 1992), other purpuric rashes with or without Koplik spots (Evans et al., 1992) and erythema multiforme (Frank et al., 1996; Lobkowicz et al., 1989).

Joint Involvement/Arthropathy

In children, B19 infection is usually mild and of short duration. However, in adults, and especially in women, there may be arthropathy in ~50% of patients (Woolf, 1990). It is now also clear, with the widespread application of B19 diagnostic tests, that the joint involvement may occur in the absence of any evidence of a rash, although there are no estimates of how frequent this is.

In adults, the most common presentation is with a sudden onset of symmetrical arthralgia and even frank arthritis affecting the small joints of the hand. Proximal interphalangeal and metacarpophalangeal joints are most often affected, followed by wrists, ankles, knees and elbows. Shoulders, cervical spine and lumbar spine as well as the hips may also be involved. There may be pain and stiffness in the joints, which may be accompanied by minor swelling or synovitis. Resolution usually occurs within a few weeks, but persistent or recurring symptoms can continue for years (Reid et al., 1985). In children the joint involvement may be asymmetrical and symptoms seem more severe than in adults and may be of longer duration.

In the absence of a history of rash, the symptoms may be mistaken for acute rheumatoid arthritis, especially as prolonged symptoms do not correlate with serological studies, such as the duration of B19 IgM response, or persistent viraemia. In addition, B19 infection can be associated with transient autoantibody production, including transient rheumatoid factor (Luzzi et al., 1985). In one large study of patients attending an 'early synovitis' clinic in England, 12% had evidence of recent infection with B19 (White et al., 1985). Three patients would have fulfilled the American Rheumatism Association's diagnostic criteria for definite rheumatoid arthritis. B19 infection should be considered as part of the differential diagnosis in any patient presenting with acute arthritis. In contrast to rheumatoid arthritis, B19 infection is not generally associated with joint destruction. However, differentiation between early rheumatoid arthritis and B19 arthropathy is important, as immunosuppressive therapy prescribed for rheumatoid arthritis is not indicated in parvovirus B19 infection.

The role of parvovirus B19 in the aetiology of chronic arthritis is unclear. Parvovirus B19 DNA has been found in the synovial fluid of a women with serologically proven B19 infection (Dijkmans et al., 1988) and in synovial fluid cells of a patient with 'reactive arthritis' (Kandolf et al., 1989). However,

PCR amplification studies should be interpreted with care: in one carefully performed controlled study, although B19 DNA was indeed detected in synovial tissue of 28% of children with chronic arthritis, it was also found in 48% of non-arthropathy controls (Soderlund et al., 1997), indicating that PCR-detectable DNA may persist in synovial tissues for months/years.

It has been postulated that B19 is involved in the initiation and perpetuation of rheumatoid arthritis leading to joint lesions (Takahashi et al., 1998), but these results have not been reproducible by other groups (El-Gabalawy, Goldbach-Mansky and Brown, unpublished observations). In addition, in one study of long-term follow-up, none of 54 patients with B19-associated arthralgia reported persistence of joint swelling or restricted motion, and no evidence of inflammatory joint disease was found (Speyer et al., 1998). It seems unlikely, though, that B19 plays a role in classic erosive rheumatoid arthritis, but understanding the pathogenesis of B19 arthropathy may provide insight into the mechanisms by which rheumatoid arthritis develops.

Transient Aplastic Crisis

Transient aplastic crisis is the abrupt cessation of erythropoiesis characterised by a fall from steady-state values of haemoglobin concentration, disappearance of reticulocytes from peripheral blood and the absence of red blood cell precursors in the bone marrow. It is classically seen in patients with haemolytic anaemia, where the B19-induced cessation of erythropoiesis lasts 5–7 days and patients present with symptoms of worsening anaemia, namely fatigue, shortness of breath, pallor, lassitude, confusion and sometimes congestive cardiac failure. The event is serious in most patients and occasionally it is fatal. Blood transfusion is required in the acute phase but after about 1 week the bone marrow recovers rapidly. There is a brisk reticulocytosis and the haemoglobin concentration returns to steady-state values.

Transient aplastic crisis was the first clinical illness associated with B19 infection. When stored sera from 600 children admitted to a London hospital were examined, six children had evidence of recent B19 infection (either antigenaemia or seroconversion). All were Jamaican immigrants with sickle cell disease presenting with aplastic crisis. There was a reduced haematocrit, and evidence of aplastic crises on their bone marrow (Pattison et al., 1981). Retrospective studies of sera from Jamaican sickle-cell patients showed that 86% of transient aplastic crises were associated with recent parvovirus infection (Serjeant et al., 1981). Studies since then have shown that more than 90% of all cases of aplastic crises in patients with chronic haemolytic anaemia are due to B19 virus infection (Anderson et al., 1982; Serjeant et al., 1993). Most cases occur in children under the age of 20 (Serjeant et al., 2001) but adults who remain susceptible to the virus infection may have B19-associated aplastic crises in later life.

B19-associated aplastic crises are not confined to patients with sickle cell anaemia, but have been described in a wide range of patients with underlying haemolytic disorders, such as hereditary spherocytosis (Kelleher et al., 1983), thalassaemia (Brownell et al., 1986), red cell enzymopathies, such as pyruvate kinase deficiency (Duncan et al., 1983), and autoimmune haemolytic anaemia (Smith et al., 1989). Aplastic crisis can also occur under conditions of erythroid 'stress', such as haemorrhage (Frickhofen et al., 1986), iron deficiency anaemia (Lefrere and Bourgeois, 1986) and following kidney (Neild et al., 1986) or bone marrow transplantation (Niitsu et al., 1990). Acute anaemia has been described in normal patients (Hamon et al., 1988) and a drop in red cell count (and reticulocytes) was seen in healthy volunteers (Anderson et al., 1985a), but usually there is sufficient haematopoietic reserve and this is not apparent clinically.

Although suffering from an ultimately self-limiting disease, patients with aplastic crisis can be severely ill. Symptoms include not only the dyspnoea and lassitude of worsening anaemia, but the patient may develop confusion, congestive heart failure, severe bone marrow necrosis (Conrad et al., 1988), cerebrovascular complications (Wierenga et al., 2001) and the illness can be fatal (Serjeant, 1992). Aplastic crisis can be the first presentation of an underlying haemolytic disease in a well-compensated patient (Cutlip et al., 1991; McLellan and Rutter, 1987).

Community-acquired aplastic crisis is almost always due to parvovirus B19 (Anderson et al., 1982) and should be the presumptive diagnosis in any patient with anaemia due to abrupt cessation of erythropoiesis, as documented by reduced reticulocytes and bone marrow appearance. In contrast to patients with erythema infectiosum, transient aplastic crisis patients are often viraemic at the time of presentation with concentrations of virus as high as 10^{14} genome copies/ml, and the diagnosis is readily made by detection of B19 DNA in the serum. As the B19 DNA is cleared from the serum, B19-specific IgM becomes detectable. Typical transient aplastic crisis is readily treated by blood transfusion. It is a unique event in the patient's life, and following the acute infection immunity is lifelong.

Transient aplastic crisis and B19 infection in haematologically normal patients is often associated with changes in the other blood lineages. There may be varying degrees of neutropenia (Doran and Teall, 1988; Saunders et al., 1986) and thrombocytopenia (Inoue et al., 1991). Transient pancytopenia is less common (Frickhofen et al., 1986; Hanada et al., 1988; Saunders et al., 1986). Haemophagocytosis, which can occur after many different viral infections, has been noted in acute (Boruchoff et al., 1990; Muir et al., 1992) and persistent B19 infection (Koch et al., 1990).

B19 Infection in Pregnancy

Animal parvoviruses are known to cause congenital infections in a variety of animals, leading to fetal loss in rodents and pigs (Mengeling, 1975) and to congenital infections in cats (Kilham and Margolis, 1966) and dogs (Jefferies and Blakemore, 1979). Thus, the potential for parvovirus B19 causing disease in pregnancy is high, and the occurrence and effects of B19 virus infection in pregnancy have always been of interest.

Initial studies of the relationship between parvovirus B19 infection and pregnancy did not show any adverse relationship. No increase in fetal malformations could be detected following clinically diagnosed outbreaks of erythema infectiosum (Ager et al., 1966) and in a study of sera taken during the first month of life from infants with birth defects, no B19 antigen or specific IgM could be detected (Mortimer et al., 1985a). However, there have been a large number of case reports of B19 infection in pregnancy leading to an adverse outcome, either miscarriage or hydrops fetalis (Anand et al., 1987). The clinical features have been remarkably similar. In cases where pathological studies were undertaken, the fetuses showed evidence of leukoerythroblastic reaction in the liver, and large pale cells with eosinophilic inclusion bodies and peripheral condensation or marginatum of the nucleus were seen. Parvovirus B19 DNA could be detected by dot–blot or in situ hybridisation, and parvovirus particles seen by electron microscopy (Field et al., 1991). There are however many more reports of favourable outcome after confirmed parvovirus B19 in pregnancy (Kinney et al., 1988).

To address the frequency of complications associated with parvovirus B19 infection in pregnancy, two prospective studies in the UK followed 190 and 255 women, respectively, with serologically confirmed B19 during pregnancy (Miller et al., 1998; Public Health Laboratory Service Working Party on Fifth Disease,

1990). In both studies there was an excess fetal loss rate (spontaneous abortion and intrauterine deaths) during the first 20 weeks of pregnancy of 9% compared to controls, with the greatest fetal loss due to B19 during weeks 9–16. The fetus was lost most frequently 4–6 weeks after the maternal infection, although there was no difference between outcomes following either asymptomatic or symptomatic maternal infection. It thus appears that B19 infection is a significant cause of second trimester fetal loss.

In seven of the cases the fetus developed hydrops fetalis and the risk of hydrops fetalis following B19 infection during weeks 9–20 was calculated at 2.9%. Three of the hydropic infants survived: two of the three were treated with intrauterine blood transfusions. Other studies have shown that spontaneous resolution of hydrops following B19 infection does occur (Pryde et al., 1992; Sheikh et al., 1992) and there are risks associated with intrauterine blood transfusions. However, several studies have shown that intrauterine blood transfusions may enhance survival: an observational study from the UK reported survival of 9/12 fetuses treated with transfusions, compared to 13/26 untreated, a significant difference after allowing for ultrasound findings and gestational age (Fairley et al., 1995).

Non-immune hydrops fetalis is rare (1:3000 births) and in approximately 50% of cases the aetiology is unknown. In a study of 50 cases, the majority were due to cardiovascular or chromosomal abnormalities, but parvovirus B19 DNA was detected by in situ hybridisation in the lungs of four fetuses despite there being no known epidemic of B19 during the study period (Porter et al., 1988). Parvovirus B19 probably causes 10–15% of all cases of non-immune hydrops (Yaegashi et al., 1998), and it is worth investigating B19 as a cause of non-immunological hydrops fetalis by specific tests for B19.

Congenital Malformations

Although sporadic case reports have noticed an association between genitourinary abnormalities (Public Health Laboratory Service Working Party on Fifth Disease, 1990; Rodis et al., 1990), cerebral abnormalities (Katz et al., 1996) and ocular malformations (Hartwig et al., 1989), the abnormalities reported are all relatively common and, without a control population, it is difficult to interpret the abnormalities as being due to B19. No systematic studies have shown evidence for congenital abnormalities following B19 infection. In the two British studies only one case with congenital malformation was seen (a ventral septal

defect) and it was concluded that the risk of congenital malformations due to B19 infection was less than 1%. In addition, no late effects of B19 infection were seen in the children followed-up at 7–10 years. In a similar study in America, again no increase in adverse long-term outcomes was observed. Thus, there is no evidence to date that B19 causes birth defects, although it should be remembered that the sample sizes in the studies have been too small to detect a rare defect, i.e. one with a rate of 1% or less. Nevertheless, there is no reason to recommend termination of pregnancies complicated by laboratory-proven B19 virus infection.

Infants born with chronic anaemia following a history of maternal B19 exposure and intrauterine hydrops have been described (Brown et al., 1994a). In three such cases, who at birth were found to have hypogamma-globulinaemia, viral DNA was present in the bone marrow although absent from the serum. One child died but the other two remained persistently anaemic in spite of immunoglobulin therapy. In a related study of bone marrow from children with Diamond–Blackfan anaemia, B19 DNA was found in 3/11 marrow smears, all from children that underwent remission of their anaemia. Thus, intrauterine B19 infection may be responsible for some cases of congenital anaemia, although the incidence is probably rare.

B19 Infection in the Immunosuppressed

A chronic B19 infection resulting in pure red cell aplasia (PRCA) occurs in immunocompromised individuals who have failed to produce neutralising antibody to the virus. Chronic infection has been reported in a wide variety of immunosuppressed patients, ranging from patients with congenital immunodeficiency (Kurtzman et al., 1987), acquired immunodeficiency (AIDS; Frickhofen et al., 1990), lymphoproliferative disorders (Kurtzman et al., 1988) and transplant patients (Frickhofen and Young, 1989). The stereotypical presentation is with persistent anaemia rather than immune-mediated symptoms of rash or arthropathy. Patients have absent or low levels of B19 specific antibody (Kurtzman et al., 1989b) and persistent or recurrent parvoviraemia, as detected by B19 DNA in the serum. Bone marrow examination generally reveals the presence of scattered giant pronormoblasts. Administration of neutralising antibody in the form of human normal immunoglobulin often leads to a fall in virus titre, reticulocytosis and in some cases rash illness presumed to be due to immune complexes (Kurtzman et al., 1988).

Table 24.3 Atypical disease presentations of parvovirus B19

Infection in the healthy host
  Neurological disorders/encephalitis
  Myocarditis
  Hepatitis
  Glomerulonephritis
  Haematological
    Thrombocytopenia
    Neutropenia
    Pancytopenia
    Haemophagocytosis
  Rheumatic diseases
    Chronic fatigue syndrome
    Fibromylagia
    Myositis
    Vasculitis
    Kawasaki disease

The prevalence of B19-induced anaemia in HIV-seropositive patients is probably higher than recognised at present. In one early study of 50 patients with AIDS, no patients with B19 viraemia were identified. In a larger cohort study, B19 DNA was found in only 1/191 (0.5%) of HIV-seropositive homosexuals. However, B19 DNA was found in 5/30 (17%) of transfusion dependent HIV-seropositive homosexuals, and when a haematocrit of < 20 was used as a criterion, 4/13 (31%) were positive (Abkowitz *et al.*, 1997). In contrast to the earlier studies, the marrow morphology need not be suggestive of PRCA and giant pronormoblasts may not be present.

In less severely immunosuppressed patients (i.e. SLE on steroid therapy), prolonged anaemia following B19 infection has also been described (Koch *et al.*, 1990). However, in these patients there was a spontaneous, albeit delayed, development of antibodies, and viraemia resolved without therapy. Presumably such patients represent one end of the spectrum of disease manifestations of B19 in patients with a compromised immune system.

Atypical Presentations

A wide variety of symptoms and diseases have been associated with parvovirus disease (Table 24.3; and see Török, 1997), generally as case reports or limited small series of patients. Determining the role of B19 in these diseases is often difficult: the diseases are rare and B19 may not be the only cause. In addition, with sensitive PCR-based assays B19 DNA can be detected in bone marrow (Cassinotti *et al.*, 1997) and other tissues (Soderlund-Venermo *et al.*, 2002; Soderlund *et al.*, 1997) from healthy individuals. When the disease is rare, large multicentre trials may be required to substantiate or disprove the causal relationship.

LABORATORY DIAGNOSIS

Aplastic crisis is the only one of the clinical syndromes that can be assumed, with some accuracy, to be due to B19 infection. Even so, in patients with chronic haemolytic anaemia moderate to severe degrees of hypoplasia may be associated with systemic bacterial infection or marrow-suppressive drugs, and anaemia in the immunocompromised may have many other causes. Illnesses associated with maculopapular rashes with or without joint involvement also have a multiplicity of causes and only a minority of cases of hydrops fetalis will prove to be due to B19 infection. Thus, accurate diagnosis of B19 infection depends upon specific laboratory tests.

Specimens

Serum is the principal specimen used for the laboratory diagnosis of B19 infection. This approach is suitable for virus detection in cases of aplastic crisis, persistent infection in immunosuppressed patients and persistent fetal infection. The detection of specific IgM antibody in serum is the cornerstone of the diagnosis of rash illness and arthropathy, and is often valuable in cases of aplastic crisis. Standard blood specimens are all that are required and no special arrangements are needed for transport to or storage in the laboratory. It should be remembered that viraemic samples may contain high titres of infectious virus, and care should be taken when handling samples, especially those taken early in the course of an aplastic crisis, to ensure that seronegative individuals in the laboratory are not infected (probable cases of laboratory-acquired infection have been described; Cohen *et al.*, 1988).

B19 assays can also be performed on tissue samples. DNA can be extracted from fresh, frozen or fixed samples for detection of parvoviral DNA. Detection of B19 virus by either immunohistochemistry or *in situ* hybridisation can also be performed on formalin-fixed, paraffin-embedded tissue, so that standard pathology protocols can be used for dealing with bone marrow or fetal tissue.

Virus Detection

The culture of parvovirus B19 in erythroid progenitor cells remains a research procedure and is not used in the routine diagnosis of B19 infections. Instead, B19 virus detection relies on the detection of either viral antigen or viral DNA. Although ELISA- and haemagglutination-based assays are being developed to detect viral antigen, this is generally in the context of blood screening (Wakamatsu *et al.*, 1999). Instead, for diagnostic purposes, DNA hybridisation and/or electron microscopy are commonly used. The common clinical situation in which these tests are applied is to the acute-phase specimen of cases of aplastic crisis or immunosuppressed patients with chronic anaemia. DNA hybridisation using cloned viral genome labelled with ^{32}P (Anderson *et al.*, 1985b) will detect about 10^4 particles/ml, in specimens taken within 24 h of the onset of an aplastic crisis this will yield positive results in 60% of cases. Immune electron microscopy is only slightly less sensitive than DNA hybridisation.

The most sensitive technique for the detection of virus requires amplification of the DNA using PCR. A variety of different primers and probes have been described, the most sensitive assays are capable of detecting 1–10 virus particles (Clewley, 1993; Patou *et al.*, 1993). This can be a very useful tool, but as with all PCR, there is also great propensity for cross-contamination and false positive results. In addition, low levels of viral DNA can be detected for months or even years after acute infection (Cassinotti *et al.*, 1997; Musiani *et al.*, 1995) and thus the detection of B19 DNA by PCR alone cannot be used to diagnose acute B19 infection.

The diagnosis of B19 infection in a fetus also depends upon the detection of virus. Maternal infection will have occurred some weeks previously and maternal serum may therefore be B19-specific IgM-negative. In most instances the fetus has also been found to be specific IgM-negative but there is frequently a persistent viraemia. Therefore, the diagnosis is best made by detection of virus in fetal blood samples by the techniques described above. Equally virus can be detected in fetal tissues taken at autopsy, from which DNA has been extracted or detected by immunohistochemistry or *in situ* hybridisation on formalin-fixed, paraffin-embedded tissue sections. Glutaraldehyde-fixed material can also be used for electron microscopy, but scattered B19 particles within cells may be more difficult to recognise, due to the large number of ribosomes of similar size.

Specific Antibody Detection

Standard solid-phase enzyme-labelled immunoassays (ELISAs) are the preferred method for the serological diagnosis of recent B19 infection, although immuno-fluorescent and Western blot assays are commercially available. Due to the inability to grow B19 in standard cell culture systems, until recently there has been a shortage of viral antigen for any diagnostic assays. Attempts have been made to develop assays based on the use of synthetic peptides or fusion proteins in *Escherichia coli*, but the epitopes presented by these products do not accurately reproduce the epitopes of the native capsids, and the practical results have generally been disappointing, with lack of specificity when used on discriminating sera. The expression of B19 capsid proteins as virion-like particles, using the baculovirus expression system (Brown *et al.*, 1991a; Kajigaya *et al.*, 1991), appears to have overcome these problems, and assays based on these antigens show excellent correlation with assays based on native virus (Kajigaya *et al.*, 1991). The antigens are relatively easy to mass-produce and are non-infectious, and therefore without hazard to laboratory workers.

The best assay to detect recent infection with B19 remains the IgM capture assay in which IgM-specific antibody in the patient's serum is bound by a solid phase coated with antibody to human μ-chains. The viral specificity of the bound antibody is determined by the addition of B19 virus antigen to the solid phase. In turn bound antigen is detected by the addition of monoclonal anti-B19 antibody, which may itself be tagged with enzyme. Alternatively, an extra step may be incorporated, whereby the bound monoclonal anti-B19 is detected by the addition of labelled anti-mouse immunoglobulin (Cohen *et al.*, 1983). IgM tests using an indirect format, are less useful for diagnosis due to their lack of both specificity and sensitivity.

Sera containing 10 au/ml or more of anti-B19 IgM are unequivocally associated with recent infection. This relatively high threshold is set because sera containing high concentrations of antirubella virus IgM may give low false positive results when tested for anti-B19 IgM, and vice versa (Kurtz and Anderson, 1985). This must be borne in mind when testing sera taken within 2 weeks of a rubelliform illness. However, high concentrations of anti-Bl9 IgM usually appear within 3–4 days of the onset of symptoms and antibody can be detected in over 90% of cases by the third day of transient aplastic crisis, or at the time of rash in erythema infectiosum. IgM antibody remains detectable for 2–3 months following infection. In patients presenting with symptoms of aplastic crisis, and occasionally in rash-like presentations, specific IgM may not appear until 7–10 days after the onset. Therefore, if a negative or equivocal result for anti-B19 IgM is obtained with a serum taken within 10 days of the onset of the illness, the serum should be tested for viral DNA and/or a second specimen to be taken about 14 days after the onset of symptoms should be requested. Specific IgM is detectable for 2–3 months after acute infection. Interpretation of equivocal low concentrations of anti-B19 IgM in sera taken after this time is difficult and in this circumstance testing for IgG may be helpful.

B19 IgG can be detected by capture assay or preferably by indirect assay. It is usually present by day 7 of illness and probably is lifelong thereafter. As more than 50% of the population have IgG antibody to B19 infection, detection of B19 IgG in a single sample is not useful for the diagnosis of acute infection, but can be used to document seroconversion.

In 1995, the WHO Expert Committee on Biological Standardization recommended that an international standard (IU/ml) be set for anti-parvovirus B19 testing. The international standard chosen correlates well with the original arbitrary unit (au) scale in the earlier literature. In the 12 months following infection, patients have relatively high (< 50 IU/ml) concentrations of anti-B19 IgG and the finding of such concentrations supports the diagnosis of infection during that time. However, there is marked individual variation in the maximum amounts of specific IgG that can be demonstrated in a patient, so that the finding of only low values (> 20 IU/ml) does not exclude recent infection. Previous infection (and therefore immunity in most individuals) is indicated by the detection of > 5 IU/ml of anti-B19 IgG. However, a negative result cannot be taken to be synonymous with susceptibility.

There is a poor humoral immune response in immunocompromised patients with chronic parvovirus infection and only low concentrations of anti-B19 IgG (and IgM) can be detected in these patients. None of the detectable antibody neutralises virus infectivity and this is taken to be an essential component of the pathogenesis of the chronic infection. The diagnosis of B19 infection in these patients is dependent on the detection of viral antigen or DNA.

TREATMENT AND PREVENTION

There is no specific antiviral chemotherapy for B19 infection. Symptomatic relief of troublesome joint symptoms may be required for B19 virus-associated arthralgia, and blood transfusion may be necessary in the acute phase of aplastic crisis.

The only specific treatment for B19 infection is the intravenous administration of human immunoglobulin in cases of persistent infection in the immunocompro-

mised. Human normal immunoglobulin preparations are a good source of neutralising antibodies to B19 virus (Takahashi et al., 1991), since at least half the adult population have been exposed to the virus. Controlled trials have not been done but on an empirical basis the administration of 0.4 g/kg body weight/day for 5–10 days has proved effective in reducing viraemia and allowing the haemoglobin to return to near-normal values (Frickhofen et al., 1990; Kurtzman et al., 1989a). Patients sometimes relapse months later but they have been shown to respond to repeat courses.

Prevention of disease by isolating susceptible individuals is impractical because infections may be subclinical, and even symptomatic individuals are most frequently infectious before any sign of illness. Theoretically, susceptible individuals with chronic haemolytic anaemia (or immunocompromised children) could be temporarily protected by the administration of human immunoglobulin, but to date this has not been put into practice.

Many animal parvovirus infections are prevented in animals by vaccination, and the prospects for a B19 parvovirus vaccine are good. The immunogen will be recombinant capsid rather than attenuated or killed virus, due to the difficulty of cultivating B19 parvovirus in vitro and the potential dangers of inadvertently modifying, for the worse, the host range of B19 parvovirus by selection in vitro. Baculovirus-produced B19 parvovirus capsids induce neutralising antibodies in experimental animals (Kajigaya et al., 1991), even without adjuvant. The presence of VP1 protein in the capsid immunogen appears critical for the production of antibodies that neutralise virus activity in vitro, and capsids with supranormal VP1 content are even more efficient in inducing neutralising activity (Bansal et al., 1993). Sera from human volunteers immunised with one candidate vaccine had neutralising antibody titres equal to or higher than those observed after natural infection. Phase I trial results appear promising, and phase II trials are planned. However, the targets for such a vaccine remain to be determined. Should only patients at high risk of severe or life-threatening disease, such as sickle cell patients be protected? Or, in view of the wide variety of disease manifestations affecting all strata of the population, should a universal vaccine policy be pursued?

REFERENCES

Abkowitz JL, Brown KE, Wood RW et al. (1997) Clinical relevance of parvovirus B19 as a cause of anemia in patients with human immunodeficiency virus infection. *J Infect Dis*, **176**, 269–273.

Agbandje M, Kajigaya S, McKenna R *et al.* (1994) The structure of human parvovirus B19 at 8 Å resolution. *Virology*, **203**, 106–115.

Ager AE, Chin TDJ and Poland JD (1966) Epidemic erythema infectiosum. *N Engl J Med*, **275**, 1326–1331.

Anand A, Gray ES, Brown T *et al.* (1987) Human parvovirus infection in pregnancy and hydrops fetalis. *N Engl J Med*, **316**, 183–186.

Anderson MJ, Davis LR, Hodgson J (1982) Occurrence of infection with a parvovirus-like agent in children with sickle cell anaemia during a two-year period. *J Clin Pathol*, **35**, 744–749.

Anderson MJ, Higgins PG, Davis LR *et al.* (1985a) Experimental parvoviral infection in humans. *J Infect Dis*, **152**, 257–265.

Anderson MJ, Jones SE, Fisher-Hoch SP *et al.* (1983) Human parvovirus, the cause of erythema infectiosum (fifth disease)? [letter]. *Lancet*, **i**, 1378.

Anderson MJ, Jones SE and Minson AC (1985b) Diagnosis of human parvovirus infection by dot–blot hybridization using cloned viral DNA. *J Med Virol*, **15**, 163–172.

Anderson MJ, Lewis E, Kidd IM *et al.* (1984) An outbreak of erythema infectiosum associated with human parvovirus infection. *J Hyg (Lond)*, **93**, 85–93.

Balfour HH (1969) Erythema infectiosum (fifth disease). Clinical review and description of 91 cases seen in an epidemic. *Clin Pediatr*, **8**, 721–727.

Bansal GP, Hatfield JA, Dunn FE *et al.* (1993) Candidate recombinant vaccine for human B19 parvovirus, *J Infect Dis*, **167**, 1034–1044.

Bartolomei Corsi O, Azzi A, Morfini M *et al.* (1988) Human parvovirus infection in haemophiliacs first infused with treated clotting factor concentrates. *J Med Virol*, **25**, 165–170.

Berns KI, Bergoin M, Bloom M *et al.* (1995) Family *Parvoviridae*. In *Virus Taxonomy. Classification and Nomenclature of Viruses* (eds Murphy FA, Fauquet CM, Bishop DHL *et al.*), pp 169–178. Springer-Verlag, New York.

Blumel J, Schmidt I, Willkommen H and Lower J (2002) Inactivation of parvovirus B19 during pasteurization of human serum albumin. *Transfusion*, **42**, 1011–1018.

Boruchoff SE, Woda BA, Pihan GA *et al.* (1990) Parvovirus B19-associated hemophagocytic syndrome. *Arch Intern Med*, **150**, 897–899.

Brass C, Elliott LM and Stevens DA (1982) Academy rash. A probable epidemic of erythema infectiosum ('fifth disease'). *J Am Med Assoc*, **248**, 568–572.

Brown CS, Van Lent JW, Vlak JM and Spaan WJ (1991a) Assembly of empty capsids by using baculovirus recombinants expressing human parvovirus B19 structural proteins. *J Virol*, **65**, 2702–2706.

Brown KE, Anderson SM and Young NS (1993) Erythrocyte P antigen: cellular receptor for B19 parvovirus. *Science*, **262**, 114–117.

Brown KE, Green SW, Antunez de Mayolo J *et al.* (1994a) Congenital anaemia after transplacental B19 parvovirus infection. *Lancet*, **343**, 895–896.

Brown KE, Hibbs JR, Gallinella G *et al.* (1994b) Resistance to parvovirus B19 infection due to lack of virus receptor (erythrocyte P antigen). *N Engl J Med*, **330**, 1192–1196.

Brown KE, Mori J, Cohen BJ and Field AM (1991b) *In vitro* propagation of parvovirus B19 in primary foetal liver culture. *J Gen Virol*, **72**, 741–745.

Brownell AI, McSwiggan DA, Cubitt WD and Anderson MJ (1986) Aplastic and hypoplastic episodes in sickle cell disease and thalassaemia intermedia. *J Clin Pathol*, **39**, 121–124.

Cassinotti P, Burtonboy G, Fopp M and Siegl G (1997) Evidence for persistence of human parvovirus B19 DNA in bone marrow. *J Med Virol*, **53**, 229–232.

Cheinisse L (1905) Une cinquième maladie éruptive: le mégal-érythème épidémique. *Sem Med*, **25**, 205–207.

Chipman PR, Agbandje-McKenna M, Kajigaya S *et al.* (1996) Cryo-electron microscopy studies of empty capsids of human parvovirus B19 complexed with its cellular receptor. *Proc Natl Acad Sci USA*, **93**, 7502–7506.

Clewley JP (1989) Polymerase chain reaction assay of parvovirus B19 DNA in clinical specimens. *J Clin Microbiol*, **27**, 2647–2651.

Clewley JP (1993) PCR detection of parvovirus B19. In *Diagnostic Molecular Microbiology: Principles and Applications*, 1st edn (eds Persing DH, Smith TF, Tenover FC and White TJ), pp 367–373. American Society for Microbiology, Washington, DC.

Cohen BJ and Buckley MM (1988) The prevalence of antibody to human parvovirus B19 in England and Wales. *J Med Microbiol*, **25**, 151–153.

Cohen BJ, Couroucé AM, Schwarz TF *et al.* (1988) Laboratory infection with parvovirus B19 [letter]. *J Clin Pathol*, **41**, 1027–1028.

Cohen BJ, Field AM, Gudnadottir S *et al.* (1990) Blood donor screening for parvovirus B19. *J Virol Meth*, **30**, 233–238.

Cohen BJ, Mortimer PP and Pereira MS (1983) Diagnostic assays with monoclonal antibodies for the human serum parvovirus-like virus (SPLV). *J Hyg (Lond)*, **91**, 113–130.

Conrad ME, Studdard H and Anderson LJ (1988) Aplastic crisis in sickle cell disorders: bone marrow necrosis and human parvovirus infection. *Am J Med Sci*, **295**, 212–215.

Cossart YE, Field AM, Cant B and Widdows D (1975) Parvovirus-like particles in human sera. *Lancet*, **i**, 72–73.

Cutlip AC, Gross KM and Lewis MJ (1991) Occult hereditary spherocytosis and human parvovirus infection. *J Am Board Fam Practit*, **4**, 461–464.

de Freitas RB, Wong D, Boswell F *et al.* (1990) Prevalence of human parvovirus (B19) and rubella virus infections in urban and remote rural areas in northern Brazil. *J Med Virol*, **32**, 203–208.

Deiss V, Tratschin JD, Weitz M and Siegl G (1990) Cloning of the human parvovirus B19 genome and structural analysis of its palindromic termini. *Virology*, **175**, 247–254.

Dijkmans BA, van Elsacker-Niele AM, Salimans MM *et al.* (1988) Human parvovirus B19 DNA in synovial fluid. *Arthrit Rheumatol*, **31**, 279–281.

Doran HM and Teall AJ (1988) Neutropenia accompanying erythroid aplasia in human parvovirus infection. *Br J Haematol*, **69**, 287–288.

Duncan JR, Potter CB, Cappellini MD *et al.* (1983) Aplastic crisis due to parvovirus infection in pyruvate kinase deficiency. *Lancet*, **ii**, 14–16.

Evans LM, Grossman ME and Gregory N (1992) Koplik spots and a purpuric eruption associated with parvovirus B19 infection. *J Am Acad Dermatol*, **27**, 466–467.

Fairley CK, Smoleniec JS, Caul OE and Miller E (1995) Observational study of effect of intrauterine transfusions on outcome of fetal hydrops after parvovirus B19 infection. *Lancet*, **346**, 1335–1337.

Field AM, Cohen BJ, Brown KE *et al.* (1991) Detection of B19 parvovirus in human fetal tissues by electron microscopy. *J Med Virol*, **35**, 85–95.

Frank R, Glander HJ and Haustein UF (1996) [Dermatologic symptoms of parvovirus B19 infections]. *Hautarzt Zeitschr Dermatol, Venerol verw Gebiete*, **47**, 365–368.

Frickhofen N, Abkowitz JL, Safford M *et al.* (1990) Persistent B19 parvovirus infection in patients infected with human immunodeficiency virus type 1 (HIV-1): a treatable cause of anemia in AIDS. *Ann Intern Med*, **113**, 926–933.

Frickhofen N, Raghavachar A, Heit W *et al.* (1986) Human parvovirus infection [letter]. *N Engl J Med*, **314**, 646.

Frickhofen N and Young NS (1989) Persistent parvovirus B19 infections in humans. *Microb Pathogen*, **7**, 319–327.

Friedman-Einat M, Grossman Z, Mileguir F *et al.* (1997) Detection of adeno-associated virus type 2 sequences in the human genital tract. *J Clin Microbiol*, **35**, 71–78.

Gao GP, Alvira MR, Wang L *et al.* (2002) Novel adeno-associated viruses from rhesus monkeys as vectors for human gene therapy. *Proc Natl Acad Sci USA*, **99**, 11854–11859.

Green SW, Malkovska I, O'Sullivan MG and Brown KE (2000) Rhesus and pig-tailed macaque parvoviruses: identification of two new members of the Erythrovirus genus in monkeys. *Virology*, **269**, 105–112.

Grilli EA, Anderson MJ and Hoskins TW (1989) Concurrent outbreaks of influenza and parvovirus B19 in a boys' boarding school. *Epidemiol Infect*, **103**, 359–369.

Halasz CL, Cormier D and Den M (1992) Petechial glove and sock syndrome caused by parvovirus B19. *J Am Acad Dermatol*, **27**, 835–838.

Hamon MD, Newland AC and Anderson MJ (1988) Severe aplastic anaemia after parvovirus infection in the absence of underlying haemolytic anaemia [letter]. *J Clin Pathol*, **41**, 1242.

Hanada T, Koike K, Takeya T *et al.* (1988) Human parvovirus B19-induced transient pancytopenia in a child with hereditary spherocytosis. *Br J Haematol*, **70**, 113–115.

Hartwig NG, Vermeij-Keers C, van Elsacker-Niele AM and Fleuren GJ (1989) Embryonic malformations in a case of intrauterine parvovirus B19 infection. *Teratology*, **39**, 295–302.

Heegaard ED, Qvortrup K and Christensen J (2002) Baculovirus expression of erythrovirus V9 capsids and screening by ELISA: serologic cross-reactivity with erythrovirus B19. *J Med Virol*, **66**, 246–252.

Heegaard ED and Taaning EB (2002) Parvovirus B19 and parvovirus V9 are not associated with Henoch–Schonlein purpura in children. *Pediatr Infect Dis J*, **21**, 31–34.

Inoue S, Kinra NK, Mukkamala SR and Gordon R (1991) Parvovirus B-19 infection: aplastic crisis, erythema infectiosum and idiopathic thrombocytopenic purpura. *Pediatr Infect Dis J*, **10**, 251–253.

Jefferies AR and Blakemore WF (1979) Myocarditis and enteritis in puppies associated with parvovirus. *Vet Rec*, **104**, 221.

Kajigaya S, Fujii H, Field A *et al.* (1991) Self-assembled B19 parvovirus capsids, produced in a baculovirus system, are antigenically and immunogenically similar to native virions. *Proc Natl Acad Sci USA*, **88**, 4646–4650.

Kandolf R, Kirschner P, Hofschneider PH and Vischer TL (1989) Detection of parvovirus in a patient with 'reactive arthritis' by *in situ* hybridization. *Clin Rheumatol*, **8**, 398–401.

Katz VL, McCoy MC, Kuller JA and Hansen WF (1996) An association between fetal parvovirus B19 infection and fetal anomalies: a report of two cases. *Am J Perinatol*, **13**, 43–45.

Kelleher JF, Luban NL, Mortimer PP and Kamimura T (1983) Human serum 'parvovirus': a specific cause of aplastic crisis in children with hereditary spherocytosis. *J Pediatr*, **102**, 720–722.

Kilham L and Margolis G (1966) Viral etiology of spontaneous ataxia of cats. *Am J Pathol*, **48**, 991–1011.

Kinney JS, Anderson LJ, Farrar J *et al.* (1988) Risk of adverse outcomes of pregnancy after human parvovirus B19 infection. *J Infect Dis*, **157**, 663–667.

Koch WC and Adler SP (1989) Human parvovirus B19 infections in women of childbearing age and within families. *Pediatr Infect Dis J*, **8**, 83–87.

Koch WC, Massey G, Russell CE and Adler SP (1990) Manifestations and treatment of human parvovirus B19 infection in immunocompromised patients. *J Pediatr*, **116**, 355–359.

Kurtz JB and Anderson MJ (1985) Cross-reactions in rubella and parvovirus specific IgM tests [letter]. *Lancet*, **ii**, 1356.

Kurtzman G, Frickhofen N, Kimball J *et al.* (1989a) Pure red-cell aplasia of 10 years' duration due to persistent parvovirus B19 infection and its cure with immunoglobulin therapy. *N Engl J Med*, **321**, 519–523.

Kurtzman GJ, Cohen B, Meyers P *et al.* (1988) Persistent B19 parvovirus infection as a cause of severe chronic anaemia in children with acute lymphocytic leukaemia. *Lancet*, **ii**, 1159–1162.

Kurtzman GJ, Cohen BJ, Field AM *et al.* (1989b) Immune response to B19 parvovirus and an antibody defect in persistent viral infection. *J Clin Invest*, **84**, 1114–1123.

Kurtzman GJ, Ozawa K, Cohen B *et al.* (1987) Chronic bone marrow failure due to persistent B19 parvovirus infection. *N Engl J Med*, **317**, 287–294.

Lefrere JJ and Bourgeois H (1986) Human parvovirus associated with erythroblastopenia in iron deficiency anaemia [letter]. *J Clin Pathol*, **39**, 1277–1278.

Lefrère JJ, Couroucé AM, Muller JY *et al.* (1985) Human parvovirus and purpura [letter]. *Lancet*, **ii**, 730.

Leruez-Ville M, Vassias I, Pallier C *et al.* (1997) Establishment of a cell line expressing human parvovirus B19 non-structural protein from an inducible promoter. *J Gen Virol*, **78**, 215–219.

Liu JM, Green SW, Shimada T and Young NS (1992) A block in full-length transcript maturation in cells non-permissive for B19 parvovirus. *J Virol*, **66**, 4686–4692.

Lobkowicz F, Ring J, Schwarz TF and Roggendorf M (1989) Erythema multiforme in a patient with acute human parvovirus B19 infection. *J Am Acad Dermatol*, **20**, 849–850.

Luo W and Astell CR (1993) A novel protein encoded by small RNAs of parvovirus B19. *Virology*, **195**, 448–455.

Luzzi GA, Kurtz JB and Chapel H (1985) Human parvovirus arthropathy and rheumatoid factor [letter]. *Lancet*, **i**, 1218.

Lyon DJ, Chapman CS, Martin C *et al.* (1989) Symptomatic parvovirus B19 infection and heat-treated factor IX concentrate [letter]. *Lancet*, **i**, 1085.

McLellan NJ and Rutter N (1987) Hereditary spherocytosis in sisters unmasked by parvovirus infection. *Postgrad Med J*, **63**, 49–50.

McOmish F, Yap PL, Jordan A *et al.* (1993) Detection of parvovirus B19 in donated blood: a model system for screening by polymerase chain reaction. *J Clin Microbiol*, **31**, 323–328.

Mengeling WL (1975) Porcine parvovirus: frequency of naturally occurring transplacental infection and viral contamination of fetal porcine kidney cell cultures. *Am J Vet Res*, **36**, 41–44.

Miller E, Fairley CK, Cohen BJ and Seng C (1998) Immediate and long term outcome of human parvovirus B19 infection in pregnancy. *Br J Obstet Gynaecol*, **105**, 174–178.

Miyagawa E, Yoshida T, Takahashi H *et al.* (1999) Infection of the erythroid cell line, KU812Ep6 with human parvovirus B19 and its application to titration of B19 infectivity. *J Virol Meth*, **83**, 45–54.

Moffatt S, Yaegashi N, Tada K *et al.* (1998) Human parvovirus B19 nonstructural (NS1) protein induces apoptosis in erythroid lineage cells. *J Virol*, **72**, 3018–3028.

Momoeda M, Wong S, Kawase M *et al.* (1994) A putative nucleoside triphosphate-binding domain in the nonstructural protein of B19 parvovirus is required for cytotoxicity. *J Virol*, **68**, 8443–8446.

Morey AL, Ferguson DJ and Fleming KA (1993) Ultrastructural features of fetal erythroid precursors infected with parvovirus B19 *in vitro*: evidence of cell death by apoptosis. *J Pathol*, **169**, 213–220.

Mortimer PP, Cohen BJ, Buckley MM *et al.* (1985a) Human parvovirus and the fetus [letter]. *Lancet*, **ii**, 1012.

Mortimer PP, Cohen BJ, Rossiter MA *et al.* (1985b) Human parvovirus and purpura. *Lancet*, **ii**, 730–731.

Mortimer PP, Luban NL, Kelleher JF and Cohen BJ (1983) Transmission of serum parvovirus-like virus by clotting-factor concentrates. *Lancet*, **ii**, 482–484.

Muir K, Todd WT, Watson WH and Fitzsimons E (1992) Viral-associated haemophagocytosis with parvovirus-B19-related pancytopenia. *Lancet*, **339**, 1139–1140.

Murray JC, Kelley PK, Hogrefe WR and McClain KL (1994) Childhood idiopathic thrombocytopenic purpura: association with human parvovirus B19 infection. *Am J Pediatr Hematol Oncol*, **16**, 314–319.

Musiani M, Zerbini M, Gentilomi G *et al.* (1995) Parvovirus B19 clearance from peripheral blood after acute infection. *J Infect Dis*, **172**, 1360–1363.

Naides SJ, Piette W, Veach LA and Argenyi Z (1988) Human parvovirus B19-induced vesiculopustular skin eruption. *Am J Med*, **84**, 968–972.

Naides SJ and Weiner CP (1989) Antenatal diagnosis and palliative treatment of non-immune hydrops fetalis secondary to fetal parvovirus B19 infection. *Prenatal Diagn*, **9**, 105–114.

Neild G, Anderson M, Hawes S and Colvin BT (1986) Parvovirus infection after renal transplant [letter]. *Lancet*, **ii**, 1226–1227.

Nguyen QT, Sifer C, Schneider V *et al.* (1999) Novel human erythrovirus associated with transient aplastic anemia. *J Clin Microbiol*, **37**, 2483–2487.

Nguyen QT, Wong S, Heegaard ED and Brown KE (2002) Identification and characterization of a second novel human erythrovirus variant, A6. *Virology*, **301**, 374–380.

Niitsu H, Takatsu H, Miura I *et al.* (1990) [Pure red cell aplasia induced by B19 parvovirus during allogeneic bone marrow transplantation]. *Jap J Clin Hematol*, **31**, 1566–1571.

Nishizawa T, Okamoto H, Konishi K *et al.* (1997) A novel DNA virus (TTV) associated with elevated transaminase levels in posttransfusion hepatitis of unknown etiology. *Biochem Biophys Res Commun*, **241**, 92–97.

O'Sullivan MG, Anderson DC, Fikes JD *et al.* (1994) Identification of a novel simian parvovirus in cynomolgus monkeys with severe anemia: a paradigm of human B19 parvovirus infection. *J Clin Invest*, **93**, 1571–1576.

Owren PA (1948) Congenital hemolytic jaundice: the pathogenesis of the 'hemolytic crisis'. *Blood*, **3**, 231–248.

Ozawa K, Ayub J, Hao YS *et al.* (1987) Novel transcription map for the B19 (human) pathogenic parvovirus. *J Virol*, **61**, 2395–2406.

Ozawa K, Ayub J, Kajigaya S *et al.* (1988) The gene encoding the nonstructural protein of B19 (human) parvovirus may be lethal in transfected cells. *J Virol*, **62**, 2884–2889.

Ozawa K, Ayub J and Young N (1988) Translational regulation of B19 parvovirus capsid protein production by multiple upstream AUG triplets. *J Biol Chem*, **263**, 10922–10926.

Ozawa K, Kurtzman G and Young N (1987) Productive infection by B19 parvovirus of human erythroid bone marrow cells *in vitro*. *Blood*, **70**, 384–391.

Ozawa K and Young N (1987) Characterization of capsid and noncapsid proteins of B19 parvovirus propagated in human erythroid bone marrow cell cultures. *J Virol*, **61**, 2627–2630.

Patou G, Pillay D, Myint S and Pattison J (1993) Characterization of a nested polymerase chain reaction assay for detection of parvovirus B19. *J Clin Microbiol*, **31**, 540–546.

Pattison JR, Jones SE, Hodgson J *et al.* (1981) Parvovirus infections and hypoplastic crisis in sickle-cell anaemia. *Lancet*, **i**, 664–665.

Paver WK, Caul EO, Ley CR *et al.* (1973) A small virus in human faeces. *Lancet*, **i**, 664–665.

Plummer FA, Hammond GW, Forward K *et al.* (1985) An erythema infectiosum-like illness caused by human parvovirus infection. *N Engl J Med*, **313**, 74–79.

Porter HJ, Heryet A, Quantrill AM and Fleming KA (1990) Combined non-isotopic *in situ* hybridisation and immunohistochemistry on routine paraffin wax embedded tissue: identification of cell type infected by human parvovirus and demonstration of cytomegalovirus DNA and antigen in renal infection. *J Clin Pathol*, **43**, 129–132.

Porter HJ, Khong TY, Evans MF *et al.* (1988) Parvovirus as a cause of hydrops fetalis: detection by in situ DNA hybridisation. *J Clin Pathol*, **41**, 381–383.

Potter CG, Potter AC, Hatton CS *et al.* (1987) Variation of erythroid and myeloid precursors in the marrow and peripheral blood of volunteer subjects infected with human parvovirus (B19). *J Clin Invest*, **79**, 1486–1492.

Pryde PG, Nugent CE, Pridjian G *et al.* (1992) Spontaneous resolution of nonimmune hydrops fetalis secondary to human parvovirus B19 infection. *Obstet Gynecol*, **79**, 859–861.

Public Health Laboratory Service Working Party on Fifth Disease (1990) Prospective study of human parvovirus (B19) infection in pregnancy. *Br Med J*, **300**, 1166–1170.

Reid DM, Reid TM, Brown T *et al.* (1985) Human parvovirus-associated arthritis: a clinical and laboratory description. *Lancet*, **i**, 422–425.

Rodis JF, Quinn DL, Gary GW Jr *et al.* (1990) Management and outcomes of pregnancies complicated by human B19 parvovirus infection: a prospective study. *Am J Obstet Gynecol*, **163**, 1168–1171.

Rouger P, Gane P and Salmon C (1987) Tissue distribution of H, Lewis and P antigens as shown by a panel of 18 monoclonal antibodies. *Rev Franç Transfus Immunohématol*, **30**, 699–708.

Saikawa T, Anderson S, Momoeda M *et al.* (1993) Neutralizing linear epitopes of B19 parvovirus cluster in the VP1 unique and VP1–VP2 junction regions. *J Virol*, **67**, 3004–3009.

Saunders PW, Reid MM and Cohen BJ (1986) Human parvovirus induced cytopenias: a report of five cases [letter]. *Br J Haematol*, **63**, 407–410.

Schwarz TF, Gürtler LG, Zoulek G *et al.* (1989) Seroprevalence of human parvovirus B19 infection in Sao Tomé and Principe, Malawi and Mascarene Islands. *Int J Med Microbiol*, **271**, 231–236.

Serjeant BE, Hambleton IR, Kerr S *et al.* (2001) Haematological response to parvovirus B19 infection in homozygous sickle-cell disease. *Lancet*, **358**, 1779–1780.

Serjeant GR (1992) *Sickle Cell Disease*, 2nd edn, p 95. Oxford University Press, Oxford.

Serjeant GR, Serjeant BE, Thomas PE *et al.* (1993) Human parvovirus infection in homozygous sickle cell disease. *Lancet*, **341**, 1237–1240.

Serjeant GR, Topley JM, Mason K *et al.* (1981) Outbreak of aplastic crisis in sickle cell anaemia associated with parvovirus-like agent. *Lancet*, **ii**, 595–597.

Servant A, Laperche S, Lallemand F *et al.* (2002) Genetic diversity within human erythroviruses: identification of three genotypes. *J Virol*, **76**, 9124–9134.

Shade RO, Blundell MC, Cotmore SF *et al.* (1986) Nucleotide sequence and genome organization of human parvovirus B19 isolated from the serum of a child during aplastic crisis. *J Virol*, **58**, 921–936.

Sheikh AU, Ernest JM and O'Shea M (1992) Long-term outcome in fetal hydrops from parvovirus B19 infection. *Am J Obstet Gynecol*, **167**, 337–341.

Shimomura S, Wong S, Brown KE *et al.* (1993) Early and late gene expression in UT-7 cells infected with B19 parvovirus. *Virology*, **194**, 149–156.

Smith MA, Shah NS and Lobel JS (1989) Parvovirus B19 infection associated with reticulocytopenia and chronic autoimmune hemolytic anemia. *Am J Pediatr Hematol Oncol*, **11**, 167–169.

Soderlund M, von Essen R, Haapasaari J *et al.* (1997) Persistence of parvovirus B19 DNA in synovial membranes of young patients with and without chronic arthropathy. *Lancet*, **349**, 1063–1065.

Soderlund-Venermo M, Hokynar K, Nieminen J *et al.* (2002) Persistence of human parvovirus B19 in human tissues. *Pathol Biol*, **50**, 307–316.

Speyer I, Breedveld FC and Dijkmans BA (1998) Human parvovirus B19 infection is not followed by inflammatory joint disease during long-term follow-up. A retrospective study of 54 patients. *Clin Exp Rheumatol*, **16**, 576–578.

Srivastava A, Bruno E, Briddell R *et al.* (1990) Parvovirus B19-induced perturbation of human megakaryocytopoiesis *in vitro*. *Blood*, **76**, 1997–2004.

St Amand J and Astell CR (1993) Identification and characterization of a family of 11 kDa proteins encoded by the human parvovirus B19. *Virology*, **192**, 121–131.

Summers J, Jones SE and Anderson MJ (1983) Characterization of the genome of the agent erythocyte aplasia permits its classification as a human parvovirus. *J Gen Virol*, **64**, 2527–2532.

Takahashi M, Koike T, Moriyama Y and Shibata A (1991) Neutralizing activity of immunoglobulin preparation against erythropoietic suppression of human parvovirus [letter]. *Am J Hematol*, **37**, 68.

Takahashi T, Ozawa K, Takahashi K *et al.* (1990) Susceptibility of human erythropoietic cells to B19 parvovirus *in vitro* increases with differentiation. *Blood*, **75**, 603–610.

Takahashi Y, Murai C, Shibata S *et al.* (1998) Human parvovirus B19 as a causative agent for rheumatoid arthritis. *Proc Natl Acad Sci USA*, **95**, 8227–8232.

Tobiasch E, Rabreau M, Geletneky K *et al.* (1994) Detection of adeno-associated virus DNA in human genital tissue and in material from spontaneous abortion. *J Med Virol*, **44**, 215–222.

Török TJ (1997) Unusual clinical manifestations reported in patients with parvovirus B19 infection. In *Human Parvovirus B19*, vol 1 (eds Anderson LJ and Young NS), pp 61–92. Basel, Karger.

Umene K and Nunoue T (1990) The genome type of human parvovirus B19 strains isolated in Japan during 1981 differs from types detected in 1986 to 1987: a correlation between genome type and prevalence. *J Gen Virol*, **71**, 983–986.

van Elsacker-Niele AM and Anderson MJ (1987) First picture of erythema infectiosum? [letter]. *Lancet*, **i**, 229.

Wakamatsu C, Takakura F, Kojima E *et al.* (1999) Screening of blood donors for human parvovirus B19 and characterization of the results. *Vox Sanguis*, **76**, 14–21.

White DG, Woolf AD, Mortimer PP *et al.* (1985) Human parvovirus arthropathy. *Lancet*, **i**, 419–421.

Wierenga KJ, Serjeant BE and Serjeant GR (2001) Cerebrovascular complications and parvovirus infection in homozygous sickle cell disease. *J Pediatr*, **139**, 438–442.

Williams MD, Cohen BJ, Beddall AC *et al.* (1990) Transmission of human parvovirus B19 by coagulation factor concentrates. *Vox Sang*, **58**, 177–181.

Woolf AD (1990) Human parvovirus B19 and arthritis. *Behring Inst Mitt*, 64–68.

Woolf AD, Campion GV, Chishick A *et al.* (1989) Clinical manifestations of human parvovirus B19 in adults. *Arch Intern Med*, **149**, 1153–1156.

Yaegashi N, Niinuma T, Chisaka H *et al.* (1998) The incidence of, and factors leading to, parvovirus B19-related hydrops fetalis following maternal infection; report of 10 cases and meta-analysis. *J Infect*, **37**, 28–35.

Yaegashi N, Shiraishi H, Takeshita T *et al.* (1989) Propagation of human parvovirus B19 in primary culture of erythroid lineage cells derived from fetal liver. *J Virol*, **63**, 2422–2426.

Yoto Y, Kudoh T, Haseyama K *et al.* (1995) Incidence of human parvovirus B19 DNA detection in blood donors. *Br J Haematol*, **91**, 1017–1018.

Young N, Harrison M, Moore J *et al.* (1984) Direct demonstration of the human parvovirus in erythroid progenitor cells infected *in vitro*. *J Clin Invest*, **74**, 2024–2032.

Zadori Z, Szelei J, Lacoste MC *et al.* (2001) A viral phospholipase A2 is required for parvovirus infectivity. *Dev Cell*, **1**, 291–302.

Human Immunodeficiency Viruses

Robin A. Weiss[1], **Angus G. Dalgleish**[2], **Clive Loveday**[3] and **Deenan Pillay**[1]

[1]*University College London and* [2]*St George's Hospital Medical School, London, and* [3]*International Clinical Virology Centre, Great Missenden, UK*

INTRODUCTION TO HUMAN RETROVIRUSES

Retroviruses occur in numerous vertebrate species and are associated with a diversity of diseases. Studies of animals have shown that retroviruses cause a wide variety of neoplasms, many with human counterparts. Leukaemia and sarcomas in chickens were first identified as having a viral aetiology from 1908, and retroviruses were later found to be associated with malignant disease in mice, cats, primates and other hosts, including fish. Apart from malignancy, retroviruses are associated with autoimmune disease, immunodeficiency syndromes, aplastic and haemolytic anaemias, bone and joint disease (osteopetrosis and arthritis) and neuropathy (Table 25.1). A comprehensive text covers most aspects of the biology and molecular biology of animal and human retroviruses (Coffin *et al.*, 1997).

Retroviruses are a single taxonomic group of RNA viruses that encode RNA-directed DNA polymerase (reverse transcriptase, RT). Upon infection, this enzyme catalyses the synthesis of a double-stranded virion DNA. The provirus subsequently becomes integrated into host chromosomal DNA and serves as a template for viral genomic and messenger RNA transcription by the host cell's RNA synthetic and processing systems (Figure 25.1). Other special features of retroviruses include a diploid RNA genome, high frequency of intermolecular recombination between related viruses and the ability to acquire host genes which encode functions responsible for neoplastic transformation (oncogenes). There also exist endogenous proviruses in the normal cellular DNA of many vertebrates (including humans), which represent 'fossil' infections of the germline suggestive of prior infection of the human species by retroviruses, and which are passed from generation to generation in a Mendelian manner.

All retroviruses carry at least three genes in the order 5'-*gag–pol–env*-3'. *Gag* encodes a precursor protein which is cleaved to yield three or four structural core and matrix proteins; *pol* encodes the reverse transcriptase, protease and integrase, synthesised from a *gag–pol* precursor; and *env* encodes a precursor cleaved to form the two envelope proteins, surface protein (SU) and transmembrane (TM). The core proteins are often named by molecular weight (e.g. p24 and p17 of HIV). The outer surface protein is glycosylated and is known as gp120 (e.g. for HIV, with an approximate molecular weight of 120 000) or gp70 (e.g. γ-retroviruses). The

Table 25.1 Diseases caused by retroviruses in animals

Disease	Species affected
Leukaemia	Avian, mouse, cat, primates
Lymphoma	Avian, mouse, cat, primates, fish
Carcinoma	Mouse (mammary), chicken (renal)
Sarcoma	Rat, chicken, fish
Anaemia, aplasia	Cat, horse
Autoimmune disorders	Cat, primates, sheep, mouse
Immune deficiency	Cat, primates
Nervous system	Sheep, goat, mouse
Osteopetrosis	Chicken
Arthritis	Goat

SLE, systemic lupus erthematosus. A wide variety of diseases are caused by animal retroviruses with familiar human counterparts of unknown aetiology. The major associations are listed above.

Principles and Practice of Clinical Virology, Fifth Edition. Edited by A. J. Zuckerman, J. E. Banatvala, J. R. Pattison, P. D. Griffiths and B. D. Schoub
© 2004 John Wiley & Sons Ltd   ISBN 0 470 84338 1

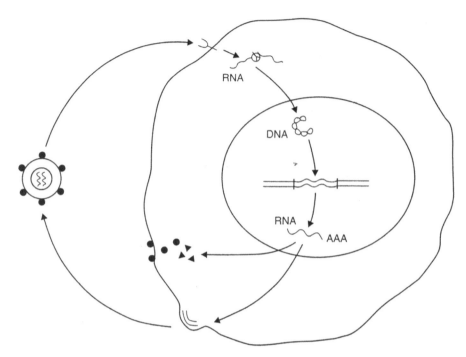

Figure 25.1 Simplified replication cycle of a retrovirus. The virion containing two RNA genome copies enters the virus via a specific cell surface receptor complex. The single-stranded RNA genome is converted into a double-stranded DNA provirus by the virion enzyme reverse transcriptase. The provirus inserts into host chromosomal DNA in the same orientation as the original virion RNA. Transcription of RNA from the integrated DNA provirus is mediated by cellular RNA polymerases, and this RNA serves both as messenger RNA for the synthesis of viral antigens and as genomic RNA, which becomes packaged into progeny virion budding from the cell surface

anchored transmembrane protein, to which the surface protein is bound, is glycosylated in some retroviruses (e.g. gp41 of HIV) but not others (e.g. p15E of gamma retroviruses). The DNA proviral genome is capped by long terminal repeats (LTRs) at both ends and the RNA form has a polyadenylate tract at the 3′ end like mRNA. The LTRs are responsible for integration of the DNA provirus with cellular DNA, and contain important promoter and enhancer sequences which bind cellular and viral proteins regulating viral gene expression.

CLASSIFICATION OF RETROVIRUSES

Retroviruses used to be taxonomically divided into three subfamilies: the *Oncovirinae*, which include those with oncogenic potential; the *Lentivirinae* or slow viruses, including HIV and the prototype Maedi–Visna virus (MVV) of sheep which causes progressive wasting disease, pneumonia and degeneration of the central nervous system; and the *Spumavirinae* or foamy

viruses, which have not been shown to be pathogenic. More recently, retroviruses of higher vertebrates have been reclassified into seven distinct genera by dividing oncoviruses into five, as they are only distantly related by genome sequence and morphology (Figure 25.2, Table 25.2). More generally, retroviruses are divided into those with 'simple' genomes, having *gag*, *pol* and *env* genes and perhaps one other, and those with 'complex' genomes. Members of the latter group possess regulatory genes, such as *tat* and *rev* of HIV and *tax* of HTLV, and accessory genes, such as *nef*, *vif* and *vpr* of HIV.

Four groups of retroviruses have been reported as human infections but only the first will be described in detail in this chapter:

1. *Human immunodeficiency virus types 1 and 2* (HIV-1 and HIV-2) are the lentiviruses that cause acquired immune deficiency syndrome (AIDS). Before the term 'HIV' was coined in 1986, HIV was called lymphadenopathy virus (LAV), HTLV-III or ARV. HIV and AIDS are the main topics of this chapter.

Table 25.2 Classification of retroviruses of vertebrates

Genus	Example	Virion morphology[a]	Genome
1. Alpha-retroviruses	*Rous sarcoma virus* *Avian leukosis virus*	Central spherical core; C-type	Simple
2. Beta-retroviruses	*Murine mammary tumour virus* *Simian retrovirus type I*	Eccentric spherical core; B-type Central spherical core; D-type	Simple
3. Gamma-retroviruses	*Murine leukaemia virus*	Central spherical core; C-type	Simple
4. Delta-retroviruses	*Human T cell leukaemia virus*	Central spherical core	Complex
5. Epsilon-retroviruses	*Fish dermal sarcoma virus*	Central spherical core; C-type	Simple
6. Lentiviruses	*Human immunodeficiency virus*	Cone-shaped core	Complex
7. Spumaviruses	*Primate foamy virus*	Central spherical core; pronounced envelope spikes	Complex

[a]Beta-retroviruses and spumaviruses have condensed cores visible in the cytoplasm of infected cells, whereas in the other retroviruses the cores condense as crescent-shaped bodies during maturation and budding at the cell membrane (see Figure 25.5).

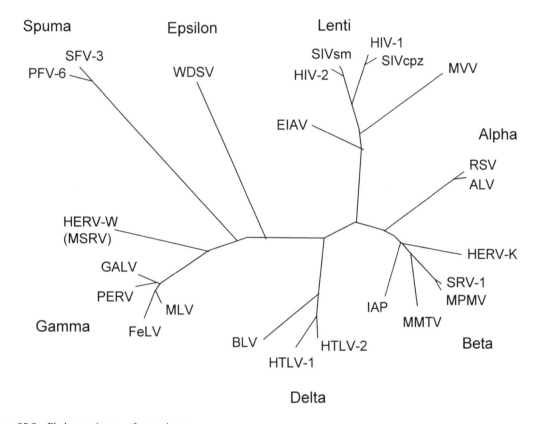

Figure 25.2 Phylogenetic tree of retroviruses

2. *Human T lymphotropic virus types 1 and 2* (HTLV-1 and HTLV-2) are deltaviruses. Type 1 causes adult T cell leukaemia and neurological disease. They are reviewed in Chapter 25A.

3. *Primate foamy virus* (PFV) is a spumavirus originally detected in cultured nasopharyngeal carcinoma of a Kenyan patient (Achong *et al.*, 1971). Because the PFV genome is indistinguishable from that of the simian foamy virus type 6 of chimpanzees, it may represent a zoonosis (Rosenblum and McClure, 1999). Serological studies indicate that spumaviruses are not endemic in human populations (Ali *et al.*, 1996), in contrast to many other primate species. Zoonotic SFV infection without

clinical symptoms has been recorded in primate handlers who have suffered bites or puncture wounds (Heneine *et al.*, 1998).

4. *Human endogenous retroviruses* (HERVs) are Mendelian loci in human chromosomes representing 'fossil' infections of the germline. These endogenous genomes derive from mammalian γ and β (HERV-K) retroviruses. No lentiviruses or spumaviruses are known to have become endogenous. HERV genomes are defective, i.e. human endogenous retroviral genomes have not been rescued in infectious form, in contrast to BaEV of baboons and PERV of pigs, which threaten the safety of human xenotransplantation from these sources (Weiss, 1998). Some HERV genomes, however, express envelope and other proteins, e.g. ERV-3 and HERV-W in the human placenta (Mi *et al.*, 2000; Venables *et al.*, 1995), HERV-K in testicular tumours and type 1 diabetes (Conrad *et al.*, 1997; Löwer *et al.*, 1996) and HERV-W (MSRV) in multiple sclerosis (Perron *et al.*, 1997). None of these viral genomes, however, has been unequivocally shown to play a causal role in disease. With the complete version of the human genome available in 2003, it has become apparent that approximately 8% of human DNA derives from fossil retroviruses.

HISTORY OF AIDS

The disease AIDS first came to the notice of physicians and epidemiologists in 1981 in the USA, when a handful of homosexual men in cities presented with *Pneumocystis carinii* pneumonia (PCP) and Kaposi's sarcoma (KS). These diseases were previously extraordinarily rare in young adults and indicated that some kind of immune deficiency was occurring in gay men. The first full case description already showed a selective depletion of CD4$^+$ T helper lymphocytes in the peripheral blood (Gottlieb *et al.*, 1981).

It was soon noted that a larger proportion of gay men suffered from generalised, extended lymphadenopathy. The disease was initially called gay-related immune deficiency (GRID). By early 1982, however, investigators at the Centers for Disease Control and Prevention in Atlanta, USA, detected similar cases of what we now call AIDS among injecting drug users, sex workers and recipients of blood transfusions and blood products, especially of pooled clotting factors administered for haemophilia. These epidemiological observations were familiar to those working with hepatitis B virus in the 1970s and led to the conclusion that AIDS was not simply a consequence of the gay lifestyle, but was caused by an infectious agent spreading both by sexual and by parenteral transmission. Similar signs and symptoms to AIDS in USA were recorded in Haiti, Europe and Africa.

Retrospective serological surveys indicated that HIV-1 began to spread among American gay men from 1977 onwards, showing a considerable incubation period before the manifestation of AIDS. The earliest known positive blood sample was collected in 1959 in Zaire (Zhu *et al.*, 1998). However, molecular clock analyses of diversity suggests a common origin for HIV-1 (Group M) dating from around 1931 (Korber *et al.*, 2000) and HIV-2 from around 1940 (Lemey *et al.*, 2003).

CLASSIFICATION OF HIV

HIV-1 was first isolated in 1983 (Barré-Sinoussi *et al.*, 1983), just 2 years after the identification of AIDS. Further HIV-1 isolates were reported in 1984 (Gallo *et al.*, 1984; Levy *et al.*, 1984; Vilmer *et al.*, 1984) which, together with serology (Cheingsong-Popov *et al.*, 1984), made a convincing case for HIV as the cause of AIDS. HIV-2 was first isolated in 1986 (Clavel *et al.*, 1986).

HIV-1 and HIV-2 represent two separate epidemics with distinct origins (Hahn *et al.*, 2000). HIV-1 probably started as a zoonosis from the chimpanzee, which harbours a related lentivirus, SIVcpz, whereas HIV-2 came from sooty mangabey monkeys in West Africa. HIV-1 is divided into three groups, the main group (M), the new group (N) and the outlier group (O). These groups may represent three separate zoonotic transfers from the chimpanzee. Groups N and O remain largely confined to a part of West Central Africa (Gabon and Cameroon), although sporadic infection through contact with persons from that region occur. Group M has radiated widely to cause the worldwide AIDS pandemic. The HIV-1 subtypes or clades lettered A–K all belong to group M. The genomic and antigenic variation manifested by HIV-1 groups and subtypes is important for diagnostic virology based on genomic and serological assays.

HIV-1 and HIV-2 strains can also be classified according to phenotype, which does not relate directly to their major genotypic classification. Thus, within each HIV-1 subtype there are virus isolates that are syncytium-inducing (SI) (Figure 25.3) or are non-syncytium-inducing (NSI) for CD4 cells *in vitro*. Most primary, transmitting HIV-1 strains have an NSI phenotype, while SI substrains tend to appear in

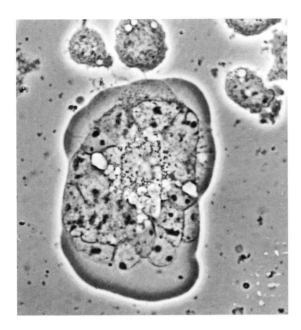

Figure 25.3 Phase-contrast micrograph of a giant syncytial cell formed 6 h after mixing, 10% HIV-1-producing H9 cells with 90% JM (Jurkat) indicator cells

Table 25.3 Global estimates of HIV infection and AIDS in adults and children (end of 2003)

People living with HIV/AIDS	Global	40.0 million
	Africa	29.4 million
	Adults	38.6 million
	Women	19.2 million
	Children	3.2 million
New HIV infections in 2003		5.0 million
Deaths due to HIV/AIDS in 2003		3.2 million
Total deaths from AIDS, 1982–2003		23.0 million
Children orphaned by AIDS		14.8 million

Data from UNAIDS (2002).

infected individuals later as they progress to AIDS. As described later, this phenotypic classification is related to cellular tropism for macrophages or T cell lines and to which kind of chemokine co-receptor the virus uses to gain entry into cells. Most NSI strains utilise the CCR5 co-receptor and are known as R5 viruses, whereas most SI strains utilise the CXCR4 co-receptor and are known as X4 viruses (Berger *et al.*, 1998).

EPIDEMIOLOGY

In the early stages of the AIDS epidemic, the main risk groups for HIV infection in Western countries were gay men practising anal sexual intercourse, men and boys with haemophilia who were exposed to contaminated clotting factors, recipients of blood transfusion, and intravenous injecting drug users. However, in Africa (where AIDS was originally recognised as 'slim' disease; Serwadda *et al.*, 1985) and when it spread to Asia, HIV has from the beginning been heterosexually transmitted, affecting men and women alike. With the rapid introduction of screening following the development of commercial antibody tests in 1985, HIV transmission through blood and blood products virtually disappeared, although this remains a problem in countries where screening is not stringent. 'Safe sex'

practices have also helped to reduce sexual transmission, and antiviral drug treatment has markedly reduced perinatal transmission from mother to child.

Nevertheless, HIV continues to spread, and 30% of new infections in developed countries and over 50% in developing countries affect women. In parts of the developing world HIV infection has been catastrophic. By the end of 2003, estimates of the global burden of HIV infection were close to 63 million cases, with 42 million living with HIV and over 23 million deaths since 1981 (UNAIDS, 2003), with an estimated 5.5 million new HIV infections and 3.2 million AIDS-related deaths in 2002 (Table 25.3 and Figure 25.4). In the UK, the epidemic has been slowly but steadily increasing over the last 5 years. This trend extrapolates to an estimate of over 49 000 people living with HIV/AIDS in the UK in 2004 and doubling by the end of the decade (Communicable Disease Surveillance Centre, 2002).

The greatest burden of AIDS falls on Africa (Figure 25.4), although there has also been rapid spread of HIV in India, the Far East, South America, Russia and Eastern Europe. Indeed, India has become the country with the second largest estimated number of infected individuals after South Africa. While HIV-1 infection first arose in Central Africa, the greatest recent increase is in southern Africa, with 30% or more young adults infected in South Africa, Botswana and Zimbabwe. There are large differences in HIV prevalence in different cities in Africa for reasons that are still not clear, although sexually transmitted diseases associated with genital ulceration, such as herpes simplex type 2 infection, and lack of male circumcision are risk factors; women become infected at younger ages than men (Auvert *et al.*, 2001).

Across the world, approximately 80% of new HIV infections among adults are heterosexually transmitted, the remainder being via homosexual transmission (6%), intravenous drug use (7%) and

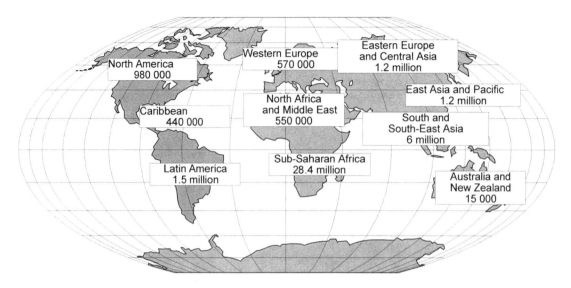

Figure 25.4 Distribution of adults and children (total 40 million) estimated to be living with HIV/AIDS at the end of 2003. Adapted from UNAIDS (2003)

other modes, including contaminated blood transfusions and contaminated hypodermic needles (7%). A recent suggestion that a higher proportion of HIV transmission results from non-sterile injection (Gisselquist *et al.*, 2003) is hotly contested (Schmid *et al.*, 2004; Walker *et al.*, 2003). In the UK, 28% of new HIV infection is homosexual, 51% heterosexual and 20% intravenous drug use. In recent years an increasing proportion has been heterosexual, with most infections caught abroad (Communicable Disease Surveillance Centre, 2004). However, this pattern may change again if a new generation of homosexuals disregard 'safe sex' practices.

Up to 10% of all HIV infection occurs in children, almost entirely among infants of infected mothers, so non-sterile injection is not a major route of transmission. Transmission is mainly perinatal, and maternal antiviral therapy shortly before birth greatly reduces transmission rates. Breast-feeding is also a significant route of HIV transmission, particularly during primary infection with high viraemia in the mother. Thus, a combination of maternal treatment, Caesarean section to reduce contact of the baby with maternal genital secretions and blood during birth, and abstinence from breast-feeding can virtually eliminate vertical transmission.

HIV-1 clades or subtypes differ in prevalence geographically. In Africa, subtypes A, C, D and F are frequent, whereas subtype B is the commonest subtype in the West. In Thailand, recombinant subtype A/E is most prevalent. In recent years various subtypes

have become more widely distributed and in the UK most subtypes currently occur (Parry *et al.*, 2001). Genetically recombinant viruses derived from more than one subtype (co-existing in the community) are becoming increasingly prevalent, and these are called circulating recombinant forms (CRFs).

HIV-2 has a lower transmission rate than HIV-1. In West Africa, where HIV-2 remains endemic, HIV-1 infection has now surpassed HIV-2 in incident infections. HIV-2 has spread elsewhere, including Europe and India. Mother-to-child transmission of HIV-2 is rare, perhaps owing to a generally lower plasma HIV-2 viral load.

VIROLOGY

HIV Culture and Isolation

HIV can be propagated in short-term cultures of CD4$^+$ peripheral blood mononuclear cells (PBMCs) stimulated by phytohaemagglutinin and interleukin 2 (IL-2). The SI strains can adapt to growth in immortal CD4$^+$ T cell lines, which become chronic virus producers. NSI strains, however, need to be propagated in PBMCs, where they are cytopathic, and in non-cytopathic macrophage culture. Virus isolation is useful for determining the phenotype of HIV strains, whether they are SI or NSI, and whether they have developed drug resistance, although genotyping is

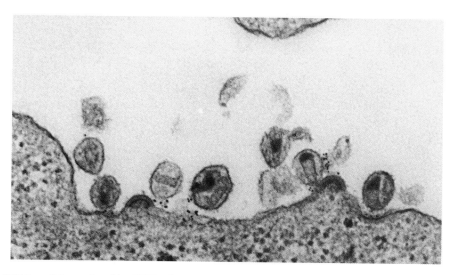

Figure 25.5   HIV-1 particles produced by CEM cells. Note the crescent-shaped core in budding particles and the condensed cone-like core in mature particles of approximately 100 nm diameter. The black spots are indirect immunogold labelling of antibody from an AIDS patient absorbed to the virus-producing cells

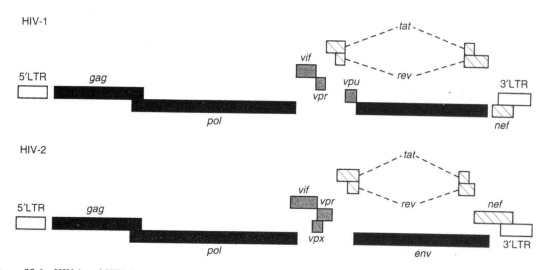

Figure 25.6   HIV-1 and HIV-2 genome maps

more rapid. Figure 25.5 shows HIV particles produced by the CEM T cell line in culture.

Isolation of HIV in cell culture can be detected by several means: (a) a cytopathic effect (CPE), including syncytia for SI strains (Figure 25.3); (b) detection of viral antigens in infected cells by antibodies, e.g. immunofluorescence, enzyme-linked immunocytology of infected cells, ELISA for p24 antigen in cells or in supernatant medium from infected cultures; (c) RT assay, either by enzyme activity or by ELISA; and (d) genome detection, using PCR or Southern blots.

HIV Genome and Proteins

Figure 25.6 shows the proviral genomes of HIV-1 and HIV-2. The gene maps are similar except that HIV-2 lacks *vpu* but carries *vpx*. The core and matrix proteins are encoded by *gag*. The Gag proteins of the mature virus are p17, p24, p7 and p6, and are processed by cleavage of the p55 precursor protein by the viral protease. The matrix antigen p17 is localised to the inner layer of the viral envelope and requires myristoylation, which allows it to be tightly bonded to the inner envelope; matrix antigen is indispensable for budding. The core shell is made of p24 capsid antigen. This is the viral protein most usually detected clinically as a measure of antigenaemia. The *pol* gene encodes the enzymes protease, reverse transcriptase and integrase. The *env* gene encodes the gp41 and gp120 envelope glycoproteins, cleaved by cellular enzymes (furins) from the gp160 precursor.

In addition to *gag*, *pol* and *env*, HIV-1 and HIV-2 carry seven regulatory and accessory genes (Emerman and Malim, 1998). The *tat* gene encodes a protein that binds to TAR RNA sequences in the 5' LTR to upregulate viral RNA transcription through complexes of cellular transcription factors and cyclin T; *rev* serves to aid export of long HIV transcripts from nucleus to cytoplasm through recognition of Rev-response elements (RREs) in unspliced or singly-spliced viral mRNA; *nef* has multiple functions in signal transduction and downmodulation of CD4 cell surface expression; *vpr* allows transport of newly infected pre-integration complexes of the HIV proviral DNA into the nucleus for integration (by integrase) into host chromosomal DNA; *vpr* also arrests cells in the G_2 phase of the mitotic cycle, enhancing virus production; *vpu* has poorly understood functions; *vif* is incorporated into virus particles and helps infection in new target cells by abrogating restriction exerted by host APOBECG3 (Sheehy *et al.*, 2003). Although SI strains of HIV-1 can be propagated in T cell lines with deletions or non-functional mutations in *nef*, *vpu* or *vif*, such mutations adversely affect HIV replication in PBMCs and macrophages, so that attenuated infection or no replication occurs. Thus, all the viral genes are required for efficient infection and pathogenesis *in vivo* (Stevenson, 2003).

HIV Serology

The major diagnostic method for determining whether a person is infected by HIV is a serological assay for specific anti-HIV antibodies. A number of ELISA assays are commercially available which are sensitive and specific (having extremely low false negative or false positive rates), and which are relatively inexpensive. Most of these assays are based on detection of antibodies bound to HIV antigens in ELISA plates and detected with enzyme-linked antiglobulin. The antigen in modern assays is generally a mixture of recombinant viral proteins, including envelope (gp41) and core (p24) antigens, or including synthetic peptides based on immunodominant epitopes. Some ELISA assays

have a competitive format, i.e. the antibody in the serum sample to be tested needs to displace an enzyme-labelled standard antibody in the test kit to score a positive result. Microparticle agglutination assays bearing crude inactivated HIV antigens are also useful. Strategies for clinical testing are discussed later.

For mass screening of sera, as in blood banks, combined tests for HIV-1, HIV-2 and sometimes other viruses are used. Differential HIV-1 and HIV-2 tests can then distinguish between the two types of HIV. Antibodies to the various subtypes of HIV-1 are detected in screening assays with different sensitivities, although current commercial assays detect all subtypes of HIV-1 group M and also the outlier group O, prevalent in Cameroon and Gabon. Group N has not been rigorously tested in commercial kits because few humans, confined so far to West Central Africa, are infected with group N viruses.

Neutralising antibodies can be measured by reduction of infectious titre of HIV in cell culture assays. Such assays are not useful for screening or diagnosis but are important for testing HIV candidate vaccines and in monitoring progression to AIDS. Immunofluorescence assays are no longer used for diagnostic purposes.

Differential assays for antibodies in sera to specific HIV antigens are generally performed by Western blot on antigens prepared from whole virions, infected cultures or recombinant viral proteins on nitrocellulose strips. In the early days of HIV diagnosis, Western blots were considered important as confirmatory to ELISA tests. They still have a place for sera yielding indeterminate results, especially at the beginning of seroconversion during primary infection, although genome detection using PCR is now preferred for such cases.

HIV Load and Resistance

Detection of viraemia was originally performed by tests for p24 antigen in plasma (antigenaemia) and more recently by detection of viral genomes. Molecular techniques for detecting HIV, quantifying viral load and typing for drug resistance have become a significant part of patient diagnosis and clinical management. Measurement of proviral DNA is of importance in detecting early HIV infection before seroconversion (although p24 antigaemia is also convenient). Measurement of plasma viral load and resistance markers are important for antiviral treatment.

The detection of viraemia through the measurement of viral genomes is performed for HIV-1 and HIV-2 by extracting RNA from virions, preparing complementary DNA and PCR amplification of the cDNA product (RT-PCR) (Berry and Tedder, 1999; Semple et al., 1993). These processes can be combined and performed with commercial kits. Alternatives to PCR, such as branched DNA (bDNA) and nucleic acid-sequence based amplification (NASBA) systems are also available. Quantification of viral load can be measured by serial dilution of the sample against a known standard, by competitive PCR, or by real-time kinetic methods of detecting amplified product.

While the sensitivity of HIV genome detection for the major HIV subtypes is well established, detection of HIV-2 viral load, and detection of minor HIV-1 groups such as groups O and N, requires further development (Berry and Tedder, 1999). The principal method of determining HIV infection by a molecular technique is the detection of proviral DNA in peripheral blood cells or other tissues. PCR amplification of proviral DNA, like RT-PCR of virions in plasma, is a sensitive technique, provided that inhibitors of the amplifying enzymes are not present in the sample. The great sensitivity of PCR amplification for any diagnostic target means that there is a danger of obtaining false positive results unless scrupulous care is taken to prevent contamination of the sample. Modern diagnostic kits incorporate high containment for the sample but the specimen must also be handled properly from the point of venepuncture or biopsy.

With the increasing use of antiretroviral therapy and the emergence of drug-resistant HIV strains and substrains, diagnostic methods are required to monitor resistance in managing HIV-infected patients and deciding upon optimal therapy. For the current drugs targeting RT and protease, certain mutations which are associated with a high frequency of drug resistance occur in the pol gene. These can either be detected phenotypically by testing drug sensitivity of HIV isolates in culture or, in a much more rapid and less laborious test, by genotypic detection of mutations associated with drug resistance, by PCR or other genomic amplification (see later).

PATHOGENESIS OF HIV INFECTION

HIV Dynamics

Primary HIV infection entails symptomatic fever and lymphadenopathy in about 50% of infections. Following seroconversion, there follows an asymptomatic phase of infection lasting 2–15 years (Figure 25.7). Virologically, however, this does not represent latent infection but rather a high turnover of HIV production (up to 10^{10} infectious particles/day) and of infected lymphocytes (about 10^8–10^9 cells/day) with equally active replenishment (Ho et al., 1995; Wei et al., 1995). Thus, it is remarkable that the overall CD4 T lymphocyte count does not decline much faster (McCune, 2001; Perelson, 2002). Generally, a high HIV load in the plasma after seroconversion is predictive of faster progression to AIDS (Mellors et al., 1996) and is known as the viral 'set point'. Lymphoid tissue is actively infected by HIV throughout the asymptomatic period (Stevenson, 2003).

The constant, high production of virus was discovered through measurement of the perturbation of viral dynamics by antiviral drug treatment (Ho, 1995; Wei et al., 1995). It helps to explain the extraordinary rate of evolution of HIV, both within one infected individual and throughout the human population, because the virus undergoes so many replication cycles, and the RT does not recognise or repair mutations. There are, however, reservoirs of stable, integrated provirus in non-proliferating memory T lymphocytes and in macrophages. These can re-supply active HIV replication when antiviral therapy ceases. Many infected cells contain more than one provirus (Jung et al., 2002), which may lead to recombinant progeny. While the high turnover of virus provides an opportunity for intervention via antiviral therapy, it also provides opportunities for selection for drug resistance, immune escape and new cell tropisms to evolve.

HIV-infected lymphocytes may be depleted in several ways (Letvin and Walker, 2003; Pope and Haase, 2003): (a) by a direct cytopathic effect of HIV, including cell fusion by SI strains; (b) by cytotoxic T lymphocytes recognising specific HIV antigenic peptides presented on MHC antigens, leading to immune destruction; and (c) by apoptosis, due to lymphocyte activation and a changed cytokine and chemokine milieu.

Although apoptosis correlates with disease progression, it is largely a late measure of activation of the affected cells. Studies on apoptosis in human rapid progressors, non-progressors and chimpanzees revealed the extraordinary association between apoptosis, non-specific activation of the immune system and progression to disease. Indeed, the most important correlates of disease progression after the virus load and CD4 count are the activation markers, and in this regard the soluble tumour necrosis factor (TNF) receptor is as accurate at predicting disease prognosis

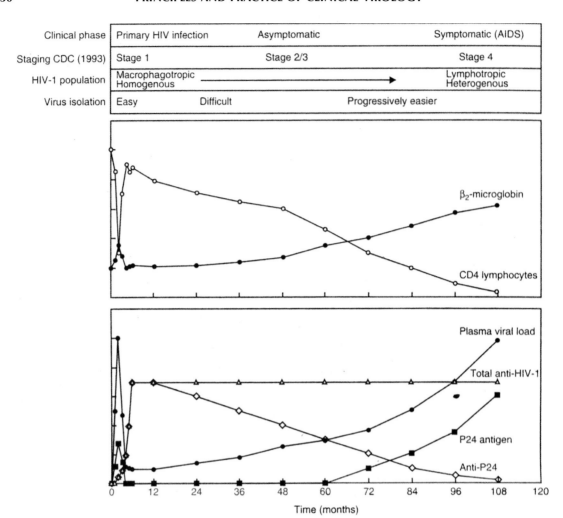

Figure 25.7 The clinical, virological and immunological phases of HIV/AIDS. The clinical phases of the disease have been staged by the Centers for Disease Control (1985, 1993) to define primary HIV infection (PHI, CDC stage 1), asymptomatic (CDC stages 2/3) and symptomatic (CDC stage 4). Viruses are easy to isolate during PHI and are generally a relatively homogenous population of macrophagotropic viruses. During the asymptomatic phase of disease viruses evolve into a heterogenous population but are difficult to isolate; this becomes progressively easier as a population of lymphotropic viruses predominate in the host in symptomatic disease. CD4 lymphocyte counts (○) show distinctive changes during disease, with a rapid, short-term decline associated with the viraemia in PHI, a recovery to near-normal levels, a gradual loss of cells during the asymptomatic phase, and finally an accelerated decline associated with late symptomatic disease. The reciprocal of these changes is shown by β_2-microglobulin (●, top panel), a plasma measure of immune activation. Plasma viral load (●) reaches a peak in PHI (mirrored by p24 antigen, ■), declines to a 'set point' during early asymptomatic disease, and then gradually increases after about 24 months of infection at 0.1–0.2 $\log_{10}$ copies/ml per year. In symptomatic disease viral load and p24 antigen increase progressively. Both viral load and CD4 cell counts in early asymptomatic disease are highly predictive of disease progression. Anti-HIV-1 antibodies (△) increase to a maximum within 3–6 months of infection and remain detectable throughout the natural course of disease. However, subpopulations of antibodies (i.e. anti-p24 antibodies, ◇) may decline in association with, and predict, disease progression. With the introduction of potent antiretroviral therapy and persistently long-term undetectable plasma virus (<50 copies/ml), the antigenic stimulus for the immune system is diminished and quantitative declines in plasma anti-HIV-1 antibodies are observed. This model of the natural history of the disease has been shown in practice to exhibit, in a minority of patients, an accelerated course where viral load remains relatively high or rises, p24 antigen remains detectable. CD4 cell counts decline rapidly and patients progress clinically in <5 years (rapid progressors), or a protracted course where the CD4 cell counts remain in the normal range and viral load low or undetectable with asymptomatic disease for >15 years (long-term non-progressors). These differences probably represent the limits of a normal distribution

as is the virus load at the time of infection. There are clear but not absolute correlates between the rate of progression to disease and the immunogenetic background of the host (Carrington and O'Brien, 2003), e.g. patients with HLA-1 B8 DR3 are unusually rapid progressors to disease, whereas in HIV-1 infected Caucasians, patients with HLA B27 are slow or non-progressors to disease.

Chronic activation and progression to disease dependent on the HLA background is seen with viruses that encode superantigens. Initial reports that HIV did so have not been confirmed and, although superantigen activity with regards to B cell epitopes have been reported, it is not thought to be sufficient to drive the panactivation seen throughout the immune system in HIV-infected patients progressing to AIDS (Westby et al., 1996). This panactivation is similar to that seen in chronic HLA mismatched transplantation, which leads to chronic graft-vs.-host disease, and it is notable that HIV incorporates many HLA molecules into its envelope. This property may enhance infectivity in vivo and could be one mechanism of activating the immune system resulting in enhancement of infection (Letvin and Walker, 2003; Westby et al., 1996). It is notable that sooty mangabey monkeys naturally infected with SIVsm have a high virus load without immune activation, and remain healthy (Silvestri et al., 2003).

Cell Tropism and HIV Receptors

HIV infects mainly CD4$^+$ cells by binding to CD4 as a receptor (Dalgleish et al., 1984). However, many of these cells are not lymphocytes, e.g. monocytes, macrophages, dendritic cells (Langerhans cells) and some brain cells, such as the microglia, express the CD4 receptor, and many are susceptible to infection by HIV. It is likely that infection of these cell types plays a major role in the pathogenesis of disease (Stevenson, 2003; Weiss, 2003). Importantly, HIV particles bind to the DC-SIGN receptor on dendritic cells without infecting them, and hence may be delivered to CD4 lymphocytes in the lymph node (Geijtenbeek et al., 2000; Pope and Haase, 2003).

The CD4 cell surface antigen is necessary but not sufficient for HIV-1 infection (Dalgleish et al., 1984; Maddon et al., 1986). While CD4 is required for high affinity binding of gp120, co-receptors are required for subsequent steps leading to fusion between the viral envelope and cell membrane. The co-receptors were identified in 1996 to be chemokine receptors and help to explain the differential tropism for lymphocytes and macrophages (Berger et al., 1999; Moore et al., 2004). Primary, NSI strains of HIV mainly utilise CCR5 (R5 strains), which is the receptor for the chemokines MIP-1α, MIP-1β and RANTES, whereas SI strains utilise CXCR4 (X4 strains), the receptor for stromal derived factor 1 (SDF-1). The discovery that chemokine receptors act as co-receptors to CD4 (Feng et al., 1996) helped to explain why these chemokines can inhibit HIV-1 infection in vitro (Cocchi et al., 1995). Modified chemokines and small molecular receptor blockers can potently inhibit HIV-1 entry and may have promise in therapy (Baba et al., 1999; Simmons et al., 1996).

The importance of the CCR5 co-receptor for NSI viruses in HIV transmission and disease progression is borne out in people with mutations in the gene for this receptor. In Caucasian populations a deletion in CCR5, rendering it non-functional, occurs frequently; people homozygous for this 'delta 32' mutation are resistant to infection by R5 strains of HIV-1, even when exposed, e.g. by regular sexual contact with an HIV carrier (O'Brien and Moore, 2000). Mutations in the promoter region of CCR5, which lower the level of CCR5 expression, delay progression to AIDS in infected individuals (An et al., 2000; Carrington and O'Brien, 2003; Kostrikis et al., 1998).

Several host factors that constrain HIV replication after virus entry but before provirus integration have also recently been discovered. A human protein, APOBECG3, that blocks HIV-1 infection, is suppressed by the viral Vif protein (Sheehy et al., 2003). A different kind of suppression mediated by Lv1 also acts at an early step in the HIV replication cycle and differentially affects HIV-1, HIV-2 and various strains of SIV (Hatziioannou et al., 2003). Another type of early restriction has been observed for HIV-2 (McKnight et al., 2001).

Sequence analysis indicates that HIV in different organs and cell types may represent different subpopulations in the various compartments of the body (Atkins et al., 1998). Thus, the dominant HIV substrains in the blood and cerebrospinal fluid (CSF) and, within the blood, between CD4$^+$ cells and in CD8$^+$ cells may differ in late stage AIDS (Livingstone et al., 1996). Whereas the depletion of CD4$^+$ cells accounts for the profound immune deficiency, and falling CD4 cell counts are a useful marker of disease progression, the wasting disease and central nervous system (CNS) disease (AIDS dementia) are probably more closely related to macrophage infection. This includes the microglial cells of the brain, which are derived from monocytes rather than neurectoderm. Astrocytes may also become latently infected, with

Table 25.4 AIDS-defining illnesses in HIV infection (defined by Centers for Disease Control in 1985, revised 1993)

Infections	Neoplasms
Pneumocysis carinii pneumonia	Kaposi's sarcoma
Cytomegalovirus (non-RE system)	Primary lymphoma (brain)
	Non-Hodgkin's lymphoma
Candidiasis (excluding oral)	Invasive cervical cancer[a]
Cryptococcosis (extrapulmonary)	
Mycobacterium avium (disseminated)	
M. kansasii (disseminated)	
M. tuberculosis (disseminated)	
M. tuberculosis (pulmonary)[a]	
Herpes simplex (>1 month, or non-orogenital)	
Cryptosporidiosis (>1 month)	
Histoplasmosis (extra pulmonary)	
Toxoplasmosis	
Nocardiosis	
Recurrent disseminated salmonella	
Strongyloidosis (non-intestinal)	
Recurrent bacterial pneumonia[a]	
Coccidioidomycosis (extrapulmonary)	
Isosporosis (>1 month)	
Primary HIV-1 dementia	
Primary HIV-1 wasting disease	

[a]Added in revisions of 1993.

Table 25.5 Centers for Disease Control (CDC): classification of the effects of HIV-1 infection (CDC, 1985, 1993)

CDC1		Acute infection with seroconversion (PHI)
CDC2		Asymptomatic infection
CDC3		Persistent generalised lymphadenopathy
CDC4	a	Constitutional disease
	b	Neurological disease
	c	Immunodeficiency
		ci CDC definitions of AIDS
		cii Infections without definition
	d	Tumours with CDC definition
	c	Others, e.g. carcinomas, interstitial pneumonia

changes to local cytokine secretion in the brain leading to neuronal loss.

HIV AND AIDS: CLINICAL DISEASE AND MANAGEMENT

HIV infection is characterised by an initial acute viral illness followed by a chronic, asymptomatic phase of disease associated with active viral replication and dissemination, and lasting as long as 5–10 years. Ultimately, immune destruction results in end-stage disease (AIDS) associated with opportunistic infections, malignancies and neurological disorders. These clinical events correlate with virological and immunological changes and are shown in Figure 25.7.

Early classification of the disease by the Centers for Disease Control and Prevention, Atlanta, USA, defined an asymptomatic phase followed by a list of symptomatic conditions that defined AIDS (Table 25.4). This was later revised to reflect the effects of HIV/AIDS infection on clinical status (Table 25.5). In 1993 it was expanded to take account of additional respiratory diseases and recently discovered malignancies, and Table 25.6 outlines the classification most widely used to define entry into contemporary clinical trials. The classification of paediatric HIV infection evolved independently to reflect the unique features of the disease in this patient group (Table 25.7).

Early Infection

Primary HIV infection (PHI) results in a well-recognised constellation of clinical, virological and immunological responses associated with rapid and widespread dissemination of virus following infection. An initial illness occurs in 50–90% of cases, is classically described as mononucleosis-like, although in practice <20% have these features. A typical presentation, in order of frequency, may include:

Table 25.6 Centers for Disease Control (CDC) AIDS surveillance case definition (CDC, 1993)

CD4 counts (× 10^6/l)	Clinical group		
	A: asymptomatic PGL or PHI	B: symptomatic but not A or C[b]	C: AIDS conditions[a]
>500	A1	B1	C1
200–500	A2	B2	C2
<200	A3	B3	C3

PGL, persistent generalised lymphadenopathy; PHI, primary HIV infection.
[a]Patients in groups C1, C2, C3, and A3 and B3 are reported as AIDS according to Table 25.4 and/or having a CD4 count below 200×10^6/l.
[b]Symptomatic but not included in C are those conditions associated with defective immunity.

Table 25.7 Centers for Disease Control (CDC) clinical categories for children with HIV-1 infection (CDC, 1994)

Category	Clinical stage	Features
N	Asymptomatic	HIV-infected but with no signs or symptoms
A	Mildly symptomatic	Children with two or more of the following conditions but none in B or C: Lymphadenopathy Hepatomegaly/splenomegaly Dermatitis Parotitis Persistent urinary tract infections
B	Moderately symptomatic	Children with conditions other than those in A or C including: Anaemia Persistent fever (>1 month) Cytomegalovirus (onset <1 month of age) Herpes simplex stomatitis (recurrent <year) Herpes simplex bronchitis/oesophagitis Disseminated varicella Hepatitis Bacterial meningitis, pneumonia or sepsis Toxoplasmosis (<1 month) Candidiasis, persistent oral after 6 months age Nocardiosis Diarrhoea, chronic Cardiomyopathy or nephropathy
C	Severely symptomatic	Cytomegalovirus (onset >1 month) Herpes simplex oral/internal >1 month Kaposi's sarcoma Candidiasis, oesophageal/pulmonary Coccidioidomycosis (disseminated) Cryptococcosis (extrapulmonary) Cryptosporidiosis (symptoms >1 month) Histoplasmosis (disseminated) *Mycobacterium tuberculosis* (disseminated) *Mycobacterium avium* or *M. kansasii* *Pneumocystis carinii* pneumonia *Salmonella* septicaemia Toxoplasmosis (CNS, <1 month age) Recurrent serious bacterial infections Encephalopathy (developmental delays) Progressive multifocal leukoencephalopathy Wasting syndrome (developmental delays)

acute onset of fever, lethargy, maculopapular rash, myalgia, headache, sore throat, cervical lymphadenopathy, arthralgia, oral ulcers, photophobia, oral candida and, rarely, meningoencephalitis. The time from exposure to onset of signs and symptoms is approximately 10–30 days.

Lymphadenopathy is a frequent event during PHI, usually in the second week of illness and is often associated with a lymphocytosis. The lymph nodes tend to decrease in size with time. The architecture remains relatively normal but HIV can be visualised in association with both lymphocytes and dendritic cells. A distinctive feature of PHI is mucocutaneous disease involving the buccal mucosa, gingiva, palate, oesophagus, anus and penis.

The commonest neurological feature is an aseptic meningoencephalitis reflecting the neurotropism associated with this group of viruses. Less frequently, myelopathy, peripheral neuropathy, facial palsy and Guillain–Barré syndrome are seen. They are usually self-limiting. HIV has been detected in the CSF soon after infection, indicating the speed at which the virus penetrates the blood–brain barrier. Marked changes in the lymphocyte count are seen. The CD4:CD8 ratio is reversed, largely due to an increase in the number of CD8 cells. An early CD4 lymphopenia is characteristic of PHI; it is associated with very high plasma viral load levels (in excess of 10^{11} copies/l) that occur in early disease prior to immunomodulation. The mechanism of this CD4 lymphopenia is explained by a 'predator–

prey model', with HIV-1 undergoing multiple rounds of replication and 'consuming' available target cells (Perelson, 2002). It is generally short-lived, but on occasions precipitous early lymphopenia does occur and is thought to be one of the aetiological factors associated with acute *Pneumocyctis carinii* pneumonia, oral and oesophageal candida and mucocutaneous ulceration. By 6 months after infection, a plasma viral load 'set point' has been reached.

The symptomatic phase of PHI lasts less than 14 days on average and is self-limiting; however, it is now clearly evident that protracted and wide-ranging symptoms, oral and/or oesophageal candida, neurological involvement, and persistently high plasma viral loads are associated with rapid disease progression. The differential diagnosis of PHI should include: Epstein–Barr virus, cytomegalovirus, herpes simplex, rubella and other acute viral infections; in addition, syphilis, disseminated gonorrhoea, toxoplasmosis and drug reactions should also be considered.

The timing of initiation of therapy in primary infection is controversial. Some investigators have demonstrated that short-term therapy at this time may preserve immune responses, with associated lower levels of proviral DNA and plasma HIV-1 RNA suppression (Kinloch *et al.*, 2003). However, others are more concerned over drug-related reduction in quality of life, with accumulation of adverse events, earlier emergence of resistance and limited future antiretroviral options. Pragmatically, the most important role of therapy at this stage is probably to limit symptoms in a severe seroconversion illness.

The Asymptomatic Phase

The period after PHI and prior to symptomatic disease has been described as the latent or asymptomatic phase. Although it is a clinically latent period, the notion of virological latency is misleading, as virus persistence and active replication and cell turnover clearly occurs throughout the lymphoreticular and other tissues (Perelson, 2002), and continual monitoring of viral load and CD4 cell counts are required. Since these individuals are infectious, advice on sexual health is required. A detailed review of the numerous factors which affect viral latency and persistence is beyond the scope of this chapter (Letvin and Walker, 2003; Levy, 1998; Stevenson, 2003). The duration of the asymptomatic phase may be variable and is related to the severity of PHI, the phenotypic characteristics of the infecting viruses, the status of the host immunity,

the lifestyle of the host and the use of antiretroviral therapies.

Clinically, patients are relatively free of symptoms, although lymphadenopathy may be a complaint in some cases. Patients are offered a clinical review every 3 months and regular plasma viral loads and CD4 lymphocyte counts are used to monitor disease status. Plasma viral loads measured 6–12 months after PHI have been shown to be a powerful predictor of subsequent disease progression (Mellors *et al.*, 1996), superseding CD4 lymphocyte counts taken at the same time; in combination, the two values are the most accurate method for determination of patient prognosis (Loveday and Hill, 1995; Mellors *et al.*, 1996). This phase of clinical care is often supportive, involves surveillance of patients for features of early progression and for the optimum time to commence antiretroviral therapy.

Symptomatic Disease and AIDS

In untreated patients, early features of symptomatic disease were often non-specific and associated with dermatological manifestations, such as eczema and human papillomavirus eruptions, as well as oral and vaginal candidiasis, recurrent chest infections, night sweats, weight loss and the appearance of lymphadenopathy. Oral lesions become more common with gingivitis, candida, herpes simplex eruptions and aphthous ulcers. 'Oral hairy leukoplakia' presents as white, ribbed lesions on the lateral margins of the tongue; it may be asymptomatic or produce soreness within the mouth. It is associated with Epstein–Barr virus infection and may respond to aciclovir therapy. All these features are far less frequent in the era of combined antiretroviral therapy. The progressive immune deficiency associated with long-term HIV/AIDS infection results in the opportunistic infections and malignancies that characterise AIDS, which are often multiple and contribute to the rapid clinical deterioration in patients.

Opportunistic Infections

Opportunistic infections seen in symptomatic HIV-1 disease (Tables 25.4 and 25.7) reflect adult and childhood exposure; hence, fungal infections such as histoplasmosis may be seen in persons who come from areas where the organisms are endemic. Infectious agents may be categorised into: (a) those that do not cause disease in the immunocompetent host, e.g.

Pneumocystis carinii; (b) those that cause mild disease in the normal host, e.g. herpes simplex virus (HSV), *Toxoplasma gondii*; (c) those that are conventional pathogens, e.g. *Mycobacterium tuberculosis*, but, as a consequence of immunosuppression associated with HIV-1 infection, produce widespread debilitating disease in the host.

Overall, the presenting features of symptomatic HIV disease may be quite distinct, according to the geographical areas in which the hosts are found, e.g. *Pneumocystis carinii* pneumonia and Kaposi's sarcoma are the commonest presenting diseases in the UK, whereas *Mycobacterium tuberculosis* and gastrointestinal infections are more frequent in Central Africa.

Pneumocystis carinii pneumonia differs from the disease seen in other groups with non-HIV-associated immunosuppression, in being characterised by subacute onset, involving a mild, persistent cough and progressive chest discomfort and fatigue of 2–10 weeks duration. It is rare when CD4 cell counts are above $200 \times 10^6/l$. Subtle bilateral infiltrations with a batwing appearance may be seen on a chest radiograph but 50% of cases are normal at presentation. Minimal hypoxia is present and diagnosis is made by detection of the pneumocystis organism in induced sputum or bronchoalveolar lavage. It is treated with co-trimoxazole or pentamidine, and the introduction of prophylaxis in patients with CD4 cell counts $< 200 \times 10^6/l$ has markedly reduced the incidence of this infection in HIV/AIDS, as have antiretroviral drugs.

Cytomegalovirus is the commonest cause of progressive chorioretinitis in AIDS. The lesions are initially asymptomatic but, as the perivascular exudates and haemorrhages involve the macula, vision becomes impaired. Interestingly, CMV pneumonitis is rare in AIDS patients because it requires active recruitment of the immune system to cause disease. In contrast, CMV retinitis is common in untreated AIDS patients, as it is an uncontained cytopathic disease not requiring immunocompetence. In addition, gastrointestinal ulceration, adrenalitis and encephalitis may occur. Progression of CMV infection can be restricted by parenteral ganciclovir or foscarnet, and the institution of antiretroviral therapies has reduced the incidence and/or severity of CMV.

Cryptococcus neoformans also causes a diffuse pneumonitis, although more commonly it causes meningitis and is widely disseminated. It may also present with fever, granulocytopenia, thrombocytopenic purpura, maculopapular rashes and ulcerating gastrointestinal lesions. It may be isolated from many sites, including throat washings, urine or blood. It is treated with fluconazole or amphotericin B.

Toxoplasma gondii causes space-occupying lesions in the CNS and is treated with combinations of antimicrobials. These patients present with fever and focal neurological signs and may have associated chorioretinitis. Serological tests for *Toxoplasma* are unreliable, and demonstration of the organism in the affected tissues by PCR may offer a more definitive diagnosis. The differential diagnosis of cerebral lymphoma may be excluded using a highly sensitive and specific PCR for Epstein–Barr virus.

Other CNS-related conditions include progressive multifocal leukoencephalopathy (PML), a condition associated with JC virus, producing oligodendritic lysis. It is diagnosed by characteristic histological changes and confirmed if possible by PCR for JC virus. No specific treatment is available. In addition, other viral encephalites (including herpes simplex) and bacterial infections are often implicated in AIDS. Overall, the use of combined antiretroviral therapy has had a dramatic impact on the frequency and severity of such conditions. Progressive HIV-associated encephalopathy involves inflammatory changes in white and grey matter and is characterised by foci of inflammatory cells, including microglia, macrophages and multinucleate giant cells with actively replicating HIV-1.

Mycobacterium avium and *M. intracellulare* (MAI) are two closely related species of ubiquitous environmental organisms which in the past had rarely been shown to cause disseminated disease. However, MAI is common in patients with symptomatic HIV infection, the bacteria being ingested or inhaled. MAI produces disseminated disease with non-specific symptoms, including fatigue, fever, night sweats, weight loss, abdominal pain and diarrhoea, in patients with $< 50 \times 10^6/l$ CD4 lymphocytes. It is diagnosed by positive blood cultures using Lowenstein–Jensen solid medium (3–4 weeks) or a non-speciating broth medium (1–2 weeks), and confirmation by PCR, in 90% of cases. Treatment and prophylaxis is with specific antituberculous combination therapy. With the advent of highly active antiretroviral therapy (HAART), these therapies need not be lifelong. Both this condition and the more classical *M. tuberculosis* have become increasingly common in HIV-infected patients in the developed as well as the developing world, and antimicrobial-resistant organisms are evident in this new tuberculosis epidemic.

Oral candidiasis is commonly seen, and oesophageal involvement may be present with dysphagia, odynophagia and retrosternal burning. Diagnosis is based on clinical findings and simple histology. Treatment is by topical antifungal agents or intravenous therapy in the event of refractory and severe disease. Other fungal infections, such as *Aspergillus*, can produce life-threatening respiratory disease, with white plaque-like colonies in the bronchi, and cavitation. Infection is diagnosed by culture and treated with itraconazole or amphotericin B; without immune restoration following antiretroviral therapy the outcome is poor, and time from diagnosis to death is short (months).

Herpes simplex virus (HSV2 > HSV1) infection commonly presents as a vesicular lesion on an erythematous base in oral, genital or perianal areas. Attacks are usually more widespread and of longer duration, with more frequent recurrences in HIV-1 infection; the lesions are associated with secondary bacterial infection and have been associated with widespread epidermal erosion, in some cases requiring skin grafts. Oesophageal and tracheobronchial involvement is described. Diagnosis is by virus culture and/ or PCR; treatment is with aggressive use of oral or intravenous aciclovir therapy, depending on the severity of the condition.

Reactivation of varicella zoster virus is common in HIV-infected patients but is less often seen in advanced symptomatic disease. Ophthalmic zoster may threaten vision, and any dermatomal presentation may become disseminated. Treatment is with high-dose aciclovir, antibiotics for secondary infection and analgesia.

Human papillomavirus (HPV-6 and -11)-induced warts and molluscum contagiosum (*Poxvirus*) are both common skin conditions in up to 25% of patients with HIV infection and may be of abnormal presentation and persistent.

Persistent or recurrent diarrhoea, which may be copious in volume and watery in content, is a frequent problem in symptomatic patients. *Giardia lamblia*, *Entamoeba histolytica*, *Shigella*, *Salmonella* and *Campylobacter* all cause symptomatic disease; however, appropriate treatment against these pathogens does not always eliminate the watery diarrhoea. *Cryptosporidium parvum*, an enteric coccidium, attaches to the epithelial surface of both small and large intestines and produces protracted and severe diarrhoea in symptomatic HIV/AIDS patients. The diagnosis is by direct modified Ziehl–Neelsen staining of stool preparations; treatment is difficult, with a wide range of antimicrobial agents demonstrating marginal success. CMV, *Mycobacterium avium* and *M. intracellulare*, *Isospora belli*, *Microsporidium encephalozitozoon* and Kaposi's sarcoma involving the bowel wall may also produce these clinical features. There is growing evidence that HIV-1 itself may cause enteropathic signs and symptoms through infection and infiltration of local target cells, when treatment of specific pathogens is unsuccessful and patients have both malabsorption and loss of weight. The clinical consequences of this condition may be profound, but HAART has been found to be of value.

The widespread use of antiretroviral therapy has reduced the incidence of many of the above opportunistic infections and there is recent evidence to indicate that a CD4 cell nadir, prior to restoration with HAART, of > 200 cells/μl is not predictive of increased risk of opportunistic infections (Miller *et al.*, 1999). However, there has been a concurrent increase in the morbidity and mortality due to hepatitis B and C infections. This is not due to an increased prevalence *per se*, but rather to the longer lifespan of HIV-infected individuals, enabling the pathogenic processes to advance. The interplay of host and viral factors in viral hepatitis pathology is complex, and it remains unclear whether antiretroviral therapy slows progression of these infections. A number of clinical trials are in progress to study the impact of HBV and HCV treatment on HIV disease progression and vice versa. Those infected with either hepatitis virus should be closely monitored by serological and quantitative molecular assays.

Many of the opportunistic infections discussed above manifest disease through an immunopathological process. It is now becoming apparent that unique presentations of these infections can occur consequent to immune reconstitution induced by retroviral therapy, e.g. cystoid macula oedema and vitritis due to cytomegalovirus may be observed in those receiving anti-HIV therapy.

AIDS-associated Malignancies

Malignancy is a common feature of AIDS as a consequence of the profound cell-mediated immunosuppression. However, only certain types of cancer are significantly increased in AIDS and HIV infection, indicating that the role of immune surveillance in preventing cancer is selective (Boshoff and Weiss, 2002). It is striking that AIDS-associated tumours mainly have a viral aetiology. Kaposi's sarcoma is the commonest AIDS-defining malignancy, with non-Hodgkin's lymphomas and anogenital squamous carcinomas next in importance. Tumours present at late stages of infection at a time of diminishing immunocompetence, although they may be the first symptom of AIDS.

Kaposi's Sarcoma

Kaposi's sarcoma (KS) is a rare vascular or lymphatic tumour (Dupin *et al.*, 1999) that has been simply classified into different epidemiological forms (see Chapter 2F; Boshoff and Weiss, 2002):

1. Classic KS is seen in Jewish, Mediterranean and Middle Eastern populations. It occurs mainly in elderly people (median 72 years) with a much greater prevalence in men than women. Classic KS typically presents in the lower limbs and follows an indolent course.
2. Transplant or iatrogenic KS in immunosuppressed patients, often of the same ethnic groups as classic KS.
3. Endemic KS in sub-Saharan Africa, presenting in adults and children. This tumour was already commonly seen before the HIV/AIDS era.
4. AIDS-associated KS. This is an aggressive form of tumour, often presenting viscerally and in the lung as well as cutaneously.

All these forms are linked to infection by Kaposi's sarcoma-associated herpesvirus (KSHV or HHV-8) and reflect the prevalence of this infection. Together with PCP, KS was the sentinel disease that alerted epidemiologists and physicians to the incipient AIDS epidemic in 1981.

Early studies of the epidemiology of the AIDS-KS defined clusters of cases in homosexual and bisexual men in the developed world, with increasing cases at sites associated with the original epidemic. Female cases were associated with bisexual male partners. The sexual practice of oral–anal contact was significantly higher in those with KS and was proposed as a route of transmission of a potential infectious agent associated with this group. The disease has a lower prevalence in transfusion-acquired AIDS (4%) and haemophiliacs (<1%), suggesting the blood-borne route as an unusual pathway for transmission.

Using representational DNA analysis, a modified PCR technique applied to substractive hybridisation, Chang et al. (1994) identified novel DNA sequences in KS that showed homology with gamma-herpesviruses such as *Herpesvirus saimiri* and EBV. The new virus was called KSHV or HHV-8. DNA from KSHV was found in all KS lesions, independent of HIV status (Chapter 2F). PCR and serological assays are available for testing for KSHV. The presence of KSHV predicts the subsequent development of KS. The increasing frequency of HHV-8 seropositivity with age (Sitas et al., 1999) suggests that horizontal transmission occurs, and paediatric studies confirm vertical transmission, probably via saliva (Boshoff and Weiss, 2002).

Histopathologically, a variety of features are seen, which suggests a multipotential mesenchymal cell of origin with markers of lymphatic endothelium in particular (Dupin et al., 1999). Vascular proliferation and spindle-shaped neoplastic cells form a network of reticulin fibres. The lesions start in the mid-dermis and extend towards the epidermis. Lesions in the gastrointestinal tract arise in the submucosa.

AIDS-KS has a wide variety of clinical presentations. Typically, single or multiple indolent lesions appear as pink macular lesions on the skin; they may evolve into reddish-purple maculopapular lesions or nodules, increasing in size and distribution. They range from benign innocuous lesions to aggressive, invasive and fungating forms over time. The lesions may occlude or invade lymphatics, producing lymphoedema.

A disseminated form occurs, with soft gastrointestinal lesions producing dysphagia or gastrointestinal bleeding. Pulmonary KS is associated with space-occupying bronchial lesions, producing wheeze and cough, dypsnoea, a typical chest X-ray picture, and life-threatening haemoptysis. In both these presentations, endoscopy and biopsy require considerable thought. The prognosis of KS is dependent upon the disease stage, the severity of HIV-associated immunosuppression and other systemic illnesses (Table 25.8).

The treatment of KS in AIDS depends on the severity of the primary disease and the extent of the KS. Broadly, in otherwise asymptomatic HIV infection, treatment of 'benign' skin lesions is only for psychological or cosmetic reasons, whereas in symptomatic or visceral disease it may be life-saving (Table 25.9). Before HAART, less than 50% responded to systemic chemotherapy and the response time was limited. Intralesional vinblastine will reduce bulk and number but leave skin pigmentation. Radiotherapy is used in large skin or oral lesions; responses are good but recurrence common. Immunotherapy using IFN-α, even in high doses, only produces a 30% response and is complicated by the systemic toxicity of this agent. In view of the causative agent, studies using cidofovir and foscarnet are being explored for therapy and prophylaxis because these anti-herpetic drugs inhibit KSHV replication. Above all, the use of HAART for the treatment of HIV/AIDS has greatly reduced the prevalence of KS in patients with symptomatic disease (Boshoff and Weiss, 2002).

Non-Hodgkin's Lymphoma (NHL)

Most of the lymphoid malignancies are high-grade Burkitt's lymphomas and immunoblastic lymphomas.

Table 25.8 TIS staging of AIDS Kaposi's sarcoma

Criteria	Good risk (0)	Poor risk (1)
Tumour bulk (T)	Limited to skin, lymph nodes or no oral involvement (T0)	Tumour-associated oedema or ulceration; + + lesions in mouth, GI tract or other organs (T1)
Immune status (I)	CD4 cell counts $>200 \times 10^6$/l (I0)	CD4 cell counts $<200 \times 10^6$/l (I1)
Systemic disease (S)	No history of OIs or candidiasis; no B symptoms[a]; Karnofsky score >70 (S0)	History of OIs, candidiasis; B symptoms; Karnofsky score <70; other AIDS-related illness (S1)

OI, opportunistic infection; Karnofsky score, clinical scale of HIV/AIDS disability in units of 10, from 0 = dead to 100 = normal, no signs or symptoms.
[a]B symptoms—see Table 25.6.

Table 25.9 Choices of treatment for AIDS Kaposi's sarcoma

Early disease (T0, I0/1 or S0/1)	Advanced disease (T1, I0/1 or S0/1)
HAART	HAART
No treatment	Radiotherapy
or	or
Intralesional vinblastine (lesions <1 cm^2)	Systemic chemotherapy
	1st line: bleomycin + vincristine
or	
	2nd line: liposomal anthracycline
Radiotherapy (lesions >1 cm^2)	+ doxil
or	
Interferon-α	

The diagnosis is 50 times more common in HIV/AIDS than in the normal population. Its age distribution is bimodal, with the former at a peak in 10–20 year-olds and the latter in 50–60 year-olds. They are usually widespread at presentation and often occur in extranodal sites, particularly the brain. Only about 50% of the lymphomas are EBV-related, although higher figures have been claimed in some populations. This suggests that the pathogenesis is more complicated than the expression of an oncogenic virus in the face of immunosuppression, although it is likely that activation of virus stimulation has a role, just as in KS. KSHV is causally associated with two rare forms of AIDS lymphoma, plasmablastic multicentric Castleman's disease (Dupin et al., 1999) and primary effusion lymphoma (Chapter 2F). In contrast to KS, NHL has become more common in HIV/AIDS, as patients live longer as a consequence of HAART and prophylaxis for opportunistic infections (Boshoff and Weiss, 2002).

Diagnosis of NHL is essentially by biopsy, but this is not routine for suspected primary cerebral disease. In the latter case, a presumptive diagnosis of a CT lesion is made in the absence of response to anti-toxoplasmal therapy, a negative thalium uptake scan and a positive EBV PCR result in CSF.

Treatment of systemic disease is stratified according to prognostic factors. Generally, those with major adverse factors, such as prior AIDS-defining illness, CD4 counts $<100 \times 10^6$/l, primary cerebral disease and low Karnofsky score (<70), receive palliative care and low-toxicity chemotherapy, focusing on quality of life. The minority, with a better prognosis, are treated with conventional 'curative' chemotherapy for non-Hodgkin's lymphoma. Primary cerebral lymphoma is associated with profound immunosuppression and very low CD4 cell counts; a brief clinical improvement is derived from brain radiotherapy and dexamethasone, but the survival time is only about 2 months.

An increased incidence of Hodgkin's disease has been reported in patients with HIV/AIDS (Boshoff and Weiss, 2002). It is associated with intravenous drug users, and is more aggressive than in the general population, with bone marrow or other extra-nodal involvement. Patients have mixed cellularity or lymphocyte-depleted histology, and a survival time of less than 1 year.

Anogenital Squamous Carcinoma

Rapidly progressive, squamous intraepithelial carcinomas develop in the cervical canals and anorectal junction of women and men, respectively, with HIV/AIDS. Each site has a squamous-columnar border and there is evidence of viral causation (Mathews, 2003). These regions are commonly infected with human papillomavirus (HPV) in these patient groups and, especially as immunosuppression increases in symptomatic disease, the HPV-encoded oncoproteins (E6 and E7) known to promote genetic instability in cells may lead to tumour formation.

Studies of those with HIV/AIDS confirm an increased risk particularly of *in situ* cervical cancer but also of invasive disease (Boshoff and Weiss, 2002), which follows a more aggressive course in this patient group. More frequent (annual) cervical screening is offered to patients with HIV/AIDS but anal cytology in men has not yet been systematically evaluated. These malignancies are treated conventionally with chemotherapy and radiotherapy.

Other Cancers

Other tumours that appear to have a high frequency in patients with HIV/AIDS include testicular tumours, squamous cell carcinoma of the oropharynx, tumours of the skin, hepatocellular carcinoma, and squamous carcinoma of the conjunctiva in Africa (Allardice *et al.*, 2003; Boshoff and Weiss, 2002). These tumours may be associated with immunosuppression and/or viral aetiology, e.g. papillomaviruses, but further evidence is awaited. An increase in liver and lung cancers in HIV/AIDS may be accounted for by increased infection with hepatitis B and C viruses and cigarette smoking, respectively, in HIV-positive persons.

Clinical HIV/AIDS in Children

Since 1982, cases of vertically transmitted paediatric HIV infection have been associated with mothers in risk groups (intravenous drug users, sex workers, partners of haemophiliacs, transfusion recipients and partners of bisexuals). Further large populations of infected children were identified in sub-Saharan Africa, the seat of the epidemic. Rates of vertical transmission varied between African (30–50%), North American (20–30%) and European (14%) studies. These differences are probably due to populations at different stages of disease being investigated.

The virus may be transmitted throughout pregnancy, during delivery and as a consequence of breast-feeding. HIV has been isolated from first/second trimester aborted fetuses; twin studies show that the first-born has a higher rate of infection, presumed to be associated with longer exposure to secretions; and breast-milk has been demonstrated to carry HIV and be infectious as a consequence of ingestion. Contemporary research evidence indicates that the majority of transmission events occur perinatally and during breast-feeding.

Strategies for interruption of vertical transmission have had a dramatic impact on the numbers of children infected with HIV-1 in the developed world. Evidence shows that treatment of the mother with zidovudine during the last trimester of pregnancy and the infant for the first 6 weeks of life produced a 60–70% reduction in vertical transmission (Study ACTG 076: 23% vs. 8% transmission in recipients of placebo; Connor *et al.*, 1994). Studies of combination therapies are now under way to optimise regimens in relation to drug toxicity and duration of treatment. However, these drugs are not available worldwide and probably less than 10% of HIV-infected mothers are in a position to benefit at present. Trials of a single dose of nevirapine given to women in labour to prevent transmission have shown very good results. However, one concern raised by these studies is the emergence of nevirapine resistance in some of these women—the rapidity of this process is probably associated with the slow decline in plasma levels following this one dose, creating an ideal selective pressure for resistance. Caesarean section gave early inconclusive results, but a recent meta-analysis of European and American studies showed a 55% reduction in risk of vertical transmission.

Avoiding breast-feeding reduces the rate of transmission and this is strongly advised in the developed world; however, in the developing world the risks to the infant of morbidity and mortality associated with gastrointestinal infections due to lack of conferred immunity from breast milk, and poor hygiene in preparation of bottle feeds, are greater than those associated with HIV infection. Besides, formula-feeding is often stigmatised as indicating that the mother is HIV-positive. Thus, at present the World Health Organization advises exclusive breast-feeding in Africa and avoidance in developed countries.

In summary, with the triple strategy of antiretroviral therapy, Caesarean section and avoidance of breast feeding, vertical transmission of HIV can be reduced to negligible levels. However, this strategy requires knowledge of maternal HIV antibody status in early pregnancy in order to accurately advise and implement preventative measures, and at present this is not universally available. In the developed world the uptake of HIV antibody testing in pregnancy is only about 50%, and in the developing world only an incomplete infrastructure exists to screen and counsel pregnant women.

Disease Presentation in Children

Paediatric HIV-1 infection exhibits some distinct qualities in relation to adult disease; the natural history has not been fully defined but infection of the host at a stage of immunological and biofunctional immaturity will clearly influence the expression of disease. Factors like time of infection, exposure to other pathogens, nutritional status, time of diagnosis and quality of care are all-important. Evidence suggests two groups of vertically infected infants: 30% with early clinical problems and life-threatening illnesses in the first year of life; and 70% with few problems in early life but who develop disease after several years. It has been proposed that these two groups represent early transplacental infection in the former and late infection in the latter. While this is plausible, one must also consider issues such as the pathogenicity of infecting viruses and immunological maturation, which may vary widely from case to case.

The CDC disease classification for children is summarised in Table 25.7. Infections are common in HIV-infected children. Herpes simplex, varicella zoster and measles viruses all produce severe forms of the recognised presentations that require prompt and prolonged therapy to avoid high morbidity and mortality. Common paediatric bacterial infections, such as *Streptococcus pneumoniae*, *Haemophilus influenzae*, *Escherichia coli* and *Salmonella* spp., exhibit unusual presentations and severity. Prompt treatment is required until culture results are available, and multiple infections should always be suspected in unresolving cases. Antimicrobial prophylaxis and immunoglobulin are instituted by some centres.

As in adults, opportunistic infections with *Pneumocystis carinii*, *Mycobacterium tuberculosis*, *M. avium* and *M. intracellulare*, CMV, cryptosporidia and non-oral candidiasis as a consequence of immunodeficiency are common. Failure to thrive is a common feature of paediatric HIV disease. The reasons are multiple: sick mothers; decreased food intake due to oral infections; decreased absorption due to intestinal disease and recurrent diarrhoea; and decreased calorie utilisation for growth, due to demands associated with inflammatory responses and tissue repair.

HIV encephalopathy usually occurs in symptomatic disease, presenting with developmental delay, motor deficits, and cognitive and behavioural disorders. It may be slow or rapid in progression, and cerebral atrophy and ventricular enlargement is seen on CT. Other infectious causes, such as *Toxoplasma*, *Mycobacteria*, *Cryptococcus* and JC virus, are unusual but should be excluded.

The use of antiretroviral therapies has improved the prognosis for all these clinical conditions. We do not know the long-term prognosis of acquiring HIV at such an early phase of host development (Pizzo and Wilfert, 1994), although there are increasing numbers of HIV-positive children surviving through to adolescence and adulthood.

Diagnosis and Monitoring of HIV Infection

Serology remains the cornerstone for the diagnosis of HIV infection in adults. ELISAs may be used alone to exclude adult infection, but a positive diagnosis involves more complex algorithms that are dependent upon the mode of transmission (horizontal or vertical) and the duration of the infection. The availability of antiretroviral therapies makes rapid diagnosis imperative and strategies have therefore been devised to include PCR in clinical algorithms.

The algorithm for diagnosis of established adult disease is summarised in Figure 25.8. After the primary screen using a sensitive HIV-1 + HIV-2 ELISA format, all negative results are reported once the 'reactive' samples in the run (those with a signal greater than the mean of the negative) are confirmed and the patient identification is assured. Reactive samples are entered into a confirmatory algorithm using three further ELISAs, with diverse HIV-1 antigens on the solid phase and different principles of action (e.g. antiglobulin, particle agglutination (PAA), competitive, etc.). A positive report is released if consensus results are obtained from all three assays (>90% of cases), and a second blood specimen is requested to confirm patient identity.

If there is non-consensus in the confirmatory tests, the clinical virologist should consider HIV-2 infection, seroconversion, non-specific reactivity or, rarely, a new non-reactive HIV subtype. The proposed algorithm for follow-up of these samples generally resolves 99.9% of cases, but a smaller number remain that often produce alarming reactivity, which may persist for life or disappear over time. These cases are often resolved by repeat negative results with diagnostic PCR of proviral HIV-1 DNA from PBMCs. The Western blot assay is relatively insensitive in relation to modern ELISAs and is reserved for difficult cases, HIV-2 confirmation, seroconverters and research.

The adult seroconverter is confounded by initial low or non-detectable levels of anti-HIV-1 antibodies, and ELISAs may be negative in the face of clinical signs and symptoms of PHI. If a clinical diagnosis of PHI is proposed, the sample is tested with all four serological assays, a p24 antigen assay and the diagnostic PCR test. In most cases a PCR-positive result is seen prior to, or associated with, low-level seroreactivity, and in approximately 50% of cases will show detectable

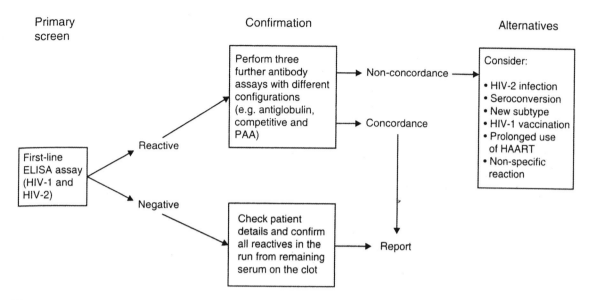

Figure 25.8 An algorithm for the diagnosis of HIV-1 infection

plasma p24 antigen. This is repeated at weekly intervals and evolving signals in the serological assays confirm seroconversion. The Western blot will demonstrate the evolution of a serological response to specific HIV antigens but that post-dates the sensitive serological assays (Table 25.10).

Patients with non-specific reactivity (presumed to have cross-reacting antibodies that signal in certain or all assays) show a distinctive virological pattern but present a difficult clinical problem. They often present through the blood transfusion service as a reactive sample on whom the donation has been withheld. The clinical follow-up usually involves establishing that

they are PCR-negative and that they have non-evolving serology. They are followed over time for reassurance, support if they proceed to any other medical investigations, repeat testing at 6-monthly intervals, and in the majority the reactivity will eventually wane.

The diagnosis of HIV-1 infection in the newborn infant is confounded by the presence of maternal antibodies in the baby's circulation from approximately 32 weeks of gestation onwards. Early diagnosis is essential for early clinical interventions and considerable effort has been applied to establishing algorithms. One approach uses Western blot and

Table 25.10 Typical serological and PCR changes associated with early primary HIV-1 infection

Time (weeks)	−6	Illness	1	2	4	12
Immunometric HIV-1 + 2 ELISA	NEG (0.4)	NEG (0.4)	NEG (0.85)	POS (2.1)	POS (6.9)	POS (10.1)
Antiglobulin HIV-1 + 2 ELISA	NEG (0.15)	NEG (0.2)	NEG (0.6)	NEG (0.85)	POS (4.6)	POS (83)
Competitive HIV-1 ELISA	NEG (0.4)	NEG (0.4)	NEG (0.9)	POS (1.1)	POS (3.7)	POS (91)
PAA	NEG (<1/16)	NEG (<1/16)	EQUIV (1/16)	POS (1/32)	POS (1/128)	POS (1/512)
Western blot	NEG (−)	NEG (—)	NEG (—)	EQUIV (p24 wk b.d.)	POS (p24/gp160)	POS
p24 antigen ELISA	NEG (<10 pg)	NEG (<10 pg)	POS (56 pg)	POS (10 pg)	NEG (<10 pg)	NEG (<10 pg)
Diagnostic PCR (*pol/gag*)	NEG (−/−)	POS (+/+)	POS (+/+)	POS (+/+)	POS (+/+)	POS (+/+)

Table 25.11a Typical serological and PCR changes from birth associated with an uninfected baby

Time	3 days	3 weeks	3 months	6 months	12 months	18 months
PAA	POS (1/600 K)	POS (1/400 K)	POS (1/48 K)	POS (1/6 K)	POS (1/200)	NEG (<1/16)
Western blot	POS (19 bands)	POS (19 bands)	POS (14 bands)	POS (5 bands)	EQUIV (2 bands)	NEG (—)
p24 antigen ELISA	NEG (<10 pg)	NEG (<10 pg)	NEG (<10 pg)	NEG (<10 pg)	NEG (<10 pg)	NEG (<10 pg)
Diagnostic PCR (*pol/gag*)	EQUIV (+/−)	NEG (−/−)	NEG (−/−)	NEG (−/−)	NEG (−/−)	NEG (−/−)

Table 25.11b Typical serological and PCR changes from birth associated with an infected baby

Time	3 days	3 weeks	3 months	6 months	12 months	18 months
PAA	POS (1/900 K)	POS (1/600 K)	POS (1/90 K)	POS (1/70 K)	POS (1/200 K)	NEG (1/980 K)
Western blot	POS (19 bands)	POS (19 bands)	POS (11 bands)	POS (6 bands)	POS (3 bands)	POS (14 bands)
p24 antigen ELISA	NEG (<10 pg)	NEG (<10 pg)	NEG (<10 pg)	POS (100 pg)	NEG (<10 pg)	NEG (<10 pg)
Diagnostic PCR (*pol/gag*)	NEG (−/−)	POS (+/+)	POS (+/+)	POS (+/+)	POS (+/+)	POS (+/+)

titrated particle agglutination assays to measure qualitatively and quantitatively antibody concentrations from 3 days of life onwards, serum p24 antigen and diagnostic PCR of infant-specific HIV-1 proviral DNA (Table 25.11). If available, PBMC culture may also be added to the algorithm. Rapid diagnosis is confirmed by two positive PCR and one positive p24 antigen result in samples taken at 3 days, 3 weeks and 3 months. Titrated serology in an uninfected baby of an HIV-infected mother should demonstrate a halving of passive antibody concentration every 28 days; if antigen (virus) is present which stimulates an immune response in an infected baby, this will be reflected in a levelling-off of the exponential decline in antibody concentrations or an increase over time. It takes up to 18 months for all passive antibody to disappear in the majority of infants and the analysis and reporting of these events involves considerable virological experience.

In the early 1990s molecular virologists modified PCR-based technologies to quantify HIV-1 RNA load (viral load) and genotypic resistance in plasma viruses (Kaye *et al.*, 1992; Semple *et al.*, 1993). These methods were useful to monitor the efficacy of antiretroviral therapy in trials (Katlama *et al.*, 1996; Schuurman *et al.*, 1995), to demonstrate their predictive value for disease progression (Loveday and Hill, 1995), to demonstrate the association between failing virological response and evolving resistance *in vivo* (Loveday

et al., 1995) and to demonstrate the rapid initial decline in plasma HIV-1 that defined the dynamics of virus replication and allowed the development of new theories of pathogenesis (Perelson, 2002). By 1994, first-generation commercial assays were available, based upon plasma HIV-1 nucleic acid capture, reverse transcription and amplification and resulting complementary DNA signalling to quantify plasma viral load.

These genome assays initially detected down to a level between hundreds and thousands of copies per ml plasma, but later second-generation assays defined cut-off values of around 20–50 (Loveday, 1999). These viral load assays were initially used experimentally to define virological efficacy in clinical trials (Brun-Vezinet *et al.*, 1997). A large cohort study revealed the predictive value of such measures for clinical outcome (Mellors *et al.*, 1996). Thus, viral load was established as an essential marker, substituting for clinical endpoints, to define the efficacy of new antiretroviral drug combinations. In clinical practice, patients have regular viral load measures to assist the determination of disease stage, monitor progression, assess responses to antiretroviral therapies, and provide evidence of early treatment failure.

Early *in vitro* studies and investigations of patients receiving monotherapies revealed that, as viral load response failed, drug-resistant viruses evolved in the plasma. These were detected using both drug-sensitive culture assays (phenotypic) and HIV RT and protease

Table 25.12 Comparison of the advantages and disadvantages of genotyping and phenotyping for the determination of antiretroviral drug resistance

	Advantages	Disadvantages
Genotyping	Widely available in laboratories Rapid PCR-based methods (days) Less technically demanding Mutations precede phenotype Quantifies the proportion of wild to mutant strains	Indirect measure Limit of detection (2–5% of population) May not correlate with phenotype Complex data generated that needs virological interpretation May be difficult to interpret Expensive ($>£200.00$/sample) If genetically diverse will not amplify
Phenotyping	Direct measure PCR-based technology gives improved variance Familiar to physicians	Restricted availability (i.e. no clinical throughput system in UK) Slow (weeks) Technically demanding, needs P3[a] Less sensitive than genotyping Very expensive ($>£400.00$/sample) No analysis of sensitivities of combination of drugs

[a]P3, high containment laboratory for the culture of certain infectious pathogens like HIV-1.

genome analysis to identify mutations associated with resistance (genotypic). These approaches were rapidly adapted for commercial assays, which allowed a wide availabilty of resistance testing in clinical virology laboratories to support patient care. The relative advantages and disadvantages of these approaches are summarised in Table 25.12. Phenotypic testing requires RT/protease genes from patient plasma viruses to be transfected into recombinant HIV viruses and their susceptibility to single antiretroviral drugs to be evaluated *in vitro*. Results are expressed as fold change in sensitivity to the drug, relative to a recombinant drug-sensitive laboratory strain of HIV-1. Clinical cut-offs for susceptibility have been derived for each drug that correlate closely with antiviral activity in humans.

Genotypic testing involves the nucleotide sequence analysis of RT/protease to identify mutations known to be associated with drug resistance. The results are described according to their codon position (e.g. M184V, the mutation associated with lamivudine resistance, involves the substitution of a methionine for valine at codon 184 in the RT gene). Tables of mutations are prepared by expert panels based on scientific and clinical experience to provide 'rules-based' advice of the relative importance of mutational patterns in any given clinical case (www.iasusa.org).

Retrospective data show that antiretroviral resistance is associated with poor virological and clinical outcomes, but prospective randomised controlled trials to demonstrate clinical utility of resistance testing vs. standard of care generally involve small patient groups with short follow-up periods. A recent meta-analysis

(Torre and Tambini, 2002) concluded that there was benefit for using genotyping but not phenotyping to support clinical care, and that expert opinion added significantly to the effect. Recently the MRC ERA trial has also demonstrated no additional benefit (in terms of virological and immunological responses) of phenotyping in addition to genotyping in patients with limited therapeutic options after 1 year of follow-up (Loveday et al., 2003).

ANTIRETROVIRAL THERAPY

Historical Context

Antiretroviral therapy, where available, has transformed HIV-1 infection into a treatable chronic condition rather than a death sentence (Pomerantz and Horn, 2003). With hindsight, many now recognise the suboptimal policies made during the early period of antiretroviral therapy. Zidovudine was the first licenced drug against HIV-1, in the late 1980s, following demonstration of clinical benefit in a placebo-controlled trial, and there was widespread demand for monotherapy at this time. Controversy was fuelled by results of the French–UK Concorde study, which showed little benefit of initiating zidovudine therapy early, compared to later in disease. In the early 1990s double therapy with ZDV and didanosine or zalcitabine (or other nucleoside analogues) proved more beneficial than single therapy, which provided the underpinning for later combination treatments using three or more drugs. Monitoring of therapy response was undertaken by CD4 cell count changes during this period, as well as the time to clinical endpoints, such as AIDS and death.

The mid-1990s marked a paradigm shift in HIV therapy, driven by two independent advances. First, assays for accurate and sensitive quantitation of plasma viraemia became commercialised and therefore widely available. Second, the results of the first clinical studies of protease inhibitors (PI) demonstrated the profound potency of this class of drugs when combined with two nucleoside analogues, defined by reductions in viral load. Since the application of plasma virus quantitation to natural history cohorts showed viral load to be predictive of disease progression (Mellors et al., 1996), a leap of logic was taken to postulate that a therapy-induced fall in viral load would lead to improved prognosis, and this was demonstrated subsequently. Since viral replication (as measured by plasma viral load) became central to theories of pathogenesis, the pendulum swung back to early initiation of therapy. This approach was exemplified by the statement at the time, 'it's the virus, stupid', and various estimates were made of the duration of therapy required to eradicate the virus from infected individuals.

Unfortunately, this optimism was tempered by two practical manifestations of therapy—adherence problems and toxicity, as well as the recognition of long-lasting reservoirs of infection within the body. Long-term PI therapy generated severe lipid abnormalities, leading to body shape changes and cardiac problems (although some of these are now also known to be associated with long-term nucleoside analogue treatment; Carr, 2003). The large pill burden of early triple therapy regimens also caused difficulty in drug compliance, and rates of therapy failure were significant. By the late 1990s, non-nucleoside reverse transcriptase inhibitors (NNRTIs), such as nevirapine and efavirenz, had started to replace PIs within first-line regimens, following encouraging clinical trial data.

More recently, there has been a move towards later initiation of therapy, in the CD4 count range of 200–350×10^6/l, based on cohort study data. This is a reflection of the remaining inadequacies of therapy, primarily with respect to adherence, toxicity and resistance issues, rather than representing an ideal approach to a chronic viral infection.

The principles currently underpinning antiretroviral therapy are as follows:

1. Drugs should be used in combination (at least three drugs), for the purposes of potency and limiting the escape of resistant mutants.

2. Following viral rebound, all components of the drug regimen should be changed, if possible, to maximise the benefit of new drugs.

3. The advantages of virological suppression should be balanced against the long-term toxicities of therapy, poor adherence and emergence of resistance, when deciding on the time of initiation of therapy. Currently, clinical cohort data suggest that starting therapy at a CD4 cell count of 200–350 cells/μl confers similar benefit to patients as starting at an earlier stage of infection (Egger et al., 2002).

Therapy of Pregnant Women and Neonates

In general, the indications for treatment of pregnant women conform to the guidelines for non-pregnant adults. Those in whom therapy is not indicated, e.g. due to a high CD4 cell count, should then initiate treatment in the late 2nd/early 3rd trimester, to prevent vertical transmission. Many such regimens include zidovudine in light of the favourable results in ACTG 076, and some prefer to use monotherapy if the viral load is low. Therapy of the neonate should continue for 4–6 weeks. Current guidance suggests that oral zidovudine should be given if the mother received this drug. Combination therapy should be considered if the risk of transmission is high, e.g. the mother starts therapy late in pregnancy.

DRUGS AND THEIR RESISTANCE PATTERNS

Below, each approved drug is briefly described, with its drug resistance patterns, since clinical virologists are increasingly required to advise clinicians on the interpretation of drug resistance test results (Table 25.13). The reader is directed to a more detailed review for discussion of resistance (D'Aquila et al., 2003) and also a recent description of recently available drugs (Gulick, 2003). Further, information on the lipodystrophic side-effects of anti-HIV-1 drugs can be found in the following reviews (Carr, 2003; John et al., 2001; Nolan et al., 2001).

Nucleoside and Nucleotide Analogues

Six nucleoside analogues and one nucleotide analogue are currently approved for use. They act to inhibit the viral RT. They all represent analogues of one of the four natural nucleosides, thymidine, cytidine, adenosine and guanosine, and become triphosphorylated

Table 25.13 Antiretroviral drugs available to treat HIV-1 infection

Drug	Dose	Viral load[a] and resistance[b]	Adverse reactions	Comments
NRTIs				
Zidovudine (ZDV)	250–300 mg b.d.	-0.5 to $0.7 \log_{10}$ codons 41, 67, 70, 215 and 219, 151	Nausea, headache, myopathy, bone marrow suppression	Prodrug Enters CNS Combivir-AZT/3TC
Didanosine (ddI)	200 mg b.d. 400 mg o.d. (no food)	-0.5 to $0.7 \log_{10}$ codons 65, 74, 75, 184, 151	Nausea, diarrhoea, rarely pancreatitis, peripheral neuropathy	Prodrug > Efficacy with hydroxyurea
Zalcitabine (ddC)	0.75 mg t.d.s.	$-0.5 \log_{10}$ codons 65, 69, 74, 75, 184, 151	Oral ulcers and peripheral neuropathy	Prodrug
Lamivudine (3TC)	150 mg b.d.	-0.5 to $0.7 \log_{10}$ codon 184	Nausea, bone marrow suppression	Prodrug Well tolerated
Stavudine (d4T)	40 mg b.d.	$0.6 \log_{10}$ codon 75	Peripheral neuropathy	Prodrug
Abacavir (1592)	300 mg b.d.	$-1.5 \log_{10}$ codons 65, 74, 115, 184	Hypersensitivity: fever, rash, and fatal rechallenge	Prodrug Rechallenge contraindicated
Tenofovir	300 mg o.d.	0.3–$1.5 \log_{10}$ codons 65, and 41/67, /210/215 together	Fanconi's syndrome—very rare	Nucleotide analogue. Well tolerated
NNRTIs				
Nevirapine	200 mg b.d. initial dose escalation	NR codons 103, 106, 108, 181, 188	Rash on induction >15%, 5% grade 3, induces cytochrome P450	Long half-life. Induction with prednisolone
Delavirdine	400 mg t.d.s. 600 mg b.d.	NR codons 103, 181, 236	Rash >20%, 5% grade 3, headache, nausea, raised LFTs	USA only Inhibits cytochrome p450
Efavirenz	600 mg nocte (minimise side-effects)	NR codons 100, 103, 108, 188, 190	Headache, dizziness, vivid insomnia, rarely psychoses, raised LFTs	Induces and inhibits cytochrome p450
Protease inhibitors (PIs)				
Indinivir	800 mg t.d.s. fasting/low fat	-1 to $2 \log_{10}$ codons 82, 46, 10 × 2nd MTs	Nausea, nephrolithiasis, haematuria, lipodystrophy, hyperlipidaemia	'Early efficacy, late toxicity' x-resistance PIs
Ritonavir	600 mg b.d. (400 in combo)	-1 to $2 \log_{10}$ codons 82 and 10 × 2nd MTs	Nausea, vomiting, taste changes, lipid and transaminase elevation	'Early toxicity' x-resistance PIs
Saquinavir (soft gel)	1200 mg t.d.s. 1800 mg b.d. (with food)	$> -1 \log_{10}$ codons 48, 90 7 × 2nd MTs	Nausea, diarrhoea, mild abdominal pain (self-limiting)	Early formulation had poor absorption x-resistance PIs
Nelfinavir	750 mg t.d.s. 1250 mg b.d. (with food)	-1 to $2 \log_{10}$ codon 30 8 × 2nd MTs	Diarrhoea: controlled by drug treatment (self-limiting)	x-resistance PIs
Amprenavir	1200 mg b.d.	$> -1 \log_{10}$ codon 50 4 × 2nd MTs	Nausea, vomiting, taste changes, paraesthesia	x-resistance PIs

LFT, liver function test; MT, mutations; NRTI, nucleoside reverse transcriptase inhibitor; NNRTI, non-NRTI; NR, not recorded; PI, protease inhibitor.
[a]Reduction of viral RNA in plasma.
[b]Position of mutations conferring resistance in reverse transcriptase (NRTIs, NNRTIs) and protease.

within the cell so that they compete with natural nucleotides as substrates for the viral RT. The nucleotide analogue, tenofovir, is a phosphonate, structurally similar to a nucleoside monophosphate.

Zidovudine was the first licenced drug against HIV-1 (Pomerantz and Horn, 2003). Together with stavudine, it is a thymidine analogue, and these two drugs are antagonistic, presumably due to competition for the same intracellular phosphorylation pathways. Since it was the first drug to demonstrate efficacy as monotherapy, it has remained a key component of combination regimens. Benefit was also observed in prevention of mother-to-child transmission in the landmark ACTG 076 study, in which drug was given from the second and third trimester of pregnancy, and to the newborn for 6 weeks following birth. The relatively high rates of toxicity observed in early studies (e.g. anaemia) have been ascribed to the large doses used at that time, and this is less of a problem with current dosing regimens.

The extensive use of zidovudine has led to a detailed appreciation of virus resistance. The acquisition of high-level zidovudine resistance requires several changes in the RT, including amino acid positions 41, 67, 70, 215 and 219. Large surveillance studies of nucleoside analogue-experienced patients identifies T215Y as the most prevalent drug resistance mutation. This is unsurprising in view of the time period over which zidovudine has been available. It has also become apparent that the mutations associated with thymidine analogue resistance cluster according to two groups, vz. that including mutations at positions 41, 67, 210 and 215 (Y), and a group including 70, 215 (F) and 219 mutations. The determinants of one or other route remain unclear. The key mechanism by which ZDV resistance mutations confer reduced susceptibility is thought to be an increase in pyrophosphorolysis, whereby a ZDV-monophosphate moiety incorporated into the growing cDNA chain is subsequently cleaved, thus allowing continued reverse transcription rather than chain termination by the drug. It is of interest that interactions between mutations are increasingly evident, such as the attenuating effect of M184V (lamivudine resistance), L74V (didanosine resistance) and Y181C (nevirapine resistance) on the phenotype of viruses containing zidovudine-resistance mutations. At least for the M184V mutation, this is due to reversal of the pyrophosphorolysis process described above.

Stavudine, a thymidine analogue, has proven efficacy within combination regimens and has good bioavailability. Concerns about toxicity focus on peripheral neuropathy and lactic acidosis, probably associated with inhibition of mitochondrial DNA polymerase-γ. For many years, stavudine resistance was thought to be associated with changes at position 75 of RT only, which were rarely observed in clinical practice. More recently, long-term stavudine therapy has been associated with the emergence of zidovudine resistance-associated mutations, as well as 'multi-drug' resistance mutations (see later), and a poor response to stavudine has been associated with the presence of zidovudine

resistance mutations. In addition, the presence of the T215Y/F/Q mutation predicted a poor short-term response to a stavudine/lamivudine combination in zidovudine-experienced patients (Montaner *et al.*, 2000). Although the phenotypic resistance to stavudine conferred by such mutations is relatively modest, small shifts in susceptibility are sufficient for this drug to lose efficacy.

Didanosine is an adenosine analogue which requires deamination prior to phosphorylation. Gastrointestinal side-effects have been reduced somewhat by the introduction of an enteric coated pill, although a major side-effect remains pancreatitis. The emergence of resistance to didanosine and zalcitabine occurs more slowly than for zidovudine *in vivo* and *in vitro*. In addition, those mutations conferring resistance, such as at positions 65, 69, 74 and 184, lead to only modest increases in IC_{50}. Longer experience with these drugs has allowed more subtle identification of cross-resistance with other nucleoside analogues. An increasing resistance to didanosine is observed as nucleoside analogue mutations are accumulated, and the clinical relevance of small changes in fold resistance may have a greater impact than previously recognised.

Zalcitabine, a cytidine analogue, is associated with peripheral neuropathy. Additionally, potency is only modest, and therefore this drug is now rarely used in clinical practice.

Lamivudine, another cytidine analogue, has potent activity against HBV as well as HIV, which makes it an important component of therapy for co-infected individuals. It is well tolerated, and has been combined within a single pill with zidovudine, as well as with zidovudine and abacavir, to improve adherence. High-level lamivudine resistance is generated by the M184V mutation within RT, and occurs within weeks on monotherapy. It is also commonly observed as the initial mutation emerging following failure of a lamivudine-containing triple regimen, suggesting that the loss of control of this drug drives the evolution of resistance against other components of the regimen. Nevertheless, some lines of evidence call into question the precise impact of this mutation. Virological analysis of the NUCA 3001 study in drug-naïve patients demonstrated that lamivudine with zidovudine effected greater viral load suppression over 24 weeks compared to zidovudine alone, despite the virtually universal emergence of M184V in the double-therapy arm. A longer-term follow-up on a similar lamivudine/zidovudine patient cohort showed phenotypic resistance to zidovudine, but not lamivudine, to be the only independent risk factor for virological failure. Similar results have been presented from other clinical trials with a lamivudine-containing arm.

A number of explanations for these observations have been put forward. First, the fitness of the M184V mutant may be reduced, thus contributing to a reduced virological rebound following emergence of lamivudine resistance. Second, this mutation enhances RT fidelity, which in turn would reduce the rate at which new mutants (including drug-resistant mutants) are generated. Third, the presence of M184V partially reverses the zidovudine resistance phenotype in the presence of zidovudine resistance mutations. Finally, pyrophosphorolysis appears to be diminished within a M184V-containing RT, thus enhancing the chain termination effect of the nucleoside analogues. All these mechanisms have been demonstrated within *in vitro* systems, often with purified RT, and may not be applicable *in vivo*. Indeed, there is conflicting evidence that reduced fitness or increased fidelity of the M184V mutant is a significant factor with infected individuals. In addition, long-term therapy with zidovudine and lamivudine lead to the emergence of novel mutations, such as at positions 43, 44, R211K, L214F and G333E/D, suggesting routes to lamivudine resistance that bypass M184V.

Abacavir is a guanosine analogue, which is converted to carbovir triphosphate as the active component. A severe hypersensitivity reaction may occur in more than 5% of patients. Since re-challenge has been associated with death, close monitoring is required when initating patients on this drug. *In vitro* selection experiments lead to a virus with reduced abacavir susceptibility associated with mutations at RT positions 65, 74, 115 and 184. Preliminary data suggest that viral rebound in patients receiving zidovudine/lamivudine/abacavir is initially associated with the appearance of M184V alone. This is likely to reflect resistance to lamivudine in these patients, as discussed above, and such viruses appear to be fully susceptible to abacavir. A more extensive analysis of the success of abacavir use within salvage therapy demonstrates that abacavir failure is associated with the presence of three or more zidovudine resistance-associated mutations at baseline. Nevertheless, even in heavily pre-treated patients, the reduced susceptibility to abacavir observed in phenotypic assays is often rather modest (<eight-fold resistant).

Tenofovir is the first nucleotide analogue to be approved for HIV treatment, which appears to be unencumbered by the renal toxicity problems of its cousin, adefovir. Like lamivudine, it is a potent inhibitor of HBV as well as HIV-1. As for many other drugs, the RT mutations associated with reduced activity in the clinic are not necessarily those selected by tenofovir in the laboratory (K65R). This is because the drug has been most widely tested in drug-experienced patients in whom resistant virus already exists and predictors of poor response can be identified. Thus, common nucleoside analogue resistance mutations, such as M41L, L210W (possibly a key marker in this respect) and T215Y, appear to reduce, although not to negate, clinical efficacy. Nevertheless, the widespread use of tenofovir in salvage therapy, and promising first-line treatment trial data, suggest that it represents an important addition to our antiretroviral armoury.

Cross-resistance between Nucleoside Analogues

There is variable cross-resistance between the five licensed drugs discussed above, such that second- or third-line therapy may be compromised following failure of first-line therapy. In addition, combination therapies may select for novel mutations or groups of mutations not observed in monotherapy studies. Some of these have been discussed above. Other examples include the constellation of A62V, V75I, F77L, F116Y and Q151M, which confer cross-resistance to all NRTIs. Of interest is that viruses containing all five of the above mutations appear more replication-competent than wild-type virus within *in vitro* competition experiments. Multi-nucleoside analogue resistance is also caused by a diverse cluster of amino acid insertions and deletions between positions 67 and 70, commonly 69S-(S-S) or 69S-(S-G), which directly influence the nucleoside triphosphate binding site of RT. To date, the prevalence of these multi-drug resistance mutations in treated patients appears low; however, this figure should be expected to rise, and is of major concern.

New Drugs for Use against Nucleoside Analogue-resistant Viruses

Amdoxovir (DAPD) is a new nucleoside analogue prodrug whose oral administration leads to a rapid *in vivo* conversion to (−)-β-D-dioxalane guanosine (DXG). Resistance to this drug in the laboratory appears to involve the K65R and L74V mutations, similar to those observed for abacavir (although abacavir failure is rarely associated with these mutations in the clinic). Phase I/II studies demonstrate a reasonable activity of this drug against nucleoside analogue-resistant viruses, although more data are needed before clarifying its potential role. FTC, a fluorinated derivative of lamivudine, has similar potency and spectrum of action to lamivudine. However, it has a long half-life and can be dosed once daily, which may provide an advantage over lamivudine.

Non-nucleoside Reverse Transcriptase Inhibitors (NNRTIs)

The NNRTIs are a structurally diverse group of compounds, of which nevirapine and efavirenz are approved for use (Table 25.13). Despite this diversity, the current drugs all bind within the same RT pocket, occupied by the side chains of amino acids at positions 181 and 188, and the 103 residue is close to the entry to this site. This pocket is not present in HIV-2, and therefore NNRTIs are ineffective against this virus. The potency of these drugs, and at least equivalence to PI-containing regimens, has led NNRTI-containing regimens to be common as first-line therapy. The most common side-effect of nevirapine is a self-limiting rash; however, a rare but severe (fulminant) hepatitis has been reported, and close monitoring of liver function is required. The major side-effect of efavirenz is insomnia and vivid dreams, especially in the first weeks after starting treatment.

In vitro selection experiments demonstrate the rapid acquisition of high-level resistance to NNRTIs. The mutations associated with resistance may vary between drugs, with variable levels of phenotypic cross-resistance. However, wide cross-resistance appears evident in clinical practice and failure of NNRTIs is often caused by a single mutation. It is likely that these variants therefore pre-exist within the viral population, as for the lamivudine resistance mutation, and can quickly emerge if viral replication is maintained on therapy.

Failure of efavirenz-containing triple regimens is associated with the K103N mutation in up to 90% of cases, producing phenotypic cross-resistance to nevirapine and delavirdine. Other mutations, such as G190S/A/E, Y188L and L100I, may also be observed and they may be acquired sequentially. This suggests that the emergence of high-level resistance with K103N does not preclude further selective pressure. The low genetic barrier to emergence of NNRTI resistance reaffirms the importance of maintaining optimal suppression of viral replication in those receiving this class of drugs.

The rapid emergence of resistance to nevirapine in monotherapy studies during the early 1990s led to a halt in further clinical development of this compound. More recently, the efficacy of this drug has been demonstrated within the context of combination regimens. The genetic pathway to resistance is dependent upon co-therapies. Thus, resistance to single therapy is usually caused by the Y181C mutation. By contrast, in the presence of zidovudine, other mutations, such as the K103N, are the preferred route. This may be explained by the *in vitro* observation that the Y181C mutation suppresses the emergence of zidovudine resistance. Thus, there may be an evolutionary bias against the emergence of the 181 mutation in such co-treated patients. The majority of patients failing a nevirapine-containing therapy will be expected to show NNRTI mutations, the most common combination being K103N and Y181C, but also including changes at codons 101, 106, 108, 179, 188 and 190. This illustrates the variability in pathways to nevirapine resistance, possibly influenced by the concurrent nucleoside analogues used.

Finally, it is noteworthy that 'naturally' occurring resistance to NNRTIs has been observed in group O HIV-1 strains, as well as HIV-2 and SIV. In addition, many non-clade B subtypes of HIV-1 contain polymorphisms at RT positions which may impact on NNRTI susceptibility, such as codons 98, 101 and 179. More work is required to delineate the precise impact of these polymorphisms, and whether they influence the genetic route to high-level NNRTI resistance.

New NNRTIs

The phenomenon of extensive cross-resistance between NNRTIs is one of the more widely accepted facts of HIV drug resistance, due to the small binding site for this group of drugs within the viral RT. The key mutations in this regard are K103N, T181C and G190A/E, all of which compromise nevirapine, efavirenz and delaviridine responses, and this cross-resistance represents a major limitation of the class as a whole. However, two new compounds, TMC125 and TMC120, appear to have activity against such resistant viruses, both *in vitro* and *in vivo*. Another compound (capravirine) demonstrated activity against a virus bearing the K103N or V106A or L100I single mutation, although high-level resistance to this drug was reported in the presence of mutations at codon 181.

It appears not so much that different patterns of resistance mutations are observed with these new

NNRTIs drugs, but rather that emergence of resistance is much slower than existing NNRTIs—note that single-dose nevirapine in pregnancy is sufficient to select for resistant mutants—and that the well-recognised NNRTI mutations have a marginal, and possibly clinically irrelevant, impact on fold susceptibility. It is argued that these properties are a function of the unique structures of these second-generation NNRTIs, in the context of binding to the RT enzyme.

Protease Inhibitors

The development of protease inhibitors (PIs) followed rapidly on from the publication of the crystal structure of HIV-1 protease in 1988 (Pomerantz and Horn, 2003). The enzyme itself is small, comprising a homodimer with 99 amino acids in each strand. Since the functional expression of protease is essential for virus replication, it was initially thought that emergence of drug resistance mutations within such a small gene would be limited. Not only has this proved incorrect but also an extensive polymorphism of this gene has been demonstrated in viruses from PI-naïve patients, such that up to 50% of the amino acids may vary within clade B viruses. This diversity widens when other HIV-1 subtypes are considered. Nevertheless, these variants do not appear to compromise *in vitro* or *in vivo* responses to PIs. All PIs are metabolised, at least partially, through the CYP 3A4 isozyme of the cytochrome p450 system. This leads to significant interactions with other drugs, and also individual differences in plasma drug levels achieved. The major limitation of this class of drugs is the syndrome of hyperlipidaemia, insulin resistance and peripheral fat wasting (lipodystrophy), the precise pathogenesis of which is under intense investigation.

Indinavir. The major side-effect is nephrolithiasis, including flank pain with or without haematuria. Early dose ranging studies of indinavir monotherapy generated detailed information on resistance-associated mutations for this drug. Sequential acquisition of mutations was observed, with changes at positions 10, 24, 46, 54, 71, 82, 84 and 90 being significantly correlated with phenotypic resistance. Nevertheless, the V82A/F/T mutation is recognised as the best predictor of reduced indinavir susceptibility occurring early in drug failure, with or without M46I/L/V (although not in themselves leading to significantly reduced susceptibilities). These changes are followed by a series of other more variable changes, which confer increasing resistance and compensate for reduced fitness. A significant advance in our understanding of protease inhibitor resistance was made following failure of indinavir therapy with the demonstration of mutations, in conjunction with protease mutations, which map outside the protease gene, but map within the enzyme's substrate, the *gag* protease cleavage sites. Changes at the *gag* p7/p1 site are most commonly observed, and mutagenesis experiments suggest that their major role is to compensate for partial replication deficiency caused by the 82 and/or 46 mutations. Similarly, some of the additional mutations acquired within the protease gene itself may also be compensatory.

Saquinavir. The bioavailability of the original hard-gel capsule of this drug was low but it has been increased by the use of the soft-gel formulation. Failure of monotherapy within clinical trials was commonly associated with the L90M mutation and rarely with the G48V, mutations which together severely reduce the catalytic efficiency of the enzyme. Although residue 48 is in an important flap loop of the enzyme, residue 90 appears distant to the active site and may lead to conformational effects on inhibitor binding.

Nelfinavir. Co-adminstration with high-fat meals increases blood levels of nelfinavir significantly, and improves antiviral efficacy. Diarrhoea remains the most important side-effect. Initial monotherapy studies with nelfinavir identified a unique mutation, D30N, as responsible for reduced drug susceptibility, without corresponding cross-resistance to other protease inhibitors. It is now apparent that failure of nelfinavir-containing triple regimens is associated with either the D30N or the L90M mutation. The 30 mutation may be associated with N88D and A71T/V, whereas the 90 mutation emerges together with changes at one or more of positions 10, 20, 46, 60 73 and 74. The constellation of mutations around L90M confers cross-resistance to saquinavir and possibly other PIs, and therefore the route taken for nelfinavir resistance may determine the success of subsequent PI therapies; however, more extensive evidence is required.

Amprenavir. In vitro selection of amprenavir-resistant virus identifies I50V as a key resistance mutation, together with other secondary mutations. However, cross-resistance of isolates from PI-experienced patients to amprenavir can be predicted by the presence of M46I/L, I54L/V, I84V and L90M. Thus, an algorithm of I84V and/or any two of the three mutations 46/54/90, allowed prediction of high-level resistance with a sensitivity of 88% and specificity of 79%. In view of the poor pharmacokinetics and high pill burden of amprenavir, a prodrug, fos-amprenavir has recently been developed.

Ritonavir. This was the first PI to be licensed in Europe. However, the frequency and severity of side-effects has limited its use as an antiviral drug in its own right. It is one of the most potent p450 inhibitors identified. This has led to it being used primarily at low dose to boost the blood concentrations of other PIs. Such dosing is not thought sufficient to confer antiviral efficacy, or to select for resistance.

Lopinavir. This is co-formulated with ritonavir to achieve drug levels sufficient to inhibit viruses with resistance mutations for many other PIs. The ratio of trough drug concentration divided by the IC_{50} value, termed the inhibitory quotient (IQ), has been introduced in order to quantify the benefit conferred by high drug levels. Such IQ measurements are currently undergoing trials to assess their clinical utility. The major side-effects of lopinavir appear to be lipid abnormalities. *In vitro* selection experiments identified lopinavir resistance-associated mutations at 84, 10, 46, 71, 32 and 47. However, it appears likely that the clinical benefit of this drug, co-administered with ritonavir, is due to the high plasma levels achieved, which may overcome reduced drug susceptibility, rather than lack of cross-resistance patterns *per se*. This drug appears to be highly effective when used as first- or second-line PI therapy, and little data are yet available on the mutations which emerge during therapy to lead to drug failure.

New PIs

Issues of resistance and cross-resistance are particularly pertinent to the protease inhibitor class of drugs. Many claims have been made on the apparent uniqueness of resistance patterns for specific drugs, based on *in vitro* data, which do not then translate into clinical benefit for that drug in PI-experienced patients. Two new PIs have now undergone initial clinical evaluation. Atazanavir demonstrated different resistance profiles when used in PI-naïve and PI-experienced patients. In the former group, resistance emerges with the I50L and A71V mutations. This is a unique combination, since amprenavir-resistance mutations include a different amino acid change at position 50 (viz. I50V), although the A71V mutation is a polymorphism (not infrequently observed in the absence of PI therapy). By contrast, in PI-experienced patients, some level of cross-resistance between atazanavir and other PIs was apparent. Since the I50L–A71V mutation combination does not appear to reduce susceptibility to other PIs, there may be advantage, from a resistance perspective, in using atazanavir as a first-line PI; however, data are required on the actual efficacy of PI treatment after atazanavir failure to fully assess the importance of the 'unique resistance pattern'. Clinical data have also been presented for tipranavir, which shows potency against viruses containing a large variety of PI-resistance mutants *in vitro*. Clinical activity was observed in PI-experienced patients, suggesting that a large number of PI-resistance mutations were required to compromise activity. More work is required to further clarify such 'clinical cut-offs', whereby clinicians can be guided on the likely effect of this new drug in a patient with existing PI-resistant virus.

Fusion Inhibitors

Following attachment of the virus to the cell membrane, the helical proteins of the gp41 molecule contract and bring the gp120 and cell receptor into close proximity, thus allowing membrane fusion to occur. The viral genome can then enter the cell. Data are now emerging from the trials of T-20 (enfuvirtide), the first fusion inhibitor to enter the clinic, which acts to inhibit this process (Lalezari *et al.*, 2003). Since the Phase III trials were undertaken in heavily pre-treated patients, it is not surprising that failure rates (lack of full suppression) were relatively high overall. However, this affords the opportunity to characterise the emergence of resistance. Data from Phase II studies demonstrate that the majority of such failure patients had mutations in the gp41 region targeted by the drug, namely between amino acids 36–45, which indeed confirms that activity of the drug is mediated through the proposed mechanism. Since variation in this region is very rare in enfuvirtide-naïve patients, including those infected with non-subtype B viruses, it can be assumed that prior RT inhibitor and PI therapy will not compromise enfuvirtide activity *per se*. The key issue with use of this drug in salvage therapy will therefore be the choice of other active drugs to combine with it. Of interest, the second-generation fusion inhibitor T-1249 appears to be active against most enfuvirtide-resistant mutants, although so far this is based on *in vitro* evidence alone. Both compounds have the disadvantage of requiring parenteral administration.

New Drug Targets

Figure 25.9 depicts the many stages of the HIV replication at which inhibition may be possible.

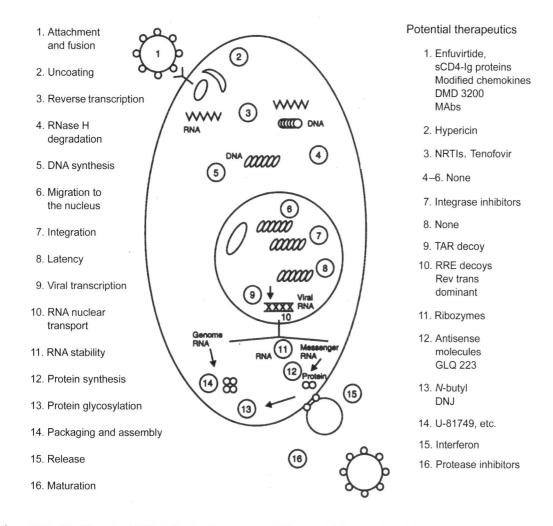

1. Attachment and fusion
2. Uncoating
3. Reverse transcription
4. RNase H degradation
5. DNA synthesis
6. Migration to the nucleus
7. Integration
8. Latency
9. Viral transcription
10. RNA nuclear transport
11. RNA stability
12. Protein synthesis
13. Protein glycosylation
14. Packaging and assembly
15. Release
16. Maturation

Potential therapeutics

1. Enfuvirtide, sCD4-Ig proteins Modified chemokines DMD 3200 MAbs
2. Hypericin
3. NRTIs, Tenofovir
4–6. None
7. Integrase inhibitors
8. None
9. TAR decoy
10. RRE decoys Rev trans dominant
11. Ribozymes
12. Antisense molecules GLQ 223
13. N-butyl DNJ
14. U-81749, etc.
15. Interferon
16. Protease inhibitors

Figure 25.9 The life cycle of HIV, indicating the stages at which potential therapeutics might act

Co-receptor antagonists have been developed to inhibit CCR5 and CXCR4 binding to virus. Concern over such compounds has focused on the detrimental effect of blockade of important stimulatory molecules, and the ability of the virus to evolve to switch co-receptor usage following the use of one particular antagonist. Promising data have been presented for the CCR5 inhibitors (Baba *et al.*, 1999; Simmons *et al.*, 1997) and clinical studies of new, small molecular weight drugs are ongoing at the time of writing.

Integrase is a unique enzyme which catalyses the integration of viral cDNA into the host cell genome. As such it is essential, and a promising target for antiviral drugs. The enzyme structure has been resolved for some years; however, it has taken longer to dissect the enzymatic components of the molecule. Lead compounds have now been developed, and clinical studies are due to start (Pomerantz and Horn, 2003).

Transmission of Drug Resistance

Epidemiological studies of acute infections or chronic untreated infections in Europe and North America demonstrate the presence of viruses containing drug resistance mutations in up to 20% of cases (UK Collaborative Group on Monitoring the Transmission of HIV Drug Resistance, 2001). This reflects *de novo* transmission of drug-resistant variants. These viruses appear to persist in the absence of therapy, and may compromise the efficacy of first-line therapy (Grant *et al.*, 2002; Little *et al.*, 2002). Therefore routine resistance testing at baseline is increasingly undertaken, to guide optimal treatment.

Novel Approaches to Management of Multi-resistant Virus Infection

A number of new strategies have been suggested as a means of dealing with multi-resistant HIV-1, some of which have been subject to pilot studies:

1. *Treatment interruption.* Since wild-type (non-resistant) virus regrows out as the majority species when treatment is stopped, it has been proposed that such a strategy will allow resensitisation of the virus to treatment (Deeks and Hirschel, 2002). A number of further reasons have been given for the potential advantage of such an approach, such as providing immune stimulation; however, there is little evidence that this provides any lasting benefit in subsequent response to therapy.
2. *GIGA-HAART.* A pilot study has been undertaken of treatment interruption in patients with low CD4 count, followed by the use of up to eight and nine drugs. It is of interest that this multiple treatment has been shown to provide some benefit (Katlama *et al.*, 2003).
3. *Continuing therapy.* Drug-resistant viruses may also have deficiencies in viral replicative capacity (fitness). This has led some to propose that continuing on therapy, to maintain the presence of drug resistance mutations, may be beneficial compared to stopping therapy. An alternative interpretation of these data is that resistance is not all or nothing, and that drugs may maintain some residual activity (Deeks and Hirschel, 2002).

Immunotherapy

The fact that HIV induces gradual immunosuppression over a long period raises the question of reconstitution of the immune system using immunotherapy (Imami and Gotch, 2002). The three major approaches tried to date are:

1. Passive immunisation with plasma selected for high neutralising antibodies.
2. Use of cytokines, such as IL-2 and GM-CSF.
3. Use of therapeutic vaccines.

Passive immunisation has been tried by a number of investigators, using either anti-HIV plasma or selective high-titre anti-HIV V3 anti-loop antibodies and, in the case of children, normal immunoglobulin. Encouraging results have been claimed with all these approaches, although a claimed correlation between high-titre anti-V3 loop antibodies and preventive mother-to-child transmission could not be duplicated by others, and no firm evidence for efficacy *in vivo* exists at present. A limitation of this approach is the availability of high-titre sera containing neutralising antibodies to the relevant HIV strain of the patient being treated. However, the success of human antibodies in the treatment of cancer, such as herceptin for breast cancer and rituximab for lymphoma, raises the possibility that the five available human monoclonal antibodies that have been found to be capable of neutralising a broad range of primary HIV-1 isolates may be better potential candidates for passive immunotherapy.

HAART has made a dramatic impact on patients who are able to receive these drugs frequently. Unfortunately, even though viral load can be reduced to undetectable levels, cessation of the drugs leads to rebound, a rising viral load and falling CD4 count in the majority of patients. Because many patients wish to cease HAART due to side-effects, there is an unmet need to use some other form of treatment to maintain the low viral state when HAART is ceased. Although the immune response to a variety of antigens recovers in patients on HAART, it is clearly not enough to induce the appropriate immune response to HIV.

The concept of enhancing an appropriate immune response and the concept of therapeutic vaccination following the partial immune improvement are actively being pursued in clinical research. Interleukin 2 (IL-2) production in patients with HIV infection is reduced leading to T-helper-1 type deficiency, whereas Th-2 type cytokines (IL-4, IL-6) are increased. Replacement by recombinant IL-2 increases the peripheral CD4 counts when given as pulsed therapy or subcutaneous injections. By causing the lymphocyte population to expand, IL-2 could increase viral production by activating cells for HIV propagation. However, a number of studies have shown that IL-2 combined with HAART leads to a substantially greater increase in CD4 count and a larger decrease in viral load than seen with HAART alone. Response to recall antigens is eight-fold higher in IL-2 recipients than in patients treated with HAART alone. However, it is not clear that this translates into enhanced responses to immunisation *in vivo*. A large randomised multi-centre study, called ESPRIT, hopes to answer whether IL-2 plus HAART genuinely improves morbidity and mortality.

Other cytokines may also have a role in the management of chronic HIV infection. Chronic granulocyte macrophage colony stimulating factor (GM-CSF) is capable of enhancing monocytes and macrophages, and can restore the allogenic stimulatory function to accessory cells in patients with AIDS. As dendritic cell function is impaired in HIV patients, a case for using GM-CSF and IL-2 in the same regimen can be made.

Therapeutic vaccines are designed to induce the immune response not normally initiated in the HIV patient for a number of different reasons (Letvin and Walker, 2003). With the ability of HAART to reduce the viral load and IL-2 to increase CD4 and NK populations, it is attractive to consider the possibility of immunising patients with dominant components of HIV. One of these, known as REMUNE, containing inactivated HIV particles, induced immune responses to HIV antigens in patients being treated with HAART. A therapeutic vaccine based on the recombinant glycoprotein 160 has been tried in asymptomatic volunteers with CD4 counts above 400. It was concluded that gp160 was safe and persistently immunogenic, although there was no evidence that this vaccine had efficacy as a therapeutic vaccine in early stage HIV infection, as measured by primary endpoints or disease progression.

In conclusion, although it has been shown that HAART plus IL-2 therapy can greatly improve the CD4 count and the immune system over time, there are still deficits in the immune response to HIV. However, it took a combination of antiretroviral drugs to achieve significant clinical efficacy over time, and it may well require judicious use of a combination of cytokines and therapy over the right time interval to induce a clinically significant and beneficial immune response.

THE PROSPECTS FOR HIV VACCINES

Many investigations of many different candidate HIV vaccines are under study at the present time (McMichael and Hanke, 2003). These agents include envelope gp120 or gp140 for humoral immunity, as well as viral vectors and DNA-based vaccines encoding Gag, Pol, Nef, Tat, Rev, and Vpu epitopes.

Early in 2003, the first results of the randomised trial of a lead HIV vaccine candidate were reported, but no protective effect was observed in a gp120 vaccine made by Vaxgen (Cohen, 2003). This failure has highlighted many doubts about the ability of HIV to be successfully contained by prophylactic vaccination. Major questions with regard to the vaccines involve whether neutralising antibody responses or cell-mediated responses are the more important and what the importance of virus variation is. With regard to the HIV envelope, the dominant antigen, the V3 loop, is very variable. Only five human monoclonal antibodies have been reported to neutralise a broad range of HIV isolates by recognising conserved epitopes across HIV-1 clades, although two of these require CD4 binding of gp120 to expose the epitope. Protection has been demonstrated in SCID mice reconstituted with human T cells, and with SIV challenge of macaques, although the titres required are high and may be impossible to achieve by current vaccination methods.

HIV induces a strong CD8 T cell response during acute viraemia and this can persist in most patients (Letvin and Walker, 2003). CD8 T cell responses can select HIV escape mutants. CD8 cells are able to protect against high-dose challenge with several viruses in experimental systems and therefore it may be possible to stimulate CD8 protection in HIV. Unfortunately, in SIV and SHIV macaque models single amino acid change can escape an effective CD8 response. Nevertheless, the presence of heavily exposed but HIV-seronegative people who have CD8 T cell responses suggest that this may contribute to protection as well as IgA neutralising responses.

There are many variations on a possible HIV vaccine, involving a range of vectors and immunogens (Table 25.14). A DNA prime, modified vaccinia

Table 25.14 Possible approaches to HIV vaccines

Immunogens
Whole killed virions
Purified protein subunits
Recombinant proteins
Synthetic peptides
Viral vectors
   Vaccinia
   Canarypox
   Alpha-virus
   Venezuelan equine encephalitis
DNA encoding HIV antigens
Live attenuated HIV

Adjuvants
Those that induce Th1 cellular immune responses

(a)   (b)

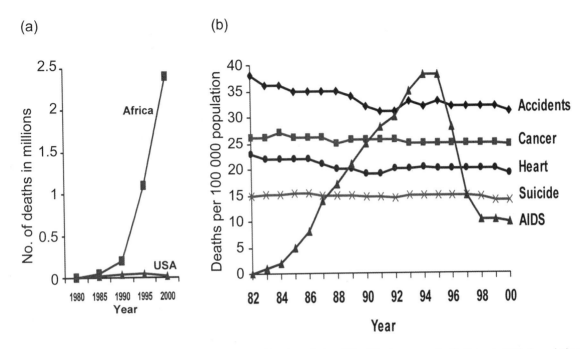

Figure 25.10 (a) Annual AIDS deaths in sub-Saharan Africa (population 640 million) compared with those in USA (population 273 million). (b) Deaths in the USA in more detail, showing the five leading causes of death in men and women aged 25–44 years. Over the course of 10 years, AIDS came to be the leading cause of death in this generally healthy age group. The sharp decline in mortality followed the introduction of HAART, although the prevalence of HIV infection has not decreased (Weiss, 2003)

Ankara boost immunisation protocol is one of the more promising approaches (McMichael and Hanke, 2003). It is clear that any vaccine will need to induce responses against more than one epitope (because of escape) and will probably need to recruit both humoral and T cell responses. Such a vaccine must either offer protection across HIV subtypes, or include antigens derived from multiple subtypes.

CONCLUSIONS AND PROSPECTS

During the 20 years since HIV-1 was first isolated and characterised (Barré-Sinoussi *et al.*, 1983), we have made immense progress in understanding HIV infection and AIDS. Early scientific research was rapidly translated to provide sensitive and accurate blood tests for HIV infection that led to the introduction of blood donor screening in 1985. Our knowledge of the molecular biology of HIV replication led directly to antiretroviral therapy. Although HAART has yet to make any impact on AIDS mortality in Africa (Figure 25.10A), it has had a profound effect in reducing mortality in Europe and USA (Figure 25.10B).

Although antiretroviral therapy is now being introduced into developing countries, and behavioural and social changes can help to reduce HIV transmission (Valdiserri *et al.*, 2003), the most important advance for controlling the HIV pandemic will be a safe and efficacious vaccine to prevent HIV infection. Unfortunately, HIV has so far defied the best scientific efforts to develop such a vaccine, but it is imperative that this goal continues to be pursued with vigour and innovation.

REFERENCES

Achong BG, Mansell PW, Epstein MA *et al.* (1971) An unusual virus in cultures from a human nasopharyngeal carcinoma. *J Natl Cancer Inst*, **46**, 299–307.

Ali M, Taylor GP, Pitman RJ *et al.* (1996) No evidence of antibody to human foamy virus in widespread human populations. *AIDS Res Hum Retrovir*, **12**, 1473–1483.

Allardice GM, Hole DJ, Brewster DH *et al.* (2003) Incidence of malignant neoplasms among HIV-infected persons in Scotland. *Br J Cancer*, **89**, 505–507.

An P, Martin MP, Nelson GW *et al.* (2000) Influence of CCR5 promoter haplotypes on AIDS progression in African-Americans. *AIDS*, **14**, 2117–2122.

Atkins M, Strappe P, Kaye S *et al.* (1998) Quantitative differences in the distribution of zidovudine resistance mutations in multiple post-mortem tissues from AIDS patients. *J Med Virol*, **55**, 138–146.

Auvert B, Buvé A, Ferry B *et al.* (2001) Ecological and individual level analysis of risk factors for HIV infection in four urban populations in sub-Saharan Africa with different levels of HIV infection. *AIDS*, **15**(suppl 4), S15–S30.

Baba M, Nishimura O, Kanzaki N *et al.* (1999) A small-molecule, nonpeptide CCR5 antagonist with highly potent and selective anti-HIV-1 activity. *Proc Natl Acad Sci USA*, **96**, 5698–59703.

Barré-Sinoussi F, Chermann JC, Rey F *et al.* (1983) Isolation of a T-lymphotropic retrovirus from a patient at risk for acquired immune deficiency syndrome (AIDS). *Science*, **220**, 868–871.

Berger EA, Doms RW, Fenyo E-M *et al.* (1998) A new classification for HIV-1. *Nature*, **391**, 240.

Berger EA, Murphy PM and Farber JM (1999) Chemokine receptors as HIV-1 co-receptors: roles in viral entry, tropism, and disease. *Ann Rev Immunol*, **17**, 657–700.

Berry N and Tedder RS (1999) HIV-1 and HIV-2 molecular diagnosis. In *HIV and the New Viruses* (eds Dalgleish AG and Weiss RA), pp 207–222. Academic Press, London.

Boshoff C and Weiss RA (2002) AIDS-related malignancies. *Nature Rev Can*, **2**, 373–382.

Brun-Vezinet F, Boucher C, Loveday C *et al.* (1997) HIV-1 viral load, phenotype, and resistance in a subset of drug-naive participants from the Delta trial. The National Virology Groups. Delta Virology Working Group and Coordinating Committee. *Lancet*, **350**, 983–990.

Carr A (2003) HIV lipodystrophy: risk factors, pathogenesis, diagnosis and management. *AIDS*, **17**(suppl 1), S141–S148.

Carrington M and O'Brien SJ (2003) The influence of HLA genotype on AIDS. *Ann Rev Med*, **54**, 535–551.

Centers for Disease Control (1985) Revision of the case definition of acquired immunodeficiency syndrome for national reporting: United States. *Morbid Mortal Wkly Rep*, **34**, 373–375.

Centers for Disease Control (1993) Review classification system for HIV infection and expanded case definition for AIDS amongst adolescents and adults. *Morbid Mortal Wkly Rep*, **43**, 1–19.

Centers for Disease Control (1994) Review classification system for human immunodeficiency virus infection in children less than 13 years of age. *Morbid Mortal Wkly Rep*, **43**, RR–12.

Chang Y, Cesarman E, Pessin MS *et al.* (1994) Identification of herpesvirus-like DNA sequences in AIDS-associated Kaposi's sarcoma. *Science*, **266**, 1865–1869.

Cheingsong-Popov R, Weiss RA, Dalgleish A *et al.* (1984) Prevalence of antibody to human T-lymphotropic virus type III in AIDS and AIDS-risk patients in Britain. *Lancet*, **2**, 477–480.

Clavel F, Brun Vezinet F, Guetard D *et al.* (1986) LAV type II: a second retrovirus associated with AIDS in West Africa. *C R Acad Sci III*, **302**, 485–488.

Cocchi F, DeVico AL, Garzino Demo A *et al.* (1995) Identification of RANTES, MIP-1α, and MIP-1β as the major HIV-suppressive factors produced by CD8$^+$ T cells. *Science*, **270**, 1811–1815.

Coffin J, Hughes SH and Varmus HE (1997) *Retroviruses*, pp 1–843. Cold Spring Harbor Laboratory Press, New York.

Cohen J (2003) HIV/AIDS. Vaccine results lose significance under scrutiny. *Science*, **299**, 1495.

Communicable Disease Surveillance Centre (2004) HIV and AIDS in the United Kingdom quarterly update: data to end December 2003. *CDR Weekly*, **14**(7). http://www.hpa.org.uk/cdr/pages/hiv.htm

Connor EM, Sperling RS, Gelber R *et al.* (1994) Reduction of maternal–infant transmission of human immunodeficiency virus type 1 with zidovudine treatment. Pediatric AIDS Clinical Trials Group Protocol 076 Study Group. *N Engl J Med*, **331**, 1173–1180.

Conrad B, Weissmahr RN, Boni J *et al.* (1997) A human endogenous retroviral superantigen as candidate autoimmune gene in type I diabetes. *Cell*, **90**, 303–313.

Dalgleish AG, Beverley PC, Clapham PR *et al.* (1984) The CD4 (T4) antigen is an essential component of the receptor for the AIDS retrovirus. *Nature*, **312**, 763–767.

D'Aquila RT, Schapiro JM, Brun-Vezinet F *et al.* (2003) Drug resistance mutations in HIV-1. *Topics HIV Med*, **11**, 92–96.

Deeks SG and Hirschel B (2002) Supervised interruptions of antiretroviral therapy. *AIDS*, **16**, S157–169.

Dupin N, Fisher C, Kellam P *et al.* (1999) Distribution of human herpesvirus-8 latently infected cells in Kaposi's sarcoma, multicentric Castleman's disease, and primary effusion lymphoma. *Proc Natl Acad Sci USA*, **96**, 4546–4551.

Egger M, May M, Chene G *et al.* (2002) Prognosis of HIV-1-infected patients starting highly active antiretroviral therapy: a collaborative analysis of prospective studies. *Lancet*, **360**, 119–129.

Emerman M and Malim MH (1998) HIV-1 regulatory/accessory genes: keys to unraveling viral and host cell biology. *Science*, **280**, 1880–1884.

Feng Y, Broder CC, Kennedy PE *et al.* (1996) HIV-1 entry cofactor: functional cDNA cloning of a seven-transmembrane, G protein-coupled receptor. *Science*, **272**, 872–877.

Gallo RC, Salahuddin SZ, Popovic M *et al.* (1984) Human T-lymphotropic retrovirus, HTLV-III, isolated from AIDS patients and donors at risk for AIDS. *Science*, **224**, 500–503.

Geijtenbeek TB, Kwon DS, Torensma R *et al.* (2000) DC-SIGN, a dendritic cell-specific HIV-1-binding protein that enhances trans-infection of T cells. *Cell*, **100**, 587–597.

Gisselquist D, Potterat JJ, Brody S *et al.* (2003) Let it be sexual: how health care transmission of AIDS in Africa was ignored. *Int J STD AIDS*, **14**, 148–161.

Gottlieb MS, Schroff R, Schanker HM *et al.* (1981) *Pneumocystis carinii* pneumonia and mucosal candidiasis in previously healthy homosexual men: evidence of a new acquired cellular immunodeficiency. *N Engl J Med*, **305**, 1425–1431.

Grant RM, Hecht FM, Warmerdam M *et al.* (2002) Time trends in primary HIV-1 drug resistance among recently infected persons. *J Am Med Assoc*, **288**, 181–188.

Gulick RM (2003) New antiretroviral drugs. *Clin Microbiol Infect*, **9**, 186–193.

Hahn BH, Shaw GM, De Cock KM *et al.* (2000) AIDS as a zoonosis: scientific and public health implications. *Science*, **287**, 607–614.

Hatziioannou T, Cowan S, Goff SP *et al.* (2003) Restriction of multiple divergent retroviruses by Lv1 and Ref1. *EMBO J*, **22**, 385–394.

Heneine W, Switzer WM, Sandstrom P *et al.* (1998) Identification of a human population infected with simian foamy viruses. *Nature Med*, **4**, 403–407.

Ho DD (1995) Time to hit HIV, early and hard. *N Engl J Med*, **333**, 450–451.

Ho DD, Neumann AU, Perelson AS *et al.* (1995) Rapid turnover of plasma virions and CD4 lymphocytes in HIV-1 infection. *Nature*, **373**, 123–126.

Imami N and Gotch F (2002) Prospects for immune reconstitution in HIV-1 infection. *Clin Exp Immunol*, **127**, 402–411.

John M, Nolan D and Mallal S (2001) Antiretroviral therapy and the lipodystrophy syndrome. *Antivir Therapy*, **6**, 9–20.

Jung A, Maier R, Vartanian JP *et al.* (2002) Multiply infected spleen cells in HIV patients. *Nature*, **418**, 144.

Katlama C, Dominguez S, Durivier C *et al.* (2003) Long-term benefit of treatment interruption in salvage therapy (GIGAHAART ANRS 097) 10th Conference on Retroviruses and Opportunistic Infections, Boston, Abst 68.

Katlama C, Ingrand D, Loveday C *et al.* (1996) Safety and efficacy of lamivudine–zidovudine combination therapy in antiretroviral-naive patients. A randomized controlled comparison with zidovudine monotherapy. Lamivudine European HIV Working Group. *J Am Med Assoc*, **276**, 118–125.

Kaye S, Loveday C and Tedder RS (1992) A microtitre format point mutation assay: application to the detection of drug resistance in human immunodeficiency virus type-1 infected patients treated with zidovudine. *J Med Virol*, **37**, 241–246.

Kinloch S, Cooper D, Lampe F *et al.* (2003) The QUEST study: treatment of primary HIV infection with quadruple HAART. National Conference of Retroviruses and Opportunistic Infections, Boston, USA, abstr 520.

Korber B, Muldoon M, Theiler J *et al.* (2000) Timing the ancestor of the HIV-1 pandemic strains. *Science*, **288**, 1789–1796.

Kostrikis LG, Huang Y, Moore JP *et al.* (1998) A chemokine receptor CCR2 allele delays HIV-1 disease progression and is associated with a CCR5 promoter mutation. *Nature Med*, **4**, 350–353.

Lalezari JP, Henry K, O'Hearn M *et al.* (2003) Enfuvirtide, an HIV-1 fusion inhibitor, for drug-resistant HIV infection in North and South America. *N Engl J Med*, **348**, 2175–2185.

Lemey P, Pybus OG, Wang B *et al.* (2003) Tracing the origin and history of the HIV-2 epidemic. *Proc Natl Acad Sci USA*, **100**, 6588–6592.

Letvin NL and Walker BD (2003) Immunopathogenesis and immunotherapy in AIDS virus infections. *Nature Med*, **9**, 861–866.

Levy JA (1998) *HIV and the pathogensis of AIDS*. American Society for Microbiology Press, Washington, DC.

Levy JA, Hoffman AD, Kramer SM *et al.* (1984) Isolation of lymphocytopathic retroviruses from San Francisco patients with AIDS. *Science*, **225**, 840–842.

Little SJ, Holte S, Routy JP *et al.* (2002) Antiretroviral-drug resistance among patients recently infected with HIV. *N Engl J Med*, **347**, 385–394.

Livingstone WJ, Moore M, Innes D *et al.* (1996) Frequent infection of peripheral blood CD8-positive T-lymphocytes with HIV-1. Edinburgh Heterosexual Transmission Study Group. *Lancet*, **348**, 649–654.

Loveday C (1999) Ultrasensitive assays for nucleic acid quantification. In *Scientific and Clinical Implications of Resistance to Antiretroviral Agents* (ed. Simmonds H). Mediscript Press.

Loveday C, Dunn D, Green H *et al.* on behalf of the ERA Steering Committee (2003) XII International HIV Drug Resistance Workshop, June 2003, Caba del Sol, Mexico, abstr *Antiviral Therapy*.

Loveday C and Hill A (1995) Prediction of progression to AIDS with serum HIV-1 RNA and CD4 count. *Lancet*, **345**, 790–791.

Loveday C, Kaye S, Tenant-Flowers M *et al.* (1995) HIV-1 RNA serum-load and resistant viral genotypes during early zidovudine therapy. *Lancet*, **345**, 820–824.

Löwer R, Löwer J and Kurth R (1996) The viruses in all of us: characteristics and biological significance of human endogenous retrovirus sequences. *Proc Natl Acad Sci USA*, **93**, 5177–5184.

Maddon PJ, Dalgleish AG, McDougal JS *et al.* (1986) The T4 gene encodes the AIDS virus receptor and is expressed in the immune system and the brain. *Cell*, **47**, 333–348.

Mathews WC (2003) Screening for anal dysplasia associated with human papillomavirus. *Topics HIV Med*, **11**, 45–49.

McCune JM (2001) The dynamics of CD4$^+$ T-cell depletion in HIV disease. *Nature*, **410**, 974–979.

McKnight A, Griffiths DJ, Dittmar M *et al.* (2001) Characterization of a late entry event in the replication cycle of human immunodeficiency virus type 2. *J Virol*, **75**, 6914–6922.

McMichael AJ and Hanke T (2003) HIV vaccines 1983–2003. *Nature Med*, **9**, 874–880.

Mellors JW, Rinaldo CR Jr, Gupta P *et al.* (1996) Prognosis in HIV-1 infection predicted by the quantity of virus in plasma. *Science*, **272**, 1167–1170.

Mi S, Lee X, Li X *et al.* (2000) Syncytin is a captive retroviral envelope protein involved in human placental morphogenesis. *Nature*, **403**, 785–789.

Miller V, Mocroft A, Reiss P *et al.* (1999) Relations among CD4 lymphocyte count nadir, antiretroviral therapy, and HIV-1 disease progression: results from the EuroSIDA study. *Ann Intern Med*, **130**, 570–577.

Montaner JS, Mo T, Raboud JM *et al.* (2000) Human immunodeficiency virus-infected persons with mutations conferring resistance to zidovudine show reduced virologic responses to hydroxyurea and stavudine-lamivudine. *J Infect Dis*, **181**, 729–732.

Moore JP, Kitchen SG, Pugach P and Zack JA (2004) The CCR5 and CXCR4 coreceptors—central to understanding the transmission and pathogenesis of human immunodeficiency type 1 infection. *AIDS Res Hu Retroviruses*, **20**, 111–126.

Nolan D, John M and Mallal S (2001) Antiretroviral therapy and the lipodystrophy syndrome, part 2: concepts in aetiopathogenesis. *Antivir Therapy*, **6**, 145–160.

O'Brien SJ and Moore JP (2000) The effect of genetic variation in chemokines and their receptors on HIV transmission and progression to AIDS. *Immunol Rev*, **177**, 99–111.

Parry JV, Murphy G, Barlow KL *et al.* (2001) National surveillance of HIV-1 subtypes for England and Wales: design, methods, and initial findings. *J Acqu Immune Defic Syndr*, **26**, 381–388.

Perelson AS (2002) Modelling viral and immune system dynamics. *Nature Rev Immunol*, **2**, 28–36.

Perron H, Garson JA, Bedin F *et al.* (1997) Molecular identification of a novel retrovirus repeatedly isolated from patients with multiple sclerosis. *Proc Natl Acad Sci USA*, **94**, 7583–7588.

Pizzo P and Wilfert C (1994) *Paediatric AIDS*. Williams and Wilkins, Baltimore, MD.

Pomerantz RJ and Horn DL (2003) Twenty years of therapy for HIV-1 infection. *Nature Med*, **9**, 867–873.

Pope M and Haase AT (2003) Transmission, acute HIV-1 infection and the quest for strategies to prevent infection. *Nature Med*, **9**, 847–852.

Rosenblum L and McClure M (1999) Non-lentiviral primate retroviruses. In *HIV and the New Viruses*, 2nd edn (eds Dalgleish AG and Weiss RA), pp 251–279. Academic Press, London.

Schmid GP, Buvé A, Mugyenyi P *et al.* (2004) Transmission of HIV-1 infection in sub-Saharan Africa and effect of elimination of unsafe injections. *Lancet*, **363**, 482–488.

Schuurman R, Nijhuis M, van Leeuwen R *et al.* (1995) Rapid changes in human immunodeficiency virus type 1 RNA load and appearance of drug-resistant virus populations in persons treated with lamivudine (3TC). *J Infect Dis*, **171**, 1411–1419.

Semple MG, Kaye S, Loveday C *et al.* (1993) HIV-1 plasma viraemia quantification: a non-culture measurement needed for therapeutic trials. *J Virol Meth*, **41**, 167–179.

Serwadda D, Mugerwa RD, Sewankambo NK *et al.* (1985) Slim disease: a new disease in Uganda and its association with HTLV-III infection. *Lancet*, **2**, 849–852.

Sheehy AM, Gaddis NC and Malim MH (2003) The antiretroviral enzyme APOBEC3G is degraded by the proteasome in response to HIV-1 Vif. *Nature Med*, **9**, 1404–1407.

Silvestri G, Sodora DL, Koup RA *et al.* (2003) Nonpathogenic SIV infection of sooty mangabeys is characterized by limited bystander immunopathology despite chronic high-level viremia. *Immunity*, **18**, 441–452.

Simmons G, Clapham PR, Picard L *et al.* (1997) Potent inhibition of HIV-1 infectivity in macrophages and lymphocytes by a novel CCR5 antagonist. *Science*, **276**, 276–279.

Simmons G, Wilkinson D, Reeves JD *et al.* (1996) Primary, syncytium-inducing humans immunodeficiency virus type 1 isolates are dual-tropic and most can use either Lstr or CCR5 as co-receptors for virus entry. *J Virol*, **70**, 8355–8360.

Sitas F, Carrara H, Beral V *et al.* (1999) Antibodies against human herpesvirus 8 in black South African patients with cancer. *N Engl J Med*, **340**, 1863–1871.

Stevenson M (2003) HIV-1 pathogenesis. *Nature Med*, **9**, 853–860.

Torre D and Tambini R (2002) Antiretroviral drug resistance testing in patients with HIV-1 infection: a meta-analysis study. *HIV Clin Trials*, **3**, 1–8.

UK Collaborative Group on Monitoring the Transmission of HIV Drug Resistance (2001) Analysis of prevalence of HIV-1 drug resistance in primary infections in the United Kingdom. *Br Med J*, **322**, 1087–1088.

UNAIDS (2003) http://www.unaids.org/en/resources/epidemiology/epidemicupdateslides.asp

UNAIDS (2003) Expert Group stresses that unsafe sex is primary mode of HIV transmission in Africa. http://www.unaids.org/whatsnew/press/eng/HIVinjections140303_en.html.

Valdiserri RO, Ogden LL and McCray E (2003) Accomplishments in HIV prevention science: implications for stemming the epidemic. *Nature Med*, **9**, 881–886.

Venables PJ, Brookes SM, Griffiths D *et al.* (1995) Abundance of an endogenous retroviral envelope protein in placental trophoblasts suggests a biological function. *Virology*, **211**, 589–592.

Vilmer E, Fischer A, Griscelli C *et al.* (1984) Possible transmission of a human lymphotropic retrovirus (LAV) from mother to infant with AIDS. *Lancet*, **2**, 229–230.

Walker PR, Worobey M, Rambaut A *et al.* (2003) Epidemiology: sexual transmission of HIV in Africa. *Nature*, **422**, 679.

Wei X, Ghosh SK, Taylor ME *et al.* (1995) Viral dynamics in human immunodeficiency virus type 1 infection. *Nature*, **373**, 117–122.

Weiss RA (1998) Xenotransplantation. *Br Med J*, **317**, 931–934.

Weiss RA (2003) HIV and AIDS: looking ahead. *Nature Med*, **9**, 887–891.

Westby M, Manca F and Dalgleish AG (1996) The role of host immune responses in determining the outcome of HIV infection. *Immunol Today*, **17**, 120–126.

Zhu T, Korber BT, Nahmias AJ *et al.* (1998) An African HIV-1 sequence from 1959 and implications for the origin of the epidemic. *Nature*, **391**, 594–597.

25A

The Human T Cell Lymphotropic Viruses

Graham P. Taylor

Imperial College, London, UK

INTRODUCTION

The HTLV-BLV viruses are a subfamily of retroviruses. They comprise human T lymphotropic virus types I and II (HTLV-I, HTLV-II); bovine leukaemia virus (BLV); and an increasing number of simian or primate T lymphotropic viruses (STLV/PTLVs) closely related to HTLV-I and -II. HTLV-I infection is usually asymptomatic but is associated with malignant and inflammatory diseases and mild or selective impairment of immune function in a minority. Disease associations with HTLV-II are less well established. STLVs have been associated with malignant disease in non-human primates, but not necessarily in the primary host species. In a small proportion of naturally infected cattle, BLV is associated with a B cell leukaemia. However, leukaemia is very common in experimentally BLV-infected sheep.

HISTORY

The discovery of HTLV-I as an important human pathogen was the result of two distinct lines of research. One, the long search for cancer-causing retroviruses in humans, was dependent on the earlier discovery and refinement of tests for reverse transcriptase, together with the identification and use in cell culture of T cell growth factor, now known as interleukin 2 (IL-2). In 1980, Gallo's team found one of their many transformed T cell lines derived from leukaemia/lymphoma patients to contain a retrovirus (Poiesz *et al.*, 1980). This virus, now known as the human T lymphotropic virus type I, is also known as the human T cell leukaemia/lymphoma virus type I. The second was the recognition (1974) and description (1977) of a new disease entity, adult T cell leukaemia-lymphoma (ATLL) by Takatsuki and colleagues, in Japan (Uchiyama *et al.*, 1997). The clustering of this disease, particularly in south-western Japan, suggested an environmental or infectious aetiology. Gallo's cell line was derived from the lymphocytes of an Afro-American patient with an aggressive form of cutaneous T cell lymphoma subsequently recognised to be cutaneous ATLL. In 1981 Miyoshi and colleagues produced an immortalised T cell line by the co-culture of peripheral blood lymphocytes from a woman with ATLL with cord blood cells from a male baby (Miyoshi *et al.*, 1981). This cell line (MT-2), which has an XY karyotype, was observed to produce numerous extracellular type C retroviral particles and was positive for adult T cell leukaemia antigen by indirect immunofluorescence (Hinuma *et al.*, 1981). Using viral antigens from MT-2 cells to develop a serological test, they demonstrated that nearly all ATLL patients and a high proportion of their relatives had antibodies to this virus (Yoshida *et al.*, 1982). Known initially in Japan as adult T cell leukaemia virus (ATLV), sequence analysis showed that ATLV was almost identical with HTLV-I. Seroprevalence studies revealed that ATLV/HTLV-I was endemic in south-western Japan, with 15% of the population seropositive, rising to 30% in some villages. In Central Japan only 1% of the population were seropositive, with higher rates again in the north. The inhabitants of central Japan are believed to have come from mainland Asia circa BC 300, displacing the 'older' population to the north and south-west. This

Principles and Practice of Clinical Virology, Fifth Edition. Edited by A. J. Zuckerman, J. E. Banatvala, J. R. Pattison, P. D. Griffiths and B. D. Schoub
© 2004 John Wiley & Sons Ltd   ISBN 0 470 84338 1

distribution suggests that the arrival of HTLV-I in Japan preceded this migration. A high seroprevalence of HTLV-I in patients in Martinique with tropical spastic paraparesis was first described in 1985 (Gessain *et al.*, 1985) and an identical condition, HTLV-I associated myelopathy (HAM), was described in Japan the following year (Osame *et al.*, 1986). This disease is commonly referred to as HAM/TSP but here the acronym HAM will be used, as the data presented refer only to HTLV-I associated myelopathy. HTLV-I-seronegative TSP occurs.

A related virus, HTLV-II was isolated from the cells of a patient with an atypical hairy cell leukaemia (HCL) in 1982 (Kalyanaraman *et al.*, 1982). Hairy cell leukaemias are usually of B cell origin; however, the infected cell line expressed T cell markers. Although HTLV-II was isolated from a second patient with HCL, subsequent extensive investigation has failed to confirm any association between HCL and HTLV-II infection. HTLV-II shares 60–70% sequence homology with HTLV-I and anti-HTLV-II antibodies are detected by HTLV-I lysate or whole virus-based assays.

Simian T lymphotropic viruses have been found in macaques and other Old World monkeys, and STLV-I appears to be more closely related to HTLV-I than to other STLV/PTLVs. HTLV-I/STLV-I strains cluster geographically rather than by host species. During the last few years a number of STLVs closely related to but discrete from HTLV-I have been characterised. These include relatives of HTLV-II (Giri *et al.*, 1994) and viruses, which cluster with neither HTLV/STLV-I nor -II. The first of these, found in an Eritrean baboon (*Papio hamadryas*), was designated PTLV-L after Leuven, where the baboon was residing and the virus was isolated (Goubau *et al.*, 1994), HTLV-III having already been used as a former name for human immunodeficiency virus type 1. STLVs isolated from wild-caught red-capped mangabeys (*Cercocebus torquatus*) from Cameroon are distinct from, but cluster with, PTLV-L in the newly designated PTLV-3 type (Meertens *et al.*, 2002).

THE VIRUS

Morphologically, HTLV-I and -II resemble C-type retroviruses (Figure 25A.1). They can be grown *in vitro* in immortalised lines obtained by culturing patients' cells with phytohaemagglutinin (PHA) and IL-2. *De novo* infection of T cells and cell lines requires co-cultivation using irradiated or mitomycin-C-treated HTLV producer cell lines. The HTLVs are not readily transmissible in cell-free form and this is reflected in the observation that only whole fresh blood transfusion and not plasma or other cell-free fractions results in transmission (Okochi *et al.*, 1984).

Susceptible cell lines can be identified by the formation of syncytia (giant multinucleated cells) upon contact with virus-producing cells. This interaction requires the presence of the HTLV-I envelope and specific cell membrane ligands (receptors). The syncytial assay has proved useful in studying HTLV-I, particularly for the detection of neutralising antibodies and cellular receptors (Clapham *et al.*, 1984). *In vitro*, many cell types from a broad range of species, including astrocytes, can be infected. *In vivo*, HTLV-I primarily infects $CD4^+$ lymphocytes whilst HTLV-II infects $CD8^+$ lymphocytes. However HTLV-I infection of $CD8^+$ lymphocytes does occur and is more common among HTLV-I specific cytotoxic $CD8^+$ lymphocytes than other $CD8^+$ cells (Hanon *et al.*, 2000). Richardson *et al.* (1990) found no evidence of HTLV-I infection of B cells, monocytes or natural killer (NK) cells *in vivo* but others have reported infection in B cells, monocytes (Koyanagi *et al.*, 1993) and NK cells (Igakura *et al.*, 2003). Whether HTLV-I infection of neural cells occurs *in vivo* remains controversial. Although the cellular receptor has not been identified the coding gene has been reportedly localised to chromosome 17. Various receptors have been proposed with neuropilin-1 (Ghez *et al.*, 2003) and GLUT-1 (Manel *et al.*, 2003) the most recent. The envelope proteins of HTLV-I and HTLV-II are the target for neutralising antibodies. Sera from British or American patients and asymptomatic carriers of HTLV-I equally neutralise viruses from other countries including Japan (Clapham *et al.*, 1984). This suggests that there is a single worldwide serotype for HTLV-I.

The 9 kb genome of HTLV-I contains the three major open reading frames (ORFs), *gag*, *pol* and *env*, of all retroviruses flanked by two long terminal repeats (LTR) with an additional regulatory region, pX (Figure 25A.2). The names, product size and functions of the genes of HTLV-I are summarised in Table 25A.1. The HTLV-II genome is very similar except that five ORFs have been identified in pX.

The LTR containing the viral promoter and other regulatory elements are divided into three regions, U3, R and U5. The U3 region contains elements that control proviral transcription, messenger RNA termination and polyadenylation.

The first major reading frame (*gag*) encodes a 429 amino acid precursor polyprotein Pr53^{Gag}. A second major reading frame within the *gag–pol* complex

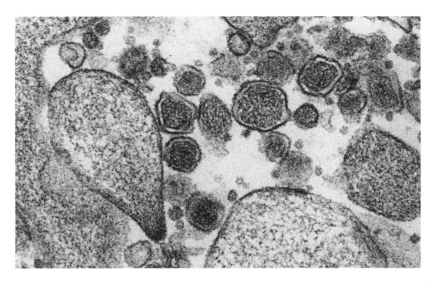

Figure 25A.1 Electron micrograph of HTLV-I particles produced by a T cell line transformed *in vitro*. Note the variable size of the particles and the diffuse spherical core

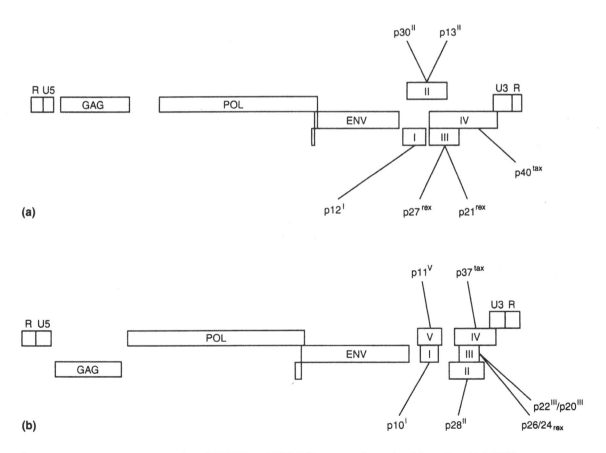

Figure 25A.2 Schematic representation of HTLV-I and HTLV-II genomes. Reproduced from Franchini (1995)

Table 25A.1 Products of HTLV-I genes

5' LTR	Contains regulatory elements essential for viral replication			
gag	*Group antigen nucleocapsid proteins*		p19	Matrix
			p24	Capsid
			p15	Nucleocapsid
pol	*Polymerase*	Reverse transcriptase	RT	Transcription of DNA from RNA
		Proteinase		Cleavage of protein precursors
		RNaseH		Digestion of RNA template
		Integrase		Integration of proviral DNA into host genome
env	*Envelope*	Surface glycoprotein	gp46	SU
		Transmembrane	gp21	TM
pX	ORF I		p12^{I}	(Rof) Infectivity
	ORF II		p13^{II}	Mitochondrial protein
			p30^{II}	(Tof) Modulation of cellular gene transcription
	ORF III		p27	Rex *Regulatory gene of 'X' region*
			p21^{rexIII}	Cytoplasmic protein unknown function
	ORF IV		p40	Tax *Trans activating gene of 'X' region*
3' LTR	Contains regulatory elements essential for viral replication			

encodes a second precursor, Pr76$^{Gag-Pro}$, which gives rise to the viral protease. This frame slightly overlaps with *gag* and is generated by a frameshift suppression of the *gag* terminator codon. During viral assembly the *gag* precursors accumulate at the inner face of the plasma membrane and are anchored there by the matrix domain. In the absence of protease, immature viral particles are released. During and early after viral budding, cleavage of Pr53^{Gag} into the three major structural proteins of the core of the virus, 19 kDa (matrix protein), 24 kDa (capsid protein) and 15 kDa (nucleocapsid protein), results in the formation of the mature virion. The viral genome is transported to the cell envelope bound to the *gag* precursor. The matrix domain of the *gag* precursor is involved in targeting of the *gag* precursor–genome complex to the plasma membrane (this also requires myristoylation of the polyprotein) and in efficient budding of the viral particle from the cell. The mature (cleaved) matrix protein also plays a role early in the replication cycle, in viral entry, as virions with defective matrix proteins have reduced infectivity even when properly released (Le Blanc *et al.*, 1999). The capsid proteins assemble during viral maturation to form the shell around the core of the nucleus. The N-terminal domain is essential for viral particle formation (Rayne *et al.*, 2001). In the viral particle the nucleocapsid protein is also a key component of the capsid and is in close contact with the genome. In the cell the nucleocapsid domain of the Gag precursor polyprotein is important for recognition and packaging of the viral genome. Retroviral Gag function is reviewed in Wills and Craven (1991).

The remaining products of *pol*, reverse transcriptase (RT) and integrase are encoded by a different open

reading frame and are cleaved from a 99 kDa precursor protein. RT transcribes the single viral RNA strand, generating first the complementary DNA strand and then using that as the template for the viral DNA version of the original RNA, which is digested by RNaseH. This double-stranded DNA is integrated into a host cell chromosome. Having no proof-reading mechanism, RT is error-prone and a high frequency of mutation would be expected to result in HTLV/STLV sequence diversity.

Env encodes a 481 amino acid protein that after glycosylation has a molecular weight of 62 kDa and is processed into an outer surface protein of 46 kDa and a transmembrane protein of 21 kDa. The envelope precursor is translated from a 4.2 kb mRNA from which *gag* and *pol* have been spliced out.

The fifth genomic region, referred to as pX, is located between *env* and the 3' LTR. The region codes for *tax* and *rex*, which are translated from a double-spliced 2.1 kb mRNA as well as three additional proteins encoded by open reading frames I, II and III, whose functions are slowly being revealed. Tax, a 40 kDa protein that is expressed early, drives viral transcription from Tax-responsive elements (21 bp repeats) in the LTR U3 and is an important upregulator of viral replication. In addition, *tax* transactivates a range of host cellular genes, through which it is thought to affect cell replication and play an important role in the pathogenesis of ATLL. The immunodominant peptides for the host cytotoxic T-lymphocyte response are also usually found in the Tax protein. This may be important both for the control of infection and in the pathogenesis of inflammatory disease associated with HTLV-I, of which the archetype is HTLV-I associated myelopathy. Rex is a

27 kDa phosphoprotein which determines the export of unspliced *gag–pol* mRNA and singly-spliced *env* mRNA from the nucleus, thereby controlling the production of viral proteins and infectious virus (Rex production results in increased export of *env* mRNA and unspliced viral RNA for the Gag/Pol proteins essential for the production of new virions and aids a shift from doubly-spliced pX RNA to *gag–pol* and *env* RNA). Thus, the overall effect of Rex may be virion production soon after infection, followed by down-regulation of viral expression. This may protect the infected cell from death due to the cytolytic effect of virion production and protect both the infected cell and the virus from the host immune response (Hidaka *et al.*, 1998).

The Tax (p37) and Rex (p26) proteins of HTLV-II are slightly smaller than those of HTLV-I. HTLV-II Tax shares 72–74% amino acid homology with HTLV-I Tax. However, the C termini of HTLV-II Tax (both HTLV-IIa and HTLV-IIb) are different from HTLV-I Tax. Tax IIa has a 22 amino acid truncation at the C terminus, whilst the C terminus of Tax IIb has 25 amino acids, which are totally different from Tax I (Lewis *et al.*, 2000). *In vitro*, HTLV-II Tax proteins activate transcription of NF-κB and the CREB pathways as well as HTLV-I Tax, although Tax from some HTLV-IIa isolates had much less transcriptional activity, possibly due to low levels of expression of Tax (Lewis *et al.*, 2002). However both Tax IIa and Tax IIb are less efficient at transforming rat fibroblast cell lines than Tax I (Endo *et al.*, 2002).

The additional proteins are p13 and p30 (ORF-II) and p12 from ORF I. p30[II] Localises to the nucleus and may modulate transcription of cellular genes. p13[II] Localises to mitochondria and *in vitro* disrupts the mitochondrial inner membrane potential. Although not essential for viral replication, these proteins are important for viral infectivity. p12[I] Exhibits weak oncogenic activity and is important in infectivity (reviewed by Ciminale *et al.*, 1996; Johnson *et al.*, 2001).

DIAGNOSIS

Detection of HTLV-I and -II infection is primarily by serology. A particle agglutination assay based on whole viral lysate is sensitive for both viruses but limited by poor specificity. First-generation commercial enzyme immunoassays (EIAs) were more specific than the agglutination assays but less sensitive particularly for HTLV-II. EIAs incorporating recom-

binant peptides are highly sensitive and specific for HTLV-I and HTLV-II. Immunofluorescence assays using fixed infected cells with uninfected cells as controls can be used to confirm and type infections, but are subjective. Peptide-based assays that discriminate between HTLV-I and HTLV-II have been developed. HTLV-I infection is usually confirmed by the detection of antibodies to Gag (p19 and p24) and Env (gp21 and gp46) by Western blot (Figure 25A.3), although radio-immune precipitation assays (RIPA), radio-immune binding assays (RIBAs), line immuno-precipitation assays (LIPAs) and competitive ELISAs can also be used. p19 Antibody is often absent in, and not required to confirm, HTLV-II infection. Recombinant Env peptides have improved the sensitivity and specificity of Western blots and type-specific antigens rgp46-I and rgp-46-II enable the infections to be discriminated without resort to molecular methods. Minimal criteria for the diagnosis of HTLV infection are the detection of antibodies to one Gag and one Env protein. Western blots which reveal some virus-specific bands but which are not sufficient to make a positive diagnosis are termed 'indeterminate'. Further investigation is then warranted, including DNA amplification using generic or type-specific primers and repeat serology after a few weeks. Viral culture may be required to confirm an infection but is costly, time consuming and must be conducted in a Category 3 laboratory (HTLV European Research Network, 1996). Although HTLV-I viral DNA load is frequently high in asymptomatic carriers very low levels, < 1 HTLV DNA copy per 100 000 PBMCs, can be found and a negative PCR does not exclude the diagnosis of HTLV infection. In European studies, HTLV-I/II infection was not confirmed in the majority of low risk subjects with WB indeterminate sera, whereas among HIV-infected injecting drug users (IDU) HTLV-II infection might be found by DNA amplification. Indeterminate WB patterns are common in the tropics, and may be more common than confirmed HTLV-I infection, even in endemic areas. In this setting antibodies to Gag proteins only have been associated with a low risk of HTLV infection (Rouet *et al.*, 2001).

The presence of the recombinant surface membrane glycoprotein (RD21 in the HTLV 2.4 WB, Genelabs, Singapore) alone may reflect recent infection and a follow-up sample should be obtained. Antibodies to the Gag proteins p19 and p24 usually appear early following seroconversion, whereas antibodies to the transmembrane glycoprotein gp46 appear later. Anti-Tax antibodies occur late or not at all (Manns *et al.*, 1994).

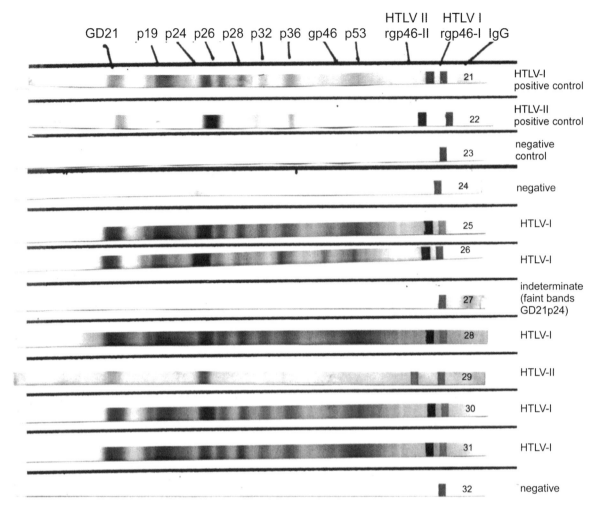

Figure 25A.3   Western blot with recombinant peptides which discriminate between HTLV-I and HTLV-II infection (Genelabs HTLV 2.4, Singapore). Courtesy of John Parry, Health Protection Agency, London, UK

VIRAL VARIATION

HTLV-I has a highly conserved genome with only about 4% sequence variation between isolates from around the world. The only exceptions are isolates from Australian aborigines and Melanesians, which form a distinct genotype or clade, HTLV-I$_{MEL}$ and which have up to 8% diversity in LTR and/or *env*. Most other isolates from Africa, Japan or the Caribbean belong to the Cosmopolitan clade, HTLV-I$_{COS}$. However, three other clades have been recognised, from Central Africa, from West Africa and from Japan (Ureta-Vidal *et al.*, 1994). In phylogenetic analyses simian T lymphotropic virus type I (STLV-I) which is almost identical to HTLV-I, clusters with

HTLV-I by geography rather than by species (Figure 25A.4). This suggests that there have been a number of simian–human transmissions (Koralnik *et al.*, 1994). HTLV-II shares 60–70% sequence homology with HTLV-I. HTLV-II isolates generally belong to genotype a or b. HTLV-IIc (Eiraku *et al.*, 1996) has to date only been described in Brazil, whilst HTLV-IId was described in Congolese pygmies (Vandamme *et al.*, 1998). A number of primate T lymphotropic virus isolates fall outside the recognised HTLV/STLV clades as described above.

The highly conserved nature of HTLV-I, HTLV-II and their simian counterparts is unexpected for a retrovirus (see discussion of reverse transcriptase, above) and quite distinct from the rapid evolution of

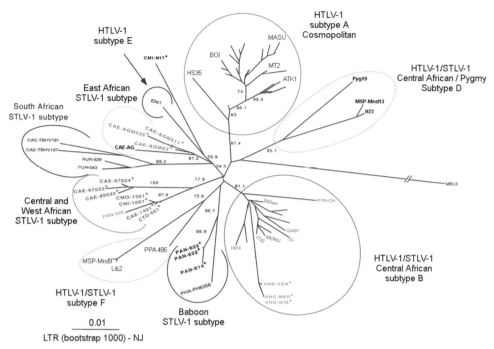

Figure 25A.4 Phylogenetic analysis showing the relationship between HTLV-I/STLV-I subtypes. Reproduced from Meertens *et al.* 2001

the human immunodeficiency viruses. RNA viruses usually evolve at 1/100–1/10 000 nucleotide substitutions/site/year, whereas HTLV-II is mutating at a rate of 1.7–7.31/10 000 000 nucleotide substitutions/site/year in the LTR. From family studies involving two or three generations it appears that HTLV-I only undergoes a few replication cycles, perhaps early following infection, in each generation (Van Dooren *et al.*, 2001). It has been shown that HTLV-II is evolving faster in IDU than in endemic populations: 2.7 nucleotide substitutions per 10 000 sites per year in IDU, which would be consistent with the virus being transmitted from one host to another after a shorter period than in the endemic populations in whom mother-to-child transmission plays an important role in maintaining the virus in the population (Salemi *et al.*, 1999).

EPIDEMIOLOGY

It has been estimated that 20 million persons worldwide are infected with HTLV-I, including 1.2 million in Japan. Other endemic areas are the Caribbean, parts of the south-eastern states of the USA, Melanesia and parts of sub-Saharan Africa, especially west and central Africa (Figure 25A.5). Recently, HTLV-I infection has been found to be relatively common in southern Africa, particularly Natal. Up to 0.5% of blood donors in Brazil are HTLV-I seropositive, with considerable interstate variation. HTLV-I infection is recognised among many native South American indigenous peoples as well as among black and Japanese immigrants. However, population mixing has been extensive and in Brazil the proportion of neurology patients with HAM/TSP is equal among the main racial groups. Northern Iran is another recently described area of HTLV-I infection with cases described in neighbouring Middle East and central Asian countries. The prevalence of HTLV-I among European Union (EU) blood donors is low (2–7/100 000) but remarkably similar across the length and breadth of the EU. Seroprevalence rates 50–100 times higher have been found among women attending antenatal clinics and among men and women attending STD clinics. However, the numbers tested are much smaller and in many countries such studies have not been conducted (Figure 25A.6). In central and eastern Europe very few studies have been conducted, but cases of HTLV-I-related pathology have been diagnosed in patients from Bulgaria, Romania and in a Georgian family. HTLV-I/II infection would appear to be rare in Hungary, although there are occasional reports of detection of deleted HTLV gene sequences

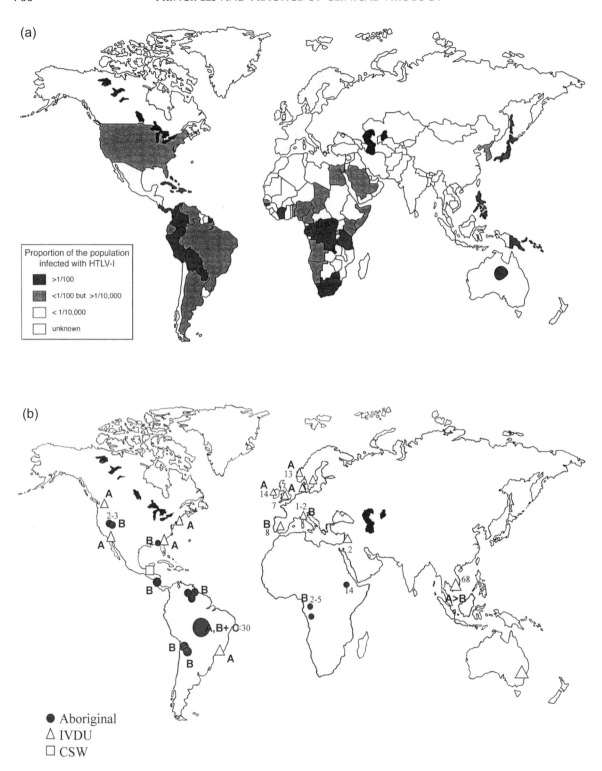

Figure 25A.5 Global seroprevalence of (a) HTLV-I and (b) HTLV-II

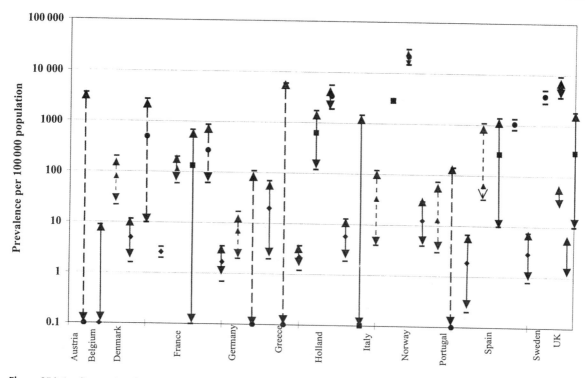

Figure 25A.6 Comparison between HTLV-I/II seroprevalence rates in different risk groups in Europe. ◆, Blood donors; ■, STD clinic attendees; σ, pregnant women; λ, IDU. Rates of HTLV-I/II among European blood donors are low but relatively uniform. Rates among the three other groups tend to have much wider 95% confidence intervals due to the smaller sample size. Compared to blood donors, the seroprevalence rate of (predominantly) HTLV-II in IDU populations is approximately 1000-fold higher; of HTLV-I among men and women attending clinics for sexually transmitted infections are approximately 100-fold higher; and of (predominantly) HTLV-I among pregnant women 10-fold higher. Data from Taylor (2002)

in seronegative subjects. Despite the importance of IDU in the spread of HIV-1 infection in former member states of the USSR, HTLV-II has not yet been detected in these high-risk populations (reviewed in Taylor, 1996). The most important recent developments in European epidemiology of HTLV infection have been: (a) the confirmation, in a large multicentre study, that HTLV-I/II infection in the EU is 10-fold more common among pregnant women than among blood donors (Taylor *et al.*, 2001); and (b) the emergence of data showing HTLV-I infection and disease (ATLL) to be relatively common in Romania. Romania can be considered to be the most recently described endemic area for HTLV-I infection and the first to be described in a Caucasian population.

HTLV-II infection is found among native American Indians in North, Central and South America and was until recently considered a New World virus. At some time prior to the AIDS epidemic, HTLV-II infection moved into, and has been spread around the 'devel-

oped' world by IDU. In Europe HTLV-II is common among IDU in Eire, Spain, Italy and Scandinavia, but rare in Germany and France. The first isolations of HTLV-II in Africa were from pygmy tribes both from Ethiopia and from West Africa (Goubau *et al.*, 1992; Gessain *et al.*, 1995). Although infection in West African prostitutes need not imply a local origin, HTLV-II has also been described in the Gabon in a male with no history to suggest exposure to an imported virus. This virus is genetically close both to the Cameroonian pygmy isolate and to a North American isolate, emphasising the conserved nature of these viruses (Letournier *et al.*, 1998). These findings, and the identification of an HTLV-II-like primate virus in Central Africa, suggest that HTLV-II, like HTLV-I, may have originated in Africa. However, a number of questions remain as HTLV-II is widely spread throughout the Americas but has been found in few populations in Africa. To date PTLVs have not been identified in New World primates and, with the exception of a report of HTLV-II in Mongolia, which may have been a recently imported infection, there is no population-based evidence of HTLV-II migrating from the Old to the New World.

TRANSMISSION

For both viruses transmission may be by three routes: from mother to child; through sexual intercourse; and through blood–blood contact. Family studies in Japan suggested that HTLV-I was mainly transmitted from mother to child (Kajiyama et al., 1986). HTLV-I was identified in lymphocytes in breast milk and transmission through breast-feeding was demonstrated in marmosets and rabbits. The mother-to-child transmission rate in Japan was 25% if babies were breast-fed, but only 5% if babies were bottle-fed. It may be that maternal anti-HTLV antibodies protect breast-feeding infants until their titre starts to decline, as in one study in Japan short-term breast-fed babies were no more likely to be infected than bottle-fed babies (Takahashi et al., 1991). Breast-feeding for 6 months is associated with higher rates of transmission, which continue to increase if weaning is further delayed. Although in one study HTLV-I was detected in cord blood, none of the cord-blood-positive babies became infected. HTLV-I has been detected but not quantified in cervico-vaginal secretions and the contribution of in utero and perinatal infections to the total infection rate is uncertain. In the Gabon the mother-to-child transmission rate was 9.7% with transmission associated with higher maternal viral load (Ureta-Vidal et al., 1999). There are conflicting data on mother-to-child transmission of HTLV-II but among the Kayapo Indians in Brazil the risk of transmission from an HTLV-II infected mother to her child was 30–50% (Ishak et al., 1995).

The aforementioned family studies also indicated that infection was likely to pass from husband to wife. In a Japanese cohort study of 100 discordant couples practising unprotected sexual intercourse, there were seven seroconversions during 5 years of observation. Uninfected females were 3.9 times more likely to become infected than uninfected males (Stuver et al., 1993). Higher rates of transmission have been reported: 60% of wives of seropositive husbands over 10 years in one study, but only 0.4% of husbands of seropositive wives; 50% of wives during 1–4 years of marriage in another. In a study of HTLV-I- and HTLV-II-infected US blood donors, those with higher HTLV-I proviral loads were more likely to have an infected partner. A similar association of transmission

with high proviral load was seen in HTLV-II, although the viral burden is generally much less than in HTLV-I (Kaplan et al., 1996). Both HTLV-I and HTLV-II are more common in females. It is reasonable to suggest that condoms will efficiently protect against transmission, but no data are available.

HTLV-I is transmitted by cell-containing blood products but not by plasma or plasma-derived products. This has been demonstrated in the rabbit model and through clinical observation. Fresh blood is more infectious than older blood, due to the short life of stored lymphocytes. Infection has occurred following transfusion of 41 ml blood. Following transfusion with HTLV-I-infected blood the median time to seroconversion was 51 days (Manns et al., 1991). The mean incubation period of HAM following infection by transfusion is 3 years, shorter than by other routes. In a post mortem study the average time to first symptoms was 8.5 months but the duration of symptoms was not different from other patients with HAM (Iwasaki, 1990). The risk of HAM was 7.7-fold higher than expected among transfusion recipients in Japan and following the introduction of blood donor screening in 1986 the incidence of HAM fell by 16%. HTLV-I is also transmitted through injecting drug use but this route is more commonly associated with HTLV-II. Indeed, outside of the endemic areas of the Americas, HTLV-II is primarily transmitted through re-use of injection paraphernalia. It seems likely that HTLV-II was introduced into the IDU population of the USA during the 1970s and into Europe slightly later.

HTLV-ASSOCIATED DISEASE

HTLV-I is recognised as a carcinogen by the International Agency for Research on Cancer (IARC Monographs on the Evaluation of Carcinogenic Risk to Humans, 1996). HTLV-I is clearly associated with ATLL and serological documentation of HTLV-I infection is an essential part of confirming this diagnosis, whereas the demonstration of clonality is only required in unusual cases. The search for sero-epidemiological evidence of an association between HTLV-I and other malignancies has been complicated by the frequent history of previous blood transfusion in patients with malignant disease included in such studies. However, two studies have demonstrated an increased rate of cervical carcinoma in patients with HTLV-I and in one of these studies patients with HTLV-I were also found to have more advanced disease. An interaction between HTLV-I and HPV directly or through an effect of HTLV-I on cell-mediated immunity is biologically plausible. However, since both HPV and HTLV-I are sexually transmitted, the association may reflect sexual activity rather than a biological interaction between two oncogenic viruses (IARC Monographs on the Evaluation of Carcinogenic Risk to Humans, 1996).

Although originally described in two patients with atypical hairy cell leukaemia, extensive studies have failed to associate HTLV-II infection with HCL. HTLV-II infection was also reported in two patients with large granular lymphocytosis and one with large granular lymphocytic leukaemia but the virus was found in the T lymphocytes and not the abnormal cells. Rare cases of $CD8^+$ lymphoproliferation in patients with HIV-1/HTLV-II co-infection have been reported, including one in which clonal expansion of HTLV-II-infected cells was demonstrated. In summary, there are as yet inadequate data to afford HTLV-II carcinogenic status, although it immortalises T cells *in vitro* (reviewed in Araujo *et al.*, 2002).

ATLL may present as acute leukaemia, chronic or smouldering leukaemia, or as a lymphoma, including a cutaneous presentation. ATLL cells are $CD3^+$ $CD4^+$ and $CD25^+$ (IL-2 receptor) and in the leukaemic form characteristic polylobed 'flower' cells (Figure 25A.7) can be easily identified. Although the cells are morphologically mature, the malignancy is aggressive and survival measured in months. The most common presentation is acute leukaemia, with lymphoma the next most common. Chronic and smouldering forms are associated with longer survival. Hypercalcaemia due to expression of PTHr peptide is a common and characteristic finding. Patients may present with acute renal failure and lytic bone lesions. Atypical presentation with opportunistic infections should also be considered.

HTLV-I is associated with a number of inflammatory conditions characterised by a lymphocytic infiltration of the target organ (Figure 25A.8). The lifetime risk of HAM in HTLV-I-infected persons is 2–7%, except in Japan where it has been estimated at 0.25%. HAM has been diagnosed in about 150 patients in the UK, mostly of Caribbean origin, but also in Caucasians. This includes at least one case following transfusion with HTLV-I-infected blood in the UK. The condition is a chronic progressive spastic paraparesis without the relapsing/remitting character of multiple sclerosis. Chronic backache, hyperactive bladder, constipation and impotence are common. Sensory signs and upper limb disease are unusual but can be found in long-standing disease. Other causes of myelopathy, including cord compression, should be

excluded (Table 25A.2). The female:male ratio is 2:1 and the onset is most common in the 3rd and 4th decades, resulting in decades of morbidity. The condition is occasionally rapidly progressive and fatal within 2 years of onset.

Uveitis is more common in HTLV-I patients than in the general population. HTLV-I-associated uveitis usually responds to treatment with topical steroids; less often systemic steroids are required. The condition is generally mild but recurs in 25% of cases (Mochizuki *et al.*, 1992). In a prospective study of 200 patients with HTLV-I in Martinique, 14.5% had uveitis, but 37% had keratoconjunctivitis sicca and interstitial keratitis was also common. (Merle *et al.*, 2002).

Polymyositis, alveolitis, arthritis and thyroiditis have been reported in subjects with HTLV-I, often in patients with HAM. Whilst these associations have not been confirmed epidemiologically, the histology/cytology characterised by lymphocytic inflammatory infiltration is consistent with an HTLV-I aetiology.

Infective dermatitis is an eczematous condition of children that only responds to long-term antibiotic treatment against *Streptococcus* and *Staphylococcus* spp., which are otherwise not usually considered pathogenic. Skin biopsies reveal an inflammatory infiltrate of $CD8^+$ lymphocytes. HTLV-associated infective dermatitis is rare outside the tropics.

Studies in Japan have repeatedly shown reduced delayed hypersensitivity to tuberculin in HTLV-I infected persons. Recently an increased adjusted odds risk of previous TB was reported in HTLV-II-positive blood donors in the USA (Murphy *et al.*, 1997b) but conversely there was no abnormality in delayed hypersensitivity skin testing to mumps virus or *Candida albicans* antigens in the same population (Murphy *et al.*, 2001). Encrusted (Norwegian) scabies has been reported in patients with HTLV-I and suggested as a marker for the development of ATLL. Failure to clear *Strongyloides stercoralis* despite appropriate treatment is also recognised with HTLV-I infection and investigation for HTLV-I is considered an essential part of the management of patients with proven strongyloidiasis. Increased rates of infection and treatment failure have also been reported for *Schistosoma mansoni* in Brazil (Porto *et al.*, 2002).

A myelopathy similar to that seen with HTLV-I has been reported in several subjects with HTLV-II infection in the absence of HIV infection (Jacobson *et al.*, 1993; Black *et al.*, 1996; Murphy *et al.*, 1997a), although some patients also have ataxia (Harrington *et al.*, 1993). Although the frequency of this condition is unknown and the causative role of HTLV-II unproven, many specialists accept that there is a growing

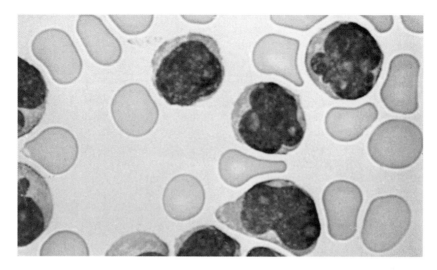

Figure 25A.7 Flower cells. A blood smear showing characteristic convoluted T cells in ATLL. Courtesy of Dr E. Matutes and Professor D. Catovsky

body of evidence to suggest that HTLV-II-associated myelopathy is a real entity.

In a cohort study of US blood donors, respiratory and urinary infections were more common among the HTLV-II infected donors than in matched controls (Murphy *et al.*, 1999).

An association between mycosis fungoides and the presence of HTLV-I tax DNA has now been refuted. There appears to be an association between HTLV-I

and Sjögren's syndrome in endemic areas but this has not yet been confirmed in properly aged-matched studies. HTLV-I-defective provirus has been amplified from the salivary glands of seronegative patients with Sjögren's syndrome. Rare cases of seronegative but PCR positive HAM/TSP are reported with defective provirus. *Tax* sequences are present in all these conditions. The absence of both humoral and cellular immune responses in these exceptional cases makes an understanding of the pathogenesis of these inflammatory conditions even more elusive.

Table 25A.2 Differential diagnosis of HAM

Compressive myelopathy
Syringomyelia
Familial spastic paraparesis
Primary lateral sclerosis
Multiple sclerosis
Transverse myelitis
Devic's disease
Motor neuron disease
Vitamin B_{12} deficiency
Folate deficiency
Syphilis
Human immunodeficiency virus
Schistosomiasis
Sarcoidosis
Neurological lupus
Behçet's disease
Sjögren's syndrome
Carcinomatous meningitis
Paraneoplastic syndrome

PATHOGENESIS

Our understanding of the pathogenesis of ATLL is incomplete, based to a large extent on *in vitro* studies of HTLV-I-infected cells and Tax constructs, and has to take into account a number of apparent discrepancies. HTLV-I can immortalise T lymphocytes *in vitro* and these cells express HTLV-I proteins, but there appears to be little expression of HTLV-I by ATL cells *in vivo*. Only a small proportion (2–4%) of those infected with HTLV-I develop ATLL and then only after many decades of infection. Indeed, the observation that only a proportion of the mothers of patients with HAM but all the mothers of ATLL patients are carriers of HTLV-I suggests that infection during infancy is important for the development of ATLL. In common with other malignancies, it is likely that transformation is a multi-step phenomenon, with the infection of a lymphocyte by HTLV-I only one of several events leading to ATLL. Since HTLV-I does not contain an oncogene and malignant transformation is not related to the integration disturbing cellular genes important in oncogenesis, the transactivating characteristics of Tax assume importance. Although adult T cell leukaemic cells contain randomly integrated (the integration site varies between subjects but is constant within a subject) HTLV-I that may be defective, *tax* is preserved.

In vitro, HTLV-I induces T cell activation and proliferation and immortalises primary human lymphocytes, which can become IL-2-independent. In these cells, as in other tumour virus models, Jak/Stat proteins are constitutively activated (Johnson *et al.*, 2001). Tax has been shown to stabilise and inactivate the tumour suppressor p53. Tax also interacts with cell cycle genes, inducing phosphorylation of cyclin D1-cdk4/6 and cyclin D3, which may contribute to the shift from G_1 to S phase in the cycle. Tax inactivates a cdk-inhibitor and the human mitotic arrest deficiency-1 protein.

Other examples of cellular genes transactivated by Tax are listed in Table 25A.3. Tax has an inhibitory effect on β polymerase, a DNA repair gene. This may increase the likelihood of mutagenesis. Tax does not act directly on the cellular genes, or on the promoter sequences in the viral LTR, but binds to a number of specific transcription factors, with resulting enhancement of their interaction with the target genes. Although others may exist, the three recognised target sequences are the cyclic AMP-response element (CRE), the NF-κB binding site and the serum-responsive element (SRE). Tax can bind to one or several members of a family of cellular transcription factors, which in turn bind to the CRE promoters. Similarly, Tax can bind to various members of the NF-κB family of transcription activators.

The interaction between the IL-2Rα gene and Tax has been of particular interest because of the high expression of IL-2R (CD25) by T lymphocytes in ATLL. IL-2Rα expression normally only occurs after antigenic stimulation by the T cell receptor. However, it appears that Tax is able to induce constitutive expression of the IL-2Rα gene. There is a 12 bp sequence in the 5′ IL-2Rα gene promoter required for *tax* transactivation, which shows homology with the NF-κB binding site. The NF-κB precursor, a p105 heterodimer, is usually found in the cytoplasm because its nuclear localisation signal is masked. Tax causes NF-κB to dissociate from its inhibitor, I-κB, which results in increased transport of NF-κB to the nucleus,

Table 25A.3 Cellular genes transactivated by HTLV-I Tax

IL-1, IL-2, IL-3, IL-6, IL-8	Interleukins
IL-2Rα	Interleukin 2 receptor α chain (CD25)
Vimentin	House-keeping gene
Class I MHC	Human leukocyte antigens
GM-CSF	Granulocyte-macrophage colony stimulating factor
NGF	Nerve growth factor
TGFb1	Transforming growth factor
PTHr-P	Parathyroid hormone related protein
TNF-α, TNF-β	Tumour necrosis factor (cachexin)
c-fos, c-myc	Cellular oncogenes (proteins localise to nucleus)
c-sis	Growth factor related to platelet-derived growth factor
PCNA	Proliferating cell nuclear antigen (cyclin)
MDR1	Multidrug resistance gene
egr-1, egr-2	Early response cellular genes
NF-κB	Nuclear factor
CRE	c-AMP response element
SRE	Serum-responsive element

where the NF-κB p50 is able to activate transcription of IL-2Rα. A secondary effect of Tax is that the dissociation of p50 from the heterodimer releases the p65 protein, which is then free to dimerise with the product of the c-Rel oncogene. This p65-Rel heterodimer is also able to activate the NF-κB motif. Thus, Tax may further enhance the activation of the many genes under the influence of NF-κB.

One theory of T cell transformation by HTLV-I has been that, by promoting activity of both IL-2R and IL-2 genes, Tax gives rise to continuous proliferation of the cells by positive feed-back—the autocrine loop theory. However, stimulation of Tax-transduced T cells can occur in an IL-2-independent manner, Tax-transfected cells continue to grow after anti-CD3 stimulation in the absence of IL-2, and not all Tax-transformed T cells express IL-2, although they all express IL-2R.

Whilst the oncogenic potential of HTLV-I has been recognised from the time of its discovery, a similar role has not been proven for HTLV-II. This could merely be a function of their different epidemiology; the HTLV-II endemic populations are small and often remote and therefore rare malignancies might be missed, whilst in industrialised states HTLV-II is mostly spread among adults who may not incubate the infection for long enough. With the exception of a few isolates of HTLV-IIa, in which Tax protein expression is low, the transactivating function of HTLV-II Tax via NF-κB does not differ significantly from HTLV-I *in vitro* (Lewis *et al.*, 2002).

The pathogenesis of HAM/TSP is also incompletely understood. It is rare to obtain histopathology at the time of the initial symptoms but a perivascular lymphocytic infiltration of the spinal cord, which is at first CD4$^+$ and later predominantly CD8$^+$ is found, followed by demyelination and atrophy. HTLV-I is rarely found in the lesions and when detected is probably in circulating CD4$^+$ lymphocytes. The peripheral lymphocyte proviral load is approximately 10-fold higher in HAM/TSP than in asymptomatic carriers although there is considerable overlap between the ranges. There appears to be a threshold of about 1 HTLV DNA copy/100 PBMCs, above which the risk of HAM increases exponentially (Nagai et al., 1998).

HTLV-I Tax-specific CTL are found in the majority of HAM/TSP patients (Jacobson et al., 1990) but also in asymptomatic carriers (Parker et al., 1992) and, by limiting dilution assays, have been found in high frequency (Daenke et al., 1996). Using MHC-peptide tetramers, as many as 10% of circulating CD8 lymphocytes have been found to recognise a single HTLV-I epitope (Bieganowska et al., 1999), although tetramer assays do not identify cytotoxic activity.

T helper responses to HTLV-I have been difficult to study but, using a short incubation ELIspot assay, higher frequencies of CD4 cells secreting interferon-γ in response to HTLV-I Env and Tax peptides have been found in patients with HAM (median 2/1000 CD4 cells) compared with asymptomatic carriers (Goon et al., 2002).

Polyclonal expansion of HTLV-I-infected lymphocytes has been reported in patients (without malignancy) with high proviral load, particularly patients with HAM/TSP. As with the oligo/monoclonal proliferation of T lymphocytes in ATLL, viral replication in these cells occurs through cell division, without the need for reverse transcription and integration. Thus, HTLV-I appears to be able to replicate through two quite distinct mechanisms, cell division and virion production. The relative contribution of 'cellular' and 'viral' replication to HTLV-I proviral load in patients with HAM/TSP and in asymptomatic carriers is uncertain. The continuous presence of a strong anti-Tax CTL response suggests continuing expression of Tax by some cells. It is possible that this may drive the proliferation of the clonally expanding cell populations. Despite the low rate of detection of HTLV-I proteins in vivo, there is now good evidence that HTLV-I-infected CD4 and CD8 cells are capable of expressing viral proteins and that such cells are lysed by HTLV-I-specific CTL. It has been proposed that the efficiency of these CTL in vivo at identifying and lysing virus protein expressing cells contributes sig-

nificantly to the apparent absence of viral expression described. Recently direct cell-to-cell spread of HTLV-I through a virus-induced synapse has been demonstrated in primary cells ex vivo (Figure 25A.9) (Igakura et al., 2003). This, if it occurs to any degree in vivo, may help explain the absence of free virions in plasma.

There are three main theories concerning HAM/TSP pathogenesis: (a) the inflammatory response is directed against virus in the CNS; (b) the inflammatory response against HTLV-I targets similar host CNS peptides; (c) CNS tissue is an innocent bystander, damaged when CTL recognise migrating, HTLV-I-expressing, CD4$^+$ cells. The latter has been considered most probable, although the potential role of HTLV-specific CD4 cells and NK cells might also be considered. Molecular mimicry between HTLV-I and the human neural ribosomal nucleoprotein A1 has, however, been reported (Levin et al., 2002). The effect of Tax on matrix metalloproteinases and on tissue inhibitors of metalloproteinases disturbing the neuronal milieu which has been reported in vitro could be implicated in the degeneration of neurons.

Although HAM/TSP is associated with high proviral load, differences in the rates of HAM/TSP per HTLV-I infected subjects in different populations suggest that other, possibly host factors, are important. Of the candidate factors, HLA types have attracted considerable interest. HLA types are known to be associated with other inflammatory diseases but could also influence outcome by controlling viral replication. In Japanese ATLL patients, HLA-A26, B61 and DR9 were found at an increased frequency, whilst HLA0A24 and HLA-Cw1 were less frequently found than in controls. Conversely, in patients with HAM/TSP HLA-Cw7, B7 and DR1 were found more commonly than in controls and patients with ATLL. It has been suggested that in Japan the A26Cw3B61DR9DQ3 haplotype is representative of ATLL and is associated with a low immune response, whilst A24Cw7B7DR1DQ1 is the representative haplotype of HAM/TSP and is associated with a high immune response. Amongst different ethnic groups HLA class I haplotypes were variable but examination of class II suggested that some haplotypes associated with disease are panethnic, whilst others are ethnospecific (Sonoda et al., 1996). In a study of Japanese blood donors and patients with HAM, possession of the HLA-A*02 and HLA-Cw*08 were found to protect against HAM through an association with lower HTLV-I viral burden, whereas HLA-B*5401 was associated with an increased risk of disease (Jeffery et al., 1999, 2000). Further studies of single nucleotide polymorphisms in the same population have revealed that TNF-963A predisposes to HAM (OR = 9.7), SDF-1 + 801A 3′UTR reduced the risk of HAM by half, whilst the IL-15 191C allele also conferred protection against HAM by being associated with lower proviral loads (Vine *et al.*, 2002).

TREATMENT

Few instances of curative treatment of ATLL have been reported and there have been no randomised controlled clinical trials. Until recently the overall management has been to treat the disease as for other malignancies and the regimens for non-Hodgkin's lymphoma, such as CHOP (cyclophosphamide, adriamycin, vincristine and prednisolone), are favoured. Although successive improvements in chemotherapy have increased remission rates to 42%, ATLL is essentially a highly drug-resistant malignancy and survival remains less than 12 months for the acute leukaemia and lymphoma presentations. Enhanced transcription of the multi-drug resistance gene (MDR1) with significant P-glycoprotein-mediated drug efflux in the T cells of HTLV-I-infected individuals, with and without malignancy, has been demonstrated, as has the ability of the HTLV-I tax protein to activate the MDR1 promoter. Other treatments, such as deoxycoformycin, interferons β and γ and topoisomerase II have been tried with limited success. Since CD25 is expressed by all ATLL cells, anti-Tac (CD25) antibodies have been tried, although with limited success. Improved remission rates (56%) were obtained with [99]Yttrium-labelled anti-Tac antibodies (Waldmann *et al.*, 1995). Successful eradication, not only of ATLL cells but also of HTLV-I infection, has been reported following bone marrow transplantation (BMT) but patients often fail to survive to or through BMT. Improved remission rates and survival have been reported, in uncontrolled studies, by three groups using the combination of interferon-α and zidovudine (Gill *et al.*, 1995; Hermine *et al.*, 1995; Matutes *et al.*, 2001). The mechanism of activity of these compounds in ATLL is not clear; they are not effective when given independently and do not appear to have a cytotoxic effect. Interest in this treatment followed anecdotal improvement in a patient with ATLL and HIV. The immune suppression seen in patients with ATLL is more severe than in other malignancies, and prophylaxis against *Pneumocystis* pneumonia is recommended. Where appropriate, infection with *Strongyloides stercoralis* should be sought and treated.

HAM/TSP is also difficult to treat, and there have to date been only two randomised controlled studies. Early reports of the use of pulsed high-dose steroids, steroid-sparing cytotoxics and plasmapheresis, all targeting the immune response, were encouraging (Osame *et al.*, 1990) but the improvements have not been long term (Matsuo *et al.*, 1989). High-dose vitamin C (Kataoka *et al.*, 1993) and oxpentifylline have also been promoted (Shirabe *et al.*, 1997). Extensive research into the treatment of HIV-1 has resulted in the licensing of four classes of antiretroviral therapy. Unfortunately, the current protease inhibitors and non-nucleoside reverse transcriptase inhibitors have no activity against HTLV-I. The nucleoside analogue reverse transcription inhibitors (NRTIs) zidovudine and zalcitabine have been shown to be active against HTLV-I *in vitro* and in animal models. Unfortunately, zalcitabine and two other NRTIs, didanosine and stavudine, are neurotoxic. Zidovudine was reported to improve mobility in ambulant patients in one study (Sheremata *et al.*, 1993) but not in another (Gout *et al.*, 1991); neither reported proviral load measurements. In the management of HAM/TSP it is important to consider that in long-standing disease demyelination and atrophy may prevent improvement, even if viral replication or the production of damaging cytokines has been reduced. Clinical improvement with a reduction in HTLV-I proviral load was reported with lamivudine (Taylor *et al.*, 1999), but in a randomised placebo-controlled study zidovudine plus lamivudine was not effective (Taylor *et al.*, 2003).

The earliest studies of interferon-α were of short duration but temporary benefit was observed (Shibayama *et al.*, 1991; Kuroda *et al.*, 1992). In a randomised study of interferon-α given for 4 weeks with 2 months follow-up, a dose-related effect was observed. Thus, the 16 patients prescribed 0.3×10^6 IU did not benefit, but a clinical response was reported in 3/17 and 6/16 patients randomised to 1×10^6 and 3×10^6 IU daily, respectively (Izumo *et al.*, 1996). Interferon-β1A for 6 months did not alter the clinical status of 12 patients in an observational study and although a reduction in CTL activity was documented in three patients, this was not specific to HTLV-I (Mora *et al.*, 2003).

Symptomatic management remains the mainstay of therapy. Bladder spasticity with urgency, frequency, nocturia and incontinence is often distressing. Some patients respond well to oxybutinin. The anabolic steroid danazol has been reported to improve these symptoms. Intravesical instillation of capsaicin has been shown to reduce the bladder spasticity in these patients, with symptomatic improvement lasting months (Dasgupta *et al.*, 1996). Intranasal antidiuretic hormone, cautiously used, may reduce nocturia in refractory cases. In a minority of patients the bladder is hypotonic and catheterisation, intermittent or permanent, is necessary to both relieve symptoms and protect renal function. A titrated dose of baclofen may reduce limb spasticity—tizanidine may be tried if baclofen is not tolerated. The combination of urinary frequency with impaired mobility is particularly frustrating for patients with HAM. Lumbar pain which has a radicular pattern is common in some, but not all, patient series. Management can be complex and long-acting local anaesthesia can be useful in more severe cases.

HTLV-I associated uveitis usually responds to non-specific therapy with corticosteroids. Patients with HTLV-I-infection and strongyloidiasis should be carefully followed after therapy with thiabendazole and/or ivermectin, as initial treatment is not always curative.

PREVENTION OF DISEASE

There is no vaccine for HTLV-I or HTLV-II infection. Although the association of HAM/TSP with high proviral load suggests that antiretroviral therapy may in the future be part of the treatment or prevention of this disease, current strategies must be directed at preventing infection. Two transmission routes can be targeted relatively easily. Many blood transfusion services now include HTLV-I/II antibody screening of all or of new donors. This was first introduced in 1986 in Japan, where blood transfusion accounted for up to 60% of seroconversions in the Kyushu region of South West Japan (Kamihira *et al.*, 1987). Blood donor screening has been standard practice in the USA and Australia for many years and more recently was introduced in South American countries. With the commercial production of suitably sensitive and specific screening assays, HTLV-I/II blood donor testing has been introduced in the majority of EU countries. In France more than 300 HTLV-I-positive blood donors have been detected since screening began in 1991. In the UK donor screening was introduced in August 2002. Prior to that, the risk of transmission was almost certainly reduced by leukodepletion, introduced in 1999 to protect recipients from the transmission of prions. Screening of blood donors undoubtedly prevents infection in recipients, but cost-effectiveness in terms of preventing HTLV-I-associated disease in them has been questioned (Tynell *et al.*, 1998). In such analyses more weight has been given to the 'cost' of developing ATLL following transfusion

rather than HAM/TSP, although the latter causes more morbidity and is a much more common consequence.

HTLV-I, and probably HTLV-II, can also be transmitted through organ donation. In endemic areas it has been suggested that donors and recipients should be matched for HTLV-I antibody status. Elsewhere the arguments that apply to blood donor screening should apply to donated organs.

Eighty per cent of mother-to-child transmission can be prevented by avoidance of breast feeding. In Japan, carrier mothers are identified through ante-natal screening programmes. In the UK the prevalence of HTLV-I/II infection in women attending metropolitan ante-natal clinics is approximately 1:200 (cf. HIV-1) but HTLV-I antibody testing has never been offered as a routine part of ante-natal care. Although breast-feeding is less common in the UK, there is now increasing concern to prevent the transmission of other viral infections by this route and recognition that when offered there is a high uptake, by the mothers, of interventions to reduce transmission. Reduction of HTLV-I transmission from mothers to their infants is likely to prevent most cases of HTLV-associated disease in the UK—ATLL by preventing infection of the infant, and HAM/TSP by both preventing early infection and reducing the pool of infected persons who will transmit HTLV-I sexually in adult life. Any effect on the incidence of disease would not be seen for several decades.

HIV AND HTLV CO-INFECTION

Co-infections with HTLV-I plus HIV-1 or HTLV-II plus HIV-1 occur where the two families of viruses occur in the same risk population. Thus, HTLV-I and HIV-1 co-infections are likely to be most common in Latin America, the Caribbean and West/Central Africa, whereas HTLV-II co-infection with HIV-1 is common among IDUs in Europe and North America.

HTLV-I and HIV-1 share tropism for $CD4^+$ lymphocytes but $CD4^+$ lymphocyte counts and CD4:CD8 ratios are normal in HTLV-I infection alone. Studies in Brazil and French Guiana have reported decreased survival in patients co-infected with HTLV-I and HIV-1 and more advanced HIV disease than anticipated from the CD4 counts. Thus, the initiation of prophylaxis against *Pneumocystis* pneumonia and/or antiretroviral therapy at CD4 levels higher than currently recommended should be considered. No effect of HTLV-II on HIV-1 outcome was found in a study of North American and Italian IDUs, whereas increased risk of sensory motor polyneuropathy has been observed with this co-infection. HTLV-I-associated myelopathy is more common in HIV-1 co-infection. HTLV-II viral load seems to be inversely related to HIV-1 viral load, although whether this association is causal is uncertain. HTLV-II infection may be more difficult to detect serologically and indeterminate Western blot results warrant further molecular investigation.

REFERENCES

Araujo A, Sheehy N, Takahashi H and Hall WW (2002) Concomitant infections with human immunodeficiency virus type 1 and human T lymphotropic virus types 1 and 2. In *Polymicrobial Diseases* (eds Brogden KA and Guthmiller J), pp 75–97. ASM Press, Washington DC.

Bieganowska K, Hollsberg P, Buckle GJ *et al.* (1999) Direct analysis of viral-specific CD8$^+$ T cells with soluble HLA-A2/Tax11-19 tetramer complexes in patients with human T cell lymphotropic virus-associated myelopathy. *J Immunol*, **162**, 1765–1771.

Black FL, Biggar RJ, Lal RB *et al.* (1996) Twenty-five years of HTLV Type II follow-up with a possible case of tropical spastic paraparesis in the Kayapo, a Brazilian Indian tribe. *AIDS Res Hum Retrovirol*, **12**, 1623–1627.

Ciminale V, D'Agostino DM, Zotti L *et al.* (1996) Coding potential of the X region of human T-cell leukaemia/lymphotropic virus type II. *J Acqu Immune Defic Syndr Hum Retrovirol*, **13** (suppl), S220–S227.

Clapham P, Nagy K and Weiss RA (1984) Pseudotypes of human T-cell leukaemia virus types 1 and 2: neutralisation by patients' sera. *Proc Natl Acad Sci USA*, **81**, 2886–2889.

Daenke S, Hall SE, Taylor GP *et al.* (1996) Cytotoxic T cell response to HTLV-I: equally high effector frequency in healthy carriers and patients with tropical spastic paraparesis. *Virology*, **217**, 139–146.

Dasgupta P, Fowler CJ, Scaravilli F *et al.* (1996) Bladder biopsies in tropical spastic paraparesis and the effect of intravesical capsaicin on nerve densities. *Eur Urol*, **30** (abstr), S2.

Eiraku N, Novoa P, da Costa Ferreira M *et al.* (1996) Identification and characterization of a new and distinct molecular subtype of human T cell lymphotropic virus type 2. *J Virol*, **1481**, 1492.

Endo K, Hirata A, Iwai K *et al.* (2002) Human T-cell leukaemia virus type 2 (HTLV-2) Tax protein transforms a rat fibroblast cell line but less efficiently than HTLV-1 Tax. *J Virol*, **76**(6), 2648–2653.

Franchini G (1995) Molecular mechanisms of human T cell leukaemia. *Blood*, **86**, 3619–3639.

Gessain A, Mauclere P, Froment A *et al.* (1995) Isolation and molecular characterisation of a human T-cell lymphotropic virus type II (HTLV-II) subtype B from a healthy pygmy living in a remote area of Cameroon: an Ancient origin of HTLV-II in Africa. *Proc Natl Acad Sci USA*, **92**, 4041–4045.

Gessain A, Vernant JC, Maurs L *et al.* (1985) Antibodies to human T-lymphotropic virus type I in patients with tropical spastic paraparesis. *Lancet*, **ii**, 407–409.

Ghez D, Lepelletier Y, Amulf B *et al.* (2003) Identification of a cell surface protein behaving as a cellular receptor for HTLV-I and HTLV-2. *AIDS Res Hum Retrovirol*, **19** (suppl), O28–S15.

Gill P, Harrington W, Kaplan J *et al.* (1995) Treatment of adult T-cell leukaemia–lymphoma with a combination of interferon α and zidovudine. *N Engl J Med*, **332**, 1744–1748.

Giri A, Markham P, Digilio L *et al.* (1994) Isolation of a novel simian T-cell lymphotropic virus from *Pan paniscus* that is distantly related to the human T-cell leukaemia/lymphotropic virus types I and II. *J Virol*, **68**, 8392–8395.

Goon P, Hanon E, Igakura T *et al.* (2002) High frequencies of Th1-type CD4$^+$ T cells specific to HTLV-1 Env and Tax proteins in patients with HTLV-1-associated myelopathy/tropical spastic paraparesis. *Blood*, **99**, 3335–3341.

Goubau P, Desmyter J, Ghesquiere J and Kasereka B (1992) HTLV-II among pygmies. *Nature*, **359**, 201.

Goubau P, Van Brussel M, Vandamme AM *et al.* (1994) A primate T-lymphocyte virus, PTLV-L, different from human T-lymphotropic viruses types I and II, in a wild-caught baboon (*Papio hamadryas*). *Proc Natl Acad Sci USA*, **91**, 2848–2852.

Gout O, Gessain A, Iba-Zizen M *et al.* (1991) The effect of zidovudine on chronic myelopathy associated with HTLV-I. *J Neurol*, **238**, 108–109.

Hanon E, Stinchcombe J, Taylor GP *et al.* (2000) Fratricide among CD8$^+$ lymphocytes naturally infected with human T-cell lymphotropic virus type I. *Immunity*, **13**, 657–664.

Harrington WJ Jr, Sheremata WA, Hjelle B *et al.* (1993) Spastic ataxia associated with HTLV-II infection. *Ann Neurol*, **33**, 411–414.

Hermine O, Bouscary D, Gessain A *et al.* (1995) Treatment of HTLV-I associated adult T-cell leukaemia–lymphoma with a combination of zidovudine and interferon-γ. *N Engl J Med*, **332**, 1749–1751.

Hidaka M, Inoue J, Yoshida M *et al.* (1998) Post-transcriptional regulator (rex) of HTLV-I initiates expression of viral structural proteins but suppresses expression of regulatory proteins. *EMBO J*, **7**, 519–523.

Hinuma Y, Nagata K, Hanaoka M *et al.* (1981) Adult T-cell leukaemia: antigen in an ATL cell line and detection of antibodies to the antigen in human sera. *Proc Nat Acad Sci USA*, **78**, 6476–6480.

IARC Monographs on the Evaluation of Carcinogenic Risk to Humans (1996) *Human Immunodeficiency Viruses and Human T-cell Lymphotropic Viruses*. IARC, Lyon.

Igakura T, Stinchcombe JC, Goon P *et al.* (2003) HTLV-I spreads between lymphocytes by virus induced polarization of the cytoskeleton. *Science*, **299**(5613), 1713–1716.

Ishak R, Harrington WJ Jr, Azevedo VN *et al.* (1995) Identification of human T cell lymphotropic virus type IIa infection in the Kayapo, an indigenous population of Brazil. *AIDS Res Hum Retrovirol*, **1**(7), 813–821.

Iwasaki Y (1990) Pathology of chronic myelopathy associated with HTLV-I infection (HAM/TSP). *J Neurol Sci*, **96**, 103–123.

Izumo S, Goto I, Itoyama Y *et al.* (1996) Interferon-α is effective in HTLV-I-associated myelopathy: a multicenter, randomized, double-blind, controlled trial. *Neurology*, **46**, 1016–1021.

Jacobson S, Lehky T, Nishimura M *et al.* (1993) Isolation of HTLV-II from a patient with chronic, progressive neurological disease clinically indistinguishable from

HTLV-I-associated myelopathy/tropical spastic paraparesis. *Ann Neurol*, **33**(4), 392–396.

Jacobson S, Shida H, McFarlin D *et al.* (1990) Circulating CD8$^+$ cytotoxic lymphocytes specific for HTLV-1 in patients with HTLV-1 associated neurological disease. *Nature*, **348**, 245–248.

Jeffery K, Nagai M, Taylor GP *et al.* (1999) HLA alleles determine human T-lymphotropic virus-I (HTLV-I) proviral load and the risk of HTLV-associated myelopathy. *Proc Natl Acad Sci USA*, **96**, 3848–3853.

Jeffery K, Siddiqui AA, Bunce M *et al.* (2000) The influence of HLV Class I alleles and heterozygosity on the outcome of human T cell lymphotropic virus type I infection. *J Immunol*, **165**, 7278–7284.

Johnson JM, Harrod R, and Franchini G (2001) Molecular biology and pathogenesis of the human T-cell leukaemia/lymphotropic virus type-1 (HTLV-1). *Int Exp Pathol*, **82**, 135–147.

Kajiyama W, Kashiwagi S, Ikematsu H *et al.* (1986) Intrafamilial transmission of adult T leukaemia virus. *J Infect Dis*, **154**, 851–857.

Kalyanaraman VS, Sarngadharan MG, Robert-Guroff M *et al.* (1982) A new subtype of human T-cell leukemia virus (HTLV-II) associated with a T-cell variant of hairy cell leukemia. *Science*, **218**, 571–573.

Kamihira S, Nakasima S, Oyakawa Y *et al.* (1987) Transmission of human T cell lymphotropic virus type I blood transfusion before and after mass screening of sera from seropositive donors. *Vox Sang*, **52**, 43–44.

Kaplan J, Khabbaz R, Murphy EL *et al.* (1996) Male-to-female transmission of human T-cell lymphotropic virus types I and II: association with viral load. The Retrovirus Epidemiology Donor Study (REDS) Group. *J Acqu Immune Defic Syndr Hum Retrovirol*, **12**, 193–201.

Kataoka A, Imai H, Inayoshi S and Tsuda T (1993) Intermittent high-dose vitamin C therapy in patients with HTLV-I associated myelopathy. *J Neurol Neurosurg Psychiat*, **56**, 1213–1216.

Koralnik IJ, Boeri E, Saxinger WC *et al.* (1994) Phylogenetic associations of human and simian T-cell leukaemia/lymphotropic virus type I strains: evidence for interspecies transmission. *J Virol*, **68**, 2693–2727.

Koyanagi Y, Itoyama Y, Nakamura *et al.* (1993) *In vivo* infection of human T-cell leukaemia virus type I in non-T cells. *Virology*, **196**, 25–33.

Kuroda Y, Kurohara K, Fujiyama F *et al.* (1992) Systemic interferon-α in the treatment of HTLV-I-associated myelopathy. *Acta Neurol Scand*, **86**, 82–86.

Le Blanc I, Rosenberg AR and Dokhélar MC (1999) Multiple functions for the basic amino acids of the human T-cell leukaemia virus type 1 matrix protein in viral transmission. *J Virol*, **73**, 1860–1867.

Letournier F, d'Auriol L, Dazza M-C *et al.* (1998) Complete nucleotide sequence of an African human T-lymphotropic virus type II subtype b isolated (HTLV-II-Gab): molecular and phylogenetic analysis. *J Gen Virol*, **79**, 269–277.

Levin MC, Lee SM, Kalume F *et al.* (2002) Autoimmunity due to molecular mimicry as a cause of neurological disease. *Nature Med*, **8**, 509–513.

Lewis MJ, Novoa P, Ishak R *et al.* (2000) Isolation, cloning and complete nucleotide sequence of a phenotypically distinct Brazilian isolate of human T-lymphotropic virus type II (HTLV-II). *Virology*, **271**(1), 142–154.

Lewis MJ, Sheehy N, Salemi M *et al.* (2002) Comparison of CREB NF-κB-mediated transactivation by human T lymphotropic virus Type II (HTLV-II) and Type I (HTLV-I) tax proteins. *Virology*, **295**, 182–189.

Manel N, Kim FJ, Kinet S *et al.* (2003) Identification of an HTLV envelope receptor and its impact on cell physiology. *AIDS Res Hum Retrovirol*, **19** (suppl), O27–S14.

Manns A, Murphy EL, Wilks R *et al.* (1991) Detection of early human T-cell lymphotropic virus type I antibody patterns during seroconversion among transfusion recipients. *Blood*, **7**(4), 896–905.

Manns A, Wilks RJ, Hanchard B *et al.* (1994) Virus-specific humoral immune responses following transfusion-related transmission of human T cell lymphotropic virus type-1 infection. *Viral Immunol*, **7**, 113–120.

Matsuo H, Nakamura M, Shibayama K *et al.* (1989) Long-term follow-up of immunomodulation in treatment of HTLV-I-associated myelopathy. *Lancet*, **1**(8641), 790.

Matutes E, Taylor GP, Bareford D, *et al.* (2001) Interferon-α and zidovudine therapy in adult T-cell leukaemia lymphoma: response and outcome in 15 patients. *Br J Haematol*, **113**, 779–784.

Meertens L, Mahieux R, Mauclere P *et al.* (2002) Complete sequence of a novel highly divergent simian T-cell lymphotropic virus from wild-caught red-capped mangabeys (*Cercocebus torquatus*) from Cameroon: a new primate T-lymphotropic virus type 3 subtype. *J Virol*, **76**, 259–268.

Meertens L, Rigoulet J, Mauclere P *et al.* (2001) Molecular and phylogenetic analyses of 16 novel simian T cell leukaemia virus type 1 from Africa: close relationship of STLV-1 from *Allenopithecus nigroviridis* to HTLV-1 subtype B strains. *Virology*, **287**, 275–285.

Merle H, Cabre P, Olindo S, *et al.* (2002) Ocular lesions in 200 patients infected by the human T-cell lymphotropic virus type 1 in Martinique (French West Indies). *Am J Ophthalmol*, **134**, 190–195.

Miyoshi I, Kubonishi I, Yoshimoto S *et al.* (1981) Type C virus particles in a cord (blood) T-cell line derived by co-cultivating normal human cord leukocytes and human leukaemic T-cells. *Nature*, **294**, 770–771.

Mochizuki M, Watanabe T, Yamaguchi K *et al.* (1992) HTLV-I uveitis: a distinct clinical entity caused by HTLV-I. *Jap J Cancer Res*, **82**, 236–239.

Mora CA, Yamano Y, Eist TP *et al.* (2003) Evaluation of the viral load and immune response in HTLV-I-associated myelopathy patients treated with recombinant human interferon-β1A. *AIDS Res Hum Retrovirol*, **19**, O25–S14

Murphy EL, Fridey J, Smith JW *et al.* (1997a) HTLV-associated myelopathy in a cohort of HTLV-1 and HTLV-II infected blood donors. The REDS investigators. *Neurology*, **48**, 315–320.

Murphy EL, Glynn SA, Fridey J *et al.* (1997b) Increased prevalence of infectious diseases and other adverse outcomes in human T lymphotropic virus types I- and II-infected blood donors. Retrovirus Epidemiology Donor Study (REDS) Study Group. *J Infect Dis*, **176**, 1468–1475.

Murphy EL, Glynn SA, Fridey J *et al.* (1999) Increased incidence of infectious diseases during prospective follow-up of human T-lymphotropic virus type II- and I-infected blood donors. Retrovirus Epidemiology Donor Study (REDS). *Arch Intern Med*, **159**, 1485–1491.

Murphy EL, Wu, Y, Ownby HE *et al.* and the NHLBI REDS Investigators (2001) Delayed hypersensitivity skin testing to mumps and *Candida albicans* antigens is normal in middle-aged HTLV-I and -II infected US cohorts. *AIDS Res Hum Retrovirol*, **17**(13), 1273–1277.

Nagai M, Usuku K, Matsumoto W *et al.* (1998) Analysis of HTLV-I proviral load in 202 HAM/TSP patients and 243 asymptomatic HTLV-I carriers: high proviral load strongly predisposes to HAM/TSP. *J Neurovirol*, **4**, 586–593.

Okochi K, Sato H and Hinuma Y (1984) A retrospective study on transmission of adult T cell leukaemia virus by blood transfusion: seroconversion in recipients. *Vox Sang*, **46**, 245–253.

Osame M, Usuku K, Izumo S *et al.* (1986) HTLV-1-associated myelopathy new clinical entity [letter]. *Lancet*, **i**, 1031–1052.

Osame M, Igata A, Matsumoto M *et al.* (1990) HTLV-I-associated myelopathy (HAM): treatment trials, retrospective survey and clinical and laboratory findings. *Hematol Rev*, **3**, 271–284.

Parker CE, Daenke S, Nightingale S and Bangham C (1992) Activated, HTLV-1-specific cytotoxic T-lymphocytes are found in healthy seropositives as well as in patients with tropical spastic paraparesis. *Virology*, **188**, 628–636.

Poiesz BJ, Ruscetti FW, Gazdar AF *et al.* (1980) Detection and isolation of type C retrovirus particles from fresh and cultured cells of a patient with cutaneous T-cell lymphoma. *Proc Natl Acad Sci USA*, **77**, 7415–7419.

Porto AF, Neva F, Braga S, *et al.* (2002) Clinical and immunological impact of the co-infection of HTLV-I/intestinal parasites. VIIth International Symposium on HTLV in Brazil, Balém, Pará, Brazil, 18–21 August.

Rayne F, Bouamr F, Lalanne J and Mamoun RZ (2001) The NH$_2$-terminal domain of the human T-cell leukaemia virus type 1 capsid protein is involved in particle formation. *J Virol*, **75**(11), 5277–5287.

Richardson JH, Edwards AJ, Cruikshank JK *et al.* (1990) *In vivo* cellular tropism of human T-cell leukaemia virus type 1. *J Virol*, **64**, 5682–5687.

Rouet F, Meertens L, Courouble GJ *et al.* (2001) Serological, epidemiological and molecular differences between human T-cell lymphotropic virus type 1 (HTLV-1) seropositive healthy carriers and persons with HTLV-I gag indeterminate WB patterns from the Caribbean. *J Clin Microbiol*, **39**, 1247–1253.

Salemi M, Lewis M, Egan JF *et al.* (1999) Different population dynamics of human T cell lymphotropic virus type II in intravenous drug users compared with endemically infected tribes. *Proc Natl Acad Sci USA*, **96**, 13253–13258.

Sheremata WA, Benedict BS, Squilacote DC *et al.* (1993) High-dose zidovudine induction in HTLV-I associated myelopathy. Safety and possible efficacy. *Neurology*, **43**, 2125–2129.

Shibayama K, Nakamura T, Nagasato *et al.* (1991) Interferon α treatment in HTLV-I-associated myelopathy. Studies of clinical and immunological aspects. *J Neurol Sci*, **106**, 186–192.

Shirabe S, Nakamura T, Tsujino A *et al.* (1997) Successful application of pentoxifylline in the treatment of HTLV-I associated myelopathy. *J Neurol Sci*, **151**, 97–101.

Sonoda S, Fujiyoshi T and Yashiki S (1996) Immunogenetics of HTLV-I/II and associated diseases. *J Acqu Immune Defic Syndr Hum Retrovirol*, **13** (suppl), S119–S123.

Stuver SO, Tachibana N, Okayama A *et al.* (1993) Heterosexual transmission of human T-cell leukaemia/lymphoma virus type I among married couples in south-western Japan: an initial report from the Miyazaki Cohort Study. *J Infect Dis*, **167**, 57–65.

Takahashi K, Talezaki T, Oki T *et al.* (1991) Inhibitory effect of maternal antibody on mother-to-child transmission of human T-cell lymphotropic virus type I. *Int J Cancer*, **49**, 673–677.

Taylor GP (1996) The epidemiology of HTLV-1 in Europe. *J Acqu Immune Defic Syndr Hum Retrivirol*, **13**, S8–S14.

Taylor GP, Hall SE, Navarette S *et al.* (1999) Effect of Lamivudine on human T-cell leukaemia virus type 1 (HTLV-1) DNA copy number, T-cell phenotype, and anti-Tax cytotoxic T-cell frequency in patients with HTLV-1 associated myelopathy. *J Virol*, **73**, 10289–10295.

Taylor GP, Goubau P, Coste J *et al.* (2001) The HTLV European Research Network International Antenatal Seroprevalence Study (HERNIAS). *AIDS Res Hum Retrovirol*, **17**(abstr), 9.

Taylor GP, Goon P, Usuku K *et al.* (2003) The Bridge Study—a double-blind, placebo-controlled trial of zidovudine plus lamivudine for the treatment of patients with HTLV-I-associated myelopathy. *AIDS Res Hum Retrovirol*, **19**, O23–S13.

The HTLV European Research Network (1996) Seroepidemiology of the human T-cell leukaemia/lymphoma viruses in Europe. *J Acqu Immune Defic Syndr Hum Retrovirol*, **14**, 68–77.

Tynell E, Andersson S, Lithander E, *et al.* (1998) Screening for human T cell leukaemia/lymphoma virus among blood donors in Sweden: cost effectiveness analysis. *Br Med J*, **316**, 1417–1422.

Uchiyama T, Yodoi J, Sagawa K *et al.* (1997) Adult T-cell leukaemia: clinical and haematological features of 16 cases. *Blood*, **50**, 481–492.

Ureta-Vidal A, Angelin-Duclos C, Tortvoye P *et al.* (1999) Mother-to-child transmission of human T-cell leukaemia/lymphoma virus type I: implication of high antiviral antibody titer and high proviral load in carrier mothers. *Int J Cancer*, **82**, 832–836.

Ureta-Vidal A, Gessain A, Yoshida M *et al.* (1994) Phylogenetic classification of human T cell leukaemia/lymphoma type I genotypes in five major molecular and geographical subtypes. *J Gen Virol*, **75**, 3655–3666.

Van Dooren S, Salemi M, Liu HF *et al.* (2001) Intrafamilial HTLV-I sequence divergence: a tool for estimating the HTLV-I evolutionary rate? *Virus Res*, **78**, 119–120.

Vandamme A-M, Salemi M, Van Brussel M *et al.* (1998) African origin of human T-lymphotropic virus type 2 (HTLV-2) supported by a potential new HTLV-2d subtype in Congolese Bambuti Efe pygmies. *J Virol*, **72**(5), 4327–4340.

Vine AM, Witkover A, Lloyd AL *et al.* (2002) Polygenic control of HTLV-I proviral load and the risk of HTLV-I-associated myelopathy/tropical spastic paraparesis (HAM/TSP). *J Infect Dis*, **186**, 932–939.

Waldmann TA, White JD, Carrasquillo JA *et al.* (1995) Radioimmunotherapy of interleukin-2R α expressing adult T-cell leukemia with Yttrium-90-labeled anti-Tac. *Blood*, **86**(11), 4063–4075.

Willis JW and Craven RC (1991) Form, function and use of retroviral Gag proteins. *AIDS*, **5**, 639–654.

Yoshida M, Miyoshi I and Hinuma Y (1982) A retrovirus from human leukemia cell lines: its isolation, characterization, and implications in human adult T-cell leukemia (ATL). *Princess Takamatsu Symposia*, **12**, 285–294.

26

Human Prion Diseases

John Collinge

University College London, London, UK

INTRODUCTION TO PRIONS AND HISTORICAL PERSPECTIVE

The prion diseases, or transmissible spongiform encephalopathies, are a closely related group of neurodegenerative conditions that affect both humans and animals. They have previously been called 'the sub-acute spongiform encephalopathies', 'slow virus diseases' and 'transmissible dementias'. The prototypic disease is scrapie, a naturally occurring disease of sheep and goats, which has been recognised in Europe for over 200 years and is present in many countries worldwide. Other animal prion diseases, described over the last few decades, include transmissible mink encephalopathy and chronic wasting disease of mule deer and elk, both principally in the USA, and since the 1980s bovine spongiform encephalopathy (BSE), first described in the UK and now seen in most European Union and some other countries. The more recently described feline spongiform encephalopathy of domestic cats and spongiform encephalopathies of an increasing number of species of zoo animals (Kirkwood *et al.*, 1990) are now also recognised as animal prion diseases.

The human prion diseases have been traditionally classified into Creutzfeldt–Jakob disease (CJD), Gerstmann–Sträussler syndrome (GSS) (also known as Gerstmann–Sträussler–Scheinker disease) and kuru. Although these are rare neurodegenerative disorders, affecting about 1 person per million worldwide per annum, remarkable attention has been focused on these diseases in recent years. This is because of the unique biology of the transmissible agent or prion, and also because of the fears that the epizootic BSE could pose a threat to public health through dietary exposure to infected tissues.

Scrapie was demonstrated to be transmissible by inoculation between sheep (and goats) following prolonged incubation periods in 1936. It was assumed that some type of virus must be the causative agent and Sigurdsson coined the term 'slow virus infection' in 1954. There was considerable interest in the 1950s in an epidemic of a neurodegenerative disease, kuru, characterised principally by a progressive ataxia, amongst the Fore linguistic group of the Eastern Highlands of Papua New Guinea. Subsequent field work, by a number of investigators, suggested that kuru was transmitted during cannibalistic feasts. In 1959, Hadlow drew attention to the similarities between kuru and scrapie at the neuropathological, clinical and epidemiological levels, leading to the suggestion that these diseases may also be transmissible. A landmark in the field was the transmission, by intracerebral inoculation with brain homogenates into chimpanzees, of first kuru and then CJD by Gajdusek and colleagues in 1966 and 1968 respectively (Gibbs *et al.*, 1968). Transmission of GSS followed in 1981. This work led to the concept of the 'transmissible dementias'. The term 'Creutzfeldt–Jakob disease (CJD)' was introduced by Spielmeyer in 1922, drawing from the case reports of Creutzfeldt (1920) and Jakob (1921), and was used in subsequent years to describe a range of neurodegenerative conditions, many of which would not meet modern diagnostic criteria for CJD. The criterion of transmissibility allowed diagnostic criteria for CJD to be assessed and refined; atypical cases could be classified as CJD on the basis of their transmissibility. All the animal and human conditions

Principles and Practice of Clinical Virology, Fifth Edition. Edited by A. J. Zuckerman, J. E. Banatvala, J. R. Pattison, P. D. Griffiths and B. D. Schoub
© 2004 John Wiley & Sons Ltd ISBN 0 470 84338 1

share common histopathological features. The classical diagnostic triad of spongiform vacuolation (affecting any part of the cerebral grey matter), neuronal loss and astrocytic proliferation may be accompanied by amyloid plaques.

The nature of the transmissible agent in these diseases has been a subject of intense and often heated debate for many years. The understandable initial assumption that the agent must be some form of virus was challenged, however, both by the failure to directly demonstrate such a virus (or any immunological response to it) and by evidence indicating that the transmissible agent showed remarkable resistance to treatment expected to inactivate nucleic acids (such as ultraviolet radiation or treatment with nucleases). Such findings had led to suggestions as early as 1966 by Alper and others that the transmissible agent might be devoid of nucleic acid (Alper et al., 1966, 1967) and to Griffith's (1967) suggestion that the transmissible agent might be a protein and his proposal of several hypothetical mechanisms for replication. Progressive enrichment of brain homogenates for infectivity resulted in the isolation of a protease-resistant sialoglycoprotein, designated the prion protein (PrP), by Prusiner and co-workers in 1982. This protein was the major constituent of infective fractions and was found to accumulate in affected brains and sometimes to form amyloid deposits. The term 'prion' (from *proteinaceous infectious particle*) was proposed by Prusiner (1982) to distinguish the infectious pathogen from viruses or viroids. Prions were defined as 'small proteinaceous infectious particles that resist inactivation by procedures which modify nucleic acids'.

The protease-resistant PrP extracted from affected brains was of 27–30 kDa and became known as PrP$^{27-30}$. N-terminal sequencing of PrP$^{27-30}$ enabled production of isocoding mixtures of oligonucleotides that were used to screen cDNA libraries prepared from scrapie-infected hamsters. These studies led to recovery of cognate cDNA clones by Weissmann and colleagues in 1985. Remarkably, PrP$^{27-30}$ was encoded by a single copy host chromosomal gene rather than by a putative nucleic acid in fractions enriched for scrapie infectivity. PrP$^{27-30}$ was found to be derived from a larger molecule of 33–35 kDa designated PrP^{Sc} (denoting the scrapie isoform of the protein; Oesch et al., 1985). The normal product of the PrP gene, however, is protease-sensitive and was designated PrP^C (denoting the cellular isoform of the protein). No differences in amino acid sequence between PrP^{Sc} and PrP^C have been identified. PrP^{Sc} is known to be derived from PrP^C by a post-translational process (Borchelt et al., 1990; Caughey and Raymond 1991).

Many of the key advances in understanding the pathogenesis of the prion diseases have come from study of the various forms of human prion disease. In particular, the recognition that the familial forms of the human diseases are autosomal dominant inherited conditions, associated with *PRNP* coding mutations (Hsiao et al., 1989; Owen et al., 1989), as well as being transmissible to laboratory animals by inoculation, strongly supported the contention that the transmissible agent, or prion, was composed principally of an abnormal isoform of prion protein.

STRUCTURAL BIOLOGY OF PRIONS

A wide body of data now supports the idea that prions consist principally or entirely of an abnormal isoform of a host-encoded protein, the prion protein (PrP), designated PrP^{Sc} (for review see Prusiner, 1991). PrP^{Sc} is derived from PrP^C by a post-translational mechanism (Borchelt et al., 1990) and no covalent differences (Caughey and Raymond 1991) between PrP^C and PrP^{Sc} have been demonstrated. It is proposed that PrP^{Sc} acts as a template which promotes the conversion of PrP^C to PrP^{Sc} and that this conversion involves only conformational change.

The conformation of the cellular isoform was first established by NMR measurements of recombinant mouse PrP (Riek et al., 1996). Since then NMR measurements on recombinant hamster, human and other mammalian PrPs have shown that they have essentially the same conformation; however, despite strenuous efforts, no group has yet determined the three-dimensional structure of PrP^C by crystallographic methods.

Following cleavage of an N-terminal signal peptide and removal of a C-terminal peptide on addition of a glycosylphosphatidylinositol (GPI) anchor, the mature PrP^C species consists of an N-terminal region of about 100 amino acids, which is unstructured in the isolated molecule in solution, and a C-terminal segment, also around 100 amino acids in length. The C-terminal domain is folded into a largely α-helical conformation (three α-helices and a short anti-parallel β-sheet) and is stabilised by a single disulphide bond linking helices 2 and 3. There are two asparagine-linked glycosylation sites (see Figure 26.1).

The N-terminal region contains a segment of five repeats of an eight-amino acid sequence (the octapeptide-repeat region), whose expansion by insertional mutation leads to inherited prion disease. While unstructured in the isolated molecule, this highly

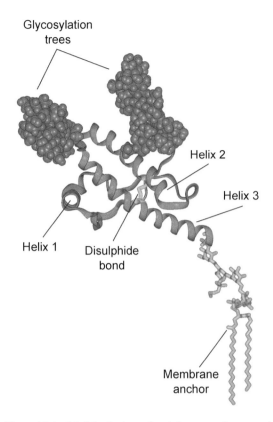

Glycosylation trees

Helix 2

Helix 3

Helix 1   Disulphide bond

Membrane anchor

Figure 26.1 Model of glycosylated human prion protein indicating positions of N-linked glycans, the single disulphide bond joined helixes 2 and 3 and GPI anchor to outer surface of cell membrane

hydrogen/deuterium exchange measurements on the human protein, which show that the overall equilibrium constant describing the distribution of folded and unfolded states is the same as the protection factor (Hosszu *et al.*, 1999). This shows that there are no partially unfolded forms or intermediates that have a population greater than the unfolded state. The data suggest that PrP^{Sc} is unlikely to be formed from a kinetic folding intermediate, as has been hypothesised in the case of amyloid formation in other systems. In fact, on the basis of population it would be more likely that PrP^{Sc} were formed from the unfolded state of the molecule.

Inherited prion diseases may produce disease by destabilising PrP^C, which would predispose the molecule to aggregate. Alternatively, a mutation could facilitate the interaction between PrP^C and PrP^{Sc} or affect the binding of a ligand or co-protein. In order to relate the folding stability of PrP^C to its propensity for forming PrP^{Sc}, several of the human mutations have been copied into the recombinant mouse protein (Liemann and Glockshuber, 1999). Although this work broadly concluded that there is no absolute correlation between stability and disease, all of the fully penetrant pathogenic mutations show significant destabilisation, while non-pathogenic polymorphisms have little effect.

PrP^{Sc} is extracted from affected brains as highly aggregated, detergent insoluble material that is not amenable to high-resolution structural techniques. However, Fourier transform infrared (FTIR) spectroscopic methods show that PrP^{Sc}, in sharp contrast to PrP^C, has a high β-sheet content (Pan *et al.*, 1993). PrP^{Sc} is covalently indistinguishable from PrP^C (Pan *et al.*, 1993; Stahl *et al.*, 1993).

The underlying molecular events during infection which lead to the conversion of PrP^C to the scrapie agent remain ill-defined. The most coherent and general model thus far proposed is that the protein, PrP, fluctuates between a dominant native state, PrP^C, and a series of minor conformations, one or a set of which can self-associate in an ordered manner to produce a stable supramolecular structure, PrP^{Sc}, composed of misfolded PrP monomers. Once a stable 'seed' structure is formed, PrP can then be recruited, leading to an explosive, auto-catalytic formation of PrP^{Sc}. Such a system would be extremely sensitive to three factors: (a) overall PrP^C concentration; (b) the equilibrium distribution between the native conformation and the self-associating conformation; and (c) complimentarity between surfaces which come together in the aggregation step. All three of these predictions from this minimal model are manifest in

conserved region contains a tight binding site for a single Cu^{2+} ion with a dissociation constant (K_d) of 10^{-14} M. A second tight copper site ($K_d = 10^{-13}$ M) is present upstream of the octa-repeat region but before the structured C-domain (Jackson *et al.*, 2001; Hornshaw *et al.*, 1995; Stöckel *et al.*, 1998). Clearly, it is possible that the unstructured N-terminal region may acquire structure following copper binding. A role for PrP in copper metabolism or transport is possible and disturbance of this function by the conformational transitions between isoforms of PrP could be involved in prion-related neurotoxicity.

The structured C-domain folds and unfolds reversibly in response to chaotropic denaturants, and recent work on the folding kinetics of mouse PrP^C (Wildegger *et al.*, 1999) demonstrates that there are no populated intermediates in the folding reaction and that the protein displays unusually rapid rates of folding and unfolding. These findings have been reinforced by

the aetiology of prion disease: an inversely proportional relationship between PrP^C expression and prion incubation period in transgenic mice (Bueler et al., 1993; Collinge et al., 1995b; Prusiner et al., 1990; Telling et al., 1995); predisposition by relatively subtle mutations in the protein sequence (Collinge, 1997); and a requirement for molecular homogeneity for efficient prion propagation (Palmer et al., 1991; Prusiner et al., 1990).

Little is known for certain about the molecular state of the protein that constitutes the self-propagating, infectious particle itself. There are examples of infectivity in the absence of detectable PrP^{Sc} (Collinge et al., 1995a; Lasmézas et al., 1997; Shaked et al., 1999; Wille et al., 1996) and different strains of prions (see below) are known to differ in their degree of protease resistance. A single infectious unit corresponds to around 10^5 PrP molecules (Bolton et al., 1982). It is unclear whether this indicates that a large aggregate is necessary for infectivity or, at the other extreme, whether only a single one of these PrP^{Sc} molecules is actually infectious. This relationship of PrP^{Sc} molecules to infectivity could, however, simply relate to the rapid clearance of prions from the brain known to occur on intracerebral challenge.

Direct in vitro mixing experiments (Bessen et al., 1995; Kocisko et al., 1994, 1995) have been performed in an attempt to produce PrP^{Sc}. In such experiments an excess of PrP^{Sc} is used as a seed to convert recombinant PrP^C to a protease-resistant form (designated PrP^{RES}). However, the relative inefficiency of these reactions has precluded determining whether new infectivity has been generated. An artificial species barrier has, however, been exploited to address this issue, and such conversion products, expected to have a different host specificity (and so can be bioassayed in the presence of an excess of starting material), have not shown any detectable infectivity (Hill et al., 1999). These results argue that acquisition of protease resistance by PrP^C is not sufficient for the propagation of infectivity. Despite the obvious limitations of such experiments, they may represent an initial step in the generation of the infectious isoform of PrP, which requires additional, as yet unknown, co-factors for the acquisition of infectivity.

The difficulty in performing structural studies on native PrP^{Sc} has led to attempts to produce soluble β-sheet-rich forms of PrP, which may be amenable to NMR or crystallographic structure determination. It is now recognised that the adage 'one sequence, one conformation' is not strictly true. Depending on solvent conditions, probably any protein chain can adopt a variety of conformations in which there is a degree of periodic order (i.e. extensive regions of secondary structure). However, such alternative states do not have precisely and tightly packed side-chains, which are the hallmark of the native state of orthodox globular proteins.

Studies on a large fragment of the human prion protein (PrP$^{91-231}$) have shown that at acidic pH PrP can fold to a soluble monomer comprised almost entirely of β-sheet in the absence of denaturants (Jackson et al., 1999). Reduction of the native disulphide bond was a prerequisite for β-sheet formation and these observations of alternative folding pathways, dependent upon solvent pH and redox potential, could have important implications for the mechanism of conversion to PrP^{Sc}. Indeed, this monomeric β-sheet state was prone to aggregation into fibrils with partial resistance to proteinase K digestion, characteristic markers of PrP^{Sc}. Unusually for a protein with a predominantly helical fold, the majority of residues in PrP$^{91-231}$ have a preference for β-conformation (55% of non-glycine/proline residues). In view of this property, it is possible that the PrP molecule is delicately balanced between radically different folds with a high-energy barrier between them; one dictated by local structural propensity (the β-conformation) and one requiring the precise docking of side-chains (the native α-conformation). Such a balance would be influenced by mutations causing inherited human prion diseases. It is also worthy of note that individuals homozygous for valine at polymorphic residue 129 of human PrP (where either methionine or valine can be encoded) are more susceptible to iatrogenic CJD (Collinge et al., 1991a), and valine has a much higher β-propensity than does methionine.

The precise subcellular localisation of PrP^{Sc} propagation remains controversial. However, there is considerable evidence implicating either late-endosome-like organelles or lysosomes (Arnold et al., 1995; Laszlo et al., 1992; Mayer et al., 1992; Taraboulos et al., 1992). The environments of these organelles are evolved to facilitate protein unfolding at low pH prior to degradation by acid-activated proteases. It is possible that the α-PrP to β-PrP conversion, caused by reduction and mild acidification, is relevant to the conditions that PrP^C would encounter within the cell, following its internalisation during recycling. Such a mechanism could underlie prion propagation and account for the transmitted, sporadic and inherited aetiologies of prion disease (see Figure 26.2). Initiation of a pathogenic self-propagating conversion reaction, with accumulation of aggregated β-PrP, may be induced by exposure to a 'seed' of

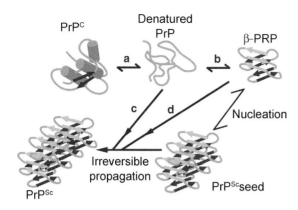

Figure 26.2 Possible mechanism for prion propagation. Largely α-helical PrP^C proceeds via an unfolded state (A) to re-fold into a largely β-sheet form, β-PrP (B). β-PrP is prone to aggregation in physiological salt concentrations. Prion replication may require a critical 'seed' size. Further recruitment of β-PrP monomers (C) or unfolded PrP (D) then occurs as an essentially irreversible process

aggregated β-PrP following prion inoculation, or as a rare stochastic conformational change, or as an inevitable consequence of expression of a pathogenic PrP^C mutant that is predisposed to form β-PrP. It remains to be demonstrated whether such alternative conformational states of the protein are sufficient to cause prion disease in an experimental host or whether other cellular co-factors are also required.

NORMAL CELLULAR FUNCTION OF PRP

While PrP plays a central role in pathogenesis of prion diseases, and mice devoid of PrP^C are resistant to scrapie and do not accumulate PrP^{Sc} or propagate infectivity (Bueler *et al.*, 1992), its normal biological function remains unclear. PrP is highly conserved amongst mammals, has been identified in marsupials, amphibians and birds, and may be present in all vertebrates. It is expressed during early embryogenesis and is found in most tissues in the adult (Manson *et al.*, 1992). However, highest levels of expression are seen in the central nervous system. The protein is found predominantly in neurons, particularly at synapses in cholesterol-rich microdomains or caveolae, known to play a central role in neuronal signalling events (for review, see Anderson, 1993). PrP is also widely expressed in cells of the immune system (Dodelet and Cashman, 1998). Mice lacking PrP as a result of gene knockout (*Prnp$^{o/o}$*) showed no gross phenotype (Bueler

et al., 1992), although they were completely resistant to prion disease following inoculation and did not replicate prions (Bueler *et al.*, 1993). However, these mice were then shown to have abnormalities in synaptic physiology (Collinge *et al.*, 1994) and in circadian rhythms and sleep (Tobler *et al.*, 1996). While none of these observations define a molecular role for PrP^C, it has been argued that PrP may act as a receptor for an as-yet unidentified extracellular ligand. Newly synthesised PrP^C is transported to the cell surface and then cycles rapidly via a clathrin-mediated mechanism, with a transit time of around an hour, between the surface and early endosomes (Shyng *et al.*, 1994).

It is possible that *Prnp$^{0/0}$* mice may be viable and healthy due to secondary compensatory mechanisms during neurodevelopment, as has been documented in other models of targeted gene knockout. The most direct approach to answering this question was by knocking out neuronal PrP expression in a developed nervous system, avoiding potential compensatory mechanisms activated during neurodevelopment, and thus to directly observe the effects of acute depletion of PrP, revealing any critical function. This has now been achieved and excludes PrP loss of function as a cause of prion neurodegeneration (Mallucci *et al.*, 2002).

PRION STRAINS

A major problem for the 'protein-only' hypothesis of prion propagation has been how to explain the existence of multiple isolates, or strains, of prions. Dickinson, Fraser and colleagues isolated multiple distinct strains of naturally occurring sheep scrapie in mice. Such strains are distinguished by their biological properties: they produce distinct incubation periods and patterns of neuropathological targeting (so-called lesion profiles) in defined inbred mouse lines (for review, see Bruce *et al.*, 1992). As they can be serially propagated in inbred mice with the same *Prnp* genotype, they cannot be encoded by differences in PrP primary structure. Furthermore, strains can be re-isolated in mice after passage in intermediate species with different PrP primary structures (Bruce *et al.*, 1994). Conventionally, distinct strains of conventional pathogen are explained by differences in their nucleic acid genome. However, in the absence of such a scrapie genome, alternative possibilities must be considered. Weissmann proposed a 'unified hypothesis' where, although the protein alone was argued to be sufficient to account for infectivity, it was proposed that strain characteristics could be encoded by a small cellular nucleic acid, or 'co-prion' (Weissmann, 1991). Although this hypothesis leads to the testable prediction that strain characteristics, unlike infectivity, would be sensitive to UV irradiation, no such test has been reported. At the other extreme, the protein-only hypothesis (Griffith, 1967) would have to explain how a single polypeptide chain could encode multiple disease phenotypes. Clearly, understanding how a protein-only infectious agent could encode such phenotypic information is of considerable biological interest.

Support for the idea that strain specificity may be encoded by PrP itself was provided by study of two distinct strains of transmissible mink encephalopathy prions which can be serially propagated in hamsters, designated hyper (HY) and drowsy (DY). These strains can be distinguished by differing physiochemical properties of the accumulated PrP^{Sc} in the brains of affected hamsters (Bessen and Marsh, 1992). Following limited proteolysis, strain-specific migration patterns of PrP^{Sc} on polyacrylamide gels were seen which related to different N-terminal ends of HY and DY PrP^{Sc} following protease treatment and implying differing conformations of HY and DY PrP^{Sc} (Bessen and Marsh, 1994).

Distinct human PrP^{Sc} types have been identified which are associated with different phenotypes of CJD (Collinge et al., 1996b; Parchi et al., 1996). The different fragment sizes seen on Western blots following treatment with proteinase K suggests that there are several different human PrP^{Sc} conformations. However, while such biochemical modifications of PrP are clearly candidates for the molecular substrate of prion strain diversity, it is necessary to be able to demonstrate that these properties fulfil the biological properties of strains. In particular, that they are transmissible to the PrP in a host of both the same and different species. This has been demonstrated in studies with CJD isolates, with both PrP^{Sc} fragment sizes and the ratios of the three PrP glycoforms (diglycosylated, monoglycosylated and unglycosylated PrP) maintained on passage in transgenic mice expressing human PrP (Collinge et al., 1996b). Furthermore, transmission of human prions and bovine prions to wild-type mice results in murine PrP^{Sc}, with fragment sizes and glycoform ratios which correspond to the original inoculum (Collinge et al., 1996b). Variant CJD is associated with PrP^{Sc} glycoform ratios, which are distinct from those seen in classical CJD. Similar ratios are seen in BSE and BSE when transmitted to several other species (Collinge et al., 1996b). These data strongly support the 'protein

only' hypothesis of infectivity and suggest that strain variation could be encoded by a combination of PrP conformation and glycosylation. Furthermore, polymorphism in PrP sequence can influence the generation of particular PrP^{Sc} conformers (Collinge et al., 1996b). Transmission of PrP^{Sc} fragment sizes from two different subtypes of inherited prion disease to transgenic mice expressing a chimaeric human mouse PrP has also been reported (Telling et al., 1996). As PrP glycosylation occurs before conversion to PrP^{Sc}, the different glycoform ratios may represent selection of particular PrP^{C} glycoforms by PrP^{Sc} of different conformations. According to such a hypothesis, PrP conformation would be the primary determinant of strain type, with glycosylation being involved as a secondary process. However, since it is known that different cell types may glycosylate proteins differently, PrP^{Sc} glycosylation patterns may provide a substrate for the neuropathological targeting that distinguishes different prion strains (Collinge et al., 1996b). Particular PrP^{Sc} glycoforms may replicate most favourably in neuronal populations with a similar PrP glycoform expressed on the cell surface. Such targeting could also explain the different incubation periods which also discriminate strains, targeting of more critical brain regions, or regions with higher levels of PrP expression, producing shorter incubation periods.

Recent work has shown strain-specific protein conformation to be influenced by metal binding to PrP^{Sc} (Wadsworth et al., 1999). Two different human PrP^{Sc} types, seen in clinically distinct subtypes of classical Creutzfeldt–Jakob disease, can be interconverted in vitro by altering the metal-ion occupancy. The dependence of PrP^{Sc} conformation on the binding of copper and zinc represents a novel mechanism for post-translational modification of PrP and for the generation of multiple prion strains.

Molecular strain typing of prion isolates can now be applied to molecular diagnosis of vCJD (Collinge et al., 1996b; Hill et al., 1997a) and to produce a new classification of human prion diseases with implications for epidemiological studies investigating the aetiology of sporadic CJD (Figure 26.3). Such methods allow strain typing to be performed in days rather than the 1–2 years required for classical biological strain typing. This technique may also be applicable to determining whether BSE has been transmitted to other species (Collinge et al., 1996b) and thereby poses a threat to human health, e.g. to sheep (Hill et al., 1998; Hope et al., 1999; Kuczius et al., 1998).

Such ability of a single polypeptide chain to encode information specifying distinct phenotypes of disease raises intriguing evolutionary questions. Do other

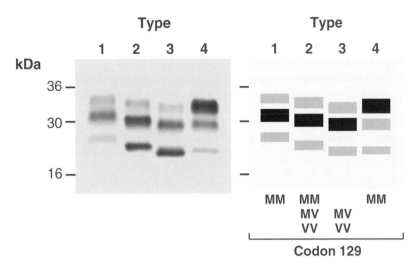

Figure 26.3 Molecular strain typing of human prions

proteins behave in this way? The novel pathogenic mechanisms involved in prion propagation may be of far wider significance and relevant to other neurological and non-neurological illnesses; indeed, other prion-like mechanisms have now been described and the field of yeast and fungal prions has emerged (Wickner, 1997; Wickner and Masison, 1996).

NEURONAL CELL DEATH IN PRION DISEASE

The precise molecular nature of the infectious agent and the cause of neuronal cell death remains unclear. The current working hypothesis is that an abnormal isoform of PrP is the infectious agent and, to date, the most highly enriched preparations contain one infectious unit per 10^5 PrP monomers (Bolton et al., 1982). Various hypotheses have been proposed to explain the mechanism of spongiform change and neuronal cell loss. These have included direct neurotoxic effects from a region of the prion protein encompassing residues 106–126 (Brown et al., 1994; Forloni et al., 1993; Tagliavini et al., 1993b) to increased oxidative stress in neurons as a result of PrP^C depletion, which has been proposed to function as an antioxidant molecule (Brown et al., 1997). Neurotoxicity of PrP 106–126 is, however, controversial (Kunz et al., 1999). It has also been suggested that PrP^C plays a role in regulating apoptosis with disturbance of normal cellular levels of PrP during infection leading to cell death (Kurschner and Morgan, 1995, 1996). Certainly there have been numerous recent reports of apoptotic cells being identified in the neuronal tissue of prion disease brains

(Williams et al., 1997). Although PrP^C expression is required for susceptibility to the disease, a number of observations argue that PrP^{Sc}, and indeed prions (whether or not they are identical), may not themselves be highly neurotoxic. Prion diseases in which PrP^{Sc} is barely or not detectable have been described (Medori et al., 1992a; Collinge et al., 1995a; Hsiao et al., 1990; Lasmézas et al., 1997). Mice with reduced levels of PrP^C expression have extremely high levels of PrP^{Sc} and prions in the brain and yet remain well for several months after their wild-type counterparts succumb (Bueler et al., 1993). Conversely, Tg20 mice, with high levels of PrP^C, have short incubation periods and yet produce low levels of PrP^{Sc} after inoculation with mouse prions (Fischer et al., 1996). In addition, brain grafts producing high levels of PrP^{Sc} do not damage adjacent tissue in PrP knockout ($Prnp^{o/o}$) mice (Brandner et al., 1996). The cause of neurodegeneration in prion diseases remains unclear. It remains possible that prion neurodegeneration is related, at least in part, to loss of function of PrP^C. That $Prnp^{o/o}$ mice (other than those associated with overexpression of the $Prnp$-like gene Dpl (Moore et al., 1999) do not develop neurodegeneration could be due to compensatory adaptations during neurodevelopment. Complete or near-complete ablation of PrP expression in an adult mouse using conditional gene expression methods has not yet been achieved. A recent study has demonstrated that mice inoculated with Sc237 hamster prions replicate prions to high levels in their brains, but do not develop clinical signs of prion disease during their normal lifespan, arguing that PrP^{Sc} and indeed prions (whether or not they are identical) may not themselves be highly neurotoxic (Hill *et al.*, 2000). An alternative hypothesis for prion-related neurodegeneration is that a toxic, possibly infectious, intermediate is produced in the process of conversion of PrP^C to PrP^{Sc}, with PrP^{Sc} present as highly aggregated material, being a relatively inert end-product. The steady-state level of such a toxic monomeric or oligomeric PrP intermediate could then determine the rate of neurodegeneration. One possibility is that Sc237-inoculated mice propagate prions very slowly and that such a toxic intermediate is generated at extremely low levels that are tolerated by the mouse (Hill *et al.*, 2000).

THE 'SPECIES BARRIER'

Transmission of prion diseases between different mammalian species is restricted by a 'species barrier' (Pattison, 1965). On primary passage of prions from species A to species B, usually not all inoculated animals of species B develop disease and those that do have much longer and more variable incubation periods than those that are seen with transmission of prions within the same species, where typically all inoculated animals would succumb with a relatively short, and remarkably consistent, incubation period. On second passage of infectivity to further animals of the species B, transmission parameters resemble within-species transmissions, with most if not all animals developing the disease with short and consistent incubation periods. Species barriers can therefore be quantitated by measuring the fall in mean incubation period on primary and second passage, or, perhaps more rigorously, by a comparative titration study. The latter involves inoculating serial dilutions of an inoculum in both the donor and host species and comparing the LD$_{50}$s obtained. The effect of a very substantial species barrier (e.g. that between hamsters and mice) is that few, if any, animals succumb to disease at all on primary passage, and then at incubation periods approaching the natural lifespan of the species concerned.

Early studies of the molecular basis of the species barrier argued that it principally resided in differences in PrP primary structure between the species from which the inoculum was derived and the inoculated host. Transgenic mice expressing hamster PrP were, unlike wild-type mice, highly susceptible to infection with Sc237 hamster prions (Prusiner *et al.*, 1990). That most sporadic and acquired CJD occurred in individuals homozygous at *PRNP* polymorphic codon 129 supported the view that prion propagation proceeded most efficiently when the interacting PrP^{Sc} and PrP^C were of identical primary structure (Collinge *et al.*, 1991; Palmer *et al.*, 1991a). However, it has been long recognised that prion strain type affects ease of transmission to another species. Interestingly, with BSE prions the strain component to the barrier seems to predominate, with BSE not only transmitting efficiently to a range of species, but maintaining its transmission characteristics even when passaged through an intermediate species with a distinct PrP gene (Bruce *et al.*, 1994). For instance, transmission of CJD prions to conventional mice is difficult, with few if any inoculated mice succumbing after prolonged incubation periods, consistent with a substantial species barrier (Collinge *et al.*, 1995b; Hill *et al.*, 1997a). In sharp contrast, transgenic mice expressing only human PrP are highly susceptible to CJD prions, with 100% attack rate and consistent short incubation periods which are unaltered by second passage, consistent with a complete lack of species barrier (Collinge *et al.*, 1995b). However, vCJD prions (again comprising human PrP of identical primary structure) transmit much more readily to wild-type mice than do classical CJD prions, while transmission to transgenic mice is relatively less efficient than with classical CJD (Hill *et al.*, 1997a). The term 'species barrier' does not seem appropriate to describe such effects and 'species–strain barrier' or simply 'transmission barrier' may be preferable (Collinge, 1999). Both PrP amino acid sequence and strain type affect the 3D structure of glycosylated PrP, which will presumably, in turn, affect the efficiency of the protein–protein interactions thought to determine prion propagation.

Mammalian PrP genes are highly conserved. Presumably only a restricted number of different PrP^{Sc} conformations (which are highly stable and can therefore be serially propagated) will be permissible thermodynamically and will constitute the range of prion strains seen. PrP glycosylation may be important in stabilising particular PrP^{Sc} conformations. While a significant number of different such PrP^{Sc} conformations may be possible amongst the range of mammalian PrPs, only a subset of these would be allowable for a given single mammalian PrP. Substantial overlap between the favoured conformations for PrP^{Sc} derived from species A and species B might therefore result in relatively easy transmission of prion diseases between these two species, while two species with no preferred PrP^{Sc} conformations in common would have a large barrier to transmission (and, indeed, transmission would necessitate a change of strain type). According to such a model of a prion transmission barrier, BSE may represent a thermodynamically highly favoured PrP^{Sc} conformation that is permissive for PrP expressed in a wide range of different species, accounting for the remarkable promiscuity of this strain in mammals. A contribution of other components to the species barrier is possible and may involve interacting co-factors which mediate the efficiency of prion propagation, although no such factors have yet been identified.

Recent data has further challenged our understanding of transmission barriers (Hill *et al.*, 2000). The assessment of species barriers has relied on the development of a clinical disease in inoculated animals. On this basis there is a highly efficient barrier limiting transmission of hamster Sc237 prions to mice. Indeed, the hamster scrapie strain Sc237 (which is similar to the strain classified as 263K; Kimberlin and Walker, 1978), is regarded as non-pathogenic for mice (with no clinical disease in mice observed for up to 735 days post-inoculation; Kimberlin and Walker, 1978) and was used in studies of species barriers in transgenic mice (Kimberlin and Walker, 1979; Prusiner *et al.*, 1990; Scott *et al.*, 1989). It was demonstrated that transgenic mice expressing hamster PrP (in addition to endogenous mouse PrP), in sharp contrast to conventional mice, were highly susceptible to Sc237 hamster prions, with consistent short incubation periods which were inversely correlated to hamster PrP expression levels (Scott *et al.*, 1989; Prusiner *et al.*, 1990). Importantly, however, these studies defined transmission using clinical criteria and did not report PrP^{Sc} levels and types, or prion titres in the brains of clinically unaffected animals. However, while not developing a clinical disease, and indeed living as long as mock-inoculated mice, Sc237-inoculated mice may accumulate high levels of prions in their brains (Hill *et al.*, 2000). Previous studies on the species barrier between hamsters and mice (using the Sc237 or 263K strain) did not report whether PrP^{Sc} and/or infectivity were present in clinically unaffected animals (Prusiner *et al.*, 1990; Scott *et al.*, 1989) or have attempted passage from mice only up to 280 days post-inoculation (Kimberlin and Walker, 1978). The barrier to primary passage appears in this case to be to the development of rapid neurodegeneration and the resulting clinical syndrome, rather than a barrier to prion propagation itself.

PATHOGENESIS

In some experimental rodent scrapie models in which prions are inoculated outside the CNS, and in natural sheep scrapie, infectivity is first detectable in the spleen and other lymphoreticular tissues (for review, see Fraser *et al.*, 1992). Spleen titres rise to a plateau early in the incubation period, a considerable period before neuroinvasion is detectable. CNS prion replication then rises to high levels and the clinical phase occurs.

The route of entry of prions following oral exposure may follow invasion of Peyer's patches and other gut lymphoid tissues; the relative protease-resistance of prions presumably allows a significant proportion of infectivity to survive the digestive tract. It is unclear how prions transit the intestinal mucosa, although M cells may be involved (Heppner *et al.*, 2001). It has been suggested that myeloid dendritic cells mediate transport within the lymphoreticular system (Aucouturier *et al.*, 2001). While mature B cells are required for peripheral prion propagation, this appears to be because they are required for maturation of follicular dendritic cells (FDCs). PrP^{Sc} accumulates in FDCs, which are a long-lived cell type, and it is thought that they are the site of prion propagation in the spleen (Mabbott *et al.*, 2000, 2003; Montrasio *et al.*, 2000). However, neuroinvasion is possible without FDCs, indicating that other peripheral cell types can replicate prions (Oldstone *et al.*, 2002; Prinz *et al.*, 2002). Neuroinvasion involves the autonomic nervous system innervating lymphoid tissue with retrograde spread to the spinal cord or via the vagus to the brainstem (Beekes *et al.*, 1998; Bencsik *et al.*, 2001). Prions have been detected in the blood at low levels in some rodent models and experimental BSE-infected primates (Bons *et al.*, 2002; Brown *et al.*, 1999; Holada *et al.*, 2002) and transmission of BSE prions between sheep by transfusion has been reported (Hunter *et al.*, 2002). Several reports of infrequent transmission from human blood to rodents have been reported (for review, see Brown, 1995).

While prominent lymphoreticular involvement is seen in some experimental models or natural prion diseases, it is undetectable in others (for review, see Fraser *et al.*, 1992). Both host and prion strain effects are relevant, e.g. infection of sheep with BSE prions results in a wide tissue distribution of infectivity but infection of cattle with this strain does not, infectivity being largely confined to the CNS. In humans infected with sporadic CJD prions, infectivity is largely confined to the CNS, while in variant CJD there is prominent involvement of lymphoreticular tissues (Hill *et al.*, 1997b, 1999; Wadsworth *et al.*, 2001). It is possible that species-barrier effects are also relevant, and it has been suggested that, on passage of prions in a new species, there is an obligate lymphoreticular phase. This would be of considerable importance with respect to human BSE infection, which can be diagnosed by tonsil biopsy (see below), as it opens the possibility that cases arising from subsequent human-to-human transmission via iatrogenic routes may not be detectable by this means.

ANIMAL PRION DISEASES

An increasing number of animal prion diseases are recognised. Scrapie, a naturally occurring disease of sheep and goats, has been recognised in Europe for over 200 years and is present endemically in many countries. Accurate epidemiology is lacking, although scrapie appears to be relatively common in some countries. Remarkably little is known about its natural routes of transmission. Transmissible mink encephalopathy (TME) and chronic wasting disease of mule deer and elk were described from the 1940s onwards, principally in the USA. It has more recently become apparent that chronic wasting disease is a common condition in wild deer and elk in Colorado. Again the routes of transmission are unclear. TME has occurred as infrequent epidemics amongst ranched mink and may result from food-borne prion exposure.

The appearance of BSE in UK cattle from 1986 onwards, which rapidly evolved to a major epidemic (Anderson et al., 1996; Wilesmith et al., 1988), was widely attributed to transmission of sheep scrapie, endemic in the UK and many other countries, to cattle via contaminated feed prepared from rendered carcasses (Wilesmith et al., 1988). However, an alternative hypothesis is that epidemic BSE resulted from recycling of rare sporadic BSE cases, as cattle were also rendered to produce cattle feed. Whether or not BSE originated from sheep scrapie, however, it was clear from 1990 onwards, with the occurrence of novel spongiform encephalopathies amongst domestic and captive wild cats, that its host range was different to that of scrapie. Many new species have developed spongiform encephalopathies coincident with or following the arrival of BSE, including greater kudu, nyala, Arabian oryx, Scimitar-horned oryx, eland, gemsbok, bison, ankole, tiger, cheetah, ocelot, puma and domestic cats. Several of these have been confirmed to be caused by a BSE-like prion strain (Bruce et al., 1994; Collinge et al., 1996b), and it is likely that most or all are BSE-related. More than 180 000 BSE cases have been confirmed in cattle in the UK, although the total number of infected animals has been estimated to be around 2 million. BSE has since been reported in many European countries, with significant epidemics reported in Switzerland and Portugal, and a number of other countries including Canada and Japan.

AETIOLOGY AND EPIDEMIOLOGY AND HUMAN PRION DISEASE

The human prion diseases have been traditionally classified into Creutzfeldt–Jakob disease (CJD), Gerstmann–Sträussler–Scheinker disease and kuru, and they can be further divided into three aetiological categories: sporadic, acquired and inherited.

Sporadic CJD makes up around 85% of all recognised human prion disease. It occurs in all countries with a random case distribution and an annual incidence of 1 per million. Hypothesised causes of sporadic CJD include spontaneous production of PrP^{Sc} via rare stochastic events, somatic mutation of PRNP or unidentified environmental prion exposure. An association with sheep scrapie is not supported by epidemiological studies, which have found a fairly uniform worldwide incidence of sporadic CJD, irrespective of scrapie prevalence (Brown et al., 1987). Although spatiotemporal groupings of sporadic CJD have been reported previously (Adikari and Farmer, 2001; Farmer et al., 1978), no direct evidence for exposure to a common source of infectious prions has been provided. Indeed, such apparent clustering of cases, while appearing to reach levels of significance when viewed in isolation, can be deemed to be expected by chance alone when analysed within the population as a whole (Collins et al., 2002). However, the lack of such evidence does not exclude the possibility that a fraction of sporadic CJD, is caused by environmental exposure to animal or human prions. There is marked genetic susceptibility in sporadic CJD in that most cases occur in homozygotes at codon 129 of PRNP, where either methionine or valine may be encoded. Heterozygotes appear significantly protected against developing sporadic CJD (Collinge et al., 1991b; Palmer et al., 1991; Windl et al., 1996). Additionally, a PRNP susceptibility haplotype has been identified indicating additional genetic susceptibility to sporadic CJD at or near to the PRNP locus (Mead et al., 2001).

The acquired prion diseases include iatrogenic CJD and kuru, and arise from accidental exposure to human prions through medical or surgical procedures or participation in cannibalistic feasts. The two most frequent causes of iatrogenic CJD occurring through medical procedures have arisen as a result of implantation of dura mater grafts and treatment with human growth hormone derived from the pituitary glands of human cadavers (Brown *et al.*, 1992, 2000). Less frequent incidences of human prion disease have resulted from iatrogenic transmission of CJD during corneal transplantation, contaminated electroencephalographic (EEG) electrode implantation and surgical operations using contaminated instruments or apparatus (Brown *et al.*, 1992, 2000). *PRNP* codon 129 genotype is also relevant to susceptibility and incubation period (see below).

Around 15% of human prion disease is inherited and all cases to date have been associated with coding mutations in the prion protein gene (*PRNP*), of which over 30 distinct types are recognised (Figure 26.3). The inherited prion diseases can be diagnosed by *PRNP* analysis and the use of these definitive genetic diagnostic markers has allowed the recognition of a wider phenotypic spectrum of human prion disease to include a range of atypical dementias and fatal familial insomnia (Collinge *et al.*, 1990, 1992; Medori *et al.*, 1992b). The protective effect of *PRNP* codon 129 heterozygosity is also seen in some of the inherited prion diseases, with a later age at disease onset in heterozygotes (Baker *et al.*, 1991; Hsiao *et al.*, 1992).

The occurrence of cases of apparently sporadic CJD in unusually young people in 1995 (Bateman *et al.*, 1995; Britton *et al.*, 1995; Tabrizi *et al.*, 1996) led to concerns that BSE transmission to humans may have occurred. Arrival of further cases in 1996 led to the recognition of a novel clinicopathological type of human prion disease, new variant CJD (vCJD) (Will *et al.*, 1996), indicating the arrival of a new risk factor for CJD in the UK (Collinge and Rossor, 1996). A link with BSE seemed highly likely on epidemiological grounds and this was strongly supported by experimental data, first from molecular strain typing studies (Collinge *et al.*, 1996b) and later by transmission studies into both transgenic and conventional mice (Hill *et al.*, 1997a; Bruce *et al.*, 1997). *PRNP* mutations are absent in vCJD, and all cases studied to date have been methionine homozygotes at codon 129 (Collinge *et al.*, 1996a; Zeidler *et al.*, 1997b and unpublished).

That vCJD is caused by the same prion strain as that causing BSE in cattle raised the possibility that a major epidemic of vCJD will occur in the UK and other countries as a result of dietary or other exposure to BSE prions, and also (Ghani *et al.*, 1999) concerns of potential iatrogenic transmission of preclinical vCJD via medical and surgical procedures. That only *PRNP* 129MM individuals are susceptible to BSE infection is questionable, since the other acquired human prion diseases, iatrogenic CJD and kuru, occur in all codon 129 genotypes as the epidemic evolves, with codon 129 heterozygotes having the longest mean incubation periods (Collinge, 1999; Lloyd *et al.*, 2002; Poulter *et al.*, 1992). Human BSE infection of other *PRNP* genotypes may simply have a longer latency (Collinge, 1999) and may also have a different phenotype (Hill *et al.*, 1997a).

Estimates of the mean incubation period of human-to-human prion transmission come from study of growth hormone-related iatrogenic CJD and kuru. The mean incubation period has been estimated in both examples to be around 12 years; in kuru, incubation periods can exceed 40 years (for review, see Collinge, 1999). The effect of a species barrier is to considerably increase mean incubation periods and the range of incubation periods, which may approach the usual lifespan of the species concerned. The cattle to mouse barrier for the BSE strain results typically in a three- to four-fold increase in mean incubation period. Mean incubation periods of human BSE infection of 30 years or more should be considered (Collinge, 1999). Furthermore, prion disease in mice follows a well-defined course with a highly distinctive and repeatable incubation time for a given prion strain in a defined inbred mouse line. In addition to the prion protein gene, a small number of additional genetic loci with a major effect on incubation period have been mapped. It can be anticipated that the human homologues of such loci may play a key role in human susceptibility to prion disease, following both accidental human prion exposure and exposure to the BSE agent. By definition, the patients identified to date with vCJD are those with the shortest incubation periods for BSE. These, in turn, given that no unusual history of dietary, occupational or other exposure to BSE has been identified, would be expected to be predominantly those individuals with short incubation time alleles at these multiple genetic loci in addition to having the codon 129 methionine homozygous *PRNP* genotype. The vCJD cases reported to date may therefore represent a distinct genetic subpopulation with unusually short incubation periods to BSE prions. It is possible, therefore, that a human BSE epidemic will be multiphasic, and that recent estimates of the size of the vCJD epidemic based on uniform genetic susceptibility may substantially underestimate the eventual size (D'Aignaux *et al.*, 2001; Ghani *et al.*, 2000). Genes involved in species barrier effects, which would further increase both the mean and range of human BSE incubation periods, are also likely to be relevant. In this context, it will be very difficult to accurately predict a human epidemic until such loci are identified and their gene frequencies in the population can be determined (Lloyd *et al.*, 2001).

CLINICAL FEATURES AND DIAGNOSIS

With the advances in our understanding of their aetiology, it now seems more appropriate to divide the human prion diseases into inherited, sporadic and acquired forms, with CJD, GSS and kuru being clinicopathological syndromes within a wider spectrum of disease. Kindreds with inherited prion disease have been described, with phenotypes of classical CJD and GSS and also with other neurodegenerative syndromes including fatal familial insomnia (Medori *et al.*, 1992b). Some kindreds show remarkable phenotypic variability which can encompass both CJD- and GSS-like cases, as well as other cases which do not conform to either CJD or GSS phenotypes (Collinge *et al.*, 1992). Cases diagnosed by PrP gene analysis have been

reported which are not only clinically atypical but which lack the classical histological features entirely (Collinge *et al.*, 1990). Significant clinical overlap exists with familial Alzheimer's disease, Pick's disease, frontal lobe degeneration of non-Alzheimer type and amyotrophic lateral sclerosis with dementia. Although classical GSS is described below, it now seems more sensible to designate the familial illnesses as inherited prion diseases and then to sub-classify these according to mutation. Acquired prion diseases include iatrogenic CJD, kuru and now vCJD. Sporadic prion diseases at present consist of CJD and atypical variants of CJD. Cases lacking the characteristic histological features of CJD have been transmitted. As there are at present no equivalent aetiological diagnostic markers for sporadic prion diseases to those for the inherited diseases, it cannot yet be excluded that more diverse phenotypic variants of sporadic prion disease exist. The key clinical features and investigations for the diagnosis of prion disease are given in Table 26.1.

Table 26.1   Diagnosis of human prion disease

Sporadic (classical) CJD	<ul><li>Rapidly progressive dementia with two or more of myoclonus, cortical bindness, pyramidal signs, cerebellar signs, extra-pyramidal signs, akinetic mutism</li><li>*PRNP* analysis: no pathogenic mutations</li><li>If brain biopsy performed: PrP immunocytochemistry or Western blot for PrP^{Sc} types 1–3</li></ul>	<ul><li>Most cases aged 45–75 Serial EEG shows pseudoperiodic complexes in most cases</li><li>CSF 14–3–3 protein usually positive</li><li>CT and MRI normal, or atrophy, or abnormal signal basal ganglia</li><li>*PRNP* analysis: most are 129 homozygotes</li></ul>
Iatrogenic CJD	<ul><li>Progressive cerebellar syndrome and behavioural disturbance, or classical CJD-like syndrome, with history of iatrogenic exposure to human prions (pituitary-derived hormones, tissue grafting or neurosurgery)</li><li>*PRNP* analysis: no pathogenic mutations</li><li>If brain biopsy performed: PrP immunocytochemistry or Western blot for PrP^{Sc} types 1–3</li></ul>	<ul><li>May be young</li><li>EEG, CSF and MRI generally less helpful than in sporadic cases</li><li>*PRNP* analysis: most are 129 homozygotes</li></ul>
Variant CJD	<ul><li>Early features: depression, anxiety, social withdrawal, peripheral sensory symptoms</li><li>EEG: non-specific slow waves</li><li>*PRNP* analysis: no pathogenic mutations</li><li>If tonsil biopsy performed: characteristic PrP immunostaining and PrP^{Sc} on Western blot (type 4t)</li></ul>	<ul><li>Cerebellar ataxia, chorea or athetosis often precedes dementia, advanced disease as sporadic CJD</li><li>Most in young adults</li><li>CSF 14–3–3 may be elevated</li><li>MRI: may be high T2-weighted signal in posterior thalamus bilaterally</li><li>*PRNP* analysis: all 129MM to date</li></ul>
Inherited prion disease	<ul><li>*PRNP* analysis: pathogenic mutations</li></ul>	<ul><li>Varied clinical syndromes between and within kindreds: should consider in all pre-senile dementias and ataxias irrespective of family history</li><li>*PRNP* analysis: codon 129 genotype may predict age at onset in pre-symptomatic testing</li></ul>

Sporadic Prion Disease

Creutzfeldt–Jakob Disease

The core clinical syndrome of classic CJD is a rapidly progressive multifocal dementia, usually with prominent myoclonus. Onset is usually in the 45–75 year age group, with peak onset between 60–65. The clinical progression is typically over weeks and may progress to akinetic mutism and death in 2–3 months. Around 70% of cases die in under 6 months. Prodromal features, present in around one-third of cases, include fatigue, insomnia, depression, weight loss, headaches, general malaise and ill-defined pain sensations. In addition to mental deterioration and myoclonus, frequent additional neurological features include extrapyramidal signs, cerebellar ataxia, pyramidal signs and cortical blindness. About 10% of cases present initially with cerebellar ataxia.

Routine haematological and biochemical investigations are normal, although occasional cases have been noted to have raised serum transaminases or alkaline phosphatase. There are no immunological markers and acute phase proteins are not elevated. Examination of the cerebrospinal fluid is normal, although raised neuronal-specific enolase (NSE), S-100 and 14–3–3 protein have been proposed as useful markers, although it is clear that they are not specific for CJD and represent markers of neuronal injury or astrocyte activation (Jimi *et al.*, 1992; Otto *et al.*, 1997; Zerr *et al.*, 1995). A positive 14–3–3 appears to be a useful adjunct to diagnosis in the appropriate clinical context (Collinge, 1996); it is also positive in recent cerebral infarction or haemorrhage and in viral encephalitis, although these conditions do not usually present diagnostic confusion with CJD. Neuroimaging with CT or MRI is essential to exclude other causes of subacute neurological illness and may also show cerebral and cerebellar atrophy. MRI scanning may demonstrate signal changes in the basal ganglia that, although not specific, can be diagnostically helpful (Schroter *et al.*, 2000). The electroencephalogram (EEG) may show characteristic pseudoperiodic sharp wave activity (Figure 26.4), which is useful in diagnosis but present only in around 70% of cases. To some extent, demonstration of a typical EEG is dependent on the number of EEGs performed and serial EEG is indicated to try to demonstrate this appearance.

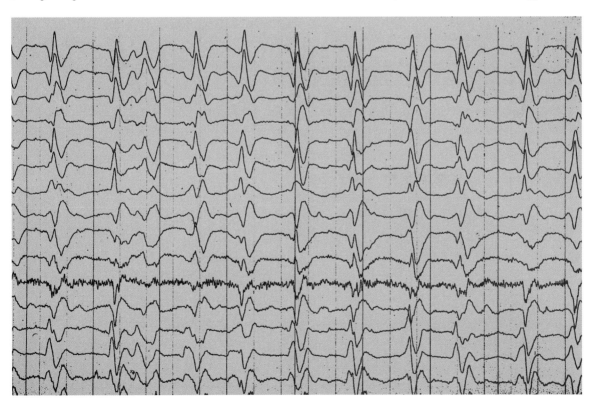

Figure 26.4 Electroencephalogram in sporadic CJD

Prospective epidemiological studies have demonstrated that cases with a progressive dementia, and two or more of the following—myoclonus; cortical blindness; pyramidal, cerebellar or extrapyramidal signs; or akinetic mutism in the setting of a typical EEG—nearly always turn out to be confirmed as histologically definite CJD if neuropathological examination is performed. Brain biopsy may be considered in selected cases to exclude alternative, potentially treatable diagnoses; inherited prion disease should be excluded prior to biopsy by gene analysis. Neuropathological confirmation of CJD is by demonstration of spongiform change, neuronal loss and astrocytosis. PrP amyloid plaques are usually not present in CJD, although PrP immunohistochemistry, using appropriate pre-treatments (Bell et al., 1997; Budka et al., 1995), will nearly always be positive (Figure 26.5). PrP[Sc], seen in all the currently recognised prion diseases, can be demonstrated by immunoblotting of brain homogenates. Genetic susceptibility to CJD has been demonstrated in that most cases of classical CJD are homozygous with respect to the common 129 polymorphism of PrP.

Atypical Forms of Creutzfeldt–Jakob Disease

Atypical forms of Creutzfeldt–Jakob disease are well recognised. Around 10% of cases of CJD have a much more prolonged clinical course, with a disease duration of over 2 years (Brown et al., 1984). These cases may represent the occasional occurrence of CJD in individuals heterozygous for PrP polymorphisms. Around 10% of CJD cases present with cerebellar ataxia rather than cognitive impairment, so-called 'ataxic CJD' (Gomori et al., 1973). Heidenhain's variant of CJD refers to cases in which cortical blindness predominates with severe involvement of the occipital lobes. The panencephalopathic type of CJD refers to cases with extensive degeneration of the cerebral white matter in addition to spongiform vacuolation of the grey matter, and has been predominately reported from Japan (Gomori et al., 1973).

Amyotrophic variants of CJD have been described with prominent early muscle wasting. However, most cases of dementia with amyotrophy are not experimentally transmissible (Salazar et al., 1983) and their relationship with CJD is unclear. Most cases are probably variants of motor neuron disease with associated dementia. Amyotrophic features in CJD are usually seen in late disease when other features are well established.

Molecular Classification of Sporadic CJD

The marked clinical heterogeneity observed in human prion diseases has yet to be explained. However, it has been clear for many years that distinct isolates, or strains, of prions can be propagated in the same host and these are biologically recognised by distinctive clinical and pathological features (Collinge, 2001; Hill and Collinge, 2001). It is therefore likely that a proportion of clinicopathological heterogeneity seen in sporadic CJD and other human prion diseases relates to the propagation of distinct human prion strains. The identification of strain-specific PrP[Sc] structural properties would thus allow an aetiology-based classification of CJD by typing of the infectious agent itself.

Four types of human PrP[Sc] have now been reliably identified using molecular strain typing (Collinge et al., 1996b; Hill et al., 1997a, 2003; Wadsworth et al., 1999) (Figure 26.3). Sporadic and iatrogenic CJD are associated with PrP[Sc] types 1–3, while type 4 human PrP[Sc] is uniquely associated with vCJD and is characterised by a fragment size and glycoform ratio that is distinct from PrP[Sc] types 1–3 observed in classical CJD (Collinge et al., 1996b; Hill et al., 1997a, 2003; Wadsworth et al., 1999). The methionine/valine polymorphism at codon 129 of PRNP is associated with different PrP[Sc] types. PrP[Sc] types 1 and 4 have so far only been detected in methionine homozygotes, type 3 cases are predominantly associated with at least one valine allele, while type 2 is seen in any PRNP codon 129 genotype (Collinge et al., 1996a, 1996b; Hill et al., 1999, 2003; Wadsworth et al., 1999). PrP[Sc] types 1 and 2 are associated with two clinically distinct subtypes of sporadic CJD and have N-terminal structures determined by the coordination of metal ions (Hill et al., 2003; Wadsworth et al., 1999). Importantly, the identification of strain-specific PrP[Sc] structural properties has enabled investigation of the influence of human PrP primary structure, in particular polymorphic residue 129, in determining PrP[Sc] structure. Transgenic mice expressing human PrP with either valine or methionine at residue 129 have revealed that this polymorphism constrains both the propagation of distinct human PrP[Sc] conformers and the occurrence of associated patterns of neuropathology (Asante et al., 2002; Collinge et al., 1996b; Hill et al., 1997a; and unpublished data). These data strongly support the biological relevance of molecular strain typing, which can now be applied to rapid molecular diagnosis of classical CJD or vCJD and to produce a new classification of human prion diseases.

Molecular strain typing has major implications for epidemiological surveillance of sporadic CJD, whose aetiology remains obscure. While spontaneous conversion of PrP^C to PrP^{Sc} as a rare stochastic event, or somatic mutation of the PrP gene resulting in expression of a pathogenic PrP mutant, are plausible explanations for sporadic CJD (Collinge, 1997), other causes for at least some cases, including environmental exposure to human or animal prions, has not been ruled out by existing epidemiological studies (Collins *et al.*, 1999). Sub-classification of sporadic CJD based upon PrP^{Sc} type immediately allows a more precise molecular classification of human prion disease, and re-analysis of epidemiological data using these molecular subtypes may reveal important risk factors obscured when sporadic CJD is analysed as a single entity. For example, it will be important to review the incidence of sporadic CJD associated with PrP^{Sc} type 2 and other molecular subtypes, in both BSE-affected and unaffected countries, in the light of recent findings suggesting that human BSE prion infection may result in propagation of either type 4 PrP^{Sc} or type 2 PrP^{Sc}(Asante *et al.*, 2002). Individuals that propagate type 2 PrP^{Sc} as a result of BSE exposure may present with prion disease that would be indistinguishable on clinical, pathological and molecular criteria from that found in classical CJD.

Acquired Prion Diseases

While human prion diseases can be transmitted to experimental animals by inoculation, they are not contagious in humans. Documented case-to-case spread has only occurred during ritual cannibalistic practices (kuru) or following accidental inoculation with prions during medical or surgical procedures (iatrogenic CJD).

Kuru

Kuru reached epidemic proportions amongst a defined population living in the Eastern Highlands of Papua New Guinea. The earliest cases are thought to date back to the early part of the century. Kuru affected the people of the Fore linguistic group and their neighbours, with whom they intermarried. Kuru predominantly affected women and children (of both sexes), with only 2% of cases in adult males (Alpers, 1987), and was the commonest cause of death amongst women in affected villages. It was the practice in these communities to engage in consumption of dead relatives as a mark of respect and mourning. Women and children predominantly ate the brain and internal organs, which is thought to explain the differential age and sex incidence. Preparation of the cadaver for consumption was performed by the women and children, such that other routes of exposure may also have been relevant. It is thought that the epidemic related to a single sporadic CJD case occurring in the region some decades earlier. Epidemiological studies provided no evidence for vertical transmission, since most of the children born after 1956 (when cannibalism had effectively ceased) and all of those born after 1959 of mothers affected with or incubating kuru, were unaffected (Alpers, 1987). From the age of the youngest affected patient, the shortest incubation period is estimated as 4.5 years, although it may have been shorter, since the time of infection was usually unknown. Currently, two or three cases are occurring annually, all in individuals aged 40 or more, consistent with exposure prior to 1956 and indicating that incubation periods can be 40 years or more (Whitfield, Alpers and Collinge, unpublished). *PRNP* codon 129 genotype has a significant effect on kuru susceptibility and most elderly survivors of the kuru epidemic are heterozygotes (Mead *et al.*, 2003). The marked survival advantage for codon 129 heterozygotes provides a powerful basis for selection pressure in the Fore. Remarkably, an analysis of worldwide haplotype diversity and allele frequency of *PRNP* coding and non-coding polymorphisms suggests that balancing selection at this locus is much older and more geographically widespread. Evidence for balancing selection (where there is more variation than expected in a gene due to heterozygote advantage) has been demonstrated in only a few human genes. Given recent biochemical and physical evidence of cannibalism on five continents, one explanation is that ancient and worldwide cannibalism resulted in a series of prion disease epidemics in human prehistory, thus imposing balancing selection on *PRNP* (Mead *et al.*, 2003).

Kuru affects both sexes and the onset of disease has ranged from age 5 to over 60. The mean clinical duration of illness is 12 months, with a range of 3 months to 3 years; the course tends to be shorter in children. The central clinical feature is progressive cerebellar ataxia. In contrast to classical CJD, dementia is much less prominent, although in the later stages many patients have their faculties obtunded (Alpers, 1987). The occasional case in which gross dementia occurs is in contrast to the clinical norm. Detailed clinical descriptions have been given by a number of observers and the disease does not appear to have changed in features at different stages of the epidemic. A prodrome and three clinical stages are recognised:

- *Prodromal stage.* Kuru typically begins with prodromal symptoms consisting of headache, aching of limbs and joint pains, which can last for several months.
- *Ambulatory stage.* Kuru was frequently self-diagnosed by patients at the earliest onset of unsteadiness in standing or walking, or of dysarthria or diplopia. At this stage there may be no objective signs of disease. However, gait ataxia worsens and patients develop a broad-based gait, truncal instability and titubation. A coarse postural tremor is usually present and accentuated by movement; patients characteristically hold their hands together in the midline to suppress this. Standing with feet together reveals clawing of toes to maintain posture. This marked clawing response is regarded as pathognomonic of kuru. Patients often become withdrawn at this stage and occasionally develop a severe reactive depression. Prodromal symptoms tend to disappear. Astasia and gait ataxia worsen and the patient requires a stick for walking. Intention tremor, dysmetria, hypotonia and dysdiadochokinesis develop. Although eye movements are ataxic and jerky, nystagmus is rarely seen. Strabismus, usually convergent, may occur, particularly in children. This strabismus does not appear to be concomitant or paralytic and may fluctuate in both extent and type, sometimes disappearing later in the clinical course. Photophobia is common and there may be an abnormal cold sensitivity with shivering and piloerection even in a warm environment. Tendon reflexes are reduced or normal and plantar responses are flexor. Dysarthria usually occurs. As ataxia progresses, the patient passes from the first (ambulatory) stage to the second (sedentary) stage. The mean clinical duration of the first stage is around 8 months and correlates closely with total duration (Alpers, 1964).
- *Sedentary stage.* At this stage patients are able to sit unsupported but cannot walk. Attempted walking with support leads to a high steppage, wide-based gait with reeling instability and flinging arm movements in an attempt to maintain posture. Hyperreflexia is seen, although plantar responses usually remain flexor with intact abdominal reflexes. Clonus is characteristically short-lived. Athetoid and choreiform movements and Parkinsonian tremors may occur. There is no paralysis, although muscle power is reduced. Obesity is

common at this stage but may be present in early disease associated with bulimia. Characteristically, there is emotional lability and bizarre uncontrollable laughter, which has led to the disease being referred to as 'laughing death'. There is no sensory impairment. In sharp contrast to CJD, myoclonic jerking is rarely seen. EEG is usually normal or may show non-specific changes (Cobb *et al.*, 1973). This stage lasts around 2–3 months. When truncal ataxia reaches the point where the patient is unable to sit unsupported, the third or tertiary stage is reached.

- *Tertiary stage.* Hypotonia and hyporeflexia develop and the terminal state is marked by flaccid muscle weakness. Plantar responses remain flexor and abdominal reflexes intact. Progressive dysphagia occurs and patients become incontinent of urine and faeces. Inanition and emaciation develop. Transient conjugate eye signs and dementia may occur. Primitive reflexes develop in occasional cases. Brainstem involvement and both bulbar and pseudobulbar signs occur. Respiratory failure and bronchopneumonia eventually lead to death. The tertiary stage lasts 1–2 months.

Iatrogenic Creutzfeldt–Jakob Disease

Iatrogenic transmission of CJD has occurred by accidental inoculation with human prions as a result of medical procedures. Such iatrogenic routes include the use of inadequately sterilised neurosurgical instruments, dura mater and corneal grafting, and use of human cadaveric pituitary-derived growth hormone or gonadotrophin. It is of considerable interest that cases arising from intracerebral or optic inoculation manifest clinically as classical CJD, with a rapidly progressive dementia, while those resulting from peripheral inoculation, most notably following pituitary-derived growth hormone exposure, typically present with a progressive cerebellar syndrome, and are in that respect somewhat reminiscent of kuru. Unsurprisingly, the incubation period in intracerebral cases is short (19–46 months for dura mater grafts) as compared to peripheral cases (typically 15 years or more). There is evidence for genetic susceptibility to iatrogenic CJD, with an excess of *PRNP* codon 129 homozygotes (Collinge *et al.*, 1991b).

Epidemiological studies have not shown increased risks of particular occupations that may be exposed to human or animal prions, although individual CJD cases in two histopathology technicians, a neuropathologist and a neurosurgeon have been

Pathogenic mutations

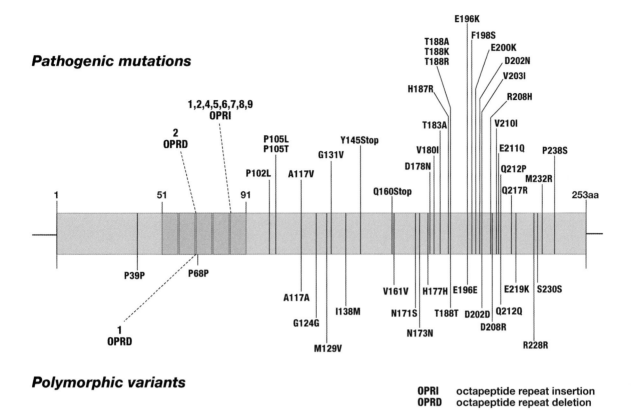

Figure 26.5 Mutations and polymorphisms in the human prion protein gene (*PRNP*)

documented. While there have been concerns that CJD may be transmissible by blood transfusion, extensive epidemiological analysis in the UK has found that the frequency of blood transfusion and donation was no different in over 200 cases of CJD and a matched control population (Esmonde *et al.*, 1993). Recipients of blood transfusions who developed CJD had clinical presentations similar to those of sporadic CJD patients and not to the more kuru-like iatrogenic cases arising from peripheral exposure to human prions. Furthermore, experimental transmission studies have shown only weak evidence for infectivity in blood (Brown, 1995), even when inoculated via the most efficient (intracerebral) route. It cannot be assumed that the same picture will hold for vCJD, as this is caused by a distinct prion strain (Collinge *et al.*, 1996b) from those causing classical CJD and has a distinct pathogenesis. It is also possible that many individuals in the UK and other countries with significant BSE exposure are sub- or pre-clinically infected with vCJD prions.

Variant CJD

In late 1995, two cases of sporadic CJD were reported in the UK in teenagers (Britton *et al.*, 1995). Only four cases of sporadic CJD had previously been recorded in teenagers, and none of these cases occurred in the UK. In addition, both cases were unusual in having kuru-type plaques, a finding seen in only around 5% of CJD cases. Soon afterwards a third very young sporadic CJD case occurred (Tabrizi *et al.*, 1996). These cases caused considerable concern and the possibility was raised that they might suggest a link with BSE. It was clearly of some importance to see whether any further such extraordinarily rare cases occurred in the UK. By March 1996, further extremely young onset cases were apparent and review of the histology of these cases showed a remarkably consistent and unique pattern. These cases were named 'new variant' CJD, although it was clear that they were also rather atypical in their clinical presentation; in fact, most cases did not meet the accepted clinical diagnostic criteria for probable CJD. Extensive studies of archival cases of CJD or other prion diseases failed to show this picture and it seemed that it did represent the arrival of a new form of prion disease in the UK. The statistical probability of such cases occurring by chance was vanishingly small and ascertainment bias seemed most unlikely as an explanation. It was clear that a new risk factor for CJD had emerged and appeared to be specific to the UK. The UK Government advisory committee on spongiform encephalopathy (SEAC) concluded that, while there was no direct evidence for a link with BSE, exposure to specified bovine offal (SBO), prior to the ban on its inclusion in human foodstuffs in 1989, was the most likely explanation. A case of vCJD was soon afterwards reported in France (Chazot et al., 1996). Direct experimental evidence that vCJD is caused by BSE was provided by molecular analysis of human prion strains and transmission studies in transgenic and wild-type mice. While it is now clear that vCJD is human BSE, it is unclear why this particular age group should be affected and why none of these cases had a pattern of unusual occupational or dietary exposure to BSE. However, very little is known about which foodstuffs contained high-titre bovine offal. It is possible that certain foods containing particularly high titres were eaten predominately by younger people. An alternative possibility is that young people are more susceptible to BSE following dietary exposure, or that they have shorter incubation periods. It is important to appreciate that BSE-contaminated feed was fed to sheep, pigs and poultry, and that although there is no evidence of natural transmission to these species, it would be prudent to remain open-minded about other dietary exposure to novel animal prions.

The clinical presentation is often, although not always, with behavioural and psychiatric disturbances, and in some cases with sensory disturbance (Will et al., 1996). Initial presentation may be to a psychiatrist and the most prominent feature is depression, but anxiety, withdrawal and behavioural change is also frequent (Zeidler et al., 1997a). Suicidal ideation is infrequent and response to antidepressants poor. Delusions, which are complex and unsustained, are common. Other features include emotional lability, aggression, insomnia and auditory and visual hallucinations. A prominent early feature in some patients is dysaesthesiae or pain in the limbs or face, or pain that is persistent rather than intermittent and unrelated to anxiety levels. A few cases have been noted to have forgetfulness or mild gait ataxia from an early stage but in most overt neurological features are not apparent until some months into the clinical course (Zeidler et al., 1997b). In the majority of patients a progressive cerebellar syndrome develops with gait and limb ataxia. Dementia usually develops later in the clinical course with progression to akinetic mutism. Myoclonus is seen in most patients, and chorea, sometimes severe, is seen in some cases. Cortical blindness develops in a minority of patients in the late stages of disease. Upgaze paresis, an uncommon feature of classical CJD, has been noted in some patients (Zeidler et al., 1997b). The age at onset, although initially in young adults, has since broadened, with a range of 12–74 years (mean 29 years) and the clinical course is relatively prolonged (9–35 months, median 14 months) compared to sporadic CJD. The EEG is abnormal, most frequently showing generalised slow wave activity, but without the pseudoperiodic pattern seen in most sporadic CJD cases. Neuroimaging by CT is either normal or shows only mild atrophy. MRI scanning has proved helpful in diagnosis of vCJD, with high signal in the pulvinar (the 'pulvinar sign'; Zeidler et al., 2000) (Figure 26.6). Although clearly of value, and reported to be present on scrutiny of scans from a high proportion

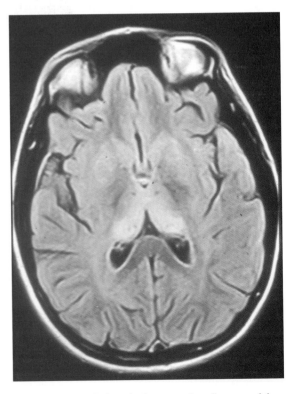

Figure 26.6 MRI signs in human prion disease: pulvinar sign in vCJD

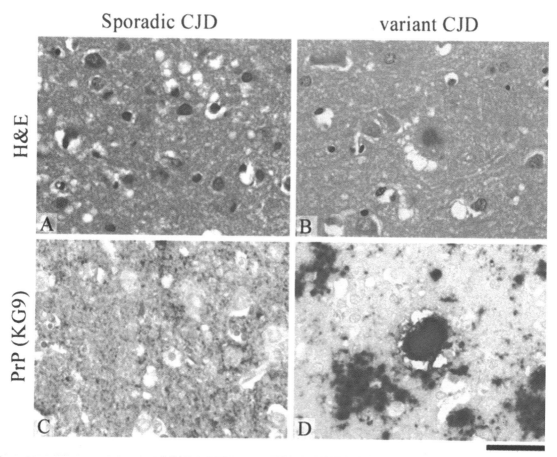

Figure 26.7 Neuropathology of sporadic and variant CJD. Mild spongiform vacuolation of the cortical grey matter is a hallmark of Creutzfeldt–Jakob disease (A). In this case there was no deposition of kuru-like plaques but widespread deposition of abnormal prion protein in a synaptic pattern (B). In contrast, variant CJD is characterised by frequent so-called florid plaque, consisting of a round amyloid core, surrounded by a daisy-like vacuolation (C). This hallmark of variant CJD can be found in several cortical areas and in the cerebellum and may be associated with vacuolar degeneration. Immunostaining for the pathological prion protein (using monoclonal antibody KG9) highlights the florid plaques but also reveals synaptic staining (D). Scale bar: 50 μm

of patients meeting clinical or neuropathological criteria for diagnosis of vCJD, its specificity and sensitivity as a diagnostic sign have not been formally evaluated in unselected series. CSF 14–3–3 protein may be elevated, but much less frequently than in sporadic CJD. *PRNP* analysis to date has demonstrated that all cases studied were homozygous for methionine at codon 129. No known or novel pathogenic mutations are found in the coding sequence (Collinge *et al.*, 1996a).

The neuropathological appearances of vCJD are striking and consistent (Figure 26.7). While there is widespread spongiform change, gliosis and neuronal loss, most severe in the basal ganglia and thalamus, the most remarkable feature was the abundant PrP amyloid plaques in cerebral and cerebellar cortex. These consisted of kuru-like, 'florid' (surrounded by spongiform vacuoles) and multicentric plaque types. The 'florid' plaques, seen previously only in scrapie, were a particularly unusual but highly consistent feature. There was also abundant pericellular PrP deposition in the cerebral and cerebellar cortex. A further highly unusual feature was the extensive PrP deposition in the molecular layer of the cerebellum. The florid plaque pathology of vCJD has been reproduced in an animal model of vCJD: transgenic mice expressing human PrP methionine 129, but not mice expressing valine 129, develop strikingly similar neuropathology when infected with either BSE or vCJD prions (Asante *et al.*, 2002).

Importantly, a clear tissue diagnosis of vCJD can now be made by tonsil biopsy with detection of characteristic PrP immunostaining and PrP^{Sc} (Collinge et al., 1997; Wadsworth et al., 2001). It has long been recognised that prion replication, in experimentally infected animals, is first detectable in the lymphoreticular system, considerably earlier than the onset of neurological symptoms. Importantly, PrP^{Sc} is only detectable in vCJD, and not other forms of human prion disease studied. The PrP^{Sc} type detected on Western blot in vCJD tonsil has a characteristic pattern designated type 4t(45) (Figure 26.8). A positive tonsil biopsy obviates the need for brain biopsy, which may otherwise be considered in such a clinical context to exclude alternative, potentially treatable diagnoses.

It is of considerable interest that some of the features of vCJD are reminiscent of kuru, in which behavioural changes and progressive ataxia predominate. In addition, peripheral sensory disturbances are well recognised in the kuru prodrome. Kuru plaques are seen in around 70% of cases and are especially abundant in younger kuru cases. The observation that iatrogenic prion disease related to peripheral exposure to human prions has a more kuru-like than CJD-like clinical picture may well be relevant and would be consistent with a peripheral prion exposure.

Other Phenotypes of BSE Infection in Humans?

The relatively stereotyped clinical presentation and neuropathology of vCJD contrasts sharply with sporadic CJD. This may be because vCJD is caused by a single prion strain and may also suggest that a relatively homogeneous genetically susceptible subgroup of the population with short incubation periods to BSE has been selected to date (Collinge, 1999). A widening of the recognised phenotypic range of vCJD from that based on the earliest patients can be anticipated and indeed is already emerging. Other phenotypic presentations of BSE prion infection in humans, particularly involving other *PRNP* genotypes, are to be anticipated (Hill et al., 1997a). It will be important to remain open-minded about such phenotypes. Recent studies in transgenic mice expressing human PrP have shown that BSE infection can result in two distinct phenotypes, one with the neuropathological and molecular phenotype of vCJD and a second with the molecular phenotype of the commonest subtype of sporadic CJD (associated with PrP^{Sc} type 2) (Asante et al., 2002). This raises the possibility that BSE infection of humans could also cause some cases of apparently sporadic CJD.

Inherited Prion Diseases

Gerstmann–Sträussler–Scheinker Disease

The first case was described by Gerstmann in 1928 and was followed by a more detailed report on seven other affected members of the same family in 1936 (Gerstmann et al., 1936). The classical presentation of GSS is with a chronic cerebellar ataxia accompanied by pyramidal features, with dementia occurring later in a much more prolonged clinical course than that seen in CJD. The mean duration is around 5 years, with onset usually in either the third or fourth decades. Histologically, the hallmark is the presence of multicentric amyloid plaques. Spongiform change, neuronal loss, astrocytosis and white matter loss are also usually present. Numerous GSS kindreds from several countries (including the original Austrian family described by Gerstmann et al., 1936) have now been demonstrated to have mutations in the PrP gene. GSS is an autosomal dominant disorder, which can now be classified within the spectrum of inherited prion disease.

Other Inherited Prion Diseases

The identification of one of the pathogenic PrP gene mutations in a case with neurodegenerative disease allows not only molecular diagnosis of an inherited prion disease but also its sub-classification according to mutation (see Figure 26.8). Pathogenic mutations reported to date in the human PrP gene consist of two groups: (a) point mutations within the coding sequence, resulting in amino acid substitutions in PrP or, in two cases, production of a stop codon resulting in expression of a truncated PrP; (b) insertions encoding additional integral copies of an octapeptide

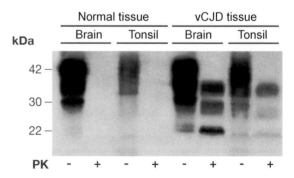

Figure 26.8 Tonsil biopsy in vCJD

repeat present in a tandem array of five copies in the normal protein. A suggested notation for these diseases is 'inherited prion disease (PrP mutation)', e.g. inherited prion disease (PrP 144 bp insertion) or inherited prion disease (PrP P102L) (Collinge and Prusiner, 1992). They are all autosomal dominantly inherited conditions. Kindreds with inherited prion disease have been described with phenotypes of classical CJD, GSS and also with a range of other neurodegenerative syndromes. Some families show remarkable phenotypic variability which can encompass both CJD- and GSS-like cases, as well as other cases which do not conform to either CJD or GSS phenotypes (Collinge et al., 1992). Such atypical prion diseases may lack the classical histological features of a spongiform encephalopathy entirely, although PrP immunohistochemistry is usually positive (Collinge et al., 1990). Progressive dementia, cerebellar ataxia, pyramidal signs, chorea, myoclonus, extrapyramidal features, pseudobulbar signs, seizures and amyotrophic features are seen in variable combinations.

Relatively little clinical or pathological information is available on some of these mutations; indeed, some have to date been described in only a single family, or indeed individual, and evidence for pathogenicity is unclear. Brief details on some of the more frequently recognised subtypes is given below.

Missense Mutations

PrP P102L. This mutation was first reported in 1989 in a UK and US family and has now been demonstrated in many other kindreds worldwide. Progressive ataxia is the dominant clinical feature, with dementia and pyramidal features. However, marked variability at both clinical and neuropathological level is apparent in some families, and has recently been extensively documented in the original Austrian GSS family (Hainfellner et al., 1995). A family with marked amyotrophic features has also been reported (Kretzschmar et al., 1992). Cases with severe dementia in the absence of prominent ataxia are also recognised. Histological examination reveals PrP immunoreactive plaques in the majority of cases. Transmissibility to experimental animals has been demonstrated.

PrP P105L. The Pro–Leu change at codon 105 has been found in four patients from three Japanese families (Kitamoto et al., 1993) and in a single UK family (unpublished). The patients presented with a history of spastic paraparesis and dementia. The

clinical duration from onset to the development of akinetic mutism was around 5 years. There was no periodic synchronous discharge on EEG but MRI scans showed atrophy of the motor cortex. On pathological examination there were plaques in the cerebral cortex, and neuronal loss but no spongiosis. Neurofibrillary tangles were variably present amongst cases and no plaques were found in the cerebellum.

PrP A117V. This mutation was first described in a French family (Doh ura et al., 1989) and subsequently in a US family of German origin (Hsiao et al., 1991b). The clinical features are presenile dementia associated with pyramidal signs, parkinsonism, pseudobulbar features and cerebellar signs. Neuropathologically, PrP immunoreactive plaques are usually present. This mutation has also been identified in a large family in the UK.

PrP Y145STOP. This mutation was detected in a Japanese patient who had a clinical diagnosis of Alzheimer's disease. She developed memory disturbance and a slowly progressive dementia at age 38. The duration of illness was 21 years. Histological examination revealed typical Alzheimer pathology without spongiform change (Kitamoto et al., 1993). Many amyloid plaques were seen in the cortex, along with diffuse neuropil threads of paired helical filaments. However, the plaques were immunoreactive with PrP antisera. A4 immunocytochemistry was negative. The clinicopathological findings in this case emphasise the importance of *PRNP* analysis in the differential diagnosis of dementias.

PrP D178N. This mutation was originally described in two Finnish families with a CJD-like phenotype, although without typical EEG appearances (Goldfarb et al., 1991c), and has since been demonstrated in additional CJD families in Hungary, The Netherlands, Canada, Finland, France and the UK. The Finnish pedigree included 15 affected members in four generations. The mean age of onset was 47 and mean duration was 27.5 months. Brain biopsy and autopsy specimens showed spongiform change without amyloid plaques.

This mutation was also reported in two unrelated families with fatal familial insomnia (FFI) (Lugaresi et al., 1986; Medori et al., 1992a). The first cases described had a rapidly progressive disease characterised clinically by untreatable insomnia, dysautonomia and motor signs, and neuropathologically by selective atrophy of the anteriorventral and mediodorsal thalamic nuclei. There is marked thalamic astrocytosis. Mild spongiform change is seen in some cases and protease-resistant PrP can be demonstrated, albeit weakly, by immunoblotting. Proteinase-K treatment of extracted PrPSc from FFI cases has shown a different sized PrP band on Western blots than PrPSc from CJD cases (Monari *et al.*, 1994), suggesting that FFI may be caused by a distinct prion strain type. In a recent study, Goldfarb *et al.*, 1992, reported that in all the codon 178 families they studied with a CJD-like disease, the codon 178 mutation was encoded on a valine 129 allele while all FFI kindreds encode the same codon 178 mutation on a methionine 129 allele. They suggested that the genotype at codon 129 determines phenotype. However, they have not demonstrated that the families they describe are unrelated and that therefore their comparison may only be based on two extended families. Insomnia is not uncommon in CJD patients and FFI and CJD may represent extremes of a spectrum of related disease phenotypes. Recently an inherited case with the E200K mutation, which is normally associated with a CJD-like phenotype, has been reported with an FFI phenotype (Chapman *et al.*, 1996). An Australian family has also been reported with the FFI genotype but in which affected family members have a range of phenotypes encompassing typical CJD, FFI and an autosomal dominant cerebellar ataxia-like illness (McLean *et al.*, 1997). It is of interest that the CJD-like codon 178 cases have frequently transmitted to experimental animals, while the FFI type did not transmit to laboratory primates (Brown *et al.*, 1994). Recently, transmission of an FFI case to mice has been reported, although this case was unusual in that a single octapeptide repeat deletion was present on the same allele (Tateishi *et al.*, 1995). This individual came from an extensive kindred in which other family members, with the same *PRNP* genotype, had a CJD-like phenotype (Bosque *et al.*, 1992). However, two cases of FFI, one a British case and the second an Italian case, both with the usual FFI genotype of D178N, 129M, transmitted to transgenic mice expressing human prion protein (Collinge *et al.*, 1995a).

PrP V180I. This mutation was identified in two Japanese patients with subacute dementia and myoclonus (Kitamoto *et al.*, 1993). The period from onset to akinetic mutism was 6–10 months. No family history was noted. EEG did not show pseudoperiodic sharp wave activity. Neuropathological examination demonstrated spongiform change, neuronal loss and astrocytosis. Interestingly, one of the patients with PrP Ile 180 also had PrP Arg 232 (see later). These were on different alleles. This disease has not been transmitted to laboratory animals.

PrP T183A. Reported in a single Brazilian family with a frontotemporal dementia of mean onset 45 years and duration 4 years (Nitrini *et al.*, 1997). Parkinsonian features were also present in some patients. Neuropathological examination revealed severe spongiform change and neuronal loss in deep cortical layers and putamen while there was relatively little gliosis. PrP immunoreactivity was demonstrated in putamen and cerebellum. No transmission studies have been reported to date.

PrP F198S. A variant form of GSS was described in a large Indiana kindred which has been traced back to 1792. Unlike other GSS patients with presenile onset of neurological disability, the Indiana kindred had widespread Alzheimer-like neurofibrillary tangles, composed of paired helical filaments, in the cortex and subcortical nuclei, in addition to amyloid plaques. The amyloid plaques were composed of PrP and not βA4. Affected individuals in this kindred have a codon 198 T–C transition, resulting in a phenylalanine to serine conversion (Dlouhy *et al.*, 1992). There is an apparent codon 129 effect with this mutation, in that individuals who were heterozygous at codon 129 had a later age of onset than homozygotes. Transmission of this disease to laboratory animals has not yet been reported.

PrP E200K. This mutation was first described in families with CJD. Affected individuals develop a rapidly progressive dementia with myoclonus and pyramidal, cerebellar or extrapyramidal signs and a duration of illness usually less than 12 months. The average age of onset for the disease is 55. Histologically, these patients are typical of CJD; plaques are absent but PrPSc can be demonstrated by immunoblotting. In marked contrast to other variants of inherited prion disease, the EEG usually shows the characteristic pseudoperiodic sharp wave activity seen in sporadic CJD. Interestingly, this mutation accounts for the three reported ethnogeographic clusters of CJD where the local incidence of CJD is around 100-fold higher than elsewhere (amongst Libyan Jews and in regions of Slovakia and Chile) (Hsiao *et al.*, 1991a; Brown *et al.*, 1992; Goldfarb *et al.*, 1990). Now that cases can be diagnosed by PrP gene analysis, atypical forms of this condition are being detected with phenotypes other than that of classical CJD. Of interest also are reports that peripheral neuropathy can occur in this disease (Neufeld *et al.*, 1992). Elderly unaffected carriers of the mutation have been reported. Chapman *et al.* (1994) have made a detailed analysis on 52 mutation-carrying patients with definite or probable CJD and 34 unaffected mutation carriers. They conclude that the cumulative penetrance reaches 50% at the age of 60 and 80% by the age of 80. However, there was a group of patients, aged 69–82, with possible CJD containing five proven and two obligate carriers of the mutation, i.e. the patients were demented but did not fulfil the clinical criteria for probable CJD. If the analysis was carried out assuming that these possible cases were actually CJD, then the penetrance reaches 100% by the age of 80. Individuals homozygous for the mutation have been identified and are phenotypically indistinguishable from heterozygotes, indicating that this condition is a fully dominant disorder (Hsiao et al., 1991a). Patients with this condition have now been reported in several other countries outside the well-recognised clusters, including the UK. At least one of the UK cases does not appear to be related to the ethnogeographic clusters mentioned above, suggesting a separate UK focus for this type of inherited prion disease (Collinge *et al.*, 1993). Goldfarb *et al.* (1991b) have found this mutation amongst 46 out of 55 CJD-affected families studied at the National Institutes of Health. The codon 129 genotype does not appear to affect age at onset of this disorder. Transmission to experimental animals has been demonstrated.

PrP Q217R. Reported to date only in a single Swedish family, the presentation is with dementia followed by gait ataxia, dysphagia and confusion (Hsiao *et al.*, 1992). As with the inherited prion disease with codon 198 serine mutation (Indiana kindred), there are prominent neurofibrillary tangles. Transmissibility to experimental animals has not yet been demonstrated in this condition.

PrP M232R. This mutation was first found on the opposite allele to a codon 180 mutation in a Japanese patient with prion disease (Kitamoto *et al.*, 1993). It was further demonstrated in two additional Japanese patients with dementia. Both of the latter cases appeared to present as sporadic cases with no family history of neurological disease. Both patients had progressive dementia, myoclonus and periodic synchronous discharges in the EEG. The mean duration of illness was 3 months. Neuropathology showed spongiform change, neuronal loss and astrocytosis. PrP immunostaining revealed diffuse grey matter staining, but no plaques.

Insertional Mutations

PrP 24 bp insertion (one extra repeat). A single octapeptide repeat insertion has been reported in a single French individual who presented at age 73 with dizziness. He later developed visual agnosia, cerebellar ataxia and intellectual impairment and diffuse periodic activity was noted on EEG. Myoclonus and cortical blindness developed and he progressed to akinetic mutism. Disease duration was 4 months. The patient's father had died at age 70 from an undiagnosed neurological disorder. No neuropathological information is available.

PrP 48 bp insertion (two extra repeats). This mutation has been reported in a single family from the USA (Goldfarb *et al.*, 1993). The proband had a CJD-like phenotype, both clinically and pathologically, with a typical EEG and an age at onset of 58. However, the proband's mother had onset of cognitive decline at age 75 with a slow progression to a severe dementia over 13 years. The maternal grandfather had a similar late onset (at age 80) and slowly progressive cognitive decline over 15 years.

PrP 96 bp insertion (four extra repeats). A 96 base pair insertional mutation, encoding four octapeptide elements, was first reported in an individual who died aged 63 of hepatic cirrhosis (Goldfarb *et al.*, 1991a). There was no history of neurological illness and it is unclear whether this finding indicates incomplete penetrance of this mutation. This is the only recorded case of a *PRNP* insertional mutation other than in an affected individual with a prion disease or an at-risk individual from an affected kindred. Two separate four octapeptide repeat insertional mutations have been reported in affected individuals, each differing in the DNA sequence from the original four-repeat insertion, although all three of the mutations encode the same PrP. Laplanche *et al.* (1995) reported a 96 bp insertion in an 82 year-old French woman who developed progressive depression and behavioural changes. She progressed over 3 months to akinetic mutism with pyramidal signs and myoclonus. EEG showed pseudoperiodic complexes. Duration of illness was 4 months. There was no known family history of neurological illness. Another 96 bp insertional mutation was seen in a patient with classical clinical and pathological features of CJD, with the exception of the unusual finding of pronounced PrP immunoreactivity in the molecular layer of the cerebellum (Campbell *et al.*, 1996).

PrP 120 bp insertion (five extra repeats). An additional five octapeptide repeat mutation was reported in a US family with an illness characterised by progressive dementia, abnormal behaviour, cerebellar signs, tremor, rigidity, hyper-reflexia and myoclonus. The age at onset was 31–45, with a clinical duration of 5–15 years (Goldfarb *et al.*, 1991a). EEG showed diffuse slowing only. Histological features were of spongiosis, neuronal loss and gliosis. Transmission has been demonstrated.

PrP 144 bp insertion (six extra repeats). This was the first PrP mutation to be reported and was found in a small UK family with familial CJD (Owen *et al.*, 1989). The diagnosis in the family had been based on an individual who died in the 1940s with a rapidly progressive illness characteristic of CJD (Meyer *et al.*, 1954). The reported duration of illness was 6 months. Pathologically there was gross status spongiosis and astrocytosis affecting the entire cerebral cortex, and this case is used to illustrate classic CJD histology in Greenfield's *Neuropathology*. However, other family members had a much longer-duration GSS-like illness. Histological features were also extremely variable. This observation led to screening of various cases of neurodegenerative disease and to the identification of a case classified on clinical grounds as familial Alzheimer's disease (Collinge *et al.*, 1989). More extensive screening work identified further families with the same mutation which were then demonstrated by genealogical studies to form part of an extremely large kindred (Collinge *et al.*, 1992; Poulter *et al.*, 1992). Clinical information has been collected on around 50 affected individuals over seven generations. Affected individuals develop, in the third to fourth decade, onset of a progressive dementia associated with a varying combination of cerebellar ataxia and dysarthria, pyramidal signs, myoclonus and occasionally extrapyramidal signs, chorea and seizures. The dementia is often preceded by depression and aggressive behaviour. A number of cases have a long-standing personality disorder, characterised by aggression, irritability, antisocial and criminal activity and hypersexuality, which may be present from early childhood, long before overt neurodegenerative disease develops. The histological features vary from those of classical spongiform encephalopathy (with or without PrP amyloid plaques) to cases lacking any specific features of these conditions (Collinge *et al.*, 1990). Age at onset in this condition can be predicted according to genotype at polymorphic codon 129. Since this pathogenic insertional mutation occurs on a methionine 129 PrP allele, there are two possible codon 129 genotypes for affected individuals, methionine 129 homozygotes or methionine 129/valine 129 heterozygotes. Heterozygotes have an age at onset which is about a decade later than homozygotes (Poulter *et al.*, 1992). Limited transmission studies to marmosets were unsuccessful. Transmission to transgenic mice expressing human prion protein has been achieved (Collinge *et al.*, in preparation). Further families with 144 bp insertions, of different nucleotide sequence, have now been reported in the UK (Nicholl *et al.*, 1995) and Japan (Oda *et al.*, 1995).

PrP 168 bp insertion (seven extra repeats). This mutation has been reported in a US family. The clinical features described include mood change, abnormal behaviour, confusion, aphasia, cerebellar signs, involuntary movements, rigidity, dementia and myoclonus. The age at onset was 23–35 years and the clinical duration 10–>13 years. EEG showed diffuse slowing in two cases; a third showed slow wave burst suppression. Neuropathological examination showed spongiform change, neuronal loss and gliosis to varying degrees (Goldfarb *et al.*, 1991a). Experimental transmission has been demonstrated.

PrP 192 bp insertion (eight extra repeats). This mutation has been reported in a French family, with clinical features which include abnormal behaviour, cerebellar signs, mutism, pyramidal signs, myoclonus, tremor, intellectual slowing and seizures. The disease duration ranged from 3 months to 13 years. The EEG findings include diffuse slowing, slow wave burst suppression and periodic triphasic complexes. Neuropathological examination revealed spongiform change, neuronal loss, gliosis and multicentric plaques in the cerebellum (Goldfarb *et al.*, 1991a; Guiroy *et al.*, 1993). Experimental transmission has been reported.

PrP 216 bp insertion (nine extra repeats). The finding of a nine-octapeptide insertional mutation was first reported in a single case from the UK (Owen *et al.*, 1992). The clinical onset was around 54 years, with falls, axial rigidity, myoclonic jerks and progressive dementia (Tagliavini *et al.*, 1993a). Although there was no clear family history of a similar illness, the mother had died at age 53 with a cerebrovascular event. The maternal grandmother died at age 79 with senile dementia. EEG was of low amplitude but did not show pseudoperiodic sharp wave activity. Neuropathological examination showed no spongiform encephalopathy but marked deposition of plaques, which in the cerebellum and the basal ganglia showed immunor-eactivity with PrP antisera (Tagliavini *et al.*, 1993a). In the hippocampus there were neuritic plaques positive for both β-amyloid protein and tau. Some neurofi-brillary tangles were also seen. In some respects, therefore, the pathology resembled Alzheimer's dis-ease. Experimental transmission studies have not been attempted. A second, German, family with a nine-octapeptide repeat insertion of different sequence has now been reported (Krasemann *et al.*, 1995).

MOLECULAR DIAGNOSIS OF PRION DISEASE

While sporadic CJD can often, following the exclusion of other causes, be diagnosed with a high degree of confidence on the basis of clinical criteria, atypical forms, which present much greater diagnostic diffi-culty, are not uncommon (Collinge, 1998). A widening of the recognised phenotypic range of vCJD from that based on the earliest patients can be anticipated and indeed is already emerging. Other phenotypic presentations of BSE prion infection in humans, particularly involving other *PRNP* genotypes, are to be anticipated. Furthermore, current clinically-based diagnostic criteria for vCJD, used for surveillance, require the evolution of disease over at least 6 months and the development of several signs indicative of extensive cerebral damage (http://www.doh.gov.uk/cjd/cjd_stat.htm). However, early diagnosis, before extensive irreversible brain damage has occurred, is crucial in such patients as they may be suffering from an alternative treatable disorder. Brain biopsy may well be considered, particularly in younger patients, to exclude such conditions as cerebral vasculitis. Early tonsil biopsy, if positive, obviates the need for further investigation. The need for early, specific diagnosis is now further emphasised by the arrival of potential therapies and clinical trials for CJD. The early clinical features of vCJD—depression, anxiety, behavioural change and sensory disturbances—are highly non-specific. Differentiation from much commoner psy-chiatric causes requires the arrival of overtly neurological features, such as ataxia, chorea and cognitive decline, although pre-existing use of neuro-leptics and other psychotropic drugs may initially delay their diagnostic recognition. While the diagnostic accuracy provided by a tonsil biopsy has to be balanced against the fact that it is an invasive procedure, early referral for investigation should allow much earlier diagnosis and access to clinical trials before extensive functional loss has occurred.

While neurologists have until recent years had to rely largely on clinical features to differentiate neuro-degenerative disorders, the major advances in molecular genetics and in understanding molecular pathogenesis increasingly enable diagnosis using cri-teria higher in the diagnostic hierarchy of pathology. Around 15% of recognised prion disease is an inherited Mendelian disorder associated with one of the more than 30 recognised coding mutations in *PRNP* (Collinge, 2001). For a single-gene inherited disorder of high penetrance, such as inherited prion disease, the diagnostic supremacy of direct demonstra-tion of causative mutation by DNA analysis is clear. Indeed, the availability of such definitive diagnostic markers has long allowed diagnosis of inherited prion disease in patients not only atypical on clinical grounds, but in whom classical neuropathological features are absent (Collinge *et al.*, 1989, 1990). Kindreds are documented in which some individuals have the classical syndromes of 'CJD' and 'Gerst-mann–Sträussler–Sheinker disease', while others do not fit these rubrics at all (Collinge *et al.*, 1992). Neuropathology in such patients is no longer the 'Gold Standard': rather, the recognised clinicopathological manifestation of a particular inherited condition simply widens. The acquired prion diseases, such as vCJD, although not contagious in humans, are infectious diseases. In infectious disease, while clinical and histopathological features may again be key, confirmation of diagnosis, not least in life-threatening conditions, is by identification of the infectious pathogen itself or a specific immune response to it. Isolation and strain typing of the pathogen is at the apex of the diagnostic hierarchy. Strain typing in particular may allow the source of an outbreak to be identified and the best available prognostic and therapeutic advice to be provided. While it is essential to balance the potential risks and discomfort involved in an invasive diagnostic test against the improved diagnostic accuracy, it will only be by progressing steadily to greater use of molecular analysis of neurological disease that we will be able to deliver the diagnostic and ultimately therapeutic advances to patients with neurodegenerative diseases that are so desperately needed.

PRESYMPTOMATIC AND ANTENATAL TESTING

Since a direct gene test has become available, it has been possible to provide an unequivocal diagnosis in patients with inherited forms of the disease. This has also led to the possibility of performing presymptomatic testing of unaffected but at-risk family members, as well as antenatal testing (Collinge *et al.*, 1991a). Because of the effect of *PRNP* codon 129 genotype on the age of onset of disease associated with some mutations, it is possible to determine within a family whether a carrier of a mutation will have an early or late onset of disease. Most of the mutations appear to be fully penetrant; however, experience with some is extremely limited. In families with the E200K mutation and in D178N (fatal familial insomnia) there are examples of elderly unaffected gene carriers who appear to have escaped the disease.

Genetic counselling in prion disease resembles that of Huntington's disease in many respects and those protocols established for Huntington's disease can be adapted for prion disease counselling. PrP gene analysis may have very important consequences for family members other than the individual tested, and it is preferable to have discussed all the issues with the family before testing commences. Following the identification of a mutation, the family should be referred for genetic counselling. Testing of asymptomatic individuals should only follow adequate counselling of individuals and will require their full informed consent. It is also important to counsel both those testing positive for mutations and those untested but at-risk that they should not be blood donors and should inform surgeons, including dentists, of their risk status prior to any procedure, as precautions should be taken to minimise risk of iatrogenic transmission (see below).

PREVENTION AND PUBLIC HEALTH MANAGEMENT

While prion diseases can be transmitted to experimental animals by inoculation, it is important to appreciate that they are not contagious in humans. Documented case-to-case spread has only occurred by cannibalism (kuru) or following accidental inoculation with prions. Such iatrogenic routes include the use of inadequately sterilised intracerebral electrodes, dura mater and corneal grafting, and from the use of human cadaveric pituitary-derived growth hormone or gonadotrophin.

Considerable concern has been expressed that blood and blood products from asymptomatic donors incubating vCJD may pose a risk for the iatrogenic transmission of vCJD. Reports of infectivity of blood

from patients with classical CJD are infrequent and have been questioned (Brown, 1995). Infectivity of blood from patients in the clinical phase of vCJD is unknown. UK policy is now to leukodeplete all whole blood, a practice already in use (for other health reasons) in some countries, and to source plasma for plasma products from outside the UK.

A further possible route of transmission of vCJD is via contaminated surgical instruments. Prions resist conventional sterilisation methods and neurosurgical instruments are known to be able to act as vectors for prion transmission: several cases of iatrogenic transmission of sporadic CJD prions via neurosurgical instruments are documented (Bernoulli *et al.*, 1977; Blattler, 2002). Recent evidence suggests that classical CJD may also be transmitted by other surgical procedures (Collins *et al.*, 1999). In the UK, all surgical instruments used on patients with suspected CJD are quarantined and not re-used unless an alternative non-prion diagnosis is unequivocally confirmed.

The pathogenesis of vCJD differs sharply from that of sporadic and other forms of 'classical' CJD. In particular, in vCJD there is extensive involvement of the lymphoreticular system (LRS) (lymph nodes, tonsil and spleen), with the highest levels of PrP^{Sc} outside the CNS being found in tonsil, where levels are typically 5–10% of brain levels (Wadsworth *et al.*, 2001). PrP^{Sc} is also detectable, at lower levels, in thymus, rectum, adrenal and retina in vCJD (Wadsworth *et al.*, 2001). This wider tissue distribution raises concerns about iatrogenic transmission of vCJD via surgical instruments previously used on patients with pre-clinical vCJD prion infection. The number of individuals incubating vCJD but currently asymptomatic is unknown, but may be substantial. Prions adhere avidly to stainless steel and transmit the disease readily in experimental models (Flechsig *et al.*, 2001). Tonsillar PrP^{Sc} is readily detectable in all cases of vCJD studied at autopsy and lymphoreticular involvement is a very early feature of natural prion infection in sheep and in experimental scrapie models, where replication in the LRS is detectable early in the incubation period and rises to a plateau, which considerably precedes, and is maintained in, the clinical phase (Fraser *et al.*, 1992). This suggests that tonsillar PrP^{Sc} has probably been present for a considerable period, perhaps years, before clinical presentation of vCJD in humans and therefore tonsil biopsy should enable diagnosis at the earliest stages of clinical suspicion. In addition, this pathogenesis forms the basis of prevalence screening of the general population for infection. Several anonymous screens of tonsil and appendix tissues, removed during routine surgery, are under way. Tonsil appears a more sensitive reporter of vCJD prion infection than appendix (Joiner *et al.*, 2002), and it is a cause for concern that a positive appendix has already been reported in these ongoing studies (Hilton *et al.*, 2002). National-scale studies are now being organised by the UK Department of Health. It is unknown as to whether there is significant prionaemia in vCJD. Blood is infectious in some rodent scrapie models and, more recently in BSE-infected sheep (which have been proposed as a model for vCJD as the tissue distribution of infectivity is similar), the disease has been transmitted by transfusion of whole blood (Hunter *et al.*, 2002).

Certain occupational groups are at risk of exposure to human prions, e.g. neurosurgeons and other operating theatre staff, pathologists and morticians, histology technicians, as well as an increasing number of laboratory workers. Because of the prolonged incubation periods to prions following administration to sites other than the central nervous system (CNS), which is associated with clinically silent prion replication in the lymphoreticular tissue (Aguzzi, 1997), treatments inhibiting prion replication in lymphoid organs may represent a viable strategy for rational secondary prophylaxis after accidental exposure. A preliminary suggested regimen is a short course of immunosuppression with oral corticosteroids in individuals with significant accidental exposure to human prions. Urgent surgical excision of the inoculum might also be considered in exceptional circumstances. There is hope that progress in the understanding of the peripheral pathogenesis will identify the precise cell types and molecules involved in colonisation of the organism by prions. The ultimate goal will be to target the rate-limiting steps in prion spread with much more focused pharmacological approaches, which may eventually prove useful in preventing disease even after iatrogenic and alimentary exposure (Collinge and Hawke, 1998).

Subclinical prion infections have been described in experimental animals, where high prion levels (comparable to those in end-stage clinically affected animals) are present in animals living a normal lifespan. While the differentiation between pre- and sub-clinical infections is perhaps semantic in diseases where the incubation period (at least when crossing species barriers) can approach the natural lifespan of the species concerned. Nevertheless, the possibility that asymptomatic carrier states of natural human and animal prion infection occurs must be considered (Asante *et al.*, 2002; Hill *et al.*, 2000).

PROGNOSIS AND TREATMENT

All forms of prion diseases that are currently recognised are invariably fatal following a relentlessly progressive course. No currently available treatment alters the clinical course of the disease and all that can be offered at present is general supportive care for the patient and family with hospitalisation in the later stages. The duration of illness in sporadic patients is very short, with a mean duration of 3–4 months. However, in some of the inherited cases the duration can be 20 years or more (Collinge *et al.*, 1990).

Various compounds, some known to bind PrP^{Sc}, including Congo red (Ingrosso *et al.*, 1995), polyene antibiotics (Pocchiari *et al.*, 1987), anthracycline (Tagliavini *et al.*, 1997), dextran sulphate, pentosan polysulphate and other polyanions (Ehlers and Diringer, 1984; Farquhar and Dickinson, 1986; Kimberlin and Walker, 1986) and β-sheet breaker peptides (Soto *et al.*, 2000) have been shown to have limited effects in animal models of prion disease. Unfortunately, most show a significant effect only if administered long before clinical onset (in some cases with the inoculum) and/or are impractical treatments due to toxicity or bioavailability. Quinacrine, an agent formerly used widely as an antimalarial agent, has been shown to block PrP^{Sc} accumulation in scrapie-infected neuroblastoma cells at concentrations that might be achievable clinically (Korth *et al.*, 2001). Clinical trials are under way or planned in several countries to evaluate any effect of this drug on disease progression.

The prion diseases are now amongst the best understood of the degenerative brain diseases and the development of rational treatments is appearing realistic. Recently, two anti-PrP monoclonal antibodies have been shown to protect mice indefinitely from developing prion disease when infected by the intraperitoneal route (White *et al.*, 2003). It is not yet known whether this approach can interfere with CNS disease, which would in any case require infusion of antibody into the CSF, but these data provide a proof of principal for antibody-based prion therapeutics and the possibility of secondary prevention by passive immunisation.

The precise molecular events which bring about the conversion of PrP^{C} to PrP^{Sc} and the molecular nature of the neurotoxic species remain ill-defined, a fact which at first sight would preclude screening for compounds which inhibit the process. However, any ligand which selectively stabilises the PrP^{C} state will prevent its rearrangement and might reasonably be expected to block prion replication (and presumably production of any putative toxic intermediate forms of PrP on the pathway to PrP^{Sc} formation). Such an approach has recently been applied to block p53 conformational rearrangements which are involved in tumorigenesis. Advances in therapeutics will have to be matched by advances in early diagnosis of prion disease to provide effective intervention before extensive neuronal loss has occurred.

CONCLUDING REMARKS

Prion diseases appear to be diseases of protein conformation and elucidating their precise molecular mechanisms may, in addition to allowing us to progress with tackling key public health issues posed by vCJD, be of wider significance in pathobiology. Common themes are emerging in neurodegenerative diseases, many of which are also associated with aggregates of misfolded protein. Also, the apparent ability of a single polypeptide chain to encode information and specify distinctive phenotypes is unprecedented and evolution may have used this mechanism in many other ways. While the protein-only hypothesis of prion propagation is supported by compelling experimental data, and now appears also able to encompass the phenomenon of prion strain diversity, the goal of the production of prions *in vitro* remains. PrP^{Sc}-like forms of PrP have recently been produced from purified recombinant material, but as yet none have been shown to be capable of producing disease in experimental animals that can be serially propagated. Success in such an endeavour would not only prove the protein-only hypothesis, it would also serve as the essential model by which the mechanism of prion propagation can be understood in molecular detail.

ON-LINE SOURCES OF INFORMATION

UK Department of Health: http://www.doh.gov.uk/cjd/
National Prion Clinic, St Mary's Hospital, London, UK: http://www.st-marys.nhs.uk/prion/
UK CJD Surveillance Unit: http://www.cjd.ed.ac.uk/

REFERENCES

Adikari D and Farmer P (2001) A cluster of Creutzfeldt–Jacob disease patients from Nassau County, New York, USA. *Ann Clin Lab Sci*, **31** 211–212.

Aguzzi A (1997) Neuro-immune connection in spread of prions in the body. *Lancet*, **349**, 742–743.

Alper T, Cramp WA, Haig DA and Clarke MC (1967) Does the agent of scrapie replicate without nucleic acid?, *Nature*, **214**, 764–766.

Alper T, Haig DA and Clarke MC (1966) The exceptionally small size of the scrapie agent. *Biochem Biophys Res Commun*, **22**, 278–284.

Alpers M (1964) *Kuru: Age and Duration Studies*. Department of Medicine, University of Adelaide.

Alpers MP (1987) Epidemiology and clinical aspects of kuru. In *Prions: Novel Infectious Pathogens Causing Scrapie and Creutzfeldt–Jakob Disease* (eds Prusiner SB, McKinley MP), pp. 451–465. Academic Press, San Diego, CA.

Anderson RG (1993) Caveolae: where incoming and outgoing messengers meet. *Proc Natl Acad Sci USA*, **90**, 10909–10913.

Anderson RM, Donnelly CA, Ferguson NM (1996) Transmission dynamics and epidemiology of BSE in British cattle. *Nature*, **382**, 779–788.

Arnold JE, Tipler C, Laszlo L, *et al.* (1995) The abnormal isoform of the prion protein accumulates in late-endosome-like organelles in scrapie-infected mouse brain. *J Pathol*, **176**, 403–411.

Asante EA, Linehan JM, Desbruslais M *et al.* (2002) BSE prions propagate as either variant CJD-like or sporadic CJD-like prion strains in transgenic mice expressing human prion protein. *EMBO J*, **21**(23), 6358–6366.

Aucouturier P, Geissmann F, Damotte D *et al.* (2001) Infected splenic dendritic cells are sufficient for prion transmission to the CNS in mouse scrapie. *J Clin Invest*, **108**(5), 703–708.

Baker HE, Poulter M, Crow TJ *et al.* (1991) Aminoacid polymorphism in human prion protein and age at death in inherited prion disease. *Lancet*, **337**, 1286.

Bateman D, Hilton D, Love S, *et al.* (1995) Sporadic Creutzfeldt–Jakob disease in a 18-year old in the UK. *Lancet*, **346**(8983), 1155–1156.

Beekes M, McBride PA, and Baldauf E (1998) Cerebral targeting indicates vagal spread of infection in hamsters fed with scrapie. *J Gen Virol*, **79**, 601–607.

Bell, JE, Gentleman, SM, Ironside, JW *et al.* (1997) Prion protein immunocytochemistry—UK five centre consensus report. *Neuropathol Appl Neurobiol*, **23**, 26–35.

Bencsik A, Lezmi S, and Baron T (2001) Autonomous nervous system innervation of lymphoid territories in spleen: a possible involvement of noradrenergic neurons for prion neuroinvasion in natural scrapie. *J Neurovirol*, **7**(5), 447–453.

Bernoulli C, Siegfried J, Baumgartner G *et al.* (1977) Danger of accidental person-to-person transmission of Creutzfeldt–Jakob disease by surgery [letter]. *Lancet*, **1**(8009), 478–479.

Bessen RA, Kocisko DA, Raymond GJ *et al.* (1995) Non-genetic propagation of strain-specific properties of scrapie prion protein. *Nature*, **375**, 698–700.

Bessen RA and Marsh RF (1992) Biochemical and physical properties of the prion protein from two strains of the transmissible mink encephalopathy agent. *J Virol*, **66**, 2096–2101.

Bessen RA and Marsh RF (1994) Distinct PrP properties suggest the molecular basis of strain variation in transmissible mink encephalopathy. *J Virol*, **68**, 7859–7868.

Blattler T (2002) Implications of prion diseases for neurosurgery. *Neurosurg Rev*, **25**(4), 195–203.

Bolton DC, McKinley MP and Prusiner SB (1982) Identification of a protein that purifies with the scrapie prion. *Science*, **218**, 1309–1311.

Bons N, Lehmann S, Mestre-Frances N *et al.* (2002) Brain and buffy coat transmission of bovine spongiform encephalopathy to the primate *Microcebus murinus* 40. *Transfusion*, **42**(5), 513–516.

Borchelt DR, Scott M, Taraboulos A *et al.* (1990) Scrapie and cellular prion proteins differ in their kinetics of synthesis and topology in cultured cells. *J Cell Biol*, **110**, 743–752.

Bosque PJ, Vnencak-Jones CL, Johnson MD *et al.* (1992) A PrP gene codon 178 base substitution and a 24-bp interstitial deletion in familial Creutzfeldt–Jakob disease. *Neurology*, **42**, 1864–1870.

Brandner S, Isenmann S, Raeber A *et al.* (1996) Normal host prion protein necessary for scrapie-induced neurotoxicity. *Nature*, **379**, 339–343.

Britton TC, Al-Sarraj S, Shaw C (1995) Sporadic Creutzfeldt–Jakob disease in a 16-year-old in the UK. *Lancet*, **346**(8983), 1155.

Brown DR, Herms J, and Kretzschmar HA (1994) Mouse cortical cells lacking cellular PrP survive in culture with a neurotoxic PrP fragment. *Neuroreport*, **5**, 2057–2060.

Brown DR, Schulz-Schaeffer WJ, Schmidt B and Kretzschmar HA (1997) Prion protein-deficient cells show altered repsonse to oxidative stress due to decreased SOD-1 activity. *Exp Neurol*, **146**, 104–112.

Brown P (1995) Can Creutzfeldt–Jakob disease be transmitted by transfusion? *Curr Opin Hematol*, **2**, 472–477.

Brown P, Cathala F, Raubertas RF, *et al.* (1987) The epidemiology of Creutzfeldt–Jakob disease: conclusion of a 15-year investigation in France and review of the world literature. *Neurology*, **37**, 895–904.

Brown P, Cervenáková L, McShane LM *et al.* (1999) Further studies of blood infectivity in an experimental model of transmissible spongiform encephalopathy, with an explanation of why blood components do not transmit Creutzfeldt–Jakob disease in humans. *Transfusion*, **39**(11–12), 1169–1178.

Brown P, Galvez S, Goldfarb LG *et al.* (1992) Familial Creutzfeldt–Jakob disease in Chile is associated with the codon 200 mutation of the PRNP amyloid precursor gene on chromosome 20. *J Neurol Sci*, **112**, 65–67.

Brown P, Gibbs CJ Jr, Rodgers Johnson P *et al.* (1994) Human spongiform encephalopathy: the National Institutes of Health series of 300 cases of experimentally transmitted disease. *Ann Neurol*, **35**, 513–529.

Brown P, Preece M, Brandel JP *et al.* (2000) Iatrogenic Creutzfeldt–Jakob disease at the millennium. *Neurology*, **55**(8), 1075–1081.

Brown P, Preece MA and Will RG (1992) 'Friendly fire' in medicine: hormones, homografts, and Creutzfeldt–Jakob disease. *Lancet*, **340**, 24–27.

Brown P, Rodgers-Johnson P, Cathala F *et al.* (1984) Creutzfeldt–Jakob disease of long duration: clinicopathological characteristics, transmissibility, and differential diagnosis. *Ann Neurol*, **16**, 295–304.

Bruce M, Chree A, McConnell I *et al.* (1994) Transmission of bovine spongiform encephalopathy and scrapie to mice: Strain variation and the species barrier. *Phil Trans R Soc Lond B Biol Sci*, **343**, 405–411.

Bruce ME, Fraser H, McBride PA *et al.* (1992) The basis of strain variation in scrapie. In *Prion Diseases in Human and Animals* (eds Prusiner SB *et al.*). Ellis Horwood, London.

Bruce ME, Will RG, Ironside JW *et al.* (1997) Transmissions to mice indicate that 'new variant' CJD is caused by the BSE agent. *Nature*, **389**, 498–501.

Budka H, Aguzzi A, Brown P *et al.* (1995) Neuropathological diagnostic criteria for Creutzfeldt–Jakob disease (CJD) and other human spongiform encephalopathies (Prion diseases). *Brain Pathol*, **5**, 459–466.

Bueler H, Aguzzi A, Sailer A *et al.* (1993) Mice devoid of PrP are resistant to scrapie. *Cell*, **73**, 1339–1347.

Bueler H, Fischer M, Lang Y *et al.* (1992) Normal development and behaviour of mice lacking the neuronal cell-surface PrP protein. *Nature*, **356**, 577–582.

Campbell TA, Palmer MS, Will RG *et al.* (1996) A prion disease with a novel 96-base pair insertional mutation in the prion protein gene. *Neurology*, **46**, 761–766.

Caughey B and Raymond GJ (1991) The scrapie-associated form of PrP is made from a cell surface precursor that is both protease- and phospholipase-sensitive. *J Biol Chem*, **266**(27), 18217–18223.

Chapman J, Arlazoroff A, Goldfarb LG *et al.* (1996) Fatal insomnia in a case of familial Creutzfeldt–Jakob disease with the codon 200^{Lys} mutation. *Neurology*, **46**, 758–761.

Chapman J, Ben-Israel J, Goldhammer Y *et al.* (1994) The risk of developing Creutzfeldt–Jakob disease in subjects with the *PRNP* gene codon 200 point mutation. *Neurology*, **44**, 1683–1686.

Chazot G, Broussolle E, Lapras CI *et al.* (1996) New variant of Creutzfeldt–Jakob disease in a 26-year-old French man. *Lancet*, **347**, 1181.

Cobb WA, Hornabrook RW and Sanders S (1973) The EEG of kuru. *Electroencephalogr Clin Neurophysiol*, **34**(4), 419–427.

Collinge J (1996) New diagnostic tests for prion diseases. *N Engl J Med*, **335**, 963–965.

Collinge J (1997) Human prion diseases and bovine spongiform encephalopathy (BSE). *Hum Mol Gen*, **6**(10), 1699–1705.

Collinge J (1998) Human prion diseases: aetiology and clinical features. In *The Dementias* (eds Growdon JH and Rossor M), pp. 113–148. Butterworth-Heinemann, Newton, MA.

Collinge J (1999) Variant Creutzfeldt–Jakob disease. *Lancet*, **354**(9175), 317–323.

Collinge J (2001) Prion diseases of humans and animals: their causes and molecular basis. *Annu Rev Neurosci*, **24**, 519–550.

Collinge J, Beck J, Campbell T, *et al.* (1996a) Prion protein gene analysis in new variant cases of Creutzfeldt–Jakob disease. *Lancet*, **348**(9019), 56.

Collinge J, Brown J, Hardy J *et al.* (1992), Inherited prion disease with 144 base pair gene insertion: II: clinical and pathological features. *Brain*, **115**, 687–710.

Collinge J, Harding AE, Owen F *et al.* (1989) Diagnosis of Gerstmann–Sträussler syndrome in familial dementia with prion protein gene analysis. *Lancet*, **2**, 15–17.

Collinge J and Hawke S (1998) B lymphocytes in prion neuroinvasion: central or peripheral players. *Nature Medicine*, **4**(12), 1369–1370.

Collinge J, Hill AF, Ironside J and Zeidler M (1997) Diagnosis of new variant Creutzfeldt–Jakob disease by tonsil biopsy—authors' reply to Arya and Evans. *Lancet*, **349**, 1322–1323.

Collinge J, Owen F, Poulter M *et al.* (1990) Prion dementia without characteristic pathology. *Lancet*, **336**, 7–9.

Collinge J, Palmer MS, Campbell TA *et al.* (1993) Inherited prion disease (PrP lysine 200) in Britain: two case reports. *Br Med J*, **306**, 301–302.

Collinge J, Palmer MS and Dryden AJ (1991b) Genetic predisposition to iatrogenic Creutzfeldt–Jakob disease. *Lancet*, **337**, 1441–1442.

Collinge J, Palmer MS, Sidle KCL *et al.* (1995a) Transmission of fatal familial insomnia to laboratory animals. *Lancet*, **346**, 569–570.

Collinge J, Palmer MS, Sidle KCL *et al.* (1995b) Unaltered susceptibility to BSE in transgenic mice expressing human prion protein. *Nature*, **378**, 779–783.

Collinge J, Poulter M, Davis MB *et al.* (1991a) Presymptomatic detection or exclusion of prion protein gene defects in families with inherited prion diseases. *Am J Hum Genet*, **49**, 1351–1354.

Collinge J and Prusiner SB (1992) Terminology of prion disease. In *Prion Diseases of Humans and Animals* (eds Prusiner SB *et al.*), pp. 5–12. Ellis Horwood, London.

Collinge J and Rossor M (1996) A new variant of prion disease. *Lancet*, **347**, 916–917.

Collinge J, Sidle KCL, Meads J *et al.* (1996b) Molecular analysis of prion strain variation and the aetiology of 'new variant' CJD. *Nature*, **383**, 685–690.

Collinge J, Whittington MA, Sidle KCL *et al.* (1994) Prion protein is necessary for normal synaptic function. *Nature*, **370**, 295–297.

Collins S, Boyd A, Fletcher A *et al.* (2002) Creutzfeldt–Jakob disease cluster in an Australian rural city. *Ann Neurol*, **52**(1), 115–118.

Collins S, Law MG, Fletcher A *et al.* (1999) Surgical treatment and risk of sporadic Creutzfeldt–Jakob disease: a case-control study. *Lancet*, **353**(9154), 693–697.

D'Aignaux JNH, Cousens SN and Smith PG (2001) Predictability of the UK variant Creutzfeldt–Jakob disease epidemic. *Science*, **294**(5547), 1729–1731.

Dlouhy SR, Hsiao K, Farlow MR *et al.* (1992) Linkage of the Indiana kindred of Gerstmann–Sträussler–Scheinker disease to the prion protein gene. *Nature Genetics*, **1**, 64–67.

Dodelet VC and Cashman NR (1998) Prion protein expression in human leukocyte differentiation. *Blood*, **91**, 1556–1561.

Doh ura K, Tateishi J, Sasaki H *et al.* (1989) Pro–leu change at position 102 of prion protein is the most common but not the sole mutation related to Gerstmann–Sträussler syndrome. *Biochem Biophys Res Commun*, **163**, 974–979.

Ehlers B and Diringer H (1984) Dextran sulphate 500 delays and prevents mouse scrapie by impairment of agent replication in spleen. *J Gen Virol*, **65**, 1325–1330.

Esmonde TFG, Will RG, Slattery JM *et al.* (1993) Creutzfeldt–Jakob disease and blood transfusion. *Lancet*, **341**, 205–207.

Farmer PM, Kane WC, and Hollenberg-Sher J (1978) Incidence of Creutzfeldt–Jakob disease in Brooklyn and Staten Island. *N Engl J Med*, **298**(5), 283–284.

Farquhar CF and Dickinson AG (1986) Prolongation of scrapie incubation period by an injection of dextran sulphate 500 within the month before or after infection. *J Gen Virol*, **67**, 463–473.

Fischer M, Rulicke T, Raeber A *et al.* (1996) Prion protein (PrP) with amino-proximal deletions restoring susceptibility of PrP knockout mice to scrapie. *EMBO J*, **15**, 1255–1264.

Flechsig E, Hegyi I, Enari M *et al.* (2001) Transmission of scrapie by steel-surface-bound prions. *Mol Med*, **7**(10), 679–684.

Forloni G, Angeretti N, Chiesa R *et al.* (1993) Neurotoxicity of a prion protein fragment. *Nature*, **362**, 543–546.

Fraser H, Bruce ME, Davies D *et al.* (1992) The lymphoreticular system in the pathogenesis of scrapie. In *Prion Diseases of Humans and Animals* (eds Prusiner SB *et al.*), Ellis Horwood, London.

Gerstmann J, Sträussler E and Scheinker I (1936) Über eine eigenartige hereditär-familiäre Erkrankung des Zentralnervensystems. Zugleich ein Beitrag zur Frage des vorzeitigen lakalen Alterns. *Zeitschr Neurol*, **154**, 736–762.

Ghani AC, Ferguson NM, Donnelly C, and Anderson RM (2000) Predicted vCJD mortality in Great Britain. *Nature*, **406**, 583–584.

Ghani AC, Ferguson NM, Donnelly CA *et al.* (1999) Epidemiological determinants of the pattern and magnitude of the vCJD epidemic in Great Britain. *Proc R Soc Lond B* **265**, 2443–2452.

Gibbs CJ Jr, Gajdusek DC, Asher DM *et al.* (1968) Creutzfeldt–Jakob disease (spongiform encephalopathy): transmission to the chimpanzee. *Science*, **161**, 388–389.

Goldfarb LG, Brown P, Little BW *et al.* (1993) A new (two-repeat) octapeptide coding insert mutation in Creutzfeldt–Jakob disease. *Neurology*, **43**, 2392–2394.

Goldfarb LG, Brown P, McCombie WR *et al.* (1991a) Transmissible familial Creutzfeldt–Jakob disease associated with five, seven, and eight extra octapeptide coding repeats in the *PRNP* gene. *Proc Natl Acad Sci USA*, **88**, 10926–10930.

Goldfarb LG, Brown P, Mitrova E *et al.* (1991b) Creutzfeldt–Jacob disease associated with the PRNP codon 200Lys mutation: an analysis of 45 families. *Eur J Epidemiol*, **7**, 477–486.

Goldfarb LG, Haltia M, Brown P *et al.* (1991c) New mutation in scrapie amyloid precursor gene (at codon 178) in Finnish Creutzfeldt–Jakob kindred. *Lancet*, **337**, 425.

Goldfarb LG, Korczyn AD, Brown P *et al.* (1990) Mutation in codon 200 of scrapie amyloid precursor gene linked to Creutzfeldt–Jakob disease in Sephardic Jews of Libyan and non-Libyan origin. *Lancet*, **336**, 637–638.

Goldfarb LG, Petersen RB, Tabaton M *et al.* (1992) Fatal familial insomnia and familial Creutzfeldt–Jakob disease: disease phenotype determined by a DNA polymorphism. *Science*, **258**, 806–808.

Gomori AJ, Partnow MJ, Horoupian DS and Hirano A (1973) The ataxic form of Creutzfeldt–Jakob disease. *Arch Neurol*, **29**, 318–323.

Griffith JS (1967) Self replication and scrapie. *Nature*, **215**, 1043–1044.

Guiroy DC, Marsh RF, Yanagihara R and Gajdusek DC (1993) Immunolocalization of scrapie amyloid in non-congophilic, non-birefringent deposits in golden Syrian hamsters with experimental transmissible mink encephalopathy. *Neurosci Letts*, **155**, 112–115.

Hadlow WJ (1959) Scrapie and kuru. *Lancet*, **ii**, 289–290.

Hainfellner JA, Brantner-Inthaler S, Cervenáková L *et al.* (1995) The original Gerstmann-Straussler-Scheinker family of Austria: divergent clinicopathological phenotypes but constant PrP genotype. *Brain Pathol*, **5**, 201–211.

Heppner FL, Christ AD, Klein MA *et al.* (2001) Transepithelial prion transport by M cells. *Nature Medicine*, **7**(9), 976–977.

Hill A, Antoniou M, and Collinge J (1999) Protease-resistant prion protein produced in vitro lacks detectable infectivity. *J Gen Virol*, **80**, 11–14.

Hill AF, Butterworth RJ, Joiner S *et al.* (1999) Investigation of variant Creutzfeldt–Jakob disease and other human prion diseases with tonsil biopsy samples. *Lancet*, **353**(9148), 183–189.

Hill AF and Collinge J (2001) Strain variations and species barriers. *Contrib Microbiol*, **7**, 48–57.

Hill AF, Desbruslais M, Joiner S *et al.* (1997a) The same prion strain causes vCJD and BSE. *Nature*, **389**, 448–450.

Hill AF, Joiner S, Linehan J *et al.* (2000) Species barrier independent prion replication in apparently resistant species. *Proc Natl Acad Sci USA*, **97**(18), 10248–10253.

Hill AF, Joiner S, Wadsworth JD *et al.* (2003) Molecular classification of sporadic Creutzfeldt–Jakob disease. *Brain*, **126**, 1333–1346.

Hill AF, Sidle KCL, Joiner S *et al.* (1998) Molecular screening of sheep for bovine spongiform encephalopathy. *Neurosci Lett*, **255**, 159–162.

Hill AF, Zeidler M, Ironside J and Collinge J (1997b) Diagnosis of new variant Creutzfeldt–Jakob disease by tonsil biopsy. *Lancet*, **349**(9045), 99–100.

Hilton DA, Ghani AC, Conyers L *et al.* (2002) Accumulation of prion protein in tonsil and appendix: review of tissue samples. *Br Med J*, **325**(7365), 633–634.

Holada K, Vostal JG, Theisen PW *et al.* (2002) Scrapie infectivity in hamster blood is not associated with platelets. *J Virol*, **76**(9), 4649–4650.

Hope J, Wood SCER, Birkett CR (1999) Molecular analysis of ovine prion protein identifies similarities between BSE and an experimental isolate of natural scrapie, CH1641. *J Gen Virol*, **80**, 1–4.

Hornshaw MP, McDermott JR, Candy JM and Lakey JH (1995) Copper binding to the N-terminal tandem repeat region of mammalian and avian prion protein: structural studies using synthetic peptides. *Biochem Biophys Res Commun*, **214**, 993–999.

Hosszu LLP, Baxter NJ, Jackson GS *et al.* (1999) Structural mobility of the human prion protein probed by backbone hydrogen exchange. *Nature Struct Biol*, **6**(8), 740–743.

Hsiao K, Baker HF, Crow TJ *et al.* (1989) Linkage of a prion protein missense variant to Gerstmann–Sträussler syndrome. *Nature*, **338**, 342–345.

Hsiao K, Dlouhy SR, Farlow MR *et al.* (1992) Mutant prion proteins in Gerstmann–Sträussler–Sheinker disease with neurofibrillary tangles. *Nature Genet*, **1**, 68–71.

Hsiao K, Meiner Z, Kahana E *et al.* (1991a) Mutation of the prion protein in Libyan Jews with Creutzfeldt–Jakob disease. *N Engl J Med*, **324**, 1091–1097.

Hsiao KK, Cass C, Schellenberg GD *et al.* (1991b) A prion protein variant in a family with the telencephalic form of Gerstmann–Sträussler–Scheinker syndrome. *Neurology*, **41**, 681–684.

Hsiao KK, Scott M, Foster D *et al.* (1990) Spontaneous neurodegeneration in transgenic mice with mutant prion protein. *Science*, **250**, 1587–1590.

Hunter N, Foster J, Chong A *et al.* (2002) Transmission of prion diseases by blood transfusion. *J Gen Virol*, **83**(11), 2897–2905.

Ingrosso L, Ladogana A and Pocchiari M (1995) Congo red prolongs the incubation period in scrapie-infected hamsters. *J Virol*, **69**, 506–508.

Jackson GS, Murray I, Hosszu LLP *et al.* (2001) Location and properties of metal-binding sites on the human prion protein. *Proc Natl Acad Sci USA*, **98**(15), 8531–8535.

Jackson GS, Hosszu LLP, Power A *et al.* (1999) Reversible conversion of monomeric human prion protein between native and fibrilogenic conformations. *Science*, **283**, 1935–1937.

Jimi T, Wakayama Y, Shibuya S *et al.* (1992) High levels of nervous system-specific proteins in cerebrospinal fluid in patients with early stage Creutzfeldt–Jakob disease. *Clin Chim Acta*, **211**(1–2), 37–46.

Joiner S, Linehan J, Brandner S *et al.* (2002) Irregular presence of abnormal prion protein in appendix in variant Creutzfeldt–Jakob disease. *J Neurol Neurosurg Psych*, **73**(5), 597–598.

Kimberlin RH and Walker CA (1978) Evidence that the transmission of one source of scrapie agent to hamsters involves separation of agent strains from a mixture. *J Gen Virol*, **39**, 487–496.

Kimberlin RH and Walker CA (1979) Pathogenesis of scrapie: agent multiplication in brain at the first and second passage of hamster scrapie in mice. *J Gen Virol*, **42**, 107–117.

Kimberlin RH and Walker CA (1986) Suppression of scrapie infection in mice by heteropolyanion 23, dextran sulfate, and some other polyanions. *Antimicrob Agents Chemother*, **30**, 409–413.

Kirkwood JK, Wells GA, Wilesmith JW *et al.* (1990) Spongiform encephalopathy in an arabian oryx (*Oryx leucoryx*) and a greater kudu (*Tragelaphus strepsiceros*). *Vet Rec*, **127**, 418–420.

Kitamoto T, Iizuka R and Tateishi J (1993) An amber mutation of prion protein in Gerstmann–Sträussler syndrome with mutant PrP plaques. *Biochem and Biophys Res Commun*, **192**(2), 525–531.

Kitamoto T, Ohta M, Doh-ura K *et al.* (1993) Novel missense variants of prion protein in Creutzfeldt–Jakob disease or Gerstmann–Sträussler syndrome. *Biochem Biophys Res Commun*, **191**(2), 709–714.

Kocisko DA, Come JH, Priola SA *et al.* (1994) Cell-free formation of protease-resistant prion protein. *Nature*, **370**, 471–474.

Kocisko DA, Priola SA, Raymond GJ *et al.* (1995) Species specificity in the cell-free conversion of prion protein to protease-resistant forms: a model for the scrapie species barrier. *Proc Natl Acad Sci USA*, **92**(9), 3923–3927.

Korth C, May BC, Cohen FE and Prusiner SB (2001) Acridine and phenothiazine derivatives as pharmacotherapeutics for prion disease. *Proc Natl Acad Sci USA*, **98**(17), 9836–9841.

Krasemann S, Zerr I, Weber T *et al.* (1995) Prion disease associated with a novel nine octapeptide repeat insertion in the PRNP gene. *Mol Brain Res*, **34**, 173–176.

Kretzschmar HA, Kufer P, Riethmuller G *et al.* (1992) Prion protein mutation at codon 102 in an Italian family with Gerstmann–Sträussler–Scheinker syndrome. *Neurology*, **42**, 809–810.

Kuczius T, Haist I and Groschup MH (1998) Molecular analysis of bovine spongiform encephalopathy and scrapie strain variation. *J Infect Dis*, **178**(3), 693–699.

Kunz B, Sandmeier E and Christen P (1999) Neurotoxicity of prion peptide 106-126 not confirmed. *FEBS Letters*, **458**(1), 65–68.

Kurschner C and Morgan JI (1996) Analysis of interaction sites in homo- and heteromeric complexes containing Bcl-2 family members and the cellular prion protein. *Brain Res Mol Brain Res*, **37**(1–2), 249–258.

Kurschner C and Morgan JI (1995) The cellular prion protein (PrP) selectively binds to Bcl-2 in the yeast two-hybrid system. *Brain Res Mol Brain Res*, **30**, 165–168.

Laplanche JL, Delasnerie Laupretre N, Brandel JP *et al.* (1995) Two novel insertions in the prion protein gene in patients with late-onset dementia. *Hum Mol Genet*, **4**(6), 1109–1111.

Lasmézas CI, Deslys JP, Robain O *et al.* (1997) Transmission of the BSE agent to mice in the absence of detectable abnormal prion protein. *Science*, **275**, 402–405.

Laszlo L, Lowe J, Self T *et al.* (1992) Lysosomes as key organelles in the pathogenesis of prion encephalopathies. *J Pathol*, **166**, 333–341.

Liemann S and Glockshuber R (1999) Influence of amino acid substitutions related to inherited human prion diseases on the thermodynamic stability of the cellular prion protein. *Biochemistry*, **38**(11), 3258–3267.

Lloyd SE, Onwuazor ON, Beck JA *et al.* (2001) Identification of multiple quantitative trait loci linked to prion disease incubation period in mice. *Proc Natl Acad Sci USA*, **98**(11), 6279–6283.

Lloyd SE, Uphill JB, Targonski PV *et al.* (2002) Identification of genetic loci affecting mouse-adapted bovine spongiform encephalopathy incubation time in mice. *Neurogenetics*, **4**(2), 77–81.

Lugaresi E, Medori R, Baruzzi PM *et al.* (1986) Fatal familial insomnia and dysautonomia, with selective degeneration of thalamic nuclei. *N Engl J Med*, **315**, 997–1003.

Mabbott NA, Mackay F, Minns F and Bruce ME (2000) Temporary inactivation of follicular dendritic cells delays neuroinvasion of scrapie. *Nature Med*, **6**(7), 719–720.

Mabbott NA, Young J, McConnell I and Bruce ME (2003) Follicular dendritic cell dedifferentiation by treatment with an inhibitor of the lymphotoxin pathway dramatically reduces scrapie susceptibility. *J Virol*, **77**(12), 6845–6854.

Mallucci GR, Ratté S, Asante EA *et al.* (2002) Post-natal knockout of prion protein alters hippocampal CA1 properties, but does not result in neurodegeneration. *EMBO J*, **21**(3), 202–210.

Manson J, West JD, Thomson V *et al.* (1992) The prion protein gene: a role in mouse embryogenesis? *Development*, **115**, 117–122.

Mayer RJ, Landon M, Laszlo L *et al.* (1992) Protein processing in lysosomes: the new therapeutic target in neurodegenerative disease. *Lancet*, **340**, 156–159.

McLean CA, Storey E, Gardner RJM *et al.* (1997) The D178N (cis-129M) 'fatal familial insomnia' mutation associated with diverse clinicopathologic phenotypes in an Australian kindred. *Neurology*, **49**, 552–558.

Mead S, Mahal SP, Beck J *et al.* (2001) Sporadic—but not variant—Creutzfeldt–Jakob disease is associated with polymorphisms upstream of *PRNP* Exon 1. *Am J Hum Genet*, **69**(6), 1225–1235.

Mead S, Stumpf MP, Whitfield J *et al.* (2003) Balancing selection at the prion protein gene consistent with prehistoric kurulike epidemics. *Science* (in press).

Medori R, Montagna P, Tritschler HJ *et al.* (1992a) Fatal familial insomnia: a second kindred with mutation of prion protein gene at codon 178. *Neurology*, **42**, 669–670.

Medori R, Tritschler HJ, LeBlanc A *et al.* (1992b) Fatal familial insomnia, a prion disease with a mutation at codon 178 of the prion protein gene [see comments]. *N Engl J Med*, **326**, 444–449.

Meyer A, Leigh D and Bagg CE (1954) A rare presenile dementia associated with cortical blindness (Heidenhain's syndrome). *J Neurol Neurosurg Psychiat*, **17**, 129–133.

Monari L, Chen SG, Brown P *et al.* (1994) Fatal familial insomnia and familial Creutzfeldt–Jakob disease: different prion proteins determined by a DNA polymorphism. *Proc Natl Acad Sci USA*, **91**, 2839–2842.

Montrasio F, Frigg R, Glatzel M *et al.* (2000) Impaired prion replication in spleens of mice lacking functional follicular dendritic cells. *Science*, **288**(5469), 1257–1259.

Moore RC, Lee IY, Silverman GL *et al.* (1999) Ataxia in prion protein (PrP)-deficient mice is associated with upregulation of the novel PrP-like protein Doppel. *J Mol Biol*, **292**(4), 797–817.

Neufeld MY, Josiphov J and Korczyn AD (1992) Demyelinating peripheral neuropathy in Creutzfeldt–Jakob disease. *Muscle Nerve*, **15**, 1234–1239.

Nicholl D, Windl O, De Silva R *et al.* (1995) Inherited Creutzfeldt–Jakob disease in a British family associated with a novel 144 base pair insertion of the prion protein gene. *J Neurol Neurosurg Psychiat*, **58**, 65–69.

Nitrini R, Rosemberg S, Passos-Bueno MR *et al.* (1997) Familial spongiform encephalopathy associated with a novel prion protein gene mutation. *Ann Neurol*, **42**, 138–146.

Oda T, Kitamoto T, Tateishi J *et al.* (1995) Prion disease with 144 base pair insertion in a Japanese family line. *Acta Neuropathol (Berl)*, **90**, 80–86.

Oesch B, Westaway D, Walchli M *et al.* (1985) A cellular gene encodes scrapie PrP 27–30 protein. *Cell*, **40**, 735–746.

Oldstone MB, Race R, Thomas D *et al.* (2002) Lymphotoxin-α and lymphotoxin-β-deficient mice differ in susceptibility to scrapie: evidence against dendritic cell involvement in neuroinvasion. *J Virol*, **76**(9), 4357–4363.

Otto M, Stein H, Szudra A *et al.* (1997) S-100 protein concentration in the cerebrospinal fluid of patients with Creutzfeldt–Jakob disease. *J Neurol*, **244**, 566–570.

Owen F, Poulter M, Collinge J *et al.* (1992) A dementing illness associated with a novel insertion in the prion protein gene. *Mol Brain Res*, **13**, 155–157.

Owen F, Poulter M, Lofthouse R *et al.* (1989) Insertion in prion protein gene in familial Creutzfeldt–Jakob disease. *Lancet*, **1**, 51–52.

Palmer MS, Dryden AJ, Hughes JT and Collinge J (1991) Homozygous prion protein genotype predisposes to sporadic Creutzfeldt–Jakob disease. *Nature*, **352**, 340–342.

Pan K-M, Baldwin MA, Nguyen J *et al.* (1993) Conversion of α-helices into β-sheets features in the formation of the scrapie prion proteins. *Proc Natl Acad Sci USA*, **90**, 10962–10966.

Parchi P, Castellani R, Capellari S *et al.* (1996) Molecular basis of phenotypic variability in sporadic Creutzfeldt–Jakob disease. *Ann Neurol*, **39**(5), 669–680.

Pattison IH (1965) Experiments with scrapie with special reference to the nature of the agent and the pathology of the disease. In *Slow, Latent and Temperate Virus Infections, NINDB Monograph 2* (eds Gajdusek CJ, Gibbs CJ, and Alpers MP), pp. 249–257. US Government Printing, Washington DC.

Pocchiari M, Schmittinger S and Masullo C (1987) Amphotericin B delays the incubation period of scrapie in intracerebrally inoculated hamsters. *J Gen Virol*, **68**, 219–223.

Poulter M, Baker HF, Frith CD et al. (1992) Inherited prion disease with 144 base pair gene insertion: I: Genealogical and molecular studies. Brain, 115, 675–685.

Prinz M, Montrasio F, Klein MA et al. (2002) Lymph nodal prion replication and neuroinvasion in mice devoid of follicular dendritic cells. Proc Natl Acad Sci USA, 99(2), 919–924.

Prusiner SB (1982) Novel proteinaceous infectious particles cause scrapie. Science, 216, 136–144.

Prusiner SB (1991) Molecular biology of prion diseases. Science, 252(14) June, 1515–1522.

Prusiner SB, Scott M, Foster D et al. (1990) Transgenetic studies implicate interactions between homologous PrP isoforms in scrapie prion replication. Cell, 63, 673–686.

Riek R, Hornemann S, Wider G et al. (1996) NMR structure of the mouse prion protein domain PrP (121–231). Nature, 382, 180–182.

Salazar AM, Masters CL, Gajdusek DC and Gibbs CJ Jr (1983) Syndromes of amyotrophic lateral sclerosis and dementia: relation to transmissible Creutzfeldt–Jakob disease. Ann Neurol, 14, 17–26.

Schroter A, Zerr I, Henkel K et al. (2000) Magnetic resonance imaging in the clinical diagnosis of Creutzfeldt–Jakob disease. Arch Neurol, 57(12), 1751–1757.

Scott M, Foster D, Mirenda C et al. (1989) Transgenic mice expressing hamster prion protein produce species-specific scrapie infectivity and amyloid plaques. Cell, 59, 847–857.

Shaked GM, Fridlander G, Meiner Z et al. (1999) Protease-resistant and detergent-insoluble prion protein is not necessarily associated with prion infectivity. J Biol Chem, 274(25), 17981–17986.

Shyng S-L, Heuser JE and Harris DA (1994) A glycolipid-anchored prion protein is endocytosed via clathrin-coated pits. J Cell Biol, 125, 1239–1250.

Soto C, Kascsack RJ, Saborío GP et al. (2000) Reversion of prion conformational changes by synthetic beta-sheet breaker peptides. Lancet, 355, 192–197.

Stahl N, Baldwin MA, Teplow DB et al. (1993) Structural studies of the scrapie prion protein using mass spectrometry and amino acid sequencing. Biochemistry, 32, 1991–2002.

Stöckel J, Safar J, Wallace AC et al. (1998) Prion protein selectively binds copper(II) ions. Biochemistry, 37, 7185–7193.

Tabrizi SJ, Scaravilli F, Howard RS et al. (1996) GRAND ROUND. Creutzfeldt–Jakob disease in a young woman. Report of a Meeting of Physicians and Scientists, St. Thomas' Hospital, London. Lancet, 347, 945–948.

Tagliavini F, Giaccone G, Prelli F et al. (1993a) A68 is a component of paired helical filaments of Gerstmann–Sträussler–Scheinker disease, Indiana kindred. Brain Res, 616, 325–328.

Tagliavini F, McArthur RA, Canciani B et al. (1997) Effectiveness of anthracycline against experimental prion disease in syrian hamsters. Science, 276, 1119–1122.

Tagliavini F, Prelli F, Verga L et al. (1993b) Synthetic peptides homologous to prion protein residues 106–147 form amyloid-like fibrils in vitro. Proc Natl Acad Sci USA, 90, 9678–9682.

Taraboulos A, Raeber A, Borchelt DR et al. (1992) Synthesis and trafficking of prion proteins in cultured cells. Mol Biol Cell, 3, 851–863.

Tateishi J, Brown P, Kitamoto T et al. (1995) First experimental transmission of fatal familial insomnia. Nature, 376, 434–435.

Telling GC, Parchi P, DeArmond SJ et al. (1996) Evidence for the conformation of the pathologic isoform of the prion protein enciphering and propagating prion diversity. Science, 274, 2079–2082.

Telling GC, Scott M, Mastrianni J et al. (1995) Prion propagation in mice expressing human and chimeric PrP transgenes implicates the interaction of cellular PrP with another protein. Cell, 83, 79–90.

Tobler I, Gaus SE, Deboer T et al. (1996) Altered circadian activity rhythms and sleep in mice devoid of prion protein. Nature, 380, 639–642.

Wadsworth JDF, Hill AF, Joiner S et al. (1999) Strain-specific prion-protein conformation determined by metal ions. Nature Cell Biol, 1, 55–59.

Wadsworth JDF, Joiner S, Hill AF et al. (2001) Tissue distribution of protease resistant prion protein in variant CJD using a highly sensitive immuno-blotting assay. Lancet, 358(9277), 171–180.

Weissmann C (1991) A 'unified theory' of prion propagation. Nature, 352, 679–683.

White AR, Enever P, Tayebi M et al. (2003) Monoclonal antibodies inhibit prion replication and delay the development of prion disease. Nature, 422(6927), 80–83.

Wickner RB (1997) A new prion controls fungal cell fusion incompatibility. Proc Natl Acad Sci USA, 94, 10012–10014.

Wickner RB and Masison DC (1996) Evidence for two prions in yeast: [URE3] and [PSI]. Curr Top Microbiol Immunol, 207, 147–160.

Wildegger G, Liemann S and Glockshuber R (1999) Extremely rapid folding of the C-terminal domain of the prion protein without kinetic intermediates. Nature Structural Biology, 6(6), 550–553.

Wilesmith JW, Wells GA, Cranwell MP and Ryan JB (1988) Bovine spongiform encephalopathy: epidemiological studies. Vet Rec, 123, 638–644.

Will RG, Ironside JW, Zeidler M et al. (1996) A new variant of Creutzfeldt–Jakob disease in the UK. Lancet, 347, 921–925.

Wille H, Zhang GF, Baldwin MA et al. (1996) Separation of scrapie prion infectivity from PrP amyloid polymers. J Mol Biol, 259, 608–621.

Williams A, Lucassen PJ, Ritchie D and Bruce M (1997) PrP deposition, microglial activation, and neuronal apoptosis in murine scrapie. Exp Neurol, 144, 433–438.

Windl O, Dempster M, Estibeiro JP et al. (1996) Genetic basis of Creutzfeldt–Jakob disease in the United Kingom: a systematic analysis of predisposing mutations and allelic variation in the PRNP gene. Human Genetics, 98, 259–264.

Zeidler M, Johnstone EC, Bamber RWK et al. (1997a) New variant Creutzfeldt–Jakob disease: psychiatric features. Lancet, 350, 908–910.

Zeidler M, Sellar RJ, Collie DA et al. (2000) The pulvinar sign on magnetic resonance imaging in variant Creutzfeldt–Jakob disease. Lancet, 355(9213), 1412–1418.

Zeidler M, Stewart GE, Barraclough CR (1997b) New variant Creutzfeldt–Jakob disease: neurological features and diagnostic tests. Lancet, 350, 903–907.

Zerr I, Bodemer M, Räcker S et al. (1995) Cerebrospinal fluid concentration of neuron-specific enolase in diagnosis of Creutzfeldt–Jakob disease. Lancet, 345, 1609–1610.

27

GBV-C and TTV

Shigeo Hino

Department of Virology, Tottori University, Yonago, Japan

INTRODUCTION

The discovery of the hepatitis A–E viruses has led to the identification of most blood-borne hepatitis viruses. In an attempt to identify any remaining such viruses, researchers are still striving to find novel blood-borne hepatitis viruses. Toward the end of the last decade, newly established molecular biological techniques were used to find two candidate viruses, known as GBV-C and TTV, although the real impact of these viruses on liver disease is still unclear. Due to the lack of a suitable cell system in which to culture these viruses, their biology remains obscure. While GBV-C is closely related to the hepatitis C virus, a member of the *Flavivirus* group, TTV, is the first human virus to be found with a single-stranded circular DNA genome similar to that of chicken anaemia virus. The prevalence of GBV-C is 1–4% in the general population, while that of TTV is over 90%. Animals have been found to harbour similar viruses that were specific to each species. Although post-transfusion hepatitis continues to occur in countries that screen blood donors for hepatitis B and C, the incidence of post-transfusion hepatitis is not sufficiently high to correlate with the high prevalence of these viruses. This review attempts to summarise the current status of the related research.

The story of the GB virus (GBV) started in 1967 (Deinhardt *et al.*, 1967). Elevation of serum transaminase levels was observed in all of four tamarins (*Saguinus* spp.) that had been inoculated with day 3 serum obtained from a surgeon (GB) who was suffering from acute hepatitis. The GB agent (GBV) that passed sequentially through the tamarins main-tained its pathogenicity. For a long time after it was first observed, however, it was not easy to distinguish GBV from the enteric hepatitis A virus. In 1995 representational difference analysis was used to iden-tify two distinct RNA viral sequences in the GB agent (Simons *et al.*, 1995a, 1995b). Both are partially related to *Hepatitis C virus* (HCV). Nevertheless, the original GB serum was found to contain another related virus, namely, GBV-C (Simons *et al.*, 1995a). An indepen-dent group discovered *Hepatitis G virus* (HGV) in the same cluster as GBV-C (Linnen *et al.*, 1996). In contrast, 1997 saw differential display technology being used to identify directly TT virus (TTV) in the serum of a hepatitis patient without any marker for known hepatitis viruses (Nishizawa *et al.*, 1997). Approximately half of the studies of these viruses have attempted to identify the pathogenicity specific to each. However, the real impact on liver disease of either of these two viruses remains uncertain. Since the prevalence of each virus in humans is significant, it is important to continue to study the true biology of these viruses.

HISTORY OF GBV-C

In 1967, Deinhardt *et al.* (1967) reported that four tamarins (*Saguinus* spp.) had been inoculated with an acute-phase serum sample obtained from a surgeon (whose initials were G.B.) suffering from acute hepatitis with jaundice. The serum transaminase levels were elevated in all four tamarins, starting at 14–53 days after the inoculation, with hyperbilirubinaemia observed in one. The agent (GBV) continued to be

Principles and Practice of Clinical Virology, Fifth Edition. Edited by A. J. Zuckerman, J. E. Banatvala, J. R. Pattison, P. D. Griffiths and B. D. Schoub
© 2004 John Wiley & Sons Ltd ISBN 0 470 84338 1

hepatogenic in the tamarins after several passages. The tamarins proved susceptible to the agent, but common marmosets (*Callithrix jacchus*) and baboons (*Papio* spp.) were not (Parks *et al.*, 1969a). In the early phases of the study, it was not easy to distinguish between GBV and *Hepatitis A virus* even though Parks *et al.* (1969a) suggested in 1969 that GBV is small, heat-labile and ether-sensitive. They also suggested that the virus is of tamarin origin, because some of the control animals exhibited similar symptoms, and the GBV-associated disease was not transmitted easily between tamarins reared in the same cage (Parks *et al.*, 1969b). However, their conclusions remain controversial (Deinhardt *et al.*, 1975). At the time, the presence of indigenous pathogens in tamarins made the results ambiguous (Parks *et al.*, 1969b). In 1989, Karayiannis *et al.* (1989) reported that only the serum and liver extracts of an infected tamarin were infectious, whereas the faeces were not.

In 1995, almost two decades after the first observation of GBV, representational difference analysis was used to identify two related RNA viral sequences in the GB agent, which came to be designated as GBV-A and GBV-B (Simons *et al.*, 1995a, 1995b). The genome of both viruses was over 9 kb long and had a limited sequence similarity to the isolates of human *Hepatitis C virus* (HCV) (Simons *et al.*, 1995a). The original serum of GB did not contain either virus, but instead contained another related virus, called GBV-C (Simons *et al.*, 1995a). Another group independently discovered a viral sequence and designated it the 'hepatitis G virus' (HGV), which was closely related, if not identical, to GBV-C (Linnen *et al.*, 1996).

GB AGENT IN ANIMALS

GBV-A was found in tamarins (*Saguinus labiatus*), mystax (*Saguinus mystax*), owl monkeys (*Aotus trivirgatus*) and common marmosets (*Saimiri* spp.), while GBV-B was found in tamarins (Leary *et al.*, 1996). GBVs from different species are divergent from each other and cluster genetically according to their original animal species, suggesting that GBV-A and GBV-B originated in New World monkeys. GBV-C was also found in chimpanzees (*Pan troglodytes*), which also cluster within the host species and which are divergent from human GBV-C (Adams *et al.*, 1998).

The natural course of a GBV-B infection in tamarins has been investigated extensively. Transient hepatitis in tamarins caused by GBV-B was confirmed by elevated liver enzyme levels and by inflammation and focal necrosis in liver biopsies (Schaluder *et al.*, 1995). Peak viraemia levels exceeded 10^9 copies/ml, after which viral clearance was achieved within 14–16 weeks. A strong protective immune response after the initial infection was suggested by the appearance of brief viraemia following a challenge by the same virus (Beames *et al.*, 2000). While some tamarins are infected persistently, the induction of chronic liver disease in tamarins has not been reported. GBV-A does not cause a significant elevation of alanine aminotransferase (ALT), even in tamarins (Schaluder *et al.*, 1995). The questions raised by the original experiments performed by Deinhardt *et al.* (1967) remain unanswered. If GBV-C does not replicate in tamarins, why did all the tamarins inoculated with the GB serum develop hepatitis? If GBV-C can replicate in tamarins, why did it disappear from the GB agent after several passages?

GENOME OF GBV

GBVs have genomes consisting of around 9.3×10^3 nucleotides, and a single large open reading frame that encodes a precursor polyprotein of around 2850 amino acids. The genome is organised much like that of HCV, with genes to encode the structural and non-structural proteins located at the 5' and 3' ends, respectively (Figure 27.1) (Simons *et al.*, 1995a, 1995b; Linnen *et al.*, 1996; Muerhoff *et al.*, 1995). The core protein of GBV-B and GBV-C seems to be truncated, while that of GBV-A is almost missing (Linnen *et al.*, 1996; Muerhoff *et al.*, 1995; Simons *et al.*, 1996). It would be interesting to know whether they produce infectious virions, either with or without a truncated core protein. The 5'-termini of GBV-A and GBV-C contain 5' non-translated sequences that are consistent with an

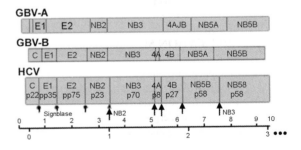

Figure 27.1 Genomic structures of GBV-A, GBV-B and HCV. Untranslated regions at the 3'- and 5'-termini are not shown

internal ribosome entry site, as in HCV (Simons et al., 1996).

The phylogenetic analysis of human GBV-Cs revealed that they could be clustered into five groups: genotype 1 (West Africa); genotype 2 (USA/Europe), genotype 3 (Asia), genotype 4 (south-east Asia) and genotype 5 (South Africa) (Tucker et al., 2000). The hypervariability of the HCV E2 protein is one of the main factors in maintaining chronic HCV infection. However, GBV-C E2 seems to be much more stable than HCV. Orii et al. (2000) studied the variability of GBV-C RNA in six patients with acute hepatitis. The average amino acid substitution rate in the E2 region of GBV-C was less than 1/100 that of HCV. No amino acid substitution in the loop domain was observed in seven additional patients with persistent GBV-C viraemia over the course of >2 years. How does GBV-C maintain persistent viraemia in some individuals without any variation in the envelope protein?

GBV IN TISSUE CULTURE

In tissue culture, GBV-C replicates in cells that originate from CD4$^+$ T cells (Ikeda et al., 1997), B cells (Shimizu et al., 1999) and hepatocytes (Seipp et al., 1999). In every case, the replication of GBV-C was not sufficiently efficient to enable classical virological analysis. In contrast, GBV-B replicates in primary cultures of normal tamarin hepatocytes with the rapid amplification of the cell-associated viral RNA and the secretion of around 10^7 copies/ml in the supernatant. In addition, the successful virus passage could be monitored by immunofluorescence staining of the GBV-B non-structural NS3 protein (Beames et al., 2000). This system may prove useful for the in vitro screening of anti-HCV drugs. However, despite a reduction in the GBV-B replication in the tissue culture system, no significant reduction in viraemia was observed in tamarins (Lanford et al., 2001).

REPLICATION SITE OF GBV-C

The in vivo replication site of GBV-C is of interest, because it may provide an insight into the possible pathogenicity of GBV-C. Fan et al. (1999) surveyed 17 patients who had undergone liver transplants and found that 70% had significantly lower GBV-C RNA titres in the liver than in the serum, while the remainder had RNA only in the serum. Shimizu et al. (2001) could not detect GBV-C RNA in the liver, colon or gall bladder, but did find it in the serum and

appendix. Tucker et al. (2000) investigated the negative-strand RNA using serum and 23 tissue samples taken from four individuals who had died in accidents. The spleen and bone marrow were invariably positive. Individual instances of a positive kidney and liver were also found. No negative strands were detected elsewhere. Radkowski et al. (2000) detected negative-strand RNA in five bone marrow samples. Although most of these studies suggest that GBV-C replicates mainly in the extrahepatic tissues, the samples were probably obtained from chronically infected people. Seipp et al. (1999) reported on the presence of negative-strand RNA in 4/6 explanted liver specimens, as well as on the hepatocyte-restricted infection caused by in situ hybridisation. Given that the hepatitis induced by GBV-B in tamarins is acute and transient, significant intrahepatic replication might occur only in the acute phase of the infection.

GBV-C IN THE HEALTHY POPULATION

Most studies of GBV-C in the healthy population have been based on voluntary blood donors, using RT-PCR for the 5'-untranslated region of GBV-C to detect the GBV-C viraemia and antibody assay against the E2 protein. Most individuals exposed to GBV-C were either RNA-positive or antibody-positive (GBV-C marker-positive). The prevalence of GBV-C viraemia has been found to be 1–4% in most countries (Table 27.1): the high rate of GBV-C viraemia is usually associated with a high rate of HCV-positive donors in the respective regions. Among those individuals with the GBV-C marker, 13–27% were GBV-C viraemic. Of the GBV-C viraemic population, 50–100% remained viraemic throughout the 1–3 year observation period. Persistence of the high viraemic rate was also observed in children (Fischler et al., 1997; Zanetti et al., 1998). This might suggest that most of the viraemic population is infected during infancy. Some genetic background, such as HLA, could have an influence on the infection, the persistence of the viraemia, or seroconversion. This alone, however, cannot explain the persistence of this virus in the human community, because the mother-to-child transmission rate is far less than 100% (discussed later).

Most reports refute the association of GBV-C infection with hepatic diseases, but Bjorkman et al. (2000) observed mild portal inflammatory lesions in 6/11 donors with persistent and isolated GBV-C viraemia, as well as steatosis in 10/13. The spouses of the viraemic population showed a high prevalence of

Table 27.1 Prevalence of GDV-C RNA viraemia among GBV-C marker-positive individuals and persistency of viraemia in healthy population

Country	% Viraemia of		Persistence	Reference
	Tested	Marker[1]		
Canada	1	13		Giulivi *et al.* (2000)
USA	1	13		Handa *et al.* (2000)
USA	2	27	100	Gutierrez *et al.* (1997)
West Indies	4	21		Cesaire *et al.* (1999)
Iceland	4	22		Love *et al.* (1999)
Norway	2	19		Nordbo *et al.* (2000)
Sweden	3		61	Bjorkman *et al.* (1998)
The Netherlands	1	27		Jongerius *et al.* (1999)
France	3	26		Mercier *et al.* (1999)
France	3	18		Cantaloube *et al.* (1999)
Poland	3	12		Brojer *et al.* (1999)
Taiwan	2		50	Wang *et al.* (1998)
Taiwan	3	27		Yu *et al.* (2001)
Japan	4	21		Akiyoshi *et al.* (1999)
South Africa	11			Casteling *et al.* (1998)
Australia	3	16	83	Hyland *et al.* (1998)
Australia	4		88	Moaven *et al.* (1996)

[1]Percentage of viraemic population among those with GBV-C markers (RNA or anti-E2 antibody).

viraemia: 7/32 spouses (22%) (Akiyoshi *et al.*, 1999) and 4/12 partners (33%) (Nordbo *et al.*, 2000). However, 5/7 spouses in the former series exhibited parenteral risk factors, such as blood transfusions, acupuncture or major surgery. Even in the apparently healthy population, people apparently at risk of parenteral infection exhibited a much higher prevalence, usually in excess of 20%. Thus, GBV-C does not seem to be efficiently transmitted via sexual intercourse.

GBV-C IN PATIENTS

Among acute non-A–E hepatitis patients, most studies found that the prevalence of GBV-C viraemia, at less than 6%, is not significantly higher than that of general population (Table 27.2). However, Frider *et al.* (1998) found 19 GBV-C viraemic cases (31%) among 62 acute non-A–E hepatitis patients. Most studies could not find evidence of significant ALT elevation, either. In a study of renal transplant recipients, De

Table 27.2 Prevalence of GBV-C and its viraemia in patients

Category	No. tested	% Viraemia of		Reference
		Tested	Marker[1]	
Acute hepatitis non-A–E	62	31		Frider *et al.* (1998)
Acute hepatitis non-A–E	53	4		Chu *et al.* (1999)
Acute hepatitis non-A–E	34	6	40	Jongerius *et al.* (1999)
HCV hepatitis	40	25	34	
Acute hepatitis non-A–E	98	3		Romano *et al.* (2000)
HCV CLD[1]	123	11	19	Hassoba *et al.* (1997)
CLD	285	9	26	Bjorkman *et al.* (2001)
Healthy	445	2	0	
CLD	100	22		Bjorkman *et al.* (2001)
Chronic haemodialysis	76	16	43	Chu *et al.* (2001)
Kidney transplantation	155	24	59	De Filippi *et al.* (2001)

[1]CLD: chronic liver disease.

Filippi *et al.* (2001) reported that 14% of the GBV-C RNA-positive and HCV-negative patients exhibited persistently elevated ALT, although 8% of the control patients who were free of GBV-C and HCV also had the same profile.

Blood transfusions are one of the major transmission pathways for GBV-C. Among those patients transfused with GBV-C RNA-positive blood, 8/21 (transmission rate, 38%) became viraemic after transfusion (Wang *et al.*, 1998). However, they reported a rate of persistent viraemia of 19% (4/21), lower than the persistency rate expected in the healthy population as quoted above. Adult infection may lead to a lower probability of persistent viraemia. The prevalence of the viraemic population in patients with chronic liver disease, chronic haemodialysis, and those who have had kidney transplants was apparently higher than that in the healthy population. The ratio of viraemic individuals to the marker-positive patient population appeared higher, especially in haemodialysis and transplant patients. Factors influencing these figures included lifestyle and associated risk factors and/or nosocomial infections. This may be explained by the fact that those patients with chronic medical interventions are more vulnerable to recent and repeated infections. Co-infection of GBV-C might moderate the course of HCV infection, since the HCV RNA levels were significantly lower in the 15 HCV/GBV-C co-infected patients than those in the 48 patients with HCV infection alone (2.2 vs. 10.8 copies/ml; $p = 0.02$; De Filippi *et al.*, 2001). The role of GBV-C in HIV infection may prove more interesting. GBV-C was not found to aggravate the course of patients with HIV infections. Moreover, carriage of GBV-C RNA was associated with the slower progression of HIV. All parameters (survival, CDC stage B/C, HIV RNA load, CD4 T cell count) showed significant differences in terms of the cumulative progression rate between those individuals who were positive and those who were negative for GBV-C RNA (Tillmann *et al.*, 2001).

MOTHER-TO-CHILD TRANSMISSION OF GBV-C

In a multicentre study conducted by Zanetti *et al.* (1998) 34/175 (19.4%) anti-HCV positive mothers were found to be positive for GBV-C RNA. All 21 (61.8%) babies to whom GBV-C was transmitted remained persistently viraemic for 3–19 months after birth, except for one who seroconverted at 18 months. Seven (35%) babies developed marginally elevated levels of ALT, excluding one dually-infected baby. Elective Caesarean section did not significantly reduce the rate of mother-to-child infection. Hino *et al.* (1998) reported a high transmission rate of 7/11 children born to mothers co-infected with HCV and GBV-C and significantly higher GBV-C RNA titres in mothers with infected children. The nucleotide sequence of the NS3 region was identical in each mother–child pair. Ohto *et al.* (2000) reported that 26/34 (77%) babies born to viraemic mothers and almost all of those born to mothers with a titre of $> 10^6$ copies/ml (23/24) were infected. They claimed that elective Caesarean section reduced the rate of transmission, but that doing so solely to avoid GBV-C transmission would not be warranted because of minimal evidence, if any, for significant pathogenicity of this virus.

In contrast, Fischler *et al.* (1997) reported that only 1/8 infants born to (HGV-GBV-C) RNA-positive mothers was persistently infected (42 months), with no signs of liver disease. Menendez *et al.* (1999) reported a transmission rate of 7/18 children born to GBV-C RNA-positive Tanzanian mothers in contrast to 4/42 children born to non-infected women ($p = 0.01$): the rate of mother-to-infant transmission was molecularly assessed in only 3/7 children born to viraemic mothers. Considering the possibility of transmission through saliva, GBV-C RNA was detected at titres of 10^{-2}–10^{-4} of that in the corresponding serum (Seemayer *et al.*, 1998).

HISTORY OF TTV

The TT virus (TTV) was found in 1997, again by the use of differential display technology (Nishizawa, 1997). The starting serum was obtained from a hepatitis patient with the initials T.T. who did not possess any markers for known hepatitis viruses. In spite of intensive studies to identify TTV-specific pathogenicity, the real impact of TTV on liver disease still remains uncertain (Moriyama *et al.*, 2001). The vast majority of virological efforts have been focused on the molecular epidemiology of the diverse spectra of the TTV genome (Biagini *et al.*, 2001; Okamoto *et al.*, 2001). The considerable diversity of TTVs and the lack of suitable conventional virological systems to study TTV limit our knowledge of TTV.

CLASSIFICATION OF TTV

The genome of TTV is the first human virus to be found with a single-stranded circular DNA genome (Mushahwar *et al.*, 1999; Miyata *et al.*, 1999). Viruses possessing single-stranded circular DNA genomes

Table 27.3 Viruses with single-stranded circular DNA genome

Family	Genus	Representative viruses	Strandedness	Number of circles
Microviridae		X174 (bacteria)	Sense	2
Geminiviridae		Maize streak virus (plant)	Ambisense	1–2
Circoviridae	*Circovirus*	Porcine circovirus (PCV)	Ambisense	2
		Psittacine beak and feather disease virus (PBFDV)		
		Pigeon circovirus (PICV)		
		Goose circovirus (GoCV)		
		Canary circovirus (CaCV)		
		Banana bunchy top virus (BBTV)		
		Coconut foliar decay virus (CFDV)		
		Subterranean clover stunt virus (SCSV)		
	Gyrovirus	Chicken anaemia virus (CAV)	Antisense	2
	Aneliovirus	TT virus (human, non-human primate, and other animals)	Antisense	3

have been known for some time, e.g. the bacterial viruses *Microviridae*, the plant viruses *Geminiviridae*, and the animal and plant viruses *Circoviridae* (Table 27.3). Members of *Geminiviridae* have more than one circular DNA genome. Within the *Circoviridae*, the genus *Circovirus* contains animal and plant viruses, such as the porcine circovirus (PCV), psittacine beak and feather disease virus (PBFDV) and the banana bunchy top virus (BBTV). The *Circovirus* has a common nine-nucleotide stem–loop structure at its replication origin. The genome of *Circovirus* is ambisense, as the largest Rep protein is coded by the genomic strand while the other two proteins are coded

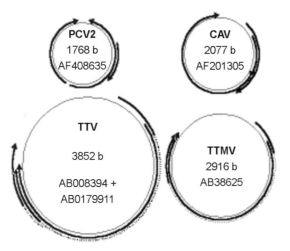

Figure 27.2 Strands of TTV and TTMV in comparison with the chicken anaemia virus (CAV, genus *Gyrovirus*) and porcine circovirus type 2 (PCV2, genus *Circovirus*). The sizes of the circles correspond to the genome size of each virus. Clockwise arrows: translations on the antigenomic strand; counterclockwise arrows: those on the genomic strand

by the antigenomic strand (Figure 27.2) (Niagro *et al.*, 1998). An earlier member of *Circovirus*, viz. chicken anaemia virus (CAV), is now classified into the genus *Gyrovirus*, since its Rep protein is coded by the antigenomic strand and the genomic strand has no significant ORFs (Pringle, 1999). CAV does not have the nine-nucleotide stem–loop structure that is common in *Circovirus*. In this sense, the genome of TTV has a feature that is common to CAV. Although the TTV and CAV genomes have a common 36 nt stretch with around 80% identity, other regions of their genomes have no significant similarity with each other. TTV differs from CAV in its genome size, 3.9 kb vs. 2.3 kb, and by its extraordinary diversity. A working group set up to establish a nomenclature for circo-viruses is working currently on a proposal to name a new genus of TTV and its related viruses *Anellovirus* (ring). The spelled-out name for TTV will be 'Torque-TenoVirus', while the TTV-like mini virus (TLMV) (Takahashi *et al.*, 2000a; Takahashi *et al.*, 2000b) will be 'TorqueTenoMiniVirus' (TTMV). The acronyms were devised to incorporate torque (necklace) and tenuis/teno (thin), while trying to retain the already widespread term, TTV. It is emphasised that the acronym TTV is based on the initials of the original patient and it is *not* an abbreviation for transfusion-transmitted virus.

GENOMIC STRUCTURE OF TTV

Okamoto *et al.* (1998) reported a sequence of linear 3739 nt as the complete genome of TTV (TA278). However, it was not likely to constitute a complete genome because of the lack of a terminal repeat. A 113 nt GC-rich stretch was added to complete its

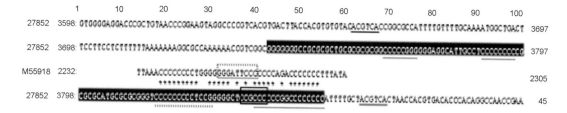

Figure 27.3 Partial genome of TTV (27852, nt 3740–3852). The GC-rich 113 nt region is shown in white with black characters. The similarity to the chicken anaemia virus (CAV, M55918) is indicated by asterisks. Multiple transcription modifier motifs include SP-1 (solid-line box), NF-κB (dotted-line box), ATF/CREB (solid underline) and AP-2 (dotted underline)

circular 3852 nt genome (Figure 27.3) (Mushahwar *et al.*, 1999; Miyata *et al.*, 1999). Within this GC-rich stretch, the 36 nt region (nt 3816–3851 of TA278) has a significant similarity to nt 2237–2272 of CAV, and no significant similarity was observed elsewhere.

This region and its immediate vicinity constituted a stem–loop structure, suggesting the origin of DNA replication (Mushahwar *et al.*, 1999; Okamoto *et al.*, 1999). One-third of the genome containing this region is non-translating, and has a high degree of similarity within the extremely divergent TTVs. Moreover, multiple transcription modifier motifs, such as ATF/CREB, AP-2, SP-1 and NF-κB binding sites, can be found in this region (Miyata *et al.*, 1999). However, the details of the biological significance of these motifs remained unclear, as no functional survey had been attempted. Detailed studies of these structures may reveal the control mechanism of TTV replication and lead to the development of a suitable target cell system.

analysis of TTMV. A single host can be infected with both virus groups, but there are some hosts with only one virus, indicating that the replications of these viruses are independent.

TTVs are composed of a variety of viruses, and are classified into at least 16 subgroups with over 30% nucleotide diversities (Okamoto *et al.*, 2000). TTMVs also share their divergent characters with TTV (Biagini *et al.*, 2001). Why and how these viruses can survive with such a wide spectrum of diversity is still unclear. A single host can be infected with different clusters of TTVs (Okamoto *et al.*, 1999; Takayama *et al.*, 1999). Do TTV and TTMV continue to mutate within a host to escape from the immunosurveillance system of the host, as is the case of HCV and *Lentivirinae*?

TTVs are prevalent in non-human primates, while the human TTV can cross-infect chimpanzees (Abe *et al.*, 2000). Furthermore, TTV sequences have been detected in 19% of chickens, 20% of pigs, 25% of cows and 30% of sheep (Leary *et al.*, 1999). The taxonomic

THE TTV GROUP

The TTV group consists of two distinct clusters; the 3.9 kb original TTV and the 2.9 kb miniature TTV (TTMV) (Figure 27.4) (Takahashi *et al.*, 2000a, 2000b). Although the genomic sizes of these two viruses are very different, they share several common features. The non-coding regions surrounding the GC-rich stretch and occupying approximately one-third of the genome are similar to each other, as is the structure of the putative replication origin. The structures of the coding regions in these two virus groups are also similar to each other. The largest, ORF1, which accounts for approximately two-thirds of the viral genome, is common to all these viruses. Two other double-spliced mRNAs have been found in TTV, and are also expected to be revealed by the DNA sequence

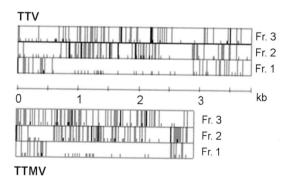

Figure 27.4 Frame and ORF structures of TTV (AB008394 + AB017911) and TTMV (AB38625). Short vertical lines represent ATGs, while long vertical lines correspond to stop codons

divergence of these animal viruses relative to human TTVs and their pathogenicity has yet to be clarified.

TARGET CELLS OF TTV

TTV was first reported as a candidate agent for non-A–E hepatitis (Nishizawa *et al.*, 1997). Ukita *et al.* found that the concentration of TTV is 10–100 times greater in bile than in peripheral blood, suggesting the replication of TTV in the liver (Ukita *et al.*, 1999). Okamoto *et al.* (2000) found the presence of the replicative form of TTV in liver and bone marrow. However, because of the wide spectrum of TTVs, the real target of each TTV remains unclear. The high prevalence and viral load of TTV in saliva suggest that TTV might also replicate in the oropharyngeal tissues and/or the salivary glands (Deng *et al.*, 2000).

Although TTV was found originally in serum, the detection of TTV in stool suggested that it is transmitted by a faecal–oral route (Okamoto *et al.*, 1998). This pathway is more consistent with its ubiquity. TTV can be transmitted by mother-to-child infection. The presence of TTV in cord blood, as reported in the literature, was 0–1% of N22 PCR (Goto *et al.*, 2000; Kazi *et al.*, 2000). Within 6 months of birth, the prevalence of TTV in children born to TTV-positive mothers was significantly higher than that of children born to TTV-negative mothers. However, once the child was 1 year old, the prevalence in children born to TTV-negative mothers caught up to that of children born to TTV-positive mothers and to that of adults, even without breast-feeding (Kazi *et al.*, 2000). This implies that the milk-borne transmission of TTV is insignificant. The low TTV titre in CSF suggested that the central nervous system is less likely to be a target of TTV replication (Maggi *et al.*, 2001).

Although 20–60% of patients with idiopathic fulminant hepatic failure (Charlton *et al.*, 1998; Simmonds *et al.* 1998) were reported to be TTV-positive, the significance of TTV in the development of fulminant hepatic failure remains questionable because of the inconsistency of the patient selection and methods used for investigation and the high prevalence of TTV in the general population. At present, the pathogenicity of TTV and TTMV remains in question. Most reports suggest that there is no significant association with liver diseases such as chronic hepatitis or hepatocellular carcinoma (Cossart, 2000). However, in addition to the original report of TTV, there have been several reports suggesting the potential aggravation of underlying hepatic diseases by TTV viraemia (Cleavinger *et al.*, 2000; Sampietro

et al., 2001). Kikuchi *et al.* (2001) suggested the possible association of TTV with aplastic anaemia, which might be interesting in conjunction with haematological disorders caused by CAV and *Parvovirus* B19. Again, the detailed genotyping of TTVs might help us to understand the pathogenicity of TTVs.

PROTEINS OF TTV

The genome configurations of TTV and CAV are similar to each other in spite of their different genome sizes (Figure 27.5). The largest ORF constitutes two-thirds of the entire genome and resides on the antigenomic strand associated with a TATA box (nt 85–90 of TA278; Accession No. AB008394) and a polyA signal (nt 3073–3079). This protein probably serves as a replicase and the major structural protein of TTV, because its N-terminus region contains a highly basic stretch consistent with other circoviral capsid proteins and several conserved Rep protein motifs (FTL and YXXK) (Niagro *et al.*, 1998; Takahashi

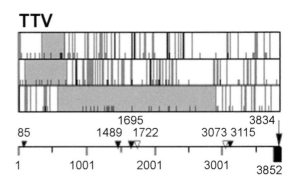

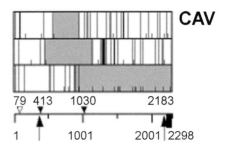

Figure 27.5 Comparative arrangement of ORFs expected from the TTV genome (AB008394 + AB017911) and CAV (AF372658). SP-1 site (arrow), TATA box (closed triangle), polyA signal (open triangle) and GC-rich region (closed box)

et al., 1998). The post-translational modification should be investigated further.

There were additional putative ORFs on the antigenomic strand without legitimate initiation codons. To explain these incomplete ORFs, the presence of several spliced mRNAs was expected with the common usage of the TATA box and the polyA signal. Kamahora *et al.* constructed a plasmid containing the promoter region through the polyA signal continuously (nt 2762–3852, 1–3770) (Kamahora *et al.*, 2000). Three species of mRNAs with sizes of 3.0, 1.2 and 1.0 kb were expressed in the transfected COS1 cells. All 15 clones obtained from the cDNA library of the polyA RNAs had the 5'-terminus at nt 123–135 adjacent to the TATA box and the 3'-terminus at 6–9 nt downstream of the polyA signal. All three species of the mRNA clones exhibited a common splicing at nt 186–276. The 3.0 kb mRNA has an initiation codon at $A^{589}TG$ downstream of the splicing and codes for the Rep protein with 770 amino acids, as expected from

the genome (Figure 27.6). The other two species of mRNA, 1.2 and 1.0 kb, had a second splicing at nt 712–2373 and 712–2566, respectively. The second exon was common to these mRNAs on ORF2 of frame 2. The third exons of the 1.2 and 1.0 kb mRNAs are located on frames 2 and 3, respectively. Our preliminary data suggested that these two mRNAs use $A^{353}TG$ as the initiation codon (as suggested by T. Kamahora). Given this assumption, we calculated an expected protein size of 286 and 290 amino acids. The real nature of these three proteins has yet to be elucidated.

Asabe *et al.* reported phosphorylation of the VP2 (ORFs 2–4) product in the COS1 cells using an expression plasmid, and claimed a similarity to NS5A of HCV (Asabe *et al.*, 2001). Yokoyama *et al.* (2002) reported on transgenic TTV mice, which expressed mRNA with a splicing corresponding to the 1.0 kb mRNA. However, the protein in the transgenic mice was corded by ORF1 on frame 1 to ORF4 on frame 2, instead of ORF2 on frame 2 to ORF5 on frame 3 in those cells that are transfected with the full-size genome. Theoretically, this type of reading frame may take place in natural infection. However, because they intentionally deleted the region including the authentic initiation codon of the natural 1.0 kb mRNA ($A^{353}TG$), their construct was forced to use $A^{589}TG$ as the initiation codon.

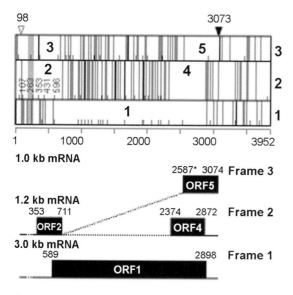

Figure 27.6 Schematic of the TTV genome (AB008394 + AB017911) and its mRNAs. Three reading frames of the genome are shown in the upper panel. The open triangle indicates the position of the cap site while the closed triangle indicates that of the polyA signal. The short and long vertical lines indicate ATGs and stop codons, respectively. Predicted ORFs are indicated by numbers. The shaded area represents the first splicing common to all mRNAs of three different sizes. The lower panel indicates the frames that are used and configurations of 3.0 kb, 1.2 kb, and 1.0 kb mRNAs. The solid lines indicate exons, the dotted lines represent introns, and the boxes indicate coding regions. Because of the alternative splicing for the 1.0 kb mRNA, the 5'-terminal nt 2567 is labelled with an asterisk

PROBLEMS WITH THE DETECTION OF TTV

In spite of the initial introduction of TTV as a putative hepatitis virus, there is little data for specifying the pathogenicity of TTV. TTV may be non-pathogenic, or only a limited genotype of TTV may be pathogenic. By applying hemi-nested PCR to the N22 region (nt 1939–216) (Okamoto *et al.*, 1998) we were able to detect genotype 1–6 TTVs, while that applied to the 5'-non-coding region (NTR; nt 26–184) (Takahashi *et al.*, 1998) can detect most genotypes. By introducing the NTR PCR, the TTV-positive population expanded from 10–30% to 90% (Okamoto *et al.*, 1999; Chan *et al.*, 2001). Some reports have claimed a higher sensitivity to NTR PCR, but were actually detecting a wider spectrum of TTVs. If only a certain genotype of TTV is pathogenic, a PCR that can detect only the responsible genotype should be used. The use of a broader assay system will dilute the possible pathogenicity, even by N22 PCR detecting genotypes 1–6. Furthermore, the sensitivities of PCR have not been carefully controlled in most studies. It may take years to determine the real pathogenicity of TTV, especially if it is noted that more than 15 years elapsed between the discovery of the porcine circovirus (PCV) (Tischer *et al.*, 1982) and the discovery of pathogenic PCV2 (Allan *et al.*, 1998).

REFERENCES

Abe K, Inami T, Ishikawa K *et al.* (2000) TT virus infection in non-human primates and characterization of the viral genome: identification of simian TT virus isolates. *J Virol*, **74**, 1549–1553.

Adams NJ, Prescott LE, Jarvis LM *et al.* (1998) Detection in chimpanzees of a novel flavivirus related to GB virus-C/hepatitis G virus. *J Gen Virol*, **79**, 1871–1877.

Akiyoshi F, Sata M, Noguchi S *et al.* (1999) Intraspousal transmission of GB virus C/hepatitis G virus in an hepatitis C virus hyperendemic area in Japan. *Am J Gastroenterol*, **94**, 1627–1631.

Allan GM, McNeilly F, Kennedy S *et al.* (1998) Isolation of porcine circovirus-like viruses from pigs with a wasting disease in the USA and Europe. *J Vet Diagn Invest*, **10**, 3–10.

Asabe S, Nishizawa T, Iwanari H *et al.* (2001) Phosphorylation of serine-rich protein encoded by open reading frame 3 of the TT virus genome. *Biochem Biophys Res Commun*, **286**, 298–304.

Beames B, Chavez D, Guerra B *et al.* (2000) Development of a primary tamarin hepatocyte culture system for GB virus B: a surrogate model for hepatitis C virus. *J Virol*, **74**, 11764–11772.

Biagini P, Gallian P, Attoui H *et al.* (2001) Genetic analysis of full-length genomes and subgenomic sequences of TT virus-like mini virus human isolates. *J Gen Virol*, **82**, 379–383.

Bjorkman P, Naucler A, Winqvist N *et al.* (2001) A case–control study of transmission routes for GB virus C/hepatitis G virus in Swedish blood donors lacking markers for hepatitis C virus infection. *Vox Sang*, **81**, 148–153.

Bjorkman P, Sundstrom G, Veress B *et al.* (2000) Assessment of liver disease and biochemical and immunological markers in Swedish blood donors with isolated GB virus C/hepatitis G virus viremia. *Vox Sang*, **78**, 143–148.

Bjorkman P, Sundstrom G and Widell A (1998) Hepatitis C virus and GB virus C/hepatitis G virus viremia in Swedish blood donors with different alanine aminotransferase levels. *Transfusion*, **38**, 378–384.

Brojer E, Grabarczyk P, Kryczka W *et al.* (1999) Analysis of hepatitis G virus infection markers in blood donors and patients with hepatitis. *J Viral Hepat*, **6**, 471–475.

Cantaloube JF, Gallian P, Biagini P *et al.* (1999) Prevalence of GB virus type C/hepatitis G virus RNA and anti-E2 among blood donors in south-eastern France. *Transfusion*, **39**, 95–102.

Casteling A, Song E, Sim J *et al.* (1998) GB virus C prevalence in blood donors and high risk groups for parenterally transmitted agents from Gauteng, South Africa. *J Med Virol*, **55**, 103–108.

Cesaire R, Martial J, Maier H *et al.* (1999) Infection with GB virus C/hepatitis G virus among blood donors and hemophiliacs in Martinique, a Caribbean island. *J Med Virol*, **59**, 160–163.

Chan PK, Chik KW, Li CK *et al.* (2001) Prevalence and genotype distribution of TT virus in various specimen types from thalassaemic patients. *J Viral Hepat*, **8**, 304–309.

Charlton M, Adjei P, Poterucha J *et al.* (1998) TT-virus infection in North American blood donors, patients with fulminant hepatic failure, and cryptogenic cirrhosis. *Hepatology*, **28**, 839–842.

Chu C, Hwang S, Luo J *et al.* (2001) Clinical, virological, immunological, and pathological significance of GB virus C/hepatitis G infection in patients with chronic hepatitis C. *Hepatol Res*, **19**, 225–236.

Chu CM, Lin SM, Hsieh SY *et al.* (1999) Etiology of sporadic acute viral hepatitis in Taiwan: the role of hepatitis C virus, hepatitis E virus and GB virus-C/hepatitis G virus in an endemic area of hepatitis A and B. *J Med Virol*, **58**, 154–159.

Cleavinger PJ, Persing DH, Li H *et al.* (2000) Prevalence of TT virus infection in blood donors with elevated ALT in the absence of known hepatitis markers. *Am J Gastroenterol*, **95**, 772–776.

Cossart Y (2000) TTV—a virus searching for a disease. *J Clin Virol*, **17**, 1–3.

De Filippi F, Lampertico P, Soffredini R *et al.* (2001) High prevalence, low pathogenicity of hepatitis G virus in kidney transplant recipients. *Dig Liver Dis*, **33**, 477–479.

Deinhardt F, Holmes AW, Capps RB and Popper H (1967) Studies on the transmission of human viral hepatitis to marmoset monkeys. I. Transmission of disease, serial passages, and description of liver lesions. *J Exp Med*, **125**, 673–688.

Deinhardt F, Peterson D, Cross G *et al.* (1975) Hepatitis in marmosets. *Am J Med Sci*, **270**, 73–80.

Deng X, Terunuma H, Handema R *et al.* (2000) Higher prevalence and viral load of TT virus in saliva than in the corresponding serum: another possible transmission route and replication site of TT virus. *J Med Virol*, **62**, 531–537.

Fan X, Xu Y, Solomon H *et al.* (1999) Is hepatitis G/GB virus-C virus hepatotropic? Detection of hepatitis G/GB virus-C viral RNA in liver and serum. *J Med Virol*, **58**, 160–164.

Fischler B, Lara C, Chen M *et al.* (1997) Genetic evidence for mother-to-infant transmission of hepatitis G virus. *J Infect Dis*, **176**, 281–285.

Frider B, Sookoian S, Castano G *et al.* (1998) Detection of hepatitis G virus RNA in patients with acute non-A–E hepatitis. *J Viral Hepat*, **5**, 161–164.

Giulivi A, Slinger R, Tepper M *et al.* (2000) Prevalence of GBV-C/hepatitis G virus viremia and anti-E2 in Canadian blood donors. *Vox Sang*, **79**, 201–205.

Goto K, Sugiyama K, Ando T *et al.* (2000) Detection rates of TT virus DNA in serum of umbilical cord blood, breast milk and saliva. *Tohoku J Exp Med*, **191**, 203–207.

Gutierrez RA, Dawson GJ, Knigge MF *et al.* (1997) Seroprevalence of GB virus C and persistence of RNA and antibody. *J Med Virol*, **53**, 167–173.

Handa A, Jubran RF, Dickstein B *et al.* (2000) GB virus C/hepatitis G virus infection is frequent in American children and young adults. *Clin Infect Dis*, **30**, 569–571.

Hassoba HM, Terrault NA, el-Gohary AM *et al.* (1997) Antibody to GBV-C second envelope glycoprotein (anti-GBV-C E2): is it a marker for immunity? *J Med Virol*, **53**, 354–360.

Hino K, Moriya T, Ohno N *et al.* (1998) Mother-to-infant transmission occurs more frequently with GB virus C than hepatitis C virus. *Arch Virol*, **143**, 65–72.

Hwang SJ, Chu CW, Lu RH *et al.* (2000) Seroprevalence of GB virus C/hepatitis G virus-RNA and anti-envelope antibody in high-risk populations in Taiwan. *J Gastroenterol Hepatol*, **15**, 1171–1175.

Hyland CA, Mison L, Solomon N *et al.* (1998) Exposure to GB virus type C or hepatitis G virus in selected Australian adult and children populations. *Transfusion*, **38**, 821–827.

Ikeda M, Sugiyama K, Mizutani T *et al.* (1997) Hepatitis G virus replication in human cultured cells displaying susceptibility to hepatitis C virus infection. *Biochem Biophys Res Commun*, **235**, 505–508.

Jongerius J, Boland G, van der Poel C *et al.* (1999) GB virus type C viremia and envelope antibodies among population subsets in The Netherlands. *Vox Sang*, **76**, 81–84.

Kamahora T, Hino S and Miyata H (2000) Three spliced mRNAs of TT virus transcribed from a plasmid containing the entire genome in COS1 cells. *J Virol*, **74**, 9980–9986.

Karayiannis P, Petrovic LM, Fry M *et al.* (1989) Studies of GB hepatitis agent in tamarins. *Hepatology*, **9**, 186–192.

Kazi A, Miyata H, Kurokawa K *et al.* (2000) High frequency of postnatal transmission of TT virus in infancy. *Arch Virol*, **145**, 535–540.

Kikuchi K, Miyakawa H, Abe K *et al.* (2001) Indirect evidence of TTV replication in bone marrow cells, but not in hepatocytes, of a subacute hepatitis/aplastic anemia patient. *J Med Virol*, **61**, 165–170.

Lanford RE, Chavez D, Guerra B *et al.* (2001) Ribavirin induces error-prone replication of GB virus B in primary tamarin hepatocytes. *J Virol*, **75**, 8074–8081.

Leary TP, Desai SM, Yamaguchi J *et al.* (1996) Species-specific variants of GB virus A in captive monkeys. *J Virol*, **70**, 9028–9030.

Leary TP, Erker JC, Chalmers ML *et al.* (1999) Improved detection systems for TT virus reveal high prevalence in humans, non-human primates and farm animals. *J Gen Virol*, **80**, 2115–2120.

Linnen J, Wages J Jr, Zhang-Keck ZY *et al.* (1996) Molecular cloning and disease association of hepatitis G virus: a transfusion-transmissible agent. *Science*, **271**, 505–508.

Love A, Stanzeit B, Gudmundsson S *et al.* (1999) Hepatitis G virus infections in Iceland. *J Viral Hepatol*, **6**, 255–260.

Maggi F, Fornai C, Vatteroni ML *et al.* (2001) Low prevalence of TT virus in the cerebrospinal fluid of viremic patients with central nervous system disorders. *J Med Virol*, **65**, 418–422.

Menendez C, Sanchez-Tapias JM, Alonso PL *et al.* (1999) Molecular evidence of mother-to-infant transmission of hepatitis G virus among women without known risk factors for parenteral infections. *J Clin Microbiol*, **37**, 2333–2336.

Mercier B, Barclais A, Botte C *et al.* (1999) Prevalence of GBV C/HGV RNA and GBV C/HGV antibodies in French volunteer blood donors: results of a collaborative study. *Vox Sang*, **76**, 166–169.

Miyata H, Tsunoda M, Kazi A *et al.* (1999) Identification of a novel GC-rich 113-nucleotide region to complete the circular, single-stranded DNA genome of TT virus, the first human circovirus. *J Virol*, **73**, 3582–3586.

Moaven LD, Hyland CA, Young IF *et al.* (1996) Prevalence of hepatitis G virus in Queensland blood donors. *Med J Aust*, **165**, 369–371.

Moriyama M, Matsumura H, Shimizu T *et al.* (2001) Histopathologic impact of TT virus infection on the liver of type C chronic hepatitis and liver cirrhosis in Japan. *J Med Virol*, **64**, 74–81.

Muerhoff AS, Leary TP, Simons JN *et al.* (1995) Genomic organization of GB viruses A and B: two new members of the Flaviviridae associated with GB agent hepatitis. *J Virol*, **69**, 5621–5630.

Mushahwar IK, Erker JC, Muerhoff AS *et al.* (1999) Molecular and biophysical characterization of TT virus: evidence for a new virus family infecting humans. *Proc Natl Acad Sci USA*, **96**, 3177–3182.

Niagro FD, Forsthoefel AN, Lawther RP *et al.* (1998) Beak and feather disease virus and porcine circovirus genomes: intermediates between the geminiviruses and plant circoviruses. *Arch Virol*, **143**, 1723–1744.

Nishizawa T, Okamoto H, Konishi K *et al.* (1997) A novel DNA virus (TTV) associated with elevated transaminase levels in posttransfusion hepatitis of unknown etiology. *Biochem Biophys Res Commun*, **241**, 92–97.

Nordbo SA, Krokstad S, Winge P *et al.* (2000) Prevalence of GB virus C (also called hepatitis G virus) markers in Norwegian blood donors. *J Clin Microbiol*, **38**, 2584–2590.

Ohto H, Ujiie N, Sato A *et al.* (2000) Mother-to-infant transmission of GB virus type C/HGV. *Transfusion*, **40**, 725–730.

Okamoto H, Akahane Y, Ukita M *et al.* (1998) Fecal excretion of a non-enveloped DNA virus (TTV) associated with posttransfusion non-A–G hepatitis. *J Med Virol*, **56**, 128–132.

Okamoto H, Nishizawa T, Kato N *et al.* (1998) Molecular cloning and characterization of a novel DNA virus (TTV) associated with posttransfusion hepatitis of unknown etiology. *Hepatol Res*, **10**, 1–16.

Okamoto H, Nishizawa T, Takahashi M *et al.* (2001) Genomic and evolutionary characterization of TT virus (TTV) in tupaias and comparison with species-specific TTVs in humans and non-human primates. *J Gen Virol*, **82**, 2041–2050.

Okamoto H, Nishizawa T, Tawara A *et al.* (2000) Species-specific TT viruses in humans and nonhuman primates and their phylogenetic relatedness. *Virology*, **277**, 368–378.

Okamoto H, Nishizawa T and Ukita M (1999) A novel unenveloped DNA virus (TT virus) associated with acute and chronic non-A–G hepatitis. *Intervirology*, **42**, 196–204.

Okamoto H, Takahashi M, Nishizawa T *et al.* (1999) Marked genomic heterogeneity and frequent mixed infection of TT virus demonstrated by PCR with primers from coding and non-coding regions. *Virology*, **259**, 428–436.

Okamoto H, Takahashi M, Nishizawa T *et al.* (2000) Replicative forms of TT virus DNA in bone marrow cells. *Biochem Biophys Res Commun*, **270**, 657–662.

Orii K, Tanaka E, Rokuhara A *et al.* (2000) Persistent infection mechanism of GB virus C/hepatitis G virus differs from that of hepatitis C virus. *Intervirology*, **43**, 139–145.

Parks WP and Melnick JL (1969b) Attempted isolation of hepatitis viruses in marmosets. *J Infect Dis*, **120**, 539–547.

Parks WP, Melnick JL, Voss WR *et al.* (1969a) Characterization of marmoset hepatitis virus. *J Infect Dis*, **120**, 548–559.

Pringle CR (1999) Virus taxonomy at the XIth International Congress of Virology, Sydney, Australia, 1999. *Arch Virol*, **144**, 2065–2070

Radkowski M, Kubicka J, Kisiel E *et al.* (2000) Detection of active hepatitis C virus and hepatitis G virus/GB virus C replication in bone marrow in human subjects. *Blood*, **95**, 3986–3989.

Romano L, Fabris P, Tanzi E *et al.* (2000) GBV-C/hepatitis G virus in acute non-A–E hepatitis and in acute hepatitis of defined aetiology in Italy. *J Med Virol*, **61**, 59–64.

Sampietro M, Tavazzi D, Martinez di Montemuros F *et al.* (2001) TT virus infection in adult β-thalassemia major patients. *Haematologica*, **86**, 39–43.

Schaluder GG, Dawson GJ, Simons JN *et al.* (1995) Molecular and serologic analysis in the transmission of the GB hepatitis agents. *J Med Virol*, **46**, 81–90.

Seemayer CA, Viazov S, Philipp T *et al.* (1998) Detection of GBV-C/HGV RNA in saliva and serum, but not in urine of infected patients. *Infection*, **26**, 39–41.

Seipp S, Scheidel M, Hofmann WJ *et al.* (1999) Hepatotropism of GB virus C (GBV-C): GBV-C replication in human hepatocytes and cells of human hepatoma cell lines. *J Hepatol*, **30**, 570–579.

Shimizu T, Moriyama M and Arakawa Y (2001) Detection of HGV RNA in digestive organs. *Intervirology*, **44**, 14–20.

Shimizu YK, Hijikata M, Kiyohara T *et al.* (1999) Replication of GB virus C (hepatitis G virus) in interferon-resistant Daudi cells. *J Virol*, **73**, 8411–8414.

Simmonds P, Davidson F, Lycett C *et al.* (1998) Detection of a novel DNA virus (TTV) in blood donors and blood products. *Lancet*, **352**, 191–195.

Simons JN, Desai SM, Schultz DE *et al.* (1996) Translation initiation in GB viruses A and C: evidence for internal ribosome entry and implications for genome organization. *J Virol*, **70**, 6126–6135.

Simons JN, Leary TP, Dawson GJ *et al.* (1995a) Isolation of novel virus-like sequences associated with human hepatitis. *Nature Med*, **1**, 564–569.

Simons JN, Pilot-Matias TJ, Leary TP *et al.* (1995b) Identification of two flavivirus-like genomes in the GB hepatitis agent. *Proc Natl Acad Sci USA*, **92**, 3401–3405.

Takahashi K, Hijikata M, Samokhvalov EI *et al.* (2000a) Full- or near-full-length nucleotide sequences of TT virus variants (Types SANBAN and YONBAN) and the TT virus-like mini virus. *Intervirology*, **43**, 119–123.

Takahashi K, Hoshino H, Ohta Y *et al.* (1998) Very high prevalence of TT virus (TTV) infection in general population of Japan revealed by a new set of PCR primers. *Hepatol Res*, **12**, 233–239.

Takahashi K, Iwasa Y, Hijikata M *et al.* (2000b) Identification of a new human DNA virus (TTV-like mini virus, TLMV) intermediately related to TT virus and chicken anemia virus. *Arch Virol*, **145**, 979–993.

Takayama S, Yamazaki S, Matsuo S *et al.* (1999) Multiple infection of TT virus (TTV) with different genotypes in Japanese hemophiliacs. *Biochem Biophys Res Commun*, **256**, 208–211.

Tillmann HL, Heiken H, Knapik-Botor A *et al.* (2001) Infection with GB virus C and reduced mortality among HIV-infected patients. *N Engl J Med*, **345**, 715–724.

Tischer I, Gelderblom H, Vettermann W *et al.* (1982) A very small porcine virus with circular single-stranded DNA. *Nature*, **295**, 64–66.

Tucker TJ, Smuts HE, Eedes C *et al.* (2000) Evidence that the GBV-C/hepatitis G virus is primarily a lymphotropic virus. *J Med Virol*, **61**, 52–58.

Ukita M, Okamoto H, Kato N *et al.* (1999) Excretion into bile of a novel unenveloped DNA virus (TT virus) associated with acute and chronic non-A–G hepatitis. *J Infect Dis*, **179**, 1245–1248.

Wang JT, Chen PJ, Liu DP *et al.* (1998) Prevalence and infectivity of hepatitis G virus and its strain variant, the GB agent, in volunteer blood donors in Taiwan. *Transfusion*, **38**, 290–295.

Yokoyama H, Yasuda J, Okamoto H *et al.* (2002) Pathological changes of renal epithelial cells in mice transgenic for the TT virus ORF1 gene. *J Gen Virol*, **83**, 141–150.

Yu ML, Chuang WL, Dai CY *et al.* (2001) The serological and molecular epidemiology of GB virus C/hepatitis G virus infection in a hepatitis C and B endemic area. *J Infect*, **42**, 61–66.

Zanetti AR, Tanzi E, Romano L *et al.* (1998) Multicenter trial on mother-to-infant transmission of GBV-C virus. The Lombardy Study Group on Vertical/Perinatal Hepatitis Viruses Transmission. *J Med Virol*, **54**, 107–112.

28

Emerging Virus Infections

Brian W. J. Mahy

National Center for Infectious Diseases, Atlanta, GA, USA

INTRODUCTION

Although infectious disease mortality declined sharply throughout the twentieth century, apart from a dramatic increase following the 1918 pandemic of influenza virus, in the last twenty years a small but noticeable increase in mortality from infectious diseases can be observed (Armstrong *et al.* 1999; Mahy, 2000; Figure 28.1). The start of this increase roughly coincides with the appearance in the population of human immunodeficiency virus (HIV) infection and associated cases of acquired immune deficiency syndrome (AIDS), but there is good evidence suggesting that many factors contributed to this situation.

In 1991, the Institute of Medicine (IOM) of the US National Academy of Sciences convened a multi-disciplinary committee to consider emerging infectious diseases and the factors responsible for them, and to make recommendations for future actions to be taken in response to their threat to public health (Lederberg *et al.*, 1992). In 2001, the IOM convened a new committee on Microbial Threats to Health in the Twenty-first Century (Smolinski *et al.*, 2003), with a similar mandate to review the situation 10 years later. It is noteworthy that during the period covered by the two sets of recommendations more than 60 new virus diseases have been recognised in the human population (Figure 28.2). These range from hepatitis C virus (HCV), first recognised in 1988, to the new human coronavirus, first recognised in 2003, which is responsible for severe acute respiratory syndrome (SARS). As with most emerging virus infections, these are examples of virus diseases that threaten public health throughout the world and are not limited in their potential geographic range. As pointed out in the first report on emerging infections, in the context of infectious diseases, there is nowhere in the world from which we are remote and no one from whom we are disconnected (Lederberg *et al.*, 1992).

FACTORS CONTRIBUTING TO EMERGENCE

Considering infectious diseases as a whole, the committee of the IOM recognised 13 factors contributory to emergence, and these are listed in Table 28.1. Some of these are natural events that can be responded to, but not prevented from occurring, such as microbial adaptation and change, and climate and weather. Others are societal and political in origin and could be eliminated, such as the breakdown of public health measures, and poverty and social inequality. Finally, 'intent to harm' refers to acts of bioterrorism, such as the deliberate release of smallpox (variola) virus (Mahy, 2003).

This chapter will consider the factors responsible for the emergence of new virus infections under four broad headings: (a) virus evolution; (b) human demographics, susceptibility to infection and behaviour; (c) improved technology for the detection of virus infection; and (d) increased contact with vectors of virus infection. By considering examples of virus emergence under each category, the factors responsible for the remarkable global increase in human virus infections over the last 15 years (Figure 28.3) will become clear.

Principles and Practice of Clinical Virology, Fifth Edition. Edited by A. J. Zuckerman, J. E. Banatvala, J. R. Pattison, P. D. Griffiths and B. D. Schoub
© 2004 John Wiley & Sons Ltd   ISBN 0 470 84338 1

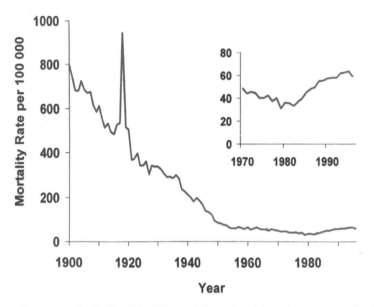

Figure 28.1   Infectious disease mortality in the USA, 1900–1996. Reproduced from Armstrong *et al.* (1999)

Virus Evolution

There are a number of different mechanisms by which viruses may evolve. In general, RNA viruses are much more likely to evolve by genome changes than DNA viruses, and this in part reflects the proof-reading functions present in the host cell that preserve the integrity of host cellular DNA. Such proof-reading

mechanisms do not exist for RNA, and so RNA viruses are much more mutable.

Mutation

The most obvious mechanisms for evolution involve point mutations in the genome RNA nucleotide

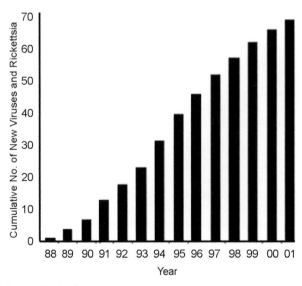

Figure 28.2   Emergence of viruses affecting humans

Table 28.1 Factors in emergence

Microbial adaptation and change
Human vulnerability
Climate and weather
Changing ecosystems
Economic development and land use
Human demographics and behaviour
Technology and industry
International travel and commerce
Breakdown of public health measures
Poverty and social inequality
War and famine
Lack of political will
Intent to harm

Reproduced by permission from Smolinski *et al.* (2003)

sequence, either random (spontaneous) or in response to a selective pressure, such as inhibition by an antibody or an antiviral drug. For example, influenza viruses undergo frequent mutations in response to humoral antibodies against influenza which exist in the general population: this phenomenon produces 'antigenic drift'.

Another example is HIV, which, in the presence of a drug which prevents DNA replication, such as zidovudine (azidothymidine), rapidly generates mutant viruses that are resistant to the drug.

Reassortment

A second mechanism for genetic change is reassortment, which is a common feature of those viruses that have a segmented genome, such as influenza viruses and rotaviruses. In cases where two viruses of distinct genetic lineage infect the same cell, it is possible for exchange of genome segments to occur, giving rise to a new reassortant virus that may have altered properties of transmission or pathogenesis. This is of particular importance clinically with the influenza viruses, and it has been clearly demonstrated that both the 1957 'Asian' influenza pandemic and the 1968 'Hong Kong' influenza pandemic resulted from viruses that were apparently generated by reassortment between human and avian influenza virus strains (Webster and Kawaoka, 1994).

Recombination

The third most common mechanism of virus evolution is recombination between the genomes of two different viruses. Although not absolutely proven, it seems most likely that rubella virus was originally generated in this way, and we see many examples of recombination in action, especially with the picornaviruses, such as poliovirus. For example, an outbreak of poliomyelitis in Hispaniola in 2001 was caused by a recombinant virus between the live Sabin poliovirus vaccine strain and an enterovirus, which restored the pathogenicity of the vaccine virus (Kew *et al.*, 2002).

As a general rule, recombination events seem to be much more common with viruses having a positive-strand RNA virus genome, and such events are rarely reported for negative-strand viruses, although they certainly can occur.

Human Demographics, Susceptibility to Infection, and Behaviour

Changes within the host population have contributed greatly to the emergence of virus diseases during the past 20 years.

Increases in World Population and Global Travel

The rapid increase in the world population has combined with the greatly enhanced opportunity for global travel to increase the opportunity for persons to come into contact with virus diseases formerly considered to be exotic to the developed world (such as Lassa fever, which causes 5000 deaths/year in West Africa), e.g. in 1989 a patient died from Lassa fever in a hospital in Chicago (Holmes *et al.*, 1990). The patient was an American citizen who had visited Nigeria to attend his mother's funeral, and became ill 2 days before his return to Chicago. Although 102 people had contact with him in the Chicago hospital, fortunately none of these contacts became infected.

Global travel also provides the opportunity for very rapid movement of a newly emerged virus, as we witnessed when severe acute respiratory syndrome (SARS) was first recognised in Guangdong Province, China, on 16 November 2002, where it had caused 300 cases of unknown aetiology and five deaths. This was reported to the World Health Organization (WHO) on 11 February 2003, and then on 26 February a WHO official working in Hanoi, Vietnam, Dr Carlo Urbani, reported an unusual case of severe acute respiratory disease to WHO. Other cases were soon identified in Hanoi and in Hong Kong, and many of these were health care workers. On 12 March WHO issued a global alert about these cases, and on 14 March cases of a similar disease syndrome were reported by Canada. Over the next few weeks it became clear that all these cases of severe respiratory disease could be linked to a hotel in Hong Kong (Hotel M), where the index case of the disease, a 65 year-old medical doctor from Guangdong Province in China, had arrived on 21 February. He had noted his onset of symptoms on 15 February, and he was hospitalised on 22 February and died the following day. Although he only stayed in the hotel one night to attend a family wedding, this single individual infected 12 other guests in the hotel, and from them several hundred persons in widely disbursed geographic areas became infected within a few weeks, resulting eventually in more than 300 deaths between February and June 2003. By the end of the epidemic in August 2003, WHO reported more than 8000 probable cases of SARS worldwide, of whom ten percent, some 800 persons, died (World Health Organization, 2003). Most of those who died were elderly patients (Centers for Disease Control and Prevention, 2003b).

Increased Numbers of Elderly Persons

This brings us to another demographic change which is affecting the emergence of infectious diseases. The elderly population is growing faster than any other segment of society in most highly developed countries, but elderly people may have impairment of normal defence mechanisms against infection, resulting in greater susceptibility to infection.

Immunosuppression

Other factors that affect susceptibility to infection include immune suppression, due to genetically inherited traits, malnutrition, use of immunosuppressive drugs following organ transplantation or as part of cancer treatment, or infection with human immunodeficiency virus (HIV). Worldwide, many millions of persons are now infected with HIV, and this has created a large segment of the global population in which emerging virus infections may spread and become amplified. In addition, a person infected with HIV may also suffer from reactivation of latent virus infections that are normally held in check by the immune system. These latent infections may include several members of the herpesvirus group, such as cytomegalovirus, or the human polyomavirus JC, which may result in progressive multifocal leukoencephalopathy.

Human Behaviour

Human behaviour is a major factor in the emergence of virus diseases. HIV, for example, would not spread within the human population if obvious precautions were taken by all individuals to prevent transmission. In addition, disease outbreaks have been recognised as resulting from unusual human behaviour. The emergence of monkeypox in the USA in 2003 is an example of a disease that only emerged because of the demand by US citizens for importation of exotic animal pets. In this case, the importer brought in giant rats from Ghana, and these rats were housed together with other animals, especially prairie dogs, burrowing rodents of the genus *Cynomys*, which are a popular pet animal in the mid-west of America. One or more of the giant rats was infected with monkeypox virus, which spread to the prairie dogs, and from them to people (Centers for Disease Control and Prevention, 2003a).

A more serious example of virus emergence due to human behaviour occurred in the early 1980s, when a decision was made to alter the production process of bovine meat and bone meal, a dietary supplement for young calves, by omitting a lipid extraction phase. As a result, a new prion disease, bovine spongiform encephalopathy (BSE), became established in the UK cattle population and eventually led to human cases of the disease, called new variant Creutzfeldt–Jakob disease (nvCJD) (Collinge *et al.*, 1996). The exact mechanism by which humans acquire this disease remains uncertain, but it is believed to be the result of eating meat from an infected bovine animal. Certainly the virus found in the brains of humans who have died of nvCJD is identical to the virus causing BSE (Almond and Pattison, 1997).

Improved Technology for Virus Detection

In recent years a variety of molecular techniques, especially the polymerase chain reaction (PCR), have been used to identify viruses causing a variety of diseases that were formerly of unknown aetiology. Examples of these are listed in Table 28.2.

Screening cDNA Expression Libraries

One of the most important discoveries that used molecular technology was the identity of the virus causing hepatitis non-A non-B, now known as *Hepatitis C virus*. It had long been recognised that an important cause of serum-transmitted hepatitis was

Table 28.2 Examples of molecular approaches to pathogen discovery

Virus	Type of approach	Reference
Hepatitis C virus	Expression library	Choo et al. (1989)
Sin Nombre virus	Consensus PCR	Nichol et al. (1993)
Human herpesvirus 8 and KS	RDA	Chang et al. (1994)
GB hepatitis viruses	RDA	Simons, et al. (1995)
TT virus	RDA	Nishizawa et al. (1997)
Human metapneumovirus	RAP-PCR	van den Hoogen et al. (2001)

due to neither hepatitis A nor hepatitis B viruses. In 1989, Bradley at the Centers for Disease Control and Prevention (CDC) collaborated with workers at Chiron Corporation. They used the blood of a chimpanzee that had been experimentally infected with a preparation known to transmit non-A non-B hepatitis. RNA extracted from the chimpanzee's blood was reverse-transcribed using random primers to make cDNAs, which were then cloned into a bacteriophage expression vector. The resultant bacterial colonies were then screened using sera from patients with non-A non-B hepatitis. Thousands of clones were screened in this way, until one was found that reacted with antibodies in the sera of infected patients. DNA from the positive clone was then used to screen other clones by DNA hybridisation, and eventually the full-length sequence of *Hepatitis C virus* was elucidated (Choo *et al.*, 1989). This enabled the development of diagnostic tests that are crucial to screening the blood supply, and to preventing transmission of hepatitis C by blood transfusion. A very similar molecular approach was used later to identify *Hepatitis E virus*, responsible for occasional large outbreaks of water-borne viral hepatitis (Purdy and Krawczynski, 1994).

Consensus PCR

Direct application of the PCR technique proved very valuable when an outbreak of cases of acute respiratory disease syndrome occurred in the south-western USA, initially on a Navajo Indian reservation. Initial serological studies suggested that the serum of patients who had experienced the disease contained antibodies that cross-reacted with *Hantaan virus*, a bunyavirus that was a known pathogen transmitted by rodents and causing haemorrhagic fever with renal syndrome (HFRS) in Asian countries such as Korea, but *Hantaan virus* was not suspected of causing fatal pulmonary disease in the USA.

Because of the serological cross-reaction, the known nucleotide sequence of *Hantaan virus* was used to make consensus primers for PCR amplification, and by this means a new group of hantaviruses, causing severe pulmonary distress syndrome, was identified (Nichol *et al.*, 1993). Once the consensus primers had amplified the RNA genome of the new hantaviruses, more specific primers could be designed, based upon sequence analysis of the new hantaviruses. The prototype virus of what has proved to be a very large group of viruses present in rodents of the subfamily *Sigmodontinae* was named *Sin Nombre virus*.

Representational Difference Analysis

In addition to PCR, sequence representational difference analysis (RDA) was used to identify *Human herpesvirus 8* (HHV8), a rhadinovirus found in association with Kaposi's sarcoma (KS), a rare skin tumour found in AIDS patients. In this technique, DNA extracted from KS tissue was compared with DNA extracted from normal tissue, and DNA sequences of a new herpesvirus were only found in the Kaposi's sarcoma tissue (Chang *et al.*, 1994; Moore *et al.*, 1996). Similar virus sequences were subsequently detected in tissue from patients with multicentric Castleman's disease and the rare primary effusion lymphoma, and HHV8 is believed to be causally associated with these tumours.

The RDA approach has also been successfully used in the identification of viruses which are apparently common human infections, but for which no clear association with disease has been found (Mushahwar, 2000). Three viruses, known as *GBV-A*, *GBV-B* and *GBV-C*, were found as a result of studies on the serum from a surgeon (George Barker) with acute non-A non-B hepatitis. When injected into marmosets (tamarins) of *Saguinus* spp., his serum caused hepatitis which could be serially passed in marmosets: the causative virus was immunologically and structurally distinct from the known *Hepatitis A, B, C* and *E* viruses. Two viruses (*GBV-A* and *GBV-B*) were isolated from serum of the infected marmoset using the RDA technique, and found to be new members of the family *Flaviviridae*, and associated with GB agent hepatitis.

A third newly discovered flavivirus, *GBV-C*, was identified in human sera by reverse transcription and consensus PCR, using primers based upon the *GBV-A*, *GBV-B* and *Hepatitis C virus* helicase gene, and appears to be identical to a virus that was independently isolated and called *Hepatitis G virus* (Simons *et al.*, 1995; Linnen *et al.*, 1996). For this reason, the virus is usually called *GB virus C/Hepatitis G virus*. This latter virus is widely distributed in the human population, but has not been shown to cause hepatitis. It seems able to infect both liver and spleen cells without causing obvious disease symptoms.

The RDA approach was also used to identify a completely different class of viruses in the human population. Once again, the initial discovery of the virus occurred during attempts to isolate a new agent causing transfusion-related hepatitis that was not due to hepatitis viruses A, B, C, D, E, or G. Using RDA, DNA clones were isolated from a patient (initials TT) before and after transfusion. The differential DNA analysis revealed a small non-enveloped virus with a DNA genome, and it was named TT virus (TTV) after the initials of the patient (Nishizawa *et al.*, 1997). Although no association of TTV has been found with any human or non-human primate disease, the virus appears to be ubiquitous in the healthy human population, with multiple variants (Mushahwar *et al.*, 1999; Okamoto *et al.*, 2000; Khudyakov *et al.*, 2000). The name *Circinoviridae* has been proposed to describe this large family of viruses that have a circular, single-stranded, negative-sense DNA genome approximately 3850 nucleotides in length. Analysis of a large collection of TT virus genomes showed nearly 50% of them to be recombinant (Worobey, 2000).

Conclusions Regarding Molecular Techniques

It seems likely that as molecular techniques continue to be applied in this manner, many more viruses that have no obvious association with pathogenesis will be found in the human population. In addition, it is likely that, using molecular approaches, a number of diseases presently of unknown aetiology will prove to be associated with causative viruses that have yet to be discovered.

Despite the availability of these sophisticated molecular approaches for the identification of emerging viruses, the most recently identified emerging virus was found to be a human coronavirus causing severe acute respiratory syndrome (SARS) by the classical technique of electron microscopy of the virus growing in cell culture (Ksiazek *et al.*, 2003). Only once the virus was discovered were molecular techniques used to establish that it was a newly identified coronavirus not hitherto suspected in the human population.

Increased Contact with Vectors of Virus Infection

As the global human population continues to expand, there is increased opportunity for human contact with natural virus vectors, such as arthropods, birds or rodents, and in recent years we have seen the emergence of a number of new virus diseases, as well as a resurgence of other diseases that were formerly well controlled. Some instances involve the invasion by humans of a new ecological niche which brings them into closer contact with the vector. As an example, in South America, deforestation of large land areas may deprive rodents carrying arenaviruses or hantaviruses of their usual habitat, resulting in infestation of houses and closer contact with the human population. Although there has been no large pandemic of influenza since 1968, it is highly likely that reassortment of an avian influenza virus with a human one, as happened in the last two pandemics, will occur again. There is a vast reservoir of influenza viruses in the avian population (Webster and Kawaoka, 1994) and our ability to control such a pandemic, if it occurs, has not significantly improved in the last 30 years.

Arthropod-borne Viruses

Another important factor that has contributed to the emergence of virus diseases is the vector population density. This is particularly true of mosquito-borne viruses. Once well-controlled, the mosquito population, including *Aedes aegypti* and *A. albopictus*, has expanded greatly since the cessation of the use of DDT, resulting in increasing cases of dengue fever worldwide (Figure 28.4) and in particular a resurgence of dengue haemorrhagic fever, a severe form of dengue involving infection with two or more serotypes of dengue virus.

Translocation of a vector-borne virus into a new geographical region can result in the emergence of a dramatic disease outbreak. In 1999 there was an outbreak of West Nile viral meningoencephalitis, first detected in New York City. This virus had only been detected previously in Africa and the Middle East, and once the virus found in New York was sequenced, it was found to be identical in sequence to a virus isolated from diseased birds in Israel. How the virus was imported into the USA is unknown—an infected person, mosquito or bird are all possibilities. However, once established in a virgin population with the appropriate vector, the virus soon spread both south and west from New York, and has now moved south into the Caribbean and Mexico and north into Canada. By 2002, *West Nile virus* had spread to 39 states and DC, and caused 2741 human cases of meningoencephalitis and 263 deaths. More than 124 000 dead birds were reported, as well as more than 12 000 cases in horses. The virus was recovered from 37 species of mosquito, and is now an endemic disease requiring considerable public health efforts for its control.

Rodent-borne Hantaviruses

In 1993 an epidemic of acute respiratory disease occurred in south-western USA, and was identified as hantavirus pulmonary syndrome (HPS), a new clinical disease of high mortality (40%), spread by a virus in the deermouse (*Peromyscus maniculatus*) population in the area. It soon emerged that climatic conditions in the summer of 1993 had favoured an explosion in the population of deermice, and this was the major factor which had contributed to a large number of HPS cases from which the epidemic became recognised. Once recognised, other hantaviruses were identified in both North and South America, many causing severe and often fatal HPS in the human population (Figure 28.5).

Although most rodents worldwide appear capable of housing and transmitting hantaviruses, the only cases of severe HPS have been associated with rodents of the subfamily *Sigmodontinae*, which is confined geographically to the Western hemisphere, North and South America. In other parts of the world hantaviruses cause milder disease, with few fatalities.

Bats as Virus Vectors

Another important group of animals that act as vectors for virus diseases are bats, which comprise a quarter of living mammalian species. In the USA, insectivorous bats are the most important vector species for human rabies, often transmitting the disease silently, by a bite of which the human is unaware.

In recent years fruit-eating bats have been recognised as important disease vectors. There are some 170 species of fruit-eating bats (Megachiroptera) in the tropical regions of Asia.

In 1994 a horse trainer and a stablehand who worked on a farm in Hendra, a suburb of Brisbane, Australia, became ill while nursing a sick pregnant mare that had recently been brought onto the property. The disease spread to other horses on the property, and 14/21 infected horses died of pulmonary disease with haemorrhagic manifestations. Of the two infected humans, the trainer died, but the stablehand survived the infection after a lengthy illness. One year later, another horse farmer died 600 miles away in Mackay, from encephalitis caused by a similar virus. The virus, named *Hendra virus*, was found to be a new paramyxovirus with a large genome, about 19 kb in length, morphologically similar to other paramyxoviruses but with a very long nucleocapsid. Subsequently, the only time this virus was recognised as causing disease again was in 1997, when it caused the death of a horse in Cairns, in the far north of Australia. However, in the meantime work carried out in the Australian Animal Health Laboratory in Geelong had identified the virus in fruit bats, and a survey revealed that a high proportion of fruit bats had antibodies against the virus.

Beginning in 1997, an outbreak of a new respiratory disease in pigs was noticed by farmers in Malaysia. In late 1998 and 1999 many farmers and other persons having close contact with pigs developed severe symptoms of encephalitis. In all there were 265 human cases, of whom 105 persons died. The disease did not appear to be transmissible between humans, and was stopped in May 1999 by the slaughter of more than a million pigs, causing great economic loss to the Malaysian pig industry. In March 1999 a virus was isolated in cell culture from the brain of a patient in Sg Nipah village, Bukit Pelandok, Malaysia. The virus caused syncytia during growth in Vero cells, and gave a positive test by immunofluorescence assay carried out at CDC using an antiserum made against *Hendra virus*. By thin-section electron microscopy of infected Vero cells, a paramyxovirus with a long nucleocapsid was found. Complete sequencing of the virus genome showed that it was a large negative-stranded RNA molecule, 18 246 nucleotides in length, with about 80% homology to the genome of *Hendra virus*. The new paramyxovirus, called *Nipah virus* (Chua et al., 2000), was subsequently found in large fruit-eating bats, and it was from these that the virus is presumed to have spread first to pigs, and then to humans in close contact with infected pigs. Curiously, the mortality rate in pigs was less than 5%, much less than was seen amongst the human cases. Pigs develop rapid, laboured breathing and an explosive non-productive cough as the main symptoms, with occasional neurological changes, such as lethargy or aggressive behaviour. Humans develop a febrile encephalitis which rapidly progresses to multisystem involvement with vasculitis and syncytial giant cell formation at various sites. Spread to the brain is by the vascular route and leads to discrete small foci of necrosis and neuronal degeneration.

Non-human Primates as Virus Vectors

It is now recognised that both HIV-1 and HIV-2 have their origin in chimpanzees and sooty mangabey monkeys, respectively (Holmes, 2001), which can be infected with these viruses but do not themselves routinely develop AIDS. The transmission of these zoonotic infections has been ascribed to the practice of killing and eating the primates (as bushmeat), and it is clear that other viruses can emerge in the same way. Viruses causing severe haemorrhagic fever, such as *Ebola virus* and *Marburg virus*, have certainly passed from non-human primates to man by this means on several occasions, but it is generally believed that another natural reservoir exists for these viruses since, like man, non-human primates are highly susceptible to both these filoviruses. Because they cause extremely high mortality in man (up to 90% of infected persons), a great deal of concern is generated when an outbreak occurs. The original outbreak of *Marburg virus* was caused by direct transmission of the virus from infected monkeys by persons handling fresh monkey tissues, but in general filovirus outbreaks are largely amplified by person–person transmission, usually in a hospital setting, as occurred in the last major outbreak caused by *Ebola virus* in Kikwit, Democratic Republic of the Congo, in 1995.

Conclusions Regarding Contact with Vectors

It is clear from the experience gained over the past 20 years that animal, bird or arthropod reservoirs are extremely important sources for the emergence of new diseases. This has led to an assumption that most newly discovered virus diseases have their origin in another species. The outbreak of SARS coronavirus may be a case in point, and suspicion has been placed on various exotic animal species that are eaten by the Chinese and may have started the epidemic in Guangdong. This remains to be proven, but it is widely believed that the next pandemic of human influenza will occur as a result of reassortment between an avian and a human influenza virus.

Only by continued global surveillance and prompt reporting to WHO can we hope to control the outcome of such an event.

REFERENCES

Almond J and Pattison J (1997) Human BSE. *Nature*, **389**, 437–438.

Armstrong GL, Conn LA and Pinner RW (1999) Trends in infectious disease mortality in the United States during the 20th century. *J Am Med Assoc*, **281**, 61–66.

Centers for Disease Control and Prevention (2003a) Update: multistate outbreak of monkeypox—Illinois, Indiana, Kansas, Missouri, Ohio, and Wisconsin. *Morbid Mortal Wkly Rep*, **52**, 561–564.

Centers for Disease Control and Prevention (2003b) Outbreak of severe respiratory syndrome worldwide. *Morbid Mortal Wkly Rep*, **52**, 226–228.

Chang Y, Cesarman E, Pessin MS *et al.* (1994) Identification of herpesvirus-like DNA sequences in AIDS-associated Kaposi's sarcoma. *Science*, **266**, 1865–1869.

Choo QL, Kuo G, Weiner A *et al.* (1989) Isolation of a cDNA clone derived from a blood-borne non-A, non-B viral hepatitis genome. *Science*, **244**, 359–362.

Chua KB, Bellini WJ, Rota PA, *et al.* (2000) Nipah virus: a recently emergent deadly paramyxovirus. *Science*, **288**, 1432–1435.

Collinge J, Sidle KCL, Heads J *et al.* (1996) Molecular analysis of prion strain variation and the aetiology of 'new variant' CJD. *Nature*, **383**, 685–690.

Holmes EC (2001) On the origin and evolution of the human immunodeficiency virus (HIV). *Biol Rev Cambr Phil Soc*, **76**, 239–254.

Holmes GP, McCormick JB *et al.* (1990) Lassa fever in the United States. Investigation of a case and new guidelines for management. *N Engl J Med*, **323**, 1120–1123.

Kew OM, Morris-Glasgow V, Landaverde M *et al.* (2002) Outbreak of poliomyelitis in Hispaniola associated with circulating type 1 vaccine-derived poliovirus. *Science*, **296**, 356–359.

Khudyakov YE, Cong M-E, Nichols B *et al.* (2000) Sequence heterogeneity of TT virus and closely related viruses. *J Virol*, **74**, 2990–3000.

Ksiazek TG, Erdman D, Goldsmith C *et al.* (2003) A novel coronavirus associated with severe acute respiratory syndrome. *N Engl J Med*, **348**, 1953–1966.

Lederberg J, Shope RE and Oaks SC (1992) *Emerging Infections. Microbial Threats to Health in the United States* (294 pp). National Academy Press, Washington, DC.

Linnen J, Wages J, Zhang-Keck ZY *et al.* (1996) Molecular cloning and disease association of hepatitis C virus: a transfusion transmissible agent. *Science*, **271**, 505–508.

Mahy BWJ (2000) The global threat of emerging infectious diseases. In *Fighting Infection in the 21st Century* (eds Andrew PW, Oyston P, Smith GL and Stewart-Tull DE), pp 1–16. Blackwell Science, Oxford.

Mahy BWJ (2003) An overview on the use of a viral pathogen as a bioterrorism agent: why smallpox? *Antiviral Res*, **57**, 1–5.

Moore PS, Kingsley LA, Holmberg SD *et al.* (1996) Kaposi's sarcoma-associated herpesvirus infection prior to onset of Kaposi's sarcoma. *AIDS*, **10**, 175–180.

Mushahwar IK (2000) Recently discovered blood-borne viruses: are they hepatitis viruses or merely endosymbionts? *J Med Virol*, **62**, 399–404.

Mushahwar IK, Erker JC, Muerhoff AS *et al.* (1999) Molecular and biophysical characterization of TT virus: evidence for a new virus family infecting humans. *Proc Natl Acad Sci USA*, **96**, 3177–3182.

Nichol ST, Spiropoulou CF, Morzunov S *et al.* (1993) Genetic identification of a novel hantavirus associated with an outbreak of acute respiratory illness in the southwestern United States. *Science*, **262**, 914–917.

Nishizawa T, Okamoto H, Konishi K *et al.* (1997) A novel DNA virus (TTV) associated with elevated transaminase levels in post-transfusion hepatitis of unknown etiology. *Biochim Biophys Res Commun*, **241**, 92–97.

Okamoto H, Nishizawa T, Tawara A *et al.* (2000) Species-specific TT viruses in humans and non-human primates and their phylogenetic relatedness. *Virology*, **277**, 368–378.

Purdy MA and Krawczynski K (1994) Hepatitis E. *Gastroenterol Clin North Am*, **23**, 537–546.

Reyes GR, Purdy MA, Kim JP *et al.* (1990) Isolation of a cDNA from the virus responsible for enterically transmitted non-A, non-B hepatitis. *Science*, **16**, 1335–1339.

Simons JN, Pilot-Matias TJ, Leary TP *et al.* (1995) Identification of two flavivirus-like genomes in the GB hepatitis agent. *Proc Natl Acad Sci USA*, **92**, 3401–3405.

Smolinski MS, Hamburg MA and Lederberg JA (eds) (2003) *Microbiol Threats to Health Emergence, Detection and Response* (306 pp). National Academies Press, Washington, DC.

van den Hoogen BG, de Jong JC, Groen J *et al.* (2001) A newly discovered human pneumovirus isolated from young children with respiratory tract disease. *Natur Med*, **7**, 719–724.

Webster RG and Kawaoka Y (1994) Influenza—an emerging and re-emerging disease. *Semin Virol*, **5**, 103–111.

World Health Organization (2003) Summary table of SARS cases by country, 1 November 2002–7 August 2003. *Wkly Epidemiol Rec*, **35**, 310–311.

Worobey M (2000) Extensive homologous recombination among widely divergent TT viruses. *J Virol*, **74**, 7666–7670.

29

Hospital-acquired Infections

INTRODUCTION

The previous chapters have covered the important clinico-pathological aspects of all the major groups of human viruses, including their epidemiology and control at a population level, yet little has been said concerning the prevention of nosocomial virus infection. This chapter aims to provide the practical knowledge and approaches required to enable microbiologists and virologists to control the spread of virus infection in hospitals. Indeed, the entire subject of nosocomial virus infection has not had the prominence it deserves and has been a largely neglected area.

This is surprising, as hospitals are a particularly easy target for several virus groups and may act as centres of virus amplification for the further spread of virus in the wider community. This has been exemplified recently in the case of SARS and previously with Ebola virus outbreaks being centred in hospitals in Africa. There is also an ever-increasing burden of extremely vulnerable patient groups, including pre-term neonates and those with immunodeficiency secondary to HIV or solid organ and bone marrow transplants. Global travel has also meant that increasingly the staff who work in health services come from all over the world. This brings with it other unique problems, such as increased susceptibility rates to chickenpox if staff are from equatorial climes.

The prevention of nosocomial virus infections requires a team effort. Very often virology is able only to prevent secondary cases where the incubation period is relatively long, e.g. 10–14 days for measles,

chickenpox, etc. Preventing the nosocomial spread of viral respiratory and gastrointestinal pathogens, however, with very short incubation periods of only hours to a few days, relies heavily on the staff admitting the patient recognising the potential for transmission and adhering strictly to basic infection control measures, such as hand-washing. The admission to single rooms of patients experiencing viral prodromes of, for example, parvovirus or measles during epidemic seasons or local upsurges, and cohort nursing are very effective but require thought from admitting teams. To facilitate this approach, clear, concise guidance from the virology, infection control and occupational health departments on how to manage individual virus infections and staff exposures to them is required.

Control of virus infections in hospitals should also be an active process. Although rapid diagnosis and excellent communication with staff in the clinical areas are essential if nosocomial infection is to be prevented, anticipating recurring problems, e.g. the annual RSV winter epidemic, by informing staff through continuous education programmes and pro-actively if local outbreaks are occurring, is of additional benefit.

In this last chapter we cover the burden of nosocomial virus infection of the most important viruses. Section A discusses blood-borne viruses, whilst section B illustrates the problems, and some of the solutions to controlling the spread of viruses by all other routes and means of contact. Practical measures that should be taken to prevent an outbreak or limit its spread and guidance on the management of staff susceptible to particular agents are also given.

Principles and Practice of Clinical Virology, Fifth Edition. Edited by A. J. Zuckerman, J. E. Banatvala, J. R. Pattison, P. D. Griffiths and B. D. Schoub
© 2004 John Wiley & Sons Ltd ISBN 0 470 84338 1

Table 29.1 Incubation periods, communicability and transmission modes for common virus infections

Virus	Mode of transmission	Incubation period	Duration of shedding	Risk of transmission in hospitals[1]	Prevention	Adverse outcomes
Rubella	Respiratory droplet	15–20 days	−7 to +2 days	Low	Screening Vaccination Reporting	Congenital Rubella Syndrome
Measles	Respiratory droplet	7–18 days	Highest before or at rash onset −2 to +5 days	Low	Screening Vaccination Reporting	SSPE Death in I/C pts
Mumps	Respiratory droplet	14–19 days	−6 to +4 days	Low (may increase in certain cohorts)	Screening Vaccination Reporting	Meningitis Deafness
Chickenpox	Respiratory droplet Physical contact Airborne	10–21 days (normally 14)	−2 to +7 days (or until scabbed)	Moderate	Screening Vaccination Reporting	Congenital chickenpox Death in I/C pts[2]
Parvovirus	Respiratory droplet	13–18 days	−6 to −3 days before symptoms	Low/moderate	Reporting	Miscarriage Aplastic crises Chronic anaemia
Enteroviruses	Faecal–oral Fomites Airborne	5–7 days	1–8 weeks	Low/moderate	Reporting	Severe neonatal disease
Influenza	Respiratory droplet Airborne	2–3 days	−1 to 7 days	High	Reporting Vaccination	Death (I/C, elderly) Ward closure
Parainfluenza	Respiratory droplet	1–7 days	7–21 days	Very high	Reporting	Ward closure Death in I/C
RSV	Respiratory droplet	1–5 days	7–21 days	High	Reporting	Death in I/C
HSV	Saliva Physical contact Fomites	Few days (mean = 6)	1–8 weeks	High if breakdown in hand washing/personal hygiene	Reporting	Death in neonates
CMV	Physical contact with virus at mucosal surfaces	1–2 weeks	Weeks	Low	Hand washing	None
Rotavirus	Faecal–oral ? Respiratory	2–4 days	6–10 days	High	Isolation Hand washing	Prolonged stay in hospital
SRSV	Faecal–oral Airborne	1–3 days	Up to 2 weeks (allow back to work 72 h after symptoms resolved)	Very high	Reporting Isolation	Ward and hospital closure

[1]Refers to overall risk of transmission, modified by level of immunity in the population.
[2]I/C pts, Immunocompromised patients.

29A

Infections Acquired by the Blood-borne Route

Anthea Tilzey

Guy's, King's and St Thomas' School of Medicine, London, UK

INTRODUCTION

The blood-borne viruses (BBVs), which are associated with persistent replication and a persistent viraemia, are well-recognised causes of nosocomial infection. The most commonly reported nosocomial BBVs are *Hepatitis B virus* (HBV), *Hepatitis C virus* (HCV) and *Human immunodeficiency virus* (HIV). Transmission may occur from patient to health care worker (HCW) or from HCW to patient; the greater risk is from the former but the greater publicity tends to surround the latter. Patient-to-patient transmission can also occur, usually only where there is a deficiency in infection control procedures.

Nosocomial infection may occur when blood, other body fluids (see Table 29A.1) (Department of Health, 1998), unfixed tissues or organs are transferred from an infected source to an uninfected recipient.

In the health care setting, transmission usually follows percutaneous exposure. The relative risk of transmission following a single percutaneous exposure is normally quoted as approximately 1/3 for HBV, with an 'e' antigen-positive source, 1/30 for HCV and 1/300 for HIV. The risk of transmission for all three will depend to a large extent on the amount of virus inoculated, and this in turn will depend on the viral load in the source and the volume and type of body fluid transferred. Mucosal exposure carries a lower risk, e.g. the risk of acquiring HIV after a single mucocutaneous exposure to blood is <1/2000 (Department of Health, 1998).

It has long been recognised that HCWs are at increased risk of BBV infection. A study among orthopaedic surgeons in the USA showed that the prevalence of markers of both HBV and HCV infection increased with age (Shapiro *et al.*, 1996). Both in this study and in a number of others, a significantly higher prevalence of HCV antibodies in HCWs compared to control volunteer blood donors has been demonstrated. For example, a survey of New York dentists (Klein *et al.*, 1991) showed an anti-HCV prevalence of 1.75% in 456 dentists compared to 0.14% in 723 blood donor controls. The prevalence was particularly high (9.3%) in 43 oral surgeons.

With regard to HIV, as of June 1999, 319 HCWs worldwide were reported to have acquired HIV infection through occupational exposure (CDSC, 1999), 102 following a documented seroconversion after a specific occupational exposure, and 217 where seroconversion was not demonstrated but no other risk factors were identified.

There have been a number of documented outbreaks of HCW-to-patient transmission of HBV, HCV and HIV. There have been over 45 reports of transmission of HBV from HCW to patient, resulting in more than 400 infected patients (Gunson *et al.*, 2003). Initially, all were associated with 'e' Ag-positive HCWs; most were associated with dental or surgical procedures, particularly cardiac surgery and obstetrics and gynaecology. Look-back exercises demonstrated transmission rates varying from 1.5% (Hadler *et al.*, 1981) to as high as 24% (Welch *et al.*, 1989). More recently there have

Principles and Practice of Clinical Virology, Fifth Edition. Edited by A. J. Zuckerman, J. E. Banatvala, J. R. Pattison, P. D. Griffiths and B. D. Schoub
© 2004 John Wiley & Sons Ltd ISBN 0 470 84338 1

Table 29A.1 Body fluids other than blood that may transmit nosocomial infection

High-risk body fluids	Low-risk body fluids
CSF	Saliva
Peritoneal fluid	Faeces
Pleural fluid	Urine
Pericardial fluid	Vomit
Synovial fluid	
Amniotic fluid	
Semen	
Vaginal secretions	
Breast milk	
Saliva in association with dentistry	
Low-risk body fluid containing visible blood	

been a number of documented transmissions of HBV from 'e' Ag-negative surgeons (Heptonstall *et al.*, 1997); all had detectable HBV DNA by nested PCR and pre-core mutants of HBV which failed to produce HBeAg.

There are also a number of reports of transmission of HCV from HCW to patients; to date, six published reports, resulting in the infection of 14 patients (Gunson *et al.*, 2003). Additional cases, as yet unpublished are under investigation. Transmission rates are lower than for HBV (0.13–0.18%) (Henderson, 2003). However, one should perhaps mention the atypical outbreak of HCV in Spain, in which a Spanish anaesthetist, who was a morphine addict, infected 171 of his patients by sharing needles and opiates with them (Henderson, 2003).

With regard to HIV, apart from the first recorded outbreak, involving a Florida dentist with AIDS who appeared to transmit infection to six of his patients (0.5% of 1100 evaluated) (Centers for Disease Control, 1991; Ciesielski *et al.*, 1992), hundreds of look-back exercises, carried out on many thousands of patients following the identification of HIV-infected HCWs, have been very reassuring and have supported the view that the risk of transmission is very small. Only two nosocomial infections have been identified in two separate look-backs—one involving an orthopaedic surgeon in France and 1000 patients tested (Lot *et al.*, 1999) and one involving the Spanish anaesthetist mentioned above.

Finally, there have been many reports of patient-to-patient transmission of BBVs, linked to a variety of medical and surgical procedures, including haemodialysis, orthopaedic, gynaecological and cardiothoracic surgery, endoscopy, colonoscopy, organ transplantation, anaesthetics, spring-loaded finger stick devices,

and contaminated immunoglobulin preparations, most resulting from inadequate infection control procedures or inadequate disinfections (Henderson, 2003).

How do we prevent or at least minimise the risk of BBV transmission in the health care setting? Prevention in this context may be divided into prevention of exposure and prevention of infection, which will apply to patient-to-HCW, patient-to-patient and HCW-to-patient transmission. Recommendations currently in place and/or under discussion to protect patients from infected HCWs are discussed below.

PREVENTION OF EXPOSURE

Preventing or minimising BBV exposure is achieved through establishing and practising high standards of infection control, i.e. general measures to minimise percutaneous or mucocutaneous exposure to blood, tissues and other body fluids.

All employing authorities should produce written protocols based on risk assessments of the work by different health care staff, and national guidelines such as those produced by the UK Health Departments or the Health and Safety Executive. The aim of such protocols is to prevent, or at least control, exposure to hazardous substances. HCWs should be trained in safe and practicable ways of performing routine tasks and these should be kept under regular review.

In the context of BBVs, 'universal precautions' should be applied, i.e. all blood, tissues and body fluids should be regarded as potentially infectious. The following general measures to reduce the risk of occupational exposure are recommended by the UK Health Departments (Department of Health, 1998).

- Wash hands before and after contact with each patient, and before putting on and after using rubber gloves.
- Change gloves between patients.
- Cover existing wounds, skin lesions and all breaks in exposed skin with waterproof dressings. Wear gloves if hands are extensively infected.
- Wear gloves where contact with blood can be anticipated.
- Avoid sharps usage where possible, and where sharps usage is essential, exercise particular care in handling and disposal.
- Avoid wearing open footwear in situations where blood may be spilt, or where sharp instruments or needles are handled.
- Clear up spillage of blood promptly and disinfect surfaces.

- Wear gloves when cleaning equipment prior to sterilisation or disinfection, when handling chemical disinfectant and when cleaning up spillages.
- Follow safe procedures for the disposal of contaminated waste.

Safe handling and disposal of sharps involves the adequate supply and positioning of sharps containers, the placing of all disposable sharps in such containers immediately after use, not overfilling such containers and avoiding resheathing needles, unless done by the single-handed technique with or without an appropriate device. Specific guidance for reducing the risk of percutaneous and mucocutaneous exposure during surgical procedures is also given in this document.

Other general measures which should be employed to prevent exposure to BBVs include adequate decontamination, i.e. sterilisation, disinfection and cleaning of equipment (Department of Health, 1996) and cleaning and disinfecting of work surfaces.

PREVENTION OF INFECTION

In addition to the general measures given above to prevent or minimise exposure to BBVs in the health care setting, there are more specific pre- and post-exposure measures whereby the risk of infection with HBV, HCV and HIV may be reduced. In addition, all

HCWs, including students, should be educated about the possible risks from occupational exposure and be made aware of the importance of seeking urgent advice following any possible exposure. Protocols on the management of such exposures should be drawn up, made readily available and health care staff should be designated to whom HCWs may be referred immediately for advice, counselling and management. HCWs who sustain an occupational exposure should have been educated about the potential risks, the recommended immediate first aid to the site of exposure, the need for prompt reporting, and the sources available for urgent advice, management and treatment, both within and outside normal working hours.

The specific pre- and post-exposure measures by which the risk of infection with BBVs in HCWs may be reduced are discussed below for the three main BBVs.

HBV

Pre-exposure

All HCWs, including students and trainees, who have direct contact with blood, tissues or other body fluids should be immunised against HBV, and have their response to vaccine checked in order to ensure an adequate response. Non-responders should be given appropriate advice regarding the management of

Table 29A.2 HBV prophylaxis for reported exposure incidents

HBV status of person exposed	Significant exposure			Non-significant exposure	
	HbsAg-positive source	Unknown source	HbsAg-negative source	Continued risk	No further risk
≤1 Dose HB vaccine pre-exposure	Accelerated course of HB vaccine* HBIG × 1	Accelerated course of HB vaccine*	Initiate course of HB vaccine	Initiate course of HB vaccine	No HBV prophylaxis Reassure
≥2 Doses HB vaccine pre-exposure (anti-HBs not known)	One dose of HB vaccine followed by second dose one month later	One dose of HB vaccine	Finish course of HB vaccine	Finish course of HB vaccine	No HBV prophylaxis Reassure
Known responder to HBV vaccine (anti-HBs ≥10 miU/ml)	Consider booster dose of HB vaccine	Consider booster dose of HB vaccine	Consider booster dose of HB vaccine	Consider booster dose of HB vaccine	No HBV prophylaxis Reassure
Known non-responder to HB vaccine (anti-HBs <10 miU/ml) 2–4 months post-vaccination	HBIG × 1. Consider booster dose of HB vaccine	HBIG × 1. Consider booster dose of HB vaccine	No HBIG. Consider booster dose of HB vaccine	No HBIG. Consider booster dose of HB vaccine	No prophylaxis Reassure

*An accelerated course of vaccine consists of doses spaced at 0, 1 and 2 months. A booster dose may be given at 12 months to those at continuing risk of exposure to HBV. Reproduced from PHLS Hepatitis Subcommittee (1992)

potential exposures, and should be investigated to identify those who may pose a risk to their patients during exposure-prone procedures (EPPs). Occupational health services are responsible for keeping accurate immunisation records for all employees and administering booster doses where appropriate.

Post-exposure

In the UK, guidance from the PHLS Hepatitis Subcommittee is summarised in Table 29A.2, which gives advice depending on the HBV status of the source and the HBV vaccination status of the recipient. Hepatitis B immune globulin (HBIG) is available as post-exposure prophylaxis (PEP) for unvaccinated individuals or non-responders.

HCV

Pre-exposure

There is currently no vaccine available for HCV.

Post-exposure

There is currently no effective post-exposure prophylaxis for HCV, and any potential exposure should be managed according to national guidelines. Close follow-up of exposed individuals is recommended with baseline and follow-up blood tests, e.g. HCV RNA PCR assays, HCV antibody tests or liver function tests (LFTs). Recommended intervals vary according to the proposed form of management. 'Watchful waiting' is likely to be replaced by pre-emptive therapy with immunomodulators as the evidence for their efficacy in reducing the risk of chronic infection accumulates (Henderson, 2003).

HIV

Pre-exposure

There is currently no vaccine available for HIV.

Post-exposure

Although the risk of infection with HIV following exposure is small, there is now evidence that post-exposure prophylaxis (PEP) with zidovudine (AZT),

with or without other anti-HIV drugs, may reduce the risk of becoming infected with HIV following a percutaneous exposure (CDC, 1998). HIV PEP, therefore, usually as a combination of three antiretroviral drugs, is recommended following percutaneous exposure or exposure of broken skin or mucous membranes to material known or strongly suspected to be infected with HIV. Details are given in the national guidelines (Department of Health, 1997; Centers for Disease Control, 1998).

PREVENTION OF HCW-TO-PATIENT TRANSMISSION

Finally, I would like to discuss measures recommended to minimise the risk of transmission of BBVs from HCWs to patients. As mentioned previously, although the risks are small, such infections attract a disproportionate amount of media publicity.

Currently, in the UK, with regard to HBV, all HCWs who carry out EPPs must be screened for HBsAg and HBeAg. All found to be eAg-positive, or eAg-negative but with HBV DNA levels of $>10^3$ genome equivalents/ml, are precluded from EPPs (Department of Health, 2003b). HCWs who feel that they may be at risk of HIV or HCV infection are encouraged to be tested. Any HCW who is HCV- or HIV-positive and found to have transmitted infection to patients must refrain from EPPs (Department of Health, 2003a). Some countries have adopted similar policies; others are less Draconian. However, in view of the ever-increasing reports of BBV transmission from HCW to patient, many countries are reviewing the situation.

In the UK, the Department of Health recently published a consultation document, *Health Clearance for Serious Communicable Diseases: New Health Care Workers*, in which it is recommended that all new HCWs who carry out EPPs will need to have standard health clearance for serious communicable diseases and additional health clearance for BBVs. It seems likely that restrictions will be imposed on the working practices of HCWs infected with any of the three main BBVs, HBV, HCV or HIV.

Increasing concern about HCW-to-patient transmission of BBVs is also evident from the recent publication of a consensus statement from a European consensus group, the aim of which is to reduce the risk of transmission of HBV and HCV from infected HCWs to patients (Gunson et al., 2003).

REFERENCES

CDSC (1999) Occupational Transmission of HIV, Summary of Published Reports, PHLS AIDS & STD Centre at the Communicable Disease Surveillance Centre and Collaborators, December 1999.

Centers for Disease Control (1987) Recommendations for prevention of HIV transmission in health care settings. *Morb Mortal Wkly Rep*, **36**, 1–8.

Centers for Disease Control (1991) Recommendations for preventing transmission of human immunodeficiency virus and hepatitis B virus to patients during exposure prone invasive procedures. *Morb Mortal Wkly Rep*, **40** (RR-8), 1–9.

Centers for Disease Control (1998) Public Health Service Guidelines for the management of health-care worker exposures to HIV and recommendations for postexposure prophylaxis. *Morb Mortal Wkly Rep*, **47** (RR-7), 1–28.

Ciesielski C, Marianos D, Ou CY *et al.* (1992) Transmission of human immunodefiency virus in a dental practice. *Ann Intern Med*, **116**, 798–805.

Department of Health (1998) *Guidance for Clinical Health Care Workers: Protection Against Infection with Bloodborne Viruses. Recommendations of the Expert Advisory Group on AIDS and the Advisory Group on Hepatitis*. UK Department of Health, London.

Department of Health (1996) *Sterilisation, Disinfection and Cleaning of Medical Equipment: Guidance on Decontamination*. Microbiology Advisory Committee to the Department of Health: Part 1, Principles. UK Department of Health, London.

Department of Health (1997) *Guidelines on Post-exposure Prophylaxis for Health Care Workers Occupationally Exposed to HIV*. UK Department of Health, London.

Department of Health (2003a) *Health Clearance for Serious Communicable Diseases: New Health Care Workers, Draft Guidance for Consultation*. UK Department of Health, London.

Department of Health (2003b) Hepatitis B-infected healthcare workers: http://www.doh.gov.uk/nhsexec/hepatitisB/html

Gunson RN, Shouval D, Roggendorf M *et al.* and the European Consensus Group (2003) Hepatitis B virus (HBV) and hepatitis C virus (HCV) infections in health care workers (HCWs): guidelines for prevention of transmission of HBV and HCV from HCW to patients. *J Clin Virol*, **27**, 213–230.

Hadler SC, Sorley DL, Acree KH *et al.* (1981) An outbreak of hepatitis B in a dental practice. *Ann Intern Med*, **95**, 133–138.

Henderson DK (2003) Managing occupational risks for hepatitis C transmission in the health care setting. *Clin Microbiol Rev*, **16**, 546–568.

Heptonstall J, on behalf of The Incident Investigation Teams (1997) Transmission of hepatitis B to patients from four infected surgeons without hepatitis B e antigen. *N Engl J Med*, **336**, 178–184.

Klein RS, Freeman K, Taylor PE and Stevens CE (1991) Occupational risk for hepatitis C virus infection among New York City dentists. *Lancet*, **338**, 1539–1542.

Lot F, Segvier JC, Fegueux S *et al.* (1999) Probable transmission of HIV from an orthopaedic surgeon to a patient in France. *Ann Intern Med*, **130**, 1–6.

PHLS Hepatitis Subcommittee (1992) *CDR Rev*, **2**, R97–R101.

Shapiro CN, Tokars JI, Chamberland ME and the American Academy of Orthopaedic Surgeons Serosurvey Study Committee, Atlanta, Georgia (1996) Use of the hepatitis B vaccine and infection with hepatitis B and C among orthopaedic surgeons, *J Bone Joint Surg*, **78-A**, 1791–1799.

Welch J, Webster M, Tilzey AJ *et al.* (1989) Hepatitis B infections after gynaecological surgery. *Lancet*, **1**, 205–207.

29B

Infections Acquired by Other Routes

Philip Rice

St George's Hospital Medical School, London, UK

HERPES SIMPLEX VIRUS (HSV)

The prevention of nosocomial HSV infections relies entirely on good standards of personal hygiene. Although virus may be shed in the genital tract and in saliva without clinical lesions, adhering to hand-washing with soap and water or alcohol-based gels is sufficient to destroy infectious virus. The main reason for concern over nosocomial HSV infections is the potential for transmission to neonates, born either pre-term or term, as neonatal HSV infection has extremely high rates of mortality and morbidity even with the prompt use of antivirals. Approximately one-third of cases of neonatal HSV infection are thought to be acquired from a non-maternal source. It is vital, therefore, that staff employed on delivery suites, postnatal wards and neonatal units understand the importance of hand-washing and of the absolute requirement to absent themselves from work if they develop an herpetic whitlow. The more commonly faced scenario, however, is of the midwife or neonatal nurse with a cold sore. The only truly safe way to manage such occurrences is to remove the individual from all clinical duties until the lesion has dried and crusted over. Although virus will still be shed in saliva, the likelihood of transmission is lower than with wet or vesicular skin lesions. One practical measure for staff who develop frequent recurrences could be to advise them to have readily available oral aciclovir, which can be started immediately prodromal symptoms appear. Such an approach, combined with strict hand-washing, will help to further reduce the risk of transmission. Additionally, if trigger factors such as sunlight can be identified, prophylaxis may be taken to cover these periods, e.g. the summer holidays.

It is important to note, however, that although nosocomial transmission has been proven by restriction enzymatic digestion analysis of cultured isolates, often the identity of the presumed common source has remained undiscovered (Linnemann *et al.*, 1978). Virus has also survived for more than 60 h on a cot that had been used for a baby who died from disseminated HSV infection. More than 60 h after this baby died, the cot was re-used without being deconta-minated. A second neonate was then nursed in it. Twelve days later this infant also died (Sakaoka *et al.*, 1986).

VARICELLA-ZOSTER VIRUS (VZV)

Preventing patients and staff from contracting chickenpox in hospitals forms a significant part of the workload of a clinical virologist. Outbreaks cause significant disruption to wards, occasionally entire hospitals, increase the workload of clinical virology laboratories at very short notice, and necessitate considerable expense when susceptible staff have to be excluded from work after exposure. Chickenpox can also occur at any age. We have personally seen primary infection in two 65 year-olds, a 78 year-old and a man of 92 years!

When a patient with varicella-zoster virus (VZV) infection is identified, all staff in contact with the case must know their immune status. A well-taken history of previous chickenpox correlates very well with

Principles and Practice of Clinical Virology, Fifth Edition. Edited by A. J. Zuckerman, J. E. Banatvala, J. R. Pattison, P. D. Griffiths and B. D. Schoub
© 2004 John Wiley & Sons Ltd   ISBN 0 470 84338 1

immunity (99%) and, even for those who are unsure whether they have had chickenpox in the past or claim never to have been infected, 60% will have evidence of past infection. Knowledge of such status is part of routine occupational health screening. Indeed, it is important for staff to appreciate the problems that VZV transmission may cause in hospital and for susceptible staff to report immediately any contact with virus. This is especially so for staff who have children, as approximately 50% of susceptible staff who ultimately develop chickenpox do so after a home exposure (Devi and Rice, 2002). For reasons unknown, individuals born in hotter climates, particularly the Indian sub-continent, Africa and the Caribbean, are much more likely to be susceptible. Indeed, of the VZV-susceptible staff employed at St George's who developed chickenpox in the last 3 years, >50% were born in these countries (Devi and Rice, 2002).

The transmission rate of chickenpox to susceptible staff from contact with VZV has been estimated to be between 4.7–29% after exposure (Myers *et al.*, 1982; Wreghitt *et al.*, 1996; Langley and Hanakowski, 2000). There are several factors that exert an effect on this rate, most of which are extremely difficult to quantify. However, there are general guidelines on the extent of exposure which can be helpful in deciding whether a real exposure has occurred. Examples of significant exposures have been defined as a face-to-face contact or being present in the same room for 1 h with an individual with chickenpox or disseminated/uncovered zoster (Salisbury and Begg, 1996). At the other end of the exposure spectrum, the likelihood of transmission taking place from cases of covered, e.g. thoraco-lumbar, zoster is remote. However, airborne transmission on open wards has been described, even, in our experience, to a susceptible neonatal unit registrar after a patient with chickenpox had been placed in a single room and with whom he had had no direct contact, the implication here being that virus escaped into the corridor.

Although chickenpox is much more infectious than zoster, most of the practical problems involved with control of infection arise from patients who have zoster. This is simply because chickenpox is easily recognisable and such patients are admitted immediately into a side room. Zoster, however, often develops days or weeks after admission and has usually been present for several days before the diagnosis is clinically suspected. Thus, many more staff and patients are exposed to VZV after contact with patients who have zoster than those with chickenpox. This was demonstrated clearly in a study from Cambridge, UK, where during a 5 year period, only 1/28 (3.6%) of susceptible staff developed chickenpox after an exposure to varicella, compared with 5/29 (17.2%) after exposure to zoster (Wreghitt *et al.*, 1996).

It is wise to remember, however, that chickenpox can be mistaken for other vesicular exanthems due to enteroviruses or even allergy, contact dermatitis or eczema. If you are presented with the information that a member of staff or a visitor/relative on the neonatal unit, for example, has developed chickenpox, the implications for the unit are considerable. Multiple doses of VZIG will almost certainly need to be administered, susceptible staff will need to be sent home, visiting may become restricted and it is possible that the unit will have to be closed to new admissions. Thus, although it is an extreme example of what might happen, before embarking on the above course of action it is essential that the diagnosis of chickenpox be confirmed by an experienced virologist or microbiologist with access to laboratory facilities capable of providing rapid results, either by direct immunofluorescence or real-time PCR on vesicular lesion scrapings.

If a susceptible member of staff has been exposed, the simplest way to manage the exposure is to send that member of staff home, commencing on day 8–10 after contact until day 21 after the first exposure. This is because cases of chickenpox are infectious 2 days prior to rash onset. Another option used quite commonly is to allow staff to remain at work, provided that they feel well and are afebrile (Josephson *et al.*, 1990; Weber *et al.*, 1996). They should be instructed to take twice daily temperatures and to remain at home if they are febrile, as this could be the first sign of a prodromal varicella illness. This measure may be used more frequently in critical members of staff whose absence from a clinical area would be detrimental to patient care. Alternatively, the individual could perform duties that do not involve patient contact, although the usefulness of this approach for an experienced ward sister, for example, is questionable. Theoretically, however, and probably practically, the most cost-effective long-term way of managing such staff is through active vaccination against VZV, either before or after an exposure (Centers for Disease Control, 1999).

Live attenuated varicella vaccine has been in use for more than 20 years in Japan and the Far East and for almost a decade in the USA, but only recently have two varicella vaccine products been licensed in the UK for susceptible individuals >12 years of age.

Both products, one from Glaxo Smith Kline, the other from Aventis-Pasteur, are highly effective at preventing chickenpox prior to exposure and produce a seroconversion rate of >95% after a two-dose schedule (Sharrar *et al.*, 2000). Although pre-exposure vaccination has been shown to be cost-effective, this has been assessed only in mathematical models (Gray *et al.*, 1997) and there are several important practical considerations before advising a staff-wide vaccination policy. These include how to manage staff working in high-risk areas, as a small proportion of vaccinees will develop a rash both at the site of vaccination and outside of the injection area, and there is also a measurable rate of breakthrough infection after exposure to wild-type virus and thus the potential for ongoing transmission.

The rate of vesicular rash post-vaccine is ca. 8% (Arbeter *et al.*, 1986). However, in the majority the rash is only maculopapular, and in the 30% where it is vesicular, the average number of lesions is only 14. The nature of the rash and the lack of evidence for pharyngeal excretion of virus probably explain why transmission of vaccine virus to another healthy susceptible individual occurs only extremely rarely. Nevertheless, to take account of this problem, staff employed in high-risk areas should take particular care in the 2 weeks after both doses and report to occupational health immediately a possible varicella-like rash develops. Breakthrough infection, however, is potentially more troublesome, as this is a long-term problem and occurs at a rate of 5–8% after an exposure (Arbeter *et al.*, 1986; Watson *et al.*, 1993). The average timing for such breakthrough infections is 30 months post-vaccination (Watson *et al.*, 1993).

Despite breakthrough cases of infection being described after contact with VZV at work, where presumably the degree of exposure is less intense compared with at home, transmission of wild-type virus from cases of breakthrough infection to susceptible contacts, even within the home, is only 12% (Watson *et al.*, 1993). This should be compared with a household transmission rate of 80–90% for natural varicella. It should also be noted that breakthrough cases have far fewer lesions, on average 31 (1–100) compared with the mean number of lesions seen in ordinary varicella of 250–500. Such breakthrough infections may occur after a documented seroconversion to VZV vaccine, but in a study by Gershon *et al.* (1988) 9/12 (75%) of staff experiencing breakthrough were shown to be seronegative after their initial vaccination. It is possible, therefore, that this group could be offered a booster dose of vaccine post-exposure and re-tested in 7 days to assess the response. If antibody were then detected, they could almost certainly continue to work uninterrupted.

VZV vaccine as a post-exposure measure is also highly effective, provided that it is given within 3 days of contact with infectious material. A study from Asano *et al.* (1977) examined 26 contacts in 21 families who were immunised within 3 days of the index case developing chickenpox. None of the vaccinees developed a rash. However, a control group of 19 unimmunised contacts in 15 families were all infected. In the same study, Asano (1977) also gave vaccine to 34 healthy siblings within 3 days of the index case rash; 2/34 (5.8%) got varicella. The protective efficacy of post-exposure vaccination is therefore >90%. Whilst this approach may not necessarily allow the member of staff to remain at work in very critical areas, such as bone marrow transplantation units, the exposure that

Table 29B.1 Arguments for and against the use of varicella vaccine for health care workers

For	Against
Eliminate natural varicella from staff	Cost £80/person
Of great use especially in high-risk areas (paediatrics, HIV, transplant, neonatal units)	Administration costs
	Uncertain durability of immunity
Reduce potential for nosocomial transmission	Vaccine-associated rash
Much lower risk of transmission to pregnant staff	Latent virus reactivation as zoster
Very good safety record: in use for 20+ years	Possible need to send off or restrict to
Lower incidence of shingles in vaccinees	non-clinical work if breakthrough
Lower rate of vaccine-related events compared with natural infection	infection occurs
Durable immunity with natural boosters	
Virtually no risk of transmission from one healthy person to another	
Less worry for final exams in students (5% intake susceptible)	
Less risk of transmission for susceptible pregnant women (c. 25% of whom are in ethnic minorities where the prevalence of adult immunity is much lower approximately 50%)	
May be used post exposure (recent US and UK license)	
Potential case for complaint or worse, if transmission of wild-type virus occurred from a susceptible staff member to vulnerable patient (e.g. a pregnant woman)	

led to the use of VZV vaccine as a post-exposure measure should be that individual's last time of needing to be sent home from work for 2 weeks.

For the 3 years 2000–2002 at St George's Hospital, all cases of varicella in staff and students notified to the medical microbiology and occupational health departments have been documented. A total of 25 cases have been notified from all staff/student disciplines. Of these 25 cases, 13/22 (59%) occurred in individuals born outside of the UK, where the country of birth was known. If pre-exposure vaccination had been adopted at St George's, even amongst only the nursing and medical staff and students, 85% of chickenpox cases would have been prevented (Devi and Rice, 2002).

One other problem with the issue of immunising staff against chickenpox is that it is a live attenuated vaccine and as such may reactivate as zoster later in life. However, the vaccine probably offers benefit over wild-type infection, because the rate of zoster with reactivated vaccine virus is about 50% lower than after wild-type infection. The key problem with a widespread staff immunisation policy, even though it is established that vaccinating susceptible staff will reduce considerably the risk to patients from nosocomial varicella, is that immunity to infection after vaccination is not guaranteed as it is after natural chickenpox, and that it is not possible to identify which staff may be at risk of breakthrough infection after an exposure.

The decision has to be made as to how to manage immunised staff in these circumstances. The data indicate, that whilst transmission of breakthrough wild-type varicella infection may occur, especially to immunosuppressed patients, this is less likely than after natural varicella. If a staff-wide vaccination policy were to be instituted, this should be accompanied by a concerted effort to immunise simultaneously the most vulnerable patient groups. Should such a policy be contemplated, the points set out in Table 29B.1 may assist in making the decision.

CYTOMEGALOVIRUS (CMV)

CMV is one of the easiest viruses to control in hospital, yet probably causes more anxiety, especially among pregnant staff, than any other virus, apart from HIV. The anxiety usually results from the identification of a baby or infant with congenital infection, often on the neonatal unit. As congenitally infected babies often excrete a high titre of virus, there are understandably concerns at the potential risk that these babies pose to pregnant members of staff. At this stage such staff are

sometimes offered CMV screening, by other staff or occasionally occupational health departments, principally as a means of providing reassurance. However, such screening tests are offered in ignorance of the data concerning the risks of transmission and are erroneously believed to be capable of determining whether a person is 'immune' to CMV infection. Moreover, the potential implications and consequences of commencing CMV antibody testing in pregnant members of staff are never considered by those requesting the tests. Indeed, the first time that a clinical virologist will be involved is when the pregnant member of staff contacts him/her to discuss the results of her own CMV serology and its significance. This is where the difficulties arise. Indeed, as discussed in the CMV chapter, the concept of CMV immunity, especially in relation to pregnancy, is incorrect, since reactivation and reinfection may lead to congenital infection and disease in newborns.

Although the CMV serology may indicate past infection or susceptibility, occasionally CMV IgM is detected, which produces considerable anxiety. Further tests, such as IgG avidity, are then required, as well as a hunt for earlier samples to try to determine, as accurately as possible, the timing of any CMV infection. Furthermore, when past infection is shown, the potential for reinfection or reactivation must then be discussed. If the member of staff is susceptible, the discussion widens to include the potential benefit and harm of follow-up testing and prenatal diagnosis and the possible outcomes for the baby if a primary infection is demonstrated.

It is obvious from this outline that screening of staff for CMV is a big undertaking and should only be done after a prolonged and informed discussion with the clinical virologist and an obstetrician. The member of staff should be advised that if she has been adhering to universal precautions and has washed her hands with soap and water or an alcohol-based solution after dealing with patients, serological testing for CMV should not be performed. This is because there are several well-conducted studies which all conclude that there is no evidence that CMV excreted by hospitalised patients pose a significant additional risk for pregnant staff (Dworsky et al., 1983; Young et al., 1983; Balfour and Balfour, 1986; Demmler et al., 1987; Balcarek et al., 1990).

The annual incidence of CMV infection in hospital staff is approximately 2% and is no different between various occupational groups within and the general population outside hospital. Balcarek et al. (1990) showed, for example, that there was no difference in the rate of infection in staff regardless of area of work, job type (nurse, doctor, support services, administrative staff) or number of patient contact hours of 10–40 h/week. Moreover, when the rates of CMV excretion by patients are known in different areas of the hospital, this does not appear to influence the rate of transmission to staff. Demmler *et al.* (1987) showed this even when rates of CMV excretion varied from 3% in newborns to 16% in a chronic care unit for children, many with severe neurological and physical handicap, a proportion of whom would have had congenital infection and be excreting high-titre virus in urine.

Further proof that patients are not the source of infection has come from studies which have examined virus strains detected in staff who are shown to seroconvert at work. In these cases either the strains of virus in staff and patient have been different or another source outside of hospital, often a sexual partner, child at home, etc., has been shown to be shedding an identical virus (Onorato *et al.*, 1985; Demmler *et al.*, 1987).

The single study that did show an increased incidence of infection among staff, demonstrated this only for student nurses on their first placement in paediatrics (Haneberg *et al.*, 1980). Such staff were reportedly observed to kiss drooling infants while feeding them. Indeed, this paper highlights the fact, as stated by others, that intimate and prolonged contact is required for CMV transmission to occur (Onorato *et al.*, 1985). This would explain the increased rate of infection seen in pregnant mothers with a young child at home or in staff employed in child day-care, where the transmission rate may be 10–25%/year (Adler, 1989).

We would certainly not advise routinely screening staff after a possible exposure occupationally to CMV, as considerable anxiety is experienced whilst waiting for the results and there can be difficulties in their correct interpretation. Indeed, when this was attempted in a hospital in the UK some years ago it was a 'disaster' and led to 'public relations, psychological and management problems' (reviewed in Young *et al.*, 1983). The key to preventing infection relies upon the education of staff about how the virus is transmitted (sexually, kissing, lapses in hand-washing, especially after changing nappies) and about the many pitfalls of antibody testing. If a staff member has requested to be tested after an exposure, ideally the virologist should see her to discuss all of the issues relating to the possible outcomes. The issues to be discussed would be the fact that CMV infection is ubiquitous, staff are at no increased risk of infection, transmission is interrupted easily by hand-washing and

CMV serology can be fraught with difficulties if low or even high level IgM is detected.

Environmentally acquired infection also does not appear to be a problem. As CMV is an enveloped virus, it does not survive well on inanimate surfaces or on hands. This was shown clearly in a study in a paediatric hospital, where virus was not isolated from any equipment, toys or hard surfaces and, although it was isolated from the dry hands of staff members, it was removed completely by hand-washing with soap and water (Demmler *et al.*, 1987). Simple hygienic measures and the washing of surfaces with household detergent is sufficient to remove infectious material from the environment.

MEASLES, MUMPS AND RUBELLA

Measles Virus

The risk of measles infection occurring in medical personnel is estimated to be 13-fold higher than in the general population (Davis *et al.*, 1986; Atkinson *et al.*, 1991). Approximately 5–10% of all notified cases of measles are reported to have been acquired in a medical setting and over one-third of cases acquired in hospitals are in health care workers, mostly (>85%) previously unvaccinated (reviewed by ACIP/HICPAC, 1997).

Measles virus infection is now a particular problem partly because of the success of MMR vaccination, because whilst this has dramatically reduced the incidence of infection in the community, the clinical skills required to diagnose measles have also waned. Moreover, as the population of immunosuppressed (organ/bone marrow transplantation, intensive care and HIV) patients has continued to grow, atypical presentations are more likely to occur and there is a higher risk of the diagnosis being missed (Kidd *et al.*, 2003). Thus, as measles virus has a reproduction rate of 14:1, it can easily re-emerge in developed countries, due largely to the importation of measles from countries with less well-developed measles vaccination programmes (Ramsay *et al.*, 2003). This becomes even more a problem if the MMR uptake rate falls, as seen recently in the UK. Once imported, measles can then circulate without the need for further outside introductions (Thomas *et al.*, 1998).

There are, however, certain clinical criteria that can assist in the diagnosis of measles. One acronym that we have found helpful is the acronym CCDC, already in use in the UK for Consultant in Communicable Disease Control (CCDC). When applied to measles it becomes cough, coryza, diarrhoea, conjunctivitis, accompanied by rash and fever. The diagnosis becomes almost certain in the context of a community-wide outbreak or an epidemiological link with other cases. Travel abroad or contact with recently returned travellers also increases the likelihood of the diagnosis, as does having had no or only one dose of MMR vaccine. Other clues to the diagnosis are lymphopaenia ($<0.6 \times 10^9$/l) and slight thrombocytopaenia ($<150 \times 10^9$/l). Patients should ideally be admitted to a negative-pressure room or, if this is not possible, to a single room, and be cared for only by staff who are aware of their measles immunity status. A strict gloves, aprons and hand-washing policy must be adhered to if further infection in staff or patients is to be avoided. Transmission is by droplet infection, although fortunately the degree of infectivity reduces quickly after the rash appears and lasts for only 3–5 days afterwards. The incubation period can be as short as 7 days, but more typically is 10–13 days. However, because it may be as long as 19 days, susceptible staff should be excluded from work for 5–21 days after contact.

Problems have arisen in the UK as at present there is no formal policy of establishing measles immunity for all staff (Mendelson et al., 2000). Guidelines already in place in the USA, however, recommend that all health care workers provide evidence of immunity to measles through either a documented physician-diagnosed measles, two doses of live attenuated measles vaccine after their first birthday or a positive measles antibody test result (Krause et al., 1994). A cut-off year of 1957 is suggested, as people born before this year are very likely to have had measles infection as a child. However, as the susceptibility rate in this age group is still 5–9%, individuals in this group who cannot provide evidence for physician-diagnosed measles must undergo antibody testing and, if susceptible, be given two doses of MMR (Braunstein et al., 1990; Smith et al., 1990; Schwarcz et al., 1992). Even this approach may not always be successful, as shown in The Netherlands, where there was measles transmission to susceptible staff even though the overall level of immunity was 98.5% (de Swart et al., 2000). Pre-exposure vaccination is known, however, to be highly efficacious, as shown by two primary school outbreaks where the attack rate in unimmunised children was 26–46% yet it was only 0.4% in children who had had MMR (Richardson and Quigley, 1994).

It is essential and, indeed, a responsibility of hospital facilities to ensure that their staff have made all practicable efforts to eliminate measles from all hospital employees. This is because, given recent falls in the uptake of MMR, we may be creating a cohort of children, at least in the UK, which will become large enough to sustain not only local virus transmission but also be a source for susceptible infants who have yet to receive MMR. This is because as most mothers now have vaccine-induced immunity, measles antibody will have disappeared in infants by 9 months and infection under 1 year of life presents a much greater risk of developing Sub-Acute Sclerosing Panencephalitis (SSPE) as an older child.

To contain measles in a hospital, the only effective measures are to isolate the patient and to maintain high uptake rates of primary measles immunisation. Even post-exposure vaccination may be of dubious merit. When administered in an epidemic setting, the efficacy can be as low as 4% (King et al., 1991). Our experience has also been very similar when attempting to prevent an outbreak in infants at a nursery. The same day the index case was notified, which was on the day the rash appeared, four of the six contacts, all aged >1 but <2 years of age and previously unimmunised with MMR, were vaccinated; 10–14 days later all six children developed clinical measles, confirmed by detection of wild-type virus in one of the vaccinees (Rice et al., 2004). Thus, it is essential to achieve the highest possible level of staff immunity as post-exposure prophylaxis, whilst advisable, should not be relied upon to prevent secondary cases. Failure to do so will eventually result in ward closure and death in unimmunised immunocompromised patients (Kidd et al., 2003).

Mumps Virus

Mumps outbreaks in closed communities, including hospitals, have been described; especially when there are many opportunities for close contact (Wharton et al., 1990). One such outbreak occurred at trading floors in Chicago in 1987, with over 100 cases (Kaplan et al., 1988). The reason for an increase in cases in young adults is again because of the success of MMR vaccination. This has led to fewer exposures for a cohort of young adults who were ineligible for immunisation, yet who have also escaped natural infection. A similar problem is also being seen in the UK, where three-quarters of reported cases have been in children and young adults aged 10–19 years (PHLS, 2003). Controlling mumps virus in hospitals is still important because of the risk of meningitis and deafness. A high index of clinical suspicion, hand-washing and admission to a single room with droplet precautions, remain the main ways that transmission is prevented in hospitals. For staff, it may become necessary to test those exposed for mumps IgG and immunise seronegative individuals. As mumps virus excretion commences 48 h prior to symptom onset and MMR vaccine given post-exposure is ineffective in preventing secondary cases, it will be necessary to send home from work staff requiring vaccination for a period of 10 days, starting 12 days after first contact (Aitken and Jeffries, 2001).

Rubella

Outbreaks of rubella in hospitals are now rare, due largely to MMR vaccination, effective staff and student antibody screening and targeted immunisation (Greaves *et al.*, 1982). The susceptibility rates in staff in the 1970s and 1980s varied from 5% to 18%, depending on age (Polk *et al.*, 1980). With such high susceptibility rates, it was possible for rubella virus to circulate in hospitals and large outbreaks were described (Polk *et al.*, 1980). However, as non-immune staff are now much less common, if transmission to a member of staff does occur it is just as likely that this merely reflects a larger community-wide outbreak. However, individuals born in developing countries where rubella vaccination programmes are non-existent are at increased risk of infection in hospital if a health care worker develops rubella. Indeed, of particular concern are women from southern Asia and Africa, where susceptibility rates may be almost 20% in those of childbearing age (Miller *et al.*, 1990; Devi *et al.*, 2002). Furthermore, infants with congenital rubella syndrome are a potential source of infection for susceptible staff and other infants, due to the excretion of high-titre virus in urine for prolonged periods, approximately 2 years (Aitken and Jeffries, 2001). Indeed, vigilance to prevent nosocomial infection must be maintained, since it was recently demonstrated that a baby with congenital rubella syndrome (CRS) infected another baby in a neighbouring cot (Sheridan *et al.*, 2002). The only way that transmission could have taken place is by non-adherence to hand-washing by staff after dealing with urine and other bodily fluids from the baby with CRS. The best way to prevent nosocomial rubella is to fully investigate staff members with rash illness, remembering that in the first 3 days after the rash has appeared they may be IgG- and IgM-negative. Once identified, colleagues in close daily contact should be tested for rubella IgG, with the focus on pregnant staff <18 weeks' gestation. Although post-exposure rubella

vaccination is ineffective in preventing infection, any non-pregnant susceptible staff should then be immunised and tested 2–3 months later for a response.

PARVOVIRUS B19

Infection with human parvovirus B19 occupies a unique place among nosocomial virus infections. This is because once a single case of symptomatic infection has been identified in a member of staff, secondary cases will have already been infectious for several days and have probably infected further tertiary cases who, in turn, will be infectious in the next few days. Thus, unlike all other virus infections, once identified, the index case poses no further risk of infection to patients or staff; the problems lie with the contacts (staff and patients), whose infectivity or immunity status is as yet unknown. It is this group which presents a significant risk in the ongoing spread of infection. There are two reasons for this. First, the typical symptoms of rash and arthralgia manifest only when virus antigen–antibody complexes are formed, so that the index case presents when no longer infectious. Second, volunteer studies have shown that the period from exposure to such symptoms is normally 13–18 days (maximum 21 days), yet the period from exposure to infectiousness is only 7 days. In addition, as an estimated 30–40% of adults are susceptible and 20–30% of adult cases are symptomless, it would appear likely that virus transmission would pose significant problems within hospitals.

Nosocomial transmission may also be especially hazardous, as there are particularly vulnerable patient groups at risk of adverse outcomes: pregnant women, the immune-compromised and those with reduced red blood cell survival, who may develop a life-threatening aplastic crisis. However, the available information suggests that whilst hospital outbreaks do occur, they are uncommon. Moreover, before ascribing cases detected within a hospital to be nosocomial, they need to be examined carefully in the context of a wider community epidemic that may be occurring concurrently. Indeed, a hospital pseudo-outbreak was described in a maternity unit after several cases among staff and patients during the preceding weeks had been notified (Dowell *et al.*, 1995). However, when cases of acute infection on other wards, different hospitals and even healthy control subjects were sought, it was demonstrated that the percentage of individuals with recent infection, both in and out of hospital, was not significantly different, being 23–30%

in all locations or wards. The most likely explanation put forward was the presence of the largest community-wide parvovirus outbreak for 18 years (Dowell *et al.*, 1995).

When hospital outbreaks have been described they appear initially to be explosive, since they are noticed only after many cases in staff and patients have occurred, often over a period of several days. This is demonstrated by the attack rate of 27–50% in susceptible individuals, both staff and patients (Bell *et al.*, 1989; Pillay *et al.*, 1992; Seng *et al.*, 1994; Miyamoto *et al.*, 2000; Lui *et al.*, 2001). What is less clear is whether or not any infection control measures can prevent further virus transmission. This is important, since the measures proposed are potentially very costly in terms of staff absences or redeployment and possible ward closure. Indeed, to limit the spread of infection some authors have proposed ward closure, transfer of only immune staff to any affected ward, and restriction of the nursing staff to working only on the affected ward (Pillay *et al.*, 1992). However, by the time that an outbreak has been notified it is highly likely that the majority of virus transmissions that are going to occur have already taken place. This was clearly demonstrated in an outbreak at a UK London teaching hospital (Seng *et al.*, 1994). Over a 1 month period on a single ward, a total of 18 cases of acute parvovirus B19 infection were detected in 15 staff, of whom 12 were symptomatic; three patients were also affected. However, of the 12 symptomatic staff and the three affected patients, all who had known dates of symptom onset, 10 either were or had recently been symptomatic prior to outbreak notification. Moreover, of the five further cases that were going to occur, four developed symptoms within 8 days of notification of the index case. Thus, only one case was possibly preventable by the institution of infection control measures (Seng *et al.*, 1994). Another outbreak on a paediatric ward demonstrated that 50% of cases might have been prevented had notification to the infection control team been made earlier (Pillay *et al.*, 1992). These hospital outbreaks mirror the experience from community outbreaks, e.g. in schools. The high transmissibility of parvovirus B19 was shown in an outbreak investigated in a UK primary school for children aged 3–11 years during the epidemic year of 1994 (Rice and Cohen, 1996). This showed that 75% of the total number of cases had already occurred by the time the first few cases had been notified and, of the remaining 25%, most would have been infected and have also been incubating the infection by this time. Any efforts aimed at limiting the spread of infection would thus have had little impact.

The high infectivity of parvovirus in an outbreak setting is also illustrated by demonstrating that after this single outbreak in the school, the prevalence of parvovirus IgG rose from 15% to 60–70%, i.e. to an adult level of immunity (Rice and Cohen, 1996). It is our experience that when single cases of infection are identified among staff, further transmission to other staff occurs probably only as a result of social contact. This was also raised as one of the reasons for the extensive ward outbreak referred to earlier (Seng *et al.*, 1994). Moreover, given the reasonably high attack rate of 50% in close, social and household contacts and the long incubation period before symptoms appear, it may be possible to detect virus in susceptible contacts by PCR or even by using standard electron microscopy. This is an additional measure which may be undertaken to limit the spread of infection, by identifying those individuals who are in the infectious phase before they have mounted an antibody response.

Nosocomial transmission is a particular problem from patients with aplastic crises, since they present earlier in the course of their illness when they are still infectious. This was clearly demonstrated in a paediatric ward outbreak, where 12 health care workers were infected, most probably as a result of a failure to recognise the patient's infection early enough (Bell *et al.*, 1989). This outbreak was, however, probably made more likely since in the two outbreaks, only 12% and 31% of staff had pre-existing immunity before the outbreak. Transmission has also been described from immunocompromised patients with chronic infection, due to an inability to clear the viraemia, and who presumably still shed oropharyngeal virus (Lui *et al.*, 2001).

As parvovirus can cause significant harm to vulnerable patient groups and pregnant staff, the following appear to be reasonable precautions to prevent virus spread:

- Patients with reduced red cell survival, especially children, should be admitted to a single room if they experience a sudden drop in haemoglobin consistent with a possible aplastic crisis. Acute infection should be assumed, especially if the reticulocyte count is normal or low, indicating a shutting down of erythropoeisis. They should not be nursed by pregnant staff and hand-washing should be re-emphasised (Bell *et al.*, 1989; Pillay *et al.*, 1992, Crowcroft *et al.*, 1999).
- Any staff with rash, and especially those with arthralgia, should be investigated for parvovirus and rubella and their household and close social contacts offered testing for recent or past infection.

However, not all laboratories offer testing and those that do may only perform them in weekly batches, and it will often be necessary to make a judgement on whether or not staff should be re-deployed or furloughed before test results are available. Those who are found to be susceptible, however, can then be tested for the presence of viraemia. Decisions may then be made about furloughing of such staff.

- Pregnant staff who are at less then 20 weeks of gestation are at an increased risk of miscarriage or fetal hydrops. They should be advised before testing of the low probability of any adverse outcome, due to the low transmissibility, moderate levels of adult immunity and low risk (ca. 12%) of miscarriage. However, advising whether an indivi-dual staff member may wish to remain at work may also be influenced by other factors, including whether or not the pregnancy was achieved using IVF.

RESPIRATORY VIRUSES

Respiratory viruses are well established as agents capable of nosocomial transmission. They are parti-cularly well suited, for many reasons. They are highly infectious, with reproduction rates of 5–15:1, can spread by both droplet and aerosol routes and have short incubation periods. Explosive outbreaks are thus possible. Furthermore, during the epidemic season high community attack rates of 10% for influenza and 40% for RSV in the groups at highest risk of infection make possible multiple introductions into hospitals. They are capable of survival on surfaces and unwashed hands for hours and among immunocompromised patients infectious virus may be shed for weeks. Finally, vaccination is available only for influenza and effective antiviral agents are available for only two agents (RSV and influenza). They represent a sig-nificant financial burden on hospitals by prolonging hospital stays, increasing mortality in vulnerable patient groups, and increasing staff absences, with the need for hiring of temporary replacements at additional cost. Ward closure may sometimes be necessary to terminate an outbreak. There are also no tests for checking the immune status of staff. Indeed, for influenza and RSV, reinfection is common.

To prevent outbreaks, close cooperation between the microbiology department and the infection control team is essential. A key element of this is rapid communication of positive results on all patients in a hospital, especially at the start of the winter season. To facilitate this, rapid diagnostic assays should be employed. A variety of methods are available, but regardless of sensitivity and specificity their proper use is the key to success in controlling infection. Near-patient testing, if used properly, has sensitivity approaching that of conventional immunofluorescent tests, but it still requires knowledgeable staff capable of collecting an adequate specimen. We undertook a small study to assess the quality of nasopharyngeal aspirates taken from an accident and emergency department. Almost one-third of samples contained insufficient cells capable of achieving a result with good negative predictive value. An alternative approach to the testing of all symptomatic infants during the RSV season, for example, would be to test those whose symptoms and presentation are atypical (Salgado et al., 2002).

Newer PCR protocols involving real-time assays are capable of providing results as fast as immunofluor-escent tests, with enhanced sensitivity. A recent paper demonstrated that real-time PCR using the light cycler could generate a result in less than 2 h after specimen receipt, and it was significantly more sensitive in older children and adults (Whiley et al., 2002). This study showed that of 77 samples positive by light cycler RT-PCR, seven were negative by immunofluorescence testing. Of these seven samples, however, six were from adults or children aged > 12 years. This is compatible with lower viral loads in these individuals, most probably as a result of reinfection. Thus, PCR may offer advantages in certain groups, e.g. less cooperative children or adults who may be harder to sample. However, immunofluorescence assays are still the simplest way to test for multiple pathogens simultaneously.

Respiratory Syncytial Virus

The most effective methods for preventing nosocomial infection with RSV are through regular hand-washing by staff, parents and visitors, the wearing of gloves and gowns and either the cohorting of infected patients or admission directly into single cubicles. This limits spread mostly by introducing an ethos among all involved in patient care, that preventing nosocomial infection and hand-washing are important. Indeed, the effectiveness of such measures has been shown by several studies. Isaacs et al. (1991) studied hospital-acquired infection among children with congenital cardiac and lung disease. They showed a nosocomial infection rate of 35% prior to the introduction of enhanced infection control measures of hand-washing and patient cohorting. Not only were they able to demonstrate a 66% reduction in the rate of nosocomial RSV, but among patients admitted for >14 days the rate was even higher. During the year prior to the intervention of 11 patients staying longer than 14 days in hospital, eight (73%) developed nosocomial RSV compared with two of 77 (2.6%) during the period of intervention.

The prevention of RSV infection is paramount on bone marrow transplant units, where the mortality from RSV lower respiratory tract infection may be 30–100% (Harrington et al., 1992). Moreover, since infected patients shed virus for longer, they act as potential reservoirs for the maintenance and cascading of infection in the ward.

Whether or not cohorting of infected patients is done on the basis of specific virus type or on respiratory symptoms alone is debatable. It was noteworthy that in the study by Madge et al. (1992), in which all children were initially cohorted on the basis of respiratory symptoms alone, they showed that no symptomatic child initially placed in an RSV infected cohort, but who was subsequently shown to be RSV-negative, became infected as a result of this contact. The underlying reason for this may in part be due to the protective effect of viral interference of a pathogen other than RSV in the upper or lower respiratory tracts. For more details on nosocomial RSV infection, please see Chapter 7.

Influenza

Influenza is a particular problem in hospitals because of the explosive nature of outbreaks and the especially vulnerable patient groups that are heavily exposed during the epidemic season. During the winter, up to 10% of the general population are infected with influenza; in hospitals during outbreaks the attack rate may be as high as 50% in patients on affected wards and up to 20% in the general hospital population. All types of wards have been affected and, whilst the mortality can be low, in geriatric wards it can be as high as 16% (Gowda, 1979) and in transplant centres mortality due directly to influenza is 30–60% (Weinstock et al., 2000). These figures are particularly worrying, since it has been estimated that up to 70% of influenza infections in transplanted patients are nosocomial in origin. The staff are also at high risk of infection, with transmission rates of 11–60% in those caring for patients with influenza (reviewed in Salgado et al., 2002). In hospitals with a particular interest in influenza and a well-developed strategy for preventing nosocomial infection, however, the attack rate in staff is significantly reduced to only 2% (reviewed in Salgado et al., 2002).

There is good evidence that most cases of influenza are originally infected by respiratory droplets of small sizes which are inhaled. The most frequently quoted paper demonstrating the airborne route concerned a 72% attack rate in passengers in the cabin of an aeroplane with an inoperative ventilation system (Moser et al., 1979). All four individuals who decided to leave the plane escaped infection. However, those that chose to remain were free to move around the passenger compartment, indicating that infection by large droplets may also have occurred. However, small particle aerosols seem to be the most important mode of infection, since volunteer studies have shown that the dose required to establish infection is 10–100-fold lower for such aerosols compared with large droplet nasal administration of virus. Furthermore, intranasally administered influenza only uncommonly leads to influenza under experimental conditions and, whilst intranasal zanamivir prevents infection introduced by the same route, in ambulatory patients who, by implication, are more likely to come into contact with aerosolised virus, zanamivir requires delivery by inhalation to prevent infection.

Influenza virus is stable for 24–48 h after aerosolisation and for at least 5 min on unwashed hands. Virus shedding begins 1 day prior to symptom onset and continues for 4–7 days in immunocompetent patients, although extended periods of virus excretion of several weeks are seen in the immune-compromised.

Preventing the spread of influenza in hospitals is difficult because of the multiple routes of entry of virus in staff, patients and visitors. However, low nosocomial rates are achievable through a concerted action by all staff and the infection control and occupational health departments. Staff must understand that they should not report for work if they are ill and that they will be sent home if they develop an influenza-like illness. The ethos should be one of protecting patients as well as working as a team.

Prior to the influenza season it is good practice for occupational health departments to actively encourage staff, especially those employed in high-risk areas (ITU, HIV, transplant, paediatrics, pathology) to be immunised against influenza. The way to achieve good uptake rates is, first, to educate staff about the benefits of vaccination and the risk that influenza poses to them, their families and their patients. This can be achieved, for example, by posters and messages via hospital e-mail or in pay slips. The final stage is to offer the vaccine in as convenient a form as possible, e.g. by immunising staff in their workplace. By adopting such an approach, uptake rates can increase from 10% to 70% (reviewed in Salgado et al., 2002).

The overall efficacy of vaccine in patients and healthy staff is 70–90%. Vaccination of staff is probably the most effective measure in reducing mortality in hospital from influenza, as shown in a study from Scotland (Carman, 2000), especially as some studies in elderly institutionalised patients have demonstrated much lower rates of vaccine efficacy of 30–40% for preventing infection.

Patients who are admitted with suspected influenza should be placed in a single room and placed on respiratory precautions, i.e. plastic apron, gloves and hand-washing. A mask should be worn because of the risk of small particle aerosols. Specimens for rapid diagnosis should be sent as soon as possible, so that cohorting may be possible if the demand for single rooms becomes too great. There is no absolute need to place such patients in negative pressure, as the experience over a 15 year period from a hospital in Virginia, USA, has been that admitting patients with influenza to private rooms at slight positive pressure has not resulted in temporally related secondary cases (reviewed in Salgado et al., 2002).

If there appears to be an increase in the number of cases of proven influenza or influenza-like illnesses on a particular ward, consideration should be given to immunising staff as rapidly as possible. Whilst this takes effect, antiviral prophylaxis should also be considered. Amantadine, the first of the antiviral agents active against influenza, was shown many years ago to be an effective prophylactic regimen. However, it does suffer from two major problems; rapid development of drug resistance and significant CNS toxicity. Even during a short treatment course of only 2–5 days, up to one-third of influenza virus isolates will have developed resistance. These are as transmissible as wild-type virus and have been known to cause fatalities. CNS toxicity is also problematic and, when compared with rimantadine, 18% of patients suffered from CNS side-effects compared with just 2% taking rimantadine. The newer neuraminidase inhibitor agents, zanamivir and oseltamivir, given by inhalation or orally respectively, have an improved side-effect profile and so are better tolerated. Furthermore, when used in the home as post-exposure prophylaxis, they are extremely effective in preventing influenza illness, with efficacies of 74% and 90%, respectively.

Parainfluenza Virus

Like other respiratory viruses, parainfluenza (PIV) virus may cause outbreaks in nurseries, neonatal units and bone marrow transplant units. Infection in high-risk patients can have considerable mortality of approximately 40–50% in bone marrow transplant (BMT) patients (Zambon et al., 1998). When outbreaks occur it is always in the context of a wider community epidemic, which for parainfluenza virus usually runs from May to September each year. Thus, it is possible that what may appear to be an outbreak is merely the result of multiple introductions of virus into the ward by patients, staff and visitors. However, the available data from two large outbreaks on a paediatric ward and a bone marrow transplant unit showed the introduction of one PIV strain and its spread and propagation from person to person (Karron et al., 1993; Zambon et al., 1998). How virus may be transmitted is not easy to determine with absolute confidence, but transmission by unwashed hands, contaminated fomites and large droplets are all possible. In a report from the UK, one of two outbreaks on a BMT unit started 9 weeks after the index case had been identified and who was still shedding infectious virus (Zambon et al., 1998). This emphasises the absolute necessity for extreme vigilance when adhering to hand-washing and for prolonged periods when patients are immune-compromised. Indeed, virus excretion for 4 months has been demonstrated in this patient group (Zambon et al., 1998). What was also clear from this study, and another in Canada, is that hospital parainfluenza virus outbreaks can, unlike those due to influenza where the median duration is only 7 days, be protracted and ultimately only terminated by closure of the unit to new admissions (Moisiuk et al., 1998). When the first case of a parainfluenza virus is discovered on a ward, especially those with high-risk patients, full adherence to all necessary infection control measures (gowns, gloves, patient cohorting and hand-washing), including reiterating the standing instructions to staff not to come to work if unwell, must be rigorously enforced.

Severe Acute Respiratory Syndrome (SARS)

The spread of SARS, now known to be caused by a previously unknown coronavirus, has highlighted the extreme dangers that are posed by emerging viruses, particularly respiratory pathogens, to virgin-soil populations. It is also unfortunate that hospitals were unwittingly involved in amplifying the spread of the epidemic (Tomlinson and Cockram, 2003). This was seen very clearly in the Prince of Wales Hospital in Hong Kong, China. Within just 3 weeks of admission of the index case, 156 further cases had been diagnosed, all capable of being traced back to this single case. The major reasons given for the spread of infection in this hospital were failure to apply appropriate isolation precautions to cases not yet identified as SARS and breaches of such precautions. Staff were also appearing for work with a mild fever, so potentially exposing other patients and staff, and of especial importance in the rapid dissemination of infection in this hospital was the use of a nebulised bronchodilator in the index case, thereby hugely increasing the droplet contamination of the patient's environment.

A case-control study in five Hong Kong hospitals demonstrated that adhering to such precautions as use of a mask, gloves, gowns and hand-washing resulted in no secondary cases in 69 staff who followed these prevention-of-infection measures. However, all of the 13 staff who became infected after caring for SARS cases reported not adhering to at least one of these measures (Seto *et al.*, 2003). When each of the four infection control measures were examined, however, only the wearing of N95 masks was shown to be essential for protection against infection. This agrees with the principal mode of spread of SARS being by respiratory droplets. Unlike most of the other respiratory viruses, however, wearing an N95 mask capable of trapping 95% of all particles adds a further level of protection to staff. The wearing of simple paper masks did not afford any additional protection.

The World Health Organization (WHO) has given recommendations to control the spread of SARS. When a suspected case enters the hospital, droplet precautions must be strictly enforced, the patient must be isolated to a negative-pressure room and, after transfer to an appropriate facility capable of handling Category 4 pathogens, rapid diagnosis with the least invasive specimen should be attempted. To prevent the spread of SARS in hospitals, patients who may represent possible cases should be given a face mask to wear, preferably one that filters exhaled air. The staff involved in the initial contact must wear a mask, e.g. N95 with 95% filter efficiency, and goggles. They must wash hands before and after contact and wear gloves. Standard disinfectant solutions, such as household bleach and alcohol gel preparations, should be readily available in the immediate vicinity of the patient. The WHO has advised that there must be strict adherence when caring for SARS patients. All precautions against airborne, droplet and contact transmission must be employed. Further infection control measures include restricting visitors and supervising those in the use of protective equipment. It has also been suggested that the wearing of footwear that can be easily decontaminated should be considered. The removal of linen should be done by staff wearing full protective equipment (goggles, N95 or N100 masks, gloves, disposable gowns/aprons). The linen must be placed in biohazard bags and destroyed by incineration. Room cleaning should then take place using a broad-spectrum disinfectant, e.g. household bleach.

SMALL ROUND STRUCTURED VIRUSES (SRSVs OR NOROVIRUSES)

Of all the viruses capable of causing nosocomial infection, noroviruses probably present the greatest challenge to clinical virologists and infection control teams. Although initially termed 'winter vomiting disease' after a school outbreak in Norwalk, Ohio in 1966, these agents are now known to circulate all year round. To an individual they are of little consequence, as the illness is short-lived, self-limiting and only in exceptional cases does it lead to any complications. In hospitals, however, when outbreaks occur, almost without exception, ward closure and occasionally the entire closure of the hospital results (Stevenson *et al.*, 1994). This is because there is often considerable spread to contacts (staff and patients), resulting in an attack rate of more than 50% (Caul, 1994). Indeed, it is our experience that by the time an outbreak is notified to the virology department, so many staff are absent from work because of illness that this alone results in ward closure. There are many factors, both host and viral, that contribute to this.

It is known from volunteer studies and outbreak investigations that the incubation period is short, often 12–48 h. Indeed, volunteers exposed to infectious virus orally have been found to be shedding virus in faeces only 15 h later (reviewed in Chadwick *et al.*, 2000). The illness commences abruptly, with projectile vomiting in over half of cases and profuse watery diarrhoea. However, because the occasional case of vomiting and diarrhoea is not unusual among patients, many of whom are debilitated, elderly or on antibiotics, this may be initially overlooked. The environment can then become contaminated quite quickly and, as the infectious dose is low (10–100 particles) and the viruses resist low-dose chlorine disinfection and a temperature of 60°C, any breakdown in hand-washing leads very quickly to secondary cases occurring via the faecal–oral route (Caul, 1994). Fomite transmission is also possible because of the environmental stability of virus and it has even been suggested, although not actually confirmed, that infection may occur via airborne transmission (Caul, 1994).

Evidence from PCR detection of viral RNA indicates that virus excretion persists for longer than previously thought. Although virus shedding in stool is maximal at 24–72 h after exposure, virus can be detected for almost 2 weeks in both symptomatic and asymptomatic persons (reviewed in Chadwick et al., 2000). The epidemiological significance of this new finding is unclear. Finally, because of the strain diversity among the noroviruses, there is incomplete cross-protection and no long-term immunity. Repeated infections throughout life are therefore common.

The main focus of the infection control effort should be that, after outbreak notification on a ward, attempts should not necessarily be made to try to stop the virus from spreading to other patients or staff already on that ward, because the transmission rate is so high. The primary consideration should be to stop it affecting other wards and parts of the hospital. Indeed, an outbreak described in Salford, UK, in 1994 is a typical case (Chadwick and McCann, 1994). By the time the problem was highlighted to microbiology, over 80% of the eventual total number of cases on the first ward to be affected were either symptomatic or incubating the infection.

Establishing an early aetiological diagnosis with laboratory techniques is often difficult with noroviruses, as the sensitivity of electron microscopy is as low as 20%. Moreover, unless stool samples are collected during the acute phase of the illness, when they are liquid or semi-solid, the detection rate declines further. Specimens from six affected persons should be tested in one batch to maximise the efficiency of electron microscopy. However, there are new EIA tests for antigen becoming available, with much better rates of virus detection, ca. 60–70%, and RT-PCR is even more sensitive. Fortunately, to counteract this key difficulty, a clinical diagnosis of a norovirus outbreak is usually reliable if the following criteria are adhered to: stool samples are negative for bacterial pathogens, the percentage of cases with associated vomiting is >50%, the duration of illness is short (1–3 days), the incubation period, if available, is only 24–48 h with both patients and staff are affected.

All affected patients should be nursed either in single rooms or cohorted together. Strict hand-washing must be observed and gloves and gowns must be worn. The risk of infection has been shown to increase in a linear fashion with the number of patient contacts or exposure to nearby vomiting. Although there is no evidence that the wearing of masks reduces the risk of infection, they could be considered for individuals who clear up and dispose of vomit and faeces. All dirty linen should be disposed of with minimal agitation (to prevent further environmental contamination), horizontal surfaces and floors should be cleaned with 1000 ppm of available chlorine, approximately equivalent to a 10% solution of household bleach. There is no need to clean the walls unless visibly contaminated. The rate of PCR detection of environmental norovirus RNA during an outbreak was found to be 30% but this was confined to the immediate vicinity of symptomatic patients, so supporting the need for patient cohorting (Green et al., 1998). This environmental cleaning should continue once the outbreak has subsided. As the number of staff affected is often high, personnel shortages may lead naturally to ward closure. If they do not, however, the ward must be closed to new admissions for a period of 72 h after the last case. Furthermore, the staff on the ward at the onset of the outbreak must not work on other wards, and neither should patients be transferred to other areas unless it is medically necessary to do so (Caul, 1994). Even then, consultation should take place with the infection control team. Staff must be made aware of the critical importance of not coming to work unless well. Visitors, too, must be made aware of the necessity for hand-washing before and after entering the ward and non-essential staff should be excluded.

ROTAVIRUSES

Rotaviruses are spread in an identical manner to noroviruses, although infection is largely restricted to young children (<5 years old) and the elderly. In the context of an outbreak, however, it is also possible for staff to not only carry virus from one patient to another on unwashed hands but also to become symptomatic cases (Cubitt and Holzel, 1980). As a group, the rotaviruses have been shown to account for approximately half of all cases of nosocomially-acquired diarrhoea in children (Ford-Jones et al., 1990). Outbreaks on neonatal units and elderly care wards are well documented, with high attack rates of 40–60%, with the elderly at particular risk of complications because of underlying disease.

Diagnosis is much easier than with noroviruses, because of the much higher titres of virus in stool and the wider availability of latex agglutination and enzyme immunoassays.

The principal reasons for the propagation of such outbreaks are lapses in basic hygienic and infection control procedures, as shown in a very protracted outbreak lasting 5 months on a neonatal unit in The Netherlands (Widdowson *et al.*, 2002). Although the detection of a novel strain of rotavirus probably contributed to the scale of the outbreak, suspicion also centred on the fact that the neonates were being fed nasogastrically by staff who were not wearing gloves. Only after the wearing of gloves was enforced and the unit was closed for 7 days was the outbreak terminated. Of additional concern was the finding that environmental contamination persisted even after cleaning (Widdowson *et al.*, 2002).

Another such outbreak demonstrated that rotavirus could be detected in stool within 5 days of infants being newly admitted to the neonatal unit (Grehn *et al.*, 1990). These outbreaks all emphasise the necessity for timely and close liaison between high-risk wards and virology at the first sign of a problem, and that this is essential for outbreaks to be controlled. Furthermore, alcohol-based solutions, handrubs and gels must be used to destroy virus infectivity; relying on hypochlorite solutions alone is not acceptable.

ENTEROVIRUSES

Overt nosocomial enterovirus outbreaks are rare. They are described most often in neonatal units and nurseries, where, because of low birth-weight, immunological immaturity and other co-morbid conditions, they suffer an increased mortality compared with healthy infants. Individual cases of enterovirus infection may be suspected based upon the clinical syndrome with which the infant presents, namely meningitis, encephalitis, myocarditis or hepatitis (Modlin, 1986). However, they may also present with a sepsis-like syndrome or a non-specific febrile illness with poor feeding, diarrhoea and apnoea, with or without a rash. Although infections tend to occur in the summer and autumn, sporadic cases are seen all year round, highlighting the need for continual vigilance.

During outbreaks in newborn nurseries, attack rates have been high (20–50%), attributed largely to the transfer of virus on unwashed hands (Modlin, 1986). The case fatality has been low (3–6%). In outbreaks where the index case could be identified, this has often been a vertically infected baby. The most common serotype noted has been *Echovirus 11* (Modlin, 1986), but other types, such as 4, 7, 9, 6 and 30, are as pathogenic and as capable of nosocomial transmission (Bailly *et al.*, 2000). As it is not always possible to provide enough single rooms to isolate neonates with suspected virus infections, rapid diagnosis of enterovirus infections by PCR has been proposed to assist in preventing transmission (Chambon *et al.*, 1999; Bailly *et al.*, 2000). Moreover, the phylogenetic analysis of VP1 sequences of *Echovirus 30* has also enabled epidemiological connections to be established over long periods where nosocomial transmission may not necessarily have been originally suspected (Bailly *et al.*, 2000). Universal precautions (rigorous hand-washing, gloves) should always be employed and as soon as a case of infection is identified on a neonatal unit, virological surveillance should commence to ascertain the degree of spread and assist in cohorting.

REFERENCES

ACIP/HICPAC (1997) Immunisation of health-care workers: recommendations of the Advisory Committee on Immunisation Practices (ACIP) and the Hospital Infection Control Practices Advisory Committee (HICPAC). *Morbid Mortal Wkly Rep*, **46**(RR-18), 1–42.

Adler SP (1989) Cytomegalovirus and child day care: evidence for an increased infection rate among day care workers. *N Engl J Med*, **321**, 1290–1296.

Aitken C and Jeffries DJ (2001) Nosocomial spread of viral disease. *Clin Microbiol Rev*, **14**, 528–546.

Arbeter AM, Starr SE and Plotkin SA (1986) Varicella vaccine studies in healthy children and adults. *Pediatrics*, **78**, 748–756.

Asano Y, Nakayama H, Yazaki T *et al.* (1977) Protection against varicella in family contacts by immediate inoculation with live varicella vaccine. *Pediatrics*, **59**, 3–7.

Atkinson WL, Markowitz LE, Adams NC and Seastrom GR (1991) Transmission of measles in medical settings—United States, 1985–1989. *Am J Med*, **91** (suppl 3B), 320S–324S.

Bailly J-L, Beguet A, Chambon M *et al.* (2000) Nosocomial transmission of *Echovirus 30*: molecular evidence by phylogenetic analysis of the VP1 encoding sequence. *J Clin Microbiol*, **38**, 2889–2892.

Balcarek KB, Bagley R, Cloud GA and Pass RF (1990) Cytomegalovirus infection among employees of a children's hospital: no evidence for increased risk associated with patient care. *J Am Med Assoc*, **263**, 840–844.

Balfour CL and Balfour HH (1986) Cytomegalovirus is not an occupational risk for nurses in renal transplant and neonatal units: results of a prospective surveillance study. *J Am Med Assoc*, **256**, 1909–1914.

Bell LM, Naides SJ, Stoffman P *et al.* (1989) Human parvovirus B19 infection among hospital staff members after contact with infected patients. *N Engl J Med*, **321**, 485–491.

Braunstein H, Thomas S and Ito R (1990) Immunity to measles in a large population of varying age. *Am J Dis Child*, **144**, 296–298.

Carman WF, Elder AG, Wallace LA *et al.* (2000) Effects of influenza vaccination of health-care workers on mortality of elderly people in long-term care: a randomised controlled trial. *Lancet*, **355**, 93–97.

Caul OE (1994) Small round structured viruses; airborne transmission and hospital control. *Lancet*, **343**, 1240–1241.

Centers for Disease Control (1999) Prevention of varicella. Updated recommendations of the Advisory Committee on Immunization Practices (ACIP). *Morb Mortal Wkly Rep*, **48** (RR-6), 1–12.

Chadwick PR, Beards G, Brown D *et al.* (2000) Management of hospital outbreaks of gastroenteritis due to small round structured viruses. *J Hosp Infect*, **45**, 1–10.

Chadwick PR and McCann R (1994) Transmission of a small round structured virus by vomiting during a hospital outbreak of gastroenteritis. *J Hosp Infect*, **26**, 251–259.

Chambon M, Bailly J-L, Henquell C *et al.* (1999) An outbreak due to echovirus type 30 in a neonatal unit in France in 1997: usefulness of PCR diagnosis. *J Hosp Infect*, **43**, 63–68.

Crowcroft N, Roth CE, Cohen BJ and Miller E (1999) Guidance for control of parvovirus B19 infection in healthcare settings and the community. *J Publ Health Med*, **21**, 439–446.

Cubitt WD and Holzel H (1980) An outbreak of rotavirus infection in a long-stay ward of a geriatric hospital. *J Clin Pathol*, **33**, 306–308.

Davis RM, Orenstein WA, Frank JA Jr *et al.* (1986) Transmission of measles in medical settings, 1980–1984. *J Am Med Assoc*, **255**, 1295–1298.

Demmler G, Yow MD, Spector SA *et al.* (1987) Nosocomial cytomegalovirus infections within two hospitals caring for infants and children. *J Infect Dis*, **156**, 9–16.

de Swart RL, Wertheim-van Dillen PM, van Binnendijk *et al.* (2000) Measles in a Dutch hospital introduced by an immunocompromised infant from Indonesia infected with a new virus genotype. *Lancet*, **355**, 201–202.

Devi R, Muir D and Rice P (2002) Congenital rubella: down but not out. *Lancet*, **360**, 803–804.

Devi R and Rice P (2002) Prevention of varicella in health care workers. *Br Med J*, **324**, 610.

Dowell SF, Torok TJ, Thorp JA *et al.* (1995) Parvovirus B19 infection in hospital workers: community or hospital acquisition? *J Infect Dis*, **172**, 1076–1079.

Dworsky ME, Welch K, Cassady G and Stagno S (1983) Occupational risk for primary cytomegalovirus infection among pediatric health care workers. *N Engl J Med*, **309**, 950–953.

Ford-Jones EL, Mindorff CM, Gold R and Petric M (1990) The incidence of viral-associated diarrhoea after admission to a pediatric hospital. *Am J Epidemiol*, **131**, 711–718.

Gershon AA, Steinberg SP, LaRussa P *et al.* (1988) Immunization of healthy adults with live attenuated varicella vaccine. *J Infect Dis*, **158**, 132–137.

Gowda H (1979) Influenza in a geriatric unit. *Postgrad Med J*, **55**, 188–191.

Gray AM, Fenn P, Weinberg J, *et al.* (1997) An economic analysis of varicella vaccination for health care workers. *Epidemiol Infect*, **119**, 209.

Greaves WL, Orenstein WA, Stetler HC *et al.* (1982) Prevention of rubella transmission in medical facilities. *J Am Med Assoc*, **248**, 861–864.

Green J, Wright PA, Gallimore CI *et al.* (1998) The role of environmental contamination with small round structured viruses in a hospital outbreak investigated by reverse-transcriptase polymerase chain reaction assay. *J Hosp Infect*, **39**, 39–45.

Grehn M, Kunz J, Sigg P *et al.* (1990) Nosocomial rotavirus infections in neonates: means of prevention and control. *J Perinat Med*, **18**, 369–374.

Haneberg B, Bertnes E and Haukenes G (1980) Antibodies to cytomegalovirus among personnel at a children's hospital. *Acta Paediatr Scand*, **69**, 407–409.

Harrington RD, Hooton TM, Hackman RC *et al.* (1992) An outbreak of respiratory syncytial virus in a bone marrow transplant center. *J Infect Dis*, **165**, 987–993.

Isaacs D, Dickson H, O'Callaghan C *et al.* (1991) Hand-washing and cohorting in prevention of hospital acquired infections with respiratory syncytial virus. *Arch Dis Child*, **66**, 227–231.

Josephson A, Karanfil L and Gomber ME (1990) Strategies for the management of varicella-susceptible health care workers after a known exposure. *Infect Control Hosp Epidemiol*, **11**, 309–313.

Kaplan KM, Marder DC, Cochi SL *et al.* (1988) Mumps in the workplace: further evidence of the changing epidemiology of a childhood vaccine-preventable disease. *J Am Med Assoc*, **260**, 1434–1438.

Karron RA, O'Brien KL, Froehlich JL and Brown VA (1993) Molecular epidemiology of a parainfluenza type 3 virus outbreak on a pediatric ward. *J Infect Dis*, **167**, 1441–1445.

Kidd IM, Booth CJ, Rigden SPA *et al.* (2003) Measles-associated encephalitis in children with renal transplants: a predictable effect of waning herd immunity? *Lancet*, **362**, 832.

King GE, Markowitz LE, Patriarca PA and Dales LG (1991) Clinical efficacy of measles vaccine during the 1990 measles epidemic. *Pediatr Infect Dis J*, **10**, 883–888.

Krause PJ, Gross PA, Barrett TL *et al.* (1994) Quality standard assurance of measles immunity among health care workers. *Clin Infect Dis*, **18**, 431–436.

Langley JM and Hanakowski M (2000) Variation in risk for nosocomial chickenpox after inadvertent exposure. *J Hosp Infect*, **44**, 224–226.

Linnemann CC, Buchman TG, Light IJ *et al.* (1978) Transmission of herpes simplex virus type 1 in a nursery for the newborn. Identification of viral isolates by DNA 'fingerprinting'. *Lancet*, **i**, 964–966.

Lohiya GS, Stewart K, Perot K and Widman R (1995) Parvovirus B19 outbreak in a developmental center. *Am J Infect Control*, **23**, 373–376.

Lui SL, Luk WK, Cheung CY *et al.* (2001) Nosocomial outbreak of parvovirus B19 infection in a renal transplant unit. *Transplantation*, **71**, 59–64.

Madge P, Payton JY, McColl JH and Mackie PLK (1992) Prospective controlled study for four infection-control procedures to prevent nosocomial infection with respiratory syncytial virus. *Lancet*, **340**, 1079–1083.

Mendelson GMS, Roth CE, Wreghitt TG *et al.* (2000) Nosocomial transmission of measles to healthcare workers. Time for a national screening and immunisation policy for NHS staff? *J Hosp Infect*, **44**, 154–155.

Miller E, Waight PA, Rousseau SA *et al.* (1990) Congenital rubella in the Asian community in Britain. *Br Med J*, **301**, 1391.

Miyamoto K, Ogami M, Takahashi Y *et al.* (2000) Outbreak of human parvovirus B19 in hospital workers. *J Hosp Infect*, **45**, 238–241.

Modlin JF (1986) Perinatal *Echovirus* infection: insights from a literature review of 61 cases of serious infection and 16 outbreaks in nurseries. *Rev Infect Dis*, **8**, 918–926.

Moisiuk SE, Robson D, Klass L *et al.* (1998) Outbreak of parainfluenza virus type 3 in an intermediate care neonatal nursery. *Pediatr Infect Dis*, **17**, 49–53.

Moser M, Bender T, Margolis H *et al.* (1979) An outbreak of influenza aboard a commercial airliner. *Am J Epidemiol*, **110**, 1–6.

Myers M, Rasley D and Hierholtzer W (1982) Hospital infection control for varicella zoster virus infection. *Pediatrics*, **70**, 199–202.

Onorato IM, Morens DM, Martone WJ and Stansfield SK (1985) Epidemiology of cytomegaloviral infections: recommendations for prevention and control. *Rev Infect Dis*, **7**, 479–497.

PHLS (2003) Laboratory-confirmed cases of measles, mumps and rubella, England and Wales: Oct–Dec 2002. *Commun Dis Rep CDR Wkly*, **12**(39) (web address: www.hpa.org.uk/cdr/PDFfiles/2003/cdr1303.pdf). Cited 27 March 2003.

Pillay D, Patou G, Hurt S *et al.* (1992) Parvovirus B19 outbreak in a children's ward. *Lancet*, **339**, 107–109.

Polk B, White JA, DeGirolami PC and Modlin JF (1980) An outbreak of rubella among hospital personnel. *N Engl J Med*, **303**, 541–545.

Ramsay ME, Jin L, White J *et al.* (2003) The elimination of indigenous measles transmission in England and Wales. *J Infect Dis*, **187** (suppl 1), S198–S207.

Rice PS and Cohen BJ (1996) A school outbreak of parvovirus B19 infection investigated using salivary antibody assays. *Epidemiol Infect*, **116**, 331–338.

Rice P, Young Y, Cohen B and Ramsay M (2004) MMR immunization after contact with measles virus. *Lancet*, **363**, 569–570.

Richardson JA and Quigley C (1994) An outbreak of measles in Trafford. *Commun Dis Rep*, **4**, R73–75.

Sakaoka H, Saheki Y, Uzuki K *et al.* (1986) Two outbreaks of herpes simplex type 1 nosocomial infection among newborns. *J Clin Microbiol*, **24**, 36–40.

Salgado CD, Farr BM, Hall KK and Hayden FG (2002) Influenza in the acute hospital setting. *Lancet Infect Dis*, **2**, 145–155.

Salisbury DM and Begg NT (eds) (1996) *Immunisation against Infectious Disease*. Department of Health/HMSO, London.

Schwarcz S, McCaw B and Fukushima P (1992) Prevalence of measles susceptibility in hospital staff. *Arch Intern Med*, **152**, 1481–1483.

Seng C, Watkins P, Morse D *et al.* (1994) Parvovirus B19 outbreak on an adult ward. *Epidemiol Infect*, **113**, 345–353.

Seto WH, Tsang D, Yung RWH *et al.* (2003) Effectiveness of precautions against droplets and contact in the prevention of nosocomial transmission of severe acute respiratory syndrome (SARS). *Lancet*, **361**, 1519–1520.

Sharrar RG, LaRussa P, Galea SA *et al.* (2000) The postmarketing safety profile of varicella vaccine. *Vaccine*, **19**, 916–923.

Sheridan E, Aitken C, Jeffries D *et al.* (2002) Congenital rubella syndrome: a risk in immigrant populations. *Lancet*, **359**, 674–675.

Smith E, Welch W, Berhow M and Wong VK (1990) Measles susceptibility of hospital employees as determined by ELISA. *Clin Res*, **38**, 183A.

Stevenson P, McCann R, Duthie R *et al.* (1994) A hospital outbreak due to Norwalk virus. *J Hosp Infect*, **26**, 261–272.

Thomas DR, Salmon RL and King J (1998) Rates of first measles–mumps–rubella immunisation in Wales (UK). *Lancet*, **351**, 1927.

Tomlinson B and Cockram C (2003) SARS: experience at Prince of Wales Hospital, Hong Kong. *Lancet*, **361**, 1486–1487.

Watson BM, Piercy SA, Plotkin SA and Starr SE (1993) Modified chickenpox in children immunised with the Oka/Merck varicella vaccine. *Pediatrics*, **91**, 17–22.

Weber DJ, Rutala WA and Hamilton H (1996) Prevention and control of varicella-zoster infections in healthcare facilities. *Infect Control Hosp Epidemiol*, **17**, 694–705.

Weinstock D, Eagan J, Malak S *et al.* (2000) Control of influenza A on a bone marrow transplant unit. *Infect Control Hosp Epidemiol*, **21**, 730–732.

Wharton M, Cochi SL, Hutcheson RH and Schaffner W (1990) Mumps transmission in hospitals. *Arch Intern Med*, **150**, 47–49.

Whiley DM, Syrmis MW, Mackay IM and Sloots TP (2002) Detection of human respiratory syncytial virus in respiratory samples by light cycler reverse transcriptase PCR. *J Clin Microbiol*, **40**, 4418–4422.

Widdowson MA, van Doornum GJ, van der Poel WH *et al.* (2002) An outbreak of diarrhea in a neonatal medium care unit caused by a novel strain of rotavirus: investigation using both epidemiologic and microbiological methods. *Infect Control Hosp Epidemiol*, **23**, 665–670.

Wreghitt T, Whipp J, Redpath C and Hollingworth W (1996) An analysis of infection control of varicella-zoster virus infections at Addenbrooke's Hospital, Cambridge, over a 5-year period, 1987–1992. *Epidemiol Infect*, **117**, 165–171.

Young AB, Reid D and Grist NR (1983) Is cytomegalovirus a serious hazard to female hospital staff? *Lancet*, **i**, 975–976.

Zambon M, Bull, T, Sadler CJ *et al.* Molecular epidemiology of two consecutive outbreaks of parainfluenza 3 in a bone marrow transplant unit. *J Clin Microbiol*, **36**, 2289–2293.

Index

Page numbers in italics indicate figures and tables.

Principles and Practice of Clinical Virology, Fifth Edition. Edited by A. J. Zuckerman, J. E. Banatvala, J. R. Pattison, P. D. Griffiths and B. D. Schoub
© 2004 John Wiley & Sons Ltd   ISBN 0 470 84338 1